The
Blackwell Dictionary
of
Neuropsychology

The Blackwell Dictionary of Neuropsychology

Edited by

J. Graham Beaumont, Pamela M. Kenealy, and Marcus J. C. Rogers

Advisory Editors
Antonio Damasio
Ennio De Renzi
Kenneth Heilman
Eran Zaidel

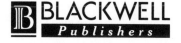

BLACKWELL
Publishers

Copyright © Blackwell Publishers Ltd, 1996, 1999

First published 1996

First published in paperback 1999

Blackwell Publishers Inc
350 Main Street
Malden, Massachusetts 02148, USA

Blackwell Publishers Ltd
108 Cowley Road
Oxford OX4 1JF, UK

Library of Congress Cataloging in Publication Data
The Blackwell dictionary of neuropsychology/edited by
  J. Graham Beaumont, Pamela M. Kenealy, and Marcus J. C. Rogers.
       p. cm.
    Includes bibliographical references.
    ISBN 0–631–17896–1 (hardcover: alk. paper)
    ISBN 0–631–21435–6 (paperback: alk. paper)
    1. Neuropsychology – Dictionaries. I. Beaumont, J. Graham.
II. Kenealy, Pamela M. III. Rogers, Marcus J. C.
    [DNLM: 1. Neuropsychology – dictionaries. WL 13 B632 1996]
    QP360.B577 1996
    612.8'03 – dc20
    DNLM/DLC   95-17884
    for Library of Congress   CIP

British Library Cataloguing in Publication Data
A CIP catalogue record for this book is available from the British Library

Typeset in 9 on 11pt Ehrhardt
at The Spartan Press Ltd, Lymington, Hampshire
Printed and bound in Great Britain
by MPG Books Ltd, Bodmin, Cornwall

This book is printed on acid-free paper

Contents

Figures

Figures

Tables

Contributors

Only entries longer than about 500 words are listed under the names of the relevant contributors. The shorter ones are all by one or other of the editors.

Roger L. Albin
University of Michigan, Ann Arbor
basal ganglia

Nancy C. Andreasen
University of Iowa College of Medicine
scan

Geoff Barrett
Centre for Human Sciences, DRA Alverstoke, Gosport
evoked potential

Jeffrey T. Barth
University of Virginia, Charlottesville
dementia

J. Graham Beaumont
Royal Hospital for Neuro-disability, London
ataxia, denial, ECT, eye movement, Ganser syndrome, LEMs, neuropsychology, perseveration, schizophrenia, tumor

D. Frank Benson
University of California, Los Angeles
alexia

Arthur Benton
University of Iowa Hospitals
body schema disturbance

Joseph E. Bogen
University of California, Los Angeles
disconnection syndrome

Jelis Boiten
University Hospital, Maastricht, The Netherlands
hemiplegia

R. A. Bornstein
Ohio State University, Columbus
stroke

Joan C. Borod
Queens College, City University, and Mount Sinai School of Medicine, New York
emotional disorders

M. I. Botez
Hôtel Dieu de Montréal, Montreal
cerebellum

Thérèse Botez
Hôtel Dieu de Montréal, Montreal
cerebellum

Patrick Bourke
University of Luton
attention

M. P. Bryden
University of Waterloo, Ontario
dichhaptic technique, dichotic listening

Daniel N. Bub
University of Victoria, British Columbia
dyslexia

Henry A. Buchtel
VA Medical Center and University of Michigan Hospitals, Ann Arbor
temporal lobe

Mario Bunge
McGill University, Montreal
mind–body problem

Contributors

Thomas Chase
National Institutes of Health, Bethesda, MD
Huntington's disease

Chris Code
University of Sydney
speech therapy for aphasia

Michael C. Corballis
University of Auckland
right–left disorientation

Deborah A. Cory-Slechta
University of Rochester School of Medicine, NY
lead poisoning

Alan Cowey
University of Oxford
blindsight

J. R. Crawford
School of Psychology, Flinders University of South Australia, Adelaide
assessment

J. L. Cummings
VA Medical Centre, Los Angeles
agraphia

Gianfranco Denes
Università degli Studi di Padova, Padua
autotopagnosia

Maureen Dennis
Hospital for Sick Children, Toronto
hydrocephalus

Ennio De Renzi
Clinica Neurologica, Modena
topographical disorders

Richard L. Doty
Smell and Tate Center, University of Pennsylvania Medical Center, Philadelphia
anosmia

Robert W. Doty
University of Rochester School of Medicine, NY
brain

P. B. Fenwick
Institute of Psychiatry, University of London
epilepsy

Hans Forssberg
Karolinska Institute, Stockholm
spasticity

John P. Fraher
University College, Cork
cranial nerves

Chris Frith
Wellcome Department of Cognitive Neurology, Institute of Neurology, University of London
blood flow studies

Uta Frith
MRC Cognitive Development Unit and University College London
spelling disorders

Guido Gainotti
Università Cattolica del Sacro Cuore, Rome
personality disorders

Alison Gallagher
MRC Cognitive Development Unit and University College London
spelling disorders

Gerald Goldstein
VA Medical Center, Pittsburgh
aging

Harold Goodglass
VA Medical Center, Boston
aphasia

Harold W. Gordon
University of Pittsburgh School of Medicine
amusia, hemisphericity

Peter W. Halligan
University Department of Clinical Neurology and Rivermead Rehabilitation Centre, Oxford
visuoperceptual disorders, visuospatial disorders

Joseph Hellige
University of Southern California, Los Angeles
divided visual field technique

C. A. Heywood
University of Durham
visual field defect

Charles Hinkin
UCLA School of Medicine and VA Medical Center, West Los Angeles
agraphia

Glyn W. Humphreys
University of Birmingham
agnosia

Nancy Hutner
Boston University School of Medicine
alcoholism

Marco Iacoboni
Università di Roma La Sapienza, Rome
subarachnoid hemorrhage

G. M. Innocenti
Université de Lausanne
maturation

Malcolm A. Jeeves
University of St Andrews
callosal agenesis

E. G. Jones
University of California, Irvine
thalamus

Robert J. Joynt
University of Rochester, NY
neurology

Jon H. Kaas
Vanderbilt University, Nashville, TN
sensorimotor cortex

Pamela M. Kenealy
Roehampton Institute London
phenylketonuria, seasonal affective disorder

Andrew Kertesz
St Joseph's Hospital, London, Ontario
localization

Marcel Kinsbourne
Sargent College, Boston University
hyperactivity

Michael D. Kopelman
United Medical and Dental School, Guy's and St Thomas's Hospital, London
Korsakoff's syndrome

Robert Lalonde
Hôtel Dieu de Montréal, Montreal
cerebellum

Lars-Erik Larsson
University Hospital, Linköping, Sweden
gait

N. J. Legg
Royal Postgraduate Medical School, University of London
encephalitis

R. N. Lemon
Institute of Neurology, University of London
pyramidal tract

Carlo Lenti
Istituto di Neuropsichiatria Infantile dell'Università, Milan
cerebral palsy

Gian Luigi Lenzi
Università di Roma La Sapienza, Rome
subarachnoid hemorrhage

T. E. Le Vere
North Carolina State University, Raleigh
plasticity

Irene Litvan
Neuroepidemiology Branch, NINDS, NIH, Bethesda, MD
Parkinson's disease

Elio Lugaresi
Istituto di Clinica Neurologica, Università di Bologna
sleep

Linda M. Luxon
University College London
postural control

Marie McCarthy
Royal Hospital for Neuro-disability, London
multiple sclerosis, neglect

Contributors

Stephen N. Macciocchi
University of Virginia, Charlottesville
dementia

William W. McKinlay
Case Management Services, Edinburgh
social behavior

Paul D. MacLean
NIMH Neuroscience Center, Washington, DC
limbic system

I. C. McManus
University College London
handedness

John C. Marshall
Department of Clinical Neurology, Radcliffe Infirmary, University of Oxford
visuoperceptual disorders

C. A. Marzi
Università di Verona
lateralization

Andrew R. Mayes
Royal Hallamshire Hospital, University of Sheffield
amnesic syndrome

Ronald Melzack
McGill University, Montreal
pain

M. Marsel Mesulam
Beth Israel Hospital, Boston
confusional state

Gabriele Miceli
Università Cattolica del Sacro Cuore, Rome
anomia

Edgar Miller
University of Leicester
hysteria

Erich Mohr
Elizabeth Bruyère Health Centre, Ottawa
Huntington's disease

Michael J. Morgan
University of Wales, Swansea
neurotransmitters

J. A. Moses Jr
Palo Alto VA Health Care System, CA
motor skill disorders

Paul D. Nussbaum
University of Pittsburgh
aging

Marlene Oscar-Berman
Boston University School of Medicine
alcoholism

Michel Paradis
McGill University, Montreal
bilingualism

A. J. Parker
University of Oxford
striate cortex

Alan J. Parkin
University of Sussex, Brighton
amnesia

Gilbert D. Pinard
McGill University, Montreal
catatonia

Michael I. Posner
University of Oregon, Eugene
attention

Bruno Preilowski
Eberhard-Karls-Universität Tübingen
commissurotomy

Fred H. Previc
Crew Technology Division, Armstrong Laboratory, Brooks Air Force Base, TX
occipital lobe

George P. Prigatano
Barrow Neurological Institute, St Joseph's Hospital, Phoenix, AZ
anosognosia

Scot E. Purdon
Alberta Hospital, Edmonton
Huntington's disease

G. Ratcliff
Harmarville Rehabilitation Center, Pittsburgh
parietal lobe

M. Jane Riddoch
University of Birmingham
simultanagnosia

Georgina M. J. Rippon
University of Warwick, Coventry
electroencephalography

Marcus J. C. Rogers
Royal Hospital for Neuro-disability, London
apraxia, hypothalamus, Pick's disease, syphilis

E. T. Rolls
Department of Experimental Psychology, University of Oxford
hippocampus

W. H. Rutherford
Royal Victoria Hospital, Belfast
postconcussion syndrome

K. Sathian
University of Chicago
tactile perception disorders

C. Semenza
Università degli Studi di Padova, Padua, and Università degli Studi di Trieste
dual task paradigm, methodological issues

Xavier Seron
Université de Louvain
acalculia

Teresa M. Sgaramella
Università degli Studi di Padova, Padua
dual task paradigm

Abigail B. Sivan
Rush-Presbyterian-St Luke's Medical Center, Chicago
body schema disturbance

Donald G. Stein
Rutgers University Graduate School, Newark, NJ
recovery of function

Mircea Steriade
Université Laval, Quebec
brain stem, reticular formation

Donald T. Stuss
Rotman Research Institute, Baycrest Centre, University of Toronto
frontal lobes

H. Gerry Taylor
Rainbow Babies and Children's Hospital, Cleveland, OH
minimal brain dysfunction

Christine Temple
University of Essex, Colchester
autism

Geoffrey Underwood
University of Nottingham
consciousness

Elliot S. Valenstein
University of Michigan, Ann Arbor
psychosurgery

Nils R. Varney
VA Medical Center, Iowa City
gestural behavior

Luigi A. Vignolo
Università degli Studi di Brescia
auditory perceptual disorders

Jean-Guy Villemure
Montreal Neurological Hospital and McGill University
hemispherectomy

J. D. Vincent
Institut Alfred Fessard, CNRS, Gif-sur-Yvette
sexuality

J. Warner-Rogers
MRC Child Psychiatry Unit, Institute of Psychiatry, University of London
congenital disorders

Anna J. Watkiss
Case Management Services, Edinburgh
social behavior

Contributors

Paul Willner
University of Wales, Swansea
depression

Barbara W. Wilson
MRC Applied Psychology Unit, Cambridge
rehabilitation

J. T. L. Wilson
University of Stirling
toxicology

Sarah L. Wilson
University of Surrey, Guildford
vegetative state

Uwe R. Windhorst
University of Calgary
reflexes

Sandra F. Witelson
McMaster University, Hamilton, Ontario
dichhaptic technique, sex differences

Lucy Yardley
University College London
postural control

Andrew W. Young
MRC Applied Psychology Unit, Cambridge
face recognition, reduplication

Dahlia W. Zaidel
University of California, Los Angeles
disconnection syndrome

Eran Zaidel
University of California, Los Angeles
disconnection syndrome

Preface

The idea for this dictionary arose out of an obvious need: the need for a comprehensive handbook and guide to contemporary neuropsychological knowledge and practice. We imagined the book that we would want to have at our elbow and set out to create it. At so many times during the course of the project, someone has said "Won't it be useful when it is published!" and we hope that will be true now.

At the outset of the project the editors were Graham Beaumont and Justine Sergent. Sadly, Justine died tragically in the spring of 1994, at which time the manuscript was still very incomplete and the editing not yet begun. Pamela Kenealy and Marcus Rogers were then recruited to the team and as a result of their efforts the project has been brought to fruition. Although Justine made a very significant contribution to the volume in its planning and in the recruitment and guidance of contributors, as a result of her unexpected death none of her writing appears in the text. The editors are listed alphabetically, and they will know the relative contributions they have made.

POTENTIAL READERS

For whom is the *Dictionary* intended? There are a number of potential groups of readers. The most obvious is the professional group of practicing clinical neuropsychologists. They will already have much of the knowledge contained in this volume, but it should nonetheless be useful both as a reference source for the more esoteric aspects of the discipline and as a guide to the current state of knowledge in selected key areas. It should also be of great value to practicing clinical psychologists who feel that their knowledge of clinical neuropsychology needs extending when they are required to serve clients who have a neuropsychological aspect to their problems. Those training and developing expertise in clinical neuropsychology should find this book invaluable as a handbook and as a guide to further study.

The *Dictionary* will also be of value to researchers and academics involved in the field of neuropsychology, for it contains some excellent contemporary reviews by neuropsychologists of international standing, the quality of which will have a significant impact and should increase general knowledge and understanding in the area. But the *Dictionary* should also be of value to those working in disciplines cognate to clinical neuropsychology, to experimental neuropsychologists and cognitive psychologists, to neuroscientists, neurologists, and those working in the care and therapy professions whose clients have neuropsychological disorders: nurses, speech and language therapists, physiother-apists, occupational therapists, music therapists, social workers and those working within rehabilitation medicine.

It is difficult to compare this *Dictionary* with previous works, as no single one has previously attempted the comprehensive coverage of neuropsychology which is the aim of the present volume. The excellent textbook by Kolb and Whishaw provides the best introductory coverage of the field, and the two handbooks by Hécaen and Albert, and Heilman and Valenstein, are invaluable for their detailed and scholarly coverage of the core aspects of the discipline. (All these works are listed in the bibliography at the end of this Preface.) Lishman's comprehensive text on organic psychiatry is also a key reference work for the clinical neuropsychologist, together with the handbook on neuropsychological assessment by Lezak. Each of these works provides considerably more detail within its chosen field of coverage than is possible within the *Dictionary*, and no doubt will be used in conjunction with it, but we hope that, if we have succeeded, this book will be the single most useful reference volume for neuropsychologists. The principle underlying its design is that if neuropsychologists need to know it then it will be mentioned here, and if there is insufficient information here then there will be a reference to a further source of information.

Preface

THE DESIGN OF THE DICTIONARY

In designing the Dictionary we were greatly assisted by the advisory editors: Antonio Damasio, Ennio De Renzi, Kenneth Heilman, and Eran Zaidel, who provided invaluable advice about the extent and balance of the appropriate coverage, although we naturally accept full responsibility for any omissions which remain. In constructing the manuscript there was inevitably a problem in striking a balance between presenting the core and enduring fundamental aspects of neuropsychology and giving coverage of the latest ideas and theories, some of which may endure while others will simply have their vogue. The temptation is always to give more attention to the ideas which currently excite and provoke, but these are also often the ideas which rapidly date. We have tried to strike a balance between these competing pressures and time will be the judge of our success. Those who have contributed the feature articles were asked to present a balanced overview of the contemporary state of knowledge in the relevant area, to adopt a broader perspective than their own personal work, but to give their personal evaluation of current concepts and theories. In general, contributors have done an excellent job in achieving this and we have tried to respect their individual views and evaluations during the editing process. Neuropsychology is a rapidly developing discipline (see the entry on NEUROPSYCHOLOGY for a survey of the current state of the discipline) and it is inevitably the case that the field will have moved on, even by the time that these words appear in print.

Inevitably, errors and omissions will have occurred in the preparation of the *Dictionary*. Given the extent of the field of neuropsychology, it is doubtful that any one person can now possess the range of knowledge needed for a project of the present kind, and even a team of editors will have lacunae in their collective expertise. We are also quite capable of human error. So, while all efforts have been made to ensure that the *Dictionary* contains accurate and valid information, we beg your forgiveness for any errors in or unreasonable omissions from the text. More important, if you detect an error or note a serious omission, any of the editors would be very grateful to know of it so that, if the *Dictionary* is revised in the future, the content can be improved.

It is also the case that, given the limited expertise that even an expert neuropsychologist may possess, in preparing the entries considerable reliance has to be placed on existing standard reference works. We freely acknowledge the debt we owe to a number of works listed below (page xix), which have provided the source for considerable parts of the shorter entries, in particular the works by Hécaen and Albert, and Heilman and Valenstein, and also those by Bannister and Lishman. Treading a path which avoids repetition of their writing has not always been easy as there are only a limited number of ways of expressing essential information concisely. I hope, however, that we have avoided any unacceptable duplication of their respective publications, while freely acknowledging the very considerable debt we owe to their prior work.

Thanks are due to all the contributors who have collaborated in this project (and especially those who submitted their text on time). We should also like to thank Alyn Shipton and Alison Mudditt of Blackwell Publishers for their enthusiasm for and stimulus to the project, and Sarah McNamee, Sandra Raphael, and all the editorial staff who have been associated with the project over the years. Without the support of all these people the book would never have appeared in print.

This project has been several years in its realization, and if we had anticipated the problems in assembling the contributions of over 120 international contributors, I doubt that we would ever have begun. Part of the reason for this slow progress was our determination to recruit only the most expert contributors for the volume, and with some topics this has required a little patience. We believe that we have succeeded and, while we are still aware of the shortcomings and limitations of the work, we hope that we have made a useful contribution to future progress in the field of human neuropsychology.

J. GRAHAM BEAUMONT
Royal Hospital for Neuro-disability
PAMELA M. KENEALY
Roehampton Institute London
MARCUS J. C. ROGERS
Royal Hospital for Neuro-disability

London, 1995

How to Use the Dictionary

Although entitled a "dictionary", this book is really more of an encyclopedia. In order to access the knowledge, the principal route is by the keyword headings which are arranged alphabetically. Having selected the most appropriate heading or subsection, further cross-references to related entries are given in the body of the text by these entries being printed in SMALL CAPITALS.

As a further aid to finding the required information, for not every topic merits an entry as a keyword, there is an index which should direct the reader to more specific information. We hope that this provides a sufficiently rich variety of routes to make the book easy to use; if you cannot find the information by one of these routes, we have almost certainly failed to provide it. If the information itself is not to be found in this volume, then the references at the end of each major article should provide an onward path for the search, or alternatively, the list of standard texts given below should help.

The *Dictionary* was also designed around a set of standard brain diagrams which contributors were encouraged to use, as an aid to the reader so that the diagrams accompanying one entry could be more easily related to those accompanying another. The reader must judge how successful this approach has been; it proved more difficult than expected to generate one set of diagrams which were adequate to the purposes of each contributing author.

BOOK LIST

This is a personal selection of books which, at the time of writing, we consider should form a basic library for the practicing neuropsychologist:

Bannister, R. (1992). *Brain and Bannister's clinical neurology*, 7th edn. Oxford: Oxford Medical Publications.

Crawford, J. R., Parker, D. M., & McKinlay, W. W. (Eds). (1992). *A handbook of neuropsychological assessment*. Hillsdale, NJ: Erlbaum.

Hécaen, H., & Albert, M. L. (1978). *Human neuropsychology*. New York: John Wiley.

Heilman, K. M., & Valenstein, E. (Eds). (1993). *Clinical neuropsychology*, 3rd edn. New York: Oxford University Press.

Kolb, B., & Whishaw, I. Q. (1995). *Fundamentals of human neuropsychology*, 4th edn. San Francisco: W. H. Freeman.

Lezak, M. D. (1995). *Neuropsychological assessment*, 3rd edn. New York: Oxford University Press.

Lishman, W. A. (1987). *Organic psychiatry: The psychological consequences of cerebral trauma*. 2nd edn. Oxford: Blackwell Scientific.

McCarthy, R. A., & Warrington, E. K. (1990). *Cognitive neuropsychology: A clinical introduction*. London: Academic Press.

Shallice, T. (1988). *From neuropsychology to mental structure*. Cambridge: Cambridge University Press.

Spreen, O., & Strauss, E. (1991). *A compendium of neuropsychological tests: Administration, norms and commentary*. New York: Oxford University Press.

A

ablation   Ablation is literally the removal of any tissue from the body. The term is used rather loosely and may, in certain contexts, be applied to almost any brain lesion in which there is a substantial and local loss of the brain substance. It is, however, more commonly applied to intentional removal of a part of the brain, usually by surgery.

absence   Absences are a form of EPILEPSY and have alternatively been known as *petit mal epilepsy* to distinguish the generalized seizures which occur from the more dramatic attacks of "grand mal" epilepsy. Absence attacks are relatively brief and are associated with a characteristic and distinctive pattern of regular waves and spikes occurring at about 3 cycles/sec. This dysrhythmia in the EEG is generalized across the cortex, and is bilaterally synchronous and symmetrical.

Absence attacks usually have their onset during early childhood and behaviorally appear as a brief suspension of activity lasting for a few seconds. The child pauses and has a rather dazed and often pale expression and may stare, but does not fall to the ground and there is no apparent convulsion. As the attack passes the child will simply resume the previous activity, and will usually have no conscious recall of the episode, although in minor forms of absence attack partial consciousness may be retained and a sense of feeling unusual will subsequently be reported. Where absence attacks are the only manifestation of the disorder, it is now generally termed *childhood absence epilepsy*; but in other cases generalized tonic-clonic (convulsive) seizures may occur, either intermixed with the absence attacks or as a development of the disorder in later life.

Absence attacks, if untreated, typically occur many times a day, and the frequency of the attacks may assist in distinguishing them from mild attacks of complex partial (temporal lobe) epilepsy which, by producing minor partial seizures, may resemble absence attacks yet occur with a much lower frequency. Absence attacks never have an onset in adult life, although, having begun in childhood, they may persist into adult life; complex partial seizures may have an onset at any age.

The characteristic wave and spike dysrhythmia in the EEG may occur without the behavioral signs of an absence attack, but these subclinical episodes are nonetheless regarded as being associated with impaired mental efficiency. The disorder, in its clinical or its subclinical form, may commonly be associated with poor educational progress, particularly where the attacks are untreated and occurring with high frequency. Absence attacks are considered to be idiopathic and a constitutional disturbance, therefore never the result of an acquired lesion, again unlike complex partial epilepsy, where the cause is commonly a small lesion of the temporal lobe. The origin of the seizure in an absence attack may be in the THALAMUS or surrounding structures.

J. GRAHAM BEAUMONT

abstract attitude   Abstract attitude is a concept employed by Gestalt theories to embody critical aspects of human thinking and reasoning. In the normal individual it may be seen in the capacity to discriminate figure from background, and it can be divided into specific functional abilities. The concept was popular in the 1940s and 1950s, and in neuropsychology it is associated with the work of Kurt Goldstein. From this perspective, brain damage causes the loss of abstract attitude and a dedifferentiation of the specific cognitive functions. This loss can be demonstrated by, for example, the loss of figure-ground perception. Influential in its period, the concept is not currently employed, following advances in the understanding of intelligence.

abulia Abulia is a loss or a deficit in the ability to make decisions. Abulic patients lack spontaneity in actions and speech, are apathetic, and show psychomotor retardation. Such patients may be temporarily roused by external stimulation, but rapidly lapse back into the anergic state once the stimulation is terminated. It is linked with AKINESIA and may be considered to be a less severe form of MUTISM; the process of recovery from akinetic mutism may pass through a stage of abulia, all being aspects of ADYNAMIA. The condition is common following many forms of severe brain damage, but is particularly to be seen following lesions (usually strokes) of the anterior cerebral artery.

acalculia Less commonly called dyscalculia, acalculia refers to all acquired disturbances in calculation and number processing, in the oral as well as in the written modality, due to a brain lesion that occurs in subjects having acquired at least an elementary training in calculation and number skills.

EARLY STUDIES

In the latter half of the nineteenth century it was often noticed that aphasic patients presented various disturbances in number processing and calculation. The idea that deficits in processing numerical material can occur independently of other cognitive or language disorders emerged progressively at the beginning of this century. The term *acalculia* was first introduced by S. E. Henschen in 1919 to designate an acquired disorder of calculation which he distinguished from a disturbance in reading and writing numbers, "cipher alexia" or "cipher agraphia." The concept of acalculia was refined in 1926 by H. Berger, who proposed a distinction between *primary* and *secondary acalculia*. In primary acalculia the disorder cannot be explained by the presence of another cognitive deficit; in contrast, in secondary acalculia the disorder could be the result of disorders associated with language, attention, spacing or memory. On the basis of a large-scale group study, Hécaen and others (1961) proposed a tripartite classification of the acalculias: *alexia and agraphia for digits and numbers* with or without alexia and agraphia for words and letters; *spatial acalculia* in which errors were due to spatial disorganization of written calculation or in the interpretation of the digit value according to

its position in a number and *anarithmetia* which consisted of a primary deficit in doing calculation. Although this classification has had a noticeable impact on the field, at present there exists no consensus concerning the existence of well delineated acalculia syndromes.

RECENT APPROACHES

Since the eighties there has been a renewal in the neuropsychological approach to numerical disorders, which is the result of an emphasis on the specific linguistic characteristics of the different number systems and of the appearance of cognitive-oriented research in the field of acalculia.

Refinements in the description of the linguistic characteristics of the different number systems (verbal, Arabic, or Roman) were made to distinguish for each system lexical and syntactical aspects (Deloche & Seron, 1987). For example, considering only the two most frequently used number systems, verbal numbers and Arabic numbers, they differ in their lexical and syntactical structures. The verbal number system is composed of three main lexical classes. The unit (or one) class from "one" to "nine" represents the basic quantities, the ten class from "ten" to "ninety" refers to the basic quantities times ten, and the "teen" class from eleven to nineteen represents quantities that combine in a sum the basic ones plus ten. The multiplier words such as "hundred," "thousand," and "million" play a specific syntactical role. They enter into sum or product relations according to their position in the word sequence (for example, "two hundreds" means two *times* a hundred whereas "a hundred and two" means a hundred *plus* two). The Arabic system is much simpler. It contains only ten lexical primitives: the digits from "1" to "9" and the "0." It is a strict positional system, which means that the value of a digit is completely determined by its position in the sequence. Lexical processing concerns the comprehension or the production of the individual lexical primitives of a numeral in the different number forms (i.e. the digit 2, the Roman V, or the words two or twenty); syntactical processing concerns the processing of the relations among the lexical primitives in order to comprehend or produce an integrated numeral (twenty-two, IX, or 102).

The adoption of a cognitive and modular perspective has led to splitting numerical processing into three main sub-components: two dealing

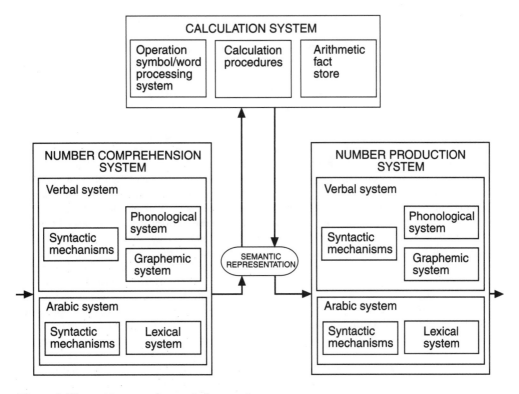

Figure 1 The architecture of numerical processing.

with comprehension and production of numbers respectively, and one devoted to calculation (McCloskey, 1992). According to McCloskey and his collaborators, the role of the number comprehension system is to translate numerical inputs into internal semantic representations, which will subsequently be used for other processing (calculation, magnitude comparison, . . .). Inversely the number production system translates internal representations of numbers into the appropriate output forms. Within these number comprehension and production mechanisms, an Arabic and a verbal component are distinguished and, within each of these sub-components, a distinction between lexical and syntactical processing is made. It should also be noted that the verbal lexicon is divided into phonological and graphemic components in both the verbal comprehension and the verbal production mechanisms.

We will use this modular architecture as a general guide to present the recent research on acalculia, because such an architecture allows us to specify the question according to different types of number processing and number representation. It must be underlined that this model is not universally accepted and that alternative architectures have been proposed (Clark & Campbell, 1991; Dehaene, 1992).

PROCESSING OF NUMBERS

Several single-case studies have shown that the different number processes (reading, writing, speaking aloud, comprehending) may be disrupted selectively, that is, the deficit may be restricted to only one number system in production or in comprehension. The clearest evidence concerns the dissociation between number comprehension and number production. Several patients have been described who were able to comprehend numbers they were unable to produce, whereas other patients could produce but not comprehend numbers. It has also been demonstrated that production errors may selectively affect lexical or syntactical mechanisms. For example, in an extensive study of the pattern of errors produced by a

3

patient HY, McCloskey et al. (1986) observed that a vast majority of errors in the reading aloud of Arabic number forms were lexical substitutions in which an incorrect number word was substituted for the correct one (for example, 17 is read as "thirteen" or 317 is read as "three hundred fourteen"). In contrast, other cases evidenced a very different pattern of errors in which the individual elements of a number were correctly processed but the number produced contained "quantity shift" errors that have been interpreted as syntactical errors (for example, "two hundred forty-nine" transcribed as "2100409").

The description of the precise functional architecture for number processing is the focus of current research. Several theoretical models have been proposed which differ with respect to the nature and organization of the hypothesized numerical semantic representations (abstract, code-dependent, or analogical); the internal structure of the cognitive architecture for number processing (modular versus distributed); and the role of semantic representations in number transcoding tasks (asemantic versus semantic transcoding algorithms have been proposed).

RETRIEVAL OF ARITHMETICAL FACTS, CALCULATION, AND OTHER NUMERICAL PROCESSING

Calculation, as well as other numerical processing (such as odd/even judgments or magnitude comparisons) may be indirectly impaired because of the presence of a deficit located in the production or comprehension processing of numbers; however, some difficulties result from deficits located beyond these encoding or production stages. Here too, fractionation of the processing domain into several interactive but relatively independent sub-components has been proposed (McCloskey & Caramazza, 1987).

Patients have been described who appear to be selectively impaired in the comprehension of arithmetical symbols (+, −, ×, and ÷). This comprehension deficit seemed highly specific since the patients were able to recognize other linguistic and non-linguistic symbols such as letters, numbers, geometrical symbols, playing cards, traffic signs, etc. (Ferro & Botelho, 1980).

Selective deficits of arithmetic fact retrieval have also been reported. For example, Warrington described the case of a patient DC, who was unable to retrieve automatically the result of simple arithmetic operations, whereas he retrieved without any difficulty other verbal non-numerical information. It thus seems highly probable that arithmetical facts constitute a separate semantic domain and that the processes involved in accessing and retrieving that specific knowledge are isolated from other thought processes (Warrington, 1982). At present, other cases of impairment of access of arithmetical facts (mainly multiplication) have been described and precise analyses of the pattern of errors have been used to evaluate the theoretical pertinence of the different models of arithmetic fact retrieval proposed to explain arithmetic performance in normal subjects.

Patients' performances have also been examined to test the abstract versus the code-dependent nature of the stored representation of arithmetical facts. This has been done by analyzing the pattern of errors made by a patient in multiplication problems presented in different number forms (i.e. "seven times four" presented in Arabic or oral modality, "7 × 4" or in dots) to be answered in Arabic or written verbal forms or in dots. Error rate and error types proved to be unaffected by stimuli presentation and response format; the present evidence thus favors a single semantic representation of arithmetical facts (Sokol et al., 1991).

There also exist reports suggesting the existence of a selective deficit in written calculation procedures, especially those concerning borrowing and carrying procedures, but the data are merely anecdotal.

NUMBER AND LANGUAGE PROCESSES

Most recent neuropsychological research has focused on calculation and number processing disorders by postulating a specific and modular functional architecture for numerical processing. However, in the present state of our knowledge, it is far from evident that number processing can be totally separated from language processing. Numbers, just like language, constitute a semiotic system. Indeed, a lexicon (the number names or the Arabic elements), a syntax (rules of succession), and semantics (the quantity represented) may be defined for the numerical domain, and many aspects of number processing, such as number reading or writing, or counting, may be considered as psycholinguistic activities. It is therefore at least plausible that numbers, when they are presented in verbal forms (either phonologic or orthographic) are processed like other verbal material, which could explain why the co-occurrence of language and numerical disorders has been so often stressed. The existence of similarities between word processing and number-word processing has been suggested in studies examining the pattern of errors produced by groups of patients presenting different aphasic disorders. It has been observed that Broca's and Wernicke's aphasics make different types of errors in written number transcoding tasks. Broca's errors consist mostly of the incorrect transcoding of teens and tens by the digits corresponding to the related unit name (e.g. "thirteen" → 3 or "sixty" → 6). These errors could result from a partial processing of the tens and teens numbers (by processing only the root information of the teens and the tens words: "*third*-teen" → 3, "*six*-ty" → 6) which could reflect a general psycholinguistic difficulty in processing the morphological structures of compound words in language in general. In contrast, Wernicke's errors consist mainly in the production of a number close to the target and belonging to the same lexical class (e.g. four → 3 or 5, or twelve → 11 or 13). These errors have been interpreted as being similar to the verbal semantic errors observed in this aphasic subgroup.

More generally, it has been proposed that number words represent a subdivision of the language lexicon which consists of semantic linear orders that are learned by rote in a conventional order during infancy. Other linguistic elements share these characteristics, such as the days, the months, the musical notes, the letters of the alphabet, and the seasons. Some cases of number processing deficits have been described with associated deficits in handling these non-numerical ordered lexicons, but at present we lack sufficient information to confirm whether these similarities in the lexical organization and learning processes result in common representations and processing (Deloche & Seron, 1984).

Another crucial question is whether Arabic numbers are processed by specific mechanisms different from those activated by letters and written verbal material. With regard to the comprehension of single digits, one may ask if the processes for encoding digits are or are not similar to those involved in the encoding of letters or words. At least two different perspectives are plausible: either digits are represented as words or as letters in a similar orthographic lexicon, or they are represented in a separate input system which would code for non-alphabetic forms of numbers and/or for other logographs. The clearest evidence showing a dissociation between the comprehension of letters or words (impaired) on one hand, and of Arabic numbers (preserved) on the other hand, comes from the observation of cases with alexia without agraphia. However, a single case of alexia with agraphia restricted to letters and words has also been described. The question of the relationship between Arabic and alphabetic number processing has also been frequently extended to the more general dichotomy between logographic and phonographic scripts. But one should be cautious with such an extension of the problem, since some dissociation strongly suggests that Kanji logographs (the Japanese alphabet) and digits cannot be equated.

In summary, at the level of single digits there is clinical evidence for single dissociation, but we lack models indicating how digits are encoded and in which way they are differentially processed from alphabetic material. More specific experiments with patients presenting difficulties in reading digits should be conducted to examine how digits are processed and in which format they are represented in an input store. It should also be underlined that if, at present, there exists some evidence indicating a better reading of digits by comparison to words or letters, the reverse dissociation is not well documented.

Little research has been done in the area of single-digit writing. However, a single case of severe agraphia for letters and words with normal written performance for digits and numbers has been reported (Anderson et al., 1990). Furthermore, results of a group study with aphasic patients confronted with counting tasks to be done orally and in the two written number forms (Arabic and alphabetic) indicated that the Arabic condition proved to be the easiest, the alphabetic condition the most difficult, and that the aphasics' performance correlated only in the oral and alphabetic conditions. The high preservation rates of aphasic performance in the Arabic condition suggest that the production of Arabic forms depends on separate production mechanisms (Seron & Deloche, 1987).

Given that the syntactic structures of sequences of digits and words were very different, one might expect differential performance in processing these inputs. Some cases have demonstrated such a dissociation but, with the exception of a well described single-case study with preservation of writing and reading of multidigit numbers with severe alexia and agraphia, no other reported cases of deficit in the production or comprehension of multidigit numbers have systematically compared numerical performance with performance on verbal material. Thus, if it seems plausible to distinguish the syntactical mechanisms for comprehension and production of Arabic numbers from those utilized in processing language, at present little empirical evidence has been gathered to support this claim.

NUMBER AND SPATIAL PROCESSES

Concerning spatial processes intervening in calculation and number processing, one has to distinguish between aspecific and potentially specific disorders. Spatial disorders not specifically restricted to the domain of numbers may interfere with the normal processing of Arabic numbers in writing, reading, or calculation. For example, it has been shown that patients with right-hemisphere lesions may neglect the left part of Arabic numbers in reading or in calculation tasks, or dots on the left side in dot-counting tasks. There is, however, a lack of studies systematically comparing the reading of words and Arabic numbers. Such a comparison may well add to our knowledge of spatial attentional aspects of reading both types of material.

At a procedural level one must consider the possibility of degradation or loss of the spatial knowledge that defines some steps of specific procedures in written calculation: for instance, to begin an addition from the column farthest left, to borrow in subtraction in the next right column, to shift to the left intermediate results in multidigit multiplication. At present there are only anecdotal reports pointing to procedural deficits of this type after a brain lesion.

Finally, it has recently been proposed that some arithmetical domains such as quantification, number comparison, and approximation resort to an analogical magnitude code for quantity representation. This analogical magnitude representation of quantities, called a number line, had been considered independent from other symbolic or abstract number representations and should be used selectively in quantification or estimation tasks (Dehaene, 1992). Some evidence favoring this hypothesis has been reported. Two single-

case studies have been described of patients presenting deficits in number processing and precise calculation while they remain able to access the approximate magnitude of numbers or the result of operations (Warrington, 1982; Dehaene & Cohen, 1986).

LOCALIZATION OF ACALCULIAS?

Franz Joseph Gall proposed in 1825 that numbers and calculation constitute an independent mental faculty located in a calculation center in the inferior frontal lobes. Since this time, no true calculation center has ever been discovered and the localization of brain mechanisms underlying arithmetical and number skills remains a largely unresolved issue. The early anatomical studies regularly stressed the role of left posterior temporal and occipital lesions. Henschen proposed a distinction between left anterior lesions which interfere with motor aspects in number production (counting or writing) and left posterior lesions which produce deficits in number reading. Yet Henschen also suggested a contribution of the right hemisphere to calculation. Several more recent group studies underlined the more dramatic effects of left hemisphere lesions (mainly posterior) on number and calculation processing; but calculation deficits, although generally less severe, have also been reported after right posterior lesions. Recent single-case studies globally reinforce the left posterior localization, but single cases with calculation or number processing deficits have also been described with frontal left lesions and right hemispheric lesions. Finally, the existence of numerical deficits after electrical stimulation of the thalamus and after subcortical lesions points to the participation of some subcortical structures in number and calculation processing.

In summary, disorders in calculation and number processing have been reported after lesions in more than one region of the brain, in both hemispheres, but especially in the left posterior areas, as well as after lesions in subcortical regions (thalamus, putamen, lenticular caudate).

However, given the absence of a precise description of the numerical disorders in most of the group studies, and given the vast differences in methodology and the diversity of arithmetical abilities which have been examined, no one conclusion can be offered at present. It is highly probable that many brain areas intervene in calculation and number processing, but the nature of the contribution of the left hemisphere in number processing, the possible contribution of the right, and the existence of acalculia disorders in the GERSTMANN SYNDROME remain largely unresolved issues (Kahn & Whitaker, 1991).

BIBLIOGRAPHY

Anderson, S. W., Damasio, A. R., & Damasio, H. (1990). Troubled letters but no numbers. Domain specific cognitive impairments following focal damage in frontal cortex. *Brain, 113,* 749–66.

Clark, J. M., & Campbell, J. J. D. (1991). Integrated versus modular theories of number skills and acalculia. *Brain and Cognition, 17,* 204–39.

Dehaene, S. (1992). Varieties of numerical abilities. *Cognition, 44,* 1–42.

Dehaene, S., & Cohen, L. (1986). Two mental calculation systems: a case study of severe acalculia with preserved approximation. *Neuropsychologia, 29,* 1045–74.

Deloche, G., & Seron, X. (1984). Semantic errors reconsidered in the procedural light of stack concepts. *Brain and Language, 21,* 59–71.

Deloche, G. & Seron, X. (1987). Numerical transcoding: a general production model. In G. Deloche & X. Seron (Eds), *Mathematical disabilities: a cognitive neuropsychological perspective* (pp. 137–70). Hillsdale, NJ: Erlbaum.

Ferro, J. M., & Botelho, M. A. S. (1980). Alexia for arithmetical signs: a cause of disturbed calculation. *Cortex, 16,* 175–80.

Hécaen, H., Angelergues, R., & Houiller, S. (1961). Les variétés cliniques acalculies au cours des lésions rétrorolandiques: approche statistique du problème. *Revue Neurologique, 105,* 85–103.

Kahn, E., & Whitaker, H. (1991). Acalculia: an historical review of localisation. *Brain and Cognition, 17,* 102–15.

McCloskey, M. (1992). Cognitive mechanisms in numerical processing: evidence from acquired dyscalculia. *Cognition, 44,* 107–57.

McCloskey, M., & Caramazza, A. (1987). Cognitive mechanisms in normal and impaired number processing and calculation. In G. Deloche & X. Seron (Eds), *Mathematical disabilities: A cognitive neuropsychological perspective* (pp. 221–34). Hillsdale, NJ: Erlbaum.

McCloskey, M., Sokol, S. M., & Goodman, R. A. (1986). Cognitive processes in verbal-number production: inferences from the performance of brain-damaged subjects. *Journal of Experimental Psychology: General, 115,* 307–30.

Seron, X., & Deloche, G. (1987). The production of counting sequences by aphasics and children: a matter of lexical processing? In G. Deloche & X. Seron (Eds), *Mathematical disabilities: a cognitive neuropsychological perspective* (pp. 171–96) Hillsdale, NJ: Erlbaum.

Sokol, S. M., McCloskey, M., Cohen, N. J., & Aliminosa, D. (1991). Cognitive representations and processes in arithmetics: inferences from the performance of brain-damaged subjects. *Journal of Experimental Psychology: Learning, Memory and Cognition, 17,* 355–76.

Warrington, E. K. (1982). The fractionation of arithmetical skills: a single case study. *Quarterly Journal of Experimental Psychology, 34A,* 31–51.

XAVIER SERON

achromatopsia Achromatopsia is the form of METAMORPHOPSIA in which objects lack color. The condition is not necessarily constant, and objects may suddenly or gradually appear to lose their color. It should be distinguished from ERYTHROPSIA in which objects appear to be of a single illusory monochrome hue; in achromatopsia no color is perceived. The nature of this and other similar visual disturbances is that its identification relies wholly on the report of the patient; it does not necessarily follow that the patient will fail a color-matching task, as it is the conscious experience of color which is affected.

The term is also applied as a synonym for acquired color blindness or color imperception. In such cases, of course, the patient will fail on objective tasks which require color matching or identification, and on the standard tests for color blindness. These patients more commonly have posterior right hemisphere lesions and are likely to have visual field defects, and it has been suggested that the anterior inferior region of the occipital lobe is the critical area explaining, on the basis of location, the observed association between color imperception and facial agnosia.

acquired dyslexia *See* DYSLEXIA.

adynamia Adynamia is a general term for flaccid paralysis resulting from muscular weakness. The term is more commonly used for the periodic form in which the patient suffers attacks which may last for minutes or hours, during which no voluntary limb movement is possible although speech is commonly spared. Various forms of periodic paralysis have been identified, mostly familial disorders, and these include adynamia episodica hereditaria.

aging   The neuropsychology of aging may be viewed as the branch of the general psychology of aging that deals with alterations of cerebral function with time. While the term may connote changes in brain function across the life span, the field has been traditionally separated from developmental neuropsychology, which deals mainly with children and adolescents, and typically covers the part of the life span extending from adulthood to old age. There is both basic scientific and clinical interest in how brain function changes with age, and brain function in the elderly is of particular interest. Indeed, there is by now a well established subdiscipline of geriatric neuropsychology (Albert & Moss, 1988). This subdiscipline can be viewed as having two aspects: a developmental one in which the focus is on changes in function with age, and a descriptive one, in which there is a particular interest in studying the behavior of elderly individuals. The first aspect utilizes longitudinal studies, thereby allowing for the observation of changes in function over time in individual subjects. The second aspect typically employs cross-sectional studies, in which older subjects are compared with younger ones, that is, age is used as the main independent variable in the design of the study. In current terminology, the longitudinal studies investigate age changes, while the cross-sectional studies investigate age differences. This distinction is of significant scientific importance.

Clinical neuropsychologists in particular utilize the important distinction between normal and abnormal aging. While this distinction appears straightforward enough, various substantive and methodological complexities make the matter less simple than it appears. Most significantly, thinking about the aging process has changed substantially during recent years. In the past, there seemed to be a general opinion that significant deterioration of cognitive function was an inevitable outcome of old age, that is, everybody who lived long enough would become "senile" in the sense of experiencing generalized cognitive impairment. More contemporary thought suggests

that this is not the case. Rather, there is a widespread belief that there is a genuine distinction between normal and abnormal aging, and that only individuals who develop some form of neuropathological process suffer significant cognitive impairment. Most of the time, this process is one of the progressive degenerative DEMENTIAS, notably Alzheimer's or PICK'S DISEASE, but there are several other causes, such as serious cerebral vascular disease, dementias associated with malnutrition, alcohol dependence, or various systemic illnesses. Another recent change in thinking is that, while it was thought in the past that most senile dementia is associated with cerebral vascular disease, there is now a consensus that most of it is actually produced by Alzheimer's disease and related degenerative disorders. In general, it appears that cognitive changes associated with normal aging are relatively benign, while those associated with dementia are devastating. It also seems unlikely that all people will develop dementia if they live long enough. In individuals without dementia, it appears that, when death occurs, it is likely to be associated with failure of some organ or organ system other than the brain, that is, the brains of very elderly individuals without dementia may look relatively normal on autopsy.

TRADITIONAL THEORIES AND THEIR DESCENDANTS

The field of aging in general is based on a conceptual framework in which there is an inseparable connection between substantive and methodological issues. Thus, neuropsychological theory about how the brain ages may vary substantially with the way experiments are designed and the data are collected. In general, aging is studied by utilizing either a longitudinal or a cross-sectional design. In longitudinal studies, the same individuals are followed over a period of time, and receive periodic evaluations. In cross-sectional designs different people varying in age are compared at the same time. Sometimes the comparison is only between old and young subjects, but sometimes subjects are divided by decades or other units of time into more than two age groups. A major dilemma of aging research is that both these designs are flawed. Longitudinal studies have the problems of attrition of subjects and the "practice effects" associated with repeated measurement using the same procedures.

Cross-sectional studies have the common problem of matching groups, but also the more serious problem of generational or cohort effects. A cohort effect is produced not by chronological age but by time of birth. For example, performance differences between 30- and 60-year-olds on a cognitive task may be associated not with aging, but with differences in educational practices between the times these 30- and 60-year-olds were in school. Longitudinal studies also have cohort effect problems; typically only a single cohort is followed and therefore it represents only individuals within a narrow range of time of birth. Methodologists, notably Schaie and colleagues (1983) have devised various mixed designs to deal with these issues, but they have not often been adopted because of major problems with implementation. Rather than adopting these complex designs, most neuropsychological investigators have instead either demonstrated the sensitivity of their tests to brain dysfunction, and the relative absence of sensitivity to education, socioeconomic status and other cultural factors, or alternatively, they have shown that longitudinal and cross-sectional studies of the same phenomena yielded essentially identical results. Another incompletely resolved methodological problem is ascertainment bias, since studies of cognitive function in elderly individuals commonly use healthy, well-educated subjects.

The discovery of the cohort effect and subsequent research have, nevertheless, altered the traditional view of the aging process. This view, initially popularized by D. Wechsler, with his curve of intelligence and vital capacity (1941), was that INTELLIGENCE QUOTIENT (IQ) peaked during the latter part of the second decade and gradually declined thereafter. Wechsler's data were cross-sectional, and it was eventually accepted that they were readily interpreted as reflecting the influence of a more or less substantial cohort effect. Wechsler also pointed out that certain abilities deteriorate substantially with age, while others are more resistant to deterioration. He called tests of the former abilities "Don't Hold" tests, and tests of the latter abilities were called "Hold" tests. An "Efficiency Quotient" was devised, contrasting the Hold tests (Information, Comprehension, Object Assembly, Picture Completion, and Vocabulary) with the Don't Hold tests (Digit Span, Arithmetic, Digit Symbol, Block Design, Similarities, and Picture Arrange-

ment) in order to reflect the degree of mental deterioration. This idea of selective deterioration of cognitive abilities has survived in various forms to the present time.

A major and still viable modification of Wechsler's theory was made by Cattell in the form of his concept of crystallized and fluid intelligence. Crystallized abilities are based on well learned information that is apparently highly resistant to extinction once learned. The lexicon is one category of information of this type, and short of the acquisition of APHASIA, remains stored in memory relatively permanently. Thus tests of vocabulary tap into crystallized intelligence. Fluid intelligence is the capacity to deal adaptively with information available in the form of conceptualization or problem solving. Problems requiring fluid intelligence are not readily solved with acquired knowledge. Thus tests of conceptual reasoning, such as sorting tasks, are largely dependent upon fluid intelligence. In addition, many tasks that require analysis and synthesis of information available for purposes of problem solving involve fluid intelligence. Thus the Wechsler Block Design test is thought to be a good measure of fluid intelligence. In a classic paper, Horn and Cattell (1967) presented the view that, while fluid intelligence deteriorates with age, crystallized intelligence remains relatively stable.

Methodological issues associated with cohort effects have led to a small number of studies with the complex mixed designs described by Schaie. Schaie and colleagues were, in fact, able to demonstrate empirically that certain abilities differ across cohort or generation, while others differ across age. These studies have suggested that the cohort effect is not only a theoretical possibility but a demonstrated reality. Since these demonstrations, it would appear that increased caution has been exercised with regard to interpreting age differences as caused by the aging process itself. Another admittedly controversial modification to traditional views concerning cognitive decline with aging relates to the belief in gradual decline from the third decade. There are some data to suggest that the decline is not at all gradual, and that elderly individuals in good health retain substantially intact cognitive function until the year preceding death. This view, called the terminal drop hypothesis, suggests that a gradual deterioration is really an artifact of grouped statistical data. Since there will be an increasing number of people in their last year of life as one goes up the age scale, mean values on tests will suggest overall deterioration with age, but they may be unduly influenced by individuals in their final year of life.

To summarize what has occurred theoretically since Wechsler's curve of intelligence and vital capacity, it would appear that the view concerning the impact of normal aging itself has become more benign. Many of the changes formerly attributed to aging itself now seem to be attributable to a combination of factors including health status or frank neurological disease, cohort or generational effects, and, possibly, statistical artifacts produced by the terminal drop phenomenon. A formulation made some time ago by Kinsbourne (1980) that age changes can be characterized in terms of decline in selective attention has received increasing support. There is now a widely held view that the essence of age-related changes in cognitive function may be a decline in the ability to maintain concentration during effortful information processing.

Furthermore, we are now inclined to separate individuals with dementia from those without it, since it now appears that dementia does not necessarily occur in every individual who lives a long life. Developments in neurodiagnostic and brain imaging technologies have significantly supported our capability of making this distinction. With regard to the etiology of dementia, it is no longer thought that most dementias are associated with cerebral vascular pathology. Rather, Alzheimer's disease, which at one time was thought to be a rare disorder, is now thought to be the most common form of senile dementia.

Much reference has been made to the "classic aging pattern" marked by preservation of verbal abilities with deterioration of what has been characterized as performance, integrative, sensory-perceptual, or psychomotor skills. This pattern has been epitomized as reflecting "Hold" and "Don't Hold" abilities, or crystallized and fluid intelligence. Apparently, language abilities only deteriorate substantially when there has been focal neuronal depletion in the language zone of usually the left cerebral hemisphere. In a study involving a factor analysis of the Halstead–Reitan battery and the WAIS, it was found that factors named "psychomotor problem solving" and "nonverbal memory" were found to be particu-

larly age-sensitive. Whether the neuronal substrata for this pattern lie in generalized depletion or selective depletion of the right hemisphere or the frontal lobe remains controversial, but there seems to be general consensus regarding the existence of some form of the classic pattern in normal aging.

NEUROPSYCHOLOGICAL THEORIES

The area of normal aging most studied, as it relates to the central nervous system, has been that of changes in cognitive functioning. The neuropsychological theories of aging are those that attempt to relate behavioral changes associated with aging to corresponding changes in brain structure and function. The earlier theories began with the phenomenon of neuronal depletion. The brain loses large numbers of neurons every day, and it was generally assumed that the depletion took place in a generalized, diffuse way. Thus, an early neuropsychological model postulated that aging produced generalized, diffuse neuronal depletion, and so was a process similar to what is found in individuals who sustain diffuse brain damage for reasons other than aging. Evidence for this view showed that neuropsychological tests that discriminated best between brain-damaged and non-brain-damaged patients also discriminated best between young and old subjects.

Theory and research built around this model also included an effort to assess the age of the brain, relative to the chronological age of the individual. Halstead and Rennick called their concept "Biological Age", while Reitan simply called it "Brain Age." Reitan invented a "Brain Age Quotient," which can be computed from tables he provides. It is based upon six tests from the Halstead–Reitan battery and one of the Wechsler Adult Intelligence Scales (Wechsler–Bellevue, WAIS, or WAIS-R); Digit Symbol and Block Design from the Wechsler, the Halstead Category Test, the total time and location components of the Halstead Tactual Performance Test, and Part B of the Trail-Making Test. These tests are thoroughly described in Reitan and Wolfson (1993), and the appropriate Wechsler scale manual. The Brain Age Quotient score itself resembles a mental age-derived IQ score computed from an intelligence test.

Rinn (1988) argued that, while a decline in mental abilities occurred with aging, the deterioration was abnormal. He proposed that age-related cognitive decline is secondary to brain pathology and is perhaps best described as a subclinical dementia. There is substantial literature to support the view that age-related decrements in cognitive functioning are secondary to age-related brain changes. Rinn noted that a small amount of cortical atrophy accompanies normal aging, beginning in the second decade, and continues until the sixth decade, with a dramatic increase occurring after age 60. In addition, normal aging is associated with reduced cerebral blood flow, beginning around age 25 and declining at increasing rates thereafter, with the most noticeable decline occurring after age 69. Rinn and others have shown that cognitive impairment correlates with brain atrophy and reduced cerebral blood flow. Albert asserted that age-related declines in intellectual processing are evident even among the most healthy elderly. While others found that comorbid physical or mental disease might also contribute to the decline in cognitive functioning, there is a well documented belief that changes in the brain occur in both normal and abnormal aging.

Reviews of the literature on age-related decrements of "normal aging" have demonstrated the existence of age-related declines in some areas of cognitive functioning, while other domains remain relatively stable until the seventh decade. Speed of cognitive processing and motor speed begin to slow at a relatively early age and are evident even in very healthy older adults. Cerella (1990) has theorized that the increased latency of information processing in older adults is attributable to defects distributed across an aging neural network. This represents a change in thinking from the previously held notion that slowed cognition might be due to a dysfunction at some particular discrete stage of information processing. Rather, it appears to pervade the entire network.

The literature has provided a relatively consistent finding of age-related cognitive decline, although the age of onset for the decline varies depending on the nature of the task demand. More recently, the idea has emerged that different domains of cognitive functioning appear to be relatively more vulnerable to the effects of aging than others. Some workers have argued against generalized age-related decline of cognitive abilities. Cognitive functions most vulnerable to aging are those that require the processing of novel information or demand the most effortful processing. Older individuals demonstrate difficulty in spontaneously engaging in deeper levels of information processing. Indeed, elderly adults perform similarly to younger adults on tasks demanding automatic processing but not effortful processing. One compensatory mechanism that assists the older adult with engaging in deeper levels of cognitive processing is the provision of external cues and organization of material.

Alternative neuropsychological theories have questioned the view that age-associated brain morphology changes are necessarily diffuse or generalized. Some time ago Kinsbourne (1980) suggested that three types of changes were possible. There may be uniform changes, but there may also be skewed depletion of neurons or very focal depletion of neurons. Skewed depletion may involve inter-hemisphere differences in the amount of depletion, and may affect various mutually inhibitory balances. Focal depletion might be associated with highly specific cognitive changes.

The concept of skewed depletion may be connected with active theorizing suggesting that there is differential depletion with normal aging. The first suggestion made was that the right hemisphere ages more rapidly than the left. This view was first stated as a clinical observation, but then received some research support. The issue is not without controversy, with some authorities suggesting that the observation is an artifact of tests sensitive to right hemisphere dysfunction tending to be more complex or more effort demanding than tests of left hemisphere function. Wechsler's "Don't Hold" tests are generally also right hemisphere tests, while most of the "Hold" tests would be viewed by neuropsychologists as left hemisphere tests. Furthermore, the selective depletion view would appear to be counterintuitive, since it would seem most likely that the brain would lose neurons in a generalized way.

Based on a review of the changes in cognitive functioning that accompany normal aging, it would also seem reasonable to speculate (as some have) that the frontal cortex of the brain is perhaps most vulnerable to the effects of aging. Squire (1987) reported that the prefrontal cortex suffers approximately 15–20 percent neuronal loss with old age, and represents an area vulnerable to the aging process. Schacter and others (1991) cautioned against overinterpretation, since the frontal lobe encompasses multiple functional and cognitive systems. The relation of frontal lobe dysfunction to specific memory and other cognitive processes demands increased investigation. For example, Boone and colleagues (1990) found little difference in frontal lobe capacity of the older adult compared to healthy middle-aged adults. Similarly, Valdois and others (1990) argued that cognitive profiles of the normal elderly are not easily related to a specific region of cortical dysfunction.

Recent studies have employed MAGNETIC RESONANCE IMAGING (MRI) technology with normal elderly (e.g. Coffey et al., 1990). Such studies might clarify the nature of structural and cognitive changes in the brain with age. Results from MRI indicate that approximately 25–30 percent of older adults without dementia demonstrate leukoaraiosis, defined as a diminution in the density of the white matter. From a review of the MRI findings, anterior cortical regions and subcortical areas, intimately connected with frontal cortex, are frequently cited as regions sensitive to changes with aging. Increased age, and the presence of hypertension, diabetes, and stroke have been found to predict the presence of leukoaraiosis in the elderly. The effect of leukoaraiosis on cognitive functioning in the older adult remains unclear.

In addition to the age-related changes of the frontal cortex, the HIPPOCAMPUS, a neuroanatomic structure important for the learning of new information, has also been found to suffer age-related neurobiological changes.

PSYCHIATRIC DISORDERS OF THE ELDERLY

Perhaps contrary to common stereotyping, most older adults are in good cognitive, behavioral, and emotional health. The situation is quite different in the case of abnormal aging. Various neurological and psychiatric disorders are thought to age in varying ways, with substantial discussion concerning the nature of aging in alcoholism, the mood disorders, SCHIZOPHRENIA, and the various dementias. Unfortunately, there is a large minority of elderly who suffer some form of psychopathology. The following section reviews some common psychiatric illnesses experienced by the elderly. This section will focus on depression since it represents the most common emotional or affective disorder of advanced age.

Depression

Prevalence estimates of major depression in the elderly vary according to the diagnostic criteria employed and whether the patient is institutionalized or not. For example, using DSM-III-R criteria, prevalence estimates of major depression in community-dwelling elderly in the USA ranged from 1 percent for men to 3.64 percent for elderly women. In contrast, 26.8 percent of community-dwelling elderly complained of dysphoric or affective symptoms. It has been argued that DSM-III criteria for major depression are not sensitive enough to capture most older adults in community populations who endorse depressive symptoms. Other studies have reported that major depression is present in approximately 4 percent and dysthymia is present in 5–8 percent of the elderly population. Prevalence estimates of major depression in institutionalized elderly are higher, ranging from 12 percent to over 40 percent.

The rate of new cases of depression in nursing home residents is estimated to be 12.6 percent, with an additional 18 percent developing new depressive symptoms over a one-year period in the USA. Major depression was found in 11.5 percent of elderly hospitalized medical patients, with a rate of 23 percent for depressive symptomatology.

Cognitive impairment in elderly depressed

Ten to 20 percent of elderly depressed suffer significant cognitive impairment. The labels pseudodementia, dementia syndrome of depression, depression-induced organic mental disorder, and depression-related cognitive dysfunction have been used to identify reversible cognitive impairment severe enough to mimic a progressive dementia in the older depressed patient. Pseudodementia occurs most frequently in older patients with depression. There have been numerous articles describing the clinical features of pseudodementia and its differences from progressive dementia. There have been several critical analyses of the label pseudodementia. While some authors have agreed that the label pseudodementia alerts clinicians to the existence of potentially treatable forms of cognitive impairment, they have argued for the abandonment of the term.

Folstein and Rabins (1991) argued that "persons who suffer from both cognitive impairment and depression have abnormalities of common

12

neural structures" (p. 37). For example, it was argued that patients with major depression, PAR-KINSON'S DISEASE, HUNTINGTON'S DISEASE, or ALZHEIMER'S DISEASE suffer a dysfunction of the cortical pathways that bridge aminergic fibers from the brain stem to the cortex. Folstein and Rabins (1991) proposed the syndrome of the aminergic nuclei (SOTAN) as an alternative to the label pseudodementia to capture the coex-istence in the older patient of changes in mood, cognition, and movement. The authors hoped that this concept would alleviate confusion within the literature and promote an understanding of the pathological mechanisms and etiology of cognitive impairment in elderly depressed.

MRI IN ELDERLY DEPRESSED

MRI has demonstrated that older depressed patients have a significantly high incidence of leukoaraiosis and subcortical pathology compared to normal controls (Coffey et al., 1990). The severity of subcortical pathology is related to the later age of onset of depression, vascular disease, presence of hypertension, smoking history, and perhaps hypercholesterolemia. One study (Figiel et al., 1991) found basal ganglia hyperintensities to occur more frequently (60 percent versus 11 percent) in late onset depressed patients (after age 60) than in early onset depressed patients (before age 60). In addition, the lesions in the late onset depressed sample were located in the dorsal aspect of the head of the caudate nucleus. Figiel and colleagues (1991) argued that the depressed patient's FRONTAL LOBE was most vulnerable to the presence of deep white matter hyperintensi-ties, while the PARIETAL and OCCIPITAL LOBES were minimally affected and the TEMPORAL LOBE was free of hyperintensities. These authors speculated that the white matter hyperintensities of the frontal lobe and CAUDATE might induce a depressed mood by disconnection of the cerebral cortex from the limbic system. This speculation would support that proposed by Folstein and Rabins (1991) providing additional evidence for a subcortical-frontal neuropathology of depression in older patients.

The clinical significance of the leukoaraiosis and subcortical pathology in the elderly depressed remains unknown. However, Coffey and coll-eagues found an association between the severity of white matter lesions and memory impairment as measured by a standard scale of verbal and figural recall. In addition, the subcortical lesions measured by CT or MRI in a sample of cogni-tively intact elderly depressed predicted later cognitive decline. Finally, the presence of multi-ple lacunar infarcts, as measured by CT, correl-ates with neuropsychological signs of frontal lobe dysfunction in older patients. These studies rep-resent early attempts to link deep white matter lesions and subcortical pathology to cognitive impairment and depressed mood.

Additional evidence for a subcortical-frontal neuropathology of late onset depression has been demonstrated in the literature on cerebrovascular disease and depression. Results from these studies have demonstrated that depressive dis-order is a common sequel of stroke. Specifically, patients with left dorsal-lateral-frontal cortical lesions and left basal ganglia lesions have been found to have a significantly higher frequency of major depression than patients with other lesion locations.

NEUROPSYCHOLOGICAL FINDINGS

A review of the neuropsychological literature of the elderly depressed suggests deficits of effortful processing, a conservative response bias, psy-chomotor slowing, reduced verbal fluency, poor concept formation, impaired abstract thinking, and poor sustained concentration. Caine (1981) asserted that depressed patients maintain cortic-ally based cognitive capacity, but suffer impair-ment of the arousal-attention-concentration sys-tem. This conclusion supports the notion of an effortful processing deficit in elderly depressed individuals. King and Caine (1990) reviewed the literature on late life depression and concluded that the basal ganglia was a primary region of neuropathology in elderly depressed with cogni-tive impairment. They also called for continued research on the neuroanatomical basis of depres-sion in older adults.

In summary, there is evidence for a neuro-anatomical basis for depression in some elderly. Specifically, depression results from lesions of the anterior cortex and basal ganglia. The existence of leukoaraiosis in elderly depressed might also contribute to the onset of the depressed mood and cognitive impairment through the disruption of cortical-subcortical neurochemical pathways. Depression, in some older adults, appears to be related to a dysfunction of the subcortical-frontal neural system.

13

Mania

Mania occurs in 5–8 percent of patients admitted to psychogeriatric hospitals in the USA (Molinari, 1991). Additionally, 13 percent of older patients diagnosed with affective disorders complain primarily of manic symptoms. It is relatively uncommon, however, for mania to occur for the first time after age 65, but older manic patients demonstrate a high rate of recidivism (Molinari, 1991).

Schizophrenia

Approximately 2 to 10 percent of geriatric psychiatric admissions carry the diagnosis of schizophrenia or other psychotic disorders not secondary to a dementia or mood disorder. A higher percentage (23 percent) of schizophrenia as a discharge diagnosis was found in a sample of geriatric male veterans, although the exclusion of dementia and mood disorders was not employed (Molinari, 1991). The prevalence of persecutory ideation is estimated to be 4 percent in a geriatric community population.

Late onset schizophrenia or "late paraphrenia" is rare but may occur. On the other hand, there are some chronic schizophrenics whose symptoms remit during old age. The view that schizophrenia is a degenerative disorder, and therefore engenders abnormal aging, has been largely discredited. There may be a relatively small subgroup of schizophrenics, characterized as the Kraepelinian type, that undergo a course of inexorable deterioration, but there is substantial evidence suggesting that the cognitive function of schizophrenics changes with age at a normal rate.

Substance abuse in the elderly

The abuse of alcohol and drugs in the elderly population is common, especially after retirement or other life stresses (Christison & Blazer, 1988; Rinn, 1988). Elderly individuals are prone to abuse prescribed medications. Older adults use more medication than younger adults. Research has found that the elderly receive nearly 25 percent of all prescribed medication and represent the largest consumers of sedative-hypnotics and tranquillizers (Christison & Blazer, 1988). Christison and Blazer reported that drug-related disorders in the elderly include abuse, intoxication, dependence/withdrawal, overmedication, drug reactions, interactions, and side effects.

Alcohol is the most frequently used drug of the older population. Nearly 10 percent of adults over the age of 60 suffer alcohol abuse or dependence and this rate increases substantially when institutional settings are considered. Molinari (1991) found the rate of discharge diagnosis of alcohol dependence to be about 3 per cent for geriatric male veterans. Atkinson and others (1990) found that 15 percent of an outpatient sample of older men (over age 59) suffered their first alcohol-related problems after age 60 and 29 percent after age 65. Compared to early onset cases, older onset alcohol problems were more mild, more circumscribed, and related to less family alcoholism and greater psychological stability. Late onset patients also demonstrated more compliance with outpatient treatment regimens (Atkinson et al., 1990).

Rinn (1988) reported that the damaging effects of alcohol on the aging brain tend to be more significant than with younger adults. Older alcoholics may develop cognitive deterioration related to an alcohol dementia, KORSAKOFF'S SYNDROME, or a toxic-metabolic confusional state. Recovery from alcohol-related brain damage is slower in older than in younger adults (Rinn, 1988). Other negative consequences of alcohol abuse in the elderly include increased risk for stroke, decreased cerebral blood flow (Shaw, 1987), severe sleep disturbance that manifests as a decrease in the rapid eye movement stage of sleep, fragmentation of sleep, and increased daytime fatigue (Rinn, 1988).

Dementia

Dementia refers to a disturbance of intellect, personality, and communication functioning. There are at least 50 different etiologies of dementia and some forms are reversible while others are progressive. The prevalence of dementia in the elderly has been estimated to be 15 percent of the population older than 65. The most frequent cause of dementia in the elderly is Alzheimer's disease (AD). Based on autopsy data (Tomlinson et al., 1970), AD alone, or with another disorder, accounts for 50 percent to 70 percent of dementia in those older than 65. A recent clinical survey (Evans et al., 1989) reported that the number of individuals with Alzheimer's disease in the USA was nearly four million. Evans and colleagues (1989) demonstrated that the risk of developing AD increases with age, and so, as longevity increases in the general population, there will be more cases. Koff (1986) reported that the number of AD patients is expected to increase to beyond eight million by the year 2050. These findings raise serious concerns for the maintenance of health care. Some authors have proposed the development of progressive special care units and alternative day-care treatment programs to assist in the care of AD patients (Berg et al., 1991; Koff, 1986). The study of AD should remain a major focus of research during the next century. Indeed, the field of geriatric neuropsychology would appear to represent a specialized area of psychology that will increase in importance with the expanding numbers in the older population.

Note Indebtedness is expressed to the Department of Veterans' Affairs for support of this work.

BIBLIOGRAPHY

Albert, M. S., & Moss, M. B. (1988). *Geriatric neuropsychology*. New York: Guilford.

Atkinson, R. M., Tolson, R. L., & Turner, J. A. (1990). Late versus early onset problem drinking in older men. *Alcoholism: Clinical and Experimental Research, 14*, 574–9.

Berg, L., Buckwalter, K. C., Chafetz, P. K., Gwyther, L. P., Holmes, D., Koepke, K. M., Lawton, M. P., Lindeman, D. A., Magasiner, J., Maslow, K., Sloane, P. D., & Teresi, J. (1991). Special care units for persons with dementia. *Journal of the American Geriatrics Society, 39*, 1229–36.

Boone, K. B., Miller, B. L., Lesser, I. M., Hill, E., & D'Elia, L. D. (1990). Performance on frontal lobe tests in healthy, older individuals. *Developmental Neuropsychology, 6*, 216–23.

Caine, E. D. (1981). Pseudodementia: current concepts and future directions. *Archives of General Psychiatry, 38*, 1359–64.

Cerella, J. (1990). Aging and the information processing rate. In J. E. Birren & K. W. Schaie (Eds), *The psychology of adult development and aging* (pp. 201–19). Washington, DC: American Psychological Association.

Christison, C., & Blazer, D. (1988). Clinical assessment of psychiatric symptoms. In M. S. Albert & M. B. Moss (Eds), *Geriatric neuropsychology* (pp. 82–99). New York: Guilford.

Coffey, E. C., Figiel, G. S., Djang, W. T., & Weiner, R. D. (1990). Subcortical hyperintensity on magnetic resonance imaging: a compar-

ison of normal and depressed elderly subjects. *American Journal of Psychiatry, 147*, 187–9.

Evans, D. A., Funkenstein, H. H., Albert, M. S., Scherr, P. A., Cook, N. R., Chown, M. J., Hebert, L. E., Hennekens, C. H., & Taylor, J. O. (1989). Prevalence of Alzheimer's disease in a community population of older adults. *Journal of the American Medical Association, 262*, 2551–6.

Figiel, G. S., Krishnan, R. R., Doraiswamy, P. M., Rao, V. P., Nemeroff, C. B., & Boyko, O. B. (1991). Subcortical hyperintensities on brain resonance imaging: a comparison between late age onset and early onset elderly depressed subjects. *Neurobiology of Aging, 26*, 245–7.

Folstein, M. F., & Rabins, P. V. (1991). Replacing pseudodementia. *Neuropsychiatry, Neuropsychology, and Behavioral Neurology, 4*, 36–40.

Horn, J. L., & Cattell, R. B. (1967). Age differences in fluid and crystallized intelligence. *Acta Psychologia, 26*, 107–29.

King, D. A., & Caine, E. P. (1990). Depression. In J. L. Cummings (Ed.), *Subcortical dementia* (pp. 218–30). New York: Oxford University Press.

Kinsbourne, M. (1980). Attentional dysfunction and the elderly: theoretical models and research perspectives. In L. W. Poon, J. L. Fozard, L. S. Cermak, D. Arenberg, & L. W. Thompson (Eds), *New directions in memory and aging* (pp. 113–29). Hillsdale, NJ: Erlbaum.

Koff, T. (1986). Nursing home management of Alzheimer's disease. *American Journal of Alzheimer's Care and Related Disorders, Summer*, 12–15.

Molinari, V. A. (1991). Demographic and psychiatric characteristics of 390 consecutive discharges from a geropsychiatric inpatient ward. *Clinical Gerontologist, 10*, 35–45.

Reitan, R. M., & Wolfson, D. (1993). *The Halstead-Reitan Neuropsychological Test Battery: theory and clinical interpretation*. 2nd edn. Tucson: Neuropsychology Press.

Rinn, W. E. (1988). Mental decline in normal aging: a review. *Journal of Geriatric Psychiatry and Neurology, 1*, 144–58.

Schacter, D. L., Kaszniak, A. W., Kihlstrom, J. F., & Valdiserri, M. (1991). The relation between source memory and aging. *Psychology and Aging, 6*, 559–68.

Schaie, K. W. (Ed.), (1983). Longitudinal

studies of adult psychological development. New York: Guilford.

Shaw, T. G. (1987). Alcohol and brain function: an appraisal of cerebral blood flow. In O. A. Parsons, N. Butters, & P. E. Nathan (Eds), *Neuropsychology of alcoholism: Implications for diagnosis and treatment* (pp. 129–54). New York: Guilford.

Squire, L. R. (1987). *Memory and brain*. New York: Oxford University Press.

Tomlinson, B. E., Blessed, G., & Roth, M. (1970). Observations on the brains of demented old people. *Journal of Neurological Science, 11*, 205–42.

GERALD GOLDSTEIN AND PAUL D. NUSSBAUM

agnosia Agnosia is the loss of recognition and identification of a previously learned stimulus. Agnosias can be found across all modalities of stimulus input, including auditory, tactile, and visual modalities. Agnosia for one input modality (e.g. for visual stimuli) need not be accompanied by agnosia for another (e.g. visual agnosic patients can have intact tactile object recognition). Agnosias are distinguished from modality-specific APHASIAS (such as optic aphasia) because the deficit is one of recognition rather than naming; thus agnosic patients are unable to produce the correct gesture or to provide correct semantic descriptions for the objects they fail to recognize. Agnosia can also occur for particular stimuli normally recognized by means of a particular input modality (e.g. for color and faces, with visual stimuli; for music, with auditory stimuli).

Visual agnosias have been studied in more detail than agnosias for stimuli presented via other input modalities. Lissauer in 1890 first distinguished between different types of agnosia. He argued for a distinction between *apperceptive* and *associative* agnosia. Apperceptive agnosia was held to reflect a problem in assembling an appropriate perceptual description of a stimulus in order for recognition to take place. Associative agnosia was held to be due to a failure to retrieve stored knowledge about objects, even though perceptual processing of the stimulus is intact.

The most common clinical test to separate apperceptive from associative agnosia is to ask the patient to copy objects that they fail to recognize; patients who succeed at copying tasks but who still fail to identify objects have been designated as associative agnosics. This simple clinical distinction is probably not adequate. Patients with very impaired visual perception may still copy objects correctly, using a slavish, line-by-line strategy, which is not dependent on intact perceptual processing. More recent work by Warrington and by Humphreys and Riddoch has thus involved attempts to develop a range of more detailed assessments of particular stages of the visual object process.

Warrington noted that patients with posterior right hemisphere lesions can have difficulty with a range of tasks assessing high-level aspects of visual perception that do not necessarily require object recognition. For instance, these agnosic patients can have problems in distinguishing a figure from a complex visual background (e.g. if a stimulus is placed among black and white "noise" squares) and in deciding whether two objects are the same when the objects are depicted in different viewpoints. This last "unusual views" task can be performed by other patients who are still agnosic, in the sense that they fail to recognize the objects involved, so it appears that the task can be performed on the basis of high-level but not stored perceptual information.

In contrast to the pattern of performance after posterior right hemisphere lesions, patients with posterior left hemisphere lesions can perform well on perceptual matching tasks (such as the "unusual views" test), but have difficulty in matching physically different exemplars of the same basic class of object (e.g. when required to match a deck chair with a rocking chair). This suggests that the left hemisphere may be relatively specialized for access to stored knowledge concerned with object functions and categories, whereas the right hemisphere is concerned with delivering high-level perceptual descriptions for the object recognition system. In line with Lissauer's original distinction, posterior right hemisphere lesions produce apperceptive type problems while left hemisphere lesions produce associative type deficits.

RECENT STUDIES

Within the general class of agnosic deficits in vision noted in patients with posterior right and posterior left hemisphere lesions, recent work has indicated that even finer-grained classifications are possible. Thus some patients appear to have problems encoding even the basic aspects of shape and so fail at tests such as the *Efron shape-matching task* in which they have to judge whether two stimuli matched for area and brightness have the same shape or not (e.g. saying yes to two squares but no to a square and a rectangle). Problems with relatively low-level tasks such as this have been noted particularly after carbon monoxide poisoning, which may produce small disseminated lesions through the visual cortex.

Patients may also use different procedures to carry out the "unusual views" matching task. Humphreys and Riddoch noted patterns of dissociation in which some patients have particular difficulty in matching objects seen from views that produce marked foreshortening of the main axis of the objects, while others are impaired if a given view masks local distinguishing features of objects. Such patterns of dissociation suggest that different types of high-level perceptual information may be derived from visually presented

objects, some concerned with local object features and some with more global properties of objects (e.g. concerning the parts of the object relative to its main axis). These two forms of visual description may be used in parallel for object recognition.

Different patterns of performance have also been noted within the general class of associative agnosic patients (with apparently intact perceptual processes but nevertheless poor object recognition). For example, some patients may perform *object decision* tasks at a normal level even though they remain impaired at matching objects on the basis of associative or functional relationships. Such object decision tasks can involve patients deciding whether a given object is real or whether it is unreal, and the difficulty of this discrimination can be altered by varying the similarity of the unreal to the real objects. When real and unreal objects have the same parts (see Figure 2), discrimination between them depends on the real object being recognized as a whole familiar shape; that is, it requires access to stored

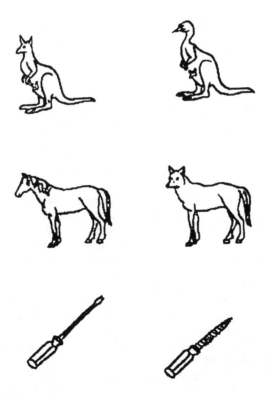

Figure 2 Examples of real and unreal objects from an object decision task. Real objects are shown on the left, unreal on the right.

knowledge about object shape. Patients have performed well on hard object decision tasks (in which unreal objects are formed by interchanging the parts of real objects), while concurrently failing on associative matching tasks, where objects must be matched by association rather than by shape. This contrast between good object decision and poor associative matching suggests that different forms of stored knowledge about objects can be distinguished; stored knowledge about the visual/perceptual properties of objects is separable from stored knowledge about the functional properties of objects. Patients can perform object decision tasks by accessing stored visual/perceptual knowledge about objects, but they can still have problems in accessing stored functional/associative knowledge.

In other cases, however, patients may perform well at high-level perceptual tasks, such as the "unusual views" matching task, but may be impaired at object decision, that is, they cannot judge whether an object that they appear to "see" normally is familiar or unfamiliar. The recognition impairment then seems to reflect either impaired visual/perceptual knowledge about objects or poor access to stored visual/perceptual knowledge from intact perceptual descriptions.

This recent work was reviewed by Humphreys and Riddoch in 1987 and 1993. The work demonstrates that different subtypes of apperceptive and associative impairment exist, reflecting breakdowns to different stages in the object recognition process. More extended classification schemes than those provided by Lissauer have thus been suggested, in which distinctions have been made between various substages in apperception and association. Such extended classification schemes have been presented by Humphreys and Riddoch, and by Warrington in 1985.

PERCEPTION AND IMAGERY

Since agnosic patients can have impaired perception of objects, such patients are relevant to the question of the relationship between perceptual and imagery processes. For instance, are perceptual and imagery processes independent, or do they depend on the same underlying medium, so that a perceptual impairment will necessarily generate problems in imaging the same perceptual information from long-term memory?

Many associative agnosics have been documented with poor recall of the visual character-istics of objects, consistent with their having problems retrieving stored visual/perceptual knowledge, whether that information is accessed directly by objects (in object recognition tasks) or indirectly in imagery tasks. In patients with perceptual rather than memorial forms of agnosia (i.e. with apperceptive rather than associative agnosia), recall from long-term visual memory for objects may be relatively good. Such patients may be far better at picture–word matching than might be expected from their ability to identify objects from vision, presumably because they can retrieve stored visual/perceptual knowledge from the word, which is then used to match against the objects. Nevertheless recent work by Young and his colleagues (1994) suggests that, given suitably sensitive testing, close correlations may be found between the perceptual impairments found in object recognition tasks and those found in imagery tasks. For example, patients whose impairment in FACE RECOGNITION seems due to poor processing of the "holistic" properties of faces (see below) may only be impaired on face imagery tasks which require the imaging of holistic facial information. Such results suggest that a common representation substrate may be used in perception and imagery.

CATEGORY-SPECIFIC DEFICITS

As noted above, patients can present with recognition problems that are more marked for some objects than for others. In 1984 Warrington and Shallice conducted the first detailed study of patients whose recognition deficits were more severe for living objects than for nonliving artifacts, following infection by the herpes simplex encephalitis virus. Numerous other cases with this same pattern of deficit have since been documented. Detailed studies of these patients suggest that the impairments for living things can reflect problems at different stages of object processing. For example, some patients are impaired at object decision tasks, particularly when required to distinguish real living objects from unreal objects made by interchanging the parts of real objects. Other patients, however, can perform at a normal level on object decision tasks but still show poor recognition of living things, for instance, failing to know when to eat fruits and vegetables. Yet other patients have been documented who seem to recognize these objects but who still show impaired naming that is more marked for living than for nonliving objects.

This contrasting set of results, across tasks used to assess different stages of object recognition, suggests that different functional impairments can underlie such category-specific problems in object processing. Living things are similar to one another on the basis of their perceptual properties (objects from the same categories tend to have common physical structures) and also their semantic properties. This means that quite fine perceptual and semantic differences may need to be derived to recognize individual exemplars from the categories, making the processing of living things relatively more vulnerable to the effects of lesioning of stored perceptual and functional knowledge than that of artifacts, where less fine perceptual and semantic differences may be needed to identify the stimulus.

Patients showing the opposite patterns of deficit (i.e. with an impairment more severe for artifacts than for living things) have also been reported, though this reverse pattern seems to be less common. Such an opposite pattern makes it difficult to argue that living things are necessarily more difficult to recognize than artifacts; it may be that the different patterns of deficit reflect problems in deriving particular types of knowledge required for recognition. Problems in recognizing artifacts may be related to difficulties in accessing functional information about motor actions and object use, for example. Stored knowledge of motor actions may be represented separately from stored knowledge of other semantic properties of objects. More work is needed to assess the precise factors involved in such category-specific recognition problems.

In 1988 McCarthy and Warrington also argued that some category-specific problems in recognition can be associated with just one input modality. For example, there may be special difficulty in deriving semantic information about living things from the name of the object, but not necessarily from a picture. From such findings they have argued that semantic memory can be further subdivided according to the modality of input, as well as perhaps according to the type of knowledge stored (e.g. knowledge of motor actions as opposed to other forms of associative knowledge). This proposal remains controversial, however, and other theorists have sought to account for the same data in terms of difficulties in accessing a supramodal semantic system from a particular modality.

One other recognition deficit specific to the class of stimulus is PROSOPAGNOSIA, the recognition deficit for faces. Recognition deficits specific to faces have been documented, and this has led to arguments for recognition procedures which are specific to the class of stimulus; the procedures for recognizing faces may thus differ from those used to recognize other classes of visual object. This specificity for face as opposed to object recognition procedures is also supported by cases showing opposite patterns of dissociation; for instance, some patients showing problems only with human faces but not animal faces (e.g. for prosopagnosic farmers), while others show the opposite deficits.

A contrasting view to this has been proposed by Farah, who has argued that visual object processing involves a continuum of visual descriptions derived from stimuli, from descriptions of non-decomposed perceptual wholes to those of the multiple local parts making up objects. Face recognition is based on non-decomposed perceptual wholes while the recognition of objects may depend either on non-decomposed perceptual wholes or on more partonomic descriptions of objects, perhaps depending upon the nature of the object (e.g. this might be one way in which living and nonliving objects differ). Another task requiring recognition of a different class of visual "object," reading, may principally involve recognition dependent on the parts of the stimulus (in this case the letters). It follows that, if all visual recognition impairments for objects are due to poor derivation of these different types of visual description, then agnosia for objects should never occur in isolation from either prosopagnosia (due to poor derivation of non-decomposed perceptual wholes) or impaired visual word recognition (ALEXIA, due to poor derivation of partonomic visual descriptions). Recent work suggests that relatively "pure" cases of agnosia for objects can occur, in the absence of alexia as well as prosopagnosia, with the object agnosia probably reflecting impaired stored knowledge for certain classes of object (Rumiati et al., 1994). Thus while the account of the types of perceptual description important for recognizing different types of object may stand, it is unlikely that all agnosias can be due to poor derivation of these descriptions. Associative agnosias, due to impairments of stored knowledge specific to certain classes of item, also exist.

OTHER ITEM-SPECIFIC AGNOSIAS WITHIN SINGLE INPUT MODALITIES

In addition to prosopagnosia, other agnosias that exist for particular items within particular input modalities are music agnosia and color agnosia. Neither disorder has been studied in great detail, and neither has had great impact on our understanding of how recognition proceeds in the brain. In each case the pattern of disorder can be understood in terms of the apperceptive–associative framework long used to understand visual object agnosia. For example, the term color agnosia is typically used to describe a form of associative impairment in which patients seem to lose stored knowledge about colors, though their basic perception and ability to match colors may be relatively intact. This may occur together with problems in remembering the stored colors of known objects, though the patients may be able to recall long-term visual knowledge about the shape of objects, suggesting some separation of stored knowledge of object color from stored knowledge of other visual properties of objects.

In general, studies of agnosic patients have been very helpful for gaining knowledge about both the perceptual information used for object recognition and the nature of our stored concepts that allow recognition to take place.

BIBLIOGRAPHY

Farah, M. J. (1990). *Visual agnosia*. Cambridge, MA: MIT Press.

Humphreys, G. W., & Riddoch, M. J. (1987). The fractionation of visual agnosia. In G. W. Humphreys & M. J. Riddoch (Eds), *Visual object processing: A cognitive neuropsychological approach* (pp. 281–306). London: Erlbaum.

Humphreys, G. W., & Riddoch, M. J. (1993). Object agnosias. In C. Kennard (Ed.), *Baillière's clinical neurology: Visual perceptual deficits* (pp. 339–59). London: Baillière Tindall.

McCarthy, R. A., & Warrington, E. K. (1988). Evidence for modality-specific meaning systems in the brain. *Nature, 334*, 428–30.

Rumiati, R., Humphreys, G. W., Riddoch, M. J., & Bateman, A. (1994). Visual object agnosia without alexia or prosopagnosia: evidence for hierarchical theories of visual recognition. *Visual Cognition, 1*, 181–226.

Warrington, E. K. (1985). Agnosia: the impairment of object recognition. In J. A. M. Frederiks (Ed.), *Handbook of clinical neurology*. Vol. 1. *Clinical neuropsychology* (pp. 333–49). Amsterdam: Elsevier.

Warrington, E. K. & Shallice, T. (1984). Category-specific semantic impairments. *Brain, 107*, 829–54.

Young, A. W., Humphreys, G. W., Riddoch, M. J., Hellawell, D., & de Haan, E. (1994). Recognition impairments and face imagery. *Neuropsychologia, 32*, 693–705.

GLYN W. HUMPHREYS

agrammatism Agrammatism is a disorder of language expression in which there are consistent defects in the syntactical structure of the output. These defects are commonly evident in the omission of the relational words: articles, prepositions, conjunctions, and minor modifiers. The resulting output is generally referred to as nonfluent APHASIA.

Not only do agrammatic patients fail to produce the relational, syntactically important elements of language, but they may also have difficulty in comprehending the relational words in understanding spoken or written language. Individuals with agrammatism therefore process relational and syntactically relevant language elements less well than they do substantive and semantically significant elements. The output produced is normally well pronounced and phonemic paraphasias, while they may be present, are less prominent and may be revealed in repetition tasks rather than in spontaneous output.

Agrammatism is classically associated with Broca's aphasia and other forms of anterior aphasia, and this supports the hypothesis that grammatical functions are associated with the more anterior cerebral components of the language system.

Agrammatism may also affect written output, when it is termed *agraphia in agrammatic aphasia*, although it may never occur as a distinct form of aphasia. As with spoken output, linguistic expression is reduced to a string of isolated nouns and verbs with a severe reduction of relational words. An attempt to convey the syntactical structure of the production is made through the order of the words within the sentence, and in writing the patient may also use punctuation. Written sentences are generally short, and all agrammatics are commonly "telegraphic" in character. However, it is uncommon for there to be a close parallel between the spoken and written forms of the agrammatism; the patient may be able to achieve better expression and employ some relational words in either spoken or written output.

Attempts have been made to conceptualize the deficit in agrammatism in linguistic terms (classically, by Tissot, Mounin, and Lhermitte in 1973). In this approach, agrammatism is seen as a syndrome of grammatic disintegration as opposed to a syndrome of phonetic disintegration. This syndrome is characterized by a reduction in language output which may be classified into three types: agrammatism with a morphological predominance; agrammatism without major morphological disturbance but with marked syntactic defects; and pseudoagrammatism with dysprosody. Only the first two of these three types represent "true" agrammatism. This view depends on a dissociation of the morphological and syntactical mechanisms of language associated respectively with deep-structure and surface-structure components.

Others have argued, on the basis of their analysis of the psycholinguistic performance of aphasics (Goodglass & Blumstein, 1973), that agrammatic disorders may not reflect a purely linguistic deficit. Such a view emphasizes performance factors and the influence of such factors as word frequency and sentence length, rather than derivational or transformational complexity, and sees agrammatism as a limitation of the ability to process language rather than an inherent defect in one or more of the component processes.
See also APHASIA

BIBLIOGRAPHY

Goodglass, H., & Blumstein, S. (1973). *Psycholinguistics and aphasia*. Baltimore, MD: Johns Hopkins University Press.
Tissot, R., Mounin, G., & Lhermitte, F. (1973). *L'Agrammatisme*. Brussels: Dessart.

J. GRAHAM BEAUMONT

agraphia Agraphia is the loss or impairment of the ability to produce written language, secondary to acquired central nervous system dysfunction.

Agraphia, a term commonly used interchangeably with dysgraphia, was first employed by Ogle in 1867 to describe a patient who, despite retaining the ability to speak, was no longer able to write. Since that time, numerous classificatory systems of agraphic disturbances have been proposed, though none has gained universal acceptance. These nosologies have largely emanated from clinical neurology and have generally attempted to classify the agraphias based on the presence or absence of accompanying symptomatology such as APHASIA, APRAXIA, or VISUOSPATIAL DISORDERS, as well as emphasizing putative anatomic substrates for these losses. One such classification upon which this entry is modelled is presented in Table 1.

Table 1   Classification of agraphias.

Aphasic agraphias

    Fluent agraphias
        with Wernicke's aphasia
        with conduction aphasia
        with transcortical sensory aphasia
        with anomic aphasia

    Nonfluent agraphias
        with Broca's aphasia
        with transcortical motor aphasia
        with mixed transcortical aphasia
        with global aphasia

    Alexia with agraphia
    Gerstmann syndrome agraphia
    Confusional state agraphia
    Pure agraphia

Nonaphasic agraphias

    Apraxic agraphias

    Motor agraphia
        Paretic agraphia
        Micrographia
        Agraphia with chorea
        Agraphia with tremor
            Essential tremor
            Exaggerated physiologic tremor
            Cerebellar tremor
            Primary writing tremor
        Writer's cramp
    Callosal agraphia
    Reiterative agraphia
    Visuospatial agraphia
    Hysterical agraphia

Recently, theorists grounded in cognitive neuropsychology have offered an alternative yet complementary framework for conceptualizing agraphia which has focused on analysis of the types and patterns of errors in writing and spelling present in agraphic disturbances (Beauvois & Derouesne, 1981; Shallice, 1981). This entry incorporates information from both the syndrome-based/anatomic approach, as well as from the information processing perspective.

While the prevalence and incidence of agraphia have been poorly specified, they are undoubtedly high. Given that writing, unlike speech, is for most a minimally practiced form of communication, it is not surprising that writing is vulnerable to a wide range of brain insults. Similarly, upon recovery from brain damage, writing is commonly among the last cognitive functions to return.

APHASIA-LINKED AGRAPHIAS

Aphasic spoken language is usually accompanied by aphasic agraphia with the pattern of writing deficits in such patients usually analogous to their oral language disturbance (e.g. fluent aphasics have a fluent agraphic output while nonfluent aphasics have nonfluent agraphic output). Despite occasional dissociation between oral and written language deficits, the aphasic agraphias can be usefully categorized using typologies borrowed from the aphasias.

Nonfluent agraphias   Like the nonfluent aphasias – Broca's aphasia, transcortical motor aphasia,

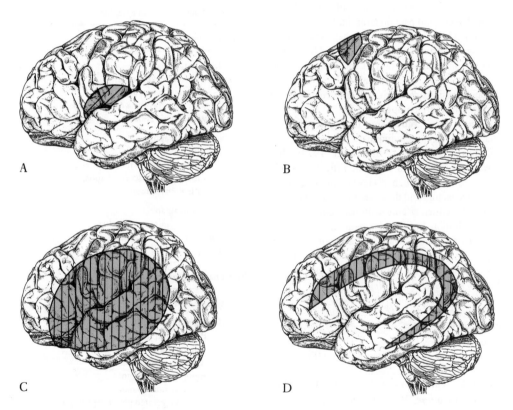

Figure 3 Characteristic lesion sites associated with nonfluent agraphia. A. The lesion site giving rise to agraphia associated with Broca's aphasia (inferior frontal gyrus and adjacent operculum and insula. B. The lesion site giving rise to agraphia associated with transcortical motor aphasia (supplementary motor area and adjacent cingulate gyrus). C. The lesion site giving rise to agraphia associated with global aphasia (entire territory of the middle cerebral artery). D. The lesion site giving rise to agraphia associated with mixed transcortical aphasia (carotid border zone or medial lesion of the anterior and posterior parasagittal structures).

global aphasia, and mixed transcortical aphasia – nonfluent agraphia is characterized by an effortful, sparse production of written output. Writing is generally large in size, scrawled and messy in nature. Patients prefer to print rather than use script, often despite explicit instructions to the contrary. In addition to impaired letter morphology, spelling and grammar are also characteristically impaired. Spelling errors are due to letter omissions, while the agrammatism of nonfluent agraphia is commonly caused by the omission of function words (e.g. prepositions, adverbs).

Among individuals with global aphasia, writing is uniformly impaired and is often limited to an unintelligible, perseverative scrawl. Patients with mixed transcortical aphasia also commonly evidence a nonfluent agraphia, though, analogous to

their retained repetition of oral speech, copying is frequently superior to spontaneous writing or writing to dictation. Nonfluent agraphia can be found with lesions to sites which give rise to the corresponding nonfluent aphasia (see Figure 3).

Fluent agraphias Fluent agraphia occurs in conjunction with the fluent aphasias such as Wernicke's aphasia, transcortical sensory aphasia, anomic aphasia, and conduction aphasia. While patients with fluent agraphia easily produce writing of normal quantity and sentence length with well-formed letter morphology, the presence of paragraphic errors along with a lack of substantive words are characteristic. Incorrect combination of letters (literal paragraphia) is more common than a substitution of semantically related phonemes or words. When asked to read their

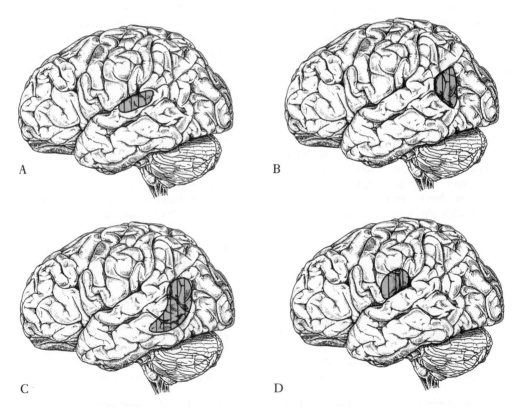

Figure 4 Characteristic lesion sites associated with fluent agraphia. A. The lesion site giving rise to agraphia associated with Wernicke's aphasia (posterior superior temporal gyrus). B. The lesion site giving rise to agraphia associated with transcortical sensory aphasia (angular gyrus or medial parietal lobule). C. The lesion site giving rise to agraphia associated with anomic aphasia (angular gyrus or adjacent areas of the posterior second temporal gyrus). D. The lesion site giving rise to agraphia associated with conduction aphasia (arcuate fasciculus in the region of the left parietal operculum).

23

own erroneous writing, patients with fluent agraphia will be able to detect their errors but may deny that the writing is their own. Lesions resulting in a fluent agraphia (see Figure 4) are commonly located in the posterior third of the dominant superior temporal gyrus and the anterior inferior parietal lobe.

Table 2 reviews the distinctive characteristics of the aphasic agraphias as well as the site of lesion associated with the above aphasic syndromes.

Pure agraphia A writing deficit in the absence of other aphasic symptomatology has been termed pure agraphia. First described by Exner (1881) in a patient with a focal lesion confined to the foot of the second and third frontal convolutions (Exner's area), this finding led Exner to contend that this was the cortical site responsible for writing. While some support for the role of Exner's area in writing has accrued, sufficient conflicting data exist to seriously undermine this contention. Others have reported the presence of pure agraphia in patients with left superior parietal lobe lesions (Brodmann's areas 5 and 7) (Auerbach & Alexander, 1981), the left centrum semiovale (Croisile et al., 1990), and, in a case of pure agraphia for Kanji (the Japanese idiogram alphabet), in the left posterior inferior temporal lobe (Soma et al., 1989).

Other etiologies for pure agraphia without aphasia include confusional state and nitrous oxide intoxication. Agraphia secondary to toxic-metabolic disorders is typically characterized by impaired calligraphy, omissions, and perseverations.

Alexia with agraphia The syndrome of alexia with agraphia, in which patients are unable to produce or understand written language, is associated with pathology of the left inferior parietal lobule – so much so that some have termed the syndrome parietal agraphia. The agraphia associated with alexia shares many of the characteristics of the fluent agraphias, such as normal quantity and ease of production with incomprehensibly ordered letters and words.

Gerstmann syndrome The agraphia associated with the Gerstmann syndrome (agraphia, finger agnosia, acalculia, and right/left confusion) is fluent in nature and is similar, if not identical, to the agraphia associated with alexia. Gerstmann syndrome occurs with lesions to the left angular gyrus (see Figure 5).

NON-APHASIC AGRAPHIA

As the syndromes listed above have illustrated, writing is intimately linked with other language functions; some degree of agraphia is almost always present in aphasic patients. However, writing is also dependent upon intact motor skill, praxis, inter-hemispheric callosal transfer, and visuospatial abilities. Disturbances in any of these realms may also lead to impaired writing.

Apraxic agraphia Praxis for writing requires the ability to correctly access, select, and execute motor programs for letter formation. In apraxic agraphia, a relatively rare phenomenon, the primary disturbance is in the correct formation of letters, especially when writing spontaneously or

Table 2   Characteristics of the agraphias associated with specific types of aphasia and the lesion site associated with each syndrome.

Aphasia type	Agraphic symptomatology	Lesion site
Broca's aphasia	Agrammatic, sparse, poor writing to dictation	Broca's area
Transcortical motor aphasia	Agrammatic, sparse, good writing to dictation	Superior to Broca's area or medial anterior left hemisphere
Global aphasia	Repetitive letters	Large, left hemisphere
Wernicke's aphasia	Fluent, few substantives, paraphasias, cannot write to dictation, cannot copy	Wernicke's area
Transcortical aphasia	Fluent, few substantives, paraphasias, can write to dictation	Angular sensory gyrus
Conduction aphasia	Fluent, few paraphasias, can copy	Arcuate fasciculus
Anomic aphasia	Fluent, reduced substantives	May be residual after any other aphasia
Mixed transcortical aphasia	Echographia only	Lesion of transcortical motor plus transcortical sensory aphasia

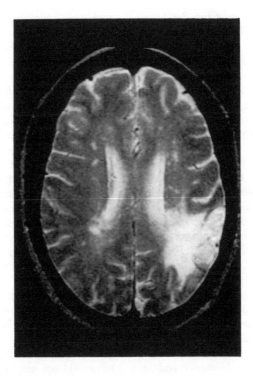

Figure 5 Magnetic resonance image of a patient with Gerstmann syndrome. The transaxial image reveals an infarction in the left angular gyrus (the left brain is on the right side of the photograph).

to dictation. Copying and spelling, especially oral spelling, are frequently, but not always, superior to writing. Though the lack of legibility characteristic of apraxic agraphia makes evaluation of written spelling difficult, the use of block letters or typing can aid in making this dissociation. The patient may or may not be apraxic for other motor acts. Lesions in either parietal lobe, to areas presumably containing letter engrams or the visuokinesthetic motor engram for letters, as well as the corpus callosum, may lead to apraxic agraphia.

Motor agraphia As detailed in Table 1, the motor agraphias consist of paretic, micrographic, hyperkinetic (i.e. associated with chorea or tremor), and reiterative types. Lesions affecting upper and lower motor neurons, the basal ganglia, cerebellum, corticospinal tracts, and the peripheral nerves and musculature may all impair writing.

Paretic agraphia Paretic agraphia results from a corticospinal tract lesion affecting the area mediating hand movements of the contralateral hemisphere or descending motor systems. The paretic

hand lacks fine motor control, is poorly coordinated, slow, and weak. There may be associated numbness if the sensory tracts, thalamus, or sensory cortex are also involved. Muscle stretch reflexes of the limb are typically hyperactive. When the patient attempts to write, the writing instrument is gripped clumsily and the written material is usually large, poorly formed, and unevenly spaced. Spelling is intact. In unusual cases, paretic agraphias may be micrographic but they do not exhibit the progressive diminution in size in a single graphic episode observed with the micrographia of basal ganglia diseases.

Micrographic agraphia Micrographia is primarily seen in Parkinsonian type basal ganglia disease and often occurs with Parkinsonian tremor, rigidity, and bradykinesia. Extrapyramidal type micrographia gets progressively smaller as graphic production proceeds across the page. In addition to progressive diminution in size, the writing of Parkinson's disease patients is often slow, crowded, and may veer off a horizontal orientation developing a left-to-right slant of the

25

lettering. The administration of anti-Parkinsonian medications such as L-Dopa usually results in at least a temporary improvement of the micrographia occurring with idiopathic Parkinson's disease. Similarly, the provision of lined paper and verbal reminders may increase letter size and improve spacing. Unfortunately, in many instances the micrographia is obligatory and resistant to such interventions.

Agraphia associated with tremor Hyperkinetic movement disorders of the upper extremities, such as action tremors, tics, and chorea also produce characteristic disorders of writing. While the resting tremor characteristic of Parkinsonism is only minimally disruptive, an action tremor renders legible writing difficult, if not impossible. Action tremors occur with idiopathic disorders such as essential, familial, and senile tremor or with exaggerated physiologic tremor. The latter can be drug-induced (e.g. by lithium, amphetamines, and tricyclic antidepressants) or may be caused by metabolic disturbances such as drug/alcohol withdrawal, uremia, hepatic encephalopathy, and hyperthyroidism. Action tremors are of small amplitude and high frequency and are particularly evident during sustained activities. There is a regular oscillation superimposed on all graphic lines. In some cases – known as primary writing tremors – the tremor is present only during the act of writing (Kachi et al., 1985). Alcohol, beta-adrenergic blocking agents, and primidone have been shown to ameliorate action tremor. Intention tremors due to cerebellar disease are generally more pronounced than action tremors and are often so severe as to preclude any semblance of legible writing.

Agraphia associated with chorea Choreiform movement disorders such as Huntington's chorea or Sydenham's chorea commonly result in a hyperkinetic motor agraphia. Writing is sloppy, large in size, and crudely formed. Often such patients encounter difficulty maintaining contact of the pen with paper; accordingly, executing fine motor movement becomes exceedingly difficult. The proximal chorea of the Huntington's patient is more likely to result in large sweeping movements which are antithetical to legible writing, whereas Sydenham's chorea is characterized by distal, small-amplitude, abrupt movements.

Writer's cramp Traditionally, writer's cramp had been thought to stem from intrapsychic conflict (though early neurologists such as Duchenne did posit a neurologic basis). However, recent evidence (Sheehy & Marsden, 1982) suggests that writer's cramp is best understood as a focal dystonia caused by disrupted basal ganglia activity.

Reiterative agraphia Reiterative agraphia, or the abnormal repetition of phrases, words, letters, or strokes, can take the form of perseverative, paligraphic, or echographic types. Perseverative behavior, including perseverative writing, is not uncommon among the DEMENTIAS, especially frontal lobe degeneration, and the aphasias, particularly fluent aphasia. Whole words, syllables (usually the final syllable of a word), letters, and parts of letters may all be reiterated. Repeating letters in a word appear especially prone to perseveration (e.g. "butter" becomes "butter"). While perseveration is common, paligraphia (the written repetition of phrases and words) and echographia (recopying of written words and phrases automatically or writing what one hears) are rare. When present, paligraphia is usually associated with severe bilateral brain disease, such as the degenerative dementias, or advanced basal ganglia disease. Echographia has been reported in large left frontotemporal injuries and in catatonia. Among patients with Gilles de La Tourette syndrome one can occasionally observe graphic analogues of verbal tics such as echographia, paligraphia, and coprographia.

Callosal agraphia Writing with one's nondominant hand necessitates that the spelling and graphemic systems of the language-dominant hemisphere have access, via the corpus callosum, to the contralateral motor strip. Lesions to the CORPUS CALLOSUM, especially to the anterior two-thirds (genu and body), disconnect the two hemispheres and result in a unilateral agraphia for the nondominant hand. Affected individuals cannot write spontaneously, or to dictation, with the nondominant hand. Copying is generally better and oral spelling is retained, as is writing with the dominant hand.

A unilateral agraphia for the nondominant hand following section of the posterior half of the corpus callosum has also been reported (Sugishita et al., 1980). In this case, the individual evidenced agraphia for the Japanese phonetic alphabet (Kana) far in excess of his agraphia for words written in the Japanese ideographic alphabet (Kanji). Dominant hand writing was intact, as was bilateral praxis and copying. The putative anatomic substrate for this syndrome was a lesion of the posterior corpus callosum, the area through which afferent fibers from the angular gyrus pass to the nondominant motor strip.

Visuospatial agraphia Lesions of the right parietal lobe, especially in the region of the temporo-parieto-occipital junction, can result in an agraphia of the visuospatial type. Patients with such an agraphia typically: (1) neglect the left side of the page with writing progressively clustered to the right; (2) veer off a horizontal orientation while writing; and (3) incorrectly slant letters, duplicate strokes, and evidence abnormal spacing of letters and syllables. This syndrome is usually accompanied by left hemineglect, hemi-inattention, and ACALCULIA of the visuospatial type.

Conversion/hysterical agraphia In rare instances, individuals with a conversion disorder may evidence an inability to write, secondary to either hysterical paralysis of the upper extremities or a hysterical tremor. In addition to the usual factors accompanying a conversion disorder, neurological examination reveals slightly diminished tone, intact muscle stretch reflexes, and variably retained sensation. Improvement following hypnotic suggestion or Amytal interview helps to confirm the diagnosis.

Hypergraphia While the syndromes previously discussed all reflect reduced and/or impaired writing, hypergraphia is defined as a pathological excess of writing production. As one of the hallmarks of the inter-ictal temporal lobe epileptic personality syndrome (along with hyper-religiosity, deepened emotion, interpersonal "stickiness," circumstantiality, and hyposexuality), the thematic content of their excessive writing commonly reflects heightened concern with religious and philosophical themes. Current evidence suggests that hypergraphia is more prevalent in patients whose epileptic foci are in the right compared to the left temporal lobe (Roberts et al., 1982).

Excessive writing, combined with bizarre content likely to reflect their thought disorder, has also been reported among schizophrenic patients. While the presence of neologisms, word salad, and tangentiality may give the appearance of a fluent agraphia, schizophrenic patients are not dysphasic unless another concomitant brain disease is present.

COGNITIVE NEUROPSYCHOLOGY AND THE AGRAPHIAS

With the advent of cognitive neuropsychology and information processing theory in the 1970s and 1980s, a number of researchers have attempted to understand the process through which writing dysfunction occurs, and by implication, how normal writing occurs. Based upon the work of Beauvois and Derouesne (1981) and Shallice (1981), it is now agreed that there exist two pathways by which words can be spelled: one based on phonology and one on lexical/orthographic representation.

Phonological agraphia The phonological approach to spelling, which relies upon phoneme-to-grapheme rules of correspondence, is the method employed when individuals attempt to "sound out" how a word is spelled. When faced with the need to write unfamiliar words or pronounceable non-words from dictation, this is the path that must be employed. Dysfunction of this system, which has been termed phonological agraphia, results in an inability to spell orthographically regular words not part of an individual's lexicon, as well as phonetically regular nonsense words (e.g. mimsy). In contrast, patients with a phonological agraphia retain the ability to spell words with which they are familiar, even if these words are highly complex or irregular. For example, Shallice (1981) has described a patient who remained able to correctly write to dictation words such as genealogy, cupola, and coniferous, despite an inability to spell unfamiliar words. It is therefore apparent that a phonological agraphia could easily be missed by all but the most thorough examination, especially in individuals with large vocabularies. When detected, however, this dissociation between the ability to write familiar words versus non-words is striking, especially to the patients, who generally remain able to identify their errors when asked to read their writing. On occasion, such subjects may even deny that the writing is their own. Though attempts at spelling non-words bear little phonetic similarity to the target word, the writing errors are commonly orthographically similar (e.g. "dollar" as "bottar"). As depicted in Figure 6, lesions to the dominant anterior inferior supramarginal gyrus and/or the insula have been implicated in this disorder (Bub & Kertesz, 1982; Roeltgen et al., 1983; Shallice, 1981).

A more severe variant of phonological agraphia, termed deep agraphia, has also been described

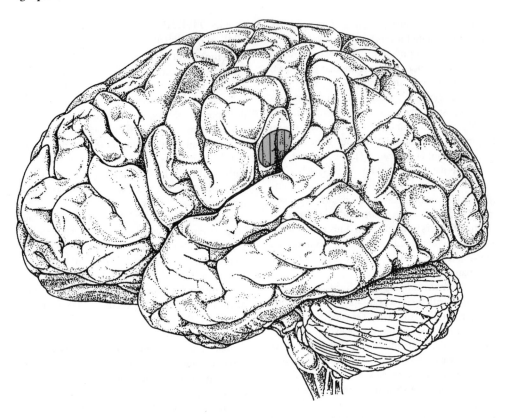

Figure 6 Site of lesion associated with phonological agraphia (dominant anterior inferior supramarginal gyrus and/or the insula immediately medial).

(Bub & Kertesz, 1982). In addition to the features present in phonological agraphia, the syndrome of deep agraphia is further marked by the presence of symptoms analogous to what is seen in deep dyslexia. Among the additional features that characterize this variant are: (1) semantic paragraphias – the substitution of semantically similar words for target words (e.g. "lynch" for "noose"); (2) difficulty spelling verbs and functors such as prepositions and adverbs; and (3) increased difficulty spelling abstract words relative to concrete, highly imageable words. An overlapping, though more extensive, lesion than the one seen in phonological agraphia typically underlies this disorder.

Lexical agraphia The alternative and probably favored method for spelling and writing is the lexical route. This pathway employs a whole-word, visual image-mediated means of retrieving words from one's lexicon and is essential for spelling phonetically irregular words that do not follow usual phoneme-to-grapheme rules of pro-

nunciation, homonyms, and ambiguous words. Disruption of this system, termed lexical or orthographic agraphia (Beauvois & Derouesne, 1981), results in an inability to spell such words against a backdrop of retained ability to spell orthographically regular words and non-words. When access to their lexicon is compromised or the lexicon itself is damaged, patients with a lexical agraphia are forced to rely on the phonological route when spelling. When attempting to write an orthographically irregular word to dictation, such patients will employ phoneme-to-grapheme rules of correspondence, thus "regularizing" the spelling of irregular words (e.g. "feign" becomes "fane"). Errors in writing homonyms and ambiguous words (e.g. pain, pane) are typical, with patients generally selecting high-frequency over low-frequency options. As depicted in Figure 7, damage to the posterior superior angular gyrus and parieto-occipital lobule have been implicated in lexical agraphia.

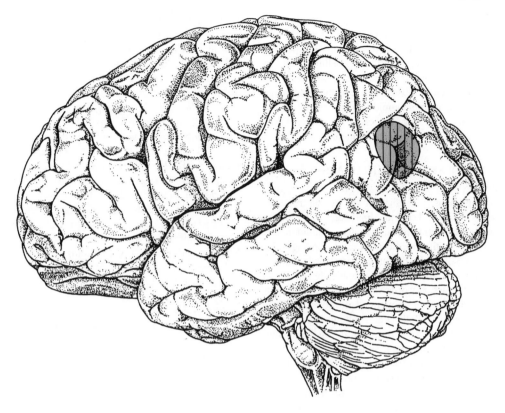

Figure 7 Site of lesion associated with lexical agraphia (posterior superior angular gyrus and parieto-occipital lobule).

Disorders of writing vs disorders of spelling Error-free writing is not only dependent upon the ability to accurately access correct spelling, but also requires the ability to graphically represent letter configurations in the correct order. This allographic procedure, through which letters are graphically generated, determines the shape, case, orientation, and sequence of written letters. Ellis (1982) has proposed three main representations of letters: (1) the grapheme – or abstract representation of a letter; (2) the allograph – which specifies the shape of the letter; and (3) the graph, or actual graphic production of the letter. Margolin (1984) alternatively compartmentalizes these steps into the letter code, the graphic motor pattern or motor engram, and the graphic code, where this motor engram is translated into specific neuromuscular output.

Disorders of the spelling assembly process can result in impaired sequencing of letters, as well as substitutions, deletions, and insertions. More common in longer words, such errors can occur at the beginning, middle, or end of the words. Among normal writers, "slips of the pen" often occur for allographically similar letters, such as M and N. Dissociations of oral spelling from written spelling have also been reported. Bub (1982) has described a patient whose oral spelling was intact, as was typing and spelling using block letters, while the writing of words was impaired. This patient was, however, able to write single letters accurately to dictation, a finding which argues that the deficit was not simply one of the graphic motor pattern.

Models based on information processing theory posit an intermediate stage between the accessing of letters of spelling (either phonologically or lexically) and the graphic production of the target word. This orthographic buffer (Margolin, 1984) can be viewed as working memory (either acoustic or a visual scratch pad) which serves several functions. Initially, one can assume that

29

both phonologic and lexical spellings of target words converge upon this buffer, at which time the individual selects the appropriate spelling. This buffer must hold the spelling code in working memory while the letter configuration is being chosen and executed. Accordingly, damage to working memory could be expected to lead to difficulty in writing, especially for longer words that tax the limits of working memory.

NEUROPSYCHOLOGICAL ASSESSMENT OF AGRAPHIA

Comprehensive evaluation of writing requires assessment of both the linguistic and motoric aspects of writing through review of spontaneous writing, writing to dictation, and copying. The patient should be presented with words that are concrete vs abstract, orthographically regular vs irregular, actual words vs nonsense words, high frequency vs low frequency, and nouns vs verbs and functors. Both oral spelling and writing, including printing, script, and, if possible, typing or use of block letters, should be evaluated. In order to identify correlative symptoms that define clinical syndromes, reading, oral speech, comprehension, repetition, recopying, praxis, visuospatial abilities, and motor/sensory function also need to be assessed. Unfortunately, no extant neuropsychological measure exists which completely captures these factors. However, use of measures such as the Boston Diagnostic Aphasia Examination (Goodglass & Kaplan, 1983) or the Western Aphasia Battery (Kertesz, 1980) in the context of a more extensive neuropsychological evaluation, should provide sufficient data for most clinical purposes. Augmenting such an approach with additional testing based upon patient-specific observations would complete the assessment.

Note The authors would like to thank Norene Hiekel, Tom Marcotte, the Department of Veterans' Affairs, and the National Institute on Aging.

BIBLIOGRAPHY

Auerbach, S. H., & Alexander, M. P. (1981). Pure agraphia and unilateral optic ataxia associated with a left superior parietal lobule lesion. *Journal of Neurology, Neurosurgery, and Psychiatry, 44*, 430–2.

Beauvois, M. F., & Derouesne, J. (1981). Lexical or orthographic agraphia. *Brain, 104*, 21–49.

Bub, D., & Kertesz, A. (1982). Deep agraphia. *Brain and Language, 17*, 146–65.

Croisile, B., Laurent, B., Michel, D., & Trillet, M. (1990). Pure agraphia after deep left hemisphere haematoma. *Journal of Neurology, Neurosurgery, and Psychiatry, 53*, 263–5.

Ellis, A. W. (1982). Spelling and writing (and reading and speaking). In A. W. Ellis (Ed.), *Normality and pathology in cognitive functions* (pp. 113–46). London: Academic Press.

Exner, S. (1881). *Untersuchungen über die Lokalisation der Funktionen in der Grosshirnrinde des Menschen*. Vienna: Wilhelm Braumuller.

Goodglass, H., & Kaplan, E. (1983). *Boston Diagnostic Aphasia Examination*, 2nd edn. Philadelphia: Lea & Febiger.

Kachi, T., Rothwell, J. C., Cowan, J. M. A., & Marsden, C. P. (1985). Writing tremor: its relationship to benign essential tremor. *Journal of Neurology, Neurosurgery, and Psychiatry, 48*, 545–50.

Kertesz, A. (1980). *Western Aphasia Battery*. London: University of Western Ontario.

Margolin, D. I. (1984). The neuropsychology of writing and spelling: semantic, phonologic, motor, and perceptual processes. *Quarterly Journal of Experimental Psychology, 36A*, 459–89.

Ogle, J. W. (1867). Aphasia and agraphia. *Report of the Medical Research Council of St George's Hospital (London), 2*, 28–122.

Roberts, J. K., Robertson, M. M., & Trimble, M. (1982). The lateralising significance of hypergraphia in temporal lobe epilepsy. *Journal of Neurology, Neurosurgery, and Psychiatry, 45*, 131–8.

Roeltgen, D. E., Sevush, S., & Heilman, K. M. (1983). Phonological agraphia: writing by the lexical-semantic route. *Neurology, 33*, 755–65.

Shallice, T. (1981). Phonological agraphia and the lexical route in writing. *Brain, 104*, 412–19.

Sheehy, M. P., & Marsden, C. D. (1982). Writer's cramp – a focal dystonia. *Brain, 105*, 461–80.

Soma, Y., Sugishita, M., Kitamura, K., Maruyama, S., & Imanaga, H. (1989). Lexical agraphia in the Japanese language. *Brain, 112*, 1549–61.

Sugishita, M., Toyokura, Y., Yoshioka, M., & Yamada, R. (1980). Unilateral agraphia after section of the posterior half of the truncus of the corpus callosum. *Brain and Language*, 9, 215–25.

CHARLES H. HINKIN AND JEFFREY L. CUMMINGS

agyria Agyria describes a developmental disorder in which there is the appearance of a smooth brain surface, that is, a failure to develop the normal gyri of the human brain. This rare congenital anomaly is seen as an element of LISSENCEPHALY and results from an arrest of brain development before the third or fourth month of gestational age. It may occur alone or in association with other developmental abnormalities which may include CALLOSAL AGENESIS and MICROCEPHALY. Besides the smooth brain surface and shallow fissures, there is decreased white matter, a thick cortex, and severe enlargement of the lateral ventricles. The condition is similar to PACHYGYRIA but in a more severe form and occurring at an earlier gestational age; it is associated with severe behavioral and cognitive abnormalities.

ahedonia, anhedonia Ahedonia or anhedonia, which is probably the more common term, refers to a loss of the ability to experience pleasure. This loss is usually inferred from the fact that the anhedonic patient exhibits very poor initiation of the normal activities of daily life, being passive and generally unresponsive, with little if any positive emotional expression.

It is presumed that the ability to experience or appreciate pleasure results in a failure of the normal motivational drive systems, so that basic consummatory responses such as eating or drinking, elementary activities such as maintaining a comfortable temperature or posture, or higher order drives such as social contact or intellectual activity, are no longer positively rewarded by the relevant goals being attained. As a result, drive strength is weakened and even well-established habitual responses are no longer expressed, or expressed with a reduced frequency.

The concept of anhedonia is most often employed following head injury, particularly trauma with frontal involvement, when the frontal regulatory systems interacting with LIMBIC SYSTEM structures are presumed to have been affected,

with a result either upon emotional tone or more directly upon the cortical regulation of reward-based drive systems. In severe frontal head injury the anhedonia may be considered to be a primary effect of the lesion, which in turn results in secondary passivity and poor initiation. In less severe head injuries the anhedonia may have less drastic results, being expressed in low motivation, reduced libido, a loss of personal interests, and social withdrawal. Psychological interventions in anhedonic patients are particularly difficult; behavioral interventions are less appropriate because of the difficulty of identifying effective rewards upon which behavioral modification can be based, and cognitive interventions cannot be organized around activities in which the patient is motivated to engage.

A related concept has been employed in the *anhedonic drive syndrome*, which is one type of the syndrome of childhood hyperactivity. Children described as suffering from this form of the syndrome are typically regarded as driven, sullen, unhappy, and remote. They can be regarded as acting driven or stimulus hungry, and restlessly search the environment as if in search of some elusive satisfaction, also showing impulsivity and a failure to sustain attention. Whether this is a valid hypothesis regarding the causes of hyperactivity in certain children is a matter of debate, but it does have some face validity in describing one subgroup of the children who manifest abnormal hyperactivity.

J. GRAHAM BEAUMONT

ahylognosia Ahylognosia is a form of tactile disorder and, more specifically, one of the four forms of tactile recognition disorder, or tactile agnosia, proposed by Delay in 1935. In Delay's classification, ahylognosia refers to an impairment in the discrimination of the distinctive properties of objects such as density, weight, texture, or thermal characteristics, and is distinct from impairment of knowledge about either the size and shape of objects (AMORPHOGNOSIS) or the identity of objects (tactile asymboly).

AIDS AIDS (acquired immune deficiency syndrome) is a progressive and potentially fatal

31

suppression of the IMMUNE SYSTEM resulting from infection by the human immunodeficiency virus (HIV). A distinction is conventionally made between HIV infection where the individual is seropositive but symptomless; ARC (AIDS-related complex), in which there are symptoms but no opportunistic infections or neoplasms; and AIDS, in which there is diagnosis of opportunistic infection, neoplasm, DEMENTIA, or ENCEPHALOPATHY.

Neurological consequences of HIV infection are extremely variable, but peripheral neuropathies occur in over a third of hospitalized AIDS patients, though demyelinating neuropathy and cranial nerve palsy also occur. Involvement of the brain in AIDS may be through direct or opportunistic infections, opportunistic TUMORS, or by complications secondary to systemic disorders. SCANS reveal focal lesions in a third to a half of AIDS patients, with only about a quarter being essentially normal, the balance being made up of cases showing cerebral atrophy.

The neuropsychological abnormalities vary with the underlying neuropathology. Some patients develop no observable neuropsychological abnormalities, and no consistent relationship between disease stage and cognitive dysfunction has been demonstrated. However, some studies have shown that cognitive decline may be demonstrated in HIV seropositive but asymptomatic individuals and it is clear that for many individuals this decline may begin early in the course of the disease, with high-level mental and motor skills being the first affected. With the onset of ARC, and subsequently AIDS, clinical impairment becomes evident in an increasing proportion of affected individuals with impairment of motor and tactile performance, receptive and expressive speech, reading, and memory. Reaction time seems to be a sensitive indicator of the course of the disease. There may well be a concomitant effect of anxiety and depression associated with the psychological distress of being an AIDS sufferer, which compounds to depress neuropsychological performance.

A specific form of AIDS, the AIDS-dementia complex (or AIDS encephalopathy; subacute encephalitis; HIV-associated cognitive-motor complex) is associated with dementia, motor deficits, and behavioral abnormalities. A classic dementia may result within a period of 6 to 12 months, with the expected symptoms of psychomotor retardation, memory deficits, apathy, and poor concentration. The course follows an increasing inability to perform activities of daily living and may result in a VEGETATIVE STATE before death.

J. GRAHAM BEAUMONT

air encephalogram (AEG)   The air encephalogram or pneumoencephalogram is a physical investigative technique which permits the ventricular system to be visualized by X-ray imaging. A large bubble of air is introduced into the CEREBROSPINAL fluid (CSF) by lumbar puncture and the patient is then manipulated on a rotating and tilting table until the bubble is located at the position within the ventricular system to be imaged, the air being differentially opaque to X-rays by contrast with the CSF. Abnormalities in the size or position of the ventricles, from which changes in the surrounding tissue such as atrophy or a space-occupying lesion may be inferred, may therefore be detected. The technique of *ventriculography* depends upon an identical principle, except that the air is directly introduced into the ventricle through a cannula inserted through the skull. As the technique is not without risk and is accompanied by a severe headache for the patient, which may persist for a day or two while the air is absorbed, it is not now commonly employed, having been largely superseded by other forms of imaging (*see* SCAN).

akathisia   Restless, fidgety changes of posture, often including movements of the legs, are known as akathisia when these abnormal movements follow the administration of psychoactive drugs, usually the phenothiazines, and are abolished on withdrawal of the drug. The movements are similar to the RESTLESS LEGS SYNDROME, but they are regarded as being neurologically distinct. Akathisia is sometimes characterized as "cruel restlessness."

akinesia   Any poverty or slowness of movement may be referred to as akinesia. It may be apparent in a blankness of facial expression, the absence of blinking, a lack of swinging the arms while walking (synergetic movements), reduced spontaneous speech, or the absence of normal postural readjustments. It may also be reflected in difficulty in performing repetitive movements, even in the absence of rigidity. It is most commonly observed in PARKINSON'S DISEASE, where almost all voluntary movement is affected by a striking slowness, but lesions of the corpus callosum by involvement of diencephalic structures may also lead to akinesia. (*See also* MUTISM, akinetic.)

alcoholism   Alcoholism is a multidimensional disorder involving ethanol ingestion, influenced by an interaction of environmental factors with specific biological components and reflected in behavior. Two aspects of problematic drinking have been recognized, *alcohol abuse* and *alcohol dependence* (NIAAA, 1993). The former emphasizes psychological or social impairments causing health problems and/or difficulties with

activities of daily living, in which alcohol consumption is implicated; the latter stresses a disability (manifested by craving, tolerance, and physical dependence) in which drinking behaviors cannot be adequately restrained. Among numerous factors influencing the expression and course of the disorder are the following: a family history of alcoholism; an individual's prenatal and perinatal environments; gender; the social and ethnic surroundings during childhood; the age of onset of alcohol consumption; the type and amount of alcohol consumed; the severity and duration of the dependency; nutritional status during periods of consumption; co-morbid medical, neurological, and psychological conditions; and the use or abuse of other psychopharmacological substances. Consequently, no single measuring instrument can establish definitive criteria for alcoholism nor for its putative neurobehavioral sequelae.

Among the most consistently reported neuropsychological consequences of long-term chronic

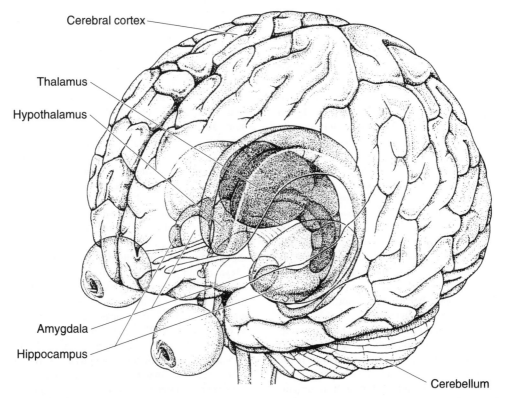

Figure 8 Brain systems important in the complex neuropsychological functions thought to be disrupted with long-term chronic alcoholism.

alcoholism are reduced VISUOSPATIAL or VISUOPERCEPTUAL capabilities, memory loss (especially short-term memory), and personality changes (diminished ability to make plans and judgments, increased rigidity in behavior, and emotional alterations). Brain systems important in these complex functions thought to be disrupted by alcoholism include the limbic lobe, the diencephalon, the basal forebrain, and neocortical regions. These key brain regions can be seen in Figure 8.

BRAIN REGIONS IMPLICATED IN ALCOHOL-RELATED IMPAIRMENTS

The LIMBIC SYSTEM is an interconnected network of structures containing the limbic lobe located deep inside the brain. Four primary parts of the limbic lobe are the CINGULATE GYRUS, the hippocampal region, the amygdaloid complex, and the septal area. Of these limbic structures, the hippocampus and amygdala in the TEMPORAL LOBES have been associated most frequently with alcohol-related neuropsychological impairments, especially changes in memory, visuospatial functions, motivation, and emotion. The role of the HIPPOCAMPUS in human memory has been recognized for decades. Bilateral neurosurgical removal of the hippocampus (along with other parts of the temporal lobes) to control intractable EPILEPSY has left patients with a severe anterograde AMNESIA similar to that seen in alcoholic KORSAKOFF'S DISEASE. Like hippocampectomized patients, patients with alcoholic Korsakoff's syndrome are permanently unable to remember new information for more than a few seconds; they can learn virtually no new information and consequently appear to live in the past. Unlike hippocampectomized patients, however, Korsakoff patients generally exhibit additional cognitive defects, presumably attributable to additional diffuse cortical atrophy. Although recent studies of hippocampal function have refined and broadened our understanding of the role of the hippocampus in behavior, its importance in memory is still generally accepted.

The role of the AMYGDALA in human memory has not been established so definitively. The amygdala receives nerve fibers from brain regions involved in processing information entering the senses. In turn, the amygdala projects information to many brain regions, including the same primary sensory areas from which it receives information.

Cross-modal functions (the ability to use one sense, e.g. vision, to learn something in another sense, e.g. touch), as well as the association of stimulus properties with reinforcement (important in learning and in emotional functioning), are thought to converge in the amygdala. A recent study of cross-modal functions in alcoholics has disclosed deficits in elderly alcoholic patients and in patients with Korsakoff's syndrome, suggesting damage to the amygdala; likewise, studies of emotional changes in alcoholics have revealed deficits attributed in part to amygdala damage (see Oscar-Berman, 1992, for review).

The DIENCEPHALON is a region of the brain nestled within the limbic system directly above the BRAIN STEM. There is controversy about the precise role of diencephalic damage in amnesia, although the involvement of this region has been clearly documented (Talland & Waugh, 1969; Victor et al., 1971). The main diencephalic structures that have been implicated are the mammillary bodies of the HYPOTHALAMUS, the dorsomedial thalamic nucleus (Figure 8), and the nerve fibers connecting these two structures. These structures have been singled out because of their anatomical relationship to the hippocampus and amygdala, and because autopsy has revealed damage there in many memory-disorder patients. Patients with acute, alcoholic WERNICKE'S ENCEPHALOPATHY (brain degeneration characterized behaviorally by general confusion, abnormal gaze and gait, and incoherent speech) who do not receive thiamine treatment, may show evidence of hemorrhagic lesions within the region around the diencephalon. THIAMINE DEFICIENCY has long been associated with neuropathology in alcoholic Korsakoff's syndrome (see reviews by Bowden, 1990, and Lishman, 1990).

The basal forebrain is located just in front of the diencephalon (see Figure 8). Damage to nuclei of the basal forebrain, including the nucleus basalis of Meynert and adjacent sites, has been linked to memory disturbances in several neurological conditions such as Alzheimer's disease, ruptured anterior communicating artery aneurysm, and alcoholic Korsakoff's syndrome. The nucleus basalis of Meynert sends fibers to various brain regions, including the hippocampus and cerebral cortex, and is a major source of the important cholinergic NEUROTRANSMITTER, acetylcholine. (Although acetylcholine deficiency has been documented in memory disorders such as alcoholic

Korsakoff's syndrome, there is evidence that catecholaminergic dysfunction of the neurotransmitters norepinepherine and dopamine may contribute to Korsakoff's syndrome as well.)

Neuroradiographical evidence has revealed a widening of the fissures and sulci over the cerebral hemispheres, and enlargement of the brain's VENTRICLES in alcoholics; these changes clearly suggest cortical atrophy, as well as damage to subcortical structures. Lishman (1990) views the brain's vulnerability to alcoholism as coming from two distinct pathological influences. The first, characterized by cortical shrinkage on CT or MRI SCANS, as well as undetected liability of basal brain regions, Lishman attributed to alcohol neurotoxicity. The second, characterized by pathology in basal brain regions as described in the preceding section, he attributed to thiamine deficiency. Alcoholics who are susceptible to alcohol toxicity alone may develop permanent or transient cognitive deficits associated with cortical shrinkage. Those who are susceptible to thiamine deficiency alone will develop a mild or transient Korsakoff state. Individuals with dual vulnerability, suffering from a combination of alcohol neurotoxicity and thiamine deficiency, will have widespread damage to basal brain structures, as well as to large regions of the cerebral cortex; these people will have severe anterograde amnesia, as well as other cognitive impairments.

Regions of the CEREBRAL CORTEX that appear to be most clearly affected by alcoholism are the FRONTAL, TEMPORAL, and PARIETAL LOBES (as measured by MRI scans of detoxified alcoholics, as well as post-mortem analyses of the brains of alcoholics). Alcoholics, especially patients with Korsakoff's syndrome, exhibit clinical signs associated with damage to the frontal cortex, for example, emotional apathy, DISINHIBITION, and abnormal response PERSEVERATION (see Oscar-Berman, 1991, 1992, for reviews). Deficits suggestive of bilateral temporal and parietal cortical atrophy have also been reported, such as difficulty in forming visual associations and spatial memories respectively. Diffusely distributed damage to cortical regions is also considered to be responsible for cognitive deficits such as poor attention, retarded perceptual processing and visuospatial abnormalities (Ellis & Oscar-Berman, 1989; Oscar-Berman, 1991). In keeping with Lishman's (1990) dual-susceptibility hypothesis, patients with alcoholic Korsakoff's

syndrome show signs of these cognitive deficits intertwined with anterograde amnesia.

NEUROPSYCHOLOGICAL IMPAIRMENTS ASSOCIATED WITH ALCOHOL-RELATED BRAIN DAMAGE

Several hypotheses have been proposed to explain the diverse neuropsychological deficits shown by chronic alcoholics: (1) chronic alcoholism selectively impairs right hemisphere functions; (2) alcoholism has selective effects on functions associated with frontal-diencephalic systems of the brain; (3) alcoholics have diffuse cortical damage that affects the functions of both hemispheres; and (4) chronic alcoholism results in premature AGING of the brain. These hypotheses are not necessarily mutually exclusive, and discussions or reviews of key hypotheses and theories can be found in papers by Bowden (1990), Ellis and Oscar-Berman (1989), Evert and Oscar-Berman (1995), Lishman (1990), and Oscar-Berman (1991, 1992), among others. Although there is considerable evidence to support and refute each of the hypotheses mentioned above, a majority of studies suggests that alcoholism results in diffusely distributed brain damage.

Certain neurological vulnerabilities are more likely to be observed in alcoholic Korsakoff patients than in non-Korsakoff alcoholics; other manifestations of neuropsychological abnormalities may overlap considerably. Dysfunctions of notable overlap include reduced attentional and visuospatial/visuoperceptual abilities that rely heavily upon cortical sensory regions and ASSOCIATION AREAS. Less consistently documented have been functional deficits with relatively little overlap. For example, Korsakoff patients have shown significantly diminished motivational and emotional abilities, as well as CONFABULATION about life events, whereas in non-Korsakoff alcoholics these deficits have been mild or nonexistent. The emotional, motivational, and confabulatory abnormalities in Korsakoff patients have been tied to pathology in limbic, diencephalic, and basal-forebrain structures, and there is evidence that these damaged brain systems are directly involved in the anterograde amnesia of alcoholic Korsakoff's syndrome.

Cognitive deficits Detoxified alcoholics perform more poorly than nonalcoholics on tasks requiring abstracting ability, strategy formulation, hypothesis testing or hand–eye speed and coordina-

35

tion. In addition, they often show subtle memory and learning deficits. Further, although they usually perform well within the normal range on standardized IQ (INTELLIGENCE QUOTIENT) tests such as the Wechsler Adult Intelligence Scale – Revised (WAIS-R), visuospatial or visuoperceptual deficiencies are prevalent. Visuospatial and visuoperceptual functions are commonly assessed with performance subtests of IQ tests. In alcoholics, scores on Digit Symbol, Object Assembly, and Block Design subtests are especially poor, and are generally inferior to scores on verbal subtests. While there is considerable evidence of intact verbal abilities in alcoholics, prudent research has revealed reliable deficits on certain verbal tasks. It has been suggested that the pattern of impairments observed in alcoholics may be influenced in part by the novelty or complexity of the tasks typically used to assess verbal and nonverbal functions. In any case, diffusely distributed cortical changes may be directly responsible for many of the diverse cognitive deficits.

Recovery Studies suggest that slow recovery of cognitive functions occurs in alcoholics who remain abstinent for at least four weeks (NIAAA, 1993), and certain CT and MRI scan parameters have been shown to improve with prolonged abstinence (Grant et al., 1987). Researchers have not established whether (or what) recovery is complete in most alcoholics, and they have not yet determined the typical length of the recovery period. Grant and others (1987, p. 322) proposed that the term "intermediate-duration organic mental disorder associated with alcoholism" be used to describe a slowly reversing subclinical neuropsychiatric syndrome that can persist for months or years in some alcoholics who remain abstinent. Other alcoholics, however, manifest even more persistent neuropsychological impairments; they display apparently irreversible deficits on specific tasks of cognitive function. The term "subacute organic mental disorder associated with alcohol abuse or alcoholism" (Grant et al., 1987, p. 322) was proposed to describe this syndrome, where subtle cognitive deficits and neuroradiological abnormalities persist after years of abstinence. Because length of abstinence has typically approximated four weeks in a majority of studies of neuropsychological deficits, past research may well have overestimated permanent neuropsychological deficits related to chronic alcohol

abuse by examining alcoholics with intermediate-duration organic mental disorder. Finally, there is evidence that older alcoholics may be less likely than younger alcoholics to completely recover from functional impairments.

Subtypes Because alcoholism is viewed as a multifaceted disorder, researchers have begun to classify subtypes of alcoholics along a variety of dimensions such as personality characteristics, family history, and gender. Although there are numerous schemes for subtyping alcoholics, research consistently suggests that specific subtypes of male alcoholics show different types of cognitive and neuropsychological deficits, e.g. antisocial vs nonantisocial, and familial vs nonfamilial. Results of studies have shown that certain familial and antisocial alcoholism subtypes are associated with early onset of alcoholism (heavy drinking before age 25) and with biological fathers who tend to be severe alcohol abusers. These men also evidence greater severity of alcoholism (which may be associated with a greater degree of neuropsychological impairment) and poorer treatment outcome than the nonfamilial and nonantisocial alcoholism subtypes.

A number of researchers have found that children of alcoholics who do not drink alcohol show deficits in neuropsychological functioning, such as impairments in verbal and abstracting abilities. Tarter (1991) reviewed evidence suggesting that children of alcoholics have problems with behavioral self-regulation, leading to characteristics such as impulsivity, emotional instability, reduced capacity for sustained goal-directed behaviors, poor language-mediated skills, and limited short-term memory. Several studies have found that children of alcoholics who do not drink alcohol can be characterized by abnormal brain electrical potentials measured from the scalp (e.g. low P3 amplitude of the event-related potential or ERP). Since abstinent alcoholics display similar electrophysiological abnormalities, researchers have inferred that these brain waves in children of alcoholics may provide a phenotypic marker for alcoholism.

Gender differences Studies indicate that females show the same pattern of deficits on neuropsychological tests as males. Females perform poorly on tests assessing visuospatial abilities, nonverbal abstracting abilities, and problem-solving abilities. Their verbal skills generally appear to be intact, but they do show impairment on tests assessing verbal abstracting and problem-solving abilities. There is evidence to suggest that chronic alcohol abuse may affect female brains in different ways from male brains. In one study, for example, although male and female alcoholic subjects showed impaired performance on neuro-psychological tests relative to control subjects, only the male alcoholics differed from controls on specific ERP amplitude measures (N1, NdA, and P3 components). In another study there was CT scan evidence of a greater degree of ventricular dilatation in female alcoholics relative to same-sex control subjects than in male alcoholics. In addition, female alcoholics were equally impaired on psychometric tests, even though they had shorter drinking histories, had consumed less alcohol, and had been abstinent for a longer period of time than the males.

Subject variables To attain greater consistency across studies than in past research endeavors, researchers should ideally use a uniform set of criteria for selecting subjects. Alcoholic and nonalcoholic groups should be matched for educational level and age, since statistical adjustments for education or age mismatch can produce misleading results. Exclusion criteria should disallow a history of head injury, coexisting psychiatric disorders, and heavy use of other drugs (unless co-morbidity is a specific focus of the research). Furthermore, there should be a consensus among researchers about how to define alcohol abuse or dependence for research purposes. For example, some researchers use DSM-III-R diagnostic criteria to classify subjects as alcoholics, while others use the amount of alcohol intake as the sole criterion (e.g. number of drinks per week and/or number of years of heavy use). If possible, researchers should use self-reported alcohol consumption measures, alcoholism screening measures, and physiological/biochemical measures of alcohol consumption (e.g. see NIAAA, 1990). Biologically based measures are especially important to confirm subjects' self-reports of abstinence in studies requiring alcoholics to be abstinent for a particular period of time before testing.

Concluding remarks Reviews of the literature on neuropsychological deficits associated with long-term alcoholism have revealed that results of alcoholism studies are often conflicting. For example, some researchers have found relationships between self-reports of drinking histories and neuropsychological findings, while others have not. Other conflicting findings in the alcoholism literature have already been mentioned. To reduce such inconsistencies, and to formulate any plausible, causal model of alcohol-associated neuropsychological deficits, a large number of important variables need to be considered. These variables include: (1) neuromedical status (e.g. disabilities existing before the onset of alcohol abuse, such as attention deficit disorder, history of head injury, presence of specific organ disease such as cirrhosis, nutritional variables, and use of other drugs); (2) age, gender, education, and social position; (3) genetic factors (e.g. family history of alcoholism); (4) personality variables such as temperament, motivation, and affect; (5) test characteristics (e.g. difficulty, complexity); (6) factors related to alcohol abuse (duration of heavy drinking, lifetime pattern of alcohol use (e.g. binge vs daily drinking), age of onset of heavy drinking, frequency of alcohol use, amount per occasion, length of abstinence, and recent drinking history); and (7) brain structure and function. Finally, careful prospective, longitudinal studies can help determine whether neuropsychological deficits precede and/or result from chronic alcoholism, and the extent to which there is recovery with abstinence.

BIBLIOGRAPHY

Bowden, S. C. (1990). Separating cognitive impairment in neurologically asymptomatic alcoholism from Wernicke-Korsakoff syndrome: is the neuropsychological distinction justified? *Psychological Bulletin, 107*, 355–66.

Ellis, R. J., & Oscar-Berman, M. (1989). Alcoholism, aging, and functional cerebral asymmetries. *Psychological Bulletin, 106*, 128–47.

Evert, D. L., & Oscar-Berman, M. (1995). Alcohol-related cognitive impairments: an overview of how alcoholism may affect the workings of the brain. *Alcohol Health and Research World, 19* (in press).

Grant, I., Reed, R., & Adams, K. M. (1987). Diagnosis of intermediate-duration and subacute organic mental disorders in abstinent alcoholics. *Journal of Clinical Psychiatry, 48*, 319–23.

Lishman, W. A. (1990). Alcohol and the brain. *British Journal of Psychiatry, 156*, 635–44.

NIAAA (1990). Alcohol and the brain. *Alcohol*

Health and Research World, 14 (whole no. 2), 81–168.

NIAAA (1993). *Eighth Special Report to the US Congress on Alcohol and Health.* Rockville, MD: US Department of Health and Human Services, Public Health Service, Alcohol, Drug Abuse, and Mental Health Administration.

Oscar-Berman, M. (1991). Clinical and experimental approaches to varieties of memory. *International Journal of Neuroscience, 58,* 135–50.

Oscar-Berman, M. (1992). The contributions of emotional and motivational abnormalities to cognitive deficits in alcoholism and aging. In L. R. Squire & N. Butters (Eds), *Neuropsychology of memory,* 2nd edn (pp. 194–202). New York: Guilford.

Talland, G. A., & Waugh, N. (Eds). (1969). *The pathology of memory.* New York: Academic Press.

Tarter, R. E. (1991). Developmental behavior-genetic perspective of alcoholism etiology. In M. Galanter (Ed.), *Recent developments in alcoholism,* Vol. 9 (pp. 69–85). New York: Plenum Press.

Victor, M., Adams, R. D., & Collins, G. H. (1971). *The Wernicke-Korsakoff syndrome.* Philadelphia: Davis.

MARLENE OSCAR-BERMAN AND NANCY HUTNER

alexia Alexia refers to an acquired disturbance in the ability to interpret written language and is adequately defined as *the loss or impairment of the ability to comprehend written or printed language caused by brain damage.*

One key to this definition is the concept of *loss;* alexia is an acquired disorder and the term is used by a majority of clinicians to designate all acquired reading impairments. By this definition, reading skills have been present and are now lost through damage to the brain. Some, however, prefer the term DYSLEXIA to signify states with partial impairment, reserving the term alexia for total loss. While rational, this usage can cause confusion as dyslexia has been widely used to designate one aspect of language retardation, an inherent inability to acquire reading skills. In this sense dyslexia is a very different disorder, an inborn defect that obviates or slows the acquisition of reading skills. Although etymologically inexact, the use of alexia for acquired reading problems

and dyslexia for inherent reading problems not only enjoys broad usage but provides some degree of precision. Others make the distinction between *developmental dyslexia* and *acquired dyslexia.*

An important component of the definition of alexia concerns the ability to comprehend. In cases with brain damage, reading out loud may be preserved while comprehension is impaired; the opposite may also occur. By definition, alexia refers only to the disorders in which comprehension is compromised.

HISTORICAL BACKGROUND

While recognized for centuries, alexia became a significant problem only in the twentieth century, after literacy became widespread. The origin of current concepts of alexia stems from two reports of single cases (Déjerine, 1891, 1892). The first describes an individual who suffered a cerebrovascular accident that caused right-sided weakness and sensory loss, a homonymous HEMI-ANOPIA and disturbed language function, including total loss of the ability to read and write. All symptoms cleared with the exception of the right visual-field defect and the acquired illiteracy. Some years later the patient expired and at post-mortem a sizable lesion that involved the left parietal lobe, particularly the angular gyrus, was demonstrated. Déjerine suggested that this area, the dominant hemisphere angular gyrus, acted as the repository for memories of written language and was essential for both reading and writing.

One year later (1892) Déjerine published a second case report that described an educated Parisian male who woke one morning to find that he was unable to read his newspaper. Ophthalmologic examination showed a right homonymous hemianopia and, although unable to comprehend written language, the patient could produce it (write) in a normal or near normal manner. At post-mortem a single lesion was demonstrated, an infarction in the left posterior cerebral artery territory that had destroyed the geniculocalcarine pathways on the left side (causing the right homonymous hemianopia) and also involved the splenium of the corpus callosum. Déjerine conjectured that, although this patient could see the written language in his intact right visual cortex, this information could not be transferred to the equally intact language area of the left hemisphere. The patient was unable to read (comprehend visual language) but writing was accomplished by the left hemisphere language area acting independently of the damaged left visual area. Although quickly accepted by ophthalmologists and neurologists, Déjerine's differentiation of alexia was lost with the rise of holistic explanations of language function. Déjerine's cases were rediscovered, republished (Geschwind, 1962) and rapidly became the established base for contemporary clinical-anatomical studies of reading. Additional case material has provided both amplification and clarification, and several significant variations of acquired reading disorder have been demonstrated in the past three decades. Several of the variations are of consequence if alexia is used to study the neural basis of reading.

MAJOR SYNDROMES OF ALEXIA

Central alexia

The core disorder, termed central alexia here, has many additional names (see Table 3) such as alexia with AGRAPHIA and parieto-temporal alexia. The basic clinical features include severe disturbance (not necessarily total) of both reading and writing, preserved ability to copy written language but in a slavish and non-comprehended manner, and loss of the ability to name letters, to comprehend spelled words, or to read out loud. Central alexia is most often accompanied by other neurological and neurobehavioral disorders including APHASIA (global, Wernicke's, transcortical sensory, or anomic), often by components of the GERSTMANN SYNDROME (finger agnosia, right/left disorientation, acalculia, and

agraphia) and some degree of hemisensory loss and/or right homonymous visual field defect (see Table 3). The essential locus of pathology includes the inferior parietal lobe of the language dominant hemisphere, centering on the angular gyrus.

Posterior alexia

This reading disorder also has many synonyms, the most frequent being alexia without agraphia. The syndrome is dramatic: although the individual has lost the ability to read, writing is almost or totally within normal limits. The written output, however, cannot be comprehended by the patient. Individuals with posterior alexia usually recognize (read) some individual letters and eventually learn to spell written words aloud and then recognize the spelled words. They write easily, both spontaneously and to dictation, but have problems when attempting to copy written language. They readily identify words spelled aloud by the examiner and can spell aloud without difficulty. The basic neurologic findings are few and variable; in most instances there is a right homonymous hemianopia and often some degree of color-naming disturbance (see Table 4). The underlying pathology is that described by Dejerine – infarction in the left posterior cerebral artery territory, including the splenium of the corpus callosum. One pathological variation, called subangular alexia, features a lesion (often tumor or hematoma) deep in the dominant hemisphere that undercuts and isolates the angular gyrus (Greenblatt, 1977).

Table 3 Three major syndromes of alexia.

Posterior alexia	Central alexia	Anterior Alexia
Associative alexia	Semantic alexia	Anterior alexia
Occipital alexia	Parieto-temporal alexia	Frontal alexia
Splenio-occipital alexia	Subangular alexia	
Postangular alexia	Angular alexia	Preangular alexia
Alexia without agraphia	Alexia with agraphia	
Agnosic alexia	Aphasic alexia	
Verbal alexia	Total (literal and verbal) alexia	Literal alexia
Optic alexia	Cortical alexia	
Word blindness	Letter and word blindness	Letter blindness
Visual alexia	Surface alexia	
Pure alexia	Acquired illiteracy	

(From Benson, 1985, with permission.)

Table 4   Clinical features differentiating the three major syndromes of alexia.

	Posterior	Central	Anterior
WRITTEN LANGUAGE			
(1) Reading	Primarily verbal alexia	Total alexia	Primarily literal alexia
(2) Writing to dictation	No agraphia	Severe agraphia	Severe agraphia
(3) Copying	Slavish (poorer than writing to dictation)	Slavish	Poor, clumsy, omissions
(4) Letter naming	Relatively good	Severe letter anomia	Severe letter anomia
(5) Comprehension of spelled words	Good	Failed	Some success
(6) Spelling aloud	Good	Failed	Poor
ASSOCIATED FINDINGS			
(1) Language output	Normal	Fluent aphasia	Nonfluent aphasia
(2) Motor	No paresis	Mild paresis	Hemiplegia
(3) Motor apraxia	None	Occasionally present	Frequently present
(4) Sensation	No sensory loss	Often hemisensory loss	Usually mild sensory loss
(5) Visual fields	Right hemianopia	Hemianopia may or may not be present	Usually intact
(6) Gerstmann syndrome	Absent	Frequently present	Absent

(From Benson, 1985, with permission.)

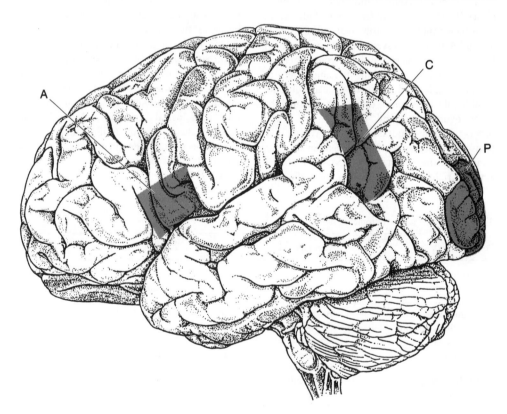

Figure 9 Primary sites of neuropathology in the three major syndromes of alexia. A, anterior; C, central; P, posterior.

Anterior alexia

Anterior alexia, although more recently described, has also acquired a number of names (Table 3). Clinically, the patient has great difficulty in naming individual letters of the alphabet but retains the ability to recognize some written words, most of which represent concrete, imageable objects. Agraphia is severe and the ability to copy written language is poor, with clumsy letter formation and a tendency to omission. Patients with anterior alexia comprehend some spelled words but are poor at spelling aloud, and careful evaluation demonstrates that they recognize some semantically meaningful words but fail to comprehend the grammatically significant function words, an agrammatism of written language. Anterior alexia most often occurs in conjunction with Broca's aphasia. The accompanying findings often include a right HEMIPLEGIA and may include unilateral sensory and/or visual-field defect (see Table 4).

Figure 9 presents a graphic outline of the general location of left hemisphere pathology in the three major syndromes of alexia.

A number of additional subtypes of acquired reading disorders have been suggested; these will be presented alphabetically. In addition, recent linguistic studies of acquired written language disturbances have introduced a linguistically oriented terminology that will be presented separately.

SUBTYPES OF ALEXIA

Agnosic alexia   An older term that was used when agnosia represented almost any inability to recognize or identify. Agnosic alexia identified an inability to recognize written language symbols.

Aphasic alexia   Another older term that refers to the disturbances in the comprehension of written language that accompany varieties of aphasia. Alexia is a defining component of both Wernicke's and the transcortical sensory aphasia syndromes and is frequent in Broca's aphasia. Aphasic alexia encompasses both the central and the anterior syndromes of alexia.

Cipher alexia   An infrequently used term that indicates difficulty in the comprehension of number language.

Global alexia   A term used to indicate total loss of the ability to understand written or printed language. Although synonymous with central alexia, global alexia indicates that the disorder is total, whereas it can be partial in central alexia.

Hemi-alexia   A condition in which an individual can read adequately in one visual field (usually the right) but not in the other visual field. The disorder has been described in cases where the posterior corpus callosum has been severed but both visual sensory areas remained intact. Thus, while the non-dominant hemisphere (usually right) visual sensory area receives appropriate signals, the information cannot be transferred to the dominant hemisphere language area in a manner analogous to the mechanism underlying posterior alexia. Tachistoscopic single-field visual presentations are necessary to demonstrate hemi-alexia.

Hemi-spatial alexia   This term has been used to denote a reading disorder in which only half a long word is read. Almost invariably, this deficit indicates a homonymous visual field and/or unilateral inattention deficit. In cases of left hemi-spatial alexia the left side of the word will be omitted (e.g. basketball will be read as "ball"), whereas the opposite occurs with right hemi-spatial neglect (e.g. basketball read as "basket"). The reading disorder of hemi-spatial alexia can be overcome by presenting words in a vertical rather than the traditional horizontal orientation.

Literal alexia   A rarely used term that defines an inability to recognize individual letters of the alphabet. Literal alexia is a significant feature of anterior alexia and is contrasted with verbal alexia.

Optic alexia   As most commonly used, optic alexia is synonymous with posterior alexia and denotes inability to comprehend visually presented language symbols. A number of additional deficits (e.g. inability to copy written language, confrontation ANOMIA, color naming disturbance, etc.) have been proposed as specific for optic alexia but none has been found consistently.

Paralexia   This term denotes substitution within written language and, almost universally, indicates substitutions made when reading aloud. Multiple variations such as literal paralexia, semantic paralexia, cipher paralexia, phonemic paralexia, etc. have been suggested. In each instance an incorrect element (letter, word, number, phoneme) has been substituted as a written word is read aloud. The incorrect substitution is often the same type of element (e.g. letter for letter, number for number) but may be a different element or a nonsense substitution (neologism).

Pseudo-alexia This term indicates an untrue claim of an inability to read. Very few cases have been recorded, almost always with psychogenic explanations offered. No consistent pattern for the reading disorder has been reported and the psychogenic explanations also lack consistency.

Spatial alexia This term denotes a disorder of reading based on difficulty in perceiving the location (place holding) of letters or words or maintaining the correct sequence of lines of print. Spatial alexia is generally considered a right hemisphere dysfunction and is usually associated with severe visual-spatial discrimination problems.

Verbal alexia This term, the opposite of literal alexia, defines a situation in which the individual can read individual letters but cannot read the full word. Verbal alexia is a striking finding of the posterior alexia syndrome.

LINGUISTIC SUBTYPES OF ALEXIA

Even more than spoken language, written language lends itself to the specific categorizations of modern linguistics. The basic concept underlying linguistic approaches to reading suggests that reading proceeds along two paths: (1) direct, in which the written word is matched to a visual word in memory; (2) indirect, in which the written word is transformed into a spoken word. Three distinct subtypes of acquired reading impairment can be devised from this concept. Most linguists tend to use the term dyslexia rather than alexia when describing acquired reading problems.

Phonological alexia (dyslexia) This disorder represents an inability to make spelling-to-sound correspondence rules. The results are visual paralexias, real words misread as visually similar words (e.g. "cat" for "car"). High frequency words are more likely to be read correctly than low frequency words and spelling is usually impaired.

Surface alexia (dyslexia) In this disorder a grapheme-to-phoneme conversion disorder produces disturbance of the ability to read words with ambiguous or irregular orthography (e.g. "tough" read as "tug") while words that follow conventional grapheme-to-phoneme conversion rules are read aloud successfully.

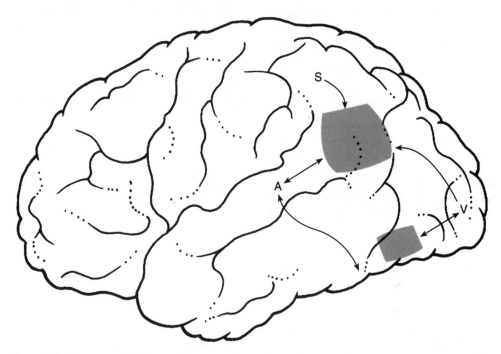

Figure 10 Two areas of left hemisphere neuropathology leading to variations of alexia in Japanese. V, visual association cortex; A, auditory association cortex; S, somesthetic association cortex. (After Iwata, 1986, with permission.)

Deep alexia (dyslexia) The prime features of this disorder are reading errors based on semantic (real word) substitutions for the target word (semantic paralexia). The substituted word may be a semantic paralexia, a totally incorrect word, or a neologism (e.g. "infant" could be read as "baby", "basement," or "garvon"). Nouns, particularly those indicating imageable objects, are more likely to be pronounced correctly than adjectives or verbs; syntactic (functional) words are almost totally omitted and pseudo-words cannot be produced.

ALEXIA IN ORIENTAL LANGUAGES

The use of pictographic characters (e.g. Chinese) or a mixture of syllabic and pictographic characters (e.g. Japanese) for writing in the Oriental languages offers potential for variations in alexia. To date, however, unique variations in the clinical presentations of alexia in the Oriental languages have not been demonstrated. It was proposed that right hemisphere damage with subsequent visual-spatial disability might interfere with the recognition of pictographic (spatial) characters, a logical theory that has not been confirmed. Studies of alexia in Japanese do suggest a pertinent distinction; however, the dominant hemisphere posterior-superior temporal region appears crucial for syllabic reading whereas the dominant inferotemporal region is more pertinent for pictographic reading; the angular gyrus appears essential for both types of reading. Figure 10 illustrates the anatomical demarcations suggested from studies of alexia in Japanese.

READING WITH THE RIGHT HEMISPHERE

Careful investigation of patients following complete section of the corpus callosum has demonstrated that the right hemisphere can comprehend selected written material, particularly words representing imageable objects. While the words can be comprehended, they cannot be "read" aloud. Thus selected nouns, adjectives, and verbs are recognized by the right hemisphere but morpheme-to-grapheme conversion is not possible and non-imageable words and pseudo-words cannot be comprehended by the right hemisphere. Right hemisphere reading resembles deep alexia except for the inability of the person affected to read aloud.

SUMMARY

Studies of alexia have been numerous for several decades. The terminological confusion has been considerable and has tended to obscure valuable findings. Nonetheless, great strides have been made in the ability to correlate the psychological and anatomical aspects of reading, and they have led to an improved ability to understand the complexities of language.

BIBLIOGRAPHY

Benson D. F. (1977). The third alexia. *Archives of Neurology*, *34*, 327–31.

Benson, D. F. (1985). Alexia. In J. A. M. Frederiks (Ed.), *Handbook of clinical neurology*. 2nd edn, Vol. 45: *Clinical neuropsychology* (pp. 433–55). Amsterdam: Elsevier.

Déjerine, J. (1891). Sur un cas de cécité verbale agraphie, suivi d'autopsie. *Mémoires de la Société Biologique*, *3*, 197–201.

Déjerine, J. (1892). Contribution à l'étude anatomoclinique et clinique des différentes variétés de cécité verbale. *Mémoires de la Société Biologique*, *4*, 61–90.

Geschwind, N. (1962). The anatomy of acquired disorders of reading. In J. Money (Ed.), *Reading disability: progress and research needs in dyslexia* (pp. 115–29). Baltimore: Johns Hopkins Press.

Greenblatt, S. (1977). Neurosurgery and the anatomy of reading: a practical review. *Neurosurgery*, *1*, 6–15.

Iwata, M. (1986). Neural mechanism of reading and writing in the Japanese language. *Functional Neurology*, *1*, 43–52.

Marshall J. C., & Newcombe F. (1973). Patterns of paralexia – a psycholinguistic approach. *Journal of Psycholinguistic Research*, *2*, 175–99.

Zaidel, E. (1985). Language in the right hemisphere. In D. F. Benson & E. Zaidel (Eds), *The dual brain: Hemispheric specialization in the human* (pp. 205–31). New York: Guilford.

D. FRANK BENSON

alexithymia A disruption of both affective and cognitive processes, alexithymia is a collection of traits rather than a psychiatric syndrome. Alexithymics are incapable of expressing emotions in the sense that, while the emotion may be experienced, the emotion cannot be associated with a mental representation and so formally expressed. Alexithymia has classically been described in patients with psychosomatic disorders, but also in alcoholics, drug addicts, and patients with traumatic stress disorders.

Alexithymia has been reported in COMMISSUROTOMY patients, and following right hemisphere STROKE. These may be regarded as primary alexithymias, while secondary alexithymias may be associated more closely with psychogenic processes of denial and repression. It has also been suggested that alexithymia reflects a variation in cerebral organization, and that this may be demonstrated by LEMS; others have proposed that alexithymia results from a functional disconnection between the cerebral hemispheres.

alien hand The "alien hand" phenomenon has two relatively distinct meanings in neuropsychology.

In cases of DEMENTIA and PARKINSON'S DISEASE, the corticobasal degeneration may result in uncontrolled dystonic posturing of an upper limb, which neurologists may term the alien hand phenomenon, indicating a hand which is outside the volitional control of the patient.

An alternative meaning is associated with callosal section in COMMISSUROTOMY or following non-surgical lesions which interrupt callosal fibers. This form of "alien hand," a translation of *la main étrangère*, relates to a change in the patient's conscious experience, so that the hand (which is usually the left) is perceived as acting outside the patient's control. This behavior may be considered "foreign" and may seem uncooperative and even hostile. The phenomenon is believed to result from a disconnection between left hemisphere language centers and the right hemisphere mechanisms responsible for control of the left hand. Whether the behavior of the hand represents some loss of volitional control, or simply a failure of conscious appreciation of the control of the hand, is a matter of debate, but a number of commissurotomy patients, and patients with callosal tumors or infarcts, do report a persisting alien hand phenomenon. It has been suggested that predisposing personality factors may play a role in the genesis of the phenomenon.

allesthesia, alloesthesia Allesthesia is a disturbance of body schema perception in the tactile modality in which stimulation at one side of the body is perceived as located on the other side of the body. The disorder is sometimes referred to as *alloesthesia* or *allochiria*. It has been linked with more general disturbances of right-left orientation, but the link between the two is not accepted as a particularly close one, and allesthesia may occur following not only cortical lesions but also spinal cord or brain-stem lesions, when right-left disorientation does not occur. Also, while allesthesia strictly refers to the mislateralization by verbal report of touch, similar phenomena may occur in other modalities or response modes, so that a patient addressed from the contralesional side may orient the head and eyes to the ipsilesional side; instructed to move an extremity touched, the patient may move the opposite limb. An alternative form of motor allesthesia may occur in hemiplegic patients who make spontaneous movements of their impaired limb, yet have the sensation that it is the contralateral limb which moves. Only specific regions of the body may be affected, and a form has been described in which the mislocation is towards the midline of the body, rather than to a homolateral region. Similar displacements may occur together in the visual and auditory modalities.

Allesthesia may be a transitory disturbance or a symptom which persists for the life of the patient. In common with other ASOMATOGNOSIAS, the disorder is normally associated with lesions of the right cortical hemisphere, and is commonly considered to be linked to the right inferior parietal region, in the area bordering the interparietal sulcus, the supramarginal gyrus, and the angular gyrus.

Optic allesthesia refers to the complex visual illusion of the displacement or mislocalization of objects in space, usually to the homolateral position in the contralateral visual field.

Allesthesia, together with hemi-attention and extinction, are all considered by some writers to be aspects of neglect, and it has been suggested that they represent a gradient of severity, so that with recovery patients pass from neglect to allesthesia to extinction. NEGLECT is a very active area of neuropsychological research, although allesthesia has received less attention in the literature than more severe forms of neglect, and there is a variety of explanations for the psychological factors underlying the phenomenon.

J. GRAHAM BEAUMONT

allochiria An alternative term for ALLES-THESIA, referring to lateral mislocalization of tactile stimuli presented to the right or left sides of the body.

Alzheimer's disease *See* DEMENTIA.

amnesia Amnesia is a general term covering any form of temporary or permanent global loss of memory. Amnesia can be divided broadly into *organic* and *psychogenic* (sometimes called functional) memory disorders (Kapur, 1994; Parkin, 1996; Parkin & Leng, 1993). In an organic disorder the patient's memory complaint can be attributed to some clearly identifiable dysfunction of the brain. In a psychogenic disorder no predisposing organic dysfunction can be identified and although, like every other aspect of behavior, it must ultimately be explained in physiological terms, the memory impairment is considered to have a psychiatric or "affective" origin.

Organic memory disorders can best be understood using a taxonomy where the first division is between *permanent* and *transient* disorders. A permanent disorder is one which does not ameliorate across time whereas a transient disorder lasts for only a specific period.

Permanent organic amnesias can themselves be further subdivided into those that are *stable* and those that are *progressive*. In the former the memory impairment does not worsen across time save for those changes expected from normal aging. In a progressive disorder the patient's memory undergoes a continuing decline. Stable organic amnesias arise from a wide number of different causes including head injury, strokes, aneurysms, tumors, metabolic deficiencies, and malnutrition, whereas progressive amnesia characterizes the various dementing illnesses such as Alzheimer's disease, multi-infarct DEMENTIA, Pick's disease, and Huntington's chorea (Kapur, 1994). A worsening global amnesia is also a characteristic of patients with acquired immune deficiency syndrome (AIDS).

THE AMNESIC SYNDROME

Permanent stable amnesia is often referred to as the AMNESIC SYNDROME. Although it has many etiologies, the amnesic syndrome is primarily associated with disruption to either one or two specific regions of the brain: the *midline* DIENCEPHALON and the *medial* TEMPORAL LOBE. Diencephalic damage is most commonly found in KORSAKOFF'S DISEASE – a condition principally associated with thiamine deficiency leading to WERNICKE'S ENCEPHALOPATHY. Most commonly the encephalopathy is a consequence of chronic alcoholism but other forms of nutritional deficiency (e.g. hyperemesis gravidarum) can also give rise to the same impairment. Diencephalic damage can also emerge following strokes (THALAMIC SYNDROME) or tumors, and there are several reports of diencephalic damage following unusual intra-nasal penetrating head injuries. The best-known of these is Case NA who became amnesic when a miniature fencing foil went up his nose and into his brain. Initially it was thought that NA had only diencephalic damage, but more detailed neurological findings indicate a more widespread pathology including the areas of the medial temporal lobe. Amnesia following medial temporal lobe damage has more widespread origins, including herpes simplex ENCEPHALITIS, certain forms of STROKE, carbon monoxide poisoning, ANOXIA, radionecrosis, and insulin overdose. The medial temporal region is commonly damaged in patients with amnesia due to CLOSED HEAD INJURY. Bilateral temporal lobectomies (LOBECTOMY) of the type that affected HM (see below) are no longer carried out.

Although the general brain regions underlying amnesia have been known for some time, the critical lesions needed to produce an amnesic syndrome have yet to be agreed upon. Within the midline diencephalon amnesia is frequently associated with damage to one or more of the following structures: MAMMILLARY BODIES, *mammillo-thalamic tract*, *peri-aqueductal grey matter*, and the *dorso-medial thalamic nucleus* (THALAMUS). Within the medial temporal region the structure most often identified is the HIPPOCAMPUS – a conclusion consistent with physiological evidence involving the hippocampus in the mechanisms of memory consolidation. Moreover, it has also been pointed out that the microanatomy of the hippocampus makes it an ideal substrate for integrating the various aspects of information assumed to make up a resulting memory trace. While most evidence points to a critical role for the hippocampus, another medial temporal structure, the AMYGDALA, has also been implicated in memory for the emotional content of stimuli.

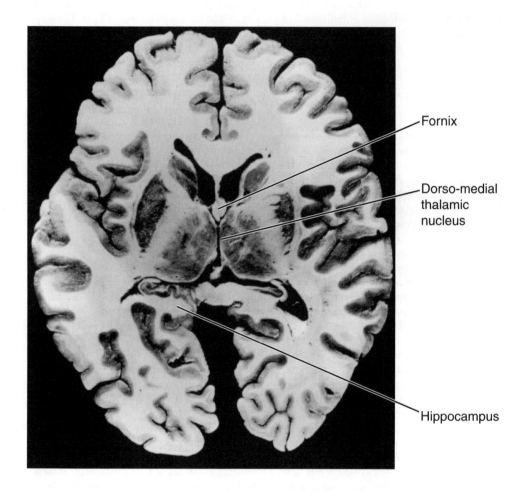

Figure 11 The principal regions of the brain implicated in the amnesic syndrome. A. Horizontal section through the thalamus. B. Coronal section through mammillary bodies. Note that all structures

The FORNIX is the major afferent pathway running from the hippocampus to the mammillary bodies and there has been some controversy concerning its role in memory function. Many early reports suggested that lesions of the fornix did not interfere with memory function to any great extent but, in a recent review, Gaffan and Gaffan (1991) have concluded that in those fornix cases with the most reliable neuroanatomical evidence there is clear evidence of substantial memory loss. Nonetheless it remains the case

that lesions of the fornix have not produced amnesic states comparable to those found with lesions to the diencephalon or the medial temporal lobe. Figure 11 shows the various anatomical structures known to be associated with memory.

The various diencephalic and medial temporal structures implicated in memory function are all part of the LIMBIC SYSTEM. Work by Mishkin and his colleagues has shown that the limbic system comprises two parallel pathways known as the *hippocampal* and *amygdalar circuits*. It has been

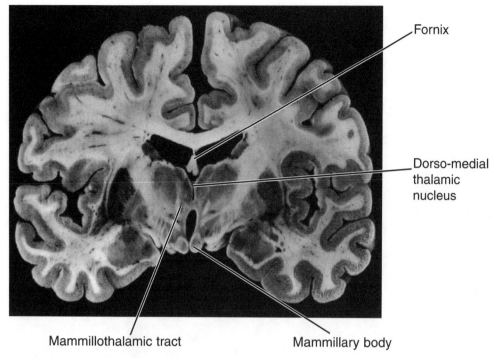

Fornix

Dorso-medial
thalamic
nucleus

Mammillothalamic tract

Mammillary body

are present bilaterally. (Adapted from Gluhbegovich and Williams, *The human brain: A photographic guide* (1980), with the permission of Harper & Row.)

suggested that for amnesia to develop both of these circuits must be interrupted. Examination of the neurological evidence suggests that most amnesic patients suffer damage to both these circuits. HM, for example, suffered bilateral removal of both hippocampal and amygdalar tissue, and Korsakoff patients also have lesions interrupting both circuits. Furthermore, studies of patients with thalamic lesions indicate that those with the greatest memory deficit have lesions in the region where the hippocampal and amygdalar circuits run most closely to one another (see Figure 12). It should be noted, however, that it may not be the amygdalar circuit that is crucial for memory. Instead the adjacent projection from the perirhinal cortex may be the critical pathway. Of those patients studied in neurological detail, only case RB (Zola-Morgan et al, 1986) and the fornix cases described above appear to have developed amnesia following damage to only one circuit (hippocampal). (See Parkin & Leng, 1993.)

BEHAVIORAL FEATURES OF THE AMNESIC SYNDROME

Although the differing lesions suffered by amnesic syndrome patients may have some implications for understanding the exact nature of their amnesic deficit (see below), these patients all suffer from certain unifying features, hence the use of the term "syndrome." These features are: intact immediate apprehension, as measured by tasks like digit span, relatively normal intelligence, and intact language abilities. Amnesic patients are also known to have intact *procedural memory*. This term is rather imprecise but can be used to describe the memory processes underlying the acquisition of skills and certain other forms of knowledge not directly accessible to consciousness, whose presence can only be demonstrated by action. Typing is a good example of procedural memory. If you are an experienced typist, try describing where your fingers must be positioned to type the word "caterpillar." A description will only be possible by performing

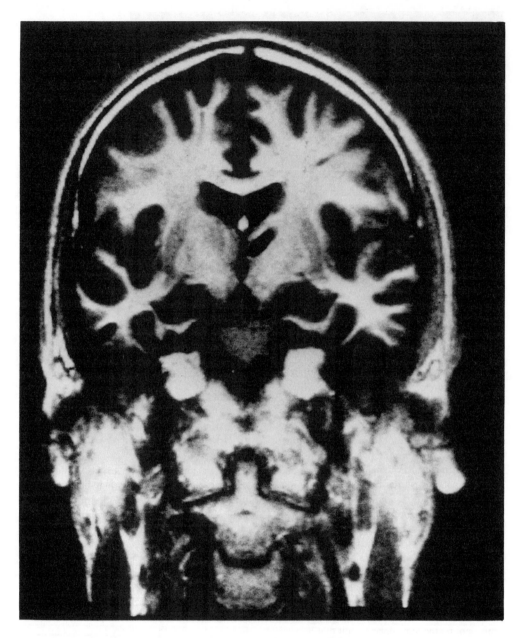

Figure 12 Neuropathological basis of diencephalic amnesia. MRI scan of patient who suffered a discrete thalamic stroke resulting in an infarction which compromised both the hippocampal and amygdalar pathways (and also projection from perirhinal cortex) in the region of the dorso-medial thalamic nucleus. The outcome was a severe amnesia for verbal information. (Reproduced from Parkin et al. (1994) with permission.)

the typing action and describing where your fingers go.

Many studies of amnesia have highlighted preserved procedural learning in amnesia. Milner and Corkin studied the amnesic patient HM, who became amnesic because of bilateral removals in the medial temporal lobes (see Corkin, 1984 for an overview of this research). HM was presented with the *pursuit rotor task*, which is essentially a test of hand–eye coordination in which a light beam emitted by a stylus must be focused on a spot which traces an erratic circular path. HM showed learning both within and across sessions but, on every occasion he was confronted with the test, he denied having done it before. HM, and many other amnesic patients, have also shown retention of *closure pictures*. These are incomplete pictures which you can suddenly see are depicting something obvious like a face or an object (see Figure 13). Once you have solved one of these pictures you are very quickly able to identify it if shown it again, even though you have no conscious access to the perceptual information you acquired in order to do that. Successful learning by amnesics can again be attributed to preserved procedural memory.

Another paradigm in which amnesic patients show procedural learning is *verbal priming*. In a prototypical experiment the patient is presented with a list of words (e.g. "watch") and after a short interval two forms of test are given, *cued recall* and *stem completion priming*. In the former the patient is given the initial letters WAT—? and asked to remember the list word that corresponded to those three letters. Performance by amnesic

patients on this test will be very poor but, if asked to say the first word that pops into mind beginning with those three letters, the patients will say "watch" at a level well above chance. This latter effect is known as *priming* and it shows that the prior learning episode (presenting the word list) can influence performance even though the patient cannot consciously recollect that episode. These types of memory task are commonly referred to as implicit memory or indirect memory. This contrasts with tests of recollection which are termed explicit or direct tests of memory (Schacter, 1987).

We have now seen three different instances of preserved procedural memory in amnesia, but it would be a mistake to think of there being a single "procedural memory system." It is much more likely that the systems subserving various abilities, such as motor skill, perceptual learning, and word recognition, have their own memory properties. What unites them is their independence fromcconscious involvement, not the sharing of a common memory system. Indeed, studies that have examined performance of several procedural memory tasks by the same subjects have failed to show any correlation between performance on those tasks.

THE NATURE OF THE AMNESIC DEFICIT

Patients with the amnesic syndrome have two major deficits: a severe *anterograde amnesia* which prevents them from acquiring any new knowledge, and *retrograde amnesia*, in which the patient is unable to remember events and knowledge learned at a time prior to the brain injury that caused the amnesia (this is known as the *premorbid period*). In cases of the amnesic syndrome anterograde amnesia is always present but retrograde amnesia can be extremely variable, with some patients showing extensive deficits and others virtually no retrograde loss at all.

Anterograde amnesia can be demonstrated in many ways. On a test involving the free recall of a 12-word list an amnesic patient would typically recall one or two words after a one-minute delay. On a test of paired-associate learning involving unrelated pairs of words (e.g. "obey–inch"), learning, if achieved at all, would be painfully slow. On a forced choice recognition test in which the patient had to choose between a previously exposed stimulus and a novel stimulus, perform-

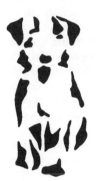 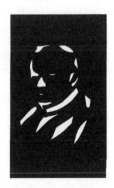

Figure 13 Examples of closure pictures.

ance would typically be at chance. On a yes–no test of recognition, performance would again be poor although the basis of this deficit can vary. Some patients tend to make lots of false positive responses whereas other patients might fail primarily because of omission errors.

So far the impression has been given that the amnesic syndrome is a neatly defined clinical entity. This is true to some extent but, because amnesia arises from brain lesions which themselves vary in severity, it is also the case that amnesia varies in its severity. This raises the awkward question, "When is a memory deficit an amnesic syndrome?" The usual approach is to use data from a patient's performance on standardized clinical tests such as the Wechsler Memory Scale Revised (WMS–R) and Wechsler Adult Intelligence Scale Revised (WAIS-R). As we have seen, the amnesic syndrome is a major impairment of memory in the presence of relatively normal intelligence. Accordingly, comparisons of a patient's scores on these two tests should give a reliable guide to the presence of amnesia. Thus a patient who scores well within the normal range on intelligence but does very badly on memory might be considered amnesic, but someone who does poorly on both tests might be considered demented. This approach is a useful rule of thumb but it can be misleading. The Wechsler Memory Scale, for example, predominantly tests verbal memory and will tend to underestimate preserved nonverbal memory which may, in the case of many patients, be a sufficient basis for functioning within normal limits in everyday situations. Most clinicians would therefore combine their judgment based on the outcome of clinical tests with their own subjective appreciation of the patient's memory capabilities.

Retrograde amnesia is harder to investigate because each person's premorbid experience is different. Psychologists try to get round this by devising retrograde memory tests which address memories one can reasonably assume most people to have acquired. Typically, these tests involve identifying people and events from different decades. The aim of these tests is to evaluate memories formed at a particular time, but they are complicated by the fact that people and events continue to be talked about long after the decade in which they initially occurred. As an alternative one can use *autobiographical cueing*, in which a patient has to date memories retrieved in response

to specific cue words. A problem here, however, is that memories will vary in their specificity and it may be difficult to authenticate much of what the person remembers.

Despite these methodological difficulties, it is clear that retrograde amnesia demonstrates a *temporal gradient*: memories formed early in life are more likely to survive than those formed during a later period. In some patients temporal gradients are absent but the reverse, greater impairment of memories formed earlier in life, has never been reported. The existence of temporal gradients has been acknowledged for a long time and is often described as reflecting Ribot's Law, which states that the vulnerability of a memory to brain injury is inversely related to its age.

Temporal gradients in retrograde amnesia have been most consistently observed in patients with KORSAKOFF'S DISEASE. On a famous faces test, for example, identification of people who came to prominence in the last 20 years of the premorbid period would be extremely poor. The patients may also be badly oriented in time, tending to estimate the current date at the point in the premorbid period for which their memory is still reasonably intact. Korsakoff's syndrome usually arises as a consequence of ALCOHOLISM. It has been suggested that the temporal gradient is due to the cumulative effects of alcoholism on learning during the premorbid period – the argument being that the alcoholism causes increasing difficulties in learning new information, particularly in the years immediately preceding the onset of amnesia proper.

There can be little doubt that chronic alcoholism does impair learning ability, but this cannot be the entire explanation of temporal gradients. It is most compelling that temporal gradients can be observed in amnesic patients who do not have a prior history of alcoholism, including the few patients studied who have developed Korsakoff's syndrome for reasons other than alcoholism. Retrograde amnesia therefore seems a distinct deficit rather than being a consequence of poor anterograde memory during the latter stages of the premorbid period.

An important issue is whether anterograde and retrograde amnesia have the same origin. It is certainly the case that they almost always co-occur (hence the clinical maxim, "No AA without RA") but it is difficult to attribute them to a common deficit. First, if they had a common origin, one would expect the severity of both disorders to be comparable, but this is not the case. HM, for example, has one of the most dense anterograde amnesias on record but his retrograde amnesia is relatively mild. Also, it has not been possible to identify factors that affect anterograde and retrograde amnesia similarly. Contextual cues, for example, can enhance the performance of amnesic patients on certain anterograde tests, but they have been found to be ineffective on tests of retrograde memory. Finally, there are a few unusual cases where retrograde amnesia seems more severe than anterograde amnesia (see *focal retrograde amnesia* below).

EXPLAINING AMNESIA

Patients with the amnesic syndrome have been studied intensively. The fact that some aspects of their memory remain intact while others are badly affected provides important information about the organization of memory. Preserved immediate apprehension, as measured by span tasks, supports the widely held distinction between short- and long-term storage processes. Intact procedural memory abilities indicate the separate existence of memories concerned with the representation of skills and related abilities but, to reiterate, there is not a single procedural memory system.

Psychologists are less agreed on how to describe the deficit in amnesia. Some (e.g. Tulving, 1989) believe that amnesics have a selective loss of *episodic memory* with preserved *semantic memory*. Episodic memory can be defined as the "autobiographical record" of our lives – that part of our memory that gives us personal continuity with the past and is used to retrieve information about specific personal events. Semantic memory corresponds to our store of knowledge about language, rules, and concepts and, although derived from specific events, it resides independent of any record of those events. Thus, in order to retrieve a specific piece of knowledge, you do not have to retrieve the original learning episode in which you acquired that knowledge.

It is certainly true that the clinical presentation of amnesic patients seems consistent with a selective impairment of episodic memory, but a finer-grained analysis does not produce such a clear picture. Amnesic patients do not, for example, acquire new vocabulary at all easily (HM is thought to have learned only six new words since his operation in 1953) and investigations of Korsakoff patients have also indicated a marked inability to learn new word meanings. Findings like these might be countered on the grounds that episodic memory is needed for the initial retention of new language until assimilation into semantic memory has occurred. More difficult is the actual nature of retrograde memory loss. Superficially, it again seems that memory for episodes is the major impairment, but this conclusion can be misleading. First, if we look at the various tests used to measure retrograde amnesia, they are predominantly tests of general knowledge (e.g. recognizing a face, describing a world event) and failure on them cannot be construed as a specific inability to remember distinct episodes. Also, the claim that amnesic patients have preserved language derives from normal performance on standardized language tests. The problem here is that these tests concentrate on the nature of language skills assumed to have been acquired in early adult life. Normal language might just reflect the known intactness of language acquired early in life, i.e. another expression of Ribot's Law. Indeed, it is now evident that when amnesic patients are asked to define words that came into use during later stages of the premorbid period (e.g. fax machine, walkman) they do very poorly.

Problems encountered in trying to describe the amnesic deficit as a selective impairment of episodic memory have led to a revised account in which the impairment is seen as one of *declarative memory* (Squire, 1987). Declarative memory can be described as any memory that is open to conscious inspection. It embraces both episodic and semantic-type knowledge and an impairment of this kind of system does characterize the amnesic deficit. However, as a description of the amnesic deficit it is very general.

Debates about the adequacy of the episodic–semantic distinction and the declarative alternative are all about how to *describe* the amnesic deficit: the next step is to explain why it has developed. There have been many attempts to explain human amnesia, but as yet there has been little progress or agreement among workers. One early idea was that amnesic patients had a deficit in *consolidation*, but this idea lost favor with the discovery that a number of learning processes remained intact in amnesia. However, a consolidation theory limited to the formation of one particular type of memory might still be viable (see below).

Another theory, current for some time, was the *retrieval deficit* theory, which held that amnesic patients had no difficulties encoding and storing information but just problems in retrieving it. However, this theory has now been dismissed, not least because of amnesic patients showing relatively intact recall from the premorbid period despite severe anterograde deficits. The *levels of processing* framework was also applied in attempts to understand amnesia. The idea here was that amnesic patients applied inadequate "shallow" encoding strategies when attempting to learn. This theory is also no longer viable, partly because of experiments showing that amnesia is not ameliorated when amnesic patients are forced to use more effective encoding strategies.

One theory gaining reasonable support argues that amnesia represents a deficit in the encoding of *contextual information* (Mayes, 1988; Parkin, 1995). Context can be defined as information associated with a specific memory that allows differentiation of that memory from other memories. In experimental terms, context is usually defined in terms of the temporo-spatial attributes associated with a stimulus. According to this theory, amnesic patients are unable to encode those contextual features of new events that are essential if those events are to be recalled at a subsequent point in time. In contrast, amnesic patients perform quite well on learning tasks which do not require the encoding of contextual information. Recognition memory in amnesic patients can, for example, show normal rates of forgetting, providing the recognition test can be performed on the basis of simply judging whether each item is or is not familiar – although one must note that this requires amnesic patients to be given far more learning trials than normal subjects. One problem, however, is that the evidence supporting the contextual theory derives almost exclusively from patients with Korsakoff's syndrome.

Earlier in this entry we saw that amnesic syndrome patients all suffer lesions of the limbic system, which comprises two parallel circuits. This neuroanatomical evidence has led some to suggest that a memory circuit or circuits exist in the brain and that, by analogy with an electrical circuit, we would expect the same outcome regardless of where the circuit was damaged. This is not a strong argument, because there is no a priori basis for assuming that each stage of the circuit carries out the same function. It is equally plausible, for example, to suppose that different parts of the circuit perform different functions and that their selective damage would result in differing patterns of memory impairment which, in turn, reflect the fractionation of the memory system.

At present there are two plausible theories of retrograde amnesia: storage deficit and retrieval deficit. It is now generally accepted that the permanent memories are stored in parts of the cortex and, in particular, within the temporal lobes. Patients with large lesions of the temporal lobes invariably show extensive retrograde amnesia, whereas those who suffer smaller lesions in the same region typically have a much less severe retrograde deficit. This relationship is most plausibly accounted for in terms of damage to storage areas. However, there are cases of extensive retrograde amnesia following diencephalic damage in which the lesion is far too small to support a storage deficit explanation. In these cases it has been suggested that some form of retrieval impairment underlies the deficit.

Whether a storage or retrieval deficit accounts best for a given pattern of retrograde amnesia, there is always a temporal gradient. However, neither type of theory has been able to offer a clear explanation of why this gradient exists. One explanation in terms of storage is that older memories have more extensive representation so are less vulnerable to partial damage. How a retrieval theory would explain temporal gradients is not clear at all.

HOW MANY TYPES OF AMNESIA?

We have already seen that retrograde amnesia may have more than one cause and this is also true for anterograde amnesia. There have been a number of studies comparing the exact nature of memory loss following temporal lobe damage as opposed to diencephalic damage. Initially there were proposals that temporal lobe damage gave rise to an amnesia which resulted in very rapid forgetting compared with diencephalic damage. Unfortunately it has proved difficult to sustain this conclusion, mainly because of methodological problems.

An alternative approach has been to look for qualitative differences between temporal lobe and diencephalic amnesics. Experiments have centered on whether the context deficit theory applies equally to both forms of amnesia. Results have shown that the context deficit theory continues to provide a good account of diencephalic amnesia. Thus, in an experiment where subjects have to distinguish previously presented targets from distractors, diencephalic patients can respond reasonably well if the discrimination can be based on whether or not items are generally familiar. However, if recognition involves discrimination that cannot be based on familiarity, i.e. one where all items are familiar and targets are defined in terms of a context such as list membership, diencephalic patients do very poorly. When presented with two lists of sentences, they may recognize the sentences quite well but be at chance on deciding which list a sentence occurred in.

Experiments with temporal lobe amnesics have yielded a different pattern. Even though these patients have an amnesia that is often more severe than diencephalic amnesia, they do not show such a disproportionate loss of memory for context. Also, when they do recognize something, there is a strong probability that they will remember the context. These results suggest that the context deficit theory does not apply to temporal lobe amnesia. As a result it has been suggested that this form of amnesia might be more readily explained as a consolidation deficit which affects all aspects of memory, not just the encoding and storage of context. This view is consistent with the proposed involvement of the hippocampus in memory consolidation (Parkin, 1992).

FOCAL RETROGRADE AMNESIA

Kapur (1993) has identified what he has termed focal retrograde amnesia (FRA). This refers to a memory impairment in which the primary deficit is a loss of remote memory, with performance on anterograde tests only mildly impaired. A problem with this type of disorder is that some of the patients may be suffering from psychogenic disorders (see below) or they may be malingering, in some way faking or dissimulating memory impairment. However, once these possibilities are discounted there is a range of case histories in which focal retrograde amnesia is presented within the context of identifiable brain injury (Kapur, 1992).

A typical case is presented by Kapur and colleagues (1994). This man performed within

normal limits on tests of anterograde memory, but his retrograde amnesia was severe. Another patient reported by Hunkin and others (1995) again showed normal anterograde memory but showed a complete inability to remember any events that happened before his head injury. Patients with FRA all have preserved hippocampal structures, but the reason for their FRA may vary. In some cases, such as that described by Kapur and colleagues (1994), retrograde amnesia may arise from damage to the cortical storage sites of long-term memory. However, others, such as that described by Hunkin's group, may have lost the ability to integrate the different components that make up retrieval of an event.

FRONTAL LOBES AND MEMORY

In the last few years there has been growing interest in the role of the FRONTAL LOBE in memory and a "frontal" profile of impaired memory has begun to be identified. There are two main strands of research. The first of these, based mainly in Montreal, has examined the effects of selective frontal removals on memory ability (Petrides, 1991; Parkin, 1995). These experiments have shown that frontal lesions can impair subjects' ability to know which of two items was presented most recently, even though recognition of those items is normal. Similarly, lesions of the frontal lobes affect the ability to estimate the frequency with which stimuli have been encountered. There are also several demonstrations of *source amnesia* in frontal patients in which retention of novel facts occurs normally without any ability to attribute the source of those facts.

A second strand of research has been based on patients who have suffered ruptured aneurysms of the anterior communicating artery (ACoA) – a disorder which very frequently gives rise to lesions in the frontal lobes and adjacent structures, such as the basal ganglia. The general impression of these patients is one of a severe recall impairment, but recognition is largely normal. Hanley and others (1994) provide a good example of a woman who performed in this manner, even though the recall and recognition tasks were matched for difficulty. (In some earlier studies it is possible that the apparent preservation of recognition was an artifact of the recognition task simply being easier.)

A contrasting case was reported by Delbecq-Derouesne and others (1990) in which recognition was impaired and characterized by high levels of false alarms. In contrast, recall was in the normal range, although the patient introduced far more irrelevant material into his recall (intrusions) than controls. Hanley and others have proposed a framework for understanding these differences which derives from a recent account of the control of action. According to this theory, most actions are controlled by schemata which, once triggered, allow a sequence of actions to be run automatically. Additional conscious control, where required, is brought about by the "executive" supervisory attentional system (SAS) which is assumed to be in the frontal cortex. With regard to memory, damage to this executive system is considered to affect the more strategic aspects of memory. Shallice (1988) has argued that the SAS is responsible for setting up retrieval strategies that will enable new information to be retrieved at a later point. In addition the SAS also determines, via a verification process, whether information accessed by these retrieval strategies is the information being sought by the system. In addition this system provides an appropriate locus of *metamemory* – our ability to monitor the contents of memory. Consistent with this are demonstrations that frontal lesions impair this ability (Janowsky et al., 1989).

Hanley and colleagues interpreted the impairments of their patient as involving ineffective generation of retrieval strategies, whereas the Delbecq-Derouesne case presented a clear instance of memory impairment due to ineffective verification. Unfortunately, this double dissociation has been questioned by the discovery that ACoA aneurysm patients showing apparently normal recognition memory do develop poor recognition, characterized by high false alarms when they are tested under more stringent conditions. The differences between these patients may therefore be quantitative and a single theory may eventually explain their memory problems (Parkin et al., 1994). It is also of interest that the possible mechanisms underlying the high false alarm rates exhibited by some frontal patients have now been implicated in accounts of false memory (Schacter & Curran, 1995).

The "dysexecutive syndrome" idea has also been invoked to account for CONFABULATION – the tendency to produce false recollections that is often observed following frontal lobe damage (so-called "honest lying"). It should be noted that the term "confabulation" tends to be used rather loosely in clinical descriptions. Most amnesic patients, if pressed to recall what they have been doing, will produce some kind of response. Usually this will have little conviction, be rather general, and entirely plausible given the patient's current circumstances. This is often termed *momentary confabulation* and is not a symptom of frontal pathology. The other, more spectacular form of confabulation is known as *fantastic confabulation* and it is this that is associated with frontal lesions. It is characterized by the production of clearly implausible memories which the patient has no doubt are true. It is interesting that these confabulated memories are unshakeable, even when the patient is directly confronted with their untruthfulness. Fantastic confabulations have much in common with the delusions shown by schizophrenic patients and frontal pathology is now implicated in both these disorders (Stuss & Benson, 1990).

Until recently there was a general view that patients with SCHIZOPHRENIA do not show any marked impairment of memory. However, recent studies have shown that many schizophrenics show levels of memory impairment comparable to that found in the amnesic syndrome. Work has only just begun to unravel the nature of schizophrenic memory impairment, but two distinct hypotheses have already emerged. From neurophysiological and neuroanatomical studies it is evident that schizophrenics suffer brain dysfunction in two areas, the basal ganglia/midline prefrontal cortex and the temporal lobes. Poor functioning in either of these brain regions would be expected to cause impaired memory. At present the small amount of evidence available tends to favor a frontal interpretation of schizophrenic memory impairment. In particular, there are several studies suggesting a disproportionate impairment of recall relative to recognition in this patient group, including an important demonstration involving tasks matched for difficulty (Calev, 1984). However, Clare and others (1993) have urged caution in interpreting these discrepancies as distinguishing schizophrenic memory loss from that encountered in the amnesic syndrome.

DEMENTING ILLNESS

There are a number of dementing illnesses (DEMENTIA) and most of them have, as a primary symptom, the development of severe amnesia.

However, there are important differences between memory loss in dementing patients and that which characterizes the amnesic syndrome.

The commonest form of dementing illness is Alzheimer's disease (AD). Neuropathological and neurochemical changes in this disease are widespread throughout the cortex. Senile plaques and neurofibrillary tangles can be found in the frontal, parietal, and temporal lobes, but there is marked sparing of the sensory cortex. Ascending cholinergic projections from the nucleus basalis of Mynert, noradrenergic projections from the locus coeruleus, and serotonergic projections from the raphe nuclei are all badly depleted (BASAL GANGLIA).

In psychological terms AD begins with a mild loss of memory but, as one might expect from the widespread neurological disturbance evident in the disease, progression leads to a far more extensive deficit than that encountered in the amnesic syndrome. Memory does deteriorate in a way comparable to the amnesic syndrome in that marked problems arise on tests such as free recall and recognition. On recognition tests there is a marked tendency for Alzheimer patients to produce high levels of false alarms and it has been suggested that this might distinguish AD from other dementing illnesses. There is also deterioration of semantic knowledge to a far greater extent than in amnesia, reflected particularly in the loss of higher level linguistic and conceptual knowledge. It is also noticeable that memory span performance, an ability usually unaffected in patients with organic memory disorders, undergoes a marked decline (see Miller & Morris, 1993; Morris, 1991).

REMEDIATION OF MEMORY DISORDER

Psychologists have recently begun to explore possible strategies for the rehabilitation of irreversibly memory-impaired people. An important issue is whether any therapy devised is aimed at restoring the impaired function or providing the patient with some alternative means of dealing with memory-based tasks. Repetitive practice is the crudest of the restorative strategies and one that is largely useless. Its use in clinical settings has largely persisted from the false belief that memory can be improved by repeated exercise, in the same way that practice might improve a weak muscle. Repetitive practice will only be effective if, through practice, the patient comes to use his or her residual memory ability more effectively, for example, by discovering a more efficient means of dealing with the information to be learned. This discovery process can be bypassed by giving the patient specific *mnemonic strategies* which will enable them to learn information more effectively. Telling a patient to form a mental image of information to be learned, for example, can often cause quite dramatic improvements in the recall of a memory-impaired person, and various other study strategies can also help patients remember more.

A major problem in using mnemonic strategies in memory rehabilitation is that patients will rarely use these strategies unless instructed to do so by someone else. This reflects a problem of metamemory: patients do not know that they have learned a strategy and therefore fail to implement it when it could be useful. Furthermore, in most situations where a mnemonic strategy would be useful, an external memory aid such as a list would be just as effective.

Failures of the restorative approach to memory disorder have resulted in an alternative strategy which attempts to use the preserved aspects of the patient's memory to overcome certain learning difficulties. We saw above that amnesic patients show relatively preserved performance on tests of implicit memory such as priming. This residual learning ability has been tapped successfully in a learning procedure known as vanishing cues (VC; Glisky & Schacter, 1988). Essentially, the technique exploits preserved priming to teach the patient a set of specific responses, such as the basic commands for operating a computer. The authors describe a number of successes, including training an amnesic woman for work as a computer operator.

Glisky and others reported that the VC procedure produced better learning than standard learning methods, but subsequent studies have failed to replicate this finding. Moreover, it has proved impossible to show effective use of implicit memory methods over standard learning methods. What is clear, however, is that, despite comparable rates of learning, amnesic patients prefer learning using methods that attempt to use implicit memory (Hunkin & Parkin, 1995). Recently an alternative approach to remediation based on the errorless learning method has produced promising results (Baddeley & Wilson, 1994).

TRANSIENT DISORDERS OF MEMORY

In a transient disorder the memory impairment is caused by some temporary brain abnormality which, when resolved, allows the patient's memory to return to normal. Most common of these disorders is *transient global amnesia* (TGA). TGA is more common in older people and more likely to be experienced by people who are also migraine sufferers. Onset of this disorder is sudden and the patient experiences both anterograde amnesia and retrograde amnesia. Language and other skills are, however, unaffected and the TGA patient can generally be considered as presenting a temporary case of the amnesic syndrome. The cause of TGA is still unknown, but its association with migraine suggests that it may have an ischemic origin, i.e. it might be due to some transient disruption of the cerebral blood supply (Hodges & Warlow, 1990).

Electro-convulsive therapy (ECT) also gives rise to a well documented memory impairment. In the days following treatment ECT patients will show marked anterograde and retrograde impairments, with the latter thought by some to convey a therapeutic advantage because it prevents patients ruminating on the events that led to their treatment! The question of whether memory returns completely to normal following ECT is a controversial one. Controlled studies of ECT provide little evidence of lasting impairment following treatment, but there is much psychiatric folklore that ECT does cause permanent brain damage. It is possible that many people complaining about memory loss following ECT do so because their medication is still having adverse effects, or because they had a bad memory before treatment but have only started to monitor their memory failures post ECT. Another factor may be that some individuals are generally susceptible to the effects of ECT but that their deficits are not picked up because of the variability inherent in large group studies (Weiner, 1984).

Concussion will normally produce a transient amnesic state known as *post-traumatic amnesia* (PTA). In PTA the patient will show both anterograde and retrograde deficits similar to TGA and post-ECT amnesia. The duration of PTA provides a rough index of the extent to which a head injury victim will show lasting impairment of memory. An interesting phenomenon in PTA is that the patient's retrograde amnesia exhibits "shrinkage" in that the patient's memories return in an orderly manner, with those from early years reappearing before those formed nearer the time of the injury. This is a temporary example of the temporal gradients characteristic of retrograde amnesia in amnesic patients. In mild cases of PTA memory is thought to return to normal, with only memory for the few minutes prior to the head injury being lost – a finding put down to the disruption of consolidation. However, there is growing evidence that even patients considered to have made a "full recovery" following concussion may have subtle memory deficits that have continuing significance for their daily lives. Patients may, for example, stop watching films because they lose track of the plot and become far more reliant on notes for remembering to do things (see Richardson, 1990 for a recent account of memory following head injury).

EPILEPSY is a complex disorder representing a set of clinical symptoms rather than being due to a specific form of brain damage. Epileptic patients show a range of memory impairments which may be due to the original illness causing epilepsy, damage caused by fits, the effects of anticonvulsant medication, and abnormal brain activity in clinical or subclinical epileptiform discharges. Memory deficits experienced by epileptic patients can be divided into the permanent or *interictal* deficits that can be detected when the patient is not experiencing epileptiform attacks and *ictal* or transient deficits that occur while an attack is occurring. Interictal deficits are variable but most pronounced in those patients whose amnesia has a temporal lobe focus. The ictal phase produces a transient disorder which is similar in some ways to TGA, although the length of the episodes tends to be a lot shorter. During the ictal phase epileptic patients sometimes exhibit aimless wandering known as *poriomania*. Kapur (1990) provides an overview of transient epileptic amnesia.

A variety of pyschoactive drugs also cause transient memory problems. Marijuana can produce quite marked memory impairments and there is also evidence of a *state-dependent effect*, i.e. the memory deficit is worse if learning and testing do not both take place under the same conditions. Some antidepressants (e.g. imipramine) also have an adverse effect on memory, but this is only found with anterograde tests. This effect, which also relates to marijuana, suggests an effect on encoding and storage rather than retrieval. The widespread use of benzodiazepines as hypnotics and anxiolytics has prompted considerable interest in their effects on memory. Single clinical doses of benzodiazepines are known to cause temporary anterograde deficits on tasks like free recall without a parallel impairment of retrograde memory – again suggesting that the locus of the drug effect is at the encoding or storage stage. Benzodiazepines also tend not to affect priming measures, although a curious exception is lorazepam, which seems to adversely affect priming relative to recall. The anterograde impairment produced by benzodiazepines is thought to be clinically useful. When used by dentists to calm down nervous patients, their memory for the procedures will be poor and thus less of a deterrent to the patient returning for more treatment. A review of drug-induced amnesia and its theoretical implications is provided by Polster (1993).

PSYCHOGENIC MEMORY DISORDERS

Psychogenic memory disorders are those which arise without any obvious organic dysfunction and thus tend to be classed as psychiatric rather than neurological deficits. The idea that our memory system can actively suppress memories that we do not wish to remember has a long history and can be traced back to nineteenth-century writers such as Freud and Janet. Freud, for example, believed that people could actively repress memories that were injurious to their ego and it was the goal of psychoanalysis to unearth these memories because, according to Freud, these repressed memories sought alternative expression via neurotic behavior. Central to Freud's theory was the concept of personal development through the oral, anal, and oedipal stages in order to reach the final sexual stage. The oedipal stage was particularly crucial because it was here that boys (Freud's theory never quite sorted out what happened in girls) had to resolve their sexual desires towards their mother with fear of their father's retribution. Normally resolution occurred because fear of the father, expressed in terms of a fear of castration, was sufficient to avert the boy from maternally based sexual feelings and allow progression into the sexual stage. For some, however, the "oedipal conflict" was not resolved but repressed, resulting in regression to either the oral or anal stage which, in turn, motivated various neurotic symptoms, as

well as, allegedly, more harmless activities such as stamp collecting!

Few people now believe that repressed memories are a characteristic of most people presenting neurotic complaints – explanations couched in behavioral terms seem perfectly sufficient without recourse to the psychodynamics that Freud envisaged. Nonetheless it would be wrong to dismiss the notion of repression completely. It may still have some relevance when we look at some of our own memory lapses (such as those Freud himself described in his book *The Psychopathology of Everyday Life*) but, more important, a concept of repression seems essential if we are to understand psychogenic memory disorders.

Perhaps the commonest form of apparent psychogenic memory loss is memory for crime. On average between 30 and 40 percent of people on trial for homicide claim to have no memory for their alleged crime (Kopelman, 1987). Many murders are committed by highly intoxicated people and it has been speculated that failure to recall might have a state-dependent aspect because alcohol has been shown to exert state-dependent effects. This hypothesis was tested in an extraordinary experiment involving convicted murderers who were allowed to get as drunk again as they were when they committed the offence. The subjects were quite loquacious but recalled nothing about their crimes.

The above study suggests that, when alcohol is involved, amnesia for crime may be due to interference with memory processes, most likely consolidation. But many murderers are not drunk, so another explanation must be found for why they are unable to remember. One possibility is that acts of violence are usually performed in states of high arousal and this may interfere with the mechanisms of learning. More likely, however, is that amnesia for crime is due to repression or, as it is more often called, motivated forgetting.

Essentially it is thought that the memory system can, under adverse circumstances, suppress memories that are extremely unpleasant for some reason. A clear example of this comes from the Moors murderer, Ian Brady, who denied for many years any knowledge of the terrible crimes he committed but quite recently remembered everything and showed police where he had buried some of his victims. Brady's amnesia can be seen as adaptive because, by suppressing memory of his awful crime, he was able to live with himself.

The existence of repressed memories was also dramatically demonstrated in studies of soldiers with *combat amnesia* – an inability to remember battle experiences. The men were given an injection of sodium amytal and then asked about the experiences they were apparently unable to remember. Under the drug the men started to relive their terrible experiences, indicating that their impaired memories arose because they were actively suppressing the information. A more dramatic but very rare form of amnesia is *fugue* –derived from the Latin *fugere* meaning "to flee" or "run away." In cases of fugue the patient loses his or her identity and typically turns up at a hospital or police station asking for help. The disorder is usually short-lived, lasting only a few days, but there are instances of fugues being maintained over long periods, with afflicted individuals starting new lives for themselves. Fugue is always precipitated by some kind of negative event, such as bereavement, and can again be seen as a form of adaptive response in which the individual dissociates him- or herself from their entire identity as a means of avoiding hurtful experience.

Perhaps the oddest of all psychogenic memory disorders is *multiple personality*. Again this is found only in people who have had extremely unpleasant lives. Estimates vary as to its incidence, with some people arguing that it is extremely rare and others claiming that it is, relatively speaking, quite common. A multiple personality has at least two different personalities, with some patients reported to have anything up to 20 or more. The personalities often have a complex interrelationship, with some personalities knowing some but not others. Typically the different personalities are used to compartmentalize different aspects of the individual's bad experiences, and a particular personality will have to be active for any given set of circumstances to be recalled. Experimental investigations of all psychogenic disorders are rare, but in multiple personality it has been shown that, despite an inability of one personality to recall information presented to another, items shown to one personality will facilitate stem completion priming (see above) in another.

At present psychogenic disorders are classified as hysterical-dissociative states and, as such, not related to possible organic disorder. However, recent work suggests that at least some forms of psychogenic loss can be plausibly attributed to some form of dysexecutive deficit (Parkin & Stampfer, 1995).

MALINGERING

A problem often faced by clinicians is malingering, i.e. deliberate faking of memory loss. This might occur in an attempt to get greater compensation following a head injury or, in the case of amnesia for crime, it might be a means of getting a more lenient sentence. Detecting malingered amnesia has become an interesting challenge for psychologists. The best approach works on the assumption that a malingerer will not be as good as an expert in knowing exactly how to portray a memory disorder. A truly amnesic person, for example, should perform around chance on a yes–no recognition test whereas malingerers, because of their attempt to fail, might respond significantly below chance. Malingerers might also underestimate the typical recall ability of someone with brain damage. The neuropsychologist Rey designed a seemingly complex-looking recall task which is, in fact, very easy for most memory-impaired people. A malingerer might not spot this and therefore put in a performance below average (see Leng & Parkin, 1995, for a review of tests for malingering).

POST-HYPNOTIC AMNESIA

In post-hypnotic amnesia manipulations subjects undergo a hypnotic induction procedure followed by suggestions that they will be temporarily unable to remember specific information. They are then given a "challenge trial" in which they are asked to recall that information. The amnesia is then cancelled and, if the information is then recalled, post-hypnotic amnesia (while in the hypnotic state) has been demonstrated. The phenomenon definitely occurs but what is the explanation? Hypnosis might result in the true dissociation of memories from the retrieval process. An alternative hypothesis, and one favored by the experimental evidence, is that hypnotized subjects tend to comply with the demands of the situation and withhold their responses. Post-hypnotic amnesia therefore has no value in our attempts to understand clinical amnesic states (Spanos, 1986).

BIBLIOGRAPHY

Baddeley, A., & Wilson, B. A. (1994). When implicit learning fails: amnesia and the problem of error elimination. *Neuropsychologia, 32,* 53–68.

Calev, A. (1984). Recall and recognition in chronic nondemented schizophrenics. *Journal of Abnormal Psychology, 93,* 172–7.

Clare, L., McKenna, P. J., Mortimer, A. M., & Baddeley, A. D. (1993). Memory in schizophrenia. What is impaired and what is preserved? *Neuropsychologia, 31,* 1225–42.

Corkin, S. (1984) Lasting consequences of medial temporal lobectomy: clinical course and experimental findings in case HM. *Seminars in Neurology, 4,* 249–59.

Delbecq-Derouesne, J., Beauvois, M. F., & Shallice, T. (1990). Preserved recall versus impaired recognition. *Brain, 113,* 1045–74.

Gaffan, D., & Gaffan, E. (1991). Amnesia in man following transection of the fornix. *Brain, 114,* 2611–18.

Glisky, E. L., & Shacter, D. L. (1988). Long-term retention of computer learning by patients with memory disorders. *Neuropsychologia, 26,* 173–8.

Hanley, J. R., Davies, A. D. M., Downes, J., & Mayes, A. R. (1994). Impaired recall of verbal material following an anterior communicating artery aneurysm. *Cognitive Neuropsychology, 11,* 543–78.

Hodges, J. R., & Warlow, C. P. (1990). The aetiology of transient global amnesia. *Brain, 113,* 639–57.

Hunkin, N. M., Parkin, A. J., Bradley, V. A., Jansari, A., & Aldrich, F. K. (1995). Focal retrograde amnesia following closed head injury. A case study and theoretical interpretation. *Neuropsychologia, 33,* 509–23.

Hunkin, N. M., & Parkin, A. J. (1995). The method of vanishing cues: an evaluation of its effectiveness in teaching memory impaired individuals. *Neuropsychologia, 33,* 509–23.

Janowsky, J. S., Shimamura, A. P., & Squire, L. R. (1989). Source memory impairment in patients with frontal lobe lesions. *Neuropsychologia, 27,* 1043–56.

Kapur, N. (1990). Transient epileptic amnesia. In H. J. Markowitsch (Ed.), *Transient global amnesia and related disorders* (pp. 140–51). Toronto: Hans Huber.

Kapur, N. (1993). Focal retrograde amnesia in neurological disease: a critical review. *Cortex, 29,* 217–34.

Kapur, N. (1994). *Memory disorders in clinical practice.* Hove: Erlbaum.

Kapur, N., Ellison, D., Parkin, A. J., Hunkin, N. M., & Burrows, E. (1994). Bilateral temporal lobe pathology with sparing of medial temporal lobe structures: lesion profile and pattern of memory disorder. *Neuropsychologia, 32,* 23–38.

Leng, N. R. C., & Parkin, A. J. (1995). The detection of exaggerated or simulated memory disorder by neuropsychological methods. *Journal of Psychosomatic Research, 39,* 767–76.

Kopelman, M. D. (1987). Amnesia: organic and psychogenic. *British Journal of Psychiatry, 150,* 428–42.

McCarthy, R. A., & Hodges, J. R. (1993). Autobiographical amnesia resulting from bilateral thalamic infarction. *Brain, 116,* 921–40.

Mayes, A. R. (1988). *Human organic memory disorders.* Cambridge: Cambridge University Press.

Miller, E., & Morris, R. (1993). *The psychology of dementia.* Chichester: Wiley.

Mishkin, M. (1982). A memory system in the monkey. *Philosophical Transactions of the Royal Society of London B, 298,* 85–95.

Morris, R. (1991). The nature of memory impairment in Alzheimer-type dementia. In J. Weinman & J. Hunter (Eds), *Memory: Neurochemical and abnormal perspectives* (pp. 163–8). London: Harwood.

Parkin, A. J. (1992). Functional significance of etiological factors in human amnesia. In L. R. Squire & N. Butters (Eds), *Neuropsychology of memory,* 2nd edn (pp. 122–9). New York: Guilford.

Parkin, A. J. (1996). *Memory and amnesia: An introduction.* 2nd edn. Oxford: Blackwell.

Parkin, A. J. (1995). *Explorations in cognitive neuropsychology.* Oxford: Basil Blackwell.

Parkin, A. J., & Leng, N. R. C. (1993). *Neuropsychology of the amnesic syndrome.* London: Erlbaum.

Parkin, A. J., & Stampfer, H. (1995). Keeping out the past. In R. Campbell & M. Conway (Eds), *Broken memories* (pp. 81–92). Oxford: Blackwell.

Parkin, A. J., Bindschaedler, C., Harsent, L., & Metzler, C. (1995). Verification impairment in the generation of memory deficit following ruptured aneurysm of the anterior communicating artery. *Brain & Cognition* (in press).

Petrides, M. R. (1991). Frontal lobes and memory. In F. Boller & J. Grafman (Eds), *Handbook of neuropsychology,* Vol. 3, section 5 (pp. 75–90). Amsterdam: Elsevier.

Polster, M. R. (1993). Drug-induced amnesia. Implications for cognitive neuropsychological investigations of memory. *Psychological Bulletin*, *114*, 477–93.

Richardson, J. T. E. (1991). *Clinical and neuropsychological aspects of closed head injury*. Basingstoke: Taylor and Francis.

Schacter, D. L. (1987). Implicit memory: history and current status. *Journal of Experimental Psychology: Learning, Memory and Cognition*, *13*, 501–18.

Schacter, D. L., & Curran, T. (1995). The cognitive neuroscience of false memories. *Psychiatric Annals* (in press).

Shallice, T. (1988). *From neuropsychology to mental structure*. Cambridge: Cambridge University Press.

Spanos, N. P. (1986). Compliance and reinterpretation of hypnotic responding. *Contemporary Hypnosis*, *9*, 7–15.

Squire, L. R. (1987). *Memory and brain*. Oxford: Oxford University Press.

Tulving, E. (1989). Memory: Performance, knowledge, and experience. *European Journal of Cognitive Psychology*, *1*, 3–26.

Weiner, R. D. (1984). Does electroconvulsive therapy cause brain damage? *Brain and Behavioural Sciences*, *7*, 1–53.

Zola-Morgan, S., Squire, L. R., & Amaral, D. G. (1987). Human amnesia and the medial temporal region. *Journal of Neuroscience*, *6*, 2950–67.

ALAN J. PARKIN

amnesic syndrome   A condition in which brain damage causes an impairment in the recall and recognition of facts and events experienced both before (retrograde amnesia) and after the onset of brain damage (anterograde amnesia) in the face of preservation of short-term memory abilities and of intelligence. The extent to which anterograde and retrograde amnesia are associated with each other is, however, controversial. The syndrome is rarely encountered in a pure form so that many patients may show additional deficits, such as minor impairments of intelligence and other kinds of memory, caused by brain lesions that do not produce amnesia. Nevertheless, amnesics typically show retention of verbal skills and well-rehearsed semantic memories. As an organic condition the amnesic syndrome should be distinguished from psychogenic amnesias such as fugues, where impaired memory is most likely to be associated with motivational and emotional factors.

The amnesic syndrome has several main causes. Most commonly, it arises from CLOSED HEAD INJURY and various kinds of vascular accident. The degree of amnesia produced by closed head injury is highly variable and other impairments such as cognitive slowing will nearly always be present. Amnesia has commonly been reported when an INFARCT affects the distribution of the posterior cerebral or paramedian arteries, as well as after the rupture and repair of anterior communicating artery aneurysms, although the specificity of this last association has been questioned. The syndrome also develops after encephalitis, particularly that associated with the herpes simplex virus, and occasionally after meningitis. Appropriately placed tumors can cause the syndrome, as can exposure to toxins, such as carbon monoxide, hypoxia associated with attempted suicide, near drownings, complications in surgical operations, and chronic alcoholism that is typically associated with malnutrition and thiamine deficiency, and even malnutrition alone (see KORSAKOFF'S SYNDROME). The amnesia arising from these causes is often severe and permanent, but partial or relatively complete recovery has been reported in a high proportion of patients with Korsakoff's syndrome. Transient amnesia is common after head injury, and occurs in some cases with any etiology. A typically mild and transient form of the syndrome is caused by electroconvulsive therapy, and a condition known as transient global amnesia exists in which severe amnesia usually lasts for well under a day before recovery occurs, although a mild memory deficit may persist for months or even permanently. This condition has been associated with migraine, and reduced metabolic activity in the medial temporal lobes or sometimes the midline thalamus has been reported during attacks, but it shows slightly different features from transient amnesia associated with temporal lobe EPILEPSY.

ANATOMY OF AMNESIA

Amnesia can be caused by damage in any one of several brain regions that most notably include the medial temporal lobes and the midline diencephalon, although recent evidence has also implicated the basal forebrain. In monkeys, lesions to the ventromedial frontal cortex, a large region comprising medial parts of the orbitofrontal cortex and the anterior half of the CINGULATE GYRUS, as well as other structures such as the gyrus rectus, have been reported to cause an anterograde recognition deficit. There is, however, no comparable evidence from humans, perhaps partly because of the size of the critical lesion. Although amnesia can be caused by lesions in different regions, this does not prove that it is a composite of several distinct functional disorders because the structures in the different regions are highly interconnected. Lesions anywhere within the regions may, therefore, disrupt processing in the same way. There is, however, some uncertainty about the precise location of the critical lesions within each region so it remains unclear whether the syndrome reflects the presence of one or several functional deficits.

Identification of amnesia's anatomy has been facilitated by the use of a monkey model of the syndrome, which involves testing animals on a delayed non-matching-to-sample task that is similar to a recognition task in humans, as well as on other tasks at which human amnesics should be impaired. Mishkin used this model to argue that severe, permanent amnesia depends on lesions to both the HIPPOCAMPUS and AMYGDALA in the medial temporal lobes, or to their projections in the midline diencephalon and ventromedial frontal cortex, or to reciprocally connected structures in the basal forebrain. If correct, this model would probably imply that two deficits underlie severe amnesia: one associated with hippocampal circuit disruption and one with amygdalar circuit disruption. Research by Zola-Morgan and his colleagues has indicated, however, that selective amygdalar lesions do not cause amnesia in monkeys or exacerbate the amnesia caused by lesions that include the hippocampus. Earlier amygdalar lesions included damage to the perirhinal polysensory association cortex, and this damage alone causes a severe recognition deficit. Monkeys with selective stereotaxic lesions of the hippocampus do show a memory deficit, although this is less severe than that found when the lesion extends into the entorhinal and parahippocampal cortices.

The human evidence is consistent with this picture because selective amygdalar lesions do not cause global amnesia and mild amnesia has been reported in a patient with bilateral damage confined to the CA1 field of the hippocampus, whereas much more severe amnesia is found in post-encephalitic patients where the medial temporal lobe damage extends into the cortex (see Squire & Zola-Morgan, 1991). The perirhinal and parahippocampal cortices receive processed sensory information from other cortical regions and project to the hippocampus via the entorhinal cortex, receiving a back-projection from the hippocampus by the same route, so it is not surprising that damage to any of these structures can cause amnesia. It is, however, unexplained why lesions of the cortical structures cause a more severe amnesia than selective hippocampal lesions. Part of the explanation may be that they project to the midline thalamus as well as to the hippocampus.

The hippocampus projects to the midline diencephalon via the FORNIX directly to the MAMMILLARY BODIES and both directly via the fornix and indirectly via the mammillothalamic tract to the anterior nucleus of the THALAMUS. The relationship of fornix lesions to amnesia has long been controversial, but patients given fornix section in order to remove colloid cysts do seem to show moderate amnesias. Patients with Korsakoff's psychosis almost invariably have mammillary body lesions, but the association of such lesions with amnesia remains controversial. Large midline thalamic lesions that include the anterior and dorsomedial nuclei cause amnesia in monkeys and humans, but there are many small nuclei in this region, so which fiber tracts and nuclei are implicated has not yet been definitively determined.

The association of basal forebrain lesions with amnesia is less well-established, but cholinergic neurons in this region do modulate hippocampal activity, and some human amnesics have been described with damage largely confined to basal forebrain structures, such as the septum and the nucleus of the diagonal band of Broca. In monkeys, Mishkin's group found that neurotoxic lesions only impaired recognition appreciably when they destroyed the basal nucleus of Meynert as well as the septum and diagonal band of Broca. The basal forebrain contains fibers of passage, so it is hard to be sure about exactly what structural damage causes amnesia.

If the medial temporal and midline diencephalic structures implicated in amnesia are serially connected and modulated by basal forebrain inputs, it remains unclear how the diencephalic structures project back to the association neocortex, where fact and event information is probably largely stored. As the involvement of frontal structures in humans remains uncertain, either back-projections or an unidentified pathway may play a role.

SINGLE OR MULTIPLE FUNCTIONAL DEFICITS

At present, knowledge of amnesia's anatomy does not give strong guidance as to whether one or several functional deficits underlie the syndrome. It is accepted, however, that left hemisphere lesions to either medial temporal lobe or midline diencephalic structures cause a verbal material-specific amnesia, whereas right-sided lesions to equivalent structures selectively disrupt recall and recognition of nonverbal materials. These material-specific amnesias are likely to be passive reflections of the verbal and nonverbal processing performed respectively by the left and right neocortices, and the disrupted mnemonic processing is therefore likely to be very similar after left- and right-sided lesions. It has been proposed that diencephalic and temporal lobe amnesia are functionally distinct from each other. Nevertheless, there is no evidence that the pattern of retrograde amnesia differs in the two conditions and much recent evidence finds normal forgetting in temporal lobe amnesics in conflict with the claim that only these patients forget pathologically fast. It remains to be shown whether direct damage to a cortico-hippocampal-cortical loop causes a memory deficit not found following midline diencephalic lesions.

Correlations between retrograde and anterograde amnesia are typically not strong, though this may partially reflect the use of different measures. A few cases of apparently selective retrograde amnesia have also been reported. It is difficult to eliminate the role of psychogenic factors in these cases, even when there is brain damage associated with amnesia, so the cases remain polemical. Claims for the converse dissociation of selective anterograde amnesia are very rare. Although the patient with the bilateral lesion of the CA1 field of the hippocampus was reported not to have a measurable retrograde amnesia, his anterograde amnesia was mild, and it seems likely that sensitive tests of his premorbid past would have identified a mild deficit with a steep temporal gradient. It remains to be shown that specific lesions cause a relatively

selective anterograde amnesia whereas others have the converse effect.

Future work may well show that amnesics with differently placed lesions show slightly different memory symptoms, but care needs to be taken to show that the differences do not result from damage incidental to the amnesia.

NATURE OF THE MEMORY DEFICITS IN THE AMNESIC SYNDROME

Amnesics do not show impairment on all kinds of memory tasks. First, they show preserved simple classical conditioning of the eye-blink response. Second, they show normal acquisition and retention of motor skills, perceptual skills such as reading mirror-reversed words, and perhaps cognitive skills for which subjects are unable to specify the basis of their success. Third, amnesics show normal perceptual learning effects, such as facilitation in perceiving random-dot stereograms after repeated exposures. Fourth, amnesics show preserved performance on a variety of item-specific implicit memory or priming tasks. These tasks tap memory indirectly for the kinds of item for which patients show impaired recall and recognition. Memory is indicated by behavioral changes that are consistent with the claim that subjects are processing individual repeated items differently from nonrepeated items. Amnesics can show these changes although they fail to recognize that items have been repeated. There is good evidence that they show preserved priming for verbal and nonverbal material that was familiar prior to the priming experience. The evidence that patients show preserved priming for material that was novel prior to the priming experience is more equivocal. Patients have been reported to perform normally on novel nonverbal priming tasks even after delays of several days, but they have not always shown preserved priming for novel verbal information. The evidence is hard to interpret because normal subjects' priming performance may not only depend on the automatic, unaware kind of retrieval processes, believed by many to underlie priming, but may also be influenced by recall either to enhance or impede performance. Future work will need to minimize these influences or estimate the strength of the automatic, unaware processes directly.

There are certain kinds of memory that some have claimed are more impaired in amnesics than is their recognition of the target material to which attention was given on an earlier occasion, despite evidence that patients encode all kinds of information normally. These claims rest on the use of a procedure that matches amnesic and control target recognition by testing the patients under easier conditions (e.g. shorter delays or more learning opportunity). Using the same conditions, if the patients are then found to do worse than their controls on another memory task, it is argued that they are more impaired at this kind of memory. The procedure is used to avoid problems associated with floor, ceiling, and scaling effects, but itself raises problems because the matching procedure may affect the two kinds of memory differently in normal controls and so artifactually give the impression of different degrees of memory impairment. Nevertheless, it has been claimed that free recall of targets is more impaired in patients than is target recognition. This effect, however, has not always been found. Recall and recognition probably depend on a different weighting of underlying processes in different tasks, and the precise conditions under which amnesics show disproportionate free recall still need to be ascertained. Amnesics have also been reported to be disproportionately impaired at various kinds of contextual memory, such as spatial and temporal location memory, memory about the source of information, and memory about the modality via which information was presented. Reports about spatial memory are conflicting and it is possible that some of the reported differential deficits, such as those with temporal position and source memory, are caused by additional damage to the frontal lobes that is unrelated to amnesia.

The major feature of retrograde amnesia that has excited interest is the relative preservation of recall and recognition for memories in proportion to how long before the occurrence of brain damage they were acquired. These temporal gradients are apparent not only to clinical impression, but also with objective tests of public information memory and formal tests of autobiographical memory. The length of the gradients varies from a scarcely measurable time in some patients to decades in others, so it seems probable that damage to more than one processing system is involved. The notion of a gradient conceals the fact that patients often show islands of preserved memory in the premorbid past, and also does not make clear whether the effect arises because older items have usually been more rehearsed or because of some other unspecified protective process. Although most patients show retrograde amnesia for autobiographical (episodic) as well as semantic information, there have been claims that impairments in memory for the two kinds of information may be dissociated in some patients.

THEORIES OF THE DEFICIT(S) UNDERLYING AMNESIA

Three main kinds of theory about the nature of the memory deficit in amnesia are currently influential. The first and perhaps most widely held view is that amnesia is caused by a failure to store recallable and recognizable information in a normal way. Such a deficit could arise for several reasons and, if different functional deficits underlie amnesia, it is possible that more than one kind of storage deficit is present in amnesics. For example, it has been suggested by Zola-Morgan and Squire (1990) that storage processes vital for fact and event memory initially occur in the hippocampus and only later is storage transferred to association neocortex. On this view, lesions to the hippocampus should disrupt new learning and cause a retrograde amnesia with a steep temporal gradient. Damage to certain midline diencephalic structures might impair storage differently by disrupting processes that facilitate the storage of fact and event information in association neocortex. Storage views do not predict either that free recall and context memory should be differentially impaired in patients or that patients prime normally to novel information, unless it can be shown that such priming involves retrieval from a different memory store from that used for recall and recognition. Storage deficits should also predict accelerated forgetting over certain delays in patients, but there is not yet convincing evidence that this occurs.

The second kind of theory is completely opposite in tenor from the storage deficit views. An earlier view, once considered by Schacter, was that amnesics store fact and event information completely normally, but that this memory system is disconnected from a conscious awareness system. An alternative possibility is that there is a special-purpose system that confers awareness only on memories and that this system has been damaged in amnesics. Evidence of preserved storage is provided by the normal performance of amnesics on priming tasks that tap memory for any kind of novel information, provided such performance can be shown to depend on automatic retrieval from the same memory system that underlies recall and recognition. This kind of theory has difficulty in explaining why some amnesics show preserved recall and recognition for older premorbid memories unless it is supposed that patients can achieve awareness of these memories because they have been transferred to a separate memory system that is not disconnected from the awareness system. Also, no attempt is made to explain how awareness is conferred.

The third kind of theory proposes that amnesics have a primary deficit in memory for the contextual information that typically falls on the periphery of attention during learning and that this causes a secondary and less severe deficit in aware memory for information to which attention was paid during learning. Variants of this kind of view identify the primary deficit as memory for particular kinds of context, such as spatiotemporal information, or background information that affects the meaningful interpretation of what is attended to during learning, or both. Also, the deficit is postulated to be one of either storage or effortful retrieval. Context views predict differential deficits in the recognition of context and the storage variant predicts impaired priming of novel contextual information. This kind of view has difficulty in explaining why the structures damaged in amnesics should normally be primarily concerned with context.

BIBLIOGRAPHY

Kapur, N. (1988). *Memory disorders in clinical practice.* London: Butterworth.

Mayes, A. R. (1988). *Human organic memory disorders.* Cambridge: Cambridge University Press.

Milner, D., & Rugg, M. (1991). *Consciousness and cognition: Neuropsychological perspectives.* London: Academic Press.

Parkin, A. J. (1987). *Memory and amnesia: An introduction.* Oxford: Blackwell.

Squire, L. R. (1988). *Memory and brain.* Oxford: Oxford University Press.

Squire, L. R., & Zola-Morgan, S. (1991). The medial temporal lobe memory system. *Science, 253,* 1380–6.

Tulving, E., & Schacter, D. L. (1990). Priming and human memory systems. *Science, 247,* 301–6.

Victor, M., Adams, R. D., & Collins, G. H. (1989). *The Wernicke–Korsakoff syndrome: Related neurological disorders due to alcoholism and malnutrition,* 2nd edn. Philadelphia: Davis.

Zola-Morgan, S., & Squire, L. R. (1990). The primate hippocampal formation: evidence for a time-dependent role in memory storage. *Science, 250,* 288–90.

ANDREW R. MAYES

amorphognosis Amorphognosis is a TACTILE PERCEPTION DISORDER and a form of tactile agnosia. In Delay's 1935 classification of impairments of tactile recognition, amorphognosis refers to an impairment in the recognition of the size and shape of objects, and is distinguished from AHYLOGNOSIA and tactile asymboly (impaired recognition of the identity of objects in the absence of amorphognosis and ahylognosia).

amorphosynthesis Amorphosynthesis is a deficit in spatial summation, leading to a loss of fine discrimination and an inability to integrate more than a few properties of a sensory stimulus. As a disorder of sensation it has been proposed as a process which might underlie the NEGLECT syndrome, and it has been associated with the function of the parietal lobes.

amusia Amusia is the inability or disability to correctly render musical expression by singing or playing an instrument; failure to apperceive musical production. The term implies an acquired condition, parallel to APHASIA.

EARLY STUDIES

Musical ability and musical disability following brain disease have been described in the medical literature since the nineteenth century. The term *amusia* was coined by A. Knoblauch in 1890 to describe a constellation of acquired disorders of musical capacity ranging from failure to recognize musical passages to distorted singing or instrumental playing. The first patients were described as having excellent musical faculties in conjunction with grossly disturbed or loss of language skills. In one early case (of Béhier, 1836) a patient could only repeat the syllable "tan" but could sing the national anthem and other well-known songs using that syllable. Similar observations of aphasics who could sing with preserved melody were echoed in later case reports. However, such patients were still classified "musically deficient" because they could not produce the words of the song along with the melody.

The cerebral mechanisms for music were considered to be parallel to those for language. Consequently, specific musical defects were hypothetically predictable from circumscribed lesions of the auditory, motor, or idea centers or their interconnecting pathways. Unfortunately there were few case reports, and therefore little evidence, to verify these predictions. Even in the current literature, symptoms of amusia are widely varied following apparently similar lesions. Such individual differences in higher cerebral processing challenge the validity of assigning any complex behavior – music is only one example – to specific neuroanatomic sites and neural mechanisms.

Case reports from the early period, and later ones up to the present, have been unequivocal in supporting one conclusion: musical ability and speech can be controlled by different, independently activated, cerebral circuitry (Gordon & Bogen, 1974). This point is not trivial since both music and language have many shared functional elements. Both require perception and comprehension of complex auditory patterns, and both use highly precise muscular control for expression. Accordingly, aspects of musical function and language function should be simultaneously affected. This would be expected for speaking and singing following damage to the motor pathways of the articulators, or for writing and instrument-playing following lesions to primary motor areas of the hand and fingers. It is the cognitive aspects – understanding, singing, speaking – which are differentially represented in the brain. The most dramatic example of this differential system is a patient who had a left HEMISPHERECTOMY to remove a recurrent, adult-acquired tumor. His speech was minimal, but he sang with remarkable ease (Smith, 1966).

RIGHT HEMISPHERE LATERALIZATION

The contribution of the right cerebral hemisphere to musical ability was first mentioned by Hughlings Jackson in 1866. His conclusion was not taken seriously until a hundred years later, when it was demonstrated systematically in patients with EPILEPSY who underwent unilateral right temporal LOBECTOMIES (Milner, 1962). These patients were selectively poorer on some tests of musical abilities, such as timbre and tonal memory, compared to patients with left lobectomies. Rhythm and pitch did not differ between the groups. This result was prophetic for subsequent studies of right and left hemisphere specialization in brain function.

Right hemisphere contribution to perception of musical stimuli was first confirmed in non-neurological subjects using a technique of simultaneous auditory presentation (DICHOTIC LISTENING) to the right and left ears (Kimura, 1964). Validated with tests of verbal material, simultaneous presentation had the functional effect of assessing hemispheric superiority by comparing the perceptual accuracy of recalled auditory stimuli presented to the contralateral ears. Thus, while more words were recalled from the right ear, more melodies were recalled from the left ear. Right ear superiority for verbal material demonstrated the known left hemisphere dominance for language function; left ear superiority demonstrated, for the first time, right hemisphere specialization for musical elements. This new paradigm provided a simple yet powerful window on hemispheric specialization for processing complex auditory stimuli. Subsequent studies confirmed the broad observation that music is more strongly associated with processes in the right hemisphere (see LATERALIZATION).

Qualifications to this generalization came almost immediately. While chords demonstrated left ear superiority confirming right hemisphere dominance (Gordon, 1980), rhythms yielded right ear superiority implying left hemisphere dominance (Gordon, 1978). One reasonable functional dichotomy explaining differential hemispheric participation in musical ability is that the left hemisphere is responsible for perception and production of temporal elements, while the right hemisphere is responsible for perception and conceptualization of "wholeness" in music (Gordon, 1983).

The contribution of the right hemisphere to musical expression (singing) was first systematically demonstrated during clinical application of (unilateral) INTRACAROTID SODIUM AMYTAL in pre-surgical patients (Bogen & Gordon, 1971). (This medical technique is necessary to determine the hemispheric contribution to speech and memory prior to major neurosurgery.) Patients were asked to sing simple songs or hum well-known melodies while one hemisphere was anesthetized, as evidenced by left hemiplegia. Singing was amelodic at a time when speaking was minimally disturbed; the reverse was never observed. By contrast, singing was less affected than speech for instances of left hemisphere anesthetization, including cases of singing when no speech was present (Gordon & Bellamy, 1991). A clearer example was a left hemispherectomy patient whose speech was limited to single words or simple phrases, while singing was initiated with little assistance (Smith, 1966). These observations confirm that there is a cerebral mechanism in the right hemisphere capable of singing better than, or exclusive of, left hemisphere mechanisms; and there are left hemisphere mechanisms that speak but cannot, or will not, sing.

Unfortunately the total picture is not so clear. Recall the historical literature in which there were repeated case reports of patients with stroke or tumor who had disturbances in both singing and speaking. There were also several cases of patients with left intracarotid amylobarbital whose singing was interrupted together with speech arrest, or who could not sing even after speech began to recover. Moreover, there are many observations of patients with right hemisphere anesthetization who could sing (and speak) without apparent impairment. These observations suggest two possibilities: either the mechanisms utilized for speech are recruited for singing in some instances, or the specialized mechanisms for singing are partially or completely operated by the left hemisphere instead of the right in some people. Once again, individual differences in these musical abilities preclude assignment of specific neural substrates to musical skills or other cognitive skills.

MUSICIANS: INDIVIDUAL DIFFERENCES

The right cerebral hemisphere is now considered to contribute most to musical behavior. However, musical training seems to modify that concept. The first report of this observation was a task to detect monaurally presented, two-note excerpts from a 12 to 18 note "melody" (Bever & Chiarello, 1974). Musicians favored their right ear (left hemisphere); non-musicians could not do the task. A second task was simply to recognize the melody itself. Non-musicians remembered more

melodies presented to their left ear (right hemisphere), confirming the standard observation. Musicians, however, remembered just as many melodies from their left ear (right hemisphere) as the non-musicians, but remembered significantly more from their right ear (left hemisphere). These group differences between musicians and non-musicians have been replicated by other studies, but results are not consistent (e.g. Zatorre, 1979). In one study there was a *bimodal* distribution (Gordon, 1980) in a task of chord recognition by professional musicians: half the subjects had a left ear superiority; half had a right ear superiority.

Differing strategies among musicians have also demonstrated shifting dominances for cerebral function. Musicians who reported a global perceptual approach to a dichotic chords recognition task, for example, had a greater left ear superiority implying right hemisphere dominance (Morais et al., 1982). But there was a significant shift toward right ear superiority when a more analytic approach (e.g. to identify individual tones) was induced (Peretz et al., 1987). The *in*consistencies among studies of lateralized brain function among musically trained persons are alarmingly *consistent*. This leaves unsettled the question of how cerebral resources are reallocated by training.

Factors of training and individual differences complicate the assessment of amusia. Complaints by a trained musician of a newly acquired musical disability would have more sophisticated implications with respect to cerebral dysfunction than would complaints by a musically immature person. For example, one musician who complains that music is now "just noise" may have lost the ability to appreciate underlying chord progressions or the relationships among note patterns. Perhaps there was a loss of analytic skill for musical substructure. Conversely, another musician with the same complaint may fail to appreciate the totality of the musical experience. In this case, perhaps, there was loss of skill for "global" perception. Musical tests, together with comprehensive neuropsychological assessment, would be needed to differentiate these disorders.

TESTS OF MUSICAL DYSFUNCTION

Assessment of musical dysfunction must be pursued with respect to the role the assessment will play, either in neuroanatomic location of the lesion or in treatment and rehabilitation of the patient. The history of testing for amusia is similar to, but a poor cousin of, the history of testing for aphasia. Auditory, visual, motor, and idea centers (and interconnecting pathways) were the only hypothesized functional units subserving musical skills. Accordingly, tests were developed to assess the result of damage to these areas. Damage to the auditory center for music, for example, would be expected to prevent appreciation (i.e. perception) of music; damage to the musical motor center would prevent singing; damage to the pathway between them would prevent repetition (singing along) of a musical passage, and so on.

Clinical tests for amusia continue to be published (e.g. Jellinek, 1956; Wertheim & Botez, 1961) and are designed according to the most current cognitive theory. In some concepts two major components, "receptive" and "productive," are recognized. Within the *receptive* component are several tests of tonal, melodic, and harmony elements for which patients are required to name, compare, and recognize tones, intervals, phrases, and melodies. There are also several subtests where patients are required to appreciate the nature of rhythms, tempi, and time. In the *production* element the patient has to produce, by singing or instrumentally, single tones, familiar or unfamiliar melodies, and musical dynamics for loudness (e.g. crescendo) and speed (e.g. ritardando). Finally, patients are tested on musical knowledge, including word definitions, note and symbol names, as well as the assignment of music to periods in history or to specific composers.

The limiting utility of any of these test batteries is the absence of a pre-morbid baseline or normative scale. For patients, it would be nearly impossible to determine a quantitative change in musical function; qualitative changes would depend on the recollection and report of the patient or family members and friends. Quantitative changes in patients with musical experience are more reliably assessed, at least for basic knowledge and ability.

Assessment of musical dysfunction is useful primarily for designing an appropriate treatment plan where rehabilitation in music would be important for restoring the quality of life for the patient. It is important that the test battery be sufficiently comprehensive to document the retained abilities for each of the elements of music. The value of musical evaluation in the non-musical patient may be to provide a clearer perspective of the patient's entire cognitive profile. In the context of other cognitive abilities and disabilities, musical dysfunction can help formulate the underlying cerebral neuropathology, and hence the range of cognitive skills retained by the patient.

SELECTED CASE HISTORIES

Maurice Ravel was one of the more notable composers who suffered from progressive brain damage resulting in aphasia and elements of amusia (Henson, 1988). His symptoms were not systematically recorded, but they included word-finding difficulty which progressed to Broca's aphasia, dysgraphia progressing to AGRAPHIA, and APRAXIA. Musical disturbances were most obvious in his inability to compose, conduct, and perform (e.g. play the piano). By contrast, there were several indications that musical perception was intact. He reportedly recognized most compositions of various composers, including all his own works. Similarly, he could appreciate tune, rhythm, tempo, and presumably, aesthetic aspects of music. Although the nature of the cerebral damage was never fully ascertained, these observations serve to demonstrate the partial separation between language and some musical functions. No autopsy was performed, but surgical intervention (which eventually killed him) revealed no grossly observable damage to the right hemisphere.

A second composer, Shebalin, had a stroke which provided a more localized (or rather lateralized) damage site (Luria et al., 1965). Right hemiparesis was observed and post-mortem examination revealed massive damage to the left temporo-parietal regions. His speech was impoverished, characterized by single words or short phrases. He also exhibited comprehension difficulties, including failure to understand names of objects. By contrast, there was virtually no disturbance reported in his ability to compose music nor to work with his pupils creatively and critically. It was not reported how he accomplished the motor task of writing the compositions, but as far as the essence of music was concerned in this patient, either the right hemisphere or areas outside the temporo-parietal regions of the left hemisphere subserved his musical ability.

Another case of a left-sided vascular injury in a trained violinist was reported (Wertheim & Botez,

67

1961) before studies of the 1960s had attributed several musical skills to the right hemisphere. This case serves to demonstrate the dangers of making observations prejudiced by preconceived notions of brain function. The patient was described as having "receptive musical function . . . much more disturbed than the verbal receptive one." Based on the reported details and hindsight, it is most likely that musical ability per se was not disturbed, but rather the patient's career was devastated. The language examination was not detailed, but it was reported that the examiner needed to utter complicated requests "slowly" for the patient to perform some tasks. Other verbal tasks were not performed because he "had no patience." Expressively, there were clear naming and word-finding difficulties, and PARAPHASIA, but these were considered "comparatively slight."

By contrast, the patient retained a wide range of musical skills. He could compare tones for accuracy, reproduce a melody with his left hand on violin strings (his right hand was paretic), recognize intentional faults in familiar melodies, distinguish chords, and appreciate musical dynamics. What the patient could *not* do was name tones, name familiar melodies or classical passages, name intervals, nor write down a simple melody. The patient also had difficulties reproducing and specifying rhythms. Singing of known melodies was not always correct, nor could he sing new melodies. This evidence suggests that a less severe indictment of amusia symptoms relative to aphasic disturbances would have been drawn had the authors devised tests excluding the burden of naming, and administered a more complete assessment of paraphasic errors and other aphasic disturbances.

SUMMARY AND CONCLUSION

Amusia is the medical term used for disturbances in musical ability acquired after cerebral injury. It may refer to defects in perception or expression of simple musical elements, or it can refer to more subtle and esoteric deficits such as failure to associate musical passages with specific composers or historical periods. The nature and importance of the deficits are dependent on the pre-morbid training and skills of the patient. Whereas many skills needed for music appear to be associated with the right cerebral hemisphere, the contribution of various brain centers may vary widely from individual to individual. Assessment of amusia is most important for rehabilitation in patients where music is a major feature in the patient's quality of life. Assessment of musical ability or disability can be useful in understanding cognitive processes, but only in conjunction with other cognitive skills and musical experiences of the examinee. Music, like language, is not innate, but "laid on" the cortical substrates of the brain through learning and experience. The challenge of neuropsychology is to discover how these basic cognitive processes are subserved by neuro-anatomical connections and neurotransmitter systems, and how cerebral mechanisms function to accommodate music as well as other higher cognitive abilities.

BIBLIOGRAPHY

Bever, T. G., & Chiarello, R. J. (1974). Cerebral dominance in musicians and non-musicians. *Science, 185,* 137–9.

Bogen, J. E., & Gordon, H. W. (1971). Musical tests for functional lateralization with intracarotid amobarbital. *Nature, 230,* 524–5.

Gordon, H. W. (1978). Left hemisphere dominance for rhythmic elements in dichotically presented melodies. *Cortex, 14,* 58–70.

Gordon, H. W. (1980). Degree of ear asymmetries for perception of dichotic chords and for illusory chord localization in musicians of different levels of competence. *Journal of Neurology, Neurosurgery and Psychiatry, 37,* 727–38.

Gordon, H. W. (1983). Music and the right hemisphere. In A. W. Young (Ed.), *Functions of the right hemisphere* (pp. 65–86). London: Academic Press.

Gordon, H. W., & Bellamy, K. (1991). Music, myelin, language, localization, speech, synapses, brain, and behavior. In *Wenner-Gren Center International Symposium Series,* Vol. 59: J. Sundberg, L. Nord, & R. Carlson (Eds), *Music, language, speech and brain* (pp. 311–17). Cambridge: University Press.

Gordon, H. W., & Bogen, J. E. (1974). Hemispheric lateralization of singing after intracarotid sodium amylobarbitone. *Journal of Neurology, Neurosurgery, and Psychiatry, 37,* 727–38.

Henson, R. A. (1988). Maurice Ravel's illness: a tragedy of lost creativity. *British Medical Journal, 296,* 1585–8.

Jellinek, A. (1956). Amusia. *Folia Phoniatrica, 8,* 124–49.

Kimura, D. (1964). Left-right differences in the perception of melodies. *Quarterly Journal of Experimental Psychology*, *16*, 355–8.

Knoblauch, A. (1890). On disorders of the musical capacity from cerebral disease. *Brain*, *13*, 317–40.

Luria, A. R., Tsvetkova, L. S., & Futer, D. S. (1965). Aphasia in a composer. *Journal of the Neurological Sciences*, *2*, 288–92.

Milner, B. (1962). Laterality effects in audition. In V. B. Mountcastle (Ed.), *Interhemispheric relations and cerebral dominance* (pp. 177–95). Baltimore, MD: Johns Hopkins Press.

Morais, J., Peretz, I., & Gudanski, M. (1982). Ear asymmetry for chord recognition in musicians and nonmusicians. *Neuropsychologia*, *20*, 351–4.

Peretz, I., Morais, J., & Bertelson, P. (1987). Shifting ear differences in melody recognition through strategy inducement. *Brain and Cognition*, *6*, 202–15.

Smith, A. (1966). Speech and other functions after left (dominant) hemispherectomy. *Journal of Neurology, Neurosurgery and Psychiatry*, *29*, 467–71.

Wertheim, N., & Botez, M. I. (1961). Receptive amusia: a clinical analysis. *Brain*, *84*, 19–30.

Zatorre, R. J. (1979). Recognition of dichotic melodies by musicians and non-musicians. *Neuropsychologia*, *17*, 607–17.

HAROLD W. GORDON

amygdala   The amygdala (or amygdaloid nucleus) is a mass of grey matter buried within the white matter of the subcortical forebrain in the region around the lateral ventricle within the temporal lobe. It is a significant component of the LIMBIC SYSTEM.

It lies immediately under the olfactory cortex and one of its nuclei fuses with the overlying olfactory cortex. The medial nuclei of the amygdala carry olfactory information to the hypothalamus (and indirectly to the thalamus) with some fibers passing directly through the stria terminalis, while others relay at the HIPPOCAMPUS and then travel via the FORNIX. The amygdala therefore contributes to autonomic and emotional responsiveness, particularly in the role which smell plays in such reactions, and the powerful links between smell and memory are also partly supported by this structure in its links with the neighbouring hippocampus.

The lateral and basal nuclei of the amygdala also have links to the hippocampus, but also to the CINGULATE GYRUS and the orbital cortex of the frontal lobes. The amygdala is rich in opiate receptors and also has a low threshold for EPILEPSY in common with other limbic structures, being implicated in temporal lobe and psychomotor seizures. The placement of surgical lesions in the amygdala (amygdalectomy) as a form of PSYCHOSURGERY has been used with some success to reduce aggressive and violent behavior but is now not commonly practiced, largely as a result of the ethical controversy surrounding psychosurgery.

amygdalectomy   Amygdalectomy is a form of PSYCHOSURGERY targeted at the AMYGDALA.

anarithmetria   *See* ACALCULIA. Anarithmetria is sometimes reserved for impairments of the process of calculation in the absence of difficulty in reading or writing numbers, or of spatial disorder. In this form it also corresponds to primary acalculia.

anarthria   Anarthria is a disorder of phonemic production for which there are a variety of alternative terms: Broca's aphasia, motor aphasia, expressive aphasia, syndrome of phonetic disintegration, efferent motor aphasia, verbal aphasia, and nonfluent aphasia (*see* APHASIA). If this were not confusing enough, some writers preserve the term anarthria as a synonym for aphemia, pure word dumbness, and subcortical motor aphasia.

In the first and broader use of the term the severely anarthric patient may be quite unable to verbalize, but it is more common to see patients who are only able to make single incoherent grunts or groans, or at best a meaningless collection of phonemes or syllables (verbal stereotypies). Broca's classic patient was known as Tantan, because all he was able to do was repeat the syllable "tan" (*see also* AMUSIA). In less severe cases verbal output is to some degree limited and may include a variety of phonemic errors. Naming of objects is commonly impossible and comprehension is variable but may be normal. Reading comprehension is unaffected, but reading aloud may be disturbed to a similar degree as spontaneous speech. Spontaneous writing and spelling are almost always impaired.

In the more restricted use of the term (equivalent to aphemia) anarthria applies more precisely to phonemic production, so the patient is acutely mute and proceeds through recovery to HYPOPHONIA, and to a soft, slow but otherwise accurate verbal output. In such cases language comprehension and the ability to read and write are all preserved. In no form of output do grammatical errors occur and ANOMIA is not present. The error is one of phonemic production and not of phonemic access. In such cases the lesion is generally in or very close to Broca's area.

anencephaly Anencephaly is a very severe congenital disorder of development which results in the absence of the cerebral hemispheres, DIENCEPHALON, and midbrain. The literal meaning of the word is "without a brain." As might be expected, although the resulting nervous sytem is viable, it produces the severest form of mental defect.

anesthesia Anesthesia, which is generally the loss of sensation, refers to two quite distinct medical entities. The first, and more commonly understood, is the procedure which makes use of specific anesthetic agents to permit various forms of surgical intervention. Local anesthetics block, by various means, the transmission of nerve impulses which would normally convey sensation or pain; general anesthetics render the patient unconscious and also produce a total amnesia, although exceptions to this have been reported when the level of anesthesia is relatively light. General anesthetic agents operate upon various structures in the brain stem mediating arousal and consciousness in order to achieve their effects.

The second meaning of anesthesia relates to sensory loss as a result of a neurological lesion. Resulting from cortical lesions, hemianesthesia for one lateral half of the body surface is the most common form, although the face may be spared. Upper limbs are more severely affected than lower limbs, and the distal parts more than the proximal. Occasionally there may be specific regions of sensory loss over limited areas of the body surface, notably on the hand around the thumb, or on the face around the lips.

Occasionally pain may be associated with sensory loss, when it is described as *anesthesia dolorosa*, most commonly as a consequence of the virus herpes zoster (shingles). When the sensory loss is restricted to pain sensation, the term "analgesia" is generally preferred, although this may also be considered a form of anesthesia.

aneurysm An aneurysm results from a deficiency in the wall of an artery so that the artery wall balloons out to form the aneurysm. These saccular aneurysms are the most common, although there are also arteriosclerotic dilatations and rare aneurysms associated with inflammatory diseases. They are therefore generally regarded as congenital in origin, although both hypertension and arterial degeneration play a role in their development.

Deficiencies in the muscle coat which forms the artery wall tend to occur at arterial junctions where the separately developed muscles fail to join adequately, and this may be one reason why the majority of aneurysms occur around the circle of Willis (the system of interconnecting arteries at the base of the brain, which receives the blood supply from the neck and distributes it to the main cerebral arteries), most being on the anterior half of the circle. Up to 15 percent of patients who have an aneurysm have additional aneurysms, and these may be at symmetrical sites.

The main significance of aneurysms is that they are likely to rupture and are the cause of over 90 percent of SUBARACHNOID HEMORRHAGES (when the origin of the hemorrhage can be traced). However, aneurysms may grow without rupturing to a size sufficient to produce displacement effects with consequent focal neurological and neuropsychological signs, and large aneurysms may also contain pools of stagnant blood which may thrombose.

Aneurysms may be neurologically silent, and often go undetected before the occurrence of a cerebrovascular accident. However, where an aneurysm is identified, as rupture of the aneurysm is a potentially life-threatening event an intervention is often indicated to try to prevent it. This may involve clipping the neck of the aneurysm or, where this is not possible, employing material to reinforce and strengthen the sac; alternatively the main supplying vessel may be occluded proximally. Similar approaches may be employed as an emergency measure even after an aneurysm has ruptured and resulted in a hemorrhage.

angiography Angiography involves the introduction of a radio-opaque contrast medium into the cerebral blood circulation for diagnostic purposes, which when imaged using X-rays produces an angiogram. The technique was formerly a widely used neurodiagnostic procedure, but its use was partly superseded by the introduction of CT SCANS and more recent developments in medical imaging.

Currently angiography, more properly termed *carotid angiography* as the medium is introduced via the carotid arteries, is used to demonstrate aneurysms and vascular malformations. By outlining these abnormalities of the cerebrovascular system on the angiogram as the structures fill with the blood carrying the contrast medium, the image can assist in determining decisions about the appropriateness of surgery, and in guiding surgical intervention when it is indicated.

Modern enhancements of the basic technique include the introduction of digital enhancement to improve image clarity and reduce the dose of radiation required, and dynamic images may be obtained using film or video recording. A technique of angiography by venous injection, rather than the traditional arterial injection, has also been developed; it is appropriate to some purposes, and dramatically reduces the risks associated with arterial angiography.

angular gyrus The angular gyrus is a region of the left cerebral cortex posterior to the posterior termination of the Sylvian fissure, and on the borders of the parietal and occipital lobes. It has traditionally been regarded as the main structure of the posterior element of the language system since its designation by Déjerine in 1914 as the center for "verbal visual images."

The crucial location of the angular gyrus was emphasized by Geschwind in his re-presentation of Déjerine's work, by its position close to the association cortices of the sensory regions for audition, vision, and somesthesis, and by its rich interconnections, which permit links between cortical areas, so supporting cross-modal associations outside the operation of the limbic system. This is regarded as a necessary basis for many aspects of human language function, and particularly for the activities of reading and writing, in addition to speech.

Nominal aphasia, a difficulty in naming objects also called "amnesic dysphasia," has been particularly associated with lesions of the angular gyrus. That the relationship between this cortical location and the diagnosis of nominal aphasia appears not to be perfect may well reflect the fact that the behavioral naming deficit may result from a variety of neuropsychological functional deficits, depending on the precise way in which the naming difficulty is assessed. Not only will the deficit depend on the nature of the task employed (naming on confrontation, naming from description, naming from an outline drawing) but it may vary in the qualitative aspects of the patient's response. It is most usual, but not invariably the case, that the patient will claim that he knows the name but cannot produce it, experiencing a sense of familiarity with the name, and he or she may well be able to accurately describe its use, or demonstrate other semantic information about the object, and will correctly accept or reject names which are offered. Nominal aphasia is commonly present in writing as in speech and may be associated with deficits in the comprehension of both written and spoken language.

When alexia occurs with agraphia, a disorder of both reading and writing in the absence of any serious disorder of speech expression or comprehension also known as "parietal alexia," the angular gyrus is considered the anatomical locus of this syndrome.

Patients who fulfilled Heilman's definition of ideational apraxia, an inability to demonstrate the use of objects in the absence of the real object, accompanied by normal performance in the presence of the object, in imitation and in recognition of movements, had lesions of the left angular gyrus. These lesions are considered to have disconnected the language areas from the motor engrams, which the patients were believed not to be able to access on the basis of language information alone.

Bilateral lesions of the angular gyrus have also been implicated in the genesis of oculomotor disorders and their role in visual agnosia (BÁLINT'S SYNDROME). While the role of frontal oculomotor centers in the control of gaze is now more commonly emphasized, there may still be a posterior element to this system. If frontal oculomotor centers exert inhibitory control over the posterior centers, then control may still be maintained in the presence of a unilateral posterior lesion, as the occipital visual centers in the two hemispheres are interconnected. However, in the presence of bilateral posterior lesions, perhaps critically involving the angular gyrus, control of voluntary visual gaze may be lost, so that fixation comes to be determined by mechanisms other than those under the indirect control of the frontal lobes. Bilateral lesions of the angular gyrus have also been noted in a case of facial agnosia.

BIBLIOGRAPHY

Geschwind, N. (1965). Disconnection syndromes in animal and man. *Brain, 88,* 237–94, 585–644.

J. GRAHAM BEAUMONT

animal studies Studies employing nonhuman animals as subjects comprise one of the methodological approaches within neuropsychology. Particularly where it is considered unethical to conduct procedures with human subjects, the study of animals may be of value. Although the ethics of animal experimentation must still be carefully considered, experiments involving invasive procedures such as surgery, the administration of drugs, and noxious stimuli may be justified for the knowledge they yield. Data obtained from the use of animal subjects should always be considered within a phylogenetic perspective, and care must be taken in extrapolating from the nonhuman to the human brain.

anomia Anomia denotes the failure to respond to a normally perceived stimulus by producing an oral or a written word. The term is commonly used in the context of picture naming. However, it applies whenever a stimulus, be it an object, an auditorily or visually presented word, or an auditorily or visually presented description of an object, fails to elicit a naming response. Omitted responses in reading aloud, writing to dictation, repetition, delayed copy, and tactile object naming should also be labelled anomias.

Anomia is the most ubiquitous naming disorder. It is observed, usually with other types of errors, in all clinical forms of aphasia, independent of etiology (vascular, traumatic, neoplastic, degenerative) in both the acute and the recovery stage. Probably because of its ubiquity, anomia is generally considered of no localizing value. However, in some studies the worst performance in object-naming tasks was obtained by patients with TEMPORAL LOBE damage, whereas patients with FRONTAL LOBE damage are often poor in action-naming tests. Sometimes anomia is the main (or the only) language deficit in an aphasic patient. In the clinical neuropsychological literature, this language deficit is called amnesic or anomic APHASIA.

The definition of anomia entails the notion that the disorder results from the inability to produce phonological or orthographic information stored in the mental lexicon. Several properties of both stimulus and target may influence the occurrence of anomia. Their effect has been documented in several single-case studies. The roles played by stimulus and response parameters will be briefly reviewed, and their implications for interpretations of anomia will be discussed.

PROPERTIES OF THE TARGET WORD AFFECTING THE PROBABILITY OF ANOMIA

Frequency of usage of the target word influences the occurrence of anomia (Kay & Ellis, 1985; Miceli et al., 1991) and of other naming errors – low-frequency words are produced incorrectly more often than high-frequency words. The role of frequency is not entirely clear and may not be the same in all tasks. At least in object naming, stimulus familiarity might be very important.

Naming performance is affected by *grammatical class*. The ability to name words of different grammatical categories can be selectively affected by brain damage. Thus, pictured objects (= nouns) are named more accurately than pictured actions (= verbs) by some patients, whereas the reverse picture is observed in other subjects (Miceli et al., 1984). The effect persists when object and action names are matched for imageability. Better performance on nouns than on verbs matched for length, frequency, and imageability is also frequently observed in so-called deep DYSLEXIA and deep dysgraphia.

Morphological structure exerts a well-documented effect on word production in aphasia (Caramazza & Miceli, 1990). The ability to produce suffixes can be selectively impaired, in the presence of normal ability to produce word roots. The effect of morphological structure is hard to demonstrate in picture naming, as only some of the appropriate target items are picturable. Selective inability to reproduce inflections, paired to normal reproduction of root morphemes, has been clearly shown in disorders of reading aloud, writing to dictation, and repetition.

Naming accuracy is affected in some cases by the *semantic category* of the stimulus. It has long been known that color, body part, and letter names can be selectively impaired by brain damage. More recently, selective deficits were demonstrated with categories such as proper names, and fruit and vegetable names. Several double dissociations have also been reported: performance on concrete words is usually more accurate than performance on abstract words, but in some cases the reverse pattern was observed; the category of animals was selectively impaired in some patients, but selectively spared in others; better performance on inanimate objects relative to living things and foods, as well as the reverse pattern was demonstrated. (For a review of semantic category effects see McCarthy & Warrington, 1990.)

EFFECTS OF STIMULUS PRESENTATION AND RESPONSE PRODUCTION MODALITY

In many cases, anomia is *independent of modality*. An object cannot be named under disparate conditions of stimulus presentation (when it is seen, or touched with eyes closed, or described by the examiner, or when the noise it produces is heard) and of response production (oral or written). This is not a general rule; anomia can be modality-specific.

In some patients anomia occurs as a function of *input modality*. Optic aphasia, auditory-specific anomia (acoustic aphasia) and tactile aphasia have been described in subjects free from elementary perceptual deficits and AGNOSIA. When an object is presented in the affected modality (visual, auditory, and tactile), the patient cannot name it but is able to demonstrate its use. When the same object is presented in unaffected modalities, the patient names it accurately. For example, a patient with optic aphasia cannot name a visually presented object, but can demonstrate its use; when

the same object is presented for tactile naming, the patient can name it, even with the eyes closed.

The occurrence of naming errors can be affected by *output modality*. In some cases, tasks requiring an oral response are disproportionately affected with respect to tasks requiring a written response; in others the reverse pattern is observed. For example, two patients (Caramazza & Hillis, 1991) were asked to read aloud and to write to dictation the same word in two different sentence contexts. The target word was a noun in one context (There is a *crack* in the mirror) and a verb in the other (Don't *crack* the nuts in here). A grammatical class effect was observed in both cases; the very same word was produced normally as a noun, but could not be produced as a verb. More important for the issue considered here, an output-modality specific effect was observed; one patient showed superior performance on nouns only in reading aloud, the other only in writing to dictation.

WHAT DO ANOMIC PATIENTS KNOW ABOUT THE WORDS THEY CANNOT NAME?

It has been claimed that, just like normal subjects in the "tip-of-the-tongue" state, anomic patients know "everything" about the target word except its pronunciation. This may be true in some patients, but is by no means the general case. Anomic patients retain different types and amounts of phonological information on the target word, perhaps also as a function of co-occurring comprehension disorders. As a consequence, performance in different patients is affected by various cues to a different degree. In some cases, phonemic cueing (presentation of the first sound or syllable of the target word) precipitates the correct response, but its effect wears out in seconds or minutes. In other cases, semantic cues result in prolonged facilitation. In yet other cases, neither phonemic nor semantic cueing help, and in at least one study semantic cueing was reported to have a detrimental effect. An anomic patient with poor word comprehension produced the correct response after phonemic cueing, but could be made to produce semantic errors when prompted with the first sound of a word semantically related to the target. Unable to name the picture of a tiger, he produced /ˈtaig / *tiger* when prompted with /t/ and /ˈɛlifˈnt/ *elephant* when presented with /ɛ/ (Howard et al.,

1985). Clearly, some anomic patients lack more than just the pronunciation of the target; they lack its meaning as well.

The inconsistent effect of various cue types suggests that the type and amount of retained information on words that are not named differ across anomic patients, and hence that the cognitive deficits underlying anomia are heterogeneous.

IMPLICATIONS FOR EXPERIMENTAL SEMANTIC-LEXICAL THEORIES OF DATA

Naming disorders can only be understood when related to explicit theories of the cognitive mechanisms involved in normal word processing. It can be assumed that performance impairments resulting from damage to a particular cognitive mechanism are constrained by the characteristics of processing structure at that level. Hence, naming deficits can be used to draw inferences on the structure of the mechanisms involved in word processing. The above-reviewed evidence severely constrains the number of viable hypotheses on the functional architecture of the semantic-lexical system. One plausible hypothesis is schematically represented in the framed portion of Figure 14.

The semantic-lexical system consists of independent semantic and lexical components. Conceptual properties of words are represented in the former, formal (linguistic) properties in the latter. The lexicon is a multicomponent system of distributed type. It consists of separate input and output components, each including independent phonological and orthographic subcomponents. In word processing, an auditorily or visually presented string activates an entry in the corresponding input lexicon, which in turn activates a conceptual representation in the semantic system. A semantic representation can be thought of as a set of functional, perceptual and other semantic features, such as [inanimate], [used for X], [has property Y], that uniquely identifies a word. It activates above the threshold corresponding entries in the output lexicons, which in turn guide the production of oral and written responses. In addition to the target word, the semantic representation also activates to a less than optimal degree lexical (output) entries that are conceptually related to the target. Under normal conditions these entries do not reach the

threshold and are not produced. In this model there is no direct link between input and output lexicons. The reasons for omitting this link, and the opposite arguments in favor of a direct, nonsemantic link between input and output lexicons, are discussed by Hillis and Caramazza (1991).

Each component of the semantic-lexical system has a composite internal organization. There is structure in the semantic system, in the form of semantic category and morphosemantic information. There is structure in the lexicon as well. In each lexical subcomponent, entries are organized by morphological structure (root morphemes and suffixes are represented independently) and by grammatical class (both root morphemes and suffixes are mark-$_{root,V}$ -ed$_{infl,V}$ for grammatical$_{Adj}$ class$_N$). High-frequency morphemes are associated with a low threshold of activation, low-frequency morphemes with a high threshold. For reviews of this hypothesis see Caramazza (1988); Caramazza and Miceli (1990).

The architecture of the lexicon sketched in Figure 14 is widely accepted (but see Allport and Funnell (1981) for a theory that rejects the distinction between input and output lexicons). The hypothesis of a single, modality-independent semantic system is more debatable. Input-modality-specific anomias have been considered as support for the alternative hypothesis of multiple, modality-specific, semantic systems – tactile, visual, verbal (Shallice, 1988; McCarthy & Warrington, 1990). In this view, a modality-specific anomia could be explained by damage to the connections between the semantic system corresponding to the affected modality and the verbal semantic system necessary for response production. In the framework of the "single semantic system" hypothesis, input-modality-specific anomias are explained by assuming that stimuli presented in different modalities activate distinct attributes in the unitary semantic system (Caramazza et al., 1990). The reader is referred to the papers quoted in this paragraph for discussions of the "single" vs "multiple" semantic system hypothesis.

The observed heterogeneity of anomia is easily accounted for by the model presented in Figure 14. Anomia is the common end-result of different underlying cognitive deficits, deriving from damage to various components of the semantic-lexical system. The overall pattern of performance in

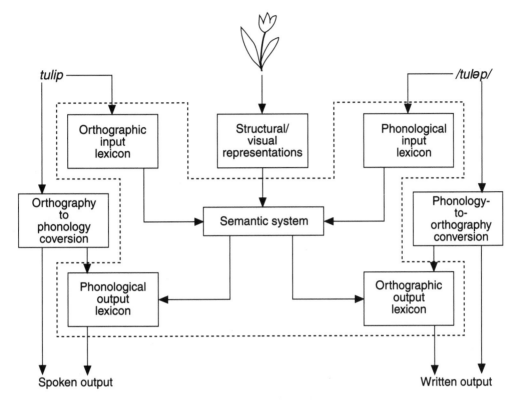

Figure 14 Schematic representation of the mechanisms involved in word processing. (Modified from Hillis & Caramazza, 1991.)

word processing tasks provides information on the locus of damage in each case. For example, anomia resulting from semantic impairment co-occurs with disorders of word comprehension, whereas anomia resulting from damage to an output lexicon affects oral and/or written naming but spares comprehension.

The term anomia, as stated above, applies to omitted responses occurring in object naming as well as in word transcoding. However, anomia occurs much more frequently in object naming than in transcoding tasks. This discrepancy is readily accounted for if the different computational demands posed by the two tasks are made explicit. This requires consideration of the components outside the frame in Figure 14. In *object naming*, abstract structural properties of the stimulus activate the corresponding representation in the semantic system and subsequently in the output lexicon. In *word transcoding*, a phonological or orthographic input string is mapped

onto an output string by lexical *and* sublexical mechanisms, working in parallel.[1] The presented string activates an entry in the input lexicon, which in turn activates a representation in the semantic system and subsequently in the output lexicon. Simultaneously, the string is parsed (by mechanisms "external" to the semantic-lexical system) in sublexical units which are then converted into phonological or orthographic output strings. The correct form for output is selected on the basis of the sum of information from lexical and sublexical conversion mechanisms (Hillis & Caramazza, 1991). There is a critical computational difference between object naming and word transcoding. Good performance in object naming relies entirely on the integrity of the semantic-lexical system, whereas good performance in word transcoding rests on both lexical and sublexical mechanisms. Thus semantic-lexical damage is sufficient to result in incorrect responses in the former but not in the latter. In word transcoding, when the semantic-lexical system is damaged, lexical and sublexical information can still interact and allow (at least in some cases) the activation of the correct but otherwise unavailable lexical form for output. As a consequence, omitted responses (anomias) occur frequently in object naming tasks, and much less often in word transcoding tasks.

The hypothesis schematically represented in Figure 14 is a reasonably satisfactory theoretical framework within which disorders of word processing can be explained. However, it is still too underspecified to account for some experimental data, such as the systematic co-occurrence of anomias with errors of other types (e.g. semantic and/or phonemic substitutions), even in very pure cases (Kay & Ellis, 1985; Miceli et al., 1991). In its present form, the theory cannot explain why, in patients with the same cognitive impairment or even in the very same patient, failure to activate a lexical entry results sometimes in anomia, sometimes in a semantic error, sometimes in a phonemic approximation. One possibility is that the form taken by an error is determined by the type and amount of residual information retained when the correct lexical form is unavailable. When semantic information is normal and phonological information, although incomplete, is sufficient to support oral output, the patient can attempt a response that is likely to result in a phonemic substitution or in a word fragment. A different situation obtains when semantic information is normal and phonological information on the target is either completely unavailable or insufficient to support oral output. In these cases the patient might opt for one of the conceptually related responses activated by semantic information in the output lexicon. Alternatively, he or she might give up all attempts at naming or provide a circumlocutory response. The same options are available when semantic information is incomplete and several words are available for output, but none to an optimal degree. In all these instances, however, why one error type is produced instead of another still remains unexplained.

IMPLICATIONS OF NEURO-PSYCHOLOGICAL DATA FOR DIAGNOSIS AND TREATMENT

Empirical observations reviewed here and the resulting theories indicate that the semantic-lexical system has a rich internal structure, and that impairments of distinct components of this system can result in failure to respond to word and picture stimuli. These conclusions have far-reaching implications for approaches to the study of anomia. Diagnostic procedures must go beyond the labelling of naming errors and the classification of a patient into a clinical category of aphasia. They should clarify, through careful analyses, the cognitive impairment responsible for the deficit in each patient. From a clinical perspective, this approach enables the neuropsychologist to diagnose aphasic disorders more accurately than has been possible so far, and to devise a REHABILITATION program most suitable for each case. From a theoretical perspective, it provides an opportunity to better understand the functioning of the components involved in normal word processing, and to clarify the relationships between these components and the neural substrate.

[1] *Dual-route theories* (such as that sketched here) are upheld by most contemporary researchers. It is hypothesized that separate lexical and sub-lexical processing mechanisms are used to process familiar and novel words respectively. Alternative, *single-route theories* have also been proposed (Glushko, 1979). According to these hypotheses, novel words are read via lexical mechanisms, by analogy to familiar words.

BIBLIOGRAPHY

Allport, D. A., & Funnell, E. (1981). Components of the mental lexicon. *Philosophical Transactions of the Royal Society, 295*, 397–410.

Caramazza, A. (1988). Some aspects of language revealed through the analysis of acquired aphasia: the lexical system. *Annual Review of Neuroscience, 11*, 395–421.

Caramazza, A., & Hillis, A. E. (1991). Lexical organization of nouns and verbs in the brain. *Nature, 349*, 788–90.

Caramazza, A., Hillis, A. E., Rapp, B. C., & Romani, C. (1990). The multiple semantics hypothesis: multiple confusions? *Cognitive Neuropsychology, 7*, 161–90.

Caramazza, A., & Miceli, G. (1990). Structure of the lexicon: functional architecture and lexical representation. In J.-L. Nespoulous & P. Villiard (Eds), *Morphology, phonology, and aphasia* (pp. 1–19). New York: Springer.

Glushko, R. J. (1979). The organization and activation of orthographic knowledge in reading aloud. *Journal of Experimental Psychology: Human Perception and Performance, 5*, 674–91.

Hillis, A. E., & Caramazza, A. (1991). Mechanisms for accessing lexical representations for output: evidence from a category-specific semantic deficit. *Brain and Language, 40*, 106–44.

Howard, D., Patterson, K. E., Franklin, S., Orchard-Lisle, V., & Morton, J. (1985). The facilitation of picture naming in aphasia. *Cognitive Neuropsychology, 2*, 49–80.

Kay, J., & Ellis, A. W. (1985). A cognitive neuropsychological case study of anomia: implications for psychological models of word retrieval. *Brain, 100*, 613–29.

McCarthy, E. A., & Warrington, E. K. (1990). *Clinical neuropsychology: A clinical introduction* (chapters 6–7, pp. 122–70). San Diego: Academic Press.

Miceli, G., Giustolisi, L., & Caramazza, A. (1991). The interaction of lexical and non-lexical processing mechanisms: evidence from anomia. *Cortex, 27*, 57–81.

Miceli, G., Silveri, M. C., Villa, G., & Caramazza, A. (1984). On the basis for the agrammatic's difficulty in producing main verbs. *Cortex, 20*, 207–20.

Shallice, T. (1988). *From neuropsychology to mental structure*. Cambridge: Cambridge University Press.

GABRIELE MICELI

anosmia Anosmia is lack of the ability to smell. In the older medical literature it was sometimes termed *olfactory anesthesia, anosphrasia*, or *parosmis expers*. In some nosological schemes anosmia is classified under the general term *dysosmia* (distorted smell function), which includes other forms of olfactory dysfunction such as distorted smell sensations (*parosmia, cacosmia*) and smell hallucinations (*phantosmia*). More commonly, anosmia and dysosmia are classified separately, with dysosmia referring specifically to strange or distorted smell sensations, rather than to the lack of smell sensations as such. *General* or *total anosmia* implies inability to smell all odorants on both sides of the nose. *Partial anosmia* implies that some, but not all, odorants are able to be sensed. In some cases, decreased ability to detect a wide range of odorants is termed partial anosmia, since such loss exceeds the threshold for only some stimuli. A better term for this phenomenon is *general hyposmia* (hyposmia = lessened smell function). *Specific anosmia* is the inability to smell one or a few odorants in the presence of an otherwise normal sense of smell. For example, nearly a fifth of the male population is unable to smell hydrogen cyanide vapors, yet responds normally to most other odorants. Unfortunately, the term specific anosmia is often a misnomer, as many so-called specific anosmics can detect the stimuli in question at very high concentrations (independent of irritating effects mediated via trigeminal free nerve endings within the nose) or following minimal training. In many cases the underlying population distribution of threshold values for such odorants is bimodal. The use of the term *specific hyposmia* to describe such cases is preferred. Individuals rarely present for medical consultation on the basis of a specific anosmia or hyposmia.

Anosmia significantly alters the quality of life and places individuals at risk to leaking natural gas, fire, and spoiled food. In a recent study of 750 consecutive patients presenting with chemosensory disturbance to a specialized taste and smell center (Deems et al., 1991), 68 percent reported that their dysfunction significantly altered their quality of life. Forty-six percent indicated that the problem changed either their appetite or body weight, and 56 percent noted that it influenced their daily living and/or psychological well-being. Interestingly, over two-thirds of the group believed they suffered from taste loss, either alone or in combination with smell loss, even though objective testing revealed that less than 4 percent evidenced such loss. This reflects the fact that the flavor of food largely depends upon stimulation of the olfactory receptors via the retronasal route. Thus, such flavors as vanilla, chocolate, strawberry, pizza, banana, onion, chicken, and steak disappear when the free flow of air from the nasopharynx to the olfactory epithelium is obstructed by a head cold or by holding the nares shut.

It has long been recognized that the sense of smell can be lost through disease or injury. For example, Theophrastus (Stratton, 1917, p. 85) stated in the third century BC that:

> it is silly to assert that those have the keenest sense of smell who inhale most; for if the organ is not in health or is, for any cause, not unobstructed, more breathing is to no avail. It often happens that a man has suffered injury [to the organ] and has no sensation at all.

77

A number of ancients, including Galen in the second century AD, attributed anosmia to obstruction of the foramina within the cribriform plate. Like Hippocrates and other Greeks before him, he believed that the smell organ was located in the ventricular system of the brain and that odorous particles had to pass through the holes in the cribriform plate of the ethmoid bone during inhalation in order to reach the organ.

Galen's views continued to the time of the Renaissance. For example, Descartes held a view about the nature of olfactory stimulation similar to Galen's and assumed that the "corporeal particles" reached the olfactory bulbs via the cribriform plate. Fifteenth- and sixteenth-century surgeons were aware that blockage of air to the cribriform plate region resulted in decreased ability to smell, as indicated in a statement by Forestus (1591; cited in Lederer, 1959) on anosmia:

> If it [anosmia] is from ethmoidal obstruction, or from the humor discharged from catarrh, the latter must first be cured. If from the flesh growing from within the nose ... it is to be cured by the surgeons by operative procedures, either with a cutting instrument, or cautery, or snare.

Considerable controversy developed in the first few decades of the 1800s as to whether olfactory function is mediated by CN I or CN V, most likely delaying informed discussions about the basis of anosmia for a number of years. Although Sir Charles Bell believed, as did a number of other authorities at that time, that the olfactory receptors were subserved by CN I (as stated in volume III of his 1812 *The Anatomy of the Human Brain*), he erroneously thought that CN I and CN V fibers were united for a portion of their projection, as indicated in his 1811 classic entitled *Idea of a New Anatomy of the Brain*. François Magendie, who was Bell's chief French rival and the major proponent of the theory that CN V mediated olfaction, published his primary arguments in 1824, along with a number of flawed physiological experiments in animals which purportedly demonstrated his point.

Magendie's conclusions received little support from other investigators and studies began to appear which were in accord with Bell's contention that CN I mediated olfactory function. In 1824 Eschricht reported that persons without an olfactory nerve or with degenerate nerves were anosmic. In 1829 Cruveilhier communicated a case to the Anatomical Society of Paris (of which he was President) in which a fungus of the dura mater had destroyed the olfactory but not the trigeminal nerves, along with sectors of the anterior cerebral lobes. In addition, the optic chiasm had been compressed. This individual was both anosmic and blind. Vidal, in 1831, reported to the same society a case of an anosmic blind person who, at autopsy, was shown to have a tumor which had destroyed the optic and olfactory nerves but not the trigeminal ones, and Bishop, in 1833, reported the case of an individual with paralysis of the trigeminal nerve who had the ability to smell. That same year Shaw wrote a scathing critique of Magendie's earlier experiments and pointed out numerous reasons why they were invalid.

Today it is widely recognized that varying degrees of olfactory loss, as well as total anosmia, can result from many different diseases or processes, including tumors and vascular disorders. In the study by Deems and others of 750 consecutive patients presenting with chemosensory dysfunction, upper respiratory infections, head trauma, and chronic nasal and paranasal sinus disease were the most common causes of alterations in the ability to smell (66 percent of 509 cases with verified olfactory dysfunction). Head trauma (22.2 percent of these cases) produced, on average, the greatest degree of loss which, in most cases, was total or near-total anosmia. In addition to idiopathic cases (17 percent), other major causes of verified anosmia or hyposmia included iatrogenic interventions (e.g. brain operations, radiation therapy, nasal operations (6.3 percent)) and toxic chemical exposures (2.4 percent). A small number of the cases (5.7 percent) were of apparent congenital origin.

It is useful heuristically to classify causes of anosmia into those related to obstruction of odorant-carrying air to the olfactory neuroepithelium (e.g. rhinitis, nasal polyposis) and those associated with damage to either the peripheral or central nervous system (CNS) structures (e.g. most forms of head trauma). In some cases, however, the relative contribution of these two classes of causes can be difficult to determine. For example, nasal and paranasal sinus disease can influence both the transport of molecules to the receptors and the functioning of the olfactory neuroepithelium. Some forms of head trauma can influence nasal airflow via changes in nasal obstruction, activation of allergic reactions that cause upper airway inflammation, and displacement of bony and cartilaginous nasal structures, as well as by trauma to the olfactory fila and to CNS structures. Indeed, the relative role of such influences can be dynamic (e.g. trauma- related inflammatory reactions and hematomas typically regress with time). It should be emphasized, however, that most cases of anosmia secondary to head trauma reflect the shearing of the olfactory nerve filaments as they course through the cribriform plate to the olfactory bulbs. Many such cases occur following blows to the back of the head which induce rapid acceleration/ deceleration of the brain relative to the cranium and are often unaccompanied by skull fractures.

Of particular interest to the neuropsychologist is the fact that decreased olfactory function is among the first signs of a number of neuro-degenerative disorders, including Alzheimer's disease (AD) and idiopathic PARKINSON'S DISEASE (PD). However, it is important to stress that considerable variability in the degree of smell dysfunction is present in such cases. Furthermore, since olfactory loss is very common in the normal elderly (over half have near-total anosmia), the use of olfactory testing as an aid to diagnosing AD in older individuals must be viewed with some caution. Nevertheless, such testing is useful to ascertain whether an individual has an olfactory problem so that guidance can be given in regard to safety and nutritional matters; furthermore, such evaluation can be helpful in the early assessment of AD and PD patients under the age of 60 years. In addition, olfactory testing may be of value in the differential diagnosis of some neurodegenerative diseases. For example, many patients with progressive supranuclear PALSY (PSP) are initially misdiagnosed as having PD. While nearly all PD patients evidence decreased olfaction relative to age- and gender-matched controls, very few PSP patients show significant olfactory loss.

Objective testing of olfactory function is necessary to (a) establish the validity of a patient's complaint, (b) characterize the specific nature of the problem, (c) objectively monitor changes in function over time, including those resulting from medical interventions or treatments, (d) detect malingering, and (e) establish compensation for permanent disability. Such measurement has important legal considerations, since anosmia is a common consequence of head injury and is often the only residual impairment from falls and motor vehicle accidents. In Great Britain, disability benefits for anosmia resulting from an injury are available under the National Insurance Acts, as discussed in detail by Douek (1974). In the United States, the *Guides to the Evaluation of Permanent Impairment* published by the American Medical Association in 1984 provide an authoritative basis for disability compensation by insurance companies, agencies of the federal government such as the Bureau of Employees Compensation of the Department of Labor for federal employees injured at work, the Social Security Administration, various state workmen's compensation agencies, and the courts. However, this document equates total anosmia with a 3 percent impairment of the whole person, a figure which is greatly exceeded in most legal settlements. Many, including the present author, view even these as insufficient.

Several tests are commonly used today to diagnose anosmia, including detection threshold tests and tests of odor identification. The most widely used clinical test is the University of Pennsylvania Smell Identification Test (UPSIT; commercially termed the Smell Identification Test™, Sensonics, Inc., Haddon Heights, NJ), which consists of four booklets containing 10 odorants apiece, one odorant per page. The stimuli are embedded in 10–50 μm diameter microencapsulated crystals located on brown strips near the bottom of each page. Above each "scratch and sniff" strip is a multiple-choice question with four response alternatives for each item. For example, one of the items reads, "This odor smells most like: (a) banana, (b) garlic, (c) cherry, or (d) motor oil," and the patient is required to choose an answer, even if none seem appropriate or no odor is perceived (i.e. the test is forced-choice). This helps to encourage the patient to carefully sample each stimulus and provides a means for detecting malingering (since chance performance is 10 out of 40, very low scores would require avoidance and hence recognition of the correct answer). Norms are provided and an individual's percentile rank established relative to a large normal group of individuals of the same age and gender. The reliability of such testing is high (test-retest Pearson $rs > 0.90$).

Treatment of patients whose anosmia is due to blockage of the airways (e.g. from allergic rhinitis, bacterial rhinitis, sinusitis, polyposis, neoplasms, and structural abnormalities in the nasal cavities) can be undertaken rationally and with optimism. Examples of treatments that have restored such function include allergic management, topical and systemic corticosteroid therapies, antibiotic therapy, and various surgical interventions. Treatment of patients with anosmia due to sensorineural problems is problematic. Although there are advocates of zinc and vitamin therapies, sound empirical evidence of their efficacy is lacking.

In summary, anosmia and other alterations in the ability to smell can be very debilitating to individuals who experience them. Recent advances in psychophysical assessment and in medical imaging (including the development of fiber-optic endoscopes through which the region near the cribriform plate can be visualized) bode well for the future treatment of a number of patients with these disorders. However, in cases which cannot be medically or surgically corrected at present, psychological benefit can be provided by adequately addressing the problem and ruling out serious causes for it, such as malignant tumors. Many patients gain psychological relief by simply being told that altered olfactory function is not an uncommon phenomenon, since they have found no medical practitioners who are knowledgeable about the problem. Nearly half of elderly patients can be consoled by informing them that, despite having decreased smell function, they are doing better than most of their peers since, by definition, half will fall above the fiftieth percentile for their age and gender-matched peers on quantitative olfactory tests.

BIBLIOGRAPHY

Deems, D. A., Doty, R. L., Settle, R. G., Moore-Gillon, V., Shaman, P., Mester, A. F., Kimmelman, C. P., Brightman, V. J., & Snow, J. B. Jr. (1991). Smell and taste disorders: a study of 750 patients from the University of Pennsylvania Smell and Taste Center. *Archives of Otolaryngology – Head and Neck Surgery*, *117*, 519–28.

Doty, R. L. (1991a). Olfactory dysfunction in neurodegenerative disorders. In T. V. Getchell, R. L. Doty, L. M. Bartoshuk & J. B. Snow, Jr. (Eds), *Smell and taste in health and disease* (pp. 735–51). New York: Raven.

Doty, R. L. (1991b). Olfactory system. In T. V. Getchell, R. L. Doty, L. M. Bartoshuk & J. B. Snow, Jr. (Eds), *Smell and taste in health and disease* (pp. 175–203). New York: Raven.

Doty, R. L. (Ed.) (1995). *Handbook of olfaction and gustation*. New York: Marcel Dekker.

Douek, E. (1974). *The sense of smell and its abnormalities*. Edinburgh: Livingstone.

Guides to the Evaluation of Permanent Impairment (1984). 2nd edn. Chicago: American Medical Association.

Lederer F. L. (1959). The problem of nasal polyps. *Journal of Allergy*, *30*, 420–32.

Magendie, F. (1824). Le nerf olfactif est-il l'organe de l'odorat? Expériences sur cette question. *Magendies Journal de Physiologie Expérimentale et Pathologique*, *4*, 169–76.

Shaw, A. (1833). *Narrative of the discoveries of Sir Charles Bell in the nervous system*. London: Longman, Orme, Brown, Green & Longmans.

Smith, D. V. (1990). Taste and smell dysfunction. In M. M. Paparella, D. A. Shumrick, J. L. Gluckman & W. L. Meyerhoff (Eds), *Otolaryngology*. Vol. III. *Head and neck*. 3rd edn (pp. 1911–34). Philadelphia: W. B. Saunders.

Stratton, G. M. (1917). *Theophrastus and the Greek physiological psychology before Aristotle*. London: George Allen & Unwin.

Wright, J. (1914). *A history of laryngology and rhinology*. Philadelphia: Lea & Febiger.

RICHARD L. DOTY

anosodiaphoria The patient with anosodiaphoria will admit to a motor or sensory impairment (usually hemiparesis or hemianopia), but be entirely unconcerned about it. The condition is considered to be allied to ANOSOGNOSIA in which the patient denies or is apparently unaware of the impairment, and both are commonly considered aspects of neglect. Anosodiaphoria may follow a period of explicit denial of illness in the process of recovery from neglect, and may persist for a protracted period.

anosognosia, anosagnosia Anosognosia refers

to the clinical phenomenon in which a brain dysfunctional patient does not appear to be aware of impaired neurological and/or neuropsychological functioning which is obvious to the clinician and other reasonably attentive individuals. The lack of awareness appears specific to individual deficits and cannot be accounted for by hypoarousal or widespread cognitive impairments.

HISTORICAL CONSIDERATIONS

The phenomenon of anosognosia has been recognized since antiquity. Citing a letter written approximately two thousand years before von Monakow's (1885) report of a patient who was not aware of loss of sight secondary to brain damage, Bisiach and Geminiani (1991) (cited in Prigatano & Schacter, 1991) provide the following excerpt which was taken from the correspondence of Seneca:

> You know that Harpastes, my wife's fatuous companion, has remained in my home as an inherited burden ... This foolish woman has suddenly lost her sight. Incredible as it might appear, what I am going to tell you is true: She does not know she is blind. Therefore, again and again she asks her guardian to take her elsewhere. She claims that my home is dark. (Bisiach & Geminiani, 1991, p. 17)

It was, however, the later observations of von Monakow (1885), Anton (1889), Babinski (1914), and Pick (1908) that brought the phenomenon to the attention of neurological clinicians (cited in Prigatano & Schacter, 1991). Babinski is credited with coining the term "anosognosia," while Pick is recognized as describing the startling case of anosognosia for hemiplegia.

Referring to Babinski's (1914) early definition, Weinstein and Friedland (1977) point out that *anosognosia* refers to a "literal lack of knowledge of disease." A central question regarding the phenomenon of anosognosia is whether or not this "lack of knowledge" is caused by neurological or psychological factors or both. Those who consider this phenomenon primarily neurological in nature tend to use such terms as "lack of awareness" or "unawareness" following brain damage (see Prigatano & Schacter, 1991). Those who consider the phenomenon to be heavily influenced or caused by psychological variables tend to use such terms as "denial of illness"

(Weinstein & Kahn, 1955) or "defensive denial" (see Prigatano & Schacter, 1991).

ANOSOGNOSIA VERSUS DENIAL OF ILLNESS

Since consciousness appears to be an emergent brain function, it would appear that disorders of brain function will influence consciousness (and self-consciousness or awareness) in predictable but undoubtedly complex ways. The work of Bisiach and colleagues (see Prigatano & Schacter, 1991) has demonstrated that patients may not only show anosognosia for hemiplegia or hemianopia, but their impaired awareness may be specific to one type of disturbance versus the other. Moreover, patients can demonstrate frank aphasia and be unaware of their language impairments (see Prigatano & Schacter, 1991).

While these classical neurological disorders have been the focus of studies on anosognosia, more recent investigators have reported impaired awareness in amnestic patients, as well as in patients with traumatic brain injury and various dementias (Prigatano & Schacter, 1991).

The early work of Weinstein and Kahn (1955) raised serious questions concerning the etiology of these disturbances. They argued that anosognosia is not determined purely by neurological variables. They persuasively point out that the apparent loss of insight into a brain-related disability may be related to the patient's premorbid personality characteristics and how they viewed their disability. They made the following astute observations:

> Our findings indicate that the various forms of anosognosia are not discrete entities that can be localized in different areas of the brain. Whether a lesion involves the frontal or parietal lobe determines the disability that may be denied, not the mechanism of denial. Thus the patterns of anosognosia for hemiplegia and blindness do not differ from those in which the fact of an operation or the state of being ill is denied. Under the requisite conditions of brain function the patient may deny the paralysis of an arm whether it results from a fracture, an injury to the brachial plexus, a brain stem or cortical lesion. The effect of the brain damage is to provide the milieu of altered function in which the patient may deny *anything* that he feels is wrong with him. Some motivation to deny illness and incapacity exists in everyone and the level of brain function determines the particular perceptual-symbolic organization, or

language, in which it is expressed. (Weinstein & Kahn, 1955, p. 123)

Weinstein (1991) has recently summarized his view of why he prefers the term "denial of illness" to that of anosognosia (see Prigatano & Schacter, 1991), yet a number of investigators believe that the phenomenon of anosognosia is an important neurological disturbance.

EXAMPLES OF THE CLINICAL PHENOMENON

Frank anosognosia and less obvious, but equally important, disorders of awareness can be readily observed in a variety of brain dysfunctional patients (McGlynn & Schacter, 1989). By far the most startling example of this phenomenon is to be seen in a patient who not only "denies" that he or she has a hemiplegic limb, but often states that the affected limb belongs to someone else (Weinstein & Kahn, 1955). While this type of disorder is almost always seen immediately after the onset of a neurological insult and progressively improves with time, there may well be "residuals" of this awareness disturbance. Just as acutely aphasic patients can improve with time, they will often show upon closer examination difficulties in such areas as naming and understanding a complex semantic. The same is true for patients who have experienced impairment in their awareness surrounding specific disabilities.

For example, traumatic brain-injured patients who are disoriented may believe that they are actually able to leave the hospital and return to work within a few days. Examination of these patients reveals not only disorientation but frank memory impairments and difficulties in abstract reasoning. Often, however, the patient does not recognize their impaired higher cerebral functioning or even the need to be in the hospital. The drawing depicted in Figure 15 illustrates this phenomenon in a traumatically brain-injured young woman 9 months postinjury. She states that "part of her head is missing" yet she is a normal person. She also wonders if she will ever "retrieve it." This paradoxical statement seems to reflect the phenomenological experience of patients suffering disorders of awareness, that is, at the very same time they both feel normal and yet sense that something has gone wrong.

There are other manifestations of this problem, as seen in patients with both focal and

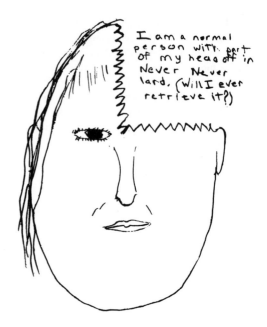

Figure 15 TBI patient drawing.

diffuse brain injury. Patients who have tumors in the frontal area of the brain often show reasonably good awareness over basic self-care activities, but may have very poor insight into how their behavior affects others in an interpersonal or social manner. In contrast, patients who have lesions involving the parietal lobe may have reasonably good insight as to their ability to socially interact with others, but lack insight into such things as their capacity to adequately dress themselves or to carry out a variety of visuospatial problem-solving tasks. These findings suggest that the awareness deficit can be quite specific and may well reveal something about the highest integration of brain function and dysfunction.

Patients with diffuse and dementing conditions also show a curious pattern of impaired awareness. In the early onset of dementia of the Alzheimer's type, it is not uncommon for the patient to be aware of subtle problems in memory, naming, and other related higher cerebral functions. As the disease progresses, however, patients often lose insight into their impairment even though those around them are painfully aware of the declining mental functions.

These clinical examples highlight the fact that disorders of awareness may indeed be more prevalent than has been previously recognized and are worthy of considerable clinical and research efforts (McGlynn & Schacter, 1989).

BRAIN LESIONS AND MECHANISMS ASSOCIATED WITH ANOSOGNOSIA

Multiple brain lesion sites can be identified in anosognostic patients. Inferior parietal cortex and frontal lobe lesions are frequently identified in cases of anosognosia for hemiplegia. Not uncommonly, the right hemisphere is implicated. Lesions involving limbic/occipital and temporal cortical connections are also reported in cases of anosognosia for cortical blindness. It has been suggested that prefrontal (and typically bilateral) lesions are common when patients lack insight into their socially inappropriate behavior.

It appears that conscious awareness is somehow distributed throughout the brain and that lesions in specific sites can lead to rather focal awareness disturbances. Various models have been proposed to explain anosognostic behavior. Some borrow heavily from the field of hemi-inattention which focuses on disturbances in perceptual systems. Disturbances in beliefs or cognitions about the self, as well as disturbances in body image, have also been suggested. Disturbances in information processing, including feedback, feedforward, and monitoring mechanisms have all been considered. There are also models which emphasize the importance of the integrative mechanisms which connect feelings with cognitions for the phenomenon of anosognostic behavior.

At this time, there is no universally agreed mechanism that accounts for anosognosia.

THEORETICAL AND DIAGNOSTIC ISSUES

From a neurological perspective, Anton raised the important point that anosognosia could exist in the presence of focal brain injury. In cases of diffuse injury, one might argue that the patient's intellectual abilities would be so compromised that a lack of insight or self-awareness would simply be an epiphenomenon of broader cognitive impairments. The fact that patients with focal brain lesions and apparent preservation of broad cognitive functioning could demonstrate unawareness of a disability suggested that the phenomenon of anosognosia is a unique one.

An important theoretical issue concerning anosognosia is whether or not the apparent unawareness is complete, that is, do patients who show anosognosia for say hemiplegia have any knowledge of their disability? Weinstein and Kahn (1955) made a distinction between "explicit verbal denial" and other more subtle forms of impaired awareness. Schacter (see Prigatano & Schacter, 1991) has recently emphasized the importance of this issue and the need to consider in future investigations how different forms and levels of altered awareness can exist following brain injury.

A second theoretical issue regarding anosognosia centers around its "time frame," that is, the phenomenon of frank anosognosia seems to exist primarily in the early or acute stages following brain injury. Generally with time there is improvement of this condition. The issue of why this is the case has not been adequately addressed.

A third and important issue from a neurological perspective is the repeated observation that anosognostic phenomena seem to be more prevalent in patients with right hemisphere damage and/or bilateral cerebral dysfunction (Weinstein & Kahn, 1955). This finding clearly underscores the importance of brain mechanisms in the etiology of impaired awareness.

From a diagnostic point of view, one is repeatedly faced with the question of establishing criteria for separating what McGlynn and Schacter (1989) referred to as "defensive denial" versus "organic" unawareness of disability. The fact that there have been no clear guidelines for doing this suggests that it may be very difficult, but not impossible, to separate these two phenomena. Clinically, one often sees differences in patients which suggest that the lack of awareness may be psychologically motivated versus directly caused by a brain insult. In the former case there is often "resistance" from the patient to obtaining insight into their difficulties. When the therapist attempts to point out to the patient how his or her behavior has changed, an active reaction on the part of the patient can be seen which discourages further communication or dialogue about the disability. In contrast, in those patients who suffer neurologically mediated impairments of awareness, particularly affecting the frontal lobes, there is often a perplexed or innocent reaction regarding what has happened to them. As they are given information in a structured and systematic way, they often appear surprised and receptive to the new information that has been obtained.

It should be emphasized that this is something that is seen clinically, but at present there have been no empirical studies investigating how one would separate defensive denial from anosognosia or organic unawareness. Further research is badly needed in this area.

METHODOLOGICAL AND DEFINITIONAL ISSUES

A major problem for studying anosognosia and/or denial of illness is the development of a clear definition of the phenomenon and appropriate methodology for investigating it. Prigatano and Schacter (1991) attempted to provide a definition of self-awareness and emphasized the importance of making a distinction between knowledge of something versus knowledge with something. Knowledge of something often refers to purely logical or perceptual phenomena. Knowledge with something often implies an element of consciousness and feeling. They state that it is exceedingly difficult, if not impossible, to provide "a clear, concise, universally acceptable definition of consciousness or awareness" (p. 13). However, they do provide the following definition:

> Self-awareness is the capacity to perceive the "self" in relatively "objective" terms while maintaining a sense of subjectivity. It is a natural paradox of human consciousness. On the one hand, it strives for "objectivity," that is, perceiving a situation, object, or interaction in a manner similar to others' perceptions while at that same time maintaining the sense of a private, subjective or unique interpretation of the experience. This latter aspect of consciousness implies a feeling state as well as a thought process. Self-awareness or awareness of higher cerebral functions thus involves an interaction of "thoughts" and "feelings." (p. 13)

Prigatano and Schacter (1991) agree with others that self-awareness appears to reflect the highest of all integrated brain functions. They argue that damage to the brain may cause specific forms of this type of dysfunction.

Prigatano (see Prigatano & Schacter, 1991) has discussed some of the methodological issues involved in researching disorders of self-awareness after brain injury. The first methodological step is to demonstrate that brain dysfunctional patients can in fact make reliable judgments or ratings about themselves. Next, studies are needed to show that different types of brain pathology may affect different types of self-reports (including ratings about the self). Third, it is important to demonstrate that patients' perceptions of themselves are uniquely affected in contrast to their perceptions of others, that is, the phenomenon of anosognosia rests on the clear demonstration that patients can be relatively objective in their perception of others, but not objective in their perception of their own specific disabilities or impairments.

To date, research has been limited primarily to reports by clinicians, verbal accounts of patients which include explicit denial of their disability, and judgments based on rating scales provided by the patients and their families.

A few studies have also focused on how cultural variables and premorbid factors may in fact affect self-reports of disability. Cultural factors have been shown to influence the degree to which "denial" is demonstrated. However, different types of impaired perceptions have also been related to lesion sites. These observations demonstrate the complexity of the anosognosia or denial of illness phenomenon and the multiple factors which appear to influence it. Further research is needed not only to understand the underlying brain mechanisms responsible for anosognosia, but also to determine what psychological and cultural variables influence the form by which this lack of insight into the self is revealed.

BIBLIOGRAPHY

McGlynn, S. M., & Schacter, D. L. (1989). Unawareness of deficits in neuropsychological syndromes. *Journal of Clinical Experimental Neuropsychology, 11*, 143–205.

Prigatano, G. P., & Schacter, D. L. (1991). *Awareness of deficit after brain injury: Clinical and theoretical issues*. New York: Oxford University Press.

Weinstein, E. A., & Friedland, R. P. (1977). *Advances in neurology*: Vol. 18. *Hemi-inattention and hemisphere specialization*. New York: Raven Press.

Weinstein, E. A., & Kahn, R. L. (1955). *Denial of illness: Symbolic and physiological aspects*. Springfield, IL: Charles C. Thomas.

GEORGE P. PRIGATANO

anoxia   The loss of oxygen in the blood carried to the brain (anoxia or its partial reduction in *hypoxia*) has rapid and serious consequences in the death of brain tissue. There are a variety of potential causes which include suffocation (mechanical, or by breathing gases other than oxygen or air), strangulation, partial drowning, exposure at high altitudes, or late resuscitation from myocardial infarction or cardiac arrest. These causes are commonly classified into four types: anoxic, anemic, stagnant and metabolic anoxia, although the type is not critical for the pathology or the neuropsychological sequelae except in that it may be associated with the period and degree of the oxygen starvation, or with the presence of other toxins or disease processes which may also have a pathological effect upon the brain (for example, in carbon monoxide poisoning or in hypoglycemia).

The human brain appears to be extremely sensitive to a reduction in the supply of oxygen by contrast with experimental studies in monkeys, where significant periods of oxygen starvation may be tolerated without significant cerebral pathology resulting. This may simply reflect the differential sensitivity of the tests which may be employed to assess the consequences of anoxia in humans and in monkeys.

Many forms of anoxia are transient events associated with impaired consciousness to a variable degree, from which there may be a full recovery with only a period of amnesia remaining. However, with prolonged hypoxia mental deterioration gradually develops and may be accompanied by personality changes. With more serious anoxic episodes, which are more likely to be survived with improved techniques of resuscitation and emergency care, a variety of neurological deficits may be apparent, accompanied by impaired memory, dementia, and even extending to prolonged coma or VEGETATIVE STATE, from which there may or may not be a partial recovery.

Anoxia appears to produce widespread degeneration and death of nerve cells throughout most of the layers of the cerebral cortex, together with cells in the cerebellum and in the STRIATUM. The GLOBUS PALLIDUS may also be bilaterally involved together with the hippocampus and surrounding areas, which may be followed by regions of subcortical demyelination which develop with increasing survival. However, when the onset of anoxia is sudden, as in cardiac arrest or myocardial infarction, "boundary zone lesions"

occur at the boundaries of the territories of the cerebral arteries, similar to the pattern seen with cerebral ISCHEMIA. The effects are greatest in the parieto-occipital regions, and the general pathology observed with other forms of anoxia is less likely to occur, although there may be severe lesions in the BASAL GANGLIA.

Carbon monoxide poisoning represents a special case, common in attempted suicide in the UK before the change to North Sea gas, but also associated with accidents involving gas heaters and vehicle exhaust fumes. If the patient survives and emerges from the resulting coma, there is likely to be a range of neuropsychological sequelae. Behaviorally there is apathy and poor initiation, and thought and speech are slow. Memory difficulties are common and a classic KORSAKOFF'S PSYCHOSIS may develop together with agnosia and constructional apraxia. Gross mental impairments may persist in a context of various neurological impairments, which may include extrapyramidal motor signs. The pathology is also distinct from other forms of anoxia, with focal areas of degeneration in the cortex, and the death of nerve cells in the globus pallidus and in Ammon's horn, a structure of the anterior temporal lobe.

J. GRAHAM BEAUMONT

anterior cerebral artery The anterior cerebral arteries, one for each cortical hemisphere, arise from the portion of the Circle of Willis known as the anterior communicating artery and project forwards under the inferior surface of the frontal lobes. Each anterior cerebral artery supplies the anterior four-fifths of the medial cortical surface of its hemisphere, extending anteriorly and superiorly around to the margins of the lateral surface of the frontal and parietal lobes.

anterior commissure The anterior commissure is one of the smaller cerebral commissures, bundles of fibers which interconnect homotopic points on the CORTEX. In humans, the CORPUS CALLOSUM is the principal commissure and interconnects most areas of the two cerebral cortices; however, substantial anterior parts of the two TEMPORAL LOBES are interconnected via the anterior commissure. It is located at the midline between the posterior end of the rostrum of the corpus callosum and the columns of the FORNIX. In the COMMISSUROTOMY operation the anterior commissure may or may not be sectioned, depending on the particular procedure adopted.

anterograde amnesia   *See* AMNESIA; AMNESIC SYNDROME.

Anton's syndrome   In Anton's syndrome, although the patient is totally blind following bilateral lesions of the visual cortex (see CORTICAL BLINDNESS), the patient denies being unable to see. Anton's syndrome is therefore the parallel of ANOSOGNOSIA in the visual modality, and presumably results from destruction of visual association areas so that the patient has no experience of being unable to see.

aphasia   Aphasia refers to a range of impairments in the use of language that are caused by injury or damaged function in the perisylvian region of the left cerebral hemisphere (Figure 16). Aphasia affects "higher language functions" in the sense that it cannot be accounted for by paralysis, weakness, or incoordination of the motor systems involved in production, by impairments of the sensory systems involved in receptive processing, nor by impairments of arousal, attention, or motivation.

The spectrum of aphasic disorders touches on virtually every aspect of linguistic knowledge or skill: the organization of articulatory movements, the comprehension of meaning at the word and sentence level, retrieval of words and grammatical forms for oral production and writing. While there are comparatively rare instances of "pure" forms of aphasia that affect a single input or output modality, the vast majority of cases involve a pattern of impairments touching on many different functions to varying degrees. A number of well-recognized patterns have been observed to occur regularly, in association with lesions at particular sites in the language zone. These have been assigned the status of named "syndromes of

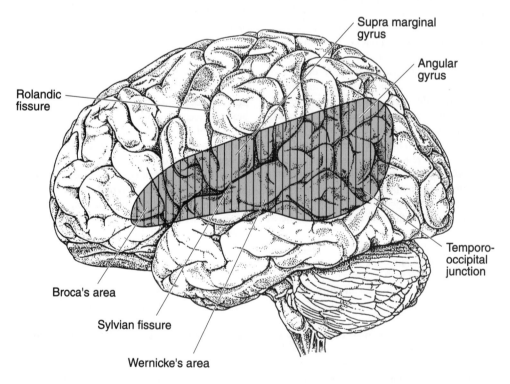

Figure 16 The perisylvian language zone, with major surface landmarks.

aphasia" and they are summarized in the final section of this entry.

SCIENTIFIC SIGNIFICANCE

Historically, it was through the investigation of the anatomical correlates of aphasia that the first insights were obtained into the organization of the brain for the mediation of language and related cognitive skills. For example, the phenomenon of cerebral LATERALIZATION was discovered through the observation that loss of language followed injury to the left hemisphere but only rarely injury to the right hemisphere. Accumulating information from post-mortem studies and, more recently, from in vivo neuroimaging has permitted progressively more accurate correlations between specific language deficits and lesions of particular brain structures that account for these deficits. In turn, inferences have been possible concerning the anatomical organization in the normal brain. It is fair to say that up to the mid-1980s, virtually all our understanding of brain organization for language had been based on the study of patients with various forms of aphasic deficit. In this regard, language differs from sensory and motor functions, where lesion studies and electrophysiological studies of animal models have been possible. While new techniques such as positron emission tomography (PET SCAN) and cortical stimulation are now being introduced for studies of brain function during the processing of normal language, the information gained through these techniques must still be interpreted in the light of observations from aphasic patients.

HISTORICAL REVIEW

There can be no doubt that aphasia, in its many guises, has been an affliction of humankind as long as speech has existed. Yet nowhere in the scattered reports prior to the Renaissance is there a sign that any observer conceived of loss of language as distinct from loss of voice or paralysis of the tongue. By the seventeenth century, case reports began to show considerable sensitivity to selective impairments in some language skills, but not others. Over the next century there was also an implicit recognition that these impairments could not be attributed to a generalized memory disorder or to paralysis of the tongue.

The modern history of aphasia is commonly regarded as beginning with Broca's (1861) anatomically supported report that aphasia was the result of a lesion destroying the foot of the third frontal convolution. Broca's observations continued, and by 1865 he was able to report that almost all of his cases involved the left hemisphere. The few exceptions to this rule were left-handers. With this report, Broca established the classical doctrine of cerebral dominance, essentially in the form that held sway until the mid-1950s. This doctrine held that there is a dominant hemisphere and a minor hemisphere. The dominant hemisphere is contralateral to the preferred hand and controls language as well.

Broca was careful to emphasize that the disorder he was describing involved the loss of articulate speech. He recognized that there was another form of language disorder that he referred to as *amnésie verbale*, but he did not offer a localization for it. It remained for Wernicke (1874) to describe the clinical picture of sensory aphasia and its anatomic basis. Wernicke's aphasia consisted of a severe impairment of auditory language comprehension, normal articulatory facility, and the production of erroneously chosen words and erroneously combined speech sounds. This syndrome resulted from destruction of the superior temporal gyrus, a region which Wernicke argued held the sound images of words that had been acquired during life.

Wernicke went on to propose an anatomical schema for spoken language that depended on two principal centers and the connection between them. Broca's area was the store for images of the motor articulatory form of words, and was the source of the innervation for the production of speech. The superior temporal convolution contained the store for auditory images of words that had been learned.

Building on Wernicke's anatomic associationism, Lichtheim proposed a slightly more elaborate model to account for seven possible aphasic syndromes. The Wernicke–Lichtheim schema (Figure 17) remains important because it provides a theoretical underpinning for the classical syndromes that are currently widely recognized. In Figure 17 M represents the center for motor articulatory images (corresponding to Broca's area), A represents the center for auditory word images (corresponding to Wernicke's area), and C represents the conceptual center. Unlike the first two centers (M and A) the conceptual center is not localized in a particular lobe or structure,

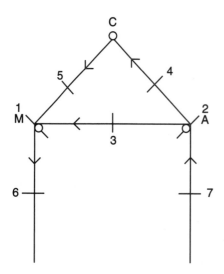

Figure 17 The Wernicke–Lichtheim schema.

but represents the stored memories of concepts that are widely distributed in the brain. The lines leading into and out of this system and connecting the centers to each other represent presumed fiber pathways providing input and output and communication between the centers. The seven numbers represent possible lesion sites that affect either a center or a particular connecting pathway. A unique pattern of deficits and spared abilities can be deduced from each lesion site, as indicated in Table 5. The labelled syndrome corresponding to each of these patterns is given in parentheses. These syndromes will be more fully described in a later section.

The Wernicke–Lichtheim schema was followed by a number of others, among them those of Charcot and Grasset. It was characteristic of all of these conceptions that they dealt only in terms of modalities of sensory input and of motor output, and the connections between them. Thus there is no provision in these schemata for anomic aphasia – a pure disorder of word retrieval.

The anatomical basis for disorders of written language was first demonstrated by Déjerine (1891, 1892), who described the syndromes of "alexia without agraphia," resulting from a specifically placed lesion of the occipital lobe, and "alexia with agraphia," resulting from a lesion of the left angular gyrus.

THE NOËTIC VIEWPOINT

Alongside the developing anatomic associationistic school, there developed a contrasting viewpoint on aphasia, one that played down the emphasis on localization of functions and emphasized instead the psychological components of the disorder. The earliest of the noëtic (or mentalistic) theorists was John Hughlings Jackson, whose papers on aphasia spanned the years 1863 to 1893. Jackson pointed out that the aphasic patient has not lost words, but rather the ability to use words to "propositionize," i.e. to convey information. As an example he could cite the commonly observed fact that aphasic patients could often use words in memorized sequences (e.g. reciting verses or prayers) or in swearing that they could not produce in voluntary communication. He regarded emotionally triggered interjections and memorized utterances as a more primitive form of language than propositional speech. He attributed the preservation of these verbalizations in aphasia to their mediation by the right cerebral hemisphere, whose limited language capacity was confined to such primitive uses of language. Jackson's distinction between automatic and propositional speech has become a basic principle in the assessment and interpretation of the behavior of aphasic patients.

A contemporary of Jackson's was Finkelnburg, who introduced the term "asymbolia" as an account of the basic disorder of aphasia. A virtually identical stance appears in the writing of Henry Head (1926), who began his two-volume work on aphasia with a diatribe against the "diagram makers" – the members of the anatomic-association school. Head defined aphasia as "a disorder of symbolic fomulation and expression" and gave examples of how this impairment was not limited to the use of language. He also introduced a typology of aphasia that eschewed reference to sensory or motor modalities which would have localizing implications. Instead he used psychological and linguistic categories: nominal aphasia, verbal aphasia, semantic aphasia, and syntactic aphasia.

Kurt Goldstein is usually associated with the noëtic approach to aphasia because of his insistence that much of the symptomatology of aphasia is a consequence of a loss of the "ABSTRACT ATTITUDE." For Goldstein, the ability to name objects implied an appreciation that the name may *stand for* the object without actually

Table 5   Aphasia: lesions and deficits.

Lesion number	Function impaired	Resulting pattern of deficits
1	Destruction of store of motor articulatory memories.	Loss of capacity to form speech sounds. Loss of ability to repeat, secondary to preceding. Normal auditory language comprehension. (Broca's aphasia.)
2	Destruction of store of auditory word images.	Loss of capacity to understand spoken language. Loss of ability to recall word sounds. Loss of the ability to recognize and correct speech errors. Loss of ability to repeat, secondary to the basic defect. (Wernicke's aphasia.)
3	Destruction of pathway between auditory and motor articulatory language centers.	Loss of ability to repeat, due to absence of a route from the auditory comprehension center to the output mechanism. Preserved auditory comprehension and articulatory facility. Preserved ability to recognize one's speech errors. (Conduction aphasia.)
4	Destruction of connections from the center for auditory comprehension and auditory word images to the knowledge stored in the rest of the brain.	Preserved perception of spoken language and perfectly preserved repetition, but without appreciation of the meaning of what has been heard. (Transcortical sensory aphasia.)
5	Destruction of connections between the center for motor articulatory images and the conceptual activity of the brain.	Inability to initiate any spoken message, in spite of preserved articulatory facility and perfectly preserved ability to repeat. Preserved auditory comprehension. (Transcortical motor aphasia.)
6	Destruction of fibers carrying outflow from the motor articulatory center to the primary motor area controlling the articulators.	Severe difficulty in forming articulatory movements, with perfectly preserved formulation of language, normal auditory comprehension, reading and writing. (Subcortical motor aphasia; also aphemia.)
7	Destruction of fibers carrying acoustic information from the primary auditory center to the center for auditory word images.	Loss of ability to understand spoken words in spite of normal hearing. Normal speech, reading, and writing. (Pure word deafness.)

being the object. The loss of this ability might result in a form of naming disorder that he termed "amnesic aphasia." Loss of the abstract attitude could also result in failure to understand the use of grammatical function words. Goldstein's "abstract attitude" had much in common with Head's "loss of symbolic formulation and expression." However, Goldstein treated this deficiency as *interacting* with aphasic impairments and he did not propose to reduce aphasia to a loss of symbol use. Aphasia primarily affected the "instrumentalities" of language – articulation, auditory comprehension, and word retrieval – and Goldstein devoted many articles, spanning the first half of the twentieth century, to the clinical manifestations of aphasia and their anatomical concomitants. Much of his lifetime's thoughts on aphasia are summed up in his book *Language and Language Disturbances* (1948).

THE REVIVAL OF ANATOMICALLY BASED APHASIA SYNDROMES: LURIA AND GESCHWIND

The Second World War brought about an intense effort to deal with the problem of the many brain-injured soldiers with language disorders. In Soviet Russia, Alexander Luria was the head of such a rehabilitation center in Moscow. His *Traumatic Aphasia*, published in Russian in 1947 and in English in 1970, was an influential statement that took into account western European "mainstream" accounts of aphasia while presenting his own distinctive viewpoint.

Luria's taxonomy of aphasia was surprisingly parallel to the contemporary version of the classical syndromes, considering that his clinical material came from wartime head injuries that were not limited to the sites of predilection for peacetime vascular lesions. Luria proposed two subtypes of motor aphasia: "afferent motor aphasia" and "efferent motor aphasia." It is the efferent type that corresponds most closely to Broca's aphasia, both in lesion site and in the prominence of articulatory breakdown as its defining symptom. Afferent motor aphasia has some features in common with the classical "conduction aphasia," although Luria did not include repetition difficulty as a primary feature. Luria's "temporal acoustic aphasia" is most similar in its symptomatology and its lesion site to Wernicke's aphasia. "Acoustic mnestic aphasia" shares features of both anomic aphasia and the classical transcortical sensory aphasia.

There is an extremely close match between Luria's "frontal dynamic aphasia" and transcortical motor aphasia. The primary feature of dynamic aphasia is the patient's inability to initiate speech or to find a way to organize his thoughts into a coherent utterance. Repetition is preserved, but for Luria this preservation is not a central feature of the syndrome.

In the United States the neurologist Norman Geschwind championed the revival of interest in the anatomic basis of aphasia, departing little from the principles laid down by Wernicke. Geschwind's special contribution was to bring to bear contemporary advances in neuroanatomy, along with well-described clinical cases, to show how the classical model could be reconciled with actual pathology. Geschwind revived interest in the understanding of the role of the CORPUS CALLOSUM as a link between the hemispheres –

particularly in providing a pathway for sensory input to the right hemisphere to gain access to the language system on the left and for language processes of the left hemisphere to gain a motor output channel to the left hand for writing and for carrying out commands given orally. In a classical paper (Geschwind, 1965) he developed the anatomical basis for interpreting both aphasia and apraxia in terms of disconnections between primary sensory and motor zones and their corresponding language association areas, and between the association areas themselves. Geschwind's writing and teaching had a great influence in promoting the detailed study of the relationship between language symptomatology in aphasia and the cerebral structures that are damaged.

THE RISE OF COGNITIVE NEURO-LINGUISTICS

While anatomical models were well suited for dealing with the contrast between impaired speech output and impaired language comprehension, there were well-recognized phenomena that lacked such a transparent relation to anatomical input or output channels. One of these was AGRAMMATISM – a pattern of speech production in which the patient seems to have lost access to the use of grammatical words and inflections and is reduced to expressing his message through short, disconnected word groupings, dominated by nouns.

But agrammatism is only one of many phenomena in aphasia that transcend the boundaries set by the sensory input or motor output modality involved, and which have to be defined and accounted for in psychological or linguistic terms. Occasionally noted but scarcely investigated prior to 1960 were specific impairments in the ability to name or to understand the names of words of particular categories – colors, numbers, parts of the body, letters of the alphabet.

Beginning in the mid-1950s, and continuing at an accelerating pace for the ensuing three decades, the field of aphasia research became host to experimentally trained neuropsychologists, linguists, and cognitive psychologists. The problems that were addressed by cognitive neurolinguists were precisely those that had escaped explanation on the basis of anatomically defined modality-specific centers. For example, in 1972, Zurif, Caramazza, and Myerson reopened the question of whether there was a central deficit that produced both agrammatism and impaired receptive processing of syntax. This paper was followed by other linguistically motivated experimental approaches to the problem of syntax.

A particularly fruitful line of investigation began when Marshall and Newcombe (1973) first described a conjunction of features that had never before been recognized as a syndrome affecting reading and which came to be referred to as "deep dyslexia." Deep dyslexia is most readily observed through oral reading behavior, in which the patient misreads words by making semantic substitutions that are often visually and phonologically unrelated to the stimulus (e.g. reading "ice" in place of the word "winter"). (See "Disorders of reading" below.)

THE SYMPTOMATOLOGY OF APHASIA

Auditory language comprehension

While some degree of reduction in the comprehension of oral language can be detected in most aphasics, severe selective impairment of auditory comprehension is usually the result of damage to the superior temporal gyrus, referred to as Wernicke's area. Even when this cortical region is not damaged, comprehension of speech may also suffer as a result of a subcortical injury of the fiber pathway from the medial geniculate body of the thalamus to the primary auditory zone (Heschl's gyrus) in the left temporal lobe. Damage to the temporal language areas affects the auditory comprehension of individual spoken words, as well as of sentences. Lexical or word comprehension nevertheless has unique features that should be treated separately from sentence comprehension.

Auditory lexical processing Impaired word comprehension is primarily a failure of the activation of lexical semantics upon the perception of the phonological form of previously known words. Although Luria (1970) argued that the underlying failure in temporal acoustic aphasia was a loss of "phonemic hearing" (i.e. of the ability to distinguish among the phonemes of one's language), other experimental evidence suggests that this impairment contributes little to aphasic comprehension loss.

Word comprehension that is defective for words spoken out of context may appear surprisingly intact when the word is used in a familiar phrase or in a lifelike context. For example,

patients who are wearing glasses almost invariably respond appropriately to the request, "May I see your glasses?" but they may pick up the wrong object when asked to select their glasses from among a group of personal possessions. Similarly, many patients respond as expected when the examiner says, "You have a smudge on your cheek," though they may not be able to point to their cheek or any other body part on request.

Category-specific comprehension disorders A phenomenon that is particularly challenging to models of lexical semantics is the selective impairment or selective preservation of comprehension for particular categories of words. In aphasia such dissociations most commonly affect the ability to identify letters of the alphabet, body parts, and numbers on hearing them named, and they are specific to auditory input. Goodglass and Budin's (1988) patient could not point to body parts on oral command, but did so perfectly in response to their written names. Except for the categories of body parts and letters of the alphabet, his comprehension of spoken object names was intact.

Dissociations in word comprehension by aphasic patients of more broadly defined semantic categories were first reported by Yamadori and Albert (1973), whose patient could not recognize the names of large objects in the room, but had no difficulty with small implements nor with outdoor objects. Warrington and Shallice (1984) and Warrington and McCarthy (1985, 1987) reported many more cases of dissociations in the comprehension of such broadly defined semantic groupings. These instances were more commonly to be found in post-encephalitic patients than in those with aphasia. In some instances the impairment appeared to affect naturally occurring objects (animals, plants, foods), while sparing manmade ones; in other cases it was the reverse.

Dissociation of categories for word comprehension almost always involves selectively *impaired* comprehension. The one exception to this observation is in the case of geographical place names, tested by having the patient find the named place on an outline map. Several investigators have found performances that were nearly intact in patients with global aphasia who failed with every other word category. The phenomenon of category-specific dissociations in word comprehension is closely related to similar dissociations in lexical production.

Comprehension disorders affecting sentences and specific syntactic tasks The correspondence between comprehension of words and of connected discourse is not one-to-one. As we have noted, the connotative information provided in a sentence may enable the processing of meaning of some words that cannot be understood out of context. A "real life" context may also permit adequate comprehension by patients who fail almost completely in formal testing with simple informational items that have no immediate personal relevance. As a general principle, the length of a sentence, the difficulty of the vocabulary employed, and the complexity of the message have a direct bearing on whether it is understood fully, partially, or not at all.

Impairments of sentence comprehension are by no means confined to patients who have difficulty with individual words. The most universally difficult syntactic manipulations are those in which a semantically reversible relationship between words is signalled either by word order, by a small grammatical morpheme, or both. By semantic reversibility, we mean that an equally plausible message may be inferred in the case of either of the two relations between the words. The most common example is the assignment of thematic roles (i.e. the subject or object of a verb) to two animate nouns. In the active voice, this is marked by word order; in the passive voice, by passive verb marking and the "by" of agency. The active (subject-verb-object) word order is canonical for English and leads to the heuristic strategy of assuming that the first noun is the actor. The interpretation of the passive requires the hearer to abandon this heuristic strategy by noting the presence of the two passive markers. Other examples of semantically reversible syntactic operations involve locative prepositions (e.g. "the chair behind the ball" vs "the ball behind the chair") and possessive relationships (e.g. "the ship's captain" vs "the captain's ship"). Luria used the term "logico-grammatical operations" to refer to this general class of semantically reversible relationships and claimed that processing difficulties for these constructions are notably severe in "semantic aphasics" – patients with lesions in the left parietal lobe. Subsequent research, however, reveals that these forms can be difficult for aphasics of all types to interpret correctly.

MOTOR ARTICULATORY PROBLEMS

Impairments of motor speech production may range in severity from total absence of voluntary control for the production of speechlike sounds to residual awkwardness on phonologically complex sound sequences. While the efforts of severely affected patients suggest a primary disorder of motor control, certain characteristic behaviors contradict such an interpretation, that is, patients who still have no useful speech output may produce stereotyped syllables or recurrent words with each effort to talk. Some patients may produce occasional relevant brief comments or interjections, while still unable to imitate or initiate any specific requested sounds. In the great majority of patients with restricted articulatory output, memorized sequences (e.g. counting) may be elicited. Articulation may be virtually normal during these productions. As recovery takes place, facility in articulation is likely to return for a small repertory of common words and expressions, while production of less accustomed and longer utterances is still impossible or very awkward.

Persistent difficulty in articulation is most likely to follow deep lesions in Broca's area. Naeser and others (1989) report that the outlook for recovery of articulation is poor when lesions encroach on the medial subcallosal fasciculus (just anterior to the frontal horn of the lateral ventricle) and also involve the middle third of the periventricular white matter. Some eventual recovery of motor speech output is the rule with less deep lesions.

Severely impaired articulation is usually part of the syndromes of global aphasia and of Broca's aphasia, where it appears in the context of very limited verbal output. However, articulatory impairment may be seen in patients who can formulate and produce sentences. A "pure" disorder of articulation without any impairment in other aspects of language (i.e. reading, writing, auditory comprehension) is an occasional result of a lesion that involves the white matter deep to the foot of the precentral gyrus and is not very extensive. This is referred to as "aphemia" or "subcortical motor aphasia."

DISORDERS OF NAMING

Disorders of naming refer to difficulty in accessing any vocabulary items that have semantic content, whether nouns, verbs, adjectives, or adverbs, but excluding access to words that have only a grammatical function, i.e. case-marking prepositions. Word-finding difficulties are present in aphasics of every type, but there are differences among types of aphasics in the prominence of naming problems in comparison to other aspects of language production, such as motor speech output and grammar. There are differences as well in the type of errors produced and in strategies for coping with word-finding failures. Finally, there are differences in the categories of words that present the greatest problems to patients of various types.

Impaired word finding as a primary feature Inability to access the high-information elements of the message – particularly nouns – may appear in patients with fluent, well articulated and grammatical speech, and relatively good auditory comprehension. This speech pattern, termed "anomic aphasia," is described in detail in the section below on the classification of aphasia.

Impaired word finding in patients with reduced speech output While word-finding difficulty stands out as the major symptom in anomic aphasia, the absolute level of word-finding impairment may be much more severe in patients with Broca's aphasia, although overshadowed by the impoverishment of output, greatly reduced grammar, and articulatory problems. Indeed, the few nouns that these patients can access may constitute most of their speech output. Word substitution errors are occasionally present. These patients are often successful in correctly completing an intended word when the first sound is provided for them.

Impaired word finding in Wernicke's aphasia Patients with the fluent but error-filled speech of Wernicke's aphasia usually have a severe or complete ANOMIA. This may be disguised in free discourse by a rambling and repetitious output, with irrelevant and syntactically incoherent structure. Semantically related or unrelated word substitutions are used, as well as partially or totally neologistic words. The same pattern of failure is observed on testing with pictures to be named. It can often be demonstrated that these patients have a poorly differentiated semantic representation of the target concepts, suggesting that the source of misnaming is at an early stage of word retrieval.

Two-way impairments of lexical processes Patients with extensive lesions in the posterior parieto-temporal zone are likely to show an inability either to retrieve words for production or to recognize

their meaning when the words are offered by the examiner. They may repeat the word aloud, without comprehension. This behavior, labelled by Luria as "alienation of word meaning," suggests a dissociation between the entire language system and the preverbal semantic structure of the corresponding concept.

Category-specific dissociations of word retrieval It is common to find that severely anomic patients may have a well-preserved ability to name numbers and/or letters of the alphabet on visual presentation. However, rare instances of other dissociations have been described. For example, Hart and colleagues (1985) have described a patient whose sole residual after a period of aphasia was an inability to retrieve the names of fruits and vegetables. Semenza and Zettin (1988) have described a patient who was incapable of retrieving any proper noun, although he was not aphasic in any other respect. In none of these cases is there a lesion locus that clearly distinguishes the patient from other patients who do not have the dissociation in question. Accounts of any of these dissociations are highly speculative and the reader is referred to the original articles for discussion.

Color naming difficulties associated with pure ALEXIA stand alone as one category-specific naming disorder for which there is an anatomical account. Among patients with isolated reading disorders resulting from occipital lesions, there is a subset who can neither name nor reliably understand the names of colors, although their color perception is normal. The lesion producing both disorders involves the left visual cortex and the splenium of the corpus callosum. (See further details below in the section on reading disorders.)

Modality-specific naming disorders Striking deficiencies in object naming that are confined to a single modality of sensory input have been described for vision (optic aphasia, Freund, 1889) and for audition (Denes & Semenza, 1975). Tactile anomia specific to left-sided tactile input is regularly observed in patients with lesions of the corpus callosum (Geschwind & Kaplan, 1962). The lesions involved in optic and acoustic anomia are both localized in or close to the association areas for their respective modalities and are presumed to interrupt the access of the sensory stimulation to the language zone. In all cases, adequate perceptual recognition in the affected sensory modality can be demonstrated by tasks that do not involve naming.

AGRAMMATISM

Agrammatism is a form of restricted speech output that is most readily defined in terms of a set of distinctive constraints affecting particular parts of speech and syntactic structures. The agrammatic speaker relies chiefly on high information words (nouns, main verbs) to convey his message, apparently unable to access for production prepositions, auxiliary verbs, or subordinating conjunctions. Agrammatic speakers often delete the article before nouns and use few pronouns. Verbs are more difficult to access than nouns and it is sometimes necessary to infer the intended verb from the context. Verbs are uninflected, appearing either as the verb stem or in the "-ing" form. A typical response by an agrammatic speaker to a question about his illness might be, "Stroke. Nine years ago. And hospital . . . Talking . . . no! Walking . . . no! Therapy, six months . . . and better." Partial recovery is expressed by more regular access to verbs and by the ability to generate some complete sentences. These, however, rarely stray from the subject –verb–object construction. Speech is referred to as "telegraphic" when the principal content words are produced but lack grammatically obligatory articles, noun and verb inflections, and other "small" grammatical words.

Agrammatism appears most often as part of the syndrome of Broca's aphasia, but it has also been reported repeatedly with parietal lobe rather than frontal lobe lesions. It is usually confined to fragmented speech in utterances one to three words in length. However, variants of agrammatism have been described in which complex syntactic constructions appear, but with deletions of articles, auxiliary verbs, and other grammatical morphemes.

While the features of agrammatism, as described by writers in most of the Western languages, appeared to be constant across languages, recent comparative cross-linguistic studies (Menn & Obler, 1990; Bates et al., 1991) have revealed a number of language-specific characteristics. For example, bound inflectional morphemes are rarely deleted in highly inflected languages, but are commonly deleted in English. Chinese, which does not use verb inflections, auxiliary verbs, or articles, accepts as correct many sentences that would be agrammatic or telegraphic in other languages.

There are a number of current explanatory accounts of agrammatism that are founded on very different preconceptions. One of the earliest of these is the theory of economy of effort. Pick regarded agrammatism as the patient's adaptation to the difficulty of producing speech; utterances are reduced to the barest essentials. Pick suggested the term "Notsprache" (emergency speech). Goldstein (1948) endorsed a similar view. Jakobson's (1956) position ascribed to agrammatism a much more fundamental change in the use of language than simply economizing effort. To him, agrammatism represented a shift toward the use of words as nominal concepts, strung together with minimal syntactic marking. Luria espoused Jakobson's account, but added that the agrammatic patient has lost the ability to predicate. The patient's inability to link subject and verb in a single statement leads him to treat them each as separate nominalized concepts. The infinitive tends to be substituted for the inflected verb form, because it serves as the name of the action.

Kolk and Heeschen (1990) proposed the view that agrammatism is the product of an avoidance strategy adopted by patients who have difficulty in the linguistic computations of accessing syntactic forms. They suggest that the agrammatic, in principle, could ultimately achieve the desired constructions, but makes a voluntary choice of simplifying his or her syntax in order to avoid an inordinately prolonged struggle. None of the foregoing theories accounts for the fact that severely agrammatic speakers have difficulty in accessing for production the phonological forms of grammatical morphemes, even when they are provided for repetition (Goodglass et al., 1967). For these patients there appears to be a link between the semantic content of a word and its accessibility to phonological realization. At this time, there is continuing active effort to arrive at a comprehensive account of agrammatism.

PARAPHASIA

In most forms of aphasia speech production errors, referred to as "paraphasia" are an integral feature of the patients' disorder. These errors may involve mistargeted phonemes (literal or phonemic paraphasia), incorrectly chosen words (verbal or semantic paraphasia), or disorganized syntax (paragrammatism). Literal paraphasia may arise at a level very close to articulatory control, particularly in Broca's aphasia. Such errors do not have the clumsy quality or the simplification of phonologically complex consonant clusters that can be attributed to awkwardness of articulation. Phonemic paraphasias involving intrusions or substitutions of totally extraneous sounds or syllables, as well as transpositions within the word, occur in "fluent aphasia" (see the following section), in a context of otherwise facile articulation.

Verbal paraphasias are heard in aphasics of every type. In most instances they involve the substitution of a semantically related word for the target or the perseverative production of a previously used word. However, verbal paraphasia involving unrelated words is not uncommon. Verbal paraphasias may be produced even when the patient has a demonstrably intact representation of the semantic properties of the intended word. In some patients, however, even the basic semantics of the intended concept are disrupted.

Paragrammatism is characteristic of fluent aphasia – particularly Wernicke's aphasia – and takes the form of syntactic constructions that are logically incoherent, sometimes involving the appearance of a verb in a noun slot or vice versa. It is distinguished from "agrammatism" by the appropriate use of grammatical morphemes (auxiliary verbs, verb and noun inflections, articles, prepositions).

FLUENCY vs NONFLUENCY

Seventy-five or eighty percent of aphasic patients can be classified on the basis of the "fluency" or "nonfluency" of their speech output pattern. Nonfluent patients are those who almost never produce a run of words, uninterrupted by a pause, exceeding three or four words in length. Fluent patients are those who commonly have uninterrupted word runs more than five words in length. Goodglass and others (1964), using a "phrase length ratio," based on a count of words per uninterrupted run, found that aphasic patients were sharply dichotomized into "long phrase dominant" (fluent) and "short phrase dominant" (nonfluent) types, with comparatively few patients who fell at an intermediate point. This observation proved to correspond well with the anterior–posterior dimension of lesion locus. Patients with post-Rolandic speech zone lesions usually have fluent forms of aphasia, while those with anterior lesions are usually nonfluent. While originally defined by Goodglass and colleagues

(1964) strictly in terms of length of word runs, the fluency concept spread to include other features of speech that were typically associated with the two types of speech output. Benson (1967) listed, among other features, anomia, paraphasia, good articulation, and good grammatical form as characteristic of "fluent aphasia," while poor articulation and agrammatism are characteristics of "nonfluent aphasia." Nonfluency is a less reliable clue to lesion locus than is fluency, because patients with large lesions and global or severe mixed forms of aphasia must be classified as nonfluent.

REPETITION

For most aphasics, the ability to repeat from an auditorily presented model is commensurate with other language skills. However, this capacity merits special attention because it may be selectively preserved in a subset of patients and selectively damaged in others. The Wernicke–Lichtheim model provides an anatomical rationale for both forms of dissociation in "transcortical sensory" and "transcortical motor" aphasia. The preservation of repetition in patients who are otherwise severely language-impaired may be quite dramatic. Not only is repetition span for sentences in the normal range, but patients are commonly able to mimic nonsense words. Repetition is not parrot-like, as it can readily be shown that patients will correct grammatical errors (e.g. "He lost him hat" → "He lost his hat"). However, they will repeat semantically nonsensical words without objection. In general they repeat only on request, but patients with transcortical aphasia characteristically re-use some or all of the words of the examiner's question in attempting to answer it. Preserved repetition is also observed in cases of hemorrhages in or close to the left thalamus (Alexander & LoVerme, 1980). While Wernicke's and Lichtheim's account of the mechanism for the preservation of repetition may not be accurate, it is the case that well preserved repetition always implies sparing of most or all of both Broca's and Wernicke's areas and the tissue between them.

Relatively impaired repetition is one of the features of conduction aphasia. However, this impairment is not as clearcut as is the preservation of repetition in the transcortical aphasias. Some authors (Dubois et al., 1964) question the definition of the impairment in conduction aphasia as specific to repetition, but Dubois and colleagues interpret the disorder as one that arises at points of maximum information load in the articulatory plan – a condition that is often present in repetition upon request, but less often in free conversation.

DISORDERS OF READING

As a rule of thumb, reading impairment for most aphasic patients parallels the severity of impairment of their auditory comprehension. This rule, however, has many exceptions that can only be specified by reference to the multiple cognitive processes that converge in reading, as well as by reference to the anatomical structures that play a part in bringing visual input into interaction with the auditorily based language system. The exceptions take the form of selective deficits related to damage to either anatomical structures or to cognitive subprocesses whose localization within the language zone is not known. The anatomical structures involved are the visual cortices and visual association areas of both hemispheres, their interconnection through the splenium of the corpus callosum, and their connection, within the left hemisphere to the region of the angular gyrus, which appears to mediate the link between visual graphic characters and auditory language. The most prominent cognitive components are the ability to recognize letter identities, to associate letter sequences with phonological strings, the ability to quickly associate familiar written lexical units to their phonology as "whole words," and the ability to derive semantic information from such lexical units, without necessarily activating their phonology at all. These are the factors generally recognized in the reading of alphabetically written languages. They are very differently weighted in idiographic languages, such as Chinese.

Aphasic alexia In the majority of aphasic patients, for whom it appears that impaired reading ability is secondary to their loss of language comprehension, there are a number of regularities that emerge from the mass of individual variations. (1) Symbol recognition is robust in the face of severe functional impairments, i.e. patients maintain the identity of individual letters across styles of print and writing, even though they can no longer name the letters. (2) The ability to read individual words is enhanced for words having strong emotional connotations, as opposed to neutral words. The appreciation of the connotative or categorical meaning of a word may persist when precise understanding is lost, with the result that words can be more readily identified within a list of mixed categories than when they appear among other words of the same category. (3) There is a slight bias in word recognition for nouns over verbs and verbs over grammatical function words. However, the persistence of whole word recognition skills and of some degree of capability for grapho-phonemic conversion has the result that part-of-speech influences on word recognition may be undetectable in many patients. (4) Comprehension of connected text in writing is subject to the same considerations of syntactic complexity as in the case of spoken sentences and paragraphs.

Alexias involving cognitive dissociations From the point of Marshall and Newcombe's (1973) description of the syndrome of "deep dyslexia," the dissociability of the cognitive components of reading has assumed a large theoretical importance. In this syndrome patients no longer attain a phonological representation on seeing a pronounceable letter string or a familiar whole word. Thus they cannot recognize the sound of a nonword (e.g. fazz) nor match a pseudohomophone like "fone" to either the written word "phone" or to a picture. They do, however, achieve a more or less accurate sense of the semantics of a written word and may verbalize it correctly. Often their verbalization is a word that is only semantically related to the stimulus, as saying "night" when shown the word "dark." The probability of accurate production of a written word is strongly linked to its semantic properties: best for picturable objects, less so for abstract nouns and verbs, and almost nil for grammatical functors. Inflectional and derivational affixes are deleted or substituted (e.g. "bake" for "bakery"). While the most salient symptoms appear during oral reading, the disorder can be demonstrated in nonverbal patients by suitable multiple-choice pointing tests. Deep dyslexia occurs most commonly in patients with agrammatic Broca's aphasia, but it may appear in patients with fluent aphasia as well.

A less common but equally interesting problem is referred to as "surface dyslexia." This is manifested as an oral reading disorder. Patients with surface dyslexia do not recognize the segmentation of syllables nor the component morphemes in a polymorphemic word. However, they can apply basic regular phonic rules to pronouncing letter strings and often apply these rules inappropriately to a wrongly segmented reading of a word. The word "home", for example, might be read as "hommee"; the word "carrot" as "car, rot." Meaning is derived from the patient's pronunciation, often leading to grossly irrelevant interpretations of written text.

Anatomically based dissociative disorders of reading Alexia without agraphia (also called "pure alexia," "pure word blindness," and "letter by letter reading") was first reported with anatomic verification by Déjerine (1892). In this disorder patients have a total or near total loss of word recognition ability, without any effect on other language functions. They may write normally and then be unable to read back their own writing. In many cases, letters can be recognized and words may then be recognized by silent spelling (hence the term "letter by letter readers"). Most cases of alexia without agraphia involve destruction of the left visual cortex, along with damage to the posterior end (splenium) of the corpus callosum. This renders the patient hemianopic in the right visual field, and also prevents the transfer of visual information from the right visual association area to the left, where it would be available to linguistic processing. In rare cases, pure alexia may be caused by a lesion within the left occipital lobe that is thought to disconnect the visual association area from access to the language-processing zone within the same hemisphere. The cerebral structures involved are within the distribution of the left posterior cerebral artery and the disorder is usually the result of an occlusion of that artery.

Since the standard anatomic account of alexia without agraphia treats it as a pure disconnection of sensory input, one would not expect to find linguistically conditioned error patterns. For example, these patients are adept at understanding words spelled orally to them and words spelled out tactilely on their fingertips. Nevertheless, semantic effects in word recognition have been observed in occasional cases (e.g. Coslett & Saffran, 1989). Farah (1990) reviews the evidence, favoring the view that pure alexia is a disorder of high-order visual perception rather than of simple disconnection.

Alexia with agraphia of the angular gyrus Déjerine was also the first to describe the symptomatology and anatomy associated with the combined disorder of reading and writing that may follow lesions of the angular gyrus. Cases that totally spare spoken language are rare, since this region is often involved in severe anomia. In these cases, the patient is unable to decode orally spelled words or to spell words aloud or in writing.

DISORDERS OF WRITING

Disruption of writing (agraphia) may result from injury at many sites within the left cerebral language zone, both anterior and posterior. The linguistic aspects of writing disorders tend to mirror those of spoken language, with respect to word retrieval, syntax, and written paraphasia in aphasic agraphia, but there are many exceptions, which will be summarized here. Writing is closely analogous to reading in that it depends on cognitive components: phono-graphemic conversion for sublexical letter strings; phono-graphemic conversion on a whole-word (lexical) basis; direct semantic activation of spelling without phonological mediation. As in the case of reading, there are selective dissociations of the phonological channel which may force patients to function imperfectly through total reliance on semantically activated spelling associations.

The graphomotor aspect of writing is extremely vulnerable to anterior speech zone lesions, with the result that severe disorders at the level of forming letters are very common, even in patients who have some capacity for speech output. Cursive writing is often replaced completely by block printing in patients with anterior lesions.

Writing (in alphabetic languages) is also unique in the fact that written word retrieval is mediated by an abstractly represented letter string that may be expressed quite as automatically in oral spelling as it is in any of a variety of graphic media, including cursive writing, printing, and typing.

Aphasic agraphia Unlike the case in other language modalities, the breakdown of writing skills usually follows a strict hierarchy from larger to smaller elements. Letter formation impairments usually presuppose a loss of spelling knowledge (except in cases of apraxic agraphia). Patients may be observed to call on every channel of association in reconstructing words in writing when they do not have access to whole-word activation of spelling, that is, sublexical phonic knowledge along with visual and graphomotor memories usually guide the first few letters, while visual memory may predominantly guide the choice of letters at the end of a word. Since visual memory is an extremely unreliable associative mode, it may lead to misplaced letters and only rarely to the complete retrieval of the letter sequence. Writing of connected text usually presupposes good recovery of single-word writing, and it is usually strictly limited by the level of spoken language.

Cognitively based dissociations in writing Phonological dysgraphia, deep dysgraphia, and surface dysgraphia are closely analogous to the reading disorders with corresponding names. Like the corresponding reading disorders, they refer to retrieval problems at the single-word level. For example, deep dysgraphia is expressed by the writing of a word that is semantically, but not structurally, related to one that has been dictated (e.g. one patient wrote "industrial" in response to the dictated word "agricultural"). As in deep dyslexia, there is an advantage for nouns over verbs and for verbs over grammatical functors. Caramazza and Hillis (1991) described a patient who had an extreme disparity between her ability to write nouns (well preserved) and verbs (severely impaired). No such disparity existed in oral production. They were able to contrast her with another patient who had a similar noun–verb disparity only in oral production, but not in writing.

Selective impairments of writing Cases of pure agraphia have been reported from a number of different anatomical lesion sites and there is currently no recognized anatomical model to account for pure agraphia. Exner (1881) proposed a site for pure agraphia in the second frontal gyrus, but this claim has had scant support. More commonly, agraphia that is disproportionately severe is observed in conjunction with parietal lobe damage. In some cases of angular gyrus lesions, associated with alexia and agraphia, the agraphia may be much more severe and long-lasting than the alexia.

CLASSIFICATION OF APHASIA

The symptoms covered in the review above tend to appear clinically in clusters. A number of these symptom clusters recur so regularly that, with minor variations, they have served as the basis for named syndromes of aphasia in the taxonomies of various authors. The following summary of syndromes is based on the widely used terminology that has developed on the basis of the Wernicke–Lichtheim schema.

Nonfluent aphasias

Broca's aphasia Severe restriction of speech output, marked by laborious articulation, very short utterances, and relatively spared auditory comprehension. Vocabulary access is usually very much restricted. Agrammatism is a common but not universal feature. Writing may be reduced to a few common words. In milder forms it may mirror the agrammatism of speech output. Reading is usually less impaired than writing. The lesion usually involves the pre-Rolandic cortical speech zone and subjacent white matter.

Transcortical motor aphasia Severe incapacity to initiate speech spontaneously or to formulate sentences in response to questions. Repetition is remarkably intact and reveals normal articulation and ability to reproduce a full range of grammatical structures. Some patients have preserved ability to name and to give brief factual answers to questions. Fluency of speech in repetition and occasional "breakthroughs" of full, well-formulated sentences make the assignment to the "nonfluent" vs "fluent" category dubious. Auditory comprehension and reading are usually well preserved. Writing is limited in the same way as speech. It is usually associated with a relatively small subcortical lesion deep to an area just anterior and superior to Broca's area, which may be partially impinged on.

Aphemia An impairment of motor speech output characterized by extremely laborious, distorted articulation, produced with syllable by syllable prosody, with assignment of the full vowel value to each syllable. Patients avoid using contractions. In other respects, there is no impairment of language function: syntax, reading, writing, and auditory comprehension are intact. It is usually caused by a small lesion involving white matter deep in the lower portion of the precentral gyrus.

Global aphasia Virtually complete abolition of motor speech output, except for short stereotyped utterances that are produced by some patients with each effort to speak. Auditory comprehension is reduced to the single word level, but simple, personally relevant comments or questions are sometimes understood. Reading and writing are below functional levels. It usually involves a large lesion that includes both frontal and temporal speech areas and extends into subcortical regions, but may also be produced by entirely subcortical lesions that extend deep to the lateral ventricle and anteriorly to the region around the frontal horn.

Fluent aphasias

Wernicke's aphasia Marked impairment of auditory language comprehension with fluent paraphasic speech. Speech errors usually include verbal and phonemic paraphasia and sentences lacking logical syntactic coherence (paragrammatism), but grammatical morphology, including appropriate use of articles, pronouns, and prepositions, is spared. Neologisms may be present or may even dominate speech. Severe cases manifest paraphasic jargon and hyperfluency, with increased speech rate and resistance to interruption. Patients are unaware of speech errors. Anomia is usually severe or complete. Reading and writing are variably affected; sometimes much superior to oral language and sometimes non-functional, depending on the extent of the lesion into the posterior (parieto-temporal) language zone. The lesion usually involves the posterior portion of the superior temporal gyrus and totally spares the anterior speech zone.

Conduction aphasia Predominantly fluent, well articulated speech, marked by sporadic instances of disrupted phonological production of words, involving transposition, substitution, or deletion of sounds or syllables (phonemic paraphasia). Production difficulties are usually marked during efforts to repeat words or sentences after the examiner. This has been defined by some authors as an aphasia for repetition, but the centrality of the repetition disorder has been disputed. Auditory comprehension is relatively unaffected and may be totally normal. Patients are usually acutely aware of their errors and may become involved in multiple attempts to repair the production of the sounds of words (*conduit d'approche*). Reading is only mildly affected and writing is usually functional, although spelling difficulties are reported. Lesions are restricted in extent and are predominantly in the supramarginal gyrus, but the clinical syndrome has also been reported with lesions elsewhere in the Sylvian zone, including the insula and the temporal lobe.

Transcortical sensory aphasia Fluent paraphasic speech with impaired auditory comprehension, but with perfect preservation of the ability to repeat sentences. Repetition may be perfect in spite of the patient's failure to grasp the meaning of what he or she is saying. Anomia is usually severe; in some instances it is characterized by "alienation of word meaning" or empty repetition of a word without any sense of its meaning. In some instances there is also "empty oral reading": fluent production of a written text, without comprehension of the words. More often, however, patients have no functional reading or writing ability. Lesions usually involve a subcortical zone extending in an arc from the area of the angular gyrus downward, deep to the temporo-occipital junction.

Anomic aphasia Fluent, well articulated, and grammatically normal speech output, marked by inability to supply the information-loaded words of the message. Nouns are the most difficult to retrieve, but all parts of speech are affected, except for grammatical words. Auditory comprehension is usually very good, and reading and writing may be unaffected. Several widely separated lesion sites may produce the disorder, notably lesions in the area of the angular gyrus, lesions of the inferior temporal gyrus, and small subcortical frontal lesions.

BIBLIOGRAPHY

Albert, M. L., Goodglass, H., Helm, N. A., Rubens, A. B., & Alexander, M. P. (1981). *Clinical aspects of dysphasia*. Vienna: Springer.

Alexander, M. P., & LoVerme, S. R. (1980). Aphasia after left hemisphere intracerebral hemorrhage. *Neurology, 30*, 1193–202.

Bates, E., Wulfeck, B., & MacWhinney, B. (1991). Cross-linguistic research in aphasia: an overview. *Brain and Language, 41*, 123–48.

Benson, D. F. (1967). Fluency in aphasia: correlation with brain scan localization. *Cortex, 3*, 373–94.

Caramazza, A., & Hillis, A. E. (1991). Lexical organization of nouns and verbs in the brain. *Nature, 349*, 788–9.

Coltheart, M., Sartori, G., & Marshall, J. C. (Eds), (1980). *Deep dyslexia*. London: Routledge and Kegan Paul.

Coltheart, M., Sartori, G., & Job, R. (Eds). (1987). *The cognitive neuropsychology of language*. Hillsdale, NJ: Erlbaum.

Coslett, H. B., & Saffran, E. M. (1989). Preserved object recognition and reading comprehension in optic aphasia. *Brain, 112*, 1091–110.

Denes, G., & Semenza, C. (1975). Auditory modality-specific anomia-evidence from a case of pure word-deafness. *Cortex, 11*, 401–11.

Dubois, J., Hécaen, H., Angelergues, R., Maufras de Chatelier, A., Marcie, P. (1964). Étude neurolinguistique de l'aphasie de conduction. *Neuropsychologia, 2*, 9–44.

Farah, M. (1990). *Visual agnosia*. Cambridge, MA: Bradford.

Geschwind, N. (1965). Disconnexion syndromes in animals and man. *Brain, 88*, 237–94, 585–644.

Geschwind, N., & Kaplan, E. (1962). A human cerebral deconnection syndrome. *Neurology, 12*, 675–85.

Goldstein, K. (1948). *Language and language disturbances*. New York: Grune and Stratton.

Goodglass, H., & Budin, C. (1988). Category and modality-specific dissociations in word comprehension and concurrent phonological dyslexia. *Neuropsychologia, 26*, 67–78.

Goodglass, H., Fodor, I., & Schulhoff, C. (1967). Prosodic factors in grammar-evidence from aphasia. *Journal of Speech and Hearing Research, 10*, 5–20.

Goodglass, H., Quadfasel, F., & Timberlake, W. H. (1964). Phrase length and the type and severity of aphasia. *Cortex, 1*, 133–53.

Hart, J., Berndt, R. S., & Caramazza, A. (1985). A category-specific naming deficit following cerebral infarction. *Nature, 316*, 338.

Head, H. (1926). *Aphasia and kindred disorders of speech*. New York: Macmillan.

Kolk, H. H. J., & Heeschen, C. (1990). Adaptation symptoms and impairment symptoms in Broca's aphasia. *Aphasiology, 4*, 221–31.

Luria, A. R. (1970). *Traumatic aphasia*. The Hague: Mouton.

Marshall, J., & Newcombe, F. (1973). Patterns of paralexia: a psycholinguistic approach. *Journal of Psycholinguistic Research, 2*, 175–99.

Menn, L., & Obler, L. (1990). *Agrammatic aphasia*. Amsterdam: Benjamins.

Naeser, M. A., Palumbo, C. L., Helm-Estabrooks, N., Stiassny-Eder, D., & Albert, M. L. (1989). Severe non-fluency in aphasia: role of the medial subcallosal fasciculus plus other white matter pathways in recovery of spontaneous speech. *Brain, 112*, 1–38.

Semenza, C., & Zettin, M. (1988). Generating proper names: a case of selective inability. *Cognitive Neuropsychology, 5*, 711–26.

Warrington, E., & McCarthy, R. (1985). Category-specific access dysphasia. *Brain, 106*, 859–78.

Warrington, E., & McCarthy, R. (1987). Categories of knowledge. *Brain, 110*, 1273–96.

Warrington, E. K., & Shallice, T. (1984). Category-specific semantic impairments. *Brain, 107*, 829–54.

Yamadori, A., & Albert, M. L. (1973). Word category aphasia. *Cortex, 9*, 83–9.

Zurif, E. B., Caramazza, A., & Myerson, R. (1972). Grammatical judgments of agrammatic aphasics. *Neuropsychologia, 10*, 405–17.

HAROLD GOODGLASS

aphasia therapy *See* SPEECH THERAPY FOR APHASIA.

aphemia *See* ANARTHRIA

apractagnosia, apractognosia Apractagnosia is a form of APRAXIA in which features of apraxia and AGNOSIA appear together. Some writers have considered the term to be synonymous with constructional apraxia, while others (Hécaen et al., 1956) have argued for a separate syndrome to be more properly termed *apractognosia for spatial relations*.

Apractognosia for spatial relations is conceived as a form of visual agnosia in which there is a disorder of the manipulation of spatial information. These disorders of the recognition and use of spatial information are closely associated with visuoconstructive deficits, spatial dyslexia, dysgraphia and dyscalculia, and with METAMORPHOPSIA and hemisomatognosia. The disorders in this group include the loss of topographical concepts (PLANATOPOKINESIA) and unilateral spatial agnosia. Unilateral spatial agnosia is phenomenologically the same as unilateral neglect, but the use of the term "agnosia" implies that the problem is semantic in nature, rather than attentional. Current views of NEGLECT more commonly reject this explanation of the phenomenon in favor of an attentional one.

Apractagnosia is associated with lesions at the parietal-occipital junction. The term is currently little used, but it is of historical importance.

BIBLIOGRAPHY

Hécaen, H., Penfield, W., Bertrand, C., & Malmo, R. (1956). The syndrome of apractognosia due to lesions of the minor cerebral hemisphere. *Archives of Neurology and Psychiatry*, *75*, 400–34.

apraxia Apraxia can be defined as an impairment in the ability to carry out voluntary movements in the absence of sensory loss, paresis, or motor weakness. It is most often apparent in situations where a person is asked to produce a motor behavior either to command or out of context. It appears to be the intentional aspect of the behavior that is critical in producing the problem. The disorder may not be apparent in those incidents when the movement is carried out fortuitously or as part of a regular routine. With this particular problem a strong dissociation exists between the testing situation and everyday life. There are some forms of apraxia that involve such circumscribed behaviors that they are rarely noticed outside the testing situation and have very little impact on normal functioning.

The term apraxia was coined by Steinthal (1871) to describe an observed difficulty with the voluntary use of objects. It was in 1890 that Meynert clarified the idea by drawing a distinction between an impairment of object recognition and a loss of the memory for motor movements. It was the work of Liepmann at the turn of the century which uncovered the true complexities of the disorder and hastened its recognition as a clinical phenomenon. In the opinion of some, the term apraxia has come to be applied rather loosely and is now being used to refer to a number of disorders whose presentation bears little resemblance to the original disorders that bore the name. It is now generally accepted that there are four major forms of apraxia, with a number of other disorders bearing the name.

IDEOMOTOR APRAXIA

Ideomotor apraxia is perhaps the best researched of all the apraxic disorders. It refers to a disorder of the execution of simple gestures, either to command or imitation, often with the ability to carry out more complex acts largely preserved. As De Renzi (1989) describes it, "The patient knows what to do but not how to do it." Gestures used to test for the presence of ideomotor apraxia include symbolic acts such as saluting or waving goodbye, object manipulation such as pretending to hammer a nail into a wall, or simply meaningless motor acts. For example, given a request to salute, a patient may be aware that his hand needs to be raised in some fashion but appears confused, being unable to either complete the movement or place the hand correctly. When asked to pretend to make use of a tool there may be body-part substitution. For example, if asked to pretend to use a comb the hand itself may be employed in place of the pretend comb.

When testing for this form of apraxia it is essential that the patient's ability to imitate the gesture should also be tested. This helps to ensure that any failure is a function of a problem other than that of poor language comprehension, language problems frequently occurring alongside apraxia. There is some debate whether the disorder is more pronounced with meaningless motor acts relative to meaningful gestures, but both should be tested. However, De Renzi (1989) feels that when imitation is being used the distinction is unimportant.

There is some conflict in the literature regarding exactly where lesions have to be placed to produce an ideomotor apraxia. However, it appears to be generally accepted that lesions in the posterior regions of the dominant hemisphere, specifically the parietal or temporoparietal region, are essential. Lesions in other areas can produce a disconnection phenomenon, a subject to be discussed below.

IDEATIONAL APRAXIA

Ideational apraxia involves a disruption of the ability to carry out acts requiring a well ordered sequencing of behaviors. The individual elements of the act may be intact but the logical ordering of the elements is disrupted. For example, a person, when asked to take a match from a box and to strike it, may misorder the elements to such a degree as to render the person unable to complete that act. There may be perseverations on one particular element, a change in sequence of the elements, or simply an omission of essential elements.

In some cases patients may demonstrate more success at tasks that have become very automatic as a result of over-learning but fail at tasks that are carried out less often, consequently requiring more thought and attention. The length and complexity of a requested act, and hence the level of attention and processing that is required, are important variables affecting success at a task. Ideational apraxia is characterized by considerable variability across tasks. The patient is sometimes able to imitate a relatively complex act, but unable to complete it on command. Equally, a patient may be able to demonstrate the use of a tool when allowed contact with that tool, but may not be able to show knowledge of the tool in an abstract context. This form of apraxia appears to result from bilateral lesions generally seen in the posterior regions of the dominant hemisphere, particularly the parietal lobe (Lishman, 1990).

Ideational apraxia has been conceptualized in a number of different ways. Some authors suggest that the deficit only becomes apparent when an actual tool is being used, so they see ideational apraxia as a problem with tool utilization (De Renzi et al., 1968; Ochips et al., 1988). Other authors, such as Lehmkuhl and Poeck (1981) believe that it is not so much a loss of conceptual knowledge related to tool use but rather a loss or disturbance in the conceptual organization of actions necessary for completion of an act. However, it is generally accepted by most researchers that this form of apraxia appears to involve a loss of the ideational plan of action when a complex sequence of acts is necessary for the successful manipulation of a tool or object.

There remains considerable debate as to whether one can draw a true distinction between ideomotor apraxia and ideational apraxia. It is relatively clear that ideomotor apraxia can occur in the absence of ideational apraxia, but it remains controversial whether or not ideational apraxia can occur in the absence of ideomotor apraxia. Liepmann (1900), in some of his first papers on the subject, felt that ideational apraxia was simply an extreme form of ideomotor apraxia. Zangwill (1960) was to raise this issue again, maintaining that the defect in tool manipulation common with ideational apraxia may simply be a function of a defect in motor programming, so not related to a conceptual defect. However, later studies have tended to confirm the presence of a dissociation between the two disorders. De Renzi and Luchelli (1988) found no correlation between the performance of 20 left-brain-damaged patients on a test requiring the coordinated use of objects and a test requiring the simple imitation of a motor movement. It has been pointed out that, in

some cases of severe ideomotor apraxia, the deficits in motor programming may be so severe as to impair the manipulation of tools or objects to such an extent as to make it extremely difficult to determine whether the errors are a function of an ideational problem or a motor programming problem.

Another issue that has brought into question the validity of ideational apraxia as an independent clinical entity is the frequency with which it has been observed to co-occur with global intellectual decline. Although there is some degree of similarity between the clinical symptoms associated with the two forms of apraxia, such as language disturbances, sensory disorders, and confusion, these are generally accepted to be more severe in those presenting with ideational apraxia. However, De Renzi and colleagues (1968) tested this idea by administering the Raven's Progressive Matrices test (a measure of visual reasoning) to a group of left-brain-damaged patients presenting with ideational apraxia. They observed little difference between the performance of this group on the test relative to a group without ideational apraxia.

It is generally considered that ideational apraxia can most readily be identified by a failure in the sequencing of acts necessary for the manipulation of multiple objects, such as the lighting of a cigarette. However, it can also be observed in the manipulation of single objects. Morlass (1928), in observing this problem, considered that ideational apraxia was in fact a form of agnosia, an agnosia for the use of objects. The person is able to name the object and describe its use but is unable to actually demonstrate physically how it is used. De Renzi (1989) considers it more accurate to view it as a semantic amnesia rather than an agnosia – the person fails to find the store for the memory engram containing the information pertaining to the use of a particular object.

CONSTRUCTIONAL APRAXIA

Constructional apraxia was first recognized as being a distinct variant of the other forms of apraxia by Kleist in 1922. Its status as an apraxia has been questioned over the years as it does not conform to many of the criteria considered important by Liepmann. Constructional apraxia involves a defect in the spatial aspects of a task within the context of an integrity of individual motor movements. The problem is not purely one of either visuoperception or voluntary action, but rather appears to be a defect in the ability to transmit information from the visuoperceptual domain to the one of voluntary action.

The defect becomes apparent when the patient is given the task of representing space in some fashion, such as the copying or drawing of simple geometric designs. Deficits are equally apparent when the person is asked to copy a simple figure or to draw one from memory. Hécaen (1978) identifies a range of errors that can be observed on these tasks, including simplification, the closing-in phenomenon where the reproduction is placed very near to the model or indeed overlaps it, misalignment on the page or spatial disorientations exemplified by reversals or rotations, or a disruption of the vertical or horizontal axis. It is also important to test construction ability in three dimensions. This can be done with tests such as Benton's Three-Dimensional Praxis Test, Koh's Block Test and the Block Design subtest of the WAIS-R. The defects may only become apparent when the task is complex or three-dimensional.

It was not until interhemispheric differences became an area of popular investigation that significant changes in thinking began to occur with regard to constructional apraxia. There was a greater focus of attention on the differences observed between individuals with right hemisphere damage relative to those with left hemisphere damage. The findings of many of the studies suggested that constructional apraxia was more frequent and severe in those with right hemisphere injuries as opposed to left. More recent reports have questioned this finding, with the focus being more on the quality of errors made by the two groups as opposed to the quantity.

Some of the qualitative differences that have been noted on tasks performed by individuals with either right or left unilateral lesions are as follows: patients with left hemisphere damage tend to simplify their constructions, with fewer lines being used than the model; they have relatively greater difficulty on tasks requiring a large amount of manipulation; the presentation of a model improves their performance and they tend to maintain the overall spatial arrangement of the design. Patients with right hemisphere damage exhibit a rather disorganized approach to their constructions; they have relatively more difficulty with complex and three-dimensional figures; the number of lines used tends to be greater with

more detail being evident in their constructions; they tend to make errors in the spatial arrangement of the various parts of the figure and evidence of left neglect is often apparent. These widespread observations have led some to conclude that there may be two dissociated factors involved in producing this form of apraxia. Constructional apraxia following right hemisphere damage appears to be a product of a perceptual impairment, whereas constructional apraxia following left hemisphere damage appears to be an impairment in executive functions, i.e. a defect in the program for the action (Warrington, 1969).

Constructional apraxia has traditionally been associated with damage to the parietal areas. As observed by McCarthy and Warrington (1990), this fits well with the nature of the errors detailed above. However, constructional apraxia has been noted in patients with more anterior lesions. Luria and others contend that frontal injuries can produce a constructional apraxia by disrupting the planning and organization necessary for the correct reproduction of a spatially complex pattern. In this case it also becomes a problem of programming and intention.

Given the nature of the damage necessary to produce constructional apraxia, it is generally associated with a number of other clinical problems. Constructional apraxia resulting from left hemisphere damage often co-occurs with impairments of more posterior-based language functions and on occasion the Gerstmann syndrome or some of its elements. With right hemisphere damage there is often an associated impairment in the recognition of corporeal and extra-corporeal space (Hécaen, 1978). Patients presenting with this form of apraxia stemming from left hemisphere damage often have an associated fluent aphasia. Mesulam (1985) suggests that a language impairment may contribute to the problem, but the association is more likely to be a function of the contiguity of the regions producing the two problems.

ORAL APRAXIA

Oral apraxia or buccofacial apraxia is characterized by an impaired ability to carry out to command skilled movements of the face, lips, cheeks, tongue, pharynx, or larynx. It was first described by Hughlings Jackson (1878). It is characterized by difficulties on tasks such as pretending to suck on a straw or to stick out the tongue. It appears not only to impair gestures having symbolic qualities, but is also seen with the imitation of meaningless actions. As pointed out by Heilman and Rothi (1985) these patients, although not improving significantly with imitation, do improve when using an actual object, such as a straw. As with the other forms of apraxia, oral apraxia is generally only evident when the movement is to command and is preserved when performed fortuitously.

In their studies of oral apraxics Tognola and Vignolo (1980) found that this impairment was associated with lesions in the frontal and central opercula and the anterior part of the insula. Other studies that have required the imitation of a sequence of three oral movements have found that failures are associated with lesions of other areas, such as the left frontal and left parietal areas. However, De Renzi (1989) believes that only single movements are appropriate for the testing of oral apraxia because of the additional and perhaps unrelated functions that are required to successfully complete a sequence. It is his contention that it is the anterior cortex which is the critical region for the planning and organization of these movements, with lesions in other areas perhaps only affecting functions such as the transfer of the motor commands.

It has now become quite common to refer to some expressive speech disorders such as Broca's aphasia as "apraxia of speech." The use of this term suggests that the deficit is somehow related to oral apraxia. Indeed, De Renzi (1989) questions whether apraxia of speech is in fact the "articulatory counterpart" of buccofacial apraxia. Various studies do suggest a close association between the two disorders, yet others show a dissociation. Given the available evidence it seems safe to assume that there are, in fact, two relatively independent mechanisms involved; as suggested by De Renzi, the observed correlations between the two disorders may be a function of the contiguity of the two motor association areas subserving buccofacial movements and the movements allowing speech production. This would tend to be confirmed by the observation that buccofacial apraxia can also be seen with conduction aphasia where output is fluent.

It has also been questioned whether a relationship exists between buccofacial and limb apraxia. Are both limb and buccofacial praxis governed by the same mechanism? Raade and others (1991) in

their study determined that they were not related. They found that the disorders presented differently according to the nature of the movement, that is, whether it was transitive or nontransitive, different error types were not proportional across the two groups and the neuropathology of the two groups was different. They concluded that the mechanisms underlying these two disorders appeared to be functionally independent.

DRESSING APRAXIA

The term apraxia has been given to other problems which appear to resemble, in some respects, the deficits characteristic of the more widely accepted forms of the disorder, such as the ideomotor and ideational types. One such problem is that of dressing apraxia, a syndrome given its name by Brain (1941). To observation the patient is unable to correctly orient items of clothing to their own body. This results in jackets being put on back to front, arms being put through neck holes, and buttons and laces, which cause particular problems, being left undone. There is a loss of all the automatic routines that allow most people to dress with little thought.

Dressing apraxia is generally seen in conjunction with deficits associated with right hemisphere lesions, such as visuospatial and constructional problems (Hécaen, 1978). It seems rarely to appear in isolation. As a result of its association with other disorders, the idea that it represents an entity independent of the other forms of apraxia has been seriously questioned. It has been speculated that it is simply a particular manifestation of an underlying problem, such as ideomotor apraxia, unilateral neglect, a disturbance of body image, or spatial disorientation. However, to reject the concept of an independent apraxia of dressing one must be able to explain why this form of apraxia can occur independently of other related problems, such as object manipulation and gesture. Anatomically, the problem is most frequently seen with either bilateral or unilateral right hemisphere lesions, particularly in the more posterior areas.

LIMB-KINETIC APRAXIA

Another disorder of voluntary action that has, by some, been termed an apraxia is that of a disturbance in the skill and delicacy of movements in actions both complex and simple (Lishman,

1990). The problem appears to be related to the psychomotor complexity of the task as opposed to the muscular complexity, and may be isolated to particular groups of muscles only. As Lishman points out, it is chiefly because it shows some characteristics of a paresis that its identification with the apraxias has been questioned.

MODELS OF APRAXIA

Even though it is now approaching 90 years since Liepmann first began to formulate his ideas on apraxia, it is still his theories with which more recent ones are compared. In brief, Liepmann believed that the many different varieties of apraxia all resulted from a disturbance of some mechanism, albeit at different levels of that mechanism. He identified three forms of apraxia: ideational apraxia, which he speculated resulted from an impairment at the stage where the concept or idea for a movement is stored or formulated; ideomotor apraxia, which he considered stemmed from an isolation of those areas of the brain responsible for formulating the plan for a movement from the area that controls the actual motor output; and finally, melokinetic apraxia, which results from a loss of the engrams for a particular movement. Liepmann's model, as described, was adopted and popularized by Geschwind (1965). He considered apraxia to be a disconnection phenomenon. Specifically he believed that a failure in the connection between the verbal-conceptual processing area and the motor association cortex of the dominant hemisphere would result in an inability of the person to carry out commands with either hand. The connection between these two areas, it is suggested, is made through the arcuate fasciculus, so when a person is told to carry out a command with his right hand it is this pathway which is used. If the command involves use of the left hand the impulse must travel across the corpus callosum from the left motor area to the equivalent area on the right. It follows from this model that lesions of the left parietal area or the arcuate fasciculus will render a person capable of understanding commands, but unable to respond motorically. However, as pointed out by Heilman and Rothi (1985), the person should still be able to imitate, but most often they cannot.

As an alternative to the above model Heilman and others (1982) raised the possibility that the left parietal lobe stores "visuokinesthetic motor engrams." These engrams provide information for a particular movement to the motor association cortex, which in turn programs the motor cortex to innervate the necessary muscles to allow a particular action to be produced. Using this model, the authors postulated that damage to the store itself would result in a person being unable to either carry out an act to command or be able to discriminate between the correct act and an incorrect act if carried out by someone else. On the other hand, if there is a disconnection between the parietal lobe and the motor association areas, the affected person should be able to distinguish an incorrectly performed act from one correctly performed, but still be unable to carry out the action to command themselves.

Based on these observations Heilman and Rothi believe there are two forms of ideomotor apraxia. The first, as described, results from lesions of the supramarginal or angular gyrus and leads to an inability to perform to command or imitation, in addition to being unable to distinguish a correctly performed action from one poorly performed. The second, resulting from a more anterior lesion, disconnecting the motor engrams from the motor cortex, can be subdivided into two different forms. It is suggested that a callosal lesion will lead to poor performance with the hand ipsilateral to the hemisphere containing the engram, despite intact performance with the contralateral hand. Patients with lesions in the hemisphere containing the motor engrams should not be able perform correctly with either hand.

McCarthy and Warrington (1990) discuss an information processing approach to apraxia which draws a sharp distinction between a failure in the completion of established acts, such as the use of a familiar object, and the inability to acquire or produce unfamiliar actions. Instead of making reference to "visuokinesthetic engrams" they use the term "schemas" to refer to a central program containing the representations of "over-learned routines." In using an object, one first needs to recognize that object and then to access the over-learned routine or schema necessary for its successful manipulation. A failure can result from inability to access information about the use of a particular object, an inability to access a relevant schema, or loss of the actual program. McCarthy and Warrington point out that poor access or damage to these schemas of over-learned behaviors cannot be used to explain ideomotor apraxia, where patients frequently show difficulty in carrying out unfamiliar actions. In these situations the person has no access to established schemas which allow a person to perform relatively complex behaviors with little thought. For a new action to be carried out, careful monitoring needs to occur and feedback from all concerned sensory modalities processed and learned. From this viewpoint, a failure to either learn or carry out an unfamiliar action, as in ideomotor apraxia, can be interpreted as a failure in selecting appropriate actions, placing them in a correct sequence, or holding them in memory.

RECOVERY FROM APRAXIA

Relatively little work has been carried out on recovery from apraxia or treatment methods. Clearly patients need to be taught alternative methods or routines for carrying out the functions they have lost, but there are, of course, some activities that have only one method of completion. Heilman and Rothi (1985) suggest that the body part as object error, often seen in those with ideomotor apraxia, is possibly a spontaneous compensatory strategy produced by the patient and as such should be encouraged. They believe the errors represent an attempt to generate a new movement by providing "an external representation for a lost or impaired internal reference from which to generate a skilled movement." One of the main reasons why there has been little emphasis upon treatment or therapy is because most forms of apraxia only become apparent under examination; the more severe forms of ideational apraxia are the exception. Research into compensatory strategies is certainly warranted as it may help to reveal some of the remaining questions that still exist regarding the mechanisms of the disorder.

Basso and others (1987) looked at the factors affecting recovery from ideomotor apraxia in acute stroke patients. They studied 26 acute patients and found the majority made a good recovery. Neurologically they observed that those with anterior lesions as opposed to posterior ones made a somewhat quicker recovery.

BIBLIOGRAPHY

De Renzi, E. (1982). *Disorders of space exploration and cognition.* New York: John Wiley.
De Renzi, E. (1989). Apraxia. In J. Boller & J. grafman (Eds), *Handbook of neuropsychology,* Vol. 2 (pp. 245–63). Amsterdam: Elsevier.
De Renzi, E., & Luchelli, F. (1988). Ideational apraxia. *Brain, 111,* 1173–85.
De Renzi, E., Pieczulo, A., & Vignolo, L. A. (1968). Ideational apraxia: a quantitative study. *Neuropsychologia, 6,* 41–52.
Basso, A., Capitani, E., Della Sala, S., Laiacona, M., & Spinnler, H. (1987). Recovery from ideomotor apraxia: a study on acute stroke patients. *Brain, 110,* 747–60.
Geschwind, N. (1965). Disconnexion syndromes in animals and man. *Brain, 88,* 237–94, 585–644.
Hécaen, H. (1978). Apraxias. In H. Hécaen & M. L. Albert (Eds), *Human neuropsychology.* New York: John Wiley.
Heilman, K. M., & Rothi, L. J. (1985). Apraxia. In K. M. Heilman & E. Valenstein (Eds), *Clinical neuropsychology* (pp. 131–50). New York: Oxford University Press.
Lehmkuhl, G., & Poeck, K. (1981). A disturbance in the conceptual organisation of actions in patients with ideational apraxia. *Cortex, 17,* 153–8.
Lishman, W. A. (1990). *Organic psychiatry: The psychological consequences of cerebral disorder,* 2nd edn. Oxford: Blackwell.
McCarthy, R. A., & Warrington E. K. (1990). *Cognitive neuropsychology: A clinical introduction.* London: Academic Press.
Mesulam, M. M. (1985). *Principles of behavioral neurology.* Philadelphia: Davis.
Ochipa, C., Rothi, L. J. G., & Heilman, K. M. (1989). Ideational apraxia: a deficit in tool selection and use. *Annals of Neurology, 25,* 190–3.
Raade, S. A., Rothi, L. J. & Heilman, K. M. (1991). The relationship between buccofacial and limb apraxia. *Brain and Cognition, 16,* 130–46.
Tognola, G., & Vignolo, L. A. (1980). Brain lesions associated with oral apraxia in stroke patients: a cliniconeuroradiological investigation with CT scan. *Neuropsychologia, 18,* 257–72.

MARCUS J.C. ROGERS

aprosodia Aprosodia is the loss of prosody in speech, prosody being the tone in the voice which conveys affective information. While, at least in right-handers, left hemisphere lesions interfere with the semantic aspects of language through APHASIA, right hemisphere lesions produce deficits in prosody.

A classification of aprosodia has been proposed, parallel to the classification of aphasias. This classification distinguishes spontaneous prosody, prosodic repetition, and prosodic comprehension, and also incorporates deficits in emotional gesturing which are closely associated with aprosody. The analysis produces motor, sensory, conduction, transcortical, and global forms similar to those identified in aphasia, which are assigned to areas in the right hemisphere homolateral to the parallel functional localization of aphasia in the left hemisphere. While this approach is attractive, it goes well beyond the available data about aprosodic deficits and should be regarded as an interesting and provocative hypothesis.

arcuate fasciculus The arcuate fasciculus (literally the "curved bundle") is a tract of fibers which connects the posterior part of the parieto-temporal junction with the frontal cortex. In the hemisphere specialized for speech it has been implicated in the language production system as one of the routes which may connect Wernicke's and Broca's areas. Lesions of the arcuate fasciculus result in a fluent dysphasia in which comprehension is relatively preserved but in which repetition is markedly defective.

Argyll Robertson pupil In this pupillary abnormality, the pupil is small and unaffected by light or shade; however, the pupil will constrict fully on convergence and dilate when convergence is relaxed. The Argyll Robertson pupil therefore reacts to accommodation but not to light, and is almost always indicative of neurosyphilis. The term is sometimes extended to other forms of abnormal reflex of the pupil in which the pupil is not necessarily smaller than normal, in which case the causes may include lesions of upper midbrain structures, and encephalitis.

arteriosclerosis Arteriosclerosis is a form of SCLEROSIS affecting the arterial blood supply to

the brain, and having the effect of producing cerebral ISCHEMIA.

The principal cause of arteriosclerosis is atheroma lining the walls of the cerebral arteries and narrowing them to a point where insufficiency of the blood supply results, or else a bolus of the atheroma lodges in the arterial supply (an *embolism*) completely occluding the supply at that point. In both cases the result is an INFARCT in the regions normally served from that point in the arterial supply. While the effects of arteriosclerosis may vary in the number and extent of the associated infarcts, the use of the term arteriosclerosis is normally employed where there is either general insufficiency throughout the cerebral supply or else diffuse multiple small occlusions, producing a generalized effect across the cerebral cortex.

The neuropsychological consequences of arteriosclerosis are a general dementia which may consist of a wide range of focal effects. There is a general reduction in cognitive abilities with impairments of memory, especially for recent events and names. Confusion and disorientation commonly occur and there may be emotional changes which include emotional lability and explosive emotional outbursts. Parkinsonian features may develop and epileptic phenomena occur in about a fifth of cases. A fluctuating course with day-to-day variability in performance is not uncommon. Progression of the disorder may lead to profound DEMENTIA, although insight and a capacity for judgment may be preserved longer than in other forms of dementia. The course of the dementia is highly variable and may be discontinuous, suggesting a pattern of repeated small strokes. The time to death is longer than in other forms of dementia.

Historically, it was conventional to classify the dementias of old age into "senile dementia" and arteriosclerotic dementia, and to differentiate these from the presenile dementias. With a recognition that the senile/presenile distinction was not a valid or helpful one, it is now conventional to classify the principal dementias as "dementia of the Alzheimer type" (with "senile dementia of the Alzheimer type" in old age) and *multi-infarct dementia* to denote dementias with a vascular origin. These multi-infarct dementias may be further classified into two types: in one there are diffuse subcortical white matter lesions with multiple small infarcts, often associated with hypertension and also called Binswanger's disease (progressive subcortical encephalopathy); in the other there are fewer, larger, cortical infarcts.

arteriovenous malformation Arteriovenous malformations (A-VMs), also known as angiomas, are congenital collections of abnormal blood vessels which result in disordered blood flow within the head. These abnormalities occur most frequently in the field of the middle cerebral artery and appear as a mass of enlarged and tortuous blood vessels located between one or more large arteries and one or more large veins. They may be associated with stroke by causing abnormal blood flow; with hemorrhage, as they are often inherently weak; and with deprivation of surrounding tissues of blood, as the blood flows almost directly from cerebral arteries into cerebral veins. Correction of these malformations may present a significant challenge to the neurosurgeon.

asomatognosia Asomatognosia is the loss of the knowledge or sense of one's own body and bodily condition. It may take many forms, which include unilateral asomatognosia, unawareness or denial of hemiplegia, most commonly on the left side following right hemisphere lesions; bilateral disorders which include GERSTMANN SYNDROME, AUTOTOPAGNOSIA, and asymbolia for pain (a reduced or absent response to painful stimulation); and bodily illusions and hallucinations, such as phantom limb and bodily distortion or displacement. These disorders are generally associated with the parietal lobe, but their independence from dysfunctions of language or spatial perception is an issue as yet unresolved.

assessment This entry provides an overview of the purposes and aims of neuropsychological assessment, outlines the information gathered in the interview component, and discusses the rationale underlying deficit measurement in clinical practice. It is concerned only minimally with the assessment of specific cognitive functions, as these functions have their own entries or are considered under entries on the neural systems which underlie them. The emphasis throughout is on practical issues in the assessment of individuals in a clinical setting.

THE AIMS OF NEUROPSYCHOLOGICAL ASSESSMENT

In the early days of clinical neuropsychology most neuropsychological assessment was aimed at answering questions concerning differential diagnosis and lesion location. With the rapid advances in brain imaging technology the importance of this aim has diminished; the focus of assessment has now moved firmly to identifying the cognitive and behavioral consequences of cerebral dysfunction whether this be for rehabilitative or medicolegal purposes. However, the neuropsychologist continues to play a valuable role in these former areas, e.g. in the diagnosis of dementing illnesses and in identifying the epileptic focus in clients who are candidates for temporal lobe resection because of intractable seizures. In addition, although most neuropsychologists work in acute neurological/neurosurgical services or rehabilitation settings, most also take direct referrals from general medical and psychiatric services. As a result of this they are often the first to establish evidence for the presence of a neurological disorder.

Medicolegal assessments constitute a significant part of many neuropsychologists' workloads. Areas in which a neuropsychological opinion is sought include issues of guardianship (e.g. is a client competent to manage his or her own financial affairs?), fitness to hold a driving licence, fitness to plead in criminal cases (i.e. could a client with known or suspected neuropsychological deficits follow a legal argument against him or her and have an appreciation of its import?), and evaluation of pleas of diminished responsibility (i.e. did pre-existing neuropsychological deficits impair a client's responsibility for his or her actions?). Most medicolegal assessment, however, arises from cases of personal injury compensation where brain injury has resulted from a road traffic or industrial accident. In such cases the clinical neuropsychologist is uniquely qualified to identify any genuine cognitive deficits that have resulted from the injury and to expose any potential exaggeration (see McKinlay, 1992).

In broad terms, neuropsychological assessment is aimed at answering the following questions:

1 Which components of the cognitive system

are dysfunctional, how severe is this dysfunction and also, just as important, which components have been spared?

2 To what extent has there been change in mood, comportment, and personality; to what extent are these likely to be a direct effect of neurological damage as opposed to a reaction to the injury or illness?

3 What are the implications of any changes in cognition, mood, and comportment for a client's everyday functioning now and in the foreseeable future?

4 Based on the pattern of cognitive strengths and weaknesses and changes in mood and comportment, what practical advice can be given regarding the design of any formal rehabilitation and what advice can be given to the client and significant others to help them adjust to any deficits?

These questions are answered by integrating information gained from an interview with the client (and whenever possible a relative or close acquaintance) and the qualitative and quantitative findings from formal neuropsychological testing.

THE NEUROPSYCHOLOGICAL INTERVIEW

Conducting a neuropsychological interview demands considerable empathy, tact, and intellectual effort. In many cases, clients will have multiple cognitive and physical disabilities and organically induced changes in mood and personality; they will also be attempting to cope with the often massive interpersonal and economic upheaval arising from their illness or injury. Added to this is the fact that a neuropsychological assessment can be anxiety-provoking because of potential threats to self-esteem or because of its medicolegal ramifications; some clients can exhibit more concern at the prospect of such an assessment than over the lengthy and sometimes painful and bewildering physical investigations they may have to undergo.

As in all clinical interviewing, time must be spent on establishing rapport and clarifying the nature and purpose of the investigation. General, open-ended, and non-threatening questions are employed, commonly followed by a request for the client to describe any problems they have been experiencing in their everyday life. The client's description of these everyday problems constitutes a principal source for the generation and refinement of clinical hypotheses which will be tested in the course of the examination. Such descriptions and follow-up questions are also crucial in establishing the degree of insight the client has into the nature and severity of his or her deficits. Lack of insight is a major barrier to effective intervention and a client's successful adjustment; a client may exhibit a cheery disregard in the face of severe deficits, coupled with grossly unrealistic expectations concerning a return to a former occupation or lifestyle; in other cases there may be a disproportionate concern with a relatively minor cognitive or physical problem when other deficits have much more serious implications.

Often the most useful clinical information from the interview is gained by asking clients about their short-, medium-, and long-term goals and how they intend to achieve them. Answers to such questions are relevant to assessing drive, mood, planning ability, and level of insight. If the client is not in competitive employment, enquiries about how they spend a typical day can also be employed to address these issues, which have implications for the approach that should be adopted in any rehabilitation or remediation attempts. As Brooks (1989) states in this latter context, "the examiner is attempting to estimate whether the patient is a passive receptor of disability or an active fighter struggling to achieve a better outcome" (p. 66).

The neuropsychologist has a large agenda to cover in the interview and will often be short of time; this necessitates a structured systematic enquiry. However, most formal neuropsychological tests also provide a structure for the client; the examiner sets out the concrete aims and rules and largely controls the pace and order of the items administered. It is therefore important that enough of the interview is minimally structured to determine the extent to which the client *initiates* and *organizes* the discussion of topics.

A detailed educational history is important in building a picture of a client's *premorbid abilities*. The history should include years of schooling (with a check on whether any of these were repeat years), the nature of any tertiary education and any further study (evening classes, day release, etc.), and formal qualifications and grades achieved. The possibility that health, economic, social, or attitudinal factors may have prevented a client achieving his or her full educational and occupational potential should be carefully explored.

Clients should be asked to describe the nature of their current and/or previous occupations, with a detailed breakdown of the duties and functions performed. The nature of their work and responsibilities provides additional clues to the general premorbid level of functioning, but also an indication of specific premorbid cognitive skills that are liable to have been strongly developed or highly practiced. The clinician should enquire about recent changes in the work environment (i.e. introduction of new technology, reorganization of duties) as such changes can often be the catalyst which exposes problems in an individual who had previously been coping despite diminished cognitive resources. A detailed breakdown is also essential for evaluating the prospects for and the timing of a return to work, and in developing recommendations regarding possible graduated resumption of former duties. The degree of detail required concerning *previous* employment history depends on the circumstances; the likely implications of current problems at work or a recent dismissal are very different for an individual with a previously solid work history than for an individual with a history of dismissals and drifting from one job to the next.

Lezak (1983) sets out a number of fundamental questions which must be addressed prior to formal testing. These include: Does the client understand the reason for referral and are there specific questions of their own they want answered? Do they understand the uses to which the information gained from the examination may be put and who will and will not have access to it (of particular importance in medicolegal contexts)? Do they know how and when feedback will be provided? Finally, do they appreciate that the assessment will largely be concerned with cognitive functioning (misperceptions abound) and are they aware of the general nature of the tests to be employed?

THE RATIONALE OF DEFICIT MEASUREMENT IN CLINICAL PRACTICE

Attempting to detect and quantify cognitive deficits in the individual case is problematic because of the wide variability in cognitive abilities within the general population. Scores on neuropsychological measures which are average or even above average can still represent a significant impairment for an individual of high premorbid skills (and may have serious implications for return to a previous occupation). Similarly, test scores which fall well below the mean do not necessarily reflect an acquired impairment. Because of this, *normative* comparison standards are of limited utility in neuropsychological assessment and must be supplemented by *individual* comparison standards when assessing acquired deficits (Crawford, 1992; Lezak, 1983; Walsh, 1991). Ideally this individual comparison standard can be obtained from psychological test scores obtained in the premorbid period. However, this is rarely a viable option; the amount of routine psychological testing conducted varies greatly between countries, so that many individuals may have had no prior formal testing. Even where such test results exist they are often difficult or impossible to obtain, the content of the tests may have limited relevance, or they may have been administered so long ago that they are of questionable value. Because of these difficulties clinicians normally have to settle for an individual comparison standard which is based on a client's current performance. The explicit rationale here is that (1) cognitive ability measures are almost invariably positively correlated, therefore performance on one measure allows some level of prediction of performance on another and (2) some abilities will be preserved, or relatively so, following most neurological injuries or illnesses. Thus the areas in which a client has performed best are used as the standards (i.e. estimates of *premorbid* ability) against which to compare performance on other measures. Large discrepancies between measures are taken as indicators of the presence and severity of acquired impairment (Lezak, 1991).

CONVERTING SCORES TO A COMMON MEASUREMENT SCALE

In constructing a neuropsychological profile of a client's strengths and weaknesses, most clinicians use instruments drawn from diverse sources. These instruments will differ from each other in the measurement scale used to express test scores; for some instruments no formal scaling will have been developed so that clinicians will be working from the means and standard deviations (SDs) of the raw scores from normative samples. The process of assimilating the information from these tests is greatly eased if the scores are all converted to a common scale of measurement.

Converting all scores to percentiles has the advantage that percentiles are easily comprehended by other health workers. However, because such a conversion involves an area transformation (i.e. the difference between a percentile score of 10 and 20 does not reflect the same underlying raw score difference as that between 40 and 50) they are not ideally suited for the rapid and accurate assimilation of information from a client's profile; percentiles are also inappropriate for use with many inferential statistical methods. One option is to convert scores to "deviation IQs" (i.e. mean 100, SD = 15) as tests commonly forming a part of the neuropsychologist's armamentarium are already expressed on this scale, e.g. memory indices from the Wechsler Memory Scale Revised (WMS-R; Wechsler, 1987) and estimates of general premorbid ability such as the National Adult Reading Test (NART; Nelson & Willison, 1991). The most common alternative is to use t scores (mean 50, SD = 10); the meaning of such scores is easy to communicate and free of the conceptual baggage associated with deviation IQs.

Regardless of which method is used, the clinician must constantly be aware that the validity of any inferences regarding relative strengths and weaknesses is heavily dependent on the degree of equivalence of the normative samples for the test results compared. Although the quality of normative data for neuropsychological tests has improved markedly over this decade, there are still tests used in practice which are standardized on small samples of convenience. Thus discrepancies in a client's profile may in some cases be more a reflection of differences between normative samples than differences in a client's relative level of functioning in the domains covered by the tests.

SPECIFIC TESTS FOR THE ESTIMATION OF PREMORBID ABILITY

Currently, the NART is the test most widely used to estimate premorbid ability. The NART is a single word, oral reading test consisting of 50 items. All the words are irregular, that is, they violate grapheme–phoneme correspondence rules (e.g. chord). Because the words are irregular, intelligent guesswork should not provide the correct pronunciation therefore the test taps *previous* word knowledge; as the test only requires the reading of single words, clients do not have to

analyze a complex stimulus and it is argued that the test therefore makes minimal demands on *current* cognitive capacity (Nelson & O'Connell, 1978). The development of the NART arose from the clinical observation that oral reading is commonly preserved in dementia (whereas reading for meaning is commonly impaired). However, the test is now used to estimate premorbid ability in a wide range of conditions.

To qualify for use as a measure of premorbid ability a test must fulfil three criteria (Crawford, 1992). First, as with any psychological test, it must possess adequate reliability. The NART has high split-half reliability/internal consistency, test-retest reliability and inter-rater reliability (see Crawford, 1992). Second, it must have high criterion validity. The NART is normally used to provide an estimate of general premorbid IQ against which current performance on the WAIS-R is compared. Thus to meet the second requirement the NART must be capable of predicting a substantial proportion of IQ variance. There has been some confusion in the literature on how to examine this issue so it is worth noting that it must necessarily be studied using unimpaired rather than clinical samples. In a clinical sample NART performance and performance on the criterion (e.g. WAIS-R) will commonly become dissociated, indeed it is the presence of such a dissociation (i.e. a large discrepancy between estimated premorbid ability and current ability in favor of the former) that is used to infer impairment. In most studies using the WAIS or WAIS-R as the criterion variable the NART predicted well over 50 percent of IQ variance. For example, in one study the NART predicted 66 percent of WAIS IQ variance in a sample of 151 healthy subjects (see Crawford, 1992).

The final criterion for a putative measure of premorbid ability is that test performance be resistant to neurological or psychiatric disorder. NART performance appears to be largely resistant to the effects of many neurological and psychiatric disorders (e.g. depression, schizophrenia, alcoholic dementia, closed head injury) and compares favorably with previously suggested alternative measures of premorbid ability such as the Vocabulary subtest of the Wechsler (e.g. Crawford et al., 1988). Mixed findings have been found in samples with probable dementia of the Alzheimer type (DAT). O'Carroll and colleagues (1987) readministered the NART to a sample of dementia cases after one year and found no change in performance, despite a significant decline on measures of dementia severity. Crawford and colleagues (1988) found that the NART performance of DAT cases did not differ significantly from matched controls, despite the presence of severe deficits on other cognitive measures and the presence of marked morphological and blood flow abnormalities on brain imaging. Stebbins and others (1988) in contrast found that NART performance was significantly impaired in DAT cases classified as moderate or severe, although impairment was not in evidence in mild cases. Any findings of impaired NART performance pose a threat to the validity of the test. However, the practical implications of impaired performance in cases of severe neurological disorder are not as serious as they may appear; in such cases the presence of deficits is unfortunately only too obvious, thereby obviating the need for the NART or a similar instrument to assist in its detection and quantification.

Most research on the NART's ability to estimate premorbid ability has used scores on IQ tests as the criterion variable. Although this is in keeping with the notion of obtaining an estimate of the general level of premorbid functioning, the NART also has the potential to provide estimates of premorbid functioning for more specific neuropsychological tests. For example, Crawford and others (1992) built a regression equation which can be used to estimate premorbid performance on the FAS verbal fluency test (this test simply requires the generation of words from initial letters under time constraints, yet it is one of the best validated measures of executive dysfunction arising from damage to the frontal cortex). Schlosser and Ivison (1989) derived a regression equation which incorporated age and NART scores to estimate performance on the Wechsler Memory Scale (WMS). These authors reported that the discrepancy between *current* WMS performance and *estimated* premorbid performance was a highly successful index for the detection and quantification of memory dysfunction in Alzheimer's disease.

RELIABILITY

Adequate reliability is a fundamental requirement for any instrument used in neuropsychology, regardless of purpose. However, when the concern is with assessing the cognitive status of an *individual* its importance is magnified, particularly as the demands of clinical practice are such that decisions must commonly be made based on information from single administrations of each instrument.

Information on test reliability is used to quantify the degree of confidence that can be placed in test scores, e.g. when comparing an individual's scores with appropriate normative data or assessing whether discrepancies between scores on different tests represent genuine differences in the functioning of the underlying components of the cognitive system as opposed to simply reflecting measurement error in the tests employed. In the latter case, i.e. where evidence for a *differential deficit* is being evaluated, it is important to consider the extent to which the tests are matched for reliability; an apparent deficit in function A with relative sparing of function B may simply reflect the fact that the measure of function B is less reliable. This point was well made in a classic paper by Chapman and Chapman (1973) in which the performance of a schizophrenic sample on two *parallel* reasoning tests was examined. By manipulating the number of test items the schizophrenic sample was made to appear to have a large differential deficit on one or other of the tests. Additional important considerations in identifying differential deficits can be found in the entry on DISSOCIATION.

Particular care should be taken in comparing test scores when one of the measures is not a simple score but a difference or ratio score. Such scores are quite commonly used in neuropsychological assessment, e.g. in the assessment of implicit memory functioning a priming score may be derived from the difference between completion of word fragments (e.g. c--pe- / carpet) from a list that has been primed in an earlier study phase and an unprimed list (performance on the unprimed list essentially controls for individual differences in verbal ability). This priming score will have poor reliability because the measurement error associated with the two lists is additive; for example, if the two lists had (equivalent) reliabilities of 0.75 and an intercorrelation of 0.6, the reliability of the priming score would be only 0.37. This compares unfavorably with the reliability of most explicit memory tests and raises the danger that the clinician may conclude that an individual has impaired explicit memory coupled with preserved implicit memory when the pattern may simply be an artifact of differences in reliability.

RELIABLE vs ABNORMAL DIFFERENCES

The distinction between the reliability and the abnormality of differences between test scores is an important one in clinical neuropsychology, particularly when assessment is conducted for medicolegal purposes. A difference between scores would normally be considered reliable if it exceeded the 95 percent confidence interval for the difference; a difference of this magnitude is unlikely to have arisen from measurement error in the instruments. Establishing if a difference is reliable is only the first step in neuropsychological profile analysis. There is considerable *intra*-individual variability in cognitive abilities in the general population, such that reliable (statistically significant) differences between tests of these different abilities are common. In evaluating the probability that a discrepancy reflects acquired impairment, it is important to consider the *abnormality* or rarity of the difference, that is, what percentage of the general unimpaired population would be expected to exhibit a difference of this magnitude?

Base rate data, which permits the clinician to assess the abnormality of test score discrepancies, is available for some neuropsychological measures. When such data is not available a simple formula can be used to estimate the abnormality of any discrepancy from the correlation between the two tests of interest. It is also possible to assess the abnormality of the discrepancy between a single test and a client's mean scores on a series of measures (Silverstein, 1984).

To highlight the distinction between the reliability and abnormality of a difference, take the example of a discrepancy between the General Memory and Attention/Concentration indices of the WMS-R. A discrepancy of 17 points would be necessary for a reliable difference ($p < 0.05$). Based on the averaged correlation between these two indices in the WMS-R standardization sample ($r = 0.51$), approximately 25 percent of the general population would be expected to exhibit a discrepancy of this magnitude; to be abnormal (operationally defined for the present purpose as a discrepancy which would occur in less than 5 percent of the general population) a 29 point discrepancy would be required.

The importance of evaluating the abnormality of discrepancies through base rate data or correlational techniques cannot be overstressed. Most clinical neuropsychologists have not had the opportunity to administer neuropsychological tests to significant numbers of individuals drawn from the general, healthy population. It is therefore possible to form a distorted impression of the degree of intra-subject variability found in unimpaired individuals. The present author's impression is that the degree of normal variability may commonly be underestimated, leading to a danger of over-interference when working with clinical populations. For example, Matarazzo and others (1988) have reported that, in the WAIS-R standardization sample, a sample presumed to be free of neurological or psychiatric disorder, the mean difference between an individual's highest and lowest WAIS-R subtest score was 6.7. For this difference (i.e. the subtest *range*) to be abnormal it would have to exceed 11 scaled score points. As subtests have an SD of 3 it can be seen that a subtest range of around 3 SDs is not unusual in individuals without acquired impairments. These considerations are just as relevant when profile analysis is carried out with more specific neuropsychological instruments. The WMS-R and WAIS-R are used here as examples simply because of the availability and quality of the relevant data.

MONITORING CHANGE

There are many situations in which the neuropsychologist needs to measure potential changes in cognitive functioning. Common examples would be to determine whether cognitive decline is occurring in an individual in whom a degenerative neurological process is suspected or to determine the extent of recovery of function following a closed head injury. In both these cases neuropsychological assessment will provide useful information to assist clients, relatives, and other health professionals to plan for the future. Monitoring the cognitive effects of surgical, pharmacological, or cognitive interventions in the individual case is also an important role for the neuropsychologist. Although the aim here is most commonly to determine if there has been any improvement, the possibility of detrimental effects can also be an issue. For example, many drugs can potentially impair cognitive functioning, particularly in the elderly; anticholinergic agents provide a good example, as they are widely used in the treatment of various conditions and can have serious cognitive effects.

In assessing the effectiveness of a rehabilitation effort it is often possible to obtain *multiple* repeated measures of an individual's performance before, during, and after intervention. A number of inferential statistical techniques can be used in this situation because there are multiple data points for the different phases (see Barlow & Hersen, 1984, for a treatment of single-case designs). However, in general clinical practice the neuropsychologist must often come to conclusions about change from only a *single* retesting. This situation will also arise in rehabilitation settings; although multiple measures may have been obtained on the training task(s), the issue of the generalizability of any improvement is often addressed by comparing single before-and-after scores on related but separate tests. Monitoring change on the basis of a single retesting is a formidable task except in cases where the level of change has been dramatic. It is rendered more formidable by the fact that many of the standard instruments currently used in clinical neuropsychology (e.g. the WMS-R, WAIS-R) do not have parallel versions. The clinician must therefore differentiate changes resulting from systematic practice effects and random measurement error from change reflecting genuine improvement or deterioration. Among other complications are the fact that (1) the magnitude of practice effects varies with the nature of the task; for example, the Performance subtests of the WAIS-R show larger practice effects than their Verbal counterparts; (2) the length of time that has elapsed between test and retest will influence the magnitude of effects; (3) a diminution of practice effects is to be expected in neurological populations, given the high prevalence of memory and learning deficits, but the expected diminution is difficult to estimate for individuals.

One approach to dealing with many of these considerable interpretive problems is to gather information from test–retest studies on the relevant neuropsychological tests. Provided that such studies report the test–retest correlations, means, and SDs, regression equations can easily be constructed to predict performance on retest from scores at initial testing. The predicted scores are then compared with the retest scores actually obtained by the client to determine if the observed gain or decline significantly exceeds that expected

(see Knight & Shelton, 1983, and McSweeny et al., 1993, for examples). The utility of this approach is determined by the extent and nature of retest studies available for a particular test. For example, the test–retest scores on memory tasks for an elderly client with suspected dementia could be compared with estimated retest scores derived from a healthy, elderly sample retested after a similar period to determine if a significant decline has occurred. For some questions test –retest data from a clinical sample may be used. For example a head-injured client's scores on measures of attention or speed of processing could be compared with estimated retest scores from a head-injured sample if the clinician suspects that the extent of recovery is atypical.

APPROACHES TO ASSESSMENT IN CLINICAL NEUROPSYCHOLOGY

Approaches to the assessment process can be characterized as falling somewhere on a continuum between what has been referred to as the "fixed, big battery" approach and a flexible, hypothesis-testing approach (Brooks, 1989; Walsh, 1991). In the former, a large comprehensive battery is routinely administered to all clients. This approach is most common in the USA and is exemplified by the Halstead–Reitan battery, which consists of a large number of specific neuropsychological measures, e.g. tests of tactual performance, sensory extinction, finger tapping, categorization, language functioning, which are often supplemented with a full-length WAIS or WAIS-R and personality inventories (see Reitan, 1986).

In the latter approach, measures are selected to test clinical hypotheses derived from the neuropsychological literature on a client's known or suspected disorder and from information gained from the interview. The process is a dynamic one; the results of preliminary testing are used to test or modify existing hypotheses and generate new ones. As a simple example, screening measures may detect problems with the organization of visual material which are consistent with spatial and/or planning deficits; follow-up measures can then be administered to evaluate these three competing possibilities.

Proponents of the flexible approach acknowledge that there is a potential danger of failing to detect a client's difficulties in some cognitive domains if the clinician focuses too rapidly on testing inadequate hypotheses. However, they argue that the fixed, big battery approach may represent an inefficient use of resources and is simply not an option in some hard-pressed services (Brooks, 1989; Walsh, 1991). Further, because of the time taken to complete an assessment, many of the measures may be administered by psychology assistants rather than clinicians. It has been argued that important clinical information may therefore be missed or misinterpreted (Brooks, 1989). It should also be noted that, because all clients and normative groups are given the same tests, services employing the fixed approach accumulate substantial data on their measures. Such databases are tremendous clinical assets. However, the very existence of this database and the resources expended to obtain it may promote a reluctance to replace existing tests with measures designed to reflect developments in neuropsychological knowledge.

Approaches to assessment can also be characterized by the emphasis placed on qualitative versus quantitative evidence. The extreme quantitative pole of this dimension is characterized by a strict statistical and actuarial methodology in which comparison of a client's test *scores* against various cutoffs is the principal focus. At the other extreme, tests are used to reveal qualitative features of a client's behavior, the emphasis being on how a task is approached rather than on empirical analysis of the test scores obtained. In the service of this end there may be major deviations from standardized test instructions, thus precluding statistical analysis in any case. Although there is no fundamental reason why this dimension should not be orthogonal to the fixed/flexible dimension, in practice they have tended to be correlated. The fixed battery approach arose from researchers working in the actuarial tradition, and the sheer number of measures administered almost demands the employment of actuarial indices to assist in the assimilation of the information obtained.

A strict quantitative methodology could be employed with the flexible hypothesis-testing approach. Indeed the term hypothesis-testing might be seen as implying this. Furthermore, influential figures in the development of this approach devoted considerable attention to quantification (Shapiro, 1973). However, many clinical proponents of this approach have tended to emphasize qualitative analysis, i.e. hypotheses may be expressed and tested in qualitative as well as quantitative terms (Walsh, 1991). It should be stressed that very few clinical neuropsychologists are at the extreme ends of this qualitative/quantitative dimension; qualitative observations are verified with quantitative instruments whenever possible, while recognizing that much important information is not easily amenable to such verification.

Qualitative observations have particular relevance in assessing the behavioral consequences of damage to the prefrontal cortex, given that changes in motivation, social comportment, and emotional regulation are the most common and serious sequelae (see Parker & Crawford, 1992). Furthermore, evaluations of formal tests which are specifically aimed at capturing the core *cognitive* problems (e.g. planning deficits, underutilization of feedback) indicate that our existing indices are of limited utility when used with individuals (Mountain & Snow, 1993). Thus considerable reliance must be placed on a careful scrutiny of a client's approach to a range of tasks to identify these cognitive difficulties. However, considerable scope exists to turn what are currently qualitative features of performance into quantitative measures. As a mundane example, error of commission on a number of neuropsychological tests (e.g. perseverative and rule-breaking errors on verbal fluency) can still only be utilized as essentially qualitative indicators. The research effort required to collect adequate normative data on the frequency of such errors would be relatively modest and would place interpretation of their occurrence in clinical populations on a sounder footing.

BIBLIOGRAPHY

Barlow, D. H., & Hersen, M. (1984). *Single case experimental designs: Strategies for studying behavior change*, 2nd edn. New York: Pergamon Press.

Brooks, D. N. (1989). Closed head trauma: assessing the common cognitive problems. In M. D. Lezak (Ed.), *Assessment of the behavioral consequences of head trauma. Frontiers of Clinical Neuroscience*, Vol. 7 (pp. 61–85). New York: Liss.

Chapman, L. J., & Chapman, J. P. (1973). Problems in the measurement of cognitive deficit. *Psychological Bulletin, 79*, 380–5.

Crawford, J. R. (1992). Current and premorbid intelligence measures in neuropsychological assessment. In J. R. Crawford, W. McKinlay, & D. M. Parker (Eds), *A handbook of neuropsychological assessment* (pp. 21–49). London: Erlbaum.

Crawford, J. R., Besson, J. A. O., & Parker, D. M. (1988). Estimation of premorbid intelligence in organic conditions. *British Journal of Psychiatry*, *153*, 178–81.

Crawford, J. R., Moore, J. W., & Cameron, I. M. (1992). Verbal fluency: a NART-based equation for the estimation of premorbid performance. *British Journal of Clinical Psychology*, *31*, 327–9.

Knight, R. G., & Shelton, E. J. (1983). Tables for evaluating predicted retest changes in Wechsler Adult Intelligence Scale scores. *British Journal of Clinical Psychology*, *22*, 77–81.

Lezak, M. D. (1983). *Neuropsychological assessment*, 2nd edn. New York: Oxford University Press.

Lezak, M. D. (1991). Identifying neuropsychological deficits. In R. G. Lister & H. J. Weingartner (Eds), *Perspectives on cognitive neuroscience* (pp. 357–67). New York: Oxford University Press.

McKinlay, W. W. (1992). Assessment of the head-injured for compensation. In J. R. Crawford, D. M. Parker, & W. W. McKinlay (Eds), *A handbook of neuropsychological assessment* (pp. 381–92). Hove: Erlbaum.

McSweeny, A. J., Naugle, R. I., Chelune, G. J., & Lüders, H. (1993). "*T* Scores for Change": an illustration of a regression approach to depicting change in clinical neuropsychology. *Clinical Neuropsychologist*, *7*, 300–12.

Matarazzo, J. D., Daniel, M. H., Prifitera, A., & Herman, D. O. (1988). Inter-subtest scatter in the WAIS-R standardization sample. *Journal of Clinical Psychology*, *44*, 940–50.

Mountain, M. A., & Snow, W. G. (1993). Wisconsin Card Sorting Test as a measure of frontal pathology: a review. *Clinical Neuropsychologist*, *7*, 108–18.

Nelson, H. E., & O'Connell, A. (1978). Dementia: the estimation of premorbid intelligence levels using the new adult reading test. *Cortex*, *14*, 234–44.

Nelson, H. E., & Willison, J. (1991). *National Adult Reading Test manual*, 2nd edn. Windsor: NFER-Nelson.

O'Carroll, R. E., Baikie, E. M., & Whittick, J. E. (1987). Does the National Adult Reading Test hold in dementia? *British Journal of Clinical Psychology*, *26*, 315–16.

Parker, D. M., & Crawford, J. R. (1992). Assessment of frontal lobe function. In J. R. Crawford, W. McKinlay, & D. M. Parker (Eds), *Handbook of neuropsychological assessment* (pp. 267–91). London: Erlbaum.

Reitan, R. M. (1986). Theoretical and methodological bases of the Halstead-Reitan Test Battery. In I. Grant & K. M. Adams (Eds), *Neuropsychological assessment of neuropsychiatric disorders* (pp. 3–30). New York: Oxford University Press.

Schlosser, D., & Ivison, D. (1989). Assessing memory deterioration with the Wechsler Memory Scale, the National Adult Reading Test, and the Schonell Graded Word Reading Test. *Journal of Clinical and Experimental Neuropsychology*, *11*, 785–92.

Shapiro, M. B. (1973). Intensive assessment of the single case. In P. E. Mittler (Ed.), *The psychological assessment of mental and physical handicaps* (pp. 645–66). London: Tavistock.

Silverstein, A. B. (1984). Pattern analysis: the question of abnormality. *Journal of Consulting and Clinical Psychology*, *52*, 936–9.

Stebbins, G. T., Wilson, R. S., Gilley, D. W., Bernard, B. A., & Fox, J. H. (1988). Use of the National Adult Reading Test to estimate premorbid IQ in dementia. *Clinical Neuropsychologist*, *4*, 18–24.

Walsh, K. W. (1991). *Understanding brain damage*, 2nd edn. Edinburgh: Churchill Livingstone.

J. R. CRAWFORD

association area Association areas are regions of the cortex which do not receive primary projections from sensory systems or have direct motor outputs. The interconnectivity of association areas is principally with other cortical regions.

The concept of association areas is a rather loose one, derived from a historical idea that all mental functions resulted from the interaction between and integration of the various sensory systems. One historical distinction is between primary projection areas of the cortex, which receive input from areas of the thalamus which have an identified origin (so-called "extrinsic" areas), while the association areas receive input from thalamic centers for which the sources of their afferents have not been identified ("intrinsic" areas).

An alternative approach is most clearly expressed in the work of Luria (1966), who described three levels of the functional cortical systems. In this scheme primary cortex receives information from sensory afferents and is therefore concerned with elementary levels of sensation; it is also the cortex from which motor afferents originate in the primary motor cortex. This primary cortex is the most highly localized, and is topographically organized for the visual, somesthetic, and motor systems. Secondary cortex is adjacent to the areas of primary cortex, and in the case of secondary sensory cortex receives input from the adjacent primary sensory cortex so that it is functionally concerned with perception, the interpretation of the elementary sensations received by primary cortex. There is some cross-modal input into the secondary sensory regions. In the case of secondary motor cortex, more complex patterns of movement are organized as opposed to the simple elementary movements which may be elicited from primary motor cortex. The evidence for this functional organization of primary and secondary cortex comes largely from studies of the stimulation of the cortex exposed at surgery (which is summarized in Penfield, 1975).

The remaining cortex in Luria's scheme is tertiary cortex and corresponds to what is generally understood to be association cortex. It is in these regions that higher-level cognitive processes of thinking, reasoning, problem solving, and the general intellectual processes are located. Because of the interconnectedness of the association areas, both within these regions and with the primary and secondary areas, there is a much lesser degree of localization of functions within these areas.

The reduced level of functional specificity within the association areas has been linked with the concept of PLASTICITY, particularly in lesions suffered by children. It is believed that plasticity, and so the potential for functional sparing and recovery, is greater following lesions of the association areas. This view is a matter of debate, and it may be invalid in that there is some confounding between the principal location of association cortex in the frontal lobes, the extent of the frontal lobes, and the particular functions

which the frontal lobes support. While there may be greater functional sparing and recovery following frontal injury in children, this may be as much due to the capacity for functional reorganization of a cognitive nature of the relevant functions associated with the frontal lobes, and the types of pathology sustained in frontal injuries, as to the fact that association cortex has been affected per se. Similar effects are not always found in non-frontal association areas.

BIBLIOGRAPHY

Luria, A. R. (1966). *Higher cortical functions in Man*. New York: Basic Books.
Penfield, W. (1975). *The mystery of the mind*. Princeton, NJ: Princeton University Press.

J. GRAHAM BEAUMONT

associationism Associationism is the term applied to a general doctrine that higher-order mental or behavioral processes result from the combination or association of simpler mental or behavioral elements. Its philosophical roots are in the British Empiricist tradition, and before that Aristotle. Scientifically, the concept has played an enduring role in many of the theories of psychology.

Within neuropsychology, the idea has been influential from the nineteenth century, particularly as a result of the writings of the neurologist Hughlings Jackson. Associationism was related to localizationist approaches, but rather than accepting the rigid localization of the cortical "diagram makers," associationists believed that certain regions of the cortex (the ASSOCIATION AREAS) were less definite in their functional specification in being the area within which the combinations of more fundamental elements were achieved. Within an association area, a lesion of a given size might have relatively indeterminate effects, particularly if it were placed towards the center of the association area; as the lesion was located closer to the boundaries of the association area, its effects would become more determinate in being influenced to a greater degree by the relative contribution of input from the adjoining area. The advantage of this conceptualization was that rough anatomical concordance between lesions that have similar psychological effects could be explained without having recourse to the existence of specific centers.

Although associationism is now infrequently referred to as a principle of cerebral organization, it is implicit in the principle of relative locationization covertly adopted by most practicing clinical neuropsychologists.

astereognosia Astereognosia (sometimes "pure astereognosia" or "tactile asymbolia") is the loss of the ability to recognize the nature of an object by touch. As such it represents the inability to appreciate the identity of an object explored by touch, even though other characteristics of the object may be perceived (i.e. in the absence of AHYLOGNOSIA and AMORPHOGNOSIS). However, there is considerable confusion in the literature as the term is also used in a broader sense, roughly equal to "tactile agnosia," and including any condition in which there is a failure of recognition in the tactile modality.

asthenopia Asthenopia (more correctly "cerebral asthenopia") is one of the recognition defects for drawn stimuli, and may be confused with SIMULTANAGNOSIA. Both are sometimes considered as "pseudoagnosias." In these disorders visual performance is broadly impaired and typically occurs after a prolonged testing session; continuation of the examination may lead to total suppression of optic function. The nature of these disorders of defective recognition of complex pictures is the subject of controversy, and their independence from related functional disorders is in doubt.

astrocytoma An astrocytoma is a tumor which develops from an astrocyte; astrocytes are the cells which form the greater part of the matrix or scaffolding in which neurons are embedded. Astrocytomas are a form of GLIOMA which infiltrate the brain substance but, being less rapid in growth than glioblastomas, they may be relatively benign and result in less dramatic neuropsychological consequences. Studies suggest that only a quarter to a third of astrocytomas result in mental changes. They may occur at any age and in either the cerebral hemispheres or the cerebellum.

asymbolia Asymbolia is a term now little used which has been subsumed within the definition of AGNOSIA. Insofar as it has any contemporary use, it is taken to be an abbreviation of *tactile asymbolia* (or *asymboly*), which is the impaired recognition of the identity of objects in the absence of more basic impairments in the recognition of basic tactile features (size, contour, density, texture, temperature). Asymbolia is therefore equivalent to tactile agnosia (see also ASTEREOGNOSIA, TACTILE PERCEPTION DISORDERS).

ataxia Ataxia is a general term used to denote incoordination, usually of voluntary movement. It is most commonly associated with lesions of the CEREBELLUM, providing there is no relevant sensory loss. The nature of the incoordination may have several aspects, so that initiation of the movement may be delayed, the course of the movement may be slow and jerky, periods of tremor may occur during the execution of the movement, there may be a failure to accurately reach the target of the movement, and subsequent limb corrections may occur. Any or all of these features may contribute to the decomposition of voluntary movements.

Specific terms are used to denote some of the abnormalities seen in ataxia. *Kinetic tremor* refers to oscillations which appear during the course of the movement, while *intention tremor* indicates the often larger oscillations which appear around the target at the termination of the movement. *Dysmetria* is the inability to eventually achieve an accurate final end position for the movement, *hypermetria* being overshoot, and *hypometria* being undershoot. DYSDIADOCHOKINESIA describes a failure to execute movements of constant force or rhythm, usually being demonstrated by tasks which require repetitive movement such as tapping. *Postural tremor* (or *static tremor*) appears when the patient is required to maintain a steady postural position, as with the arms extended. Ataxia of GAIT (*gait ataxia*) is a common sign in which the patient walks with a broad-based gait, often appearing as if drunk. Indeed, as alcohol affects the function of the cerebellum, the intoxicated individual is actually demonstrating cerebellar gait ataxia. Walking heel to toe is also difficult for ataxic patients, and the "heel-shin test," in which the patient is asked to run the heel of one foot down the shin of the other leg while sitting or lying, is commonly employed and results in poor performance. All of these symptoms may be exacerbated if the patient is directed to close the eyes and is thereby deprived of visual feedback, but this is less true of purely cerebellar ataxias than of lesions which also involve other structures, particularly the dorsal columns of the spinal cord. NYSTAGMUS may also occur.

Dysarthria often accompanies ataxia as a result of incoordination of the speech musculature following damage to the vermis of the cerebellum or to brain-stem cerebellar connections. There is a tendency for syllables to be slurred and abnormally separated, a phenomenon known as *syllabic* or *scanning speech*. Neurologists may demonstrate the dysfunction by requiring repetition of the phrase "baby hippopotamus." When severe, this form of dysarthria may result in explosive speech accompanied by violent grimaces, more commonly seen in ataxia resulting from multiple sclerosis and in the hereditary ataxias (see below), but it may also occur in association with CHOREA and ATHETOSIS.

The pathophysiology underlying ataxia is, in the great majority of cases, associated with the cerebellum. Damage to the medial zones of the cerebellum results in disorders of stance and gait, while damage to the lateral zones may result in ataxia of the arms, although gait may also be affected to a lesser degree. Ataxic deficits may, however, also follow from interruption of the afferent and efferent connections of the cerebellum, as in the spinocerebellar ataxias, which include most notably Friedreich's ataxia (see below), and in MULTIPLE SCLEROSIS. The history of the medical approach to gait ataxia has been presented by Schiller (1995), while the pathophysiology of ataxia is discussed by Diener and Dichgans (1992) and Thompson and Day (1993).

Optic ataxia, in which the patient is unable to perform coordinated voluntary conjugate lateral eye movements when these are solely under visual control, is also known as BÁLINT'S SYNDROME. It results from lesions which disconnect visual input from the appropriate regions of motor cortex, and is not therefore an ataxia in the more common usage of that term. Cortical lesions of the parieto-occipital areas may result in optic ataxia, and it is generally accepted that bilateral lesions are a prerequisite for the disorder.

A form of AGRAPHIA has also been historically referred to as *ataxic agraphia* but the term has been superseded by *apraxic agraphia*. In early discussions of agraphia a relatively severe form, in which the ability to form even single letters is lost, was described as ataxic, probably because the resulting attempts at writing appeared as a series of up and down strokes which bear no clear resemblance to letters. This deficit is now recognized as an APRAXIA.

Frontal ataxia is also a construct which is the subject of debate. As with ataxic agraphia, the disorder is probably more correctly considered as an apraxia, although this has not been unanimously accepted. The term *frontal gait disturbance* has been proposed as a less contentious alternative. The disorder is evident in an abnormal gait in which it appears as if the ground exerts a magnetic effect upon the feet, the disturbance being not simply ataxic, but involving tonic phenomena, oppositional rigidity, abnormal reflex activity, and particular difficulties of initiation. The disorder may extend beyond gait to more global whole-body movements such as lying down, rolling over, or getting up (*truncal* or *trunco-pedal* ataxia or apraxia). When standing, there may be a tendency to fall backward rather than to the side. This disorder, it is recognized, is not typical of frontal lobe lesions affecting motor function, and it is assumed that it involves frontopontine cerebellar circuits in some way that is still not clearly understood.

There are a number of other forms and causes of ataxia which should be noted. PARIETAL LOBE lesions of the somatosensory cortex may result in ataxia as a result of sensory loss, and these will routinely be excluded in considering a cerebellar origin for an ataxic disturbance. Ataxia may also result from polyneuropathy of the peripheral nerves with respect to either their motor or their sensory functions. A form of tropical ataxic neuropathy has also been described in a region of southern Nigeria: a generalized neuropathy which has been linked to a diet of cassava, which may have the effect of increasing levels of plasma cyanide, so interfering with vitamin B_{12} metabolism.

Historically, before the introduction of penicillin, one of the major causes of ataxia was neurosyphilis in the form of *tabes dorsalis*. The characteristic disorder in these patients of a broad-based gait, high lifting of the feet, and their heavy implantation upon the ground may be due both to a loss of postural functions and deficits in the higher level of control of posture and movement.

All forms of general paresis (GPI) may produce some form of ataxia, either in gait or in clumsy and uncoordinated use of the hands.

Ataxia may also be a feature of mild to moderate post-encephalitic states, although in the most severe states it is replaced or overlaid by muscular rigidity. There is a variant of the Guillain-Barré syndrome, characterized by ataxia, ophthalmoplegia, and loss of tendon reflexes, generally regarded as an inflammatory neuropathy but with possible central nervous system involvement, which is called *Miller Fisher Syndrome*. Ataxia may also be a prominent feature of WILSON'S DISEASE, and may be the defining symptom of one subgroup of patients with this disorder who have, predominantly, focal thalamic lesions. An interesting group of patients suffer contralateral ataxia following unilateral thalamic lesions, leading to the identification of the *thalamic ataxia syndrome* (Solomon et al., 1994). In such patients the lesions are generally in the ventral lateral and posterior nuclei of the THALAMUS, presenting with marked similarities to a true cerebellar syndrome.

In children, certain forms of cerebral palsy (*see* CONGENITAL DISORDERS) are associated with ataxia. When the clinical picture includes weakness and ataxia, then about one third of the children will also have visual field defects, and it is assumed that this form has some component of cerebellar involvement. *Ataxial diplegia* is most commonly seen, with the legs more severely affected than the arms, often first brought to attention through a developmental delay in the child walking.

FRIEDREICH'S ATAXIA

This condition is the commonest of the spinocerebellar ataxias and, while rare, one of the commonest of the hereditary disorders of the nervous system. An autosomal or rarely sex-linked condition, degeneration of the spinocerebellar tracts leads to cerebellar ataxia, dysarthria, nystagmus, and dysdiadochokinesis. Parallel disturbances in the corticospinal tracts lead to weakness and abnormal reflexes, and there is also peripheral nerve damage so that tendon reflexes are depressed, and dorsal column degeneration results in loss of postural sense. The disorder normally appears before the age of 20 and through a slowly progressive course results in death, usually by the age of 50 years.

Friedreich's ataxia is accompanied by generalized intellectual impairment in some, but not all, cases. Personality disturbances have also been described, but these may in part be secondary consequences of the diagnosis and the disability rather than primary effects of the disease process. Occasionally a schizophrenia-like disturbance with paranoid delusions and periods of excitement, labelled as "Friedreich's psychosis," has been described, but it is possible that this is a concurrent but independent disorder in those affected.

There are other forms of hereditary cerebellar ataxia, and these include: olivopontocerebellar atrophy, Refsum's syndrome (a chronic polyneuropathy), late-onset hereditary cerebellar degeneration, hereditary dentatorubral degeneration, progressive myoclonic ataxia, Angelman's syndrome, and some forms of hereditary spastic paraplegia (Campanella et al., 1992; Filla et al., 1992). Certain of these disorders may also be accompanied by intellectual impairment.

BIBLIOGRAPHY

Bannister, R. (1992), *Brain and Bannister's Clinical neurology*, 7th edn. Oxford: Oxford Medical Publications.

Campanella, G., Filla, A., & De Michele, G. (1992). Classifications of hereditary ataxias: a critical overview. *Acta Neurologica Napoli, 14*, 408–19.

Diener, H.-C., & Dichgans, J. (1992). Pathophysiology of cerebellar ataxia. *Movement Disorders, 7*, 95–109.

Filla, A., De Michele, G., Marconi, R., Bucci, L., Carillo, C., Castellano, A. E., Iorio, L., Kniahynicki, C., Rossi, F., & Campanella, G. (1992). Prevalence of hereditary ataxias and spastic paraplegias in Molise, a region of Italy. *Journal of Neurology, 239*, 351–3.

Lishman, W. A. (1987). *Organic psychiatry: The psychological consequences of cerebral trauma*. Oxford: Blackwell Scientific.

Rothwell, J. (1994). *Control of human voluntary movement*, 2nd edn. London: Chapman and Hall.

Schiller, F. (1995). Staggering gait in medical history. *Annals of Neurology, 37*, 127–35.

Solomon, D. H., Barohn, R. J., Bazan, C., & Grissom, J. (1994). The thalamic ataxia syndrome. *Neurology, 44*, 810–14.

Thompson, P. D., & Day, B. L. (1993). The

anatomy and physiology of cerebellar disease. *Advances in Neurology*, *61*, 15–31.

J. GRAHAM BEAUMONT

atherosclerosis Atherosclerosis is a pathological process in which cholesterol and other deposits (*atheroma*) are laid down within the walls of arteries, forming plaques which may subsequently ulcerate. The result is insufficiency of the cerebral blood supply (ISCHEMIA) which may eventually lead to a CEREBROVASCULAR ACCIDENT such as a STROKE

athetosis Athetosis is an abnormal involuntary (athetoid) movement consisting of slow writhing, particularly of the peripheral segments of the limbs. The condition may extend to one or both halves of the body, but when it is bilateral (and usually in this form congenital) the distribution of the cranial nerves is more severely affected, and includes facial grimacing, dysarthria, and dysphagia. In the unilateral form the upper limbs are more affected than the lower, and the patient may try to restrain the affected side with the unaffected hand. The movements interfere with the voluntary use of the limb, but may diminish as the patient lies down, and even disappear during sleep. Athetosis is considered to result from corticostriatal fiber degeneration leading to the release of alternating grasp and avoidance reactions.

atrophy, cerebral Cerebral atrophy describes physical shrinkage of the brain, and may be demonstrated by a variety of physical investigations, notably SCANS. As the brain shrinks, the additional space within the skull fills with additional cerebrospinal fluid. The potential causes of the shrinkage are various, but all essentially have the effect of the loss of either nerve cells or the supporting cells and tissues. The atrophy may be diffuse and generalized, or it may be concentrated in one region of the brain.

Cerebral atrophy may follow the resolution of the acute changes immediately following head injury, as a secondary result of contusions and hemorrhage, cerebral edema, and anoxia. The atrophy may be in the regions principally affected by the acute changes or may be more diffuse, affecting large areas of the cortex with widening of the sulci, accompanied by enlargement of the ventricles. If the atrophy is relatively localized, other distortions of the brain mass may occur.

Diffuse atrophy of the cortex will invariably be associated with a general dementia, although the amount of space visualized over the cortex does not correlate very highly with the degree of dementia. Conversely, an important indicator in the diagnosis of dementia is the presence of atrophy on physical investigation. Localized atrophy (for example, over the frontal lobes) may present with more focal neuropsychological findings.

A particular form of cerebral atrophy has been described in those who have pursued a career in boxing, associated with the "punch-drunkenness" of retired boxers, although modern medical controls have made the occurrence of this syndrome less common. Besides neurological disabilities which notably include motor disorders, both intellectual and personality changes have been described. The prime effects are on memory, where a chronic amnesic state may occur, together with a generalized dementia. The changes in personality include irritability, apathy, and uncontrolled outbursts of anger and violence (which may also be seen following moderate to severe head injury), but also frank psychotic states. Impotence may also occur. Pathologically, widespread changes occur, but the distinctive feature appears to be rupture of the septum and its associated regions.

Chronic alcoholism may also be associated with marked cerebral atrophy, associated with a picture of "alcoholic dementia" which includes social deterioration, difficulties with recent memory, and a progressive decline in the ability to manage affairs of everyday life, although it may be difficult to dissociate the primary neuropsychological effects from the secondary psychosocial effects of the alcohol dependence. The memory disturbances may be broadly similar to those seen in KORSAKOFF'S PSYCHOSIS, but it has been argued that these two forms of the AMNESIC SYNDROME can be distinguished. In chronic alcoholism the atrophy appears to be principally subcortical rather than cortical and presents with ventricular enlargement rather than as shrinkage around the cortex, although the latter does occur, where it tends to be greater around the frontal regions. This is consonant with the known pathology of the amnesic syndrome.

J. GRAHAM BEAUMONT

attention Two aspects of attention are defined. Attention is the selection of information for conscious processing and action, and also the maintenance of the alert state required for attentive processing. Those aspects of attention closest to aspects of neuropsychology will be stressed here.

HISTORY

The problem of understanding the process of selective attention is one of the oldest in psychology. William James wrote at the turn of the century, "Everyone knows what attention is. It is the taking possession by the mind in clear and vivid form of one out of what seem several simultaneous objects or trains of thought" (James, 1907).

The dominance of behavioral psychology postponed research into the internal mechanisms of selective attention in the first half of this century. The finding that the integrity of the brain stem reticular formation was a necessity to maintain the alert state added some anatomical reality to the study of an aspect of attention (Moruzzi & Magoun, 1949). The quest for information-processing mechanisms to support the more selective aspects of attention began following the Second World War, with studies of selective listening. A filter was proposed which was limited for information (in the formal sense of information theory) and located between highly parallel sensory systems and a limited-capacity perceptual system (Broadbent, 1958).

Selective listening experiments supported a view of attention that suggested early selection of the relevant message, with nonselective information being lost to conscious processing. However, on some occasions it was clear that unattended information was processed to a high level, since there was evidence that an important message on the unattended channel might interfere with the selected channel.

In the 1970s psychologists began to distinguish between automatic and controlled processes. It was found that words could activate other words similar in meaning (their semantic associates),

even when the person had no awareness of the words' presence. These studies indicated that the parallel organization found for sensory information extended to semantic processing. Thus selecting a word meaning for active attention appeared to suppress the availability of other word meanings. Attention was viewed less as an early sensory bottleneck and more as a system for providing priority for motor acts, consciousness, and memory (Posner, 1978).

Another approach to the problem of understanding selectivity arose in work on the orienting reflex (Kahneman, 1973). The use of slow autonomic systems (e.g. skin conductance) as measures of orienting made it difficult to analyze the cognitive components and neural systems underlying orienting. During the last 15 years there has been a steady advance in our understanding of the neural systems related to visual orienting from studies using single-cell recording in alert monkeys. This work showed a relatively restricted number of areas in which the firing rates of neurons were enhanced selectively when monkeys were trained to attend to a location. At the level of the superior colliculus (i.e. the midbrain), selective enhancement could only be obtained when eye movement was involved, but in the posterior parietal lobe of the cerebral cortex, selective enhancement occurred even when the animal maintained fixation. An area of the thalamus, the lateral pulvinar, was similar to the parietal lobe in containing cells with the property of selective enhancement (Wurtz et al., 1980).

Until recently, there has been a separation between human information-processing and the neuroscience approaches to attention using non-human animals. The former tended to describe attention either in terms of a bottleneck which prevented limited-capacity central systems from overload or as a resource that could be allocated to various processing systems in a way which is analogous to the use of the term in economics. On the other hand, neuroscience views emphasized several separate neural mechanisms that might be involved in orienting and maintaining alertness. Currently there is an attempt to integrate these two within a cognitive neuroscience of attention. For example, studies of visual search have incorporated a modern neuroscience view of a multichannel visual system with separate mechanisms for dealing with color, form, and motion, with the cognitive idea of a separate visual attention system needed for integrating information from these channels when the target requires it. We emphasize this integrated viewpoint (Treisman & Schmidt, 1982).

CURRENT KNOWLEDGE

Methods

An impressive aspect of current developments in this field is the convergence of evidence from various methods of study. These include performance studies using reaction time, dual-task performance studies, recording from scalp electrodes and lesions in humans and animals, as well as various methods for imaging and recording from restricted brain areas, including individual cells.

Current progress in understanding the anatomy of the attention system rests most heavily on two important methodological developments. First, the use of microelectrodes with alert animals allowed evidence for the altered activity of cell populations with attention. Second, anatomical (e.g. computerized tomography or MAGNETIC RESONANCE IMAGING) and physiological (e.g. positron emission tomography, magnetic resonance spectroscopy) methods of studying parts of the brain allowed more meaningful investigations of the localization of cognitive function in normal people. The future should see the use of localizing methods together with methods of tracing the time course of brain activity in the human subject. This combination should provide a convenient way to trace the rapid time-dynamic changes that occur in the course of human information processing. (See PET SCAN, SCAN.)

Principles

Three fundamental working hypotheses characterize the current state of efforts to develop a combined cognitive neuroscience of attention. First, there exists an attentional system of the brain that is anatomically separate from various data-processing systems and which can be activated passively by visual and auditory input. Second, attention is carried out by a network of anatomical areas. It is neither the property of a single brain area nor is it a collective function of the total brain working as a whole. Third, the brain areas involved in attention do not carry out the same function, but specific computations (supporting attentional functions) are assigned to different anatomical areas (Posner & Petersen, 1990).

It is not possible to specify the complete attentional system of the brain, but something is known about the areas that carry out three major attentional functions: orienting to sensory stimuli, particularly locations in visual space; detecting target events, whether sensory or from memory; and maintaining the alert state.

ORIENTING

Usually we define visual orienting in terms of the foveation of a stimulus. By foveation is meant a movement of the eyes that places the stimulus on the central part of the eye (fovea) which has the highest acuity. Foveation improves the efficiency of processing targets in terms of acuity, but it is also possible to change the priority, given a stimulus, by attending to its location covertly, without any change in eye or head position. When a person or a monkey is cued to attend to a location, events that occur at that location are responded to more rapidly, give rise to enhanced scalp electrical activity, and can be reported at a lower threshold. This improvement in efficiency is found within the first 150 msec after an event occurs at the location to which the subject is to attend. Similarly, if people are asked to move their eyes to a target, an improvement in efficiency at the target location begins well before the eyes move. This covert shift of attention appears to function as a way of guiding the eyes to appropriate areas of the visual field. Brain injury to any of the three areas that have been found to show selective enhancement of neuronal firing rates causes a reduction in this ability to shift attention covertly. However, each area seems to produce a somewhat different deficit. Damage to the posterior parietal lobe has its greatest effect on the ability to disengage from attentional focus to a target located in a direction opposite to the side of the lesion.

The effects of the parietal lobes of the two cerebral hemispheres are not identical (De Renzi, 1982). Damage to the right parietal lobe has a greater overall effect than does damage to the left parietal lobe. There is dispute about the reasons for the asymmetries. One account supposes that the right parietal lobe is dominant for spatial attention and controls attention to both sides of space, while the left parietal lobe plays a subsidiary role. According to another account, the right parietal lobe is influenced more by the global aspects of figures, while the left parietal lobe is more influenced by local aspects. A third view argues that the ability to disengage is handled symmetrically by each hemisphere, but the maintenance of the alert state is asymmetrical. Of course, more than one theory could be correct.

Lesions of the superior colliculus and the surrounding midbrain areas also affect the ability to shift attention. In this case the shift is slowed whether or not attention is first engaged elsewhere. This finding suggests that a computation involved in moving to the target is impaired. In addition, patients with damage in this midbrain area also return to former target locations as readily as to fresh locations that have never been attended to. Normal subjects and patients with parietal and other cortical lesions show a reduced probability of returning attention to a location already examined.

Patients with lesions of the thalamus and monkeys with chemical lesions of one thalamic nucleus (the pulvinar) also show difficulty in covert orienting. This difficulty appears to be in selective attention to a target on the side opposite the lesion, so as to avoid responding in error to distracting events that occur at other locations. A study of patients with unilateral lesions of this thalamic area showed a slowing of responses to a cued target on the side opposite the lesion, even when the subject had plenty of time to orient there. This contrasted with the results found with parietal and midbrain lesions, in which responses are nearly normal on both sides once attention has been cued to the location. Alert monkeys with chemical lesions of this area made faster than normal responses when cued to the side opposite the lesion, irrespective of the side of the cue. Data from normal human subjects, required to filter out irrelevant visual stimuli, showed selective metabolic increases in the pulvinar opposite the stimulus being attended (see THALAMUS).

These findings make two important points. First, they confirm the idea of anatomical areas carrying out individual cognitive operations. Second, they suggest a particular hypothesis of the circuitry involved in covert attention shifts. The parietal lobe first disengages attention from its present focus, then the midbrain is active to move the index of attention to the area of the target, and the pulvinar is involved in restricting input to the indexed area.

While the circuitry described above remains speculative, it is clear that patients with parietal lesions have difficulties in pattern recognition,

implying that somehow the parietal lobe damage comes to affect the processing of patterns (De Renzi, 1982). The dorsal pathway extending from the primary visual cortex to the parietal lobe appears to mediate selective visual attention. Considerable anatomical data suggest that a second ventral cortical pathway, leading from the striate cortex to the infratemporal cortex, is involved in processing color and form during pattern recognition. There is evidence from single-cell recording in alert monkeys that visual spatial attention affects this pattern recognition system. Attention to a visual location affects the processing of stimuli within the receptive fields of neurons of the V4 area. This area lies along the ventral pattern recognition pathway known to be active when monkeys are processing color and form information. While it is not known how attention gains access to V4, one likely candidate is via the pulvinar, which has close connections to both the parietal system and V4 (see CORTEX; Posner & Petersen, 1990).

Cognitive studies of normal humans have been important in exploring how attention influences pattern recognition processes. A major distinction is between the processing of simple features (e.g. line orientation and color) and that of items defined by a combination of features (e.g. a red vertical line). Simple features appear to be processed in parallel, that is, the search time is not affected by the number of nontarget items in the display. When targets are defined by a combination of attributes (e.g. the red vertical line) located within displays of highly similar nontargets (e.g. red horizontal lines and green vertical lines), the search appears to be a serial process and takes longer as the number of distractors increases. There is evidence that the visual orienting system described above is also involved in visual search.

One theory of how attention affects pattern recognition is that it works to combine separate features into unitary percepts. According to this view, simple features are not combined until one orients attention to them. It is for this reason that attention is necessary to search for a conjunction of features. When a target is made of features that are also present in distractors, there can be illusory conjunctions, due to an improper conjunction of elements from different locations. It is to avoid such illusory combinations that one attends selectively to each item present in the array (Treisman & Schmidt, 1982).

There is a second aspect to the visual orienting attention system. Just as we can attend to a spatial location, we can also attend to a small or large object. If one views a large letter composed of small ones, it is possible to attend either to the overall form or to its constituents. The size of the feature selected is a general property of visual system cells that relate to the type of sine wave to which they will be most sensitive (spatial frequency). When attending to local objects, people are relatively good at detecting high spatial frequency probes, but when attending to global objects they do relatively better for low-frequency stimuli.

There is evidence from both normal people and patients that the right hemisphere is biased toward global processing and the left toward local processing. When given a large letter made of small letters, patients with right parietal lesions copy the local letter but miss the global organization, while patients with left hemisphere lesions copy the global orientation while missing the local constituents (Robertson et al., 1988).

We have concentrated on visual orienting, since that has been the area in which integration between cognitive and neuroscience studies has been most advanced. However, the earliest studies of selective attention used the ears or both the eyes and the ears as channels for the presentation of sensory information. There is good evidence that one can bias processing toward one ear or one particular frequency. When this is done, the electrical signal from the selected channel is amplified with respect to information on unselected channels. When required to do so, subjects do quite well in attending to several channels at once. However, an exception to this generally good parallel processing arises when targets occur on more than one channel. The interference between targets can happen between as well as within sensory channels. The reasons for this form of sensory interference are discussed in the next section.

LIMITS ON ATTENTION

There are limits on how much we can attend to at one time. In perception, people are more successful at attending to different aspects of the same object than attending to those aspects of different objects. In performance, some of the limitations that arise in attending to different tasks simultaneously are related to the similarity of the information to which they must attend. It is more difficult to attend to sources of information when both are presented to the same modality than when they are presented to separate modalities. In a similar way, tasks that must be transformed into similar codes or which deal with similar semantic content are more difficult to attend to simultaneously than is the case when contents or codes are different. Over and above this, there is a more general limitation on how much one can attend to at one time.

This general limitation can be shown most clearly when all the specific sources of interference are removed. The reason for this limitation is unresolved. One important circumstance in which this limitation occurs is when people are required to detect two targets that occur simultaneously. In this situation there is a great deal of interference. This effect can be seen even when targets occur in separate modalities or when the only task is to decide if one or two targets have been presented. This finding underlies the idea that some limited system is involved whenever a signal (sensory or memorial) is to be consciously noted. There is also a good deal of evidence that the storage of recently presented information, the generation of ideas from long-term memory, and the development of complex schema all interfere with the detection of new signals (Duncan, 1980).

Perhaps because of these limitations, much of perceptual input goes unattended while some aspects become the focus of attention. Thus attending is jointly determined by environmental events and current goals and concerns. When appropriately balanced, these two kinds of input will lead to the selection of information relevant to the achievement of goals and lend coherence to behavior. The system, however, must remain sufficiently flexible to allow goals and concerns to be re-prioritized on the basis of changing environmental events. This balance appears to be adversely affected by major damage to the frontal lobes.

There is some evidence that areas of the frontal lobe may underlie this general attentional phenomenon. Some areas have been found to be active during both language and spatial tasks. Studies of blood flow and metabolism have shown frontal activation during tasks involving language and spatial imagery. Studies of normal subjects processing individual words show changes in blood flow for frontal midline areas, including the cingulate gyrus and the supplementary motor area, when subjects were required to process the input actively. Moreover, experimental studies show that the degree of blood flow in the anterior cingulate increases regularly as the number of targets to be detected increases. Thus this area appears to be sensitive to the mental operations of target detection.

The anterior cingulate has an internal organization that shows alternating bands of cells with close connections to the dorsolateral frontal cortex and the posterior parietal lobe (Goldman-Rakic, 1988). This organization suggests an integrative role because studies have implicated the lateral frontal cortex in semantic processing while, as we have seen, the posterior parietal lobe is important for spatial attention. The anterior cingulate might provide an important connection between widely different aspects of attention (e.g. attention to semantic content and visual location). Unfortunately, both cognitive and anatomical theories of this type of cognitive control remain highly speculative.

A persistent issue in cognitive psychology is whether one should think of an executive exercising voluntary control. In one sense this raises the issue of a homunculus and the possibility of an infinite regress. Despite this problem, there appears to be little doubt that there is some central control over our behavior and thought patterns. In particular, the study of human expertise in problem solving and other behavior has always considered a central executive system that can describe at least a significant portion of the mental operations involved in problem solving. The issue arises as to how close the central system exercising control of voluntary behavior is to the system exhibiting properties of limited capacity discussed above. There is no question that one can dissociate attention in the sense of awareness from voluntary control. During dreams while in rapid eye movement sleep, for example, we are well aware of events going on in a dream, but we seem unable to exercise voluntary control over them. On the other hand, lesions of the anterior cingulate can produce evidence for a lack of control over our own behavior. Patients may think that someone else controls the activity of their arms or that someone else controls their thought processes. A major area for the neuropsychology of attention will be understanding the complex relationship between awareness, limited capacity, and control from higher levels of cognition.

ALERTING

The earliest anatomy of attention involved maintenance of the alert state. Cognitive psychologists have studied changes in alerting, both by using long boring tasks with low target probability, such as is required by the military when monitoring radar screens for possible enemy planes or missiles, and by the use of warning signals, such as those used in foot races to get the runners to prepare to move quickly from the start position. In both of these situations, there is evidence that an increase in alertness improves the speed of target detection. The trade-off between improved speed and reduced accuracy with warning signals has led to a view that alerting does not act to improve the buildup of information concerning the nature of the target, but instead acts on the attentional system to enhance the speed of actions taken toward the target (Posner, 1978).

There has been some improvement in our understanding of the neural systems related to alerting over the last few years. Patients with lesions of the right frontal area have difficulty in maintaining the alert state. In addition, experimental studies of blood flow in normal people during tasks that demand sustained vigilance show right frontal activation.

The NEUROTRANSMITTER norepinephrine appears to be involved in maintaining the alert state. This norepinephrine pathway arises in the midbrain, but the right frontal area appears to have a special role in its cortical distribution. Among posterior visual areas in the monkey, norepinephrine pathways are selective for areas involved in visual spatial attention. At least one study shows that, during the maintenance of vigilance, the metabolic activity of the anterior cingulate is reduced over a resting baseline value. These anatomical findings would support the subjective observation that, while waiting for infrequent visual signals, one has to be prepared to orient, but one also has to empty one's head of any ideas that might interfere with detection (Posner & Petersen, 1990).

APPLICATIONS AND FUTURE DIRECTIONS

Much remains unknown concerning the macroanatomy of attention, particularly the anterior portions of the system. Studies of blood flow and metabolism in normal people should be adequate to provide candidate areas involved in aspects of attention. It will then be possible to further test the general proposal that these constitute a unified system and that constituent computations are localized.

We have made a start on understanding the circuitry that underlies the posterior attention system. However, more detailed cellular studies in monkeys are necessary to test these hypotheses and to understand more completely the time course and the control structures involved in covert shifts of attention. Even more fascinating is the possibility that the microstructure of areas involved in attention may somehow be different in organization from those areas carrying out passive data processing. Such differences could give us a clue to the way in which brain tissue might relate to subjective experience. Even in our current state of knowledge, ideas about attention have proved useful in integrating aspects of social developmental psychology with psychopathology.

The idea of attention as a network of anatomical areas makes relevant the study of both the comparative anatomy of these areas and their development in infancy. In the first few months of life, infants develop nearly adult abilities to orient to external events, but the cognitive control produced by the anterior attention system requires many months or years of development. Studies of orienting and motor control are beginning to lead to an understanding of this developmental process. As more about the maturational processes of brain and transmitter systems is understood, it could be possible to match developing attentional abilities with changing biological mechanisms. The neural mechanisms of attention must support not only common development among infants in their regulatory abilities, but also the obvious differences among infants in their rates and success of attentional control.

There are many disorders which are often supposed to involve attention, including neglect, closed head injury, schizophrenia, and attention deficit disorder. The specification of attention in terms of anatomy and function might be useful in clarifying the underlying bases for these disorders. The development of theories of deficits might also foster the integration of psychiatric and higher-level neurological disorders, both of which might affect the brain's attentional system.

BIBLIOGRAPHY

Broadbent, D. E. (1958). *Perception and communication*. London: Pergamon.

De Renzi, E. (1982). *Disorders of space exploration and cognition*. New York: Wiley.

Duncan, J. (1980). The locus of interference in the perception of simultaneous stimuli. *Psychological Review, 87*, 272–300.

Goldman-Rakic, P. S. (1988). Topography of cognition: parallel distributed networks in primate association cortex. *Annual Review of Neuroscience, 11*, 137–56.

James, W. (1907). *Psychology*. New York: Holt, Rinehart & Winston.

Kahneman, D. (1973). *Attention and effort*. Englewood Cliffs, NJ: Prentice Hall.

Moruzzi G., & Magoun, H. V. (1949). Brainstem reticular activation of the EEG. *Electroencephalography and Clinical Neurophysiology, 1*, 445–73.

Posner, M. I. (1978). *Chronometric explorations of mind*. Hillsdale, NJ: Erlbaum.

Posner, M. I., & Petersen, S. E. (1990). The attention system of the human brain. *Annual Review of Neuroscience, 13*, 25–42.

Robertson, L. C., Lamb, M. R., & Knight, R. T. (1988). Effects of temporal-parietal junction on perceptual and attentional processing in humans. *Journal of Neuroscience, 8*, 3757–69.

Treisman, A., & Schmidt, H. (1982). Illusory conjunctions in the perception of objects. *Cognitive Psychology, 14*, 107–41.

Wurtz, R. H., Goldberg, M. E., & Robinson, D. L. (1980). Behavioral modulation of visual responses in the monkey: stimulus selection for attention and movement. *Progress in Psychobiology and Physiological Psychology, 9*, 43–83.

MICHAEL I. POSNER AND PATRICK BOURKE

attention deficit disorder *See* HYPERACTIVITY.

Aubert's phenomenon The Aubert phenomenon is produced by seating the subject in a darkened room in a chair which can be tilted to the left or right. In front the subject sees a luminous rod which is to be set to the vertical. Normal subjects show an effect of head and body tilt so that the rod is misaligned away from the vertical in the opposite direction to that of the subject's tilt; this is the normal Aubert phenomenon.

Certain patients with frontal lesions, particularly in the prefrontal cortex, exhibit a greatly exaggerated Aubert phenomenon, and it has been suggested that this can be explained by COROLLARY DISCHARGE. These patients fail to generate appropriate corollary discharges in compensation for the muscular tonus which occurs during tilt, leading to a faulty perception of where the vertical should be. By extension, the patient is failing to keep proper track of where his or her body is located in space and so cannot accurately relate the external world to her or his own body. This may underlie the observed deficits in the judgment of egocentric space made by patients with prefrontal lesions.

auditory agnosia *See* AGNOSIA; AUDITORY PERCEPTUAL DISORDERS.

auditory evoked potential *See* EVOKED POTENTIAL.

auditory perceptual disorders Following damage of the forebrain in humans, auditory perceptual disorders encompass (1) a number of often overlapping clinical syndromes due to circumscribed and mostly bilateral lesions of the upper posterior temporal lobes and (2) several impairments in processing specific acoustic stimuli in apparently normally hearing patients with unilateral hemispheric lesions.

Current knowledge of these disorders relies on several single-case reports and on a few experimental studies of large series of patients. The evidence derived from the former is unsatisfactory, in spite of the relative wealth of clinical observations, because of confusion in terminology, heterogeneous testing conditions, and incomplete anatomical data. The evidence derived from experimental studies is scanty and the most sophisticated and recent findings concern the perception of music. The reader is referred to previous reviews (e.g. Ombrédane, 1944; Vignolo, 1969; Bauer & Rubens, 1985; Lechevalier et al., 1992) for discussions of this topic (*see also* AMUSIA).

EVIDENCE FROM SINGLE CASES

Clinical cases previously described cannot be precisely compared with one another, due to the lack of standard criteria of examination and categorization of the syndromes. Some investigators label the clinical pictures as if they were discrete entities (e.g. word deafness, sound deafness, etc.) while others, following Freud (1891), employ the general term of auditory agnosia and then proceed to distinguish verbal from nonverbal auditory agnosia. Cortical deafness, pure word deafness (auditory verbal agnosia), auditory nonverbal agnosia, and mixed or incomplete auditory agnosia will be described here on the basis of 70 records published in 30 main neurological and neuropsychological journals from 1969 to 1992. Case reports have been analyzed and allotted to one of the above-mentioned syndromes, irrespective of the label actually given to them by the authors. Clinical cases of AMUSIA are not included in this series.

Cortical deafness is an auditory disorder due to hemispheric (cortical and/or subcortical) damage, clinically defined by the lack of recognition of spoken language, of nonverbal sounds and noises, and of music. The case reports published from 1969 to 1992 amount to about two cases per year on average (40 cases). It is found in both males and females of all ages (range 13–82 years, mean 48, SD 15.34) and in right- as well as left-handed individuals. It is more frequent in male (about 3 to 2), right-handed (about 3 to 1, some unspecified), middle-aged persons (mean 48 years). Cortical deafness follows a cerebral vascular accident in about three-quarters of cases, but it can occasionally be due to trauma, encephalitis, or other causes. Damage usually involves the temporo-parietal region bilaterally (about three-quarters of cases), though it may be occasionally confined to the same areas unilaterally (right or left).

In the typical patient the bilateral lesions develop in two stages. The first, often transient and neglected, cerebrovascular accident (usually involving the left temporal lobe) is followed by a second stroke in the right temporal lobe, which provokes cortical deafness. The opposite, right–left sequence is less frequent. This temporal pattern of damage is found in all bilateral clinical cases of auditory perceptual disorders. Following an acute phase in which loss of consciousness, mental confusion, and aphasia may be present,

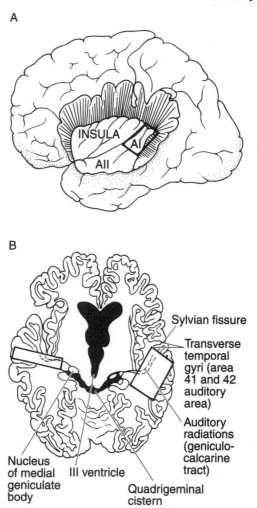

A

INSULA

AI

AII

B

Sylvian fissure

Transverse temporal gyri (area 41 and 42 auditory area)

Auditory radiations (geniculo-calcarine tract)

Nucleus of medial geniculate body

III ventricle

Quadrigeminal cistern

Figure 18 Approximate extent of the crucial areas of damage in the clinical case reports of perceptual disorders. Lesions, usually bilateral, either destroy or disconnect the auditory cortical areas – Heschl's gyri. (Modified after *Gray's Anatomy*, (Edinburgh: Churchill Livingstone), 1980, A, and after Mendez & Geehan, 1988, B, with permission.)

patients tend to improve, but they remain oddly unable to understand spoken language and to recognize noises and music. They may explain that they do hear but do not understand (almost one-third of cases) and in one case out of five they show the characteristic mimicry of a deaf person while, in fact, they are not deaf: they volunteer that they find themselves in a "strange" situation. Some of the patients' statements surprisingly recur in most published case reports, irrespective of the language community to which they belong; for example, "I hear the sounds bang within my head," or "everything I hear is strident like a baby crying." Voices may sound uniformly flat, ugly, and without the usual melody of speech, and music becomes an annoying and monotonous noise, like "somebody cutting cardboard." Occasionally patients say they feel as if they had a piece of cloth or a veil covering the ears. Patients frequently perceive all acoustic stimuli as dull and repetitious speech-like sounds, described, for example, as AOUAOUA or TA TA TAA. In rarer instances, patients say that they cannot hear their own voices. ANOSOGNOSIA for the disturbance is a

129

rare occurrence, while in more than half of patients the so-called acoustic inattention is present, i.e. the lack of the normal startle reaction following an unexpected, outstandingly loud noise. Surprisingly, patients sometimes do perceive the noise, so much so that, after a while, they volunteer that they have heard it, but they are not frightened by it in the least. The intellectual level is mildly defective in about 15 percent of cortical deaf people, probably due to the cerebral damage, since the impairment occurs independently of educational factors. The definition of cortical deafness implies that language outside the auditory input modalities is entirely spared. In fact, speech is mildly defective in about half the cases, due to the extension of the lesion to Wernicke's area. A follow-up study of the disorders has been made in only half the patients; of these, half have improved and the other half have remained stable or have become worse, in that the condition has been aggravated by auditory hallucinations and depression with paranoid ideas. Whenever improvement occurs, its extent is variable: sounds are mostly recognized before words and music, while in a few patients words are the first to recover. Occasionally improvement is limited to nonverbal sounds and noises.

In cortical deafness, the pure tone audiogram is often mildly impaired, though never to such an extent as to justify the clinical picture. Examinations of the middle ear are always normal, while the vocal audiogram score is nil. The acoustic evoked potentials selectively point to hemispheric dysfunction. Some recent authors emphasize the absence of wave Pa as selectively designating cortical deafness, though in two well-studied cases the whole range of the auditory evoked potentials was normal.

Pure word deafness (auditory verbal agnosia) is characterized by faulty recognition of speech with otherwise preserved language and with preserved recognition of nonverbal sounds, noises, and music. It is an infrequent syndrome. Out of 70 cases of auditory cerebral imperception found in the recent literature, only 6 can be defined as pure word deafness; two of them, moreover, could be so labelled only after the regression of the presenting aphasia. The patients are all right-handed, 4 males and 2 females, with age ranging between 24 and 69 years. The cerebral vascular accident is brought about by bilateral temporo-parietal lesions in 3 cases out of 6, left temporo-parietal lesions in 2, and purely left subcortical lesions in one. The typical patient with this syndrome is clinically less conspicuous than the cortical deaf; for example, he or she rarely behaves like a peripheral deaf person and only occasionally might show acoustic inattention. Patients claim that they do not understand spoken language, and sometimes volunteer that speech sounds like a foreign language (a fact which, by contrast, is virtually absent in Wernicke's aphasia). Patients sometimes complain that people talk too fast, and indeed discrimination is at its worst when the incoming speech is artificially accelerated or distorted, while it improves markedly when it is slowed down. By contrast, speaking aloud with increased volume has no beneficial effect. Patients often recognize the speaker's sex and mood by his or her voice and prosody, in spite of understanding nothing of what is being said to them. They usually recognize familiar noises and music.

The pure tone audiogram is normal or mildly impaired, a vocal audiogram cannot even be performed, middle-ear tests are perfect, and auditory evoked potentials point to lesions confined to the cerebral hemispheres.

Auditory nonverbal agnosia consists in the inability to recognize nonverbal noises, both familiar and meaningful or non-familiar and meaningless. This defect may or may not be associated with faulty perception of music. The disorder is clinically very rare: 3 cases out of the total sample of 70 under review. All of them are male, right-handed, their ages ranging between 55 and 65. The damage is centered upon the temporal lobe of the right hemisphere.

Clinically these patients are unable to grasp common noises: an automobile in motion is mistaken for a train or applause, a door repeatedly banging may be perceived as someone walking on a wooden floor, the tinkling of a bunch of keys may become a doorbell ringing. An examination of the type of errors discloses that most of them are "apperceptive" rather than "associative" in nature (according to Lissauer's terminology, 1890) in the sense that the noise is mistakenly perceived in place of another which is structurally and acoustically similar, rather than belonging to the same category of meaning. Finally, these patients have no problems in understanding speech, while their performance with respect to music is variable.

Mixed and/or incomplete auditory agnosia A number of clinical cases of auditory agnosia do not fit exactly into the previously discussed "pure" syndromes, either because they are not "pure" or because they are incompletely reported. This condition occurs in almost one-third of cases of cerebral auditory imperception. While incompleteness is self-explanatory, mixed syndromes are intended here as a superimposition of traits of the "pure" syndromes.

About half such patients (10 patients; 5 males, 5 females; all right-handed, with mean age 55 years, age range 36 to 64) fail to understand spoken language and to recognize nonverbal noises but lack the characteristics of full-blown cortical deafness. The lesion is temporo-parietal, bilateral in 8 cases, left unilateral in one case; it is not reported in one case. Etiology, whenever mentioned, is stroke in 7 cases and herpetic encephalitis in one.

The remaining half (9 patients; 7 males, 1 female, 1 unspecified; all right-handed, with mean age 65 years, age range 32 to 76) fail to understand spoken language and to recognize music in its various forms. The lesion, mostly due to stroke, is centered upon the temporo-parietal area and is bilateral in 5 cases, left unilateral in 3, and right unilateral in 1.

Careful perusal of all these case reports does not add further information to what emerges from the "pure" syndromes, except to alert the researcher about the often stressed difficulty of labelling clinical auditory imperception of hemispheric origin.

Rarer occurrences deserve mention. There are patients, such as those affected by the biopercular syndrome, whose main deficit is motor in nature, since it depends on bilateral vascular lesions placed in the frontal opercula; some of these lesions extend posteriorly so as to involve the temporal lobes and hence impair auditory recognition as well. Other uncommon cases, with unilateral left hemisphere lesion post-stroke, show right hemi-anacousis and auditory hemi-inattention. The interpretation of these symptoms is still controversial.

EVIDENCE FROM EXPERIMENTAL STUDIES

While the behaviorally conspicuous defects of auditory processing are mostly due to bilateral temporal lesions, several more discrete impairments which escape notice on a clinical examination may be disclosed by subtler, more specific auditory tests administered to series of unilateral hemisphere-damaged patients and controls for purposes of comparison. Such experimental investigations are still comparatively rare. They are designed to correlate the defective recognition of nonverbal auditory patterns with lesions in the right vs left hemisphere, in the temporal vs nontemporal and in the frontal vs nonfrontal lobes.

Milner in 1962 pioneered studies on series of patients (lobectomized epileptics) using musical tests; findings indicate that the anatomical structures subserving the recognition of nonverbal and perceptually complex auditory patterns belong to the right temporal lobe. These suggestions were supported by Shankweiler's (1966) research on brain-damaged patients and indirectly by Kimura (1964), who employed the DICHOTIC LISTENING technique in normal subjects.

Faglioni and colleagues (1969) investigated the relationship of nonverbal auditory agnosia to the hemispheric side of the lesion by means of two tasks, one requiring the discrimination of two "meaningless" sounds and the other requiring the association of a "meaningful" nonverbal sound to its meaning (e.g. *barking* with a picture of a *dog*). The performances of sizable samples of right and left hemisphere-damaged patients (with and without aphasia) and of normal controls were compared. Results indicated that poor discrimination of meaningless sounds (akin to Lissauer's 1890 "apperceptive" agnosia) was concomitant with right hemispheric damage, whereas poor association of meaningful sounds to their meaning ("associative" agnosia) was closely linked to those lesions of the left hemisphere which also brought about aphasia, particularly aphasia with poor comprehension.

Subsequent studies, carried out mostly on lobectomized patients by means of more refined auditory stimuli (see Samson and Zatorre, 1994, for recent data and references) convincingly support the hypothesis that integrity of the right hemisphere, particularly of the right superior temporal gyrus, is necessary for processing complex auditory patterns, such as melodic sequences, spectral features, and certain components of musical timbre. This view is consistent with the observation that blood flow increases in the right superior temporal gyrus when normal subjects listen to tonal sequences. The finding that, in commissurotomized patients, sound discrimination is performed by the right hemisphere points in the same direction.

AUDITORY PERCEPTUAL DISORDERS AND APHASIA

The concomitance of aphasia with Lissauer's "associative" level of nonverbal auditory recognition impairment (i.e. matching *barking* with the picture of a *cat* instead of a *dog*) seems well established (see Schnider et al., 1994) and is probably conceptual rather than perceptual in nature (see Vignolo, 1989, for discussion). By contrast, aphasic patients, even those with poor comprehension, are generally unimpaired at tasks, such as that used by Faglioni and others (1969), requiring the discrimination of meaningless noises and hence selectively tapping Lissauer's "apperceptual" level of nonverbal auditory perceptual disorders. This finding is puzzling, as one would expect a sound recognition defect to be at the origin of the auditory language comprehension impairment. And, in effect, a more complex picture is obtained when more sophisticated auditory stimuli are used. For example, it has been found that perceiving the succession of tones and clicks (Efron, 1963) is worse in left temporal lesions producing aphasia. A crucial element here seems to be the rapid change of acoustic information in nonverbal stimuli, such as complex tones; in other words, at least part of the comprehension deficit of aphasic patients reflects a disorder in auditory processing of discrete acoustic events rapidly following one another. A different line of research has focused on speech perception or "phonematic hearing," a field which conceptually lies at the interface of auditory perception and speech decoding. Inspired by the work of Luria (1970), several Western investigators (e.g. Blumstein et al., 1977; Basso et al., 1977) have studied aphasics' and nonaphasics' ability to grasp the distinctive acoustic features of incoming phonemes. Studies on the disorders of phonemic discrimination and categorization (as measured, for example, with voice-onset time: VOT) have shown that, while aphasics as a group are indeed more affected than normal and brain-damaged controls, the disorder is not specifically associated with impairment of auditory verbal comprehension. The scant evidence to date suggests that phonemic identification defects are associated with another aphasic feature, i.e. the number of *phonemic errors* in speech production, irrespective of the degree of comprehension of spoken language.

BIBLIOGRAPHY

Basso, A., Casati, G., & Vignolo, L. A. (1977). Phonemic identification defect in aphasia. *Cortex*, *13*, 85–95.

Bauer, R. M., & Rubens, A. B. (1985). Agnosia. In K. M. Heilman and E. Valenstein (Eds), *Clinical neuropsychology* (pp. 209–17). New York: Oxford University Press

Blumstein, S. E., Cooper, W. E., Zurif, E., & Caramazza, A. (1977). The perception and production of voice-onset time in aphasia. *Neuropsychologia*, *15*, 371–83.

Efron, R. (1963). Temporal perception, aphasia and déjà vu. *Brain*, *86*, 403–24.

Freud, S. (1953). *On aphasia: A critical study*. London: Imago (original work published in 1891).

Lechevalier, B., Lambert, J., & Eustache, F. (1992). Agnosie uditives et syndromes voisins (surdité corticale, surdité verbale pure). In *Encyclopédie médico-chirurgicale*. Paris: Éditions techniques.

Lissauer, H. (1988). A case of visual agnosia with a contribution to theory (translated by M. Jackson). *Cognitive Neuropsychology*, *5*, 157–92 (original work published in 1890).

Luria, A. R. (1970). *Traumatic aphasia: Its syndromes, psychology and treatment*. The Hague, Paris: Mouton.

Mendez, M. F., & Geehan, G. R., Jr. (1988). Cortical auditory disorders: clinical and psychoacoustic features. *Journal of Neurology, Neurosurgery and Psychiatry*, *51*, 1–9.

Ombrédane, A. (1944). L'Agnosie acoustique. In *Études de psychologie médicale, I: Perception et langage* (pp. 163–86). Rio de Janeiro: Atlantica Editora.

Samson, S., & Zatorre, A. R. (1994). Contribution of the right temporal lobe to musical timbre discrimination. *Neuropsychologia*, *32*, 231–40.

Schnider, A., Benson, F. D., Alexander, D. N., & Schnider-Klaus, A. (1994). Non-verbal environmental sound recognition after unilateral hemispheric stroke. *Brain*, *117*, 281–7.

Vignolo, L. A. (1969). Auditory agnosia: a review

and report of recent evidence. In A. L. Benton (Ed.), *Contributions to clinical neuropsychology* (pp. 172–208). Chicago: Aldine.

Vignolo, L. A. (1989). Non verbal conceptual impairment in aphasia. In F. Boller and J. Grafman (Eds), *Handbook of neuropsychology*, Vol. 2 (pp. 185–206). Amsterdam: Elsevier.

LUIGI A. VIGNOLO

autism In 1943 Kanner described early childhood autism. Autistic children have difficulty in relating to people early in life. In some cases this is evident from birth. The babies may not assume an anticipatory posture when they are about to be picked up, but rather arch away from their parents when held in their arms. For other autistic infants the disorder becomes evident during the second year of life, with social isolation and delay in language development. A further set of autistic children appears to have normal development initially but there is a regression during the second year.

Not all syndrome characteristics are shown by all autistic children, but a significant proportion are present in the majority of children with autism. There are clear language difficulties. Some children do not learn to speak at all. If language develops it may be used for naming and repeating rather than for communication. There is also an absence of the effective use of gesture in communication. Speech is characterized by literal repetition of phrases heard by the children, called ECHOLALIA, and by extreme literalness in the use of words. Eating difficulties are common during the first year of life. There can be extreme fear of certain noises and objects. There is minimal variety in spontaneous activity, with repetitions of noises or movements. An obsessive desire for sameness is associated with anxiety and distress if routines are altered. The children may have good relations with objects and may be fascinated by aspects of them for extended periods. Objects may be handled with skill and with fine dexterous motor movements. However, objects and toys are not played with imaginatively. The children may have excellent rote memories and a small number have highly developed precocious skills in certain narrowly defined areas. These highly developed skills, however, are not extrapolated to applications in more practical situations. Facial expressions are often serious but may be tense in the presence of others. Placid smiles may appear in a child's interaction with objects. Physical development in autism is broadly normal and the children's appearance is often bright and attractive.

DIAGNOSIS

Rutter has considered that in relation to the different aspects of autism there are four essential criteria for the syndrome diagnosis.

1. There should be onset of the syndrome before the age of 30 months.
2. Social development is impaired in ways which are not predicted from the child's general cognitive level of development.
3. Language development is delayed and deviant, also in ways not predictable from the overall level of the child's intellectual development.
4. There is an insistence on sameness, as shown by stereotyped play and abnormal preoccupations or resistance to change.

In the diagnostic system of the American Psychiatric Association (DSM-III-R) autistic disorder appears on axis 2 as a pervasive developmental disorder. The disorder is seen as distinct from a childhood version of schizophrenia, since there is absence of hallucination, delusions, and incoherence. In the DSM-III-R taxonomy, autism is characterized by a reduction in social interaction; impaired verbal and nonverbal communication with absence of imaginative play; and a restricted repertoire of interest. Characteristic behaviors are listed in relation to each of these groups, and where a critical number of the behaviors are manifest the clinician may diagnose autism. The DSM-III-R classification has been criticized as over-inclusive in comparison with previous criteria. The incidence of autism is generally quoted as 5 per 10,000 but narrow referral criteria may reduce the figure to 1 per 10,000. Diagnosis based on screening all children may raise the reported incidence to 16 per 10,000. There is a sex ratio in favor of males of approximately 3 or 4 to 1. Only a quarter to a third of autistic children attain IQ scores of above 70. For low-functioning children, IQ is predictive of outcome but for high-functioning children it is not.

INFANCY

While some autistic babies are placid and easy to manage, crying rarely, others are at the opposite extreme and will be restless and disruptive. There can be erratic sleep and feeding patterns and later there may be prolonged rocking and head-banging. A lack of interest in any social interaction may be evident early on and a responsiveness to the human voice may be reduced in relation to other children. While smiling and chuckling may develop at normal times, the responses are most easily elicited by the physical stimulation of tickling or bouncing rather than a social approach. The children's exploration of the environment is not normal. They do not point to things they want and do not attract the attention of parents to share an interest. An appearance of self-containment and contentedness in manipulating a limited number of toys in a repetitive way becomes apparent. Sometimes there is an intense fascination with early sensory experiences. They may gaze at one object or pattern for an extended period of time.

Studies of the noises made by autistic babies indicate that they can express emotions but have an idiosyncratic way of doing it, which mothers are able to learn and identify, but unlike the pattern with normal children they are not sufficiently universal to be comprehensible to carers who are unfamiliar with the child. The associated features linked to language development may also be abnormal. Facial expressions may be wooden or display extremes of emotion which are not appropriate to the social situation and context. While the child may physically move the adult to try to get something, they do not use gesture and pointing in a normal way. Attempts to teach autistic children sign language have had limited success. The vocal delivery of speech can be jerky, with poor control of pitch and intonation. At times the quality of speech resembles some of the articulatory patterns of those who have congenital hearing defects.

SPEECH DEVELOPMENT

It is suggested that even the early babbling patterns of autistic children may be abnormal, with greater monotony and less variation in pattern. About 50 percent of autistics remain mute all their lives. The amount of speech which develops may be related to intellectual development. Sometimes basic words can be learnt within conditioning paradigms when the child is reinforced for particular noises or sounds. When words begin to develop they tend not to have the same definition of lexical and semantic content as normal. Often there is not the rapid generalization to the category typical of normals. Nor is there the rapid acceleration of naming skills which characterizes normal child language development. When speech is produced it may consist predominantly of echolalia. Often the repetitions are with exactly the same inflections and accent as the original speaker. Normal children imitate adults by modifying grammatical rules to those the children are able to utilize themselves by missing out complicated aspects of language. The autistic child echoes verbatim. Some children begin to use appropriately phrases which are copied from others. Pronominal reversal in which the pronouns "you" and "me" are used instead of "I" was thought to reflect lack of awareness of personal identity and a rejection of self. However, it is now thought that the pattern of pronouns is linked to echolalic behaviors in which the ends of sentences tend to be echoed more frequently and the first personal pronouns occur less commonly in end positions. Autistic children vary in the amount of spontaneous speech which they produce. Often it requires great effort to produce speech and its character may be of immature or abnormal syntactic structure. There can also be a telegrammatic aspect to speech. The content of conversation is often restricted in range, with the use of stereotypical phrases and limited themes. Conversation is often linked to concrete pieces of information. There is an absence of the use of colloquial speech.

From early on there is a marked lack of interest in speech and there may be limited understanding of spoken language. Comprehension of language may be poorer than productive skills suggest. Idiomatic expressions tend to be taken literally. Problems of pronunciation are common. The use of inner language and imaginative play is absent. Those children for whom language develops tend to be less handicapped by the range of other associated social and behavioral disturbances. Autistic children's language may be distinguished from that of children who have developmental aphasic disorders (see APHASIA) by the absence of the use of spontaneous gesture and by the dominance of echolalic language within language production.

SENSORY RESPONSES

Variable and inconsistent responses to sensory

stimulation are common. Sometimes parents wonder if the child is deaf because of the lack of response to loud noises, yet a very subtle rustle of paper or a quiet noise may create a violent reaction. There may be over-sensitivity to certain noises, while other sensory stimulation produces an exaggerated fascination and delight. Some autistic children give the impression of having difficulty with recognition processes, and it may be difficult to determine whether the child has an agnosic aspect associated with their perceptual skills. People may ask whether the child is blind as well as deaf. Particular movements such as spinning and rotation may be of interest to the child. In some cases there is sensitivity to bright lights. An absence of conventional response to pain or temperature is sometimes noted. Excessive reactions to gentle touch may occur, with temper tantrums in response to conventional interactional situations such as hair-brushing and dressing. There may be food fads and bizarre dietary preferences suggesting possible anomalies in both taste and smell. Paradoxical responses are also sometimes observed, with children covering their eyes in response to a distressing sound.

Some autistic children appear to use peripheral rather than central vision and give the impression of not looking in the direction in which they are moving. Active avoidance of looking at faces is seen. This is thought to relate to social and behavioral interactions rather than to the nature of the perceptual stimulus itself.

SECONDARY BEHAVIOR PROBLEMS

Apparent social aloofness and indifference may be inferred by the observer because of the communication problems, gaze aversion, and dislike of touch. The absorption in concrete items rather than people may result in the exclusion of others. These aspects of behavior may be less marked in very familiar settings with well-known adults. Some aspects of social development may become established with language development. A lack of responsiveness is marked in relation to other children. There is resistance to change and excessive attachment to objects and routines. It may be difficult to predict which changes are accepted and which will cause distress. Management difficulties may occur where families are unable to modify or alter established routines in the face of changed circumstances without causing extreme distress to their child. There are

inappropriate emotional reactions with an absence of fear in situations which might be anticipated to elicit fear, such as height and danger. Laughter, crying, and giggling can also appear in inappropriate social situations. There is an absence of imaginative play, despite the focus of attention on playing with objects. Brighter children may be attracted by jigsaws and mechanical puzzles. There is socially immature and difficult social behavior with temper tantrums, screaming, and disruptive behavior, which may make it difficult for the family to move socially in the outside world with the child.

MOTOR PROBLEMS

Autistic children may experience difficulty in copying movements, with confusions of up and down, back and front, and right and left. They may have abnormal motor behaviors with jumping, flapping limbs, rocking, and grimacing, which may be exacerbated if the children are excited or absorbed. Sometimes there is a spring tiptoed walk without the appropriate swinging of the arms. An odd posture can be seen, standing with head bowed and arms flexed. Spontaneous large movements and fine skill movements may be clumsy in some children yet graceful in others. They find it difficult to acquire information by imitation and in the instruction of motor skills it is sometimes necessary to move the child's limbs through the procedures required, for example, to button clothing.

SPECIAL SKILLS

Some children have highly developed special skills. These tend to take the form of highly automated and rule-based behavior in which there is very good expression but sometimes an absence of basic comprehension and understanding. The precocious skills may take the form of unusual ability to conduct mathematical calculations; memory for prose or verbal listings; memory for music; and graphic and artistic skills. Cases where exceptional skills declined when speech developed have raised questions about whether the exaggerated skills present in autism reflect in part the absence of the involvement of certain brain regions in conventional activities. Many of the precocious skills of autistic children appear to give them extreme pleasure but cannot always be channelled in a constructive way that has a direct impact on other aspects of their life activity.

THEORIES OF ETIOLOGY AND THEORETICAL EXPLANATION

Family characteristics

Kanner stressed the high intelligence, educational and occupational achievement of parents of children with autism, though it is now established that autism occurs across social classes and cultures. Parental obsessiveness and coldness was noted along with low rates of severe mental disorder. It was suggested that cold, rejecting parents could precipitate autism in a genetically vulnerable infant. Other studies suggest that parental attitudes may reflect responses to having an abnormal child, rather than being causal. It has also been suggested that some of the rigidity in the behavior of Kanner's parents may have been related to the social circumstances of the time. The suggestion of family involvement in the etiology of the disorder, which was pervasive for some time, led in many cases to marked feelings of parental responsibility for the appearance of the disorder, which caused further distress and may not have facilitated the most constructive management of the autistic child. Interest in family characteristics has resurfaced with the development of broad-based genetic theories.

Genetics

A genetic contributant to autism is substantiated by the increased incidence of autism in the siblings of autistics with a 2–3 percent chance of a further affected sibling. Folstein and Rutter (1977) conducted an analysis of 21 pairs of twins for whom one was autistic. There were 11 monozygotic pairs and 10 dizygotic pairs. Among the 11 monozygotic pairs, 4 sets of twins were concordant for autism, a 36 percent concordance rate. Among the children who were discordant for autism, many of the nonautistic twins had some other form of congenital abnormality, with cognitive impairment, delayed speech, or problems saying words. A concordance for some form of developmental disorder occurred in 82 percent of the twin pairs for the monozygotes. Among the 10 pairs of dizygotic children there was no concordance for autism. One child did have a developmental cognitive impairment, so that there was a 10 percent concordance for a developmental

abnormality. This study indicates that heredity has a contributory role in autism, but the inherited abnormality may include but not be restricted to an autistic predisposer. For pairs of twins in which there is a discordance for autism there may be evidence of organic damage in the autistic twin.

Biological aspects

There is an increased risk of autism in a number of childhood physical disorders, and this has increased suggestions of a physical basis to the disorder. An increased risk of autism is seen following maternal rubella, cytomegalovirus, tuberous sclerosis, neurofibromatosis, untreated PKU (PHENYLKETONURIA), and, though with less overlap than had been thought, Fragile X. By the age of 18, 25–35 percent of autistics have seizures. Tics are also common. Early reports of hyperarousal of EEG and brain-stem EP abnormalities have not been substantiated. Recent EEG studies suggest abnormalities in P300 and a frontal negative component. Proposed oculovestibular abnormalities have also not been substantiated. CT is most commonly normal, though a small subgroup may have enlarged ventricles. Courchesne and others (1988) report cerebellar abnormalities on MRI and an abnormality in brain stem; cerebellar circuitry or limbic system continues to receive discussion. Bauman and Kemper, in a series of papers starting in 1985, report histological abnormalities at post-mortem in forebrain and cerebellum with abnormal neuronal dendritic trees. No replicable abnormalities are reported in PET studies but 3IP-NMR has implicated dorsal prefrontal cortex. In 30–50 percent of cases there are high blood serotonin levels.

Cognitive theories

Rutter (1978) has emphasized the importance of the linguistic deficit. The relative preservation of spatial over verbal skills once argued for a left-hemisphere cognitive deficit, but this has not been substantiated. Hobson (1990) has emphasized the importance of the social and affection deficits and the understanding of emotional signals. Others have discussed difficulties with the integration of multiple sensory inputs, attention difficulties, or reasoning difficulties associated with integrating higher-order information. The child's focus of attention on only part of a toy or part of a social situation might be related to a higher-order cognition integrative deficit. The biological abnormalities have suggested that there may be incomplete development of the distributed networks, which in current theory may underlie the representation of many cognitive systems.

Current developmental theories have discussed autism in relation to a deficit in "theory of mind." This is believed to underlie the ability to attribute a belief to a person, and at a higher level to predict what a person thinks about another person's beliefs. In the first classic experiment Wimmer and Perner's (1983) paradigm using two dolls, Sally and Anne, was employed. While Sally is absent from the room, Anne moves Sally's marble out of the basket where Sally had put it and hides it instead in Anne's own box. The examiner checks that the child remembers where the marble was in the beginning and where the marble is now. The child is then asked, "where will Sally look for the marble?" (This is a test of "conceptual perspective-taking.") Normal 3–4-year-olds understand that Sally's belief about the position of the marble differs from the reality of its new hiding place. Autistic children at a comparable intellectual level have a high error rate (Baron-Cohen et al., 1985), making reality-based judgments. Further experiments support the proposal of difficulty in reasoning about beliefs, desires, and mental states. Leslie (1987) calls the failure in the development of theory of mind a problem with metarepresentations which link the child's difficulties with pretence, social interaction, and communication. However, the theory remains controversial.

BIBLIOGRAPHY

Baron-Cohen, S., Leslie, A. M., & Frith, U. (1985). Does the autistic child have a "theory of mind"? *Cognition, 21,* 37–46.

Bauman, M. L., & Kemper, T. L. (1985). Histoanatomic observations of the brain in early infantile autism. *Neurology, 35,* 866–74.

Courchesne, E., Yeung-Courchesne, R., Press, G. A., Hesselink, J. R., & Jernigan, T. L. (1988). Hypoplasia of cerebellar vermal lobules VI and VII in autism. *New England Journal of Medicine, 318,* 1339–54.

Folstein, S., & Rutter, M. (1977). Infantile autism: a genetic study of 21 twin pairs. *Journal of Child Psychology and Psychiatry, 18,* 297–321.

Hobson, R. P. (1990). On acquiring knowledge about people, and the capacity to pretend: a response to Leslie. *Psychological Review, 97,* 114–21.

Leslie, A. M. (1987). Pretence and representation: the origins of "theory of mind". *Psychological Review, 94,* 412–26.

Rutter, M. (1978). Language disorder and infantile autism. In M. Rutter & E. Schopler (Eds), *Autism: A reappraisal of concepts and treatment* (pp. 85–104). New York: Plenum.

Wimmer, H., & Perner, J. (1983). Beliefs about beliefs: representation and constraining function of wrong beliefs in young children's understanding of deception. *Cognition, 13,* 103–218.

CHRISTINE M. TEMPLE

autocriticism Autocriticism has been described as a feature of callosal COMMISSUROTOMY in which patients produce frequent expressions of astonishment at the capacity of their left hand to behave independently of their conscious volition. Even at a considerable time from operation, some patients may express surprise when the left hand carries out some well-coordinated or obviously well-informed act, apparently outside conscious control by the patient.

automatism "Automatism" is one of a variety of names for complex behavioral and experiential manifestations of an ongoing epileptic discharge. Specifically it is a state of clouding of consciousness which occurs during or immediately after a seizure, during which the individual retains control of posture and muscle tone, but performs simple or complex movements or actions without being aware of what is happening. Amnesia for the period of the automatism is the prominent subjective feature. The epileptic basis for the automatism may be confirmed by simultaneous electroencephalographic recording, which most commonly reveals abnormality within the medial temporal lobe structures. The period of the automatism, and the complexity and apparent purposefulness of the behavior during the automatism, are all highly variable (*see* EPILEPSY).

autotopagnosia (autotopoagnosia) At the beginning of this century Pick (1922) described in

autotopagnosia (autotopoagnosia)

Table 6   Summary of neurological and neuropsychological findings in patients with autotopagnosia.

	Aphasia	Body part naming	Neuropsychological findings	Functional deficit	Site	Etiology
(1)	–	? Loss of orientation	Apraxia Dementia	Loss of mental body image	–	Hydrocephalus
(2)	–	?	Left parietal signs Inability to draw a human figure human figure	Loss of mental body image	Left parietal	?
(3)	Semantic aphasia	+(O)	Left parietal signs	Inability to analyze a whole into details	Left parietal	Tumor
(4)	Semantic aphasia	+ (O)	Left parietal signs	Inability to analyze a whole into details	Left parietal	Tumor
(5)	–	+ (O)	Left parietal signs	Inability to analyze a whole into details	Left parietal	Hematoma
(6)	–	+ (O, E, M)	Left parietal signs	Loss of discrete body image	Left parietal	Tumor
(7)	Mild aphasia	± (HP)	Left parietal signs	Loss of conceptual representation	Left parietal	Metastatic tumor
(8)	–	± (O, M)	Amnesia Mild dementia	Loss of body visuospatial represen- tation	–	Dementia

(1) Pick, 1922; (2) Engerth, 1933; (3) De Renzi & Faglioni, 1963; (4) De Renzi & Scotti, 1970; (5) Poncet et al., 1971; (6) Ogden, 1985; (7) Semenza, 1988; (8) Sirigu et al., 1991.
Key: Body part naming: (O) = own; (E) = examiner; (M) = mannikin; (HP) = human picture; + = spared; – = impaired; ± = mildly impaired.

two demented patients a dissociation between a spared ability to name their own body parts singled out by the examiner and an almost absolute inability to point to the same body parts on verbal command. This symptom was term *autotopagnosia* (AT), literally meaning lack of spatial knowledge about one's own body.

Despite the scarcity of reported cases (see Table 6) autotopagnosia ranked very high in popularity among neurologists and psychologists, being considered proof of the existence of a specific cognitive function involved in the representation (*Vorstellungbild*, Pick, 1922) of the body, with a neuronal substratum whose lesion would give rise to the symptom.

Clinical aspects   Difficulty in pointing to body parts on verbal command is not an uncommon finding among neuropsychological patients; most aphasic patients fail because of the task demand, which requires verbal mediation. Equally, right-hemisphere brain-damaged patients with lack of awareness of the contralateral space may fail to point to those parts of the body lying in the hemineglected field (personal neglect, see NEG-LECT). Attentional deficits, mental deterioration, and reaching disorders can equally interfere in the body pointing tasks; a detailed neurological and neuropsychological examination must therefore be carried out with the aim of disentangling the effects of more general factors.

The symptom   From the analysis of the reported cases it appears that autotopagnosia involves a difficulty in pointing to one's body parts, as well as those of the examiner or of a human picture. Given the nonselectivity of the deficit to one's own body parts, the term autotopagnosia seems not to be adequate, but *somatotopoagnosia* has not gained popularity.

The defective localization is equally evident in nonverbal tasks; patients are unable to point on their own body to the part corresponding to that touched by the examiner on her or his body, or to indicate on their body the part corresponding to an isolated drawing.

When faced with animal drawings some patients do not show any difficulty (Ogden, 1985) while others, although able to point correctly to the typical somatic elements (snout, tail), are unable to indicate the body parts shared with humans (e.g. eye, ear).

Autotopagnosia contrasts dramatically with implicit knowledge and use of body parts; in their daily life activities patients show a perfect orientation on their bodies. The same patients who are unable to point to their eyes may wear their spectacles perfectly. Dressing apraxia has been reported in some patients (Ogden et al., 1985; Sirigu et al., 1991), but skills involved in dressing are so numerous that a specific body knowledge deficit at the basis of dressing failure is not advocated.

Equally striking is sparing of naming body parts, ranging from perfect (Ogden, 1985) to mildly impaired (Semenza, 1988; Sirigu et al., 1991). The last dissociation is between a spared functional description of body parts and an inability to spatially define the same segments, despite being allowed to inspect her or his body.

Error analysis: random errors Following the examiner's command, the patient gropes uncertainly along her or his body, claiming that the target has disappeared, or points to items not belonging to his or her body.

Contiguity errors The patient touches a body part close to the target (hand–wrist; cheek–chin) or moves her or his hand around the target, claiming that the latter should be "around here."

Semantic errors The patient touches a body part functionally related to the target (ankle–wrist; hand–foot).

Finally, the significant effects of two factors must be remembered; the first is linguistic, the second perceptual.

Independently of the testing condition (verbal, nonverbal), the possibility of correctly locating a body part is linked to its lexical frequency (Semenza & Goodglass, 1985; Semenza, 1988).

Body parts that are perceptually well-defined, for example, the nose or the navel, are identified more easily than body parts without specific boundaries (e.g. joints or cheeks).

Accompanying symptoms On the basis of the frequent occurrence of autotopagnosia following left parietal lesion (see below) it is not surprising to find calculation and writing disorders, right –left disorientation, and apraxia (either ideomotor or ideatory) in most of the reported cases of autotopagnosia.

It is worth mentioning the fact that finger recognition deficits are absent in a consistent minority of the reported cases (De Renzi & Scotti, 1970) (*see* GERSTMANN SYNDROME and finger AGNOSIA).

Testing procedure In the last 30 years, numerous test batteries have been compiled with the aim of exploring the capacity for localizing body parts excluding the effect of possible concomitant factors. The batteries typically include the following tests (modified from Semenza & Goodglass, 1985):

(A) Tests requiring verbal mediation:

(1) subject points to their own body parts on verbal command;
(2) subject points to body parts of a sketch or a doll on verbal command;
(3) on verbal command, the subject points to a drawing of a single body part in isolation, presented in a multiple-choice paradigm.

(B) Nonverbal tests:

(4) the subject points to the examiner's body or to a drawing of a part which the examiner has touched on the subject's body;
(5) the subject points on her or his own body to the part which the examiner has shown as a single-part drawing.

Localizing value In some patients autotopagnosia appears in the context of the initial phase of a dementing illness (Pick, 1922, Sirigu et al., 1991), thus preventing any clinico-anatomical correlation. Most of the reported cases (see Table 6) have been affected by a left parietal lesion, almost always tumoral, primitive or metastatic, in nature. However, in clinical practice the vast majority of acquired cognitive disorders are vascular in origin. This may be because, in most cases, vascular damage involves not only the parietal but also the temporal lobe. As a result the concurrent appearance of aphasia and other neuropsychological signs complicates the picture.

EXPERIMENTAL INVESTIGATIONS AND THEORETICAL IMPLICATIONS

Most of the earlier case reports of autotopagnosia were re-examined in the sixties and seventies and several methodological problems were found: the observations were often anecdotal and, more important, the influence of concomitant factors was not adequately taken into account. This led some authors (e.g. Poeck and Orgass, 1971) not only to deny an autonomous status to the symptom, which was considered an artifact of the testing situation, but also to seriously question the existence and psychological reality of the concept of the Body Schema.

In the last 20 years, however, a series of single-case studies has convincingly shown that autotopagnosia cannot always be ascribed to the effect of more general impairments, mostly aphasia, and two hypotheses have been advanced in trying to elucidate the nature of the symptom: a spatial deficit hypothesis and a conceptual linguistic hypothesis.

The spatial deficit hypothesis If we consider the human body a finite set, the process of singling out a specific body part calls for the capacity of building and maintaining a clear image of how single parts are spatially related to one another within the set. If this process is disrupted by brain damage, autotopagnosia appears.

The next logical step is to see if autotopagnosia patients have lost this capacity only in regard to the human body or whether the deficit applies to any other cognitive operation that calls for dividing a whole into its components.

De Renzi and colleagues (De Renzi & Faglioni, 1963; De Renzi & Scotti, 1970) offer experimental support for the latter hypothesis; their patients were unable to point to parts of a bicycle or describe the relative position of the various parts of a car. More interestingly, although they were neither aphasic nor amnesic, they showed a striking difficulty in recalling the details of a complex scene or a well-known story in a logical sequence. If, however, they were asked definite and circumscribed questions, their performance was flawless. In the praxic sphere the same behavior appeared; use of single objects was correct, while carrying out a complex sequence of gestures was defective. According to De Renzi and Scotti (1970), this pattern of behavior was suggestive of a supramodal deficit reminiscent of Head's (1920) semantic aphasia and characterized by "a loss of power to appreciate or to formulate the logical conclusion of a train of thought." This impairment extends to a number of nonlinguistic performances, such as drawing

and topographical memory. Unfortunately autotopagnosia was not tested in Head's patients. The same line of thought can be seen for defective performance in recalling an itinerary, finding a town in an outline map of France, and oral spelling, in the autotopagnosic patient described by Poncet and others (1971).

De Renzi and others' conclusions did not stay unchallenged for long; at least three patients have been described in which autotopagnosia could not be ascribed to a general inability to analyze a whole into its details.

Ogden's (1985) patient was able to point correctly to different parts of real objects or pictures, even some as complex as the human body, or even more difficult in relation to spatial memory. He did not show any difficulty, for example, in putting the names of towns on an outline map of New Zealand. Similar findings were reported by Semenza (1988). The body part specificity of the spatial memory deficit in autotopagnosia was convincingly shown by Sirigu and others (1991). They attached ten small objects (e.g. a toy car) to different parts of the patient's body and the patient was asked to point, on command or on imitation, to a body part or an object attached in the same location. A striking dissociation was again evident; while unable to locate body parts even in the presence of the objects, the patient was able to locate perfectly the various objects. This ability was not dependent on a visual search strategy, since he was able to remember the exact location of the objects even when removed and after a long interval. This dissociation between body parts and object and picture pointing has been interpreted in various ways. According to Ogden (1985), autotopagnosia was a consequence of a loss of a "discrete body image," the characteristics of which were unspecified. An effort to clarify this issue was made by Semenza (1988) and Sirigu and others (1991).

The conceptual linguistic hypothesis In a series of group studies (Goodglass et al., 1986; Selecki & Herron, 1965) it was found that body part comprehension and naming can be selectively spared or impaired in aphasia in comparison with other semantic categories, suggesting a functional and structural link between knowledge of body parts and language processing abilities. An effort to clarify this issue was made by Semenza and Goodglass (1985). A group of aphasic patients was submitted to a body part localization task in

140

either verbal or nonverbal conditions. They found that a common factor underlies identification of body parts independently of testing conditions; the greater its lexical frequency, the higher the probability of its being correctly identified and standing out as a whole even in a nonverbal context. They therefore proposed that body parts are conceptually organized in a hierarchical way, determined by their frequency of use in language. In other words, the strength and precision of the representation of the body part as an isolated concept seems to be linguistically determined.

The concept of semantic organization of body parts as opposed to topographical representation was further reinforced by analysis of the errors made by the above authors' patients, regardless of testing modality (verbal versus nonverbal). Functional similarity errors (joint for joint, toe –thumb interchanges) and location similarities accounted for the majority of incorrect responses. In their study, however, no single patient showed body part identification impairment as a prominent neuropsychological symptom, nor did the authors compare body part identification tasks with other object or part-of-object identification tasks. However, this problem was recently overcome by the observation of a patient (Semenza, 1988) who, following a left parietal lesion and in the absence of significant aphasia, showed an almost isolated deficit in pointing to body parts as opposed to parts of other complex objects. This deficit was independent of the testing modality (verbal versus nonverbal) and a substantial proportion of her errors were semantically related.

The multiple representation theory Within the framework of cognitive neuropsychology (Shallice, 1988) the existence of a semantic system specific for the knowledge of body parts is hardly surprising, but it calls for a further analysis of its peculiarities and internal organization. This endeavor was elegantly accomplished by Sirigu and others (1991). They described a patient in the initial phase of a dementing illness, in many aspects similar to those reported by Ogden (1985) and Semenza (1988). The patient's errors in body part pointing tasks were mostly of two types: contiguity and functional substitution (*conceptual* according to Semenza & Goodglass, 1985). Through a statistical procedure, the authors checked the proportion of errors against the probability of occurrence by random pointing. Suppose that the target is a wrist; adopting a

random strategy, the possibility of pointing to a contiguous part (hand, forearm) is lower in respect to the possibility of making a functional substitution error (there are many joints). Correcting for this factor, they found that contiguity errors were the most frequent ones in all testing conditions. Moreover, *conceptual* errors were higher in the verbal condition, while the proportion of errors in the nonverbal condition did not differ from the chance level.

On the basis of this finding and those from the previous literature, they proposed that body knowledge can be represented in two systems, the first containing semantic and lexical information, organized according to linguistic and functional criteria, the second storing a body-specific visuospatial representation. These two systems can be selectively impaired following brain damage.

If the first system is damaged, a dissociation between impaired naming and spared localization tasks should appear; this was precisely what was found in a single-case study by Dennis (1976). If the body part visuospatial system is selectively damaged, a dissociation between "what tasks" and "where tasks" should necessarily take place, the *conceptual* errors reflecting the work of the verbal system which could reduce the range of choices to those body parts functionally related to the target.

BIBLIOGRAPHY

Dennis, M. (1976). Dissociated naming and locating of body parts after left anterior temporal lobe resection: an experimental case study. *Brain and Language, 3,* 147–63.

De Renzi, E., & Faglioni, P. (1963). L'autotopoagnosia. *Archivio Psicologia di Neurologia e Psichiatria, 24,* 289–319.

De Renzi, E. & Scotti, G. (1970). Autotopoagnosia: fiction or reality? *Archives of Neurology, 23,* 221–7.

Engerth, G. (1933). Zeichenstörungen bei Patienten mit Autotopoagnosie. *Zeitschrift für Neurologie, 143,* 381–402.

Goodglass, H., Wingfield, A., Hyde, M. R., & Theurkauf, J. C. (1986). Category specific dissociations in naming and recognition by aphasic patients. *Cortex, 22,* 87–102.

Head, H. (1920). Aphasia and kindred disorders of speech. *Brain, 43,* 89–165.

Ogden, J. A. (1985). Autotopoagnosia. Occurrence in a patient without nominal aphasia and with an intact ability to point to parts of animals and objects. *Brain*, *108*, 1009–22.

Pick, A. (1922). Störung der Orientierung am eigenen Körper. *Psychologische Forschungen*, *1*, 303–18.

Poeck, K., & Orgass, B. (1971). The concept of the body schema: a critical review and some experimental results. *Cortex*, *7*, 254–77.

Poncet, M., Pellissier, J. F., Sebahoun, M., & Nasser, C. J. (1971). A propos d'un cas d'autotopoagnosie secondaire à une lésion pariéto-occipitale de l'hémisphère majeur. *Encéphale*, *60*, 110–23.

Selecki, B. R., & Herron, J. T. (1965). Disturbances of the verbal body image: a particular syndrome of sensory aphasia. *Journal of Nervous and Mental Diseases*, *141*, 42–52.

Semenza, C. (1988). Impairment in localization of body parts following brain damage. *Cortex*, *24*, 443–9.

Semenza, C., & Goodglass, H. (1985). Localization of body parts in brain injured subjects. *Neuropsychologia*, *23*, 161–75.

Shallice, T. (1988). *From neuropsychology to mental structure*. Cambridge: Cambridge University Press.

Sirigu, A., Grafman, J., Bressler, K., & Sunderland, T. (1991). Multiple representations contribute to body knowledge processing. *Brain*, *114*, 629–42.

GIANFRANCO DENES

average evoked potential   *See* EVOKED POTENTIAL.

avocalia   The selective apraxia which involves the inability to sing, whistle, or hum may be referred to as avocalia or "motor amusia." The dysfunction occurs either in spontaneous production or on imitation, both for isolated notes and for melodies, and is assumed to result from an apraxia of the face, tongue, and larynx. There is a suggestion that a dissociation can occur for the reproduction of isolated musical sounds and the rhythm of melodies. There is little agreement on the location of lesions which may result in avocalia.

axial dementia   *See* DEMENTIA.

B

Babinski response The Babinski response (or *reflex*) is an alternative term for the extensor plantar reflex, more commonly and graphically referred to as "upgoing toe."

In normal adults there is a flexor plantar reflex to stimulation of the sole of the foot (particularly the outer border), but the presence of a corticospinal tract lesion results in an extensor movement of the toe; it turns upwards. It is, in fact, part of a more general reflex flexor response of the whole lower limb to a potentially harmful stimulus. In the first year of life the extensor plantar reflex is entirely normal, possibly because the corticospinal tracts are incompletely developed during this period. After this period, it is a significant neurological sign and is part of the standard neurological examination.

Bálint's syndrome The syndrome, first described by Bálint in 1909, consists of three symptoms. The first is that, presented with an array of stimuli, the patient gazes 35 to 40 degrees to the right and neglects not only the left visual field, but also other elements in the right visual field, even though spontaneous undirected gaze is directly ahead. Second, once an object has been identified, all other objects will be neglected. Third, there is a deficit in reaching under visual guidance (OPTIC ATAXIA). The syndrome occurs in the absence of cognitive deficits, without visual field defect, and the patient may use and name real and drawn objects normally, although there may be difficulty in reading. It is considered to be associated with bilateral lesions of the inferior parietal lobe, and is consequently rare.

barognosis The somesthetic deficit of the loss of tactile pressure sensitivity is barognosis. All disorders of tactile sensation are rare following

cortical lesions, and barognosis has been little studied as a dissociable function. Any deficit is more likely to be observed as a variability of response, rather than as a complete loss of ability. As with other disorders of the SOMESTHETIC SYSTEM, it is associated with lesions of the parietal lobe.

basal ganglia The basal ganglia are a group of interconnected subcortical nuclei in the forebrain and midbrain. It is known from pathological studies of some human neurologic diseases that abnormalities of the basal ganglia are associated with profound disturbances of the control of movement. Because of their involvement in human diseases, the basal ganglia have been the subject of intensive investigation by neurobiologists. These studies have revealed that the organization of the basal ganglia is quite complex.

DEFINITION AND CONNECTIONAL ANATOMY

The basal ganglia are composed of the STRIATUM, the GLOBUS PALLIDUS, the subthalamic nucleus, the ventral tegmental area, and the SUBSTANTIA NIGRA. The striatum is the main afferent structure of the basal ganglia. It lies beneath the cerebral cortex and receives massive input from the cerebral cortex. In addition, the striatum receives substantial input from the intralaminar nuclei of the THALAMUS, and an important input from the substantia nigra. In many mammals the striatum is a single structure, but in primates and some other orders the striatum is divided by a thick wall of fibers into two portions, the CAUDATE NUCLEUS and the PUTAMEN. The striatum sends its outputs to the globus pallidus and the substantia nigra. The primate globus pallidus is divided by a thin wall of fibers into an external segment and internal segment. In most mammals the internal globus pallidus is widely separated from the external globus pallidus and is termed the entopeduncular nucleus and, in animals with an entopeduncular nucleus, the external globus pallidus is simply termed the globus pallidus. The external globus pallidus projects primarily to the subthalamic nucleus. The subthalamic nucleus projects to the external globus pallidus, the internal globus pallidus, and the substantia nigra. The internal globus pallidus also receives direct input from the striatum and the internal segment of the globus pallidus projects to ventral and medial nuclei of the thalamus. The substantia nigra consists of two parts. The so-called pars reticulata is similar to the internal globus pallidus in that it receives input from the striatum and the subthalamic nucleus, and sends its output to the thalamus. In addition to projecting to the thalamus, the substantia nigra pars reticulata also projects to the superior colliculus, a midbrain structure particularly important in primates for the control of eye movements. Like the pars reticulata, the other portion of the substantia nigra, the pars compacta, receives striatal and subthalamic input. In contrast, it does not project outside the basal ganglia but rather sends its major projection to the striatum.

It is now recognized that the borders of the basal ganglia are larger than previously appreciated. The nucleus accumbens and olfactory tubercule, two brain structures ventral to the striatum proper, are now known to be ventral extensions of the striatum. Unlike the striatum proper, this ventral striatum receives its main input not from the cortex but rather from limbic system structures like the HIPPOCAMPUS, the AMYGDALA, and the primary olfactory cortex. The ventral striatum also receives a major input from the ventral tegmental area, a small midbrain nucleus that is analogous to the substantia nigra pars compacta. The ventral striatum projects to the substantia nigra and the ventral pallidum, a distinct region ventral to the globus pallidus. The ventral pallidum has some features of both the external and internal segments of the globus pallidus. Like the external segment of the globus pallidus, the ventral pallidum projects to the subthalamic nucleus. Like the internal segment of the globus pallidus, the ventral pallidum projects to the THALAMUS. The ventral pallidum also projects directly to both portions of the substantia nigra, the ventral tegmental area, and the hypothalamus.

THE CORTICO-STRIATAL-PALLIDAL-THALAMIC-CORTICAL LOOP

The basal ganglia can be conceptualized as functioning as an extensive recurrent loop emanating from and terminating within the cortex. The striatum proper receives input from virtually all areas of cortex and this input has a complicated pattern of termination within the striatum. In general, however, a given area of cortex projects to the closest region of the striatum, giving this projection a topographic character. Within the striatum, the terminals of cortical projections from distinct cortical areas do not intermingle, forming what may be distinct functional zones within the striatum. The pattern of projections to the ventral striatum is less clearly arranged. Those structures projecting to the ventral striatum are part of the so-called LIMBIC SYSTEM, a subsystem of brain thought to be involved in the control of motivation, arousal, and emotions. The hippocampus and amygdala are two important units of the limbic system and occupy positions within it analogous to the position occupied by the cortex in the control of movement, sensation, and higher-order cognition.

Since the basal ganglia receive input from all

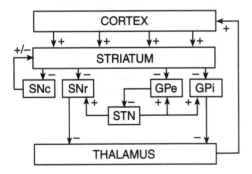

Figure 19 Schematic drawing of basal ganglia connections; SNc, substantia nigra pars compacta; SNr, substantia nigra pars reticulata; GPe, external segment of the globus pallidus; GPi, internal segment of the globus pallidus; STN, subthalamic nucleus; + excitatory projection; − inhibitory projection; +/− excitatory and inhibitory projection.

regions of cortex and analogous limbic structures, it is likely that the basal ganglia receive information pertaining to virtually all aspects of brain function. In contrast, the outputs of the basal ganglia are directed to a very limited number of targets. While there are some projections to the brain stem, notably the superior colliculus, the majority of output goes to certain nuclei of the thalamus. The internal globus pallidus projects to the ventral tier nuclei, while the substantia nigra pars reticulata and ventral pallidum project to the mediodorsal nucleus of the thalamus. These thalamic nuclei have distinctive projection targets. The ventral tier nuclei project to the motor cortex, the supplementary motor cortex, and the premotor cortex, all areas important in the control of movement. The ventral tier nuclei also project to the frontal eye fields, an area important in the control of eye movements. The mediodorsal nucleus of the thalamus projects to frontal cortical areas anterior to the motor and premotor cortices (prefrontal cortex) and these cortical areas have been implicated in higher cortical function. The basal ganglia funnel information derived from a broad variety of sources to a select group of cortical areas.

In terms of physiological function, the action of the basal ganglia may be to influence the level of activity of the cortical regions that receive projections from the ventral tier and mediodorsal nuclei of the thalamus. The projection from the thalamus to the cortex is excitatory while the projection from the basal ganglia to the thalamus is inhibitory. The basal ganglia output to the thalamus can consequently influence the level of activity in the cortex by varying the degree of inhibition of thalamic activity. This idea is undoubtedly a gross simplification of the effect of basal ganglia output on cortical function but it does provide a basis for thinking about basal ganglia function.

THE ORGANIZATION OF THE STRIATUM

The striatum is now known to be a very complicated structure. There are two major types of neurons within the striatum. At least 90 percent of the neurons within the striatum belong to one major type, the so-called medium spiny neuron. These neurons are characterized by their intermediate size and the presence of small knobby projections called spines on their dendritic arbors. Medium spiny neurons are projection neurons whose axons terminate outside the striatum, i.e. within the globus pallidus or the substantia nigra. In addition to the primary terminal outside the striatum, medium spiny neurons also have recurrent collateral axons that terminate within the striatum. Striatal medium spiny neurons appear to be divided into different subpopulations by the termination target of their primary axon. Medium spiny neurons project to one of the segments of the globus pallidus or one of the divisions of the substantia nigra without sending collaterals to any other segment of the globus pallidus or division of the substantia nigra.

The remainder of the striatal neurons lack spines, do not project outside the striatum (and are consequently termed interneurons), and are of varying size. There are large striatal neurons without spines but with extensive dendritic and axonal arbors and medium-sized to small striatal neurons with less extensive axonal and dendritic arbors.

One major advance in the past few years has been the discovery that the striatum is divided into two major compartments. One of these, termed the "patch" or "striosome" compartment, consists of tubular domains running through the surrounding "matrix" compartment. These two compartments are distinguished by differences in the content of neurotransmitter-related molecules including neurotransmitter receptors, neurotransmitter-related enzymes, neuropeptides, and neurotransmitters themselves. These two compartments also receive inputs from different areas and layers of the cortex, different parts of intralaminar/midline thalamic nuclei, and different neurons within the substantia nigra pars compacta. Medium spiny neurons within the patches tend to send their primary projections to the pars compacta of the substantia nigra, while those in the matrix send their primary projections to either segment of the globus pallidus to the pars reticulata of the substantia nigra. The functional significance of this compartmentation is not yet known.

NEUROTRANSMITTERS, NEUROMODULATORS AND NEUROTRANSMITTER RECEPTORS OF THE BASAL GANGLIA

The basal ganglia are richly endowed with a variety of neurotransmitters, neuromodulators, and neurotransmitter receptors. The primary neurotransmitter of the cortical projections to the basal ganglia is the excitatory amino acid glutamate. The primary neurotransmitter of striatal neurons projecting to the globus pallidus and substantia nigra is the inhibitory amino acid gamma-aminobutyric acid (GABA). Internal and external globus pallidus neurons, and substantia nigra neurons projecting to the thalamus also use GABA as their neurotransmitter. The identity of the neurotransmitter of thalamic neurons projecting to the cortex is unknown but is probably the excitatory amino acid glutamate. The primary neurotransmitter of the neurons projecting from the substantia nigra pars compacta to the striatum and of ventral tegmental area neurons projecting to the ventral striatum is dopamine.

Accompanying the primary neurotransmitters within neurons are a variety of peptides that probably play a role in the modulation of neuronal function. The presence of certain peptides seems to distinguish specific pools of striatal medium spiny projection neurons. Striatal neurons containing the opioid peptide enkephalin tend to project to the external globus pallidus, while striatal neurons projecting to the internal globus pallidus contain both the excitatory peptide substance P and the opioid peptide dynorphin. Striatal neurons projecting to the substantia nigra pars reticulata also contain substance P and dynorphin. Similarly, peptides are found within some neurons projecting to the striatum. Some substantia nigra and ventral tegmental area dopamine neurons also contain the peptide cholecystokinin. Large striatal interneurons without spines use acetylcholine as their primary neurotransmitter, while medium-sized to small neurons without spines contain a variety of peptides. The best characterized of these peptidergic striatal interneuron populations is a population of interneurons containing both the peptides somatostatin and neuropeptide Y. Uniquely among striatal neurons, these somatostatin/neuropeptide Y interneurons also possess the enzyme to produce the novel neuromodulator nitric oxide.

The basal ganglia are also endowed with receptors for most of the neurotransmitters and neuromodulators found within them. Complementing the rich variety of neurotransmitters within the central nervous system is an even richer assortment of neurotransmitter/neuromodulator receptors, with each type of neurotransmitter receptor possessing distinct subtypes. These receptor subtypes usually possess different functional features. The striatum and other nuclei of the basal ganglia are endowed with a variety of glutamate, dopamine, GABA, opioid, acetylcholine, and peptide receptor subtypes. The diversity of receptor subtypes within the basal ganglia indicates that synaptic information processing within the basal ganglia is likely to be complex.

MOVEMENT DISORDERS

Disorders of the basal ganglia are referred to by clinical neurologists as "movement disorders." This term is used to denote those diseases which do not have primary abnormalities of strength, sensation, or cerebellar function. Movement disorders were originally divided into a number of subtypes based on their clinical appearance. Recent analysis suggests a more rational division on the basis of their clinical appearance and clinical pharmacology into three broad categories: hyperkinetic movement disorders, hypokinetic movement disorders, and dystonic disorders.

Hyperkinetic movement disorders are characterized by an excess of involuntary movement and the fact that the movements are reduced by treatment with drugs that block the action of dopamine. There is a considerable range of abnormal movements in hyperkinetic disorders. The most violent and rarest of these disorders is HEMIBALLISM, which results from destruction of the subthalamic nucleus. Victims of hemiballism initially have wild flinging movements of the limbs contralateral to the destroyed subthalamic nucleus. In many cases hemiballistic movements subside into CHOREA, another form of hyperkinetic movement disorder characterized by milder, random, rapid movements which often have a writhing or sinuous character. The prototype choreic disease is HUNTINGTON'S CHOREA, an autosomal dominantly inherited disorder characterized by the presence of chorea, dementia, and degeneration of the striatum, especially the caudate nucleus. Underscoring the relationship between chorea and hemiballism is the fact that some Huntington's chorea patients with violent chorea have movements resembling hemiballism. The final hyperkinetic movement disorder is TIC. Tics are characterized by rapid, stereotyped movements which are often relatively complex motor acts. The prototype tic disorder is Tourette's syndrome (GILLES DE LA TOURETTE SYNDROME), a familial disorder known for motor and vocal tics.

Hypokinetic movement disorders are characterized by slowness of movement, loss of associated movements, rigidity, tremor, and impairment of postural reflexes. The classic hypokinetic movement disorder is PARKINSON'S DISEASE, an idiopathic degeneration of the pars compacta of the substantia nigra. The characteristic features of Parkinson's disease may be reproduced in normal individuals by drugs that block dopamine effect or deplete dopamine in the central nervous system, or by toxins that destroy midbrain dopamine neurons. Dopaminergic drugs reduce the symptoms of Parkinsonism and usually exacerbate the symptoms of hyperkinetic movement disorders.

The final category of movement disorders is dystonia. This movement disorder may affect the whole body, one side of the body, or just a small number of muscle groups. Most dystonias are idiopathic though some are due to focal brain injury or systemic disorders. Dystonic movements are fixed postures of the involved body part lasting from seconds to hours. These abnormal involuntary movements are distinct from those of hyperkinetic disorders and are not suppressed by drugs that block dopamine effect. Unlike Parkinsonism, dopaminergic drugs lack therapeutic benefit in the case of dystonic disorders.

THE PATHOPHYSIOLOGY OF MOVEMENT DISORDERS

The challenge of explaining the neural basis of movement disorders has been to explain why such a wide variety of abnormal movements accompany damage to the closely interconnected nuclei of the basal ganglia. It has also been difficult to explain how such similar movement disorders as hemiballism and chorea result from injury to different parts of the basal ganglia. Recent advances in understanding the anatomy and physiology of the basal ganglia have made it possible to construct models that can explain how such disparate clinical phenomena result from basal ganglia injury.

Hemiballism has historically been the only hyperkinetic movement disorder with a clear anatomic localization. Huntington's chorea is associated with striatal degeneration, but efforts to produce choreic movements by lesioning the striatum in animals failed, leaving investigators uncertain about the anatomic basis of chorea. The realization that hemiballism and chorea belonged to the same class of movement disorders and shared a common clinical pharmacology led to insight into the pathophysiology of hyperkinetic movement disorders. Destruction of the subthalamic nucleus removes a potent excitatory input to the internal globus pallidus and substantia nigra pars reticulata. As these two nuclei give rise to inhibitory projections to excitatory thalamic neurons projecting to the cortex, the thalamic neurons become more active and excessively activate their cortical targets. It has been shown in Huntington's chorea that there is selective degeneration of striatal neurons projecting to the external globus pallidus. This striatal-external pallidal projection is inhibitory and its loss means that the external globus pallidus is excessively active. As the external segment of the globus pallidus gives rise to an inhibitory projection to the subthalamic nucleus, the end effect is excessive inhibition of the subthalamic nucleus, a state analogous to the destruction of the subthalamic nucleus that underlies hemiballism. As with hemiballism, the final pathway is deficient activation of the internal globus pallidus and substantia nigra pars reticulata, resulting in excessive thalamic and cortical activity. The beneficial effects of drugs that block dopamine effect can be explained by the fact that these agents tend to increase the activity of striatal neurons projecting to the external globus pallidus, indirectly potentiating the activity of the subthalamic nucleus.

The probable explanation of the pathophysiology of Parkinsonism is equally complex. Since blocking dopamine action produces Parkinsonism, the challenge has been to explain the action of dopamine in the striatum. Recent evidence indicates that dopamine affects different populations of striatal neurons in markedly different ways. Dopamine appears to excite some striatal neurons while inhibiting others. Striatal neurons projecting to the external globus pallidus are inhibited by dopamine, while those projecting to the internal globus pallidus or the substantia nigra are excited by dopamine. In Parkinsonism, where dopamine is absent from the striatum or its effects are blocked, striatal neurons projecting to the external globus pallidus are more active and those projecting to the internal segment of the globus pallidus or substantia nigra are less active. These changes result in higher activity of the internal globus pallidus and substantia nigra neurons, and excessive inhibition of the thalamus. The ultimate result is inhibition of the thalamocortical projection and less activity in the cortex. The decrease in cortical activation found in Parkinsonism is the opposite of the increase in cortical activation characteristic of hyperkinetic movement disorders.

Dystonic disorders are harder to explain and a completely satisfactory model has yet to be described. In some cases, it appears that dystonia results from gross cessation of basal ganglia output.

BIBLIOGRAPHY

Albin, R. L., Young, A. B., & Penney, J. B. (1989). The functional anatomy of basal ganglia disorders. *Trends in Neurosciences, 12,* 366–75.

Parent, A. (1986). *Comparative neurobiology of the basal ganglia.* New York: Wiley.

Swanson, G. (Ed.). (1990). Special issue: basal ganglia research. *Trends in Neurosciences, 13,* 241–308.

Wilson, C. J. (1990). The basal ganglia. In G. M. Shepherd (Ed.), *The synaptic organization of the brain* (pp. 279–316). New York: Oxford University Press.

ROGER L. ALBIN

basolateral circuit   The basolateral circuit is part of the LIMBIC SYSTEM, and is formed of the AMYGDALA, the dorsomedial nucleus of the THALAMUS, and the orbitofrontal, insular, and anterior temporal regions of the cortex. It is commonly distinguished from the more medial components of the limbic system, and studies in animals suggest that it may be involved in self-preservation by fight or flight.

BEAM   *See* ELECTROENCEPHALOGRAPHY.

bilingualism   Bilingualism is the ability to use two languages with the fluency characteristic of a native speaker. The basic question in the neuro-

psychology of bilingualism has been whether the cerebral representation of language in bilinguals differs from that in unilinguals, and if so, in what specific ways. Models have been developed in an attempt to explain the various patterns of recovery of bilingual and multilingual aphasic patients and, by inference, the way in which two languages are organized in one brain.

Six basic patterns of recovery have been described over the past century: parallel, when all languages are recovered at the same time and to the same extent; differential, when one is recovered better than the other(s); successive, when one language is not recovered at all until the other(s) have been maximally recovered; selective, when one language is never recovered; antagonistic, when an initially recovered language is eventually replaced by another language; and mixed, when two languages are systematically mixed intrasententially (and even sometimes intramorphemically) at the level of phonology, morphology, syntax, and/or the lexicon (Paradis, 1977, 1989). The available language in some cases of antagonistic recovery has been reported to alternate over periods ranging from 24 hours to 3 weeks (Paradis et al., 1982; Nilipour & Ashayeri, 1989) or even 8 months (Paradis & Goldblum, 1989). These six patterns are not mutually exclusive. A recovery may change from one pattern into another over time, and different patterns may coexist relative to different languages. Selective aphasia (aphasia in one language with no measurable deficits in the other(s)) and selective recovery (when one language remains permanently inaccessible) have been interpreted as representing opposite poles on a continuum of differential aphasia (Paradis & Goldblum, 1989).

In addition, three cases have been interpreted as exhibiting differential aphasia, i.e. a different aphasic syndrome in each language (Albert & Obler, 1978; Silverberg & Gordon, 1979). However, one of them (Silverberg & Gordon, case 1) can be considered a standard case of selective recovery. The patient is reported to have exhibited conduction aphasia in his native Russian and global aphasia in the little Hebrew he had attempted to acquire with very little success over the previous few years. The other two patients were believed to present with Broca's aphasia in one language and Wernicke's aphasia in the other. In both cases Hebrew was the language in which the patients were said to have exhibited Wernicke's aphasia, as reflected by their paraphasias in Hebrew. Their respective native languages were English and Spanish, in which they exhibited typical agrammatism. However, a closer look at these cases suggests that the patients may have exhibited agrammatism in both their languages, and that the symptoms of substitution in Hebrew were erroneously interpreted as evidence of paragrammatism (see Paradis, 1988). It is also possible that the apparent dissociation of aphasic symptoms might have reflected the patient's differential mastery of the various components of each language before the aphasia. Indeed, the foreign language of some speakers without brain damage closely resembles that of Broca or Wernicke patients.

These various recovery patterns raise three questions that have not always been kept distinct: (1) How are these patterns possible in the first place? (2) Why does one particular pattern obtain rather than another in a given patient? (3) Why is one specific language (say, English) preferentially recovered rather than another (say, Japanese)? More specifically, one may ask what neurophysiological mechanisms are responsible for the fact that one language can be temporarily or permanently unavailable while the other(s) remain(s) relatively accessible; how is it possible that only one language is accessible for a period of time and subsequently only the other language is; and what provokes systematic mixing? Assuming that we have a satisfactory explanation for the very possibility of the occurrence of all recovery patterns, the next step is to ascertain under what circumstances which of the possible recovery patterns will obtain. Then we may further ask, given any nonparallel pattern, why one specific language is preferentially recovered rather than the other. Most early studies have attempted to answer the third question. A few have attempted to answer the first. None has addressed the second, except, possibly, those that have tried to localize a switch mechanism (see below).

The first substantive monograph on aphasia in polyglots was that of A. Pitres in 1895 (translated in Paradis, 1983, pp. 26–49). Pitres addressed two questions. How are the various patterns possible and what determines which language will be recovered first or best? Most of the literature of the subsequent 80 years has concentrated on his contribution to the latter question. On the basis of his review of the literature and of eight cases of his own, Pitres concluded that, contrary to what his precursor T. Ribot had proposed in a two-line incidental remark in a book otherwise devoted to diseases of memory, the language preferentially recovered is not the native language (by virtue of the fact that its acquisition is less recent), but is the one most familiar to the patient at the time of insult. This language in many cases indeed happens to be the mother tongue, but then it is recovered not because it was the first acquired, but because it happens also to be the most familiar. This came to be known as "Pitres's rule" and was then contrasted with "Ribot's rule" in a lively debate for years to come. Papers that claimed to refute either Ribot's or Pitres's rule, or both, appeared in quick succession, and other tentative explanations for patterns of loss and recovery were then proposed. It was thus suggested that the language to be preferentially recovered was the one for which the patient had the strongest positive affective ties (Minkowski, 1927, 1928, translated in Paradis, 1983, pp. 205–32 and 274–9), the language most needed by the patient, or the language of the environment, most often that of the hospital. However, while some patients recovered the language of the environment rather than their mother tongue or their most fluent language, just as many did not recover the language of the environment even if it was both their native and most familiar language.

With respect to the first question, namely how the various patterns are possible, although no one had actually proposed that different languages were represented in different locations in the brain, Pitres argued at length against the mere hint of such hypothetical new centers specifically assigned to each of the languages learned by polyglot subjects, and many authors continued to argue against this view for a long time, until the notion was revived in a slightly different form by Albert and Obler (1978), who suggested that there was greater participation of the right hemisphere in the acquisition and use of a second language, and by Ojemann and Whitaker (1978), who hypothesized that both languages share the core areas of the classical language zone, but that the less automatic language is also represented in additional areas at the periphery of the language area. However, there is only contradictory experimental evidence and no clinical evidence in support of the differential lateralization of language in bilinguals (Mendelsohn, 1988; Solin,

1989; Paradis, 1990), and it may be premature, for methodological reasons, to interpret Ojemann and Whitaker's electrocortical stimulation results as indicative of differential localization.

Rejecting the notion of a different location for each particular language, O. Pötzl proposed in 1925 (translated in Paradis, 1983, pp. 176–98) that there was a cerebral distributing device allowing transition from one language to another. Based on observed correlations between selective recovery and damage to the left supramarginal gyrus and the adjacent temporo-parietal area, he concluded in 1930 (translated in Paradis, 1983, pp. 301–16) that this area subserved a switch mechanism. O. Kauders (1929, translated in Paradis, 1983, pp. 286–300) and A. Leischner (1948, translated in Paradis, 1983, pp. 456–502) reached similar conclusions: damage to this switch mechanism causes a patient either to be able to speak only one language or to switch uncontrollably between languages. Yet patients with switching difficulties or mixing in the context of a lesion in the anterior language area and an intact temporo-parietal region, as well as patients without switching disturbances in the context of a damaged temporo-parietal area, have been reported. Thus, if there is a specific bilingual switch mechanism, it is not likely to be localized in the supramarginal gyrus or the adjacent temporo-parietal area. In fact, there is no need to postulate an anatomical localization or even a type of functional language organization specific to bilinguals, other than that which allows every unilingual speaker to switch between registers or to select a passive over a cleft sentence construction.

Pitres proposed a different explanation, namely that the unrecovered language is not lost, but temporarily or permanently inhibited. This hypothesis allows for two or more languages to be subserved by the same cortical areas, while remaining neurofunctionally distinct and even possibly subserved by different neural circuits, though inextricably intertwined within the same gross anatomical area. The inaccessibility of one of the languages would thus not be caused by the physical destruction of its substrate, but by the neurophysiological inhibition of its neural network. This account has the merit of being compatible with a wide range of data. In fact, it is compatible with all bilingual aphasia recovery patterns. It may also be used to explain normal bilingual verbal behavior, such as the ability to speak one language at a time, to switch between them, and to mix them at will.

In addition, it may be assumed that inhibition is not an all or nothing phenomenon. The underlying cerebral substrate of a given item is unable to "fire" (i.e. be activated) when inhibition exceeds a certain level. When a language item is selected for production, it receives excitatory impulses while its competitors are inhibited, or, more accurately, the activation threshold of its competitors is raised (i.e. more excitatory impulses are necessary to cause these items to fire). It may be further assumed that the activation threshold of an item is lower for comprehension than for production (i.e for a response to an external stimulus in contrast to self-activation). The integration of the Subsystems Hypothesis (Paradis, 1981), the Activation Threshold Hypothesis (Paradis, 1984, 1985), and Green's (1986) Activation, Control, and Resource Model should help account for all reported clinical as well as normal (i.e. nonpathological) phenomena, and shed some light on how a speaker-hearer has control over two language systems and avoids interference while retaining the ability to mix at will and to translate from one language to another.

At least four hypotheses have been formulated with respect to the way in which two languages are organized in their neuroanatomical and neurophysiological representation (Paradis, 1981). The Extended System Hypothesis holds that the languages are undifferentiated in their representation. The bilingual system is in all respects similar to a single language system except that it simply contains more phonemes, morphemes, lexical entries, and syntactic rules. The Dual System Hypothesis holds that each language is subserved by an altogether different neural system, that is, an independent network of neural connections underlies each language. The Tripartite System Hypothesis holds that those items which are identical in both languages are represented in a common underlying neural substrate, while those that are different are represented in their respective language-specific neural substrates. The Subsystems Hypothesis holds that each language is subserved as a subsystem of the larger system known as linguistic competence. Language functions form a cognitive system separate from other cognitive systems, and each language forms a distinct subset of that system. Language as a system is susceptible to inhibition as a whole, but each subsystem is also susceptible to selective inhibition (as well as parts of each subsystem). It is important to note that the subsystems hypothesis is the only one compatible with all the observed phenomena. While it is compatible with all patterns of recovery as well as with the ability to keep languages separate and to mix them at will, it nevertheless needs additional experimental and/or clinical support.

The Activation Threshold Hypothesis holds that comprehension and production are subserved by the same neural substrate, but that it takes more "energy" (or more numerous neural impulses) to voluntarily self-activate a trace (or "engram" or "address," depending on one's preferred metaphor) than to activate it as a result of impulses triggered by external stimuli. In the normal course of events, the threshold of activation (i.e. the propensity to be activated) of any given trace is a function, among other factors, of frequency and recency of activation. The more frequently a given trace is used, the lower its threshold of activation, hence the easier it is to activate it again (i.e. the less the amount of energy needed to activate it). The longer it has been since a trace was last activated, the higher its threshold of activation, that is, the more difficult it is to activate, and the greater the amount of energy needed to activate it. However, pathology may disrupt the normal pattern of activation threshold.

All things being equal, when an item is not activated, its threshold slowly rises until it is activated again, at which time the threshold is lowered and starts rising slowly again from that point on. If the item is not activated for a very long time, its threshold becomes too high for self-activation, but it can still be activated by external stimulation, thus allowing for comprehension though not for voluntary recall. When a whole language system has not been used for many years, as can occur when one emigrates, for instance, the speaker is generally said to have retained a "passive knowledge" of that language, namely the ability to understand it without necessarily being able to speak it anymore (because of massive word-finding difficulty as well as morphosyntactic interference from the currently used language). If the period of disuse has not been too lengthy, and if that system is sufficiently reactivated through extensive interaction with speakers of that language, it will again become active, namely its activation threshold will be

sufficiently lowered to allow it to be self-activated. If the period of disuse has extended beyond a certain length, the activation threshold will have been raised so high that the subject will have lost even the ability to understand that language. The length of time may vary with the age at which the speaker ceased using the language – in subjects who ceased using the language at a younger age, the language has been reported to have become permanently unavailable after shorter periods of time than in subjects who used it until an older age.

It is assumed that the selection of a particular item requires that its activation exceed that of any possible alternatives (Luria, 1973; Green, 1986). In order to ensure this, its competitors must be inhibited, i.e. their activation threshold must be raised. Thus, as an item is targeted for activation, its competitors' activation threshold is simultaneously raised and consequently more energy is required to activate them (though it is not usually raised so high as to prevent comprehension of incoming signals). In other words, the appropriate item is activated by the raising of the activation threshold of competing items (i.e. all other possible candidates) as much as by actually activating it. Since the availability of an item is a function of the frequency and recency of its activation (Luria, 1974), expressions may be more available (because they have been activated more often and/or more recently) in one language than in another. A word (or any other linguistic item) must reach a certain level of activation in order to become available for use. The activation threshold for the internal representation of specific words (or independently for their semantic and morphosyntactic properties on the one hand, and for their phonological form on the other), or of any other item (e.g. a syntactic or morphological rule) may differ from that of other items within the system.

It is further assumed that when a bilingual speaker elects to speak one language rather than another, the nonselected language is partly deactivated, that is, the activation threshold of the nonselected language is raised. In cases of aphasia, it sometimes becomes impossible to disinhibit (i.e. to sufficiently lower the activation threshold of) one of the languages, either permanently (as in selective recovery), temporarily (as in successive recovery), or alternatingly (as in antagonistic recovery). The activation threshold may be higher for one language than for the other (differential recovery). Deactivation of one language (raising its activation threshold) may be difficult, resulting in abundant inadvertent mixing or hybridization.

Nonparallel recovery in bilingual aphasia has been postulated since Pitres not to be the result of selective destruction of the cerebral representation of one language system, but of its temporary or permanent inhibition. Green (1986) argues in favor of this position and underscores the energy dimension of cerebral control over the use of language systems. He proposes that regulation of inhibition/disinhibition (or, in our terms, the respective activation threshold) involves the use (and hence possible depletion) of energy resources.

The model assumes the following. When an utterance is produced, the appropriate item comes to dominate other possible candidates by reducing their level of activation, i.e. by inhibiting them (Luria, 1973; Luria & Hutton, 1977; Green, 1986). When a bilingual speaker elects to speak one language rather than another, the nonselected language is not completely deactivated (Green, 1986; Grosjean & Soares, 1986); in other words, the threshold of activation is raised sufficiently to prevent interference during production, but not sufficiently to preclude borrowing and mixing, or comprehension in the other language. Practice could probably make a difference. Individuals used to mixing must have developed a lower activation threshold for the nonselected language than individuals who always speak each language to different unilingual groups of people and thus never have occasion to mix, in which case the two languages are rigorously kept separate at all times and hence the threshold of the nonselected language is likely to be high.

Green (1986) then goes on to assume that words possess particular "tags" that label each item as belonging to one or the other language. Alternatively, we may consider that items in a given language are part of a specific subsystem, and items of another language part of a different subsystem, each subsystem being subserved by a different neural network. These different networks need not be represented in different anatomical locations; they are indeed more likely to be intricately interwoven within the same cortical areas. In any case, Green rightly points out that selection of items in a particular language is partly a matter of increasing the activation of that language but also a matter of suppressing the activation of items in the other language.

Within Green's (1986) framework, it is assumed that brain damage may limit the availability of the means both to excite and to inhibit a system. The kinds of output produced depend on the relative balance of the means to excite or inhibit a system. Resources are not available for language in general but independently for each specific language, so that the use of one language does not deplete the resources available to the other language(s). The inhibitory system of each language is thus susceptible to selective impairment.

The question that remains unanswered is why the (partially depleted) available resources are sometimes equally distributed among the two languages (as in parallel recovery), sometimes more in one than in the other (as in differential recovery), sometimes all in one and none in the other (as in selective recovery), or sometimes alternating between one and the other (as in successive and antagonistic recovery). What determines the type of pattern? In addition, in nonparallel cases, why does, say, Turkish lack resources rather than German (or vice versa)? On what basis are resources assigned to one language rather than to the other, or on what basis are resources shared equally between them? In addition to the question of means (resource, energy), there is the question of automatic control. How, and on what basis, does the mechanism that controls the distribution of inhibitory resources function? These two fundamental questions remain unanswered. But they can now be rephrased as follows: What factors induce the control mechanism to assign all resources to one language and not the other (instead of distributing them equally), and why to German rather than to Turkish? Inhibitory resources allow the regulation of active systems. But what is it that regulates and assigns inhibitory resources? And what assigns them in one way rather than in another (reflecting a specific pattern of recovery), and once the pattern is determined, what determines that one language rather than another will be allocated more inhibitory resources?

The nonrecovered language remains active in some bilingual aphasic patients but not in others, that is, either comprehension is retained in the absence of production, or both are unavailable. In cases when not even comprehension is possible in one of the languages (i.e. when that language is not active, in Green's terms), it may be assumed that the threshold of activation for that language has been raised so high that it even prevents activation from outside stimuli. Indeed, some patients have been reported to have lost access to one of their premorbidly fluent languages to such an extent that it appeared as though they had never been acquainted with it before, not only having lost comprehension, but not even being able to repeat sentences in that language any better than someone who was hearing the language for the first time.

While some patterns of recovery are indeed explained by inhibition/disinhibition phenomena (i.e. the raising and lowering of the activation threshold), it must be conceded that, in some cases, when the neural substrate subserving the grammar has been physically destroyed or surgically removed, the grammar (i.e linguistic competence, the implicit knowledge of the language) is simply no longer there. It is extremely unlikely, however, that this could result in the loss of only one of the patient's languages, as there is no evidence that two languages are not subserved by circuits within the same (macro-)anatomical area (i.e. in terms of cubic millimeters), even if we allow for possible micro-anatomical differences (in terms of cubic microns), and a fortiori if the very same neurons are involved, albeit as part of a different neural network.

Green's model, in conjunction with the activation threshold hypothesis, offers a reasonable account of how the various observed phenomena can occur. Why one rather than any other phenomenon does occur remains to be explained. We may hope that the assessment of large numbers of bilingual aphasic patients, permitting correlational analyses of recovery patterns and the numerous linguistic, physiological, and pathological variables, will eventually provide us with sufficient data to arrive at an answer.

The collection of data obtained with tests that are linguistically equivalent in all of the patients' languages (Paradis & Libben, 1987) should allow us to determine whether the organization of two languages in one brain is a function of the structural distance between the languages concerned, and/or of their context of acquisition and/or use, the relative degree to which they have been mastered, the type of aphasia, the severity of the insult, or of any other variable that has been suspected of playing a potential role. It should also

eventually give us some indications as to whether two languages are represented in the brain as an extended system, two separate systems, a tripartite system, or as two subsystems of the language system. A more extensive treatment of this issue may be found in Paradis (1993).

BIBLIOGRAPHY

Albert, M. L., & Obler, L. K. (1978). *The bilingual brain*. New York: Academic Press.

Green, D. (1986). Control, activation, and resource: a framework and a model for the control of speech in bilinguals. *Brain and Language, 27*, 210–23.

Grosjean, F., & Soares, C. (1986). Processing mixed language: some preliminary findings. In J. Vaid (Ed.), *Language processing in bilinguals* (pp. 145–79). Hillsdale, NJ: Erlbaum.

Luria, A. R. (1973). Two basic kinds of aphasic disorders. *Linguistics, 115*, 57–66.

Luria, A. R. (1974). Basic problems of neurolinguistics. In T. A. Sebeok (Ed.), *Current Trends in Linguistics*, Vol. 12 (pp. 2561–93). The Hague: Mouton.

Luria, A. R., & Hutton, J. T. (1977). A modern assessment of the basic forms of aphasia. *Brain and Language, 4*, 129–51.

Mendelsohn, S. (1988). Language lateralization in bilinguals: facts and fantasy. *Journal of Neurolinguistics, 3*, 261–92.

Nilipour, R., & Ashayeri, H. (1989). Alternating antagonism between two languages with successive recovery of a third in a trilingual aphasic patient. *Brain and Language, 36*, 23–48.

Ojemann, G. A., & Whitaker, H. A. (1978). The bilingual brain. *Archives of Neurology, 35*, 409–12.

Paradis, M. (1977). Bilingualism and aphasia. In H. Whitaker & H. A. Whitaker (Eds), *Studies in neurolinguistics*, Vol. 3 (pp. 65–121). New York: Academic Press.

Paradis, M. (1981). Neurolinguistic organization of a bilingual's two languages. *LACUS Forum, 7*, 486–94.

Paradis, M. (Ed.). (1983). *Readings on aphasia in bilinguals and polyglots*. Montreal: Marcel Didier.

Paradis, M. (1984). Aphasie et traduction. *Meta: Translators' Journal, 29*, 57–67.

Paradis, M. (1985). On the representation of two languages in one brain. *Language Sciences, 7*, 1–39.

Paradis, M. (1988). Recent developments in the study of agrammatism: their import for the assessment of bilingual aphasia. *Journal of Neurolinguistics*, *3*, 127–60.

Paradis, M. (1989). Bilingual and polyglot aphasia. in F. Boller and J. Grafman (Eds), *Handbook of neuropsychology*, Vol. 2 (pp. 117–40). Amsterdam: Elsevier.

Paradis, M. (1990). Language lateralization in bilinguals: Enough already! *Brain and Language*, *39*, 576–86.

Paradis, M. (1993). Multilingualism and aphasia. In J. Dittmann (Ed.), *Handbooks of linguistics and communication science*, Vol. 8, *Linguistic Disorders* (pp. 278–88). Berlin and New York: Walter De Gruyter.

Paradis M., & Goldblum, M.-C. (1989). Selected crossed aphasia in a trilingual aphasic patient followed by reciprocal antagonism, *Brain and Language*, *36*, 62–75.

Paradis, M., Goldblum, M.-C., & Abidi, R. (1982). Alternate antagonism with paradoxical translation behavior in two bilingual aphasic patients. *Brain and Language*, *15*, 55–69.

Paradis, M., & Libben, G. (1987). *The assessment of bilingual aphasia*. Hillsdale, NJ: Erlbaum.

Silverberg, R., & Gordon, H. W. (1979). Differential aphasia in two bilingual individuals. *Neurology*, *29*, 51–5.

Solin, D. (1989). The systematic misrepresentation of bilingual crossed aphasia data and its consequences. *Brain and Language*, *36*, 92–116.

MICHEL PARADIS

Binswanger's disease *See* LACUNAR STATE.

bletharospasm Bletharospasm is a focal form of DYSTONIA in which there is a prolonged spasm of the orbicularis muscles of the eyes. The disorder is also known as Bruegel's syndrome. The result is prolonged twitching which may appear similar to voluntary winking but, unlike hemifacial spasm, it is bilateral and there is no associated clonic twitching in lower facial muscles. In more severe cases it results in involuntary eye closure. It may be associated with other disorders of the PYRAMIDAL TRACT, and is more common in elderly women. There may be a family history of the disorder.

blindsight The ability to detect and identify visual stimuli by forced-choice guessing when the stimuli are presented in blind portions of the visual field and are not consciously perceived is known as blindsight.

Since the late nineteenth century it has been known that damage to the striate cortex, at the back of the brain, produces a VISUAL FIELD DEFECT. If the damage is incomplete some vision may persist within the defective region. Severe damage permanently abolishes vision within the defect, which is then called a SCOTOMA. Patients with a scotoma caused by cortical damage provided the first evidence that the striate cortex is the primary representation of the retina and that it is indispensable to visual awareness.

Throughout this period of research there were occasional reports of patients who could detect some visual stimuli in what seemed to be scotoma, especially if the stimulus moved or was intense, leading a few investigators to question whether damage to the striate cortex ever caused *total* blindness in the field defect. Unfortunately this claim was difficult to evaluate because intense stimuli can produce enough scattered light within the eye for them to be detected by the intact part of the eye. Of course, the patient should literally see such scattered light, but the early reports do not make clear whether the patient really saw anything or just "felt" that something had occurred. A further problem is that it was not known whether the striate cortical damage was complete or whether the slight residual sensitivity stemmed from the impoverished activity of some remaining tissue.

What had seemed a sterile controversy in a backwater of research on the brain was transformed by a series of new reports in the 1970s. In 1973 Whitman Richards at the Massachusetts Institute of Technology (MIT) showed that an invisible visual stimulus presented within the scotoma in one eye could influence judgments about similar stimuli seen in the intact part of the visual field of the other eye. When the same patients were asked to move their eyes to where an unseen target had been briefly presented, Pöppel and colleagues found that the direction and extent of the eye movement was correlated with the position of the target. The following year, Weiskrantz and colleagues (1974) demonstrated that patient DB could localize targets much more accurately by pointing to their position within the field defect rather than moving his eyes. But even more remarkably, he could tell whether a line was vertical or horizontal and say whether a shape was X or O. All this was achieved despite repeated assertions by the patient that he was only guessing and never saw any of the stimuli. It was this paradoxical contrast between visual performance and visual experience that prompted the term "blindsight." Since its discovery, blindsight has attracted the interest of neuroscientists and philosophers, the former because the characteristics of blindsight indicate the properties of other visual pathways that survive damage to the striate cortex, the latter because it indicates something about the neural basis of visual consciousness. These are considered below, but first it is necessary to deal with assertions that blindsight is trivial and/or artifactual.

IS BLINDSIGHT GENUINE?

Not all patients with a scotoma have blindsight. Nor should this surprise us if, as discussed below, the other pathways that underlie blindsight are also damaged in such patients. However, it was found by Campion and colleagues (1983) that patients who initially showed little evidence of blindsight began to detect visual stimuli within the field defect by sensing cues such as scattered light. This led them to propose that blindsight might depend on any of three artifacts, namely: (1) the subject is detecting light scattered within the eye on to the intact retina; (2) normal subjects can tell better than expected by random guessing when a stimulus is close to the threshold for detection and the subject actually believes he or she is merely guessing. Blindsight is therefore like normal vision at threshold; (3) surviving striate cortex, even though damaged, mediates blindsight, which does not therefore reveal the properties of nonstriate pathways.

These objections were shown to be misplaced in certain patients (although they may well be true for others) by showing that (1) the same stimulus positioned on the highly reflective natural blindspot of the retina cannot be detected, despite scattering even more light; (2) in normal vision a stimulus that is not seen when just above the detection threshold as determined by forced-choice guessing is always visible when its intensity is raised to supra-threshold levels, but in blindsight the paradoxical invisibility persists, even at supra-threshold levels where detection is fault-

less; blindsight is therefore not just like normal vision at threshold; (3) when the optic tract is severed by an accident that destroys all inputs from the eye into one side of the brain, blindsight is absent, yet when an entire cerebral hemisphere is removed, sparing the THALAMUS and midbrain, some aspects of blindsight survive. Therefore blindsight cannot depend totally on the remaining striate cortex.

Properties of blindsight In addition to detecting and localizing spots of light and discriminating the orientation of lines, abilities that could hardly be described as taxing for even a simple visual system, subsequent investigations showed that some patients with blindsight had a much greater range of abilities. Detection and discrimination of movement, speed, and flicker can be present, and VISUAL ACUITY, although reduced, is still better than that of a normal cat. Outlines confined to the scotoma can influence judgments of the shape of other outlines in the immediately adjacent normal visual field. Two patients could adjust their grasp so that it matched the shape and size of an unseen object, and there was even evidence that they could use the meaning of unseen words flashed in their blind fields in order to choose a related word from a pair of words then presented in the intact field. These abilities have been reviewed by Weiskrantz (1986) and Cowey and Stoerig (1991a, b).

Despite this impressive range of unacknowledged visual accomplishments, blindsight is not merely an overall reduction in visual performance, for shape and color are notably more impaired. Although the first reports with patient DB indicated that he could discriminate between X and O, it was later shown that this was really an orientation discrimination. If two shapes with identical orientations of their component outlines, such as a square and a rectangle, were presented, DB could no longer detect the difference. Genuine shape discrimination seems to be absent in blindsight. Initial reports indicated that color (used here as a shorthand for hue and wavelength) was not registered in blindsight, but Stoerig (1987) found that six of ten patients with blindsight could discriminate between a green and a red target and that this ability could not be attributed to an "apparent" brightness difference between them. Since then it has been shown in a subset of the same patients (Stoerig & Cowey, 1991) that their spectral sensitivity (i.e. their sensitivity to light of different wavelengths) is reduced overall by about 1 log unit but, more important, the curves for both photopic (light-adapted) and scotopic (dark-adapted) viewing have the normal shape. This implies that both rods and cones are effective in blindsight, that dark and light adaptation occurs, and that color-opponent signals are transmitted at bright levels of illumination. The latter presumably underlies the successful color discrimination.

How good is the color discrimination? After all, mid-green and deep red narrow-band colors are more than 100 nanometres apart, but in normal vision differences of a few nanometres are detectable. Again with the same patients it has been shown that the color threshold in this part of the spectrum is about 20–30 nanometres, better than hitherto expected but still very impaired.

Pathways mediating blindsight There are at least eight pathways by which signals from the eye reach the brain. Largely as a result of experiments on animals, it is believed that all the routes except that to the dorsal lateral geniculate nucleus (dLGN) are involved in reflex or noncognitive functions, such as daily and seasonal rhythms in relation to light, the control of the pupil of the eye, eye movements to visual targets, and postural adjustments to movements of large parts of the visual field (optic flow). Only the signals reaching the striate cortex via the dLGN were thought to initiate visual awareness; hence the blindness when striate cortex is damaged.

Which of the remaining pathways mediate blindsight? It is possible that all or most of them contribute, depending on the visual stimuli that have been detected, but the strongest candidate is the superior COLLICULUS. This midbrain structure receives about 100,000 optic fibers from each eye in mammals as different as rats, cats, and primates. When a small hole was made in the striate cortex of a monkey, the animal could still detect visual targets and move its eyes towards them, but this was abolished when a hole was subsequently made in the corresponding part of the superior colliculus (Mohler & Wurtz, 1977). Although the superior colliculus may well be the principal structure mediating blindsight in patients with hemispherectomies, other routes may underlie some of the more remarkable abilities in blindsight, notably discrimination of direction or speed of movement, or color, which do not survive hemispherectomy.

The conclusion that parts of the cortex might be involved in "blind" movement discrimination is supported by recent electrophysiological experiments on monkeys. Cells in cortical area MT are exquisitely sensitive to the direction and speed of moving targets, and MT is often called the motion area. Its chief visual input is from striate cortex, but it also receives signals from the superior colliculus, via the pulvinar. When striate cortex in macaque monkeys was removed or reversibly inactivated by cooling it, Rodman and colleagues showed that many neurons in cortical area MT retained their sensitivity and selectivity for moving stimuli.

There is little physiological evidence that the retinal input to the superior colliculus could mediate discrimination between similar colors that is genuinely based on wavelength. However, other routes are possible. It is known that in primates only the P beta retinal ganglion cells transmit color opponent signals. The parvocellular layers of the dLGN receive this color opponent input and project to the striate cortex. When striate cortex is damaged the dLGN degenerates, as do about 80 percent of the retinal P beta cells. Why do 20 percent survive? Anatomical experiments, reviewed by Cowey and Stoerig (1991a), show that some of them can innervate the rare dLGN cells that also survive destruction of striate cortex and which project directly to other cortical visual areas, notably areas V2 and V4, where cells selectively responsive to colors are common. In monkeys P beta cells also innervate the ventral dLGN, which has many further anatomical connexions, and perhaps the pulvinar nucleus. Whether these projections survive striate cortical damage is unknown.

A final piece of evidence that visual signals from blind parts of the visual field can reach the cerebral cortex comes from the study of visually EVOKED POTENTIALS or VEPs, which have been recorded in some patients with blindness caused by occipital lobe damage. Although the latency and waveform of the potentials indicate cortical activity, they have not been localized to any particular cortical area. Nor is it yet known whether colored stimuli are effective.

Do nonhuman animals have blindsight? Long before the discovery of blindsight it was known that removing the striate cortex in monkeys did not destroy their ability to detect and discriminate visual stimuli although, as in human patients, form and color vision were conspicuously disrupted. In order to explain the striking contrast between residual vision in monkeys and the blindness experienced by human patients it was assumed that vision in monkeys was less dependent on the striate cortex. However, although there is good anatomical evidence for this in rats and cats, the visual pathways of monkeys look remarkably like ours. One possible explanation of the paradox is that striate cortical damage in monkeys produces a scotoma, and that their impressive residual abilities are based on blindsight. Attempts are now being made to demonstrate whether monkeys with field defects are "guessing" when they respond to visual stimuli confined to their defect or whether they are aware of and even genuinely "see" the stimulus.

If the removal of the striate cortex abolishes the conscious experience of vision, which to us is vision's most vivid quality, is it possible that some animals never see in the way we do? For example, fish have little or no neocortex (which includes the visual cortex) and insects have no cortex at all. Despite their often superb range of responses to visual stimuli their world might be sightless, like that sensed in blindsight.

Why is blindsight blind?   A common answer to this question is that blindsight is mediated subcortically and that the cerebral cortex is the organ of conscious awareness. If the striate cortex is the only gateway by which visual signals can reach other cortical regions, its removal or disconnexion will abolish visual awareness. This simple view is increasingly difficult to maintain. For example, as already mentioned, VEPs can be detected in cortex when visual stimuli are presented in blind areas of the visual field, and visual stimuli continue to evoke activity in the cortical motion area (MT) of monkeys when the route through striate cortex is blocked.

Several other possibilities have been proposed (see Cowey & Stoerig, 1991a, for review). (1) The visual signals that reach nonstriate cortex are too weak to be consciously perceived. This is unlikely, given that they can be recorded from the scalp, and that in normal vision stimulation initially confined to just a few receptors in the eye can be consciously appreciated. (2) The effective operation of the cerebral cortex depends on a delicate balance between excitation and inhibition. If the balance between the cerebral hemispheres is disturbed by damage to the visual areas of one side

the remaining cortex on that side may be inhibited. A major problem with this hypothesis is that bilateral damage can produce total blindness, yet it should yield no imbalance. (3) Perceptual awareness requires a precise time- and phase-locked pattern of discharge among cortical cells. Destruction of the striate cortex might permanently disrupt this pattern in extra-striate visual areas of the damaged hemisphere so that even signals reaching the cortex might not be perceived. This could be tested by stimulating these areas electrically to see whether the subject reports any visual sensation. (4) Striate cortex sends massive projections to other, secondary, visual areas, but it also receives an equally prominent back-projection from them. These back-projections might underlie visual awareness. If so, blindsight may follow damage to back-projections that leaves the visual input to striate cortex intact. This could account for the VEPs described in some patients with a scotoma.

Related phenomena   It would be strange if unacknowledged detection of stimuli were confined to vision. Other sensory modalities have not been extensively examined, but "unfeeling touch" and "deaf hearing" have both been reported in patients with damage to somatosensory or auditory cortex respectively. Implicit awareness is a phenomenon in which an unacknowledged stimulus or a detected but unidentified stimulus can be shown to produce bodily responses appropriate to its identity and/or to influence judgments in an appropriate manner. For example, patients with a permanent inability to recognize faces or even to distinguish familiar from novel faces (PROSOPAGNOSIA) following cortical brain damage, can nevertheless show different electrodermal responses or reaction times to familiar and unfamiliar faces. One patient with severe object AGNOSIA could not visually discriminate the shape and orientation of seen objects, but her hand movements when reaching for them under visual control were appropriately adjusted to the orientation and size. Patients with severe anterograde AMNESIA that prevents them from recognizing or remembering any new material or events can nevertheless be shown to have stored information about them, e.g. by forced-choice "guessing" between correct and incorrect choices. In similar vein, some subjects with acquired aphasia can be shown to have implicit knowledge of words that they are unable to read.

As many of these examples of covert knowledge involve aspects of perception, memory, and cognition that are customarily attributed to the cerebral cortex, e.g. recognition of faces or words, they bolster the view that blindsight may also involve cortical processes that are divorced from awareness.

Possible applications Quite apart from its importance in relation to our ideas about the nature of awareness and the information conveyed by non-striate visual pathways, blindsight has several potential practical applications. The chief of these involves REHABILITATION after brain damage. Although the vast majority of patients with a scotoma are so adept at using their intact visual fields to compensate for their defect that there is no need to "train" them to exploit signals from the blind region, e.g. to avoid obstacles, their ability to do so could be a model for assessing the effectiveness of different rehabilitation procedures. More important, blindsight could be used to assess measures designed to limit the physical consequences of brain damage. For example, cortical damage is followed by degeneration of brain cells in other cortical areas and in the thalamus, and in the case of damage to striate cortex even cells in the eye degenerate. Procedures to limit this degeneration, which are already being developed and assessed pharmacologically, could be evaluated by studying their effects on the quality of blindsight.

See also OCCIPITAL LOBE

BIBLIOGRAPHY

Campion, J., Latto, R., & Smith, Y. M. (1983). Is blindsight an effect of scattered light, spared cortex, and near threshold vision? *Behavioural and Brain Sciences*, *6*, 423–48.

Cowey, A., & Stoerig, P. (1991a). The neurobiology of blindsight. *Trends in Neurosciences*, *14*, 140–5.

Cowey, A., & Stoerig, P. (1991b). Reflections on blindsight. In D. Milner & D. Rugg (Eds), *The neuropsychology of consciousness* (pp. 11–37). New York: Academic Press.

Mohler, C. W., & Wurtz, R. H. (1977). Role of striate cortex and superior colliculus in visual guidance of saccadic eye movements in monkeys. *Journal of Neurophysiology*, *40*, 74–94.

Stoerig, P. (1987). Chromaticity and achromaticity: evidence of a functional differentiation in visual field defects. *Brain*, *110*, 869–86.

Stoerig, P., & Cowey, A. (1991). Increment-threshold spectral sensitivity in blindsight. Evidence for colour opponency. *Brain*, *114*, 1487–1512.

Weiskrantz, L. (1986). *Blindsight: A case study and implications*. Oxford: Oxford University Press.

Weiskrantz, L., Warrington, E. K., Sanders, M. D., & Marshall, J. (1974). Visual capacity in the hemianopic field following a restricted cortical ablation. *Brain*, *97*, 709–28.

ALAN COWEY

blood flow studies It is generally accepted that regional cerebral blood flow (rCBF) reflects synaptic activity (see Raichle, 1987). Local increases in blood flow are necessary to replace the energy consumed by maintenance of synaptic ionic gradients. These changes in blood flow have been shown to be tightly coupled to changes in neural activity in both space and time. However, it is not possible to tell directly whether this activity is excitatory or inhibitory. There are a number of techniques available for measuring rCBF in the living human brain. Currently, Positron Emission Tomography (PET) provides the best sensitivity and spatial resolution, but in the next few years there are likely to be important developments in the use of magnetic resonance imaging (MRI) to measure rCBF changes. It remains to be seen whether the sensitivity of MRI will be sufficient to detect the changes in rCBF associated with higher cortical function.

When a positron collides with an electron, the resulting annihilation reaction releases two oppositely directed gamma rays. By using pairs of detectors, these coincident events can be distinguished from random background radiation so that a high-resolution image can be obtained after tomographic reconstruction.

In order to measure rCBF using PET, the positron emitting isotope of oxygen (^{15}O) is introduced into the blood stream either in the form of CO_2 breathed in air or as H_2O injected intravenously. ^{15}O has a very short half-life (2.05 minutes) so that volunteers can be rescanned at 10-minute intervals. At current radiation safety levels, between 6 and 12 scans can be performed in a single session, depending on the sensitivity of the camera. Using such a paradigm, normal volunteers can be scanned once a year.

On the basis of recordings from electrodes

implanted in single nerve cells, we know that there are discrete brain areas for which a specific behavior is associated with an increase in neural activity. In particular, the visual system and the motor system have been studied intensively in this way. For example, there is the well-known somatotopy associated with the cortical motor strip, illustrating that one part of this strip will become active when the fingers are moved and that every part of the body maps onto different parts of the strip. In studies of vision, it has been shown that there are discrete brain regions in extra-striate cortex which increase their activity in response to attributes of the visual world, such as form, color, and motion respectively (Zeki, 1978). The same technique has also been applied to higher-level processes. For example, shifting attention to a different part of the visual field is associated with increased firing in the posterior parietal cortex (Wurtz et al., 1982). Studies of humans and animals with discrete brain lesions tell essentially the same story. In principle, these studies provide a rich database for validating rCBF studies. In most cases, increased information processing of whatever kind is associated with increased neural activity and should therefore be reflected by changes in rCBF. However, data from lesion studies must be treated with caution. Removal of tissue can demonstrate that a discrete brain area is necessary for processing a certain type of information. It does not follow that, in the intact brain, this area will show a general increase in activity when the same information is processed.

A number of studies have confirmed that rCBF patterns tell the same story as electrophysiological and lesion studies. In these studies rCBF while the subject is carrying out a control task is subtracted from rCBF while the subject is performing the experimental task of interest. The difference image indicates which parts of the brain become active when the task is performed. For example, Colebatch and others (1991) showed that moving the fingers activated a different part of the motor strip from flexing the shoulder. However, they did not find any difference between fine and gross finger movements. Zeki and others (1991) compared rCBF when passively looking at a colored image with rCBF looking at the same image in black and white. The comparison revealed that processing color activated a discrete area of the lingual and

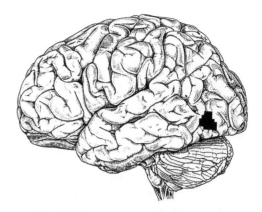

Figure 20 Location of increased blood flow when volunteers passively view moving stimuli (drawn from Zeki et al., 1991). The blood flow increases (black area) are shown on a lateral view of the left hemisphere.

fusiform gyri. This was the first study to identify the human analogue of the monkey area V4. Using a similar strategy, comparing the viewing of stationary and moving dots, Zeki and colleagues were also able to identify an area at the junction of occipital and parietal cortices that responded to movement (the equivalent of V5).

These studies confirm in humans what was already known from studies of animals. They are a very important validation of the ability to detect changes in neural activity using rCBF images measured by PET. However, these studies are not simply validations. The technique employed is the only one currently available for localizing function in the intact human brain.

The major interest in PET studies of rCBF arises because this technique makes it possible to study brain function associated with higher-order mental processes, such as those associated with thought and language. These processes cannot be studied in nonhuman animals.

Roland and his colleagues conducted many early rCBF studies on these topics using [133]Xe (radioactively labelled xenon gas). Their studies were important in that they demonstrated that pure "mental" activity that was not associated with any overt behavior was associated with detectable changes in blood flow. For example, Roland and Friberg (1985) comment that the largest changes observed in prefrontal cortex occurred when volunteers imagined all the objects in their living room. In these studies it was also observed that several distantly situated brain areas would become active simultaneously during the performance of complex tasks.

METHODOLOGICAL PROBLEMS

The changes in blood flow observed with PET are typically of the order of 4 percent of baseline flow. Such changes are usually too small to distinguish from background noise in a single scan. It is therefore necessary to combine data from many scans. Given the restrictions on the number of scans that can be taken from a single volunteer, scans from different volunteers must be combined. This raises a number of methodological problems (see Friston & Frackowiak, 1991). In order to combine scans it is necessary to take account of differences in brain shape and brain size. The outside of the brain can be relatively easily detected in the rCBF image, permitting assessment of brain position and size. Because of the marked difference in blood flow between grey and white matter, an rCBF image contains sufficient information about brain structure for various internal landmarks to be detected also.

A number of techniques have been developed which use this structural information to translate and "distort" the rCBF images from a volunteer to give the best fit to a standard template. These templates are usually linked to extant brain atlases (e.g. Talairach & Tournoux, 1988) so that brain areas can be specified in terms of x, y, z coordinates. Such specification is extremely important for comparing studies from different PET centers. An alternative approach to brain "normalization" is to coregister PET and magnetic resonance (MRI) images, since the latter provide much more detailed structural information. Even if rCBF images from different volunteers can be registered perfectly in terms of structure, it is likely that there will still be individual differences in the location of function. Smoothing the rCBF image is used to enlarge these areas so that there is a greater likelihood of overlap across volunteers. Using this technique, it is inevitable that the limits of resolution of the rCBF images are determined largely by individual variation in brain physiology, rather than the resolution of the PET camera. It is possible that the sensitivity of a new generation of cameras will be sufficient for changes in rCBF to be detected

in single volunteers. This should dramatically increase the resolution of the technique.

Once we have measured blood flow in two or more conditions in a series of volunteers, then, in principle, we can test for significant differences between conditions using repeated measures analysis of variance. However, there are very likely to be differences between volunteers in average blood flow across the whole brain (global flow). Within individual volunteers, there are also likely to be changes in global flow from one condition to another. Differences in global flow can be allowed for by expressing regional flow as a proportion of global flow or by using global flow as a covariate in the analysis of variance. A more intractable problem arises because of the very large number of comparisons that can be made in an rCBF image (or any other brain image). If every pixel in the image is to be studied, then several thousand comparisons will be made. Inevitably, many comparisons will be highly significant by chance. There are a number of strategies for coping with this problem. The "omnibus test" answers the question, "Are there significantly more significant differences than would be expected by chance?" Another approach is to apply a Bonferroni-like correction which takes account of the number of comparisons made. If this technique is used, then it is necessary to take account of the smoothness of the image, since the number of independent comparisons is likely to be much smaller than the number of pixels in the image. The simplest and best solution to these problems is to repeat the study with a new group of volunteers.

rCBF AND COGNITIVE PSYCHOLOGY

One of the major tenets of cognitive psychology is that behavior, including performance of a psychological task, is dependent upon many different underlying cognitive processes. The major task for cognitive psychologists is to specify what these components are and to devise ways of examining how they function. The group at the St Louis PET center was the first to report a study in which this cognitive approach was used to design the activation paradigms used during the PET scan and to interpret the resulting rCBF images (Petersen et al., 1988). In these studies it was assumed, first, that the operation of a discrete cognitive process would be associated with changed activity in a localized brain area. Secondly, it was assumed that, if more than one independent cognitive process was involved, then the effects on neural activity would be additive. It follows from these assumptions that it should be possible to link brain areas to cognitive processes. If task X involves processes A and B, while task Y involves processes A, B, and C, then the subtraction of rCBF in task X from that in task Y should reveal the brain region associated with cognitive process C. This has been called the *method of subtraction*.

The St Louis group chose to study single-word processing because there is an extensive empirical and theoretical literature on this topic. They assumed that single-word processing involved three major independent systems: an input system (visual and auditory word forms), a semantic system (word meanings), and an output system (articulatory word forms). Three tasks were devised that would permit isolation of these three systems by subtraction. Passive looking at or listening to words would activate the input word forms, simply repeating words would activate the input and output word forms, while generating a suitable verb for a noun (e.g. cake – eat) would activate the semantic system as well. Thus, comparison of rCBF images for generating verbs with repeating words should reveal areas activated when the semantic system is involved. On the basis of this approach, the St Louis group identified an area of extra-striate cortex to be associated with visual input word forms, an area of temporo-parietal cortex to be associated with auditory input word forms, areas of motor and premotor cortex associated with word output, and areas of inferior prefrontal cortex associated with semantic processing. Many of these conclusions have been questioned in subsequent studies, but the basic paradigm has been adopted widely. Disagreements have largely concerned the segregation of the tasks into their cognitive components. Perhaps the greatest problem is to design suitable control tasks which will highlight the cognitive process of interest when subtracted from the experimental task. There has been relatively little disagreement about the complex problems of PET technology and statistical analysis.

LANGUAGE

Wise and others (1991) have also carried out a number of studies in which sequences of words were presented in an attempt to distinguish different processing stages, such as the auditory input lexicon, the semantic system, and the speech output lexicon. Listening to nonwords and monitoring noun pairs for a semantic relationship both activated the superior temporal gyrus bilaterally, but surprisingly, no difference was observed between these two tasks. Comparisons of other word-processing tasks have highlighted the left posterior superior temporal gyrus (PSTG): for example, reading aloud lists of words compared to repeating the same word to every new nonsense stimulus. Wise and his colleagues conclude that the PSTG has a major role in the inner lexicon, but they feel unable, from results available at present, to specify this role more precisely. These authors make the important point that, even if psychological experiments have demonstrated the existence of independent processing stages, it does not follow that these processing stages must be instantiated in different brain locations. Independent processes might exist independently within the same neural network.

ATTENTION

Corbetta and others (1991) have studied the effects of selectively attending to different aspects of the same visual stimulus. In this study, volunteers observed complex visual displays in which changes occurred in color, velocity, or shape of the elements. Conditions in which volunteers selectively attended to one of these dimensions of change were contrasted with a condition in which changes in any of the three dimensions had to be detected. Selective attention enhanced blood flow in different parts of extra-striate visual cortex. For example, attention to movement enhanced activity in the inferior parietal lobule, while attention to color enhanced activity in a region between the lingual and fusiform gyri. These areas are close to those identified by Zeki and colleagues (1991) from their studies of passive viewing of colored or moving stimuli. Corbetta suggests that this study is revealing the modulation of the visual system during selective attention by a "top-down" signal.

Pardo and his colleagues (1990) studied selective attention using the Stroop paradigm. In the control condition volunteers named the color of the ink of congruent color words (e.g. the word RED written in red). In the experimental condition the color names were incongruent (e.g. the word RED written in blue). In this condition, volunteers had to select one of two competing responses: naming the color rather than reading the word. The largest increase in blood flow in the Stroop paradigm occurred in the anterior cingulate cortex.

"FRONTAL" FUNCTION

Blood flow studies are likely to be particularly informative in the study of the function of the frontal cortex (Frith, 1991). This occupies about one-third of the total cortical area in humans, a much greater proportion than in any other animal. There is much evidence from studies of patients with lesions in this area that frontal cortex is concerned with high-level supervisory functions. However, attempts to delineate specific functions for different parts of the frontal cortex in Man have met with little success so far. Using the ^{133}Xe inhalation method, Weinberger and his colleagues (1986) have shown that performance of the Wisconsin card sorting test (the classic neuropsychological test of frontal functioning) is associated with increased activity in dorsolateral prefrontal cortex.

Frith and others (1991a) have studied rCBF during performance of verbal fluency ("say as many words as you can beginning with A"), another classic "frontal" test. This task was also associated with increased activity in the dorsolateral prefrontal cortex, but on the left side only, as well as increases in the anterior cingulate cortex. In this study there was evidence that the increase in frontal activity associated with word generation was coupled with a decrease in activity in the superior temporal cortex (Wernicke's area). On the basis of this observation, Friston and others (1991) have suggested that internal or "willed" generation of actions depends upon mechanisms by which frontal cortex modulates posterior structures concerned with routine actions. These studies illustrate one of the particular strengths of rCBF measures of brain activity: the ability to detect interactions between distant brain regions.

Deiber and others (1991) studied the free generation of movements. In response to a signal, subjects had to move a joystick in one of four possible directions "at will." rCBF in this task was contrasted with that obtained when the joystick movements were predetermined. Significant increases were found in prefrontal cortex, bilaterally and in the anterior cingulate cortex. Frith and others (1991b) used a similar paradigm in which subjects selected to move one of two fingers at random on each trial. This task was also as-

sociated with activation in prefrontal cortex and the anterior cingulate cortex. On the basis of these experiments, it has been proposed that certain areas of prefrontal cortex are specifically concerned with "willed" action: the selection of one among many possible actions when all are equally motivated by external circumstances and internal desire.

THE FUTURE OF rCBF STUDIES

In this entry I have listed only a few of the early studies on the topic of rCBF in neuropsychology

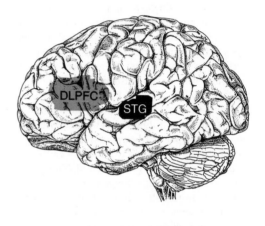

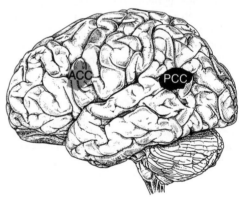

Figure 21 Locations of change in blood flow when word generation is compared with word repetition (drawn from Frith et al., 1991b). The upper figure shows a lateral view of the left hemisphere with increases in blood flow in the dorsolateral prefrontal cortex (DLPFC) and decreases in the superior temporal gyrus (STG). The lower one shows a medial view with increases in the anterior cingulate cortex (ACC) and decreases in the posterior cingulate cortex (PCC).

from a time when PET was available to a very small number of research groups. At the time of writing, many new PET centers are just becoming operational all over the world. In the next few years there will be a dramatic increase in publications combining rCBF and cognitive activations. These studies will revolutionize our understanding of the relationships between mind and brain.

BIBLIOGRAPHY

Colebatch, J. G., Deiber, M.-P., Passingham, R. E., Friston, K. J., & Frackowiak, R. S. J. (1991). Regional cerebral blood flow during voluntary arm and hand movements in human subjects. *Journal of Neurophysiology*, *65*, 1392–401.

Corbetta, M., Miezin, F. M., Dobmeyer, S., Shulman, G. L., & Petersen, S. E. (1990). Attentional modulation of neural processing of shape, color, and velocity in humans. *Science*, *248*, 1550–9.

Deiber, M.-P., Passingham, R. E., Colebatch, J. G., Friston, K. J., Nixon, P. D., & Frackowiak, R. S. J. (1991). Cortical areas and the selection of movement: a study with positron emission tomography. *Experimental Brain Research*, *84*, 393–402.

Friston, K. J., & Frackowiak, R. S. J. (1991). Imaging functional anatomy. In N. A. Lassen, D. H. Ingvar, M. E. Raichle, & L. Friberg. (Eds), *Brain work and mental activity* (pp. 267–77). Copenhagen: Munksgaard.

Friston, K. J., Frith, C. D., Liddle, P. F., & Frackowiak, R. S. J. (1991). Investigating a network model of word generation with positron emission tomography. *Proceedings of the Royal Society of London, Series B*, *244*, 101–6.

Frith, C. D. (1991). Positron emission tomography studies of frontal lobe function: relevance to psychiatric disease. In CIBA, *Exploring brain functional anatomy with positron tomography* (Ciba Foundation Symposium 163, pp. 181–97). Chichester: John Wiley.

Frith, C. D., Friston, K. J., Liddle, P. F., & Frackowiak, R. S. J. (1991a). A PET study of word finding. *Neuropsychologia*, *29*, 1137–48.

Frith, C. D., Friston, K. J., Liddle, P. F., & Frackowiak, R. S. J. (1991b). Willed action and the prefrontal cortex in man: a study with PET. *Proceedings of the Royal Society of London, Series B*, *244*, 241–6.

Pardo, J. V., Pardo, P. J., Janer, K. W., & Raichle, M. E. (1990). The anterior cingulate cortex mediates processing selection in the Stroop attentional conflict paradigm. *Proceedings of the National Academy of Sciences USA*, *87*, 256–9.

Petersen, S. E., Fox, P. T., Posner, M. I., Mintun, M., & Raichle, M. E. (1988). Positron emission tomographic studies of the cortical anatomy of single-word processing. *Nature*, *331*, 585–9.

Raichle, M. E. (1987). Circulatory and metabolic correlates of brain function in normal humans. In American Physiology Society, *Handbook of physiology. The nervous system. Higher functions of the brain* Sect. 1, Vol. V, Part 2 (pp. 643–74). Bethesda, MD: American Physiology Society.

Roland, P. E., & Friberg, L. (1985) Localisation of cortical areas activated by thinking. *Journal of Neurophysiology*, *53*, 1219–43.

Talairach, J., & Tournoux, P. (1988). *Co-planar stereotaxic atlas of the human brain*. Stuttgart: Thieme.

Weinberger, D. R., Berman, K. F., & Zec, R. F. (1986). Physiological dysfunction of the dorsolateral prefrontal cortex in schizophrenia. I. Regional cerebral blood flow (rCBF) evidence. *Archives of General Psychiatry*, *43*, 114–25.

Wise, R., Hadar, U., Howard, D., & Patterson, K. (1991). Language activation studies with positron emission tomography. In CIBA, *Exploring brain functional anatomy with positron tomography* (Ciba Foundation Symposium 163, pp. 128–234). Chichester: John Wiley.

Wurtz, R. H., Goldberg, M. E., & Robinson, D. L. (1982). Brain mechanisms of visual attention. *Scientific American*, *246*, 124–35.

Zeki, S. (1978). Functional specialisation in the visual cortex of the rhesus monkey. *Nature*, *274*, 423–8.

Zeki, S., Watson, J. D. G., Lueck, C. J., Friston, K. J., Kennard, C., & Frackowiak, R. S. J. (1991). A direct demonstration of functional specialisation in human visual cortex. *Journal of Neuroscience*, *11*, 641–9.

CHRIS FRITH

body image   *See* BODY SCHEMA DISTURBANCE.

body schema disturbance   The terms "body schema" and "body image" denote the detailed spatially organized mental model of one's body possessed by normal adults. The terms are usually employed synonymously. However, a distinction is sometimes drawn between the body schema as an unconscious representation and the body image as a conscious representation of the underlying model. Broadly speaking, "body schema" is the preferred term in neurological studies while "body image" is relatively more frequent in the psychiatric literature.

The concept of the body schema arose from observations of patients with neurological and psychiatric disease that seemed to be explained most readily by postulating the existence of a spatially organized mental model which formed the basis upon which perceptual, motor, and judgmental reactions directed towards one's body took place. Diverse phenomena such as the PHANTOM LIMB, impairment in pointing to parts of one's body (AUTOTOPAGNOSIA), defective discrimination of the left and right sides of the body (RIGHT–LEFT DISORIENTATION), disturbed awareness and denial of physical disability (ANOSOGNOSIA), defective localization of stimuli applied to the skin surface (ALLESTHESIA), and delusional thinking about the body and the self (DEPERSONALIZATION) have been regarded as expressions of disturbances in the body schema. Limited disabilities such as finger AGNOSIA have been interpreted as arising from circumscribed defects in the body schema. Even the occurrence of ACALCULIA and AGRAPHIA in some patients has been attributed by a few authors to a disturbance of the body schema.

The body schema is a multidimensional concept in the sense that, while some authors have regarded it as a primarily visual representation, others have viewed it as being primarily somatosensory in nature. The explanatory value of the concept has been disputed, one school of thought maintaining that it is merely an umbrella term covering all perceptual and judgmental responses relating to one's body. However, if it is only a label, it is a useful one because dissociation between performances relating to one's body as opposed to identical performances relating to external space are commonly observed. For example, many patients with visuospatial defects with respect to external space, such as inaccurate localization of objects, show intact ability to localize their body parts. Conversely, many patients with impaired right-left orientation or finger localization show intact orientation to ob-

jects in external space (Benton, 1959; De Renzi, 1982). Some aphasic patients show a disproportionately severe defect in naming (or understanding the names of) body parts as opposed to other classes of objects (Goodglass et al., 1966).

The illusion of the phantom limb is extraordinarily frequent among amputees, with more than 90 percent of adult patients reporting the experience. (In passing, it should be noted that amputation of other parts of the body, such as the breast and the penis, can also give rise to phantoms.) Usually arising immediately after amputation, the illusion persists for a long period, often permanently if it is accompanied by pain. The phantom limb is felt as a mobile member in different positions and directions of movement. It may be experienced as a painful contracture. There are generally changes in the experienced size and shape of the phantom, usually in the direction of foreshortening. The introduction of a prosthesis (an artificial limb) has varying effects. Upper-limb amputees generally distinguish between the phantom and the prosthesis; conversely, the phantom and the prosthesis are likely to merge in lower-limb amputees. The phenomenon of the phantom limb provides the most compelling reason for postulating the existence of a "body schema." It is not so much an expression of a disturbance of the schema, but rather the reflection of an intact schema that persists in spite of peripheral somatic changes. The cerebral basis for the phenomenon is confirmed by the finding, first noted by Head and Holmes (1911), that unilateral lesions of the parietal lobe may completely abolish or materially alter the phantom in a contralateral limb.

Finger agnosia, i.e. impairment in the ability to identify the fingers on either one's own hands or those of another person, has been viewed as the behavioral expression of a partial dissolution of the body schema or alternatively as one element of a broad syndrome of spatial disorientation. The disability is the core component of the GERSTMANN SYNDROME, the other elements of which are right-left disorientation, acalculia, and agraphia. The syndrome has long been the subject of controversy, the main questions being whether it actually exists in a pure form unaccompanied by other behavioral defects indicative of brain disease; whether it implies the presence of a focal lesion in the posterior parietal region of the language-dominant hemisphere; and whether this combination of symptoms in fact reflects an underlying single basic deficit, such as a disturbance of the body schema. Recent case reports indicate that on rare occasions the syndrome is encountered in a more or less pure form and that in these cases a focal lesion in the posterior parietal territory of the language-dominant hemisphere is usually found. However, the syndrome can also be produced by focal lesions in other areas of the brain. Moreover, a number of other symptom combinations containing one or more elements of the syndrome have the same implications with respect to lesional localization. Thus it is doubtful that the Gerstmann combination warrants a special status (Benton, 1992).

"Finger recognition" comprises a number of performances that differ in complexity and level of difficulty and that make demands on different abilities. In its simplest form it is assessed by asking the subjects to show their thumb or little finger or to name or otherwise indicate which finger the examiner has pointed to or touched. The task may be made more complicated in various ways. Subjects may be required to localize their fingers without the aid of vision by pointing to a touched finger or identifying it on a schematic representation of the hand (Figure 22). They may be required to identify two simultaneously touched fingers, to imitate finger movements of the examiner, or to indicate on one hand the finger(s) touched on the other hand. Obviously, a variety of stimulus-response situations, which

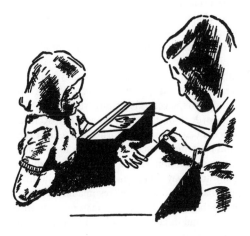

Figure 22 Arrangement for identification of fingers on a schematic representation of the hand.

make differential demands on sensory, perceptuomotor, and language capacities, are involved in these tasks.

The development of finger recognition in childhood has been the subject of detailed study, the conclusion being that the adult level of performance is reached only at the age of 12–13 years. One cognitive skill that appears to mature rather late in childhood is visuospatial representational thinking, as reflected in identifying fingers on an external schematic model instead of on one's own hand. There are indications that verbal encoding of sensory information may play a significant role in the performances of young children. The observation that the mentally retarded generally perform below expectations for their low mental age suggests that there are aspects of finger recognition which require high-level cognitive skills that are beyond their capacities. The pediatric neuropsychological significance of finger recognition is reflected in the findings that many brain-injured children of adequate intelligence level show impairment on the task and that defective finger recognition in kindergarten children is one predictor of reading failure in the early school years (Fletcher et al., 1982).

Taken by itself, finger agnosia in adult patients with brain disease does not appear to have specific localizing implications. Gainotti, Cianchetti, and Tiacci (1972) found that bilateral finger agnosia was equally frequent in patients with left and right hemisphere disease; most of the patients with left hemisphere lesions were aphasic while most of those with right hemisphere lesions showed general mental impairment. Similar results were obtained by Benke, Schelosky, and Gerstenbrand (1988), who concluded that bilateral defects in finger recognition reflected impairment in higher level cognitive processes rather than a specific disability. Poeck's (1975) studies led him to classify finger agnosia as one of a number of "neuropsychological symptoms without independent significance."

RIGHT–LEFT DISORIENTATION is a familiar symptom to neurologists. First described as simply an expression of general mental impairment, the disability attracted greater interest when it was found that it was closely allied to aphasic disorder and that it could be produced by a focal lesion in the left posterior parietal region of the left hemisphere in nonaphasic patients. "Right–left orientation" is a very broad concept that refers to performances on different levels of complexity, each performance making demands on different abilities and different types of response (Benton & Sivan, 1993). There is a linguistic component in performance in that the meaning of the labels, "right" and "left," and of the syntactic structures inherent in verbal commands must be understood. A somatosensory component, quite possibly a continuous asymmetric pattern of excitation from the muscles and joints of the body, must also be involved. Presumably, it is this "right–left gradient" of the body schema that forms the basis for the intuitive awareness of the difference between the two sides of the body which most normal persons possess (Benton, 1959). A third component is of a conceptual nature. A firm understanding of the relativistic nature of the "right–left" concept is required for correct identification of the lateral body parts of a confronting person and the simultaneous manipulation of the "own body" and "confronting person" orientational systems. Finally, a visuospatial component may be brought into play when pointing to body parts of a confronting person or to objects on the left or right.

In keeping with the hierarchical nature of the abilities involved, the development of right–left orientation in childhood follows a fixed course. The majority of 6-year-old children are able to identify single lateral parts on their body but are not likely to be able to execute double commands or to identify lateral parts on the body of a confronting person. Successful execution of crossed and uncrossed double commands is achieved by the age of 9 years. The majority of 12-year-old children can identify the lateral body parts of a confronting person and are successful in performing combined orientation tasks (e.g. "put *your* left hand on *my* left ear").

Defective right–left orientation has traditionally been related to disease of the left hemisphere and aphasic disorder. However, clinical studies indicate that there are differential associations depending upon what aspect of orientation is assessed. While defective "own body" performance is shown by aphasic patients with left hemisphere disease, it is rarely seen in nonphasic patients with lesions in either hemisphere. On the other hand, nonphasic patients with right hemisphere disease, as well as aphasic and demented patients, may show defects both on "confronting

person" tasks and in imitating right–left movements. Patients exhibiting the syndrome of NEGLECT or hemi-inattention are likely to show a "unilateral" impairment in right–left orientation in that they will consistently fail to point to parts of the neglected side of their body and to the side of the body of a confronting person corresponding to the neglected side of their own body.

ALLESTHESIA is a singular disorder of the body schema in which a patient with disease of the brain or spinal cord grossly mislocalizes tactile stimulation. The patient may report feeling a stimulus on the affected side of his or her body as being on the opposite healthy side, e.g. a stimulus to the volar surface of the left forearm is felt on the right forearm, or a stimulus to the distal part of a limb may be felt on the proximal part or on the trunk. Sometimes a single stimulus is perceived as two stimuli, one on each side of the body. These patients often exhibit a variety of other perceptual defects and many patients with brain disease prove to be demented to a greater or lesser degree. However, since patients with spinal-cord disease also report these forms of sensory displacement, their occurrence cannot be simply ascribed to general mental impairment.

Broadly speaking, two types of mechanism have been postulated to account for the phenomenon of allesthesia. One explanation, particularly applicable to spinal-cord cases, implicates an abnormal condition of the afferent sensory pathways which is characterized by impaired conduction in the normal crossed pathway together with hyperexcitability of the uncrossed pathway. A more global explanation, particularly applicable to patients with brain disease, invokes a gross disturbance of the body schema that produces a lateral shift in perception of which allesthesia is only one expression. Quite possibly, each explanation is valid for patients with different types of injury to the central nervous system.

Disorders of the body image in psychiatric patients take a variety of forms, range in severity from moderately excessive concern to delusional thinking, and appear in a number of conditions. They are always emotionally charged with interpersonal implications. Overestimation of the size of the body is a prominent feature of anorexia nervosa and in fact is considered to be a defining characteristic of the disease. Extremely negative evaluation of one's body is common in mood disorders, social phobias, and obsessive-compulsive disorders. Frank delusions about one or another aspect of the body are frequently expressed by patients, not all of whom are judged to be psychotic or even to have a psychiatric disease. "Body dysmorphic disorder" is now recognized as a distinctive entity in psychiatric diagnosis (Barsky, 1989).

BIBLIOGRAPHY

Barsky, A. J. (1989). Somatoform disorders. In H. H. Kaplan & B. J. Sadock (Eds), *Comprehensive textbook of psychiatry*, 5th edn (pp. 1009–27). Baltimore: Williams & Wilkins.

Benke, T., Schelosky, L., & Gerstenbrand, F. (1988). A clinical investigation of finger agnosia. *Journal of Clinical and Experimental Neuropsychology, 10,* 335.

Benton, A. L. (1959). *Right-left discrimination and finger localization: Development and pathology.* New York: Hoeber-Harper.

Benton, A. L. (1992). Gerstmann's syndrome. *Archives of Neurology, 49,* 445–7.

Benton, A. L., & Sivan, A. B. (1993). Disturbances of the body schema. In K. M. Heilman & E. Valenstein (Eds), *Clinical neuropsychology* (3rd edn) (pp. 123–40). New York: Oxford University Press.

De Renzi, E. (1982). *Disorders of space exploration and cognition.* New York: Wiley.

Fletcher, J. M., Taylor, H. G., Morris, R., & Satz, P. (1982). Finger recognition skills and reading achievement: a developmental neuropsychological perspective. *Developmental Psychology, 18,* 124–32.

Gainotti, G., Cianchetti, C., & Tiacci, C. (1972). The influence of hemispheric side of lesion on nonverbal tests of finger localization. *Cortex, 8,* 364–81.

Goodglass, H., Klein, B., Carey, P., & Jones, K. (1966). Specific semantic word categories in aphasia. *Cortex, 2,* 74–89.

Head, H., & Holmes, G. (1911). Sensory disturbances from cerebral lesions. *Brain, 34,* 102–254.

Poeck, K. (1975). Neuropsychologische Symptomen ohne eigenstaendliche Bedeutung. *Aktuelle Neurologie, 2,* 199–208.

ABIGAIL B. SIVAN AND ARTHUR BENTON

bradykinesia Bradykinesia is one of the primary symptoms of PARKINSON'S DISEASE, and is a retardation in initiating and executing movements and speech. There is a loss of facial expression, resulting in a mask-like face, a reduction in "associated movements" such as arm swinging, and a shuffling gait with flexed trunk. This "festinant gait" may appear as if the patient is one step behind him- or herself. Bradykinesia cannot be attributed to muscular rigidity. The alternative term "hypokinesia" is also employed.

brain Nothing overtly betrays the brain as giving rise to mind. For millennia the stuff inside the skull was viewed merely as a reservoir of bone marrow, a culinary bounty (Doty, 1965) or, by its similarity to semen in consistency and coloration, as a potent source of the male principle, as evidenced in the antlers of the stag and other commonly hunted artiodactylids (La Barre, 1984). It was thus unique in human history that Alkmaion, a pupil of Pythagoras in Kroton (Crotona) ca. 500 B.C. deduced that, since the eyes are connected to the brain, the latter must have some role in perception. Within another 50 years this recognition of the brain as the source of the intellect had entered the Hippocratic corpus and it has been a matter of faith in Western civilization since that time.

Phylogenetically, brains become a valuable component of organisms that move through space, since a brain provides a focal point for detection and decision, for selecting whether to advance, retreat, or turn. Interestingly, our distant progenitors some billion years ago solved the problem of turning by developing a brain on each side to assay the better choice. This bilateral symmetry, of course, has problems of its own, in that the two brains must reach some *modus operandi* via commissural connections whereby their decisions are coordinated, else chaotic choice would prevail (*see* LATERALIZATION).

BASIC PROPERTIES

Just like this arrangement of bilateral symmetry, so too have the basic constructs of neural action remained remarkably similar across all organisms possessing a nervous system (e.g. Figure 23). Since the primary function of a brain is to achieve a coordinated behavioral decision, its elements must be in communication with each other, and a mechanism for decision or selection must be at

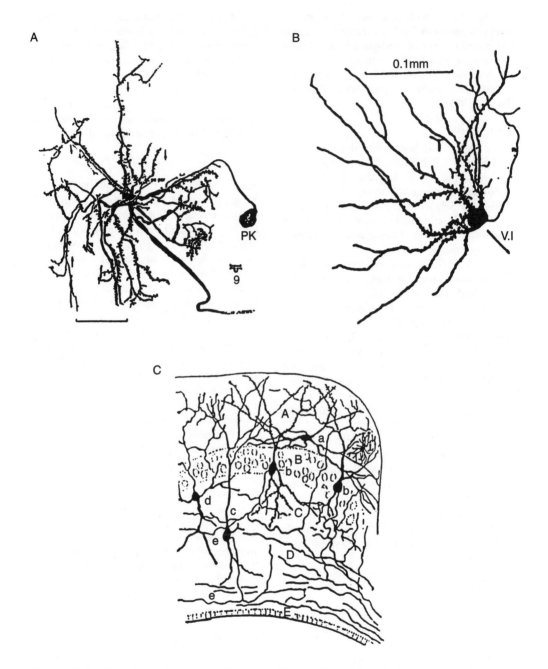

Figure 23 A. Giant descending neuron from visual brain of the drone fly, *Eristalis tenax*. B. Large, multipolar neuron from the archipallium of the frog, *Rana pipiens*. C. Selected cells drawn from cerebral cortex of a lizard. D. Types of neurons in the cerebral cortex of the hedgehog. E. Neurons in "motor" cortex of a month-old child. Note the presence of spines and the similarity of form in these various examples, the insect neuron being peculiar in having the cell body (to the right, PK) eccentric to dendrites and axon. In C, D, and E only a very few neurons have been represented from the great mat of cells within which they are embedded. (A, from Strausfeld; B, Clairambault and Derer; C and E, Cajal; D, Poliakov.)

D

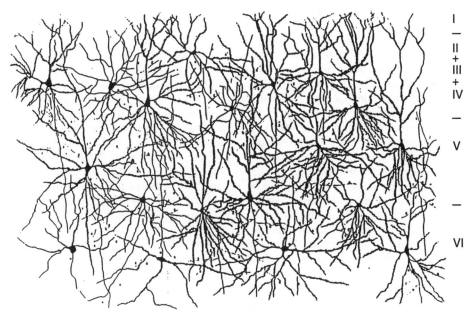

I
—
II
+
III
+
IV
—
V
—
VI

E

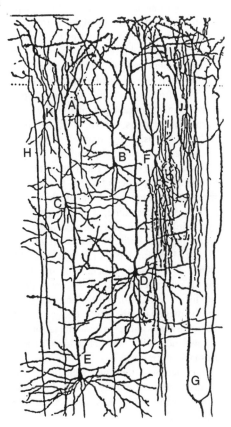

hand. Communication takes two forms, a rapid signal conveyed by an electrical flux, the *action potential*, over the surface of the constituent elements, the *neurons*; and a much slower passage of chemical signals between the neural elements. The latter signals, conveyed bidirectionally as "axoplasmic flow" within the neuronal extensions, the *axons*, appear to determine both the pattern and effectiveness of the connections among neurons; and the electrical signal, transmitted rapidly to the termination of the axon, in its turn effects the release of chemical signals (*transmitters* and *modulators*, see below) at the terminus to achieve a short-term, computational input to the recipient neuron, as well as modulating the long-term character of the connection.

As organisms grew in size and complexity, these requirements of communication and computation dictated the bizarre form of neurons, balloon-shaped cell bodies from which sprout numerous branches, the *dendrites*, covered with excrescences or "spines" (Figure 23; in mammals commonly numbering in the thousands), each in receipt of one or more connections, *synapses*, from other neurons. A single axon extends from the cell body to convey the electrochemical signals to other neurons (or muscles, or glands) upon which it terminates. In larger mammals such as Man, some of these axons attain lengths 20,000 times

169

the diameter of the parent cell. In other words, if the neurons that reach from the human brain far into the spinal cord were proportionally enlarged to the size of a tall man, the dendrites would then span some 30 m, and the axon, a tube 3 m in diameter, would wander off for almost 30 km!

In effect, each neuron is a point of decision. Throughout its vast extent the cell membrane bears an electrical charge which, when sufficiently reduced locally, gives rise to a self-propagating action potential along the axon, conveying a given neuron's "digital" output to all the other neurons with which it is in contact. The input to each neuron is the sum of the many axonal inputs it receives at the synapses on its dendrites (and cell body), each of which will briefly move the local electrical potential of the membrane toward or away from the electrical level, the *threshold*, required to produce an axonal signal. From such an arrangement it can be seen that a neuron sums its input, "positive" and "negative," at any given instant from the axons playing upon its synapses, and in turn sends out its own axonal signal when and if the threshold is attained.

MAPS, COLUMNS, AND LAMINAE

It is the richness and precision of interconnectivity which gives a nervous system its computational power. The precision of the connections is achieved and maintained by the subtleties of the electrochemical signals passed between neurons. As brains become larger, however, the extent of interconnectivity within them is inevitably limited by demands of space and time (Ringo, 1991). A variety of compromises have evolved to cope with this problem. In mammals the cerebral neocortex is organized, first, along topographical lines, so that the sensorial surfaces (skin, retina, cochlea; Figure 24) are mapped onto this sheet of neurons in a manner such that adjacent points within each sensory modality are contiguous. The advantages of adjacency are further extended by stacking the neuronal elements into a compact "column" that will perform the computing and abstracting of the information presented at any given point on the receptor surfaces; and this columnar organization holds throughout the mammalian neocortex.

The exact nature of the operations carried out by this arrangement are not known, but the outlines of the circuitry are apparent. There are, roughly, six "layers" of cells, although in more complex cases they can reasonably be still further subdivided. The afferent input from the thalamus is targeted principally upon the middle layer, IV, with less abundant input to layer VI. From layer IV the processing passes into layers II and III, whence fibers convey output primarily to other cortical areas and across the corpus callosum to the other hemisphere, giving off as they exit collateral axons into layer V. Layers V and VI are also strongly efferent in nature, layer V sending axons subcortically, especially into brain stem or spinal cord, while layer VI provides feedback onto the thalamic nuclei. In other words, each "column" can be viewed as a miniature computational module, processing an input signal and distributing outputs to a variety of loci.

TRANSMITTERS AND MODULATORS

The amino acids glutamate and aspartate serve as the major excitatory substances released at synaptic terminals; whereas glycine, primarily in the spinal cord, and γ-amino-butyric acid (GABA) elsewhere in the CNS serve as inhibitory transmitters (see NEUROTRANSMITTER). It must be emphasized that the respective effects, depolarization or hyperpolarization of the neuronal membrane, are a consequence not of the transmitter per se but of the subjacent postsynaptic receptors of the recipient cell; and in the details of their behavior there are a bewildering variety of receptors. The effect is also highly dependent upon the level of transmembrane potential in the recipient neuron. Such factors, in turn, can also be influenced by an extensive inventory of substances that "modulate", i.e. augment, prolong, or qualitatively change the effect of the transmitters. Many of these agents are peptides, e.g. the opioids and various hormones, but four of them, acetylcholine, noradrenaline, 5-hydroxytryptamine (serotonin), and dopamine, form distinct systems innervating the entire forebrain (Doty, 1989; Foote & Morrison, 1987). The exact role of these systems in neuronal functioning and behavior remains obscure, but their constant presence from fish to Man, with greatly increasing importance in mammals, the profuseness of their intracortical axons and a vast assemblage of suggestive evidence offer tantalizing hints as to their cardinal importance.

Consonant with their phylogenetic history, the noradrenergic, serotonergic, and dopaminergic neurons giving rise to these projections into the forebrain all lie in pons and/or mesencephalon;

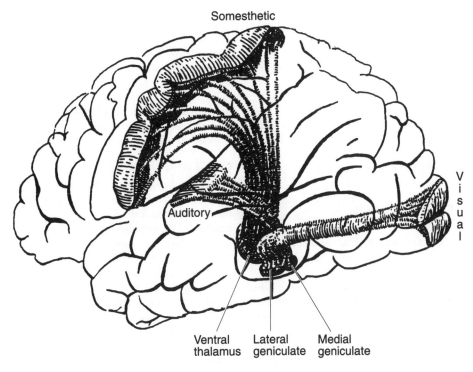

Somesthetic

Auditory

Visual

Ventral   Lateral   Medial
thalamus   geniculate   geniculate

Figure 24 Projections from the thalamus to the human neocortex for the three major sensory systems. The perspective does not accurately depict the amount of cortex allotted to the respective systems. (From Krieg.)

and these, plus cholinergic neurons in this region, also project onto the fourth, cholinergic system lying within the basal forebrain. Some further appreciation of the import of these brain-stem efferents to the forebrain is gained from the fact that a defect about the size of a cherry pit interrupting the projection from this critical mid-brain area can render the unfortunate human victim permanently unconscious, despite an otherwise intact brain. It has become clear that the cholinergic and serotonergic systems control the electrical activity (the EEG) of the cerebral cortex and hippocampus, and the firing pattern of these "modulatory" neurons changes drastically in sleep, particularly the rapid eye movement (REM) stage when dreaming occurs.

The locus coeruleus, totalling about 50,000 highly pigmented neurons in the human pons, gives rise to noradrenergic fibers with a remark-able diffuseness of termination, at least as measured in lower mammals, e.g. axonal branches from a single cell ending both in cerebellum and cerebral cortex. The serotonergic system is much more numerous, in the order of 500,000 cells in Man, mostly scattered along the midline of pons and midbrain. There are at least two subpopulations having differing types of axons; and it seems likely that some of their synaptic terminals contain glutamate as a trans-mitter as well as the modulator serotonin. The system is uniquely bilateral in its connections, for each side has neurons projecting to both sides of the brain; and the afferent fibers controlling this system are equally unique in the bilaterality of their exchange. Thus, in addition to such promi-nent commissural systems as the corpus callosum, this serotonergic system of the raphé probably plays a significant role in unifying action between the two cerebral hemispheres (Doty, 1989).

The human dopaminergic system is composed of roughly one million cells, many of them so highly pigmented as to have been long recognized as the "substantia nigra." The latter project prominently into the BASAL GANGLIA, and their

171

loss characterizes the pathology of Parkinsonism (see PARKINSON'S DISEASE). A more diffuse group, scattered in the ventral tegmental area, projects to the cerebral cortex and other areas of the forebrain. Both receive powerful input from the serotonergic system.

Lastly, the cholinergic system projecting to the cerebral cortex and hippocampus in Man constitutes about half a million large neurons variously distributed through the basal forebrain, most prominently in the nucleus basalis of Meynert. Loss of neurons in this system is particularly prevalent in ALZHEIMER'S DISEASE.

DENSITY AND ENERGY REQUIREMENTS

It is difficult to comprehend the sheer complexity of the mammalian brain. While the pinnacle of neuronal density is achieved in the million-neuron brains of bees or cockroaches, some 10–20 times greater even than that of the mammalian cerebral cortex, density in the latter is by no means meager, some 90,000 neurons/mm^3. Braitenberg and Schüz (1991) calculate that for the mouse, whose cerebral cortex is prototypically mammalian as is that of Man, there are some 4 km of axons within this cubic millimeter, serving the 700,000,000 synapses in that volume! Schüz determined that to achieve that richness of connection a rat within the first 26 days of its life must on average form 500,000 synaptic spines *per second*. Such spines, incidentally, may well be labile, since their size, number, and shape can be experimentally altered within a few days, and within as little as 2 hours for a squirrel awakening from hibernation.

These enormous numbers of elements imply an equally extraordinary extent of cellular membrane that must be sustained, plus the secretory output of each neuron at its axonal termination, all requiring metabolic support. Thus the demand of the brain for fuel, oxygen, and glucose is huge and incessant. Within a moderate-sized neuron reside about 1,500 metabolic engines, the *mitochondria*; and each mitochondrion processes some 10 atoms of oxygen per microsecond. Ten seconds without oxygen and the brain ceases to function, consciousness is lost. Constituting some 2 percent of the body mass, the brain takes 20 percent of the resting blood flow, continuously extracting energy equivalent to 20 watts (*see* BLOOD FLOW STUDIES).

Between the brain and the blood is a membran-

ous sheet, the blood–brain barrier, which precisely controls what substances gain access to the neurons. This arrangement holds even for invertebrates; and while it is common to ascribe a protective function to this barrier in relation to microorganisms, which it undoubtedly serves, an at least equally important *raison d'être* may be its protection of the milieu in which neurons conduct the subtleties of the chemical interchanges that regulate their connectivity and excitability.

INPUT AND OUTPUT

As noted above (Figure 24), input from the sensorial surfaces ultimately gains access to the cortex, following a roughly topographical arrangement. There are, however, many stages prior to this at which the incoming signal undergoes various transformations. In general, the brain controls the afferent portals, and in certain instances, e.g. pain, can largely curtail the input altogether. It seems probable that, among other things, the control exerted at these way stations to the cortex is related to various aspects of the phenomenon of ATTENTION.

One of the unsuspected features of sensorial analysis is that to a significant degree it must be "learned." This has been demonstrated most dramatically in the visual system, where individuals gaining clear vision only later in life must "learn to see" and, indeed, may be largely incapable of doing so. Animal experimentation shows that there is an extensive modelling of synaptic relations among neurons that is dependent upon experience early in life, and that if it is absent or abnormal, so too are the interconnections; the situation may be irreversible.

On the other hand, many sensory inputs have immediate motoric output, i.e. reflexes, and these can be of great complexity even while proceeding subconsciously. Particularly notable in this regard is the integration of input from skin, muscles, inner ear, and vision that subserves the human peculiarity of bipedal locomotion; but there are many others. For instance, rat and Man have clearly comparable "visuomotor programs" guiding the posture of the digits as they approach an object to be grasped. Many such programs are organized at midbrain level, so that a kitten, having no brain above this level, may still respond with typical cat-hunting behavior and pounce upon a source of faint rustling sounds. The forebrain can selectively utilize and fractionate these brain-stem programs and, in the case of certain reflexes of infancy, may suppress them lifelong. When the forebrain is severely damaged, as in Alzheimer's disease, some of these reflexes may again be released, such as the "rooting reflex" to find the teat when the skin around the mouth is touched.

Not all input and output concerns the external world. The autonomic nervous system and its central components regulate digestive, cardiovascular, immunological, and reproductive functions. Via these channels, plus the HYPOTHALAMUS and its manufacture of hormonal agents released through the pituitary gland, the brain exerts its mastery over the entire body economy.

APPETITES, EVALUATION, AND MEMORY

Phylogenetically, in the dark of the sea, the olfactory sense provided the early vertebrates with the major clue for what should be sought or avoided, food and a mate versus a variety of dangers; and it has thus been around the olfactory system (see OLFACTION) that the neuronal circuitry for evaluating what to approach or avoid has evolved. Even in Man, the AMYGDALA (Aggleton, 1992), with strong olfactory connections, serves these primitive purposes and their emotional accompaniments. It is of considerable significance that the air streams in the human nose remain sufficiently separate for each nostril to provide a unilateral input; and in primates the amygdalae on the two sides of the brain have little or no direct interconnection. The peculiar situation thus arises that each hemisphere has its "own" emotional system and, as is sometimes revealed with unilateral neocortical lesions, the two hemispheres may have somewhat differing emotional propensities.

While the amygdala is a focal point, evaluation of the beneficence or danger posed by any given input proceeds at many levels throughout the brain.

Crudely, there are two systems: the LIMBIC SYSTEM, so called because of its looping course around the middle of the brain, which deals with input from external sources, e.g. vision, taste, olfaction, in relation to feeding, mating, and avoidance of predators; and a much more diverse set of circuits dealing with a variety of "internal" signals, such as pain, warmth, hunger, and various other "appetites." In all cases, whether the input is external or internal, the appetitive-evaluative process is closely coupled to the autonomic-hormonal systems of the hypothalamus and pituitary gland and, presumably, in nonhuman animals as well as in Man, produces a correlated emotional state of hunger, contentment, rage, fear, and so on. The nature of the neuronal activity underlying the various "appetites," which create a restless state until terminated by specific stimuli, remains a major unsolved problem.

The survival of the individual and species promoted by these appetitive-evaluative systems is abetted by monitoring the organism's position in its environment. Evidence suggests that the HIPPOCAMPUS, a major part of the limbic system, serves this role. It would appear that, whenever the animal moves through space, the hippocampus somehow registers and stores (probably in the neocortex) the multisensorial input that subsequently enables the animal to retrace its path. In primates this hippocampal role may have been expanded to make it an essential mediator of mnemonic storage and retrieval of unique stimulus patterns, i.e. those that can be tagged with time and/or location of occurrence.

THE MIND–BRAIN LINK

As is apparent from Figure 23, the great similarity of the neurons in Man and lizards indicates that the quality of human mentation does not lie with any peculiarity in the elements of the brain producing it. Rather, it must be a function of their number and connectivity. A human microcephalic, with a brain no larger than a chimpanzee's, can nevertheless utter a few words, an ability not in the nature of chimpanzee brains. Yet chimpanzees can make mental inferences that are beyond the capacity of speaking 3-year-old children. Such inferential outcomes represent a type of brain activity for which there are at present no clues as to mechanism.

As is so readily apparent in this volume, the brain–mind relation displays a detailed parcelling of abilities among various neuronal areas. This distribution, and its consequent temporal dispersion, presents the major theoretical and philosophical puzzle as to how the unity of mental experience is achieved from these disparate assemblies of stuff, no matter how complex. That the unity is achieved by neural processes seems undeniable, since each hemisphere produces a largely independent mental life (save for the all-important brain-stem connections) following transection of the forebrain commissures (*see* COMMISSUROTOMY, CORPUS CALLOSUM).

The ingenious experiments of Libet (1985) have defined two essential features of the conscious process: (1) that it may take a surprisingly long time, up to half a second, for neuronal activity to produce a conscious result, and (2) that even in neocortex clear evidence of neuronal activity may proceed without conscious effect. In other words, there is in many instances a distinct difference between neuronal processes that lead to a conscious outcome and those that do not. It would seem that the only serious hope of comprehending how such an ethereal effect as mental experience can be produced by the flux of ions across neuronal membranes is to pursue these leads, that is, to investigate which neuronal patterns produce the effect, and which do not (*see* MIND–BODY PROBLEM).

BIBLIOGRAPHY

Aggleton, J. P. (Ed.). (1992). *The amygdala*. New York: Wiley-Liss.

Braitenberg, V., & Schüz, A. (1991). *Anatomy of the cortex: Statistics and geometry*. Berlin: Springer.

Dennett, D. C. (1991). *Consciousness explained*. Boston: Little, Brown.

Doty, R. W. (1965). Philosophy and the brain. *Perspectives in Biology and Medicine, 9*, 23–34.

Doty, R. W. (1989). Schizophrenia: a disease of interhemispheric processes at forebrain and brainstem levels? *Behavioural Brain Research, 34*, 1–33.

Foote, S. L., & Morrison, J. H. (1987). Extra-thalamic modulation of cortical function. *Annual Review of Neuroscience, 10*, 67–95.

La Barre, W. (1984). *Muelos: A Stone Age superstition about sexuality*. New York: Columbia University Press.

Libet, B. (1985). Unconscious cerebral initiative and the role of conscious will in voluntary action. *Behavioral and Brain Sciences, 8*, 529–66.

Paxinos, G. (Ed.). (1990). *The human nervous system*. San Diego: Academic Press.

Ringo, J. L. (1991). Neuronal interconnections as a function of brain size. *Brain Behavior and Evolution, 38*, 1–6.

Siegel, G. J., Agranoff, B. W., Albers, R. W., &
Molinoff, P. B. (Eds). (1989). *Basic neurochemistry: Molecular, cellular and medical aspects*, 4th edn. New York: Raven.

Strausfeld, N. J. (1976). *Atlas of an insect brain*. Berlin: Springer.

ROBERT W. DOTY

brain electrical activity mapping (BEAM)
See ELECTROENCEPHALOGRAPHY.

brain stem   The brain stem is located between the spinal cord and the diencephalon. This part of the encephalon comprises three major regions: the medulla (in direct continuation of the spinal cord), the pons, and the midbrain (that continues rostrally with the thalamus, subthalamus, and hypothalamus). The brain stem has sensory and motor functions and it also regulates complex behavioral states of vigilance through modulatory systems with widespread projections to other brain structures.

The brain stem contains: (a) long axonal bundles originating in the spinal cord and projecting to the thalamus, as well as descending fiber tracts arising in diencephalic structures or the cerebral cortex and projecting to lower structures (such as the cerebellum and spinal cord); (b) nuclear groups giving rise to sensory and motor cranial nerves that innervate structures of the head and neck; (c) integrative nuclei, mostly subserving motor functions, interposed between the cerebral cortex, basal ganglia, cerebellum, and spinal cord; and (d) a collection of cell aggregates using different transmitters and having important regulatory functions in setting the excitability level of other structures (spinal cord, diencephalon, and forebrain) for the control of global behavioral states.

This entry discusses the role of brain stem regulatory systems in the modulation of states of vigilance (see above, point (d)) and particularly in promoting dreaming sleep. The role of the brain stem reticular formation in controlling arousal is discussed elsewhere (*see* RETICULAR FORMATION.

BEHAVIORAL STATES OF VIGILANCE AND THE DUAL NATURE OF SLEEP

There are three major behavioral states of vigilance: waking; sleep with low-frequency and

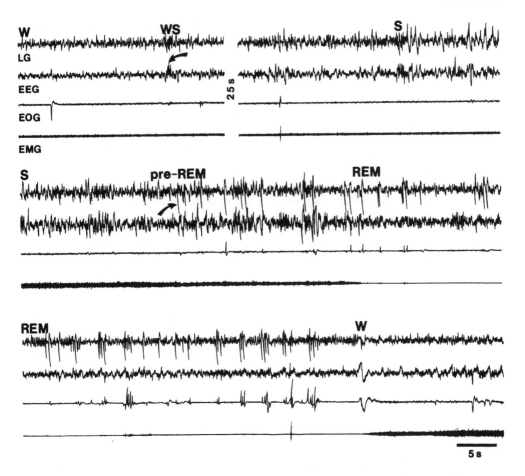

Figure 25 Distinguishing features of full-blown and transitional epochs of the waking–sleep cycle. The four ink-written traces depict the activity of lateral geniculate (LG) thalamic nucleus, EEG rhythms, ocular movements (EOG), and activity of neck muscles (electromyogram, EMG). W, waking; S, EEG-synchronized sleep; WS, transitional epoch between W and S, beginning with the first EEG spindle sequence (indicated by arrow; 25 sec elapsed between the two portions of WS leading to S); pre-REM transitional epoch between S and REM beginning with the first thalamic PGO wave (indicated by arrow).

high-amplitude synchronized waves of the electroencephalogram (hereafter called EEG-synchronized, quiet, or resting sleep); and the brain-activated state of sleep with rapid eye movements (REMs) and oneiric episodes (hereafter called REM, dreaming, or active sleep). A completely specified behavioral state would include the potentially infinite set of variables describing a system or organism. As this can never be achieved for biological systems, each of the behavioral states of vigilance is distinguished by a set of limited physiological variables. These con-

sist of three cardinal signs: the EEG, eye movements (associated with sharp bioelectrical events in thalamocortical systems), and muscular tone (Figure 25).

Wakefulness (with erect posture, open eyes, and purposeful motor acts) is apparently opposite to the whole period of sleep, when subjects are recumbent, with eyes closed, and motor behavior is reduced or absent. However, sleep is not a monolithic behavior. It consists, in fact, of two quite distinct states. The fact that a phase of sleep is characterized in animals and humans by flurries of limb twitches, by contrast to a motionless phase of sleep, was observed a long time ago. During the 1950s Aserinski and Kleitman (1953) and Dement (1958) described the state of sleep with REMs, its association with human dreaming, and its periodic occurrence in the sleep of cats. In independent studies Jouvet (1967) added two important signs that fully characterized REM sleep: the muscular atonia and the pontogeniculo-occipital waves, the latter being considered as the physiological correlate of dreaming. The dream during REM sleep is an emotionally colored experience, with predominantly visual hallucinations and spatio-temporal distortion of images.

As the physiological signs of REM sleep are basically similar in humans and cats, the species of choice for experimental studies on sleep, the question arises whether or not it is possible that the REM sleep of animals is accompanied by dreaming. Since dreams do not necessarily depend on abstract thought and language, it can be assumed that some features of the oneiric behavior may apply to subhuman species. A positive answer to this question was provided by an animal model that enters REM sleep *without* motor atonia. As discussed below, muscular atonia during REM sleep is regulated by a brain stem network inhibiting motoneurons in the spinal cord. The interruption of this circuit is followed by the absence of muscular atonia during REM sleep. This would imply that, after such lesions, animals may enter REM sleep and are able to exhibit the motor behavior accompanying dreams. It was indeed demonstrated that after adequate lesions in the pons, the cat had a dramatic oneiric behavior during REM sleep, seeming to fight against imaginary enemies or to play with an absent mouse, striking out with forelimbs, and manifesting fear reactions associated with vegetative signs. During all this hallucinatory behavior, the nictitating membrane and the pupils were myotic, indicating that the animal was in sleep.

Thus REM sleep is a state with dreaming mentation and a series of neuronal signs indicating that the brain is in a state of increased excitability, but with a concomitant inability to produce motor responses. In other words, this is an aroused yet paralyzed state. This unusual association led to the term *paradoxical sleep* for this state of vigilance. The similarity between arousal and REM sleep in terms of neuronal activities in cholinergic brain stem nuclei, as well as in various thalamic nuclei and different areas of the cerebral cortex, was demonstrated experimentally (Steriade, 1991).

It has been shown that, with the exception of muscular atonia (that specifically characterizes REM sleep, as opposed to both waking and EEG-synchronized sleep) and neurons using monoamines as neurotransmitters, the brain is similarly active during REM sleep and waking, and both these brain-activated behavioral states are opposed to quiet sleep.

BRAIN STEM NEURONS AND PHYSIOLOGICAL SIGNS OF DREAMING SLEEP

1. EEG activity. The EEG rhythms vary with different states of vigilance. (a) During quiet sleep, EEG waves have high amplitudes and low frequencies (below 15 Hz). This bioelectrical pattern reflects the synchronization of large neuronal populations in the thalamus and cerebral cortex. There are three types of oscillations during EEG-synchronized sleep: *spindle* waves (7–14 Hz), the epitome of EEG synchronization at sleep onset; *delta* waves (1–4 Hz), prevailing during late sleep stages; and a *slow* (0.1–0.9 Hz) rhythm grouping spindle and/or delta waves in sequences recurring periodically every 2 to 10 seconds. The major cellular events underlying spindle and delta oscillations are inhibitory processes. They account for the blockage of signals from the outside world. The inhibition of synaptic transmission through the thalamus and the cerebral cortex creates a closed (disconnected) brain from the very onset of EEG-synchronized sleep, a prerequisite for falling asleep. (b) During REM sleep as well as during arousal, the EEG activity shifts from low-frequency oscillations toward waves with high (20–40 Hz) frequency, generally termed *beta* and *gamma* waves. The long-lasting inhibitory processes in large neuronal ensembles, which generate synchronization of electrical activity during quiet sleep, are blocked upon arousal and during REM sleep. Then the synchronizing networks are decoupled. Desynchronization is the term used for the fast and relatively low-amplitude EEG waves during brain activation. It implies that most diencephalic and cortical neurons discharge at high rates, but their activity is generally not synchronous. However, some

synchronizing processes exist during wakefulness to create coherent cell ensembles, possibly the bases of pattern recognition functions. Whether or not this conjunction factor is also present during REM sleep has not yet been demonstrated, but this is expected. Indeed, the 40 Hz rhythm is potentiated in the cerebral cortex by setting into action mesopontine cholinergic neurons, and these cells discharge at high rates during both waking and dreaming sleep.

The neurons producing EEG activation pro-cesses are located at the junction between the pons and the midbrain, in the more rostral part of the midbrain, and in some diencephalic and forebrain structures (posterior hypothalamus and nucleus basalis). Most neurons inducing patterns of EEG activation have firing rates at least as high during REM sleep as during arousal, significantly more during both these states than during EEG-synchronized sleep (*see* RETICULAR FORMA-TION). An important exception to this rule is the group of monoamine-containing neurons in the

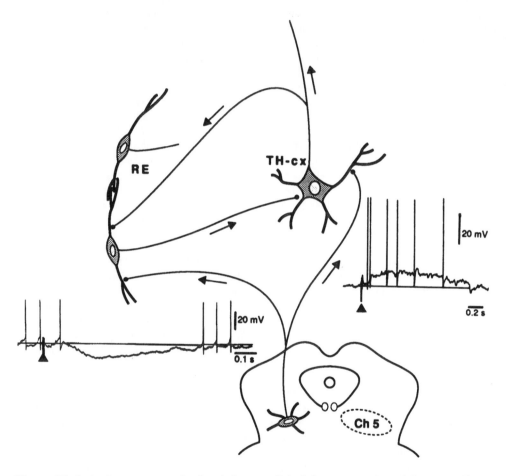

Figure 26 Activation processes in the thalamus, elicited by mesopontine cholinergic afferents. Recurrent inhibitory thalamic loop, consisting of thalamocortical cell (TH-cx) whose axonal collateral drives GABAergic inhibitory reticular thalamic (RE) cell which, in turn, projects back to TH-cx. In the brain stem only one group (Ch 5) of mesopontine cholinergic nuclei is depicted. In insets, intracellularly recorded activities of TH-cx and RE neurons are illustrated in response to Ch 5 stimulation (arrowheads). Ch 5 induces a depolarization (excitation) of TH-cx cell and a hyperpolarization (inhibition) of RE cell. Thus the direct excitation of TH-cx neurons is accompanied by their disinhibition, through inhibition of inhibitory RE neurons.

brain stem (locus coeruleus and dorsal raphé) and the tubero-infundibular hypothalamic region. These cells discharge tonically during waking, slow down their firing rates during quiet sleep, and virtually stop firing during REM sleep. The mechanisms of this decreased activity of monoaminergic neurons during resting sleep, leading to their virtual silence during REM sleep, have not yet been demonstrated. Some metabolic processes taking place inside monoaminergic nuclei may be the cause of the diminished and eventually suppressed activity during sleep stages, as a consequence of their tonic neuronal activity during wakefulness. Although the mechanisms of the suppressed activity of monoamine-containing neurons during REM sleep are not known, this phenomenon was used by McCarley and Hobson (1975) to propose a model for the genesis of dreaming sleep, which was recently revised.

The cellular mechanisms underlying EEG activation have been revealed by recording the neuronal activity in the thalamus and the cerebral cortex. They consist of an increased excitation of thalamic neurons projecting to the cerebral cortex and of cortical neurons projecting to distant structures. In addition, the activation process includes an inhibition of most inhibitory cells in the thalamus (Figure 26). Because of this "inhibition of inhibition" (i.e. suppressed activity of inhibitory neurons), thalamic neurons with cortical projections undergo an additional excitation through a disinhibitory process (removal of inhibition). The enhanced excitation of thalamic cells is transmitted to the cerebral cortex and assists in producing similar changes in cortical neurons.

Since many electrophysiological signs of dreaming sleep are so similar to those of full alertness, what are the distinguishing phenomena between these two brain-active behavioral states? This has not been entirely answered. Among many investigated processes in thalamic and neocortical neurons that are paradoxically alike in both these states, the inhibition is characteristically less effective during REM sleep than in the waking state. This may explain some bizarreries of dreaming mentation. Another difference seems to be the abolition, during dreaming sleep, of late cortical potentials elicited by sensory signals, i.e. those response components having a latency longer than 100 msec. This distinguishing feature led Llinás and Paré (1991) to suggest that the

REM sleep activity prevents the early message along thalamocortical pathways from being incorporated into the intrinsic cognitive world.

2. Muscular atonia. While thalamic and cortical neurons are at their highest excitability level during dreaming sleep, at the opposite pole of the central nervous system, in the spinal cord, motoneurons are strongly inhibited during the same state. This phenomenon explains why powerful central commands are blocked at the periphery, with the consequence of muscular atonia during REM sleep.

This phenomenon was described in the late 1950s. Cats which enter REM sleep undergo a spectacular melting of postural tone. However, during REMs, stereotyped twitching movements, especially of distal extremities, appear on this atonic background, probably because the commands from higher centers are effective enough to overwhelm the inhibition of spinal motoneurons. The inhibition of mono- and polysynaptic spinal reflexes during REM sleep has been intensively studied by Pompeiano (1967), and the intracellular aspects of motoneuronal inhibition have been more recently explored in naturally sleeping animals by Chase and Morales (1983).

It was found that, on transition from quiet to REM sleep, motoneurons undergo a tonic hyperpolarization of their membrane that lasts throughout REM sleep. Data indicated that this phenomenon is not due to removal of excitatory influences (disfacilitation), but to active inhibition mediated by synapses located both on the cell body and on more distal parts of the dendrites. Glycine is the probable transmitter involved in the inhibition. The inhibition of motoneurons is initiated in the brain stem, in a zone just ventral to the locus coeruleus. A pathway links this pontine area to the medulla, from where another projection, probably relayed by inhibitory spinal interneurons, leads to motoneuronal inhibition. The interruption of this circuit by lesions in the brain stem is followed by absence of muscular atonia during REM sleep (see above for comments on motor behavior during cats' dreams).

3. Ponto-geniculo-occipital (PGO) waves. These sharp field potentials (see Figure 25) are probably "the stuff that dreams are made of." They represent corollary discharges of ocular saccades to central structures. In other words, they signal to the brain the direction of eye movements during REM sleep. The relation

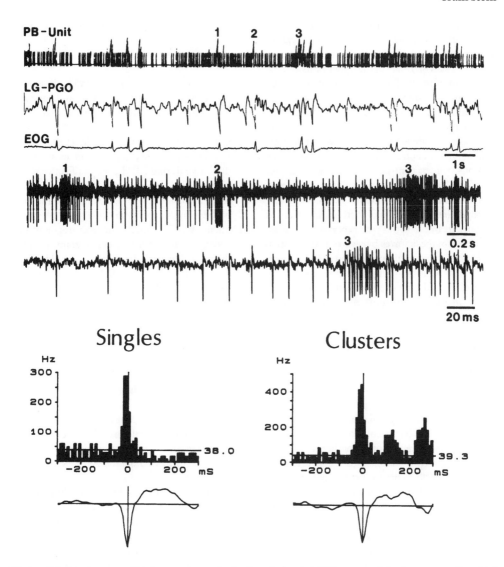

Figure 27 Discharges of brain stem neurons lead to thalamic PGO waves. A brain stem peribrachial (PB) cell is illustrated. The top three ink-written traces depict cell firing, PGO waves recorded from the lateral geniculate (LG) thalamic nucleus, and electro-oculogram (EOG). Epoch with spike bursts indicated by 1, 2 and 3 on the top trace is depicted below, with original discharges, and spike burst 3 is again expanded below to show the acceleration of spontaneous discharges leading to the PGO-related burst. Below, peri-PGO histogram of PB-cell discharges related to single PGO waves and clusters of PGO waves. Time 0 is the peak deflection of the LG-PGO wave. Note increase in firing rate of PB neuron 40–50 ms before the peak of PGO wave. Horizontal lines indicate the rate of spontaneous firing (38 Hz, 39.3 Hz).

between eye movement direction and gaze direction during dreaming was described in earlier studies and was recently confirmed.

PGO waves originate in the upper pons and the lower part of the midbrain in a variety of cellular types; they are transferred to the thalamus and especially to the visual lateral geniculate nucleus; and finally they reach the occipital cortex and other cortical areas. The PGO event is mainly cholinergic in nature, that is, most mesopontine neurons which contribute to its genesis use acetylcholine as the neurotransmitter. The origin of PGO waves in the cholinergic nuclei at the mesopontine junction and surrounding areas is supported by a series of experimental data: elicitation of these waves by electrical stimulation in that brain stem region; abolition of PGO waves by cellular lesions of mesopontine cholinergic aggregates; and evidence for neuronal discharges in cholinergic mesopontine nuclei reliably preceding the PGO wave recorded from the thalamus or the cerebral cortex (Figure 27).

PGO waves or their waking correlates, eye-movement potentials, probably have more than one function. It was proposed that these spiky events represent orienting reactions to messages from inside the brain during dreaming sleep or to external stimuli during wakefulness. This idea is supported by the habituation of PGO responses with repeated stimulation. Another hypothesis considers that the endogenous PGO activity is necessary for the correct expression of innate programs and that it plays an important role in structural maturation, especially during the early period of ontogenesis when REM sleep episodes occupy most of the sleep cycle. In favor of this hypothesis, it was found that the cellular body of visual thalamic cells of kittens with brain stem lesions (which eliminate PGO waves but not other signs of REM sleep) has a smaller size than in control animals. If maturation especially applies to early infancy, some of the functions of dreaming sleep in adult life may be involved in learning processes, especially in the consolidation of memory traces acquired during wakefulness. However, the opposite idea was also advanced, namely a function of REM sleep in negative learning, in forgetting, as parasitic modes of overloaded cortical networks might be removed by random stimulation of the brain during REM sleep. It is fair to state that the function of dreaming sleep is far from being understood and

that all these hypotheses have to be seriously tested.

BIBLIOGRAPHY

Aserinski, E., & Kleitman, N. (1953). Regularly occurring periods of eye motility, and concomitant phenomena during sleep. *Science, 118,* 273–4.

Chase, M. H., & Morales, F. R. (1983). Subthreshold excitatory activity and motoneuron discharge during REM periods of active sleep. *Science, 221,* 1195–8.

Crick, F., & Mitchison, G. (1983). The function of dreaming sleep. *Nature, 304,* 111–14.

Dement, W. C. (1958). The occurrence of low voltage, fast, electroencephalogram patterns during behavioral sleep in the cat. *Electroencephalography and Clinical Neurophysiology, 10,* 291–6.

Jouvet, M. (1967). Neurophysiology of the states of sleep. *Physiological Review, 47,* 117–77.

Llinás, R. R., & Paré, D. (1991). Of dreaming and wakefulness. *Neuroscience, 44,* 521–35.

McCarley, M., & Hobson, J. A. (1975). Neuronal excitability modulation over the sleep cycle: a structural and mathematical model. *Science, 189,* 58–60.

McCarley, R. W., & Massaquoi, S. G. (1992). Neurobiological structure of the revised limit cycle reciprocal interaction model of REM cycle control. *Journal of Sleep Research, 1,* 132–7.

Pompeiano, O. (1967). The neurophysiological mechanisms of the postural and motor events during desynchronized sleep. *Proceedings of the Association for Research into Nervous and Mental Diseases, 45,* 351–423.

Steriade, M. (1991). Alertness, quiet sleep, dreaming. In A. Peters and E. J. Jones (Eds), *Cerebral cortex* (Vol. 9, pp. 279–357). New York: Plenum Press.

Steriade, M., & McCarley, R. W. (1990). *Brainstem control of wakefulness and sleep.* New York: Plenum Press.

Steriade, M., Paré, D., Datta, S., Oakson, G., & Curró Dossi, R. (1990). Different cellular types in mesopontine cholinergic nuclei related to ponto-geniculo-occipital waves. *Journal of Neuroscience, 10,* 2560–79.

Steriade, M., Nuñez, A., & Amzica, F. (1993). Intracellular analysis of relations between the slow (< 1 Hz) neocortical oscillation and other sleep rhythms of the electroencephalogram. *Journal of Neuroscience, 13*, 3266–83.

MIRCEA STERIADE

brain stem evoked potential   *See* EVOKED POTENTIAL.

Broca's aphasia   *See* APHASIA.

Brodmann's cytoarchitectonic maps   Cyto-architectonic maps describe the cerebral cortex, not in terms of its apparent physical features but in terms of regions in which a particular type of cell is found. Brodmann's cytoarchitectonic maps, published between 1903 and 1908, have been the most influential, and his classification of the cortex into over 50 regions in which a particular distinctive type of cell is to be found, is still in use today. For example, the striate cortex at the occipital pole which forms the primary visual cortex is referred to as "area 17."

Historically, the use of cytoarchitectonic maps was most important in the period between the two World Wars, when the Localizationists attempted to ascribe psychological functions to the cerebral cortex on the basis of maps such as Brodmann's.

Bruegel's syndrome   *See* BLETHAROSPASM.

buccofacial apraxia   *See* APRAXIA.

buffoonery syndrome   A term given to the clowning, fatuous jocularity, bizarre inaccurate replies to questions, and dramatic failure on cognitive tests which may occur in the GANSER SYNDROME, as well as in certain functional states.

butterfly glioma   A malignant tumor of the CORPUS CALLOSUM which develops laterally to invade both frontal lobes may be given the term "butterfly glioma" from its radiological appearance. It has been associated by some with a degree of apathy and unresponsiveness to command, presumably from the involvement of frontal rather than callosal tissue.

C

café au lait   As the name suggests, café au lait spots are light brown marks upon the skin, of variable size, which may be present at birth or may develop in adult life. In the skin they are benign, but they may be associated with neuro-fibromatosis (Von Recklinghausen's disease), tumors of peripheral nerves, or with tuberous sclerosis, a congenital condition associated with epilepsy and mental retardation. Both of these disorders are genetically determined by auto-somal dominant genes.

callosal agenesis   Agenesis of the corpus callosum means that, for whatever reason, no identi-fiable CORPUS CALLOSUM is present. It is a com-plex malformation of neural development occur-ring in isolation or combined with other cerebral anomalies. There are degrees of dysgenesis vari-ously referred to as partial agenesis or hypogene-sis. There is also a condition in which the corpus callosum is present but thinned out in parts, sometimes referred to as hypoplasia of the corpus callosum (Ruach & Jinkins, 1993). Each of these categories, agenesis, hypogenesis, and hypo-plasia, is likely to be associated with a different neuropsychological profile. In each case the pre-cise details will further depend upon the presence and degree of other anomalies in the brain.

More than 50 different disorders have been reported associated with callosal agenesis. Of these there are five disease entities almost always associated with agenesis: Aicardi syndrome, Andermann syndrome, Shapiro syndrome, acrocallosal syndrome, and Menkes disease. The reported incidence of agenesis depends upon the population studied and the diagnostic techniques employed. Among all children the incidence is .0005 percent to 0.7 percent; among develop-mentally disabled 2.2 percent to 2.4 percent. Recently (Cioni et al., 1993) a surprisingly high incidence of 0.81 percent cases of partial or complete callosal agenesis has been reported from a study of 1,359 infants born either pre-maturely or at full term, but presenting risk conditions for the CNS.

The widespread incidence of associated cere-bral anomalies with callosal agenesis must be set alongside the increasing number of cases, detected using noninvasive neuroradiological procedures such as CT and MRI, *without* gross neurological dysfunction and with normal, or near normal, mental status.

NEUROPSYCHOLOGICAL PROFILE

The more dramatic cognitive and behavioral consequences of cerebral COMMISSUROTOMY are not evident to superficial inspection in callosal agenesis. When either their mental status is normal or they are not grossly subnormal, acal-losals may remain indistinguishable in social situations. Usually only detailed investigations reveal specific cognitive and behavioral deficits. Under the influence of commissurotomy studies, earlier investigations of acallosals tended to focus largely, though not exclusively, on two issues: first, their ability to integrate sensory input arriv-ing initially in different cerebral hemispheres; second, their ability to produce smoothly ex-ecuted coordinated activity of the arms and hands. In addition, the specialized functions of the two cerebral hemispheres have been studied, follow-ing claims that acallosals possess bilateral repre-sentation of functions which are normally lateral-ized. More recently there have been studies of language and memory where performances dis-tinguishable from those of normals have been reported. The principal features of the neuropsy-chological profile found in individuals without associated gross anomalies of other brain structures may be summarized under the follow-ing headings.

Midline sensory integration

It is generally agreed that the corpus callosum is involved in "midline fusion" thus producing continuity of sensation across somatosensory, visual, and auditory space. This essential callosal function follows from anatomical and physiological studies showing that the sensory systems mentioned project exclusively or preferentially to contralateral brain structures. Several studies have shown that, as regards the visual system, acallosals have difficulties when required to undertake midline fusion in stereopsis (Jeeves, 1991). In the somatosensory system they have difficulty on a two-point discrimination task applied in axial regions. Most recently, Lepore (1993) has reported a difficulty encountered by acallosals when localizing sound sources at the interaural plane. Their generally poorer than normal performance was not, in this instance, limited to central auditory space.

Acallosals can correctly match visual stimuli presented independently to the two visual fields with an accuracy comparable with that of normals. However, their speed of response when making such judgments is significantly slower than that of normals. A similar finding applies when they are required to perform intermanual matching of objects and cut-out shapes.

Motor coordination

That acallosals have difficulty in performing skilled movements was noted early on by clinicians and subsequently validated in experimental studies by neuropsychologists. Thus they or their carers may report difficulty experienced as children in learning to tie shoe laces and button up coats. If they are presented with a task such as a child's "Etch-a-Sketch," which demands integration of the coordinated activity of the two hands, they perform less well than normals and with great difficulty if the task is covered from view so that visual feedback is denied. Such performances would normally be regarded as signs of *frontal* disconnection. A recent (Sauerwein et al., 1993) careful study of 8 patients with total agenesis, 6 of whom suffered from the Andermann syndrome, found that on the task most indicative of perceptuomotor deficits, the initial learning with the dominant hand, as well as intermanual transfer and bimanual execution of the task, were impaired in the acallosal group. The strong evidence for difficulty in motor coordination in callosal

agenesis fits well with the now frequently reported finding of greatly lengthened interhemispheric transmission times in acallosals. Normally this is measured by flashing a spot of light briefly to the left or right of a central fixation point and asking the subject to press a key as quickly as possible when the flash appears. When a dominant right-hand response is made to a flash in the right visual field both sensory input and motor output are within the same hemisphere, whereas when a left-hand response is called for a callosal crossing is involved. There are good reasons for believing that this is a motor crossing. Whereas for normals the average interhemispheric transmission time is 2 to 3 msecs, for acallosals it ranges from 10 to 40 msecs. These lengthened times in acallosals have also been reported using EVOKED POTENTIAL techniques.

Cognitive functioning

As would be expected, the level of cognitive functioning is strongly related, not only to the degree of absence of the corpus callosum, but also to the severity of any coexisting CNS defects. Thus where there are multiple associated malformations, for instance in the Aicardi syndrome, and where these include extensive abnormalities of limbic structures, it seems likely that these subcortical malformations may be at the root of the mental deficiencies found in so many syndromes that include callosal agenesis. However, with the widespread use of noninvasive neuroradiological procedures such as CT and MRI, increasing numbers of acallosals are being detected without gross neurological dysfunction and with normal or near normal mental status. The study by Sauerwein and colleagues (1993) referred to earlier compared a group of 8 acallosals, 6 of whom suffered from the Andermann syndrome, with a group of IQ-matched controls from special education centers and a further group of normal IQ controls from regular schools. Both control groups were matched on the basis of age, gender, and handedness. Sauerwein and her colleagues evaluated intellectual capacities, attention and concentration, memory, language, perceptual abilities, motor skills, perceptuomotor integration and somatosensory functions. They concluded that individuals born without the corpus callosum can have normal cognitive abilities but tend to function at the lower end of the normal range. Their level of functioning may, on selected tasks, be still lower because of associated structural abnormalities in the CNS in specific cases. Even so, they do still differ from IQ-matched peers on some forms of sensorimotor learning and transfer and it seems that these deficits cannot easily be surmounted by practice or compensatory mechanisms (see below). However, such deficits may only become evident under very special, highly artificial testing. Testing on an auditory verbal learning task indicated problems in retrieval in cases of total agenesis, but these were not evident in a case with partial agenesis sparing the anterior part of the callosum.

Language

Studies of a small number of acallosal children of normal intelligence have revealed specific cognitive deficits in the language domain and in visuospatial skills (Temple & Ilsey, 1993). An early study had suggested that acallosals might have a specific deficit in using or understanding the syntactic-pragmatic component of language. Later studies partially confirmed the earlier findings and also demonstrated difficulty in some phonological tasks. The acallosal subjects studied showed clear articulation of speech which was well formed and thus showed no gross phonological impairment. Nonetheless there was a significant impairment in their ability to pronounce aloud nonwords, i.e. meaningless letter strings which conformed to the orthographic rules of language. Despite this difficulty they showed no overall impairment in reading levels in terms of word recognition. Current psycholinguistic theory would suggest that the acallosals' phonological reading route is developmentally impaired while the lexical reading route is normal. This finding was further compared with tests of phonemic discrimination. The same acallosals had difficulties with some tasks requiring visuo-constructional skills such as constructing jigsaws and formboards.

Cerebral hemisphere specialization

In order to explain the apparent lack of the disconnection effects evident in commissurotomized patients, it was suggested that the brains of acallosals failed to develop normal hemispheric specialization and instead possessed bilateral control of speech and other functions. Others (e.g. Chiarello, 1980) argued that such bilateral representation had not been demonstrated. Since then the evidence has increasingly strengthened this viewpoint. (1) Of 8 acallosals reported to have been given the Wada amytal test (INTRACAROTID SODIUM AMYTAL), all but two have shown normal lateralization of speech in the left hemisphere. (2) In word recognition tests a normal right visual half field advantage is found. (3) Summarizing the results of testing 29 acallosals on DICHOTIC LISTENING, Chiarello (1980) concluded there was clear evidence for a small but reliable asymmetry, a result supported by later studies. (4) Most of the acallosal patients on whom studies have been reported have been right-handed; this right-hand (left hemisphere) dominance also extends to skilled motor activity. (5) The limited evidence currently available, though more equivocal, points to right hemisphere specialization for visuospatial functions in acallosals (Jeeves, 1990). It remains an open question whether the degree of lateralization in acallosals is the same as in normals.

Compensatory mechanisms in callosal agenesis

Sperry's convincing demonstration of the importance of the forebrain commissures in integrating activity in the two cerebral hemispheres and for transferring information from one hemisphere to the other needs an answer to the question of how it is that someone born without the corpus callosum (and in some instances also without the anterior commissure) achieves interhemispheric integration and transfer so as to appear normal or near normal on tasks showing clear disconnection effects in the surgically split-brain patients. Early attempts to account for the seemingly remarkable compensation of the acallosal brain laid great weight upon two possibilities: first, bilateral representation of functions normally lateralized; second, a significantly increased role for the anterior commissure when present. As we have seen, the evidence does not support the bilateral representation hypothesis. As regards the anterior commissure, early reports that it was bigger than normal in acallosals gave credence to its likely increased role. However, subsequent detailed morphometric studies gave no support to the view; while 10 percent of the agenesis cases studied by Ruach and Jinkins (1993) showed an enlarged anterior commissure, equally 10 percent of the cases showed a smaller one. There is, however, evidence that in some cases where the corpus callosum is absent, putative callosal fibers pass through the anterior commissure. If, as seems probable, they exhibit normal topography, that would suggest a compensatory role. It seems likely that while the anterior commissure carries visual pattern information, a plausible view since the temporal lobes are interconnected through the anterior commissure, it is likely that the integration of visual spatial information is mediated by the intertectal commissure. Indeed, it seems likely in the light of the work of Sergent (1990) that more visual information is transferred subcortically than had previously been suspected.

The enhanced development of ipsilateral sensory and motor pathways would help to explain the unexpected success of some acallosal patients on tasks of tactile discrimination (including between-hand comparisons) while performing poorly on tactile localization and fine motor control. This possibility receives support from EVOKED POTENTIAL studies which showed that, while in normals there was a strong contralateral scalp response to stimulation of the wrist, with little or no ipsilateral response, in acallosals there was a strong ipsilateral response, presumed to come through the enhanced ipsilateral pathways.

There are several possible reasons why acallosals benefit from the compensatory mechanisms outlined above, whereas adult surgical split-brain patients do not. First, since cerebral plasticity is closely linked to the degree of functional maturity at the time of the injury or insult, the acallosal brain may develop alternative pathways prenatally and onwards. Second, many cortical connections undergo a state of exuberant growth before synaptic stabilization occurs in late adolescence. This means that when, as in callosal agenesis, the insult occurs early in the formative stage, connections which would otherwise have been eliminated during the critical period of axon retraction and synaptic elimination may persist. Third, it is possible that in agenesis the normal period of cerebral plasticity may be extended.

Despite these putative compensatory processes in callosal agenesis, deficits occur. It may be that in total agenesis these processes, individually or in combination, are insufficient to ensure the normal combination of the hypothetical modular subcomponents of complex tasks, especially of the kind used by Temple (1993) in her studies of phonological skills. In contrast, partial agenesis, which seems to reveal fewer and less severe

deficits, may do so largely because the remnant of the callosum which is present contains fibers which exhibit the normal widespread topographic linking of the two cerebral hemispheres, albeit with drastically reduced numbers of fibers to each cortical region so connected.

Is there a behavioral phenotype?

Perhaps because of the diversity of abnormalities associated with callosal agenesis, there has hitherto been little attempt to find out whether there may be a definable behavioral phenotype in callosal agenesis. Recently O'Brien (1993) has suggested that there may be increasing behavioral and developmental consequences from partial through total agenesis to the Aicardi syndrome. There is, for example, a clear step-wise increasing prevalence of epilepsy as one moves from partial to total agenesis and to the Aicardi syndrome. O'Brien (1993) also notes that in the children he studied emotional non-communicativeness was evident. Thus parents typically report it difficult or well-nigh impossible to know at any one time what their child is feeling or experiencing emotionally. This is not simply because the children are retarded, because the same is not commonly reported by the parents of mentally handicapped children. Thus aspects of callosal agenesis so far little studied, but which for management and rehabilitation purposes may be of potentially major importance, would include studies of social behavior, e.g. lack of empathy and of communication difficulties which may be linked to subtle language deficits of the kind noted earlier. It is possible that the missing or reduced putative function of the corpus callosum most involved here is not integration but inhibition. Several researchers using EEG measures have noted changes in coherence patterns between homologous cortical areas in acallosals, which they have attributed to a disruption of the inhibitory and facilitatory interactions between the hemispheres, normally mediated through the corpus callosum.

Arguments that the corpus callosum plays an essential inhibitory function in the development of normal cerebral lateralization must be weakened by the failure to find evidence for bilateral representation in acallosals, as well as by the findings noted earlier of evidence *for* cerebral specialization. It remains an open question, however, whether the degree of cerebral specialization in acallosals is as clear-cut as in normals.

Furthermore, the deficits in aspects of bimanual coordination and of reaching and grasping found in acallosals have plausibly been interpreted as being, in part, due to the absence of the normal inhibitory role of the callosum in preventing unwanted competition between crossed and uncrossed sensory and motor pathways.

The results of some of the studies of acallosals (Lassonde & Jeeves, 1993) lend support to the callosum normally playing a facilitative function in both intrahemispheric and interhemispheric processes. The observation that deficits in the performances of acallosals on visual and visuomotor tasks are not limited to *inter*hemispheric processing, but that *intra*hemispheric processing is also affected, may be attributed to the lack of normal callosal influx. This absence or reduction of the normal modulating or facilitatory influence of the corpus callosum has clinical implications. It helps to understand how commissurotomy not only abolishes interhemispheric propagation of seizure discharges but may also reduce activity in the initial focus. This modulating action of the corpus callosum may be actively involved in the functional reorganization that occurs after brain injury. If this is so, then an acallosal suffering further brain injury may face reduced prospects of functional reorganization. It also remains possible that one global effect of the absence of this modulating activity in acallosals is that neither hemisphere develops its full potential, hence the widely reported generally lower intellectual status in acallosals.

BIBLIOGRAPHY

Chiarello, C. (1980). A house divided? Cognitive functioning with callosal agenesis. *Brain and Language, 11*, 128–58.

Cioni, G., Bartalena, L., Biagioni, E., & Boldrini, A. (1993). The normal absent and abnormal corpus callosum: postnatal sonographic findings. In M. Lassonde & M. A. Jeeves (Eds), *Callosal agenesis: The natural split brain* (pp. 69–76). New York and London: Plenum.

Jeeves, M. A. (1990). Agenesis of the corpus callosum. In F. Boller & J. Grafman (Eds), *Handbook of neuropsychology*, Vol. 4 (pp. 99–114). Amsterdam: Elsevier.

Jeeves, M. A. (1991). Stereoperception in callosal agenesis and partial callosotomy. *Neuropsychologia, 29*, 19–34.

Lassonde, M., & Jeeves, M. A. (1993). *Callosal agenesis: The natural split brain*. New York and London: Plenum.

O'Brien, G. (1993). The behavioural and developmental consequences of corpus callosal agenesis and Aicardi syndrome. In M. Lassonde & M. A. Jeeves (Eds), *Callosal agenesis: The natural split brain* (pp. 235–46). New York and London: Plenum.

Ruach, R. A., & Jinkins, J. R. (1993). MR imaging in callosal dysgenesis. In M. Lassonde & M. A. Jeeves (Eds), *Callosal agenesis: The natural split brain* (pp. 83–95). New York and London: Plenum.

Sauerwein, H. C., Nolin, P., & Lassonde, M. (1993). Cognitive functioning in callosal agenesis. In M. Lassonde & M. A. Jeeves (Eds), *Callosal agenesis: The natural split brain* (pp. 221–33). New York and London: Plenum.

Sergent, J. (1990). Furtive incursions into bicameral minds: integrating and coordinating role of subcortical structures. *Brain, 109*, 537–68.

Temple, C., & Ilsey, J. (1993). Sounds and shapes: language and spatial cognition in callosal agenesis. In M. Lassonde & M. A. Jeeves (Eds), *Callosal agenesis: The natural split brain* (pp. 261–73). New York and London: Plenum.

MALCOLM A. JEEVES

callosal section *See* COMMISSUROTOMY.

caloric stimulation (also **calimetry**) Caloric vestibular tests are employed to investigate the function of the labyrinth, by irrigating the ear with either hot or cold water, so stimulating the labyrinth. Under standard conditions, the time between the onset of irrigation and the end of the resulting nystagmus is measured, and may indicate abnormalities of the labyrinth, the eighth cranial nerve, or lesions of the vestibular areas of the brain stem or cerebral hemispheres.

Capgras syndrome Capgras syndrome is a rare disorder in which the patient believes that members of the family, or close friends and neighbors, have been replaced by physically identical imposters, usually with some sinister intent (*see* REDUPLICATION).

carbon monoxide poisoning   Carbon monoxide poisoning is one of the principal causes of coma. Before the conversion of the UK gas supply from town gas to North Sea gas, it was relatively common in attempted suicide, and it may still be a feature of failed suicide using a vehicle exhaust. Accidents involving vehicle fumes, defective gas heaters (and previously coke braziers), and occupational accidents may all involve carbon monoxide poisoning.

The effects are related to those of general ANOXIA but have additional characteristics. During exposure, reducing mental efficiency and drowsiness lead directly to loss of consciousness, then rapidly into coma, with a characteristic neurological picture. The length of coma is variable but may be prolonged, and on emergence from coma there is commonly a loss of orientation and confusion, followed by apathy and poor initiation. There may be a prolonged period of delirium, and memory disturbances are common, although it may be difficult to distinguish between primary effects upon the memory and the effects of poor motivation and initiation. Other neuropsychological effects which may be apparent during the course of recovery include constructional apraxia, agnosia, and aphasic difficulties. Recovery from both the neurological and neuropsychological disturbances can in some cases be very considerable, although it may occur rather gradually over a protracted period of months. Occasionally a relapsing course is to be observed, with a latent period either between the emergence from coma and the onset of other symptoms, or after a period of considerable recovery.

While recovery from carbon monoxide poisoning may be remarkable, many patients are left with enduring neuropsychological deficits, particularly if the coma persists beyond a few hours. These deficits may include continuing memory dysfunction, some general cognitive impairment, and personality changes. A correlation has been suggested between the amnesic difficulties and the changes in personality. These changes, sometimes described as "affective incontinence," are increased irritability, moodiness, and impulsive verbal aggression and violence. These effects are similar to the enduring effects which may follow closed head injury, which suggests that these enduring effects of carbon monoxide poisoning are the result of somewhat diffuse mild damage to the brain.

A debate continues about the effects of chronic exposure to carbon monoxide. Besides specific neurological signs, psychological symptoms including depression, restlessness, anxiety, and cognitive impairments, all of which are typical of chronic exposure to industrial toxins, have been reported. However, as carbon monoxide rapidly clears from the blood and does not act as a cumulative poison (unlike heavy metals, for example), some doubt the validity of attributing these effects to the carbon monoxide exposure.

The pathological changes which follow carbon monoxide poisoning are bilaterally in the globus pallidus, in Ammon's horn within the temporal lobe, and patches of nerve cell death in the cortex, although not the widespread laminar changes in the cortex which are characteristic of other forms of anoxia. Changes also occur in cerebral white matter and in the cerebellum, but not in the Purkinje cells, again in contrast to a typical picture of anoxia. There are also vascular lesions, which may be the basis of the rather specific changes seen in certain structures. That the pathology differs from that of general anoxia suggests a specific toxic effect of the carbon monoxide, in addition to the restriction of oxygen in the blood.

J. GRAHAM BEAUMONT

case study   *See* LOCALIZATION; METHODOLOGICAL ISSUES.

CAT scan   Computerized axial tomography (CAT) is a form of medical imaging (*see* SCAN). The term CAT scan was adopted on the introduction of this technique, but has more generally now been replaced by CT scan (computerized tomography).

catalepsy   Catalepsy is a term for the movement disorder, common in PARKINSON'S DISEASE, characterized by muscular rigidity, in which posture is maintained but voluntary movements are reduced or absent. As a significant term, it is not commonly employed.

cataplexy   The cataplectic patient suffers complete loss of movement and posture during which muscle tone is absent, yet consciousness and memory for events during the attack are spared. Of sudden onset, so that the consequent fall may result in injury, the attacks occur more commonly at times of emotional excitement. Partial attacks of weakness or sagging at the knees may also occur, and all attacks are brief with rapid recovery. Cataplexy is commonly regarded as a disorder of sleep, and authorities differ as to whether it is a form of NARCOLEPSY or whether narcolepsy must involve loss of consciousness.

tends to emphasize the complaint, while the patient with an organic disorder may tend to minimize or be partly unaware of their difficulties, although this is a generalization to which there are frequent exceptions, catastrophic reactions are considered to be an indicator of cerebral pathology, being very rarely seen in neurotic disorders.

J. GRAHAM BEAUMONT

catastrophic reaction   The catastrophic reaction is an inappropriate and explosive outburst of emotion in the form of anger, anxiety, or tears. It is considered to occur in response to a stress, or mental demands, with which the individual is unable to cope, and is a general characteristic of all cerebral disorders, but especially of progressive disorders, although it is not uncommon during the period of recovery following head injury. It may occur within a context in which the patient more generally shows a reduction of emotional response and flatness of affect.

In the classic form, first described by Goldstein, the catastrophic reaction may occur without warning, but more often it is the culmination of increasing tension and anxiety. The patient looks dazed and starts to fumble, after which the intense outburst occurs, accompanied by the autonomic signs of sweating, trembling, and flushing. The period of the outburst may be followed by a sudden aimless restlessness.

The reaction may be elicited during cognitive assessment, especially if the examiner persists with tasks which are particularly demanding for the patient, and for this reason it may in some cases be appropriate to exercise care in the order of test administration, interspersing tests which the subject finds particularly difficult with those on which success might be more easily achieved. Tests which limit the number of items which may be failed, such as the Wechsler tests, are less likely to provoke a catastrophic reaction than tests on which persistent and repeated failure may induce great stress for the patient (most notably, the Wisconsin Card Sorting Test in its unmodified form).

It has been claimed that the catastrophic reaction is an important sign in making the distinction between neurotic and organic reactions. Besides the fact that the neurotic patient

catatonia   Originally described by Kahlbaum in 1874, catatonia was referred to as an illness with a recurrent periodic pattern that he wanted to differentiate from general paresis. He considered its most noteworthy features to be psychomotor symptoms, akinetic and hypertonic symptoms, and a deteriorating course that developed progressively through different stages which included melancholia, mania, stupor, and eventually dementia.

The typical syndrome involves a combination of the following symptoms:

1 Psychomotor negativism: refusal of movement, food, conversation, MUTISM.
2 Psychomotor inertia: attitudes of passivity and suggestibility to the extent that it may evolve into echolalia, echopraxia.
3 Stereotypy: repetition of movements, the most typical being rhythmic oscillations of the head or upper body, mannerisms with or without grimaces, contortions.
4 Bizarre intonations, intense theatrical dramatization.
5 Impulsions: inappropriate, periodic discharges of intense violence which come in complete rupture with the previously akinetic behavior.
6 CATALEPSY: since Kahlbaum, plasticity, fixity of attitude, "waxy flexibility" have been described as being characteristic of catatonia; this refers to a rigidity of muscular masses with active resistance as well as retention of posture. It may be passive, such as when the arm defies gravity by remaining in a position given to it by an observer (*signe de Lasèque*) or elicited by the patient, i.e. he or she retains an extended arm and open hand as if to shake hands once the observer has retracted his or hers.

HISTORICAL DIMENSIONS

In his classic attempt at psychiatric classification, Kraepelin (1908) grouped catatonic symptoms within dementia praecox but recognized that some of the symptoms could appear in other states, such as manic and melancholic psychoses, as well as in postictal epilepsy. When describing the group of schizophrenias, Bleuler, in 1911, made catatonia a specific subtype because he thought it also demonstrated the four primary symptoms of schizophrenia: autism, ambivalence, disturbance in thought associations and affects. In 1932, Gjessing published his remarkable studies on catatonia and considered it a disorder resulting from periodic imbalances in nitrogen metabolism. He treated his patients with desiccated thyroid extract with some success. Baruk and Claude, in the 1920s, also published on experimental production of catatonia with bulbocapnine and thus opened the way for experimental paradigms. These studies raised further doubts about the inclusion of catatonia in the concept of schizophrenia.

Nonetheless, catatonia has continued to be classified as a subtype of schizophrenia, both in the different editions of the Diagnostic Statistic Manual of the American Psychiatric Association and in the International Classifications of Diseases (World Health Organization).

CLINICAL FEATURES

A classic phenomenological preneuroleptic description of the features is offered by Baruk. Primarily, it portrays a patient folded on himself in an attitude like Rodin's *Thinker*, without expression on his face, a loss of vitality in the eyes, and a rigidity of the muscles, which retain positions for indeterminate periods of time. Patients exhibit *gegenhalten*, where the examiner encounters resistance of equal strength to his or her attempts at posture manipulation. There is a loss in psychomotor initiatives to the point of catalepsy, including the persistence of dramatic attitudes of ecstasy or crucifixion, which Kahlbaum labelled "patheticismus." Patients will sometimes repeat a question modelled on that of the interviewer's, sometimes be completely mute or, seemingly without reason, will emit incoherent, disconnected, rather simple repetitive speech (verbigeration). This may be accompanied by inappropriate chuckles, strange sounds or expressions. Periodically, there will be periods (usually brief) of extreme agitation and excitement with incoherent verbal expression, incessant shouting, violent and destructive clastic outbursts, with unprovoked attacks on personnel or other patients. Patients may roam about with no seeming purpose, go sleepless for several nights, refuse food and drink, and be extremely resistant to sedation.

Some authors have argued that, during the catatonic stupor, patients remain sufficiently aware of the environment to be able to retain memory of events. It has been my experience that patients have a narrowing of consciousness but retain some very clear memories of specific events and, once the episode is over, they will remember some details with great accuracy. Other authors have reported that, during the stupor, the patient is beset with flamboyant "oneiroid" delusional and hallucinatory experiences. It has been hypothesized that these specific cases may be toxic in origin. In other instances, patients are given to command-hallucinations encouraging aggressive acts or inappropriate behaviors and they "are forced to freeze" to prevent acting out. While I interviewed a mute and cataleptic patient medicated with sodium amobarbital, he suddenly spat in the air splattering his face and uttered, "I am rotten. If I don't become as solid as steel, I will despoil my sister. I am damned forever." Interestingly enough, several months later, following a period of remission, this patient had perfect memory of the content of his delusion and attributed his hallucinations to his conscience reproaching him for his fantasies. Obviously, emotional conflicts are also part of the experience of these patients. The refusal of food and drink in some cases may be related to the delusion of damnation and be a form of self-punishment.

PRESENT STATUS AND DIAGNOSIS

In the recent fourth edition of the Diagnostic Statistic Manual of the American Psychiatric Association, three issues have been raised:

1 Because of its present apparent rarity, should this diagnosis be retained?
2 Should it continue to be listed under the schizophrenias or in another category, such as mood disorders?
3 Are the present diagnostic criteria representative of the current presentations by patients?

The authors of the new edition have also considered a secondary catatonic disorder having the same symptomatology but relating to non-psychiatric medical conditions. The International Classification of Diseases (ninth edition) retains catatonia as a type of schizophrenia.

Many authors at present consider that several cases of functional catatonia do not represent a schizophrenic disorder but rather a severe psychotic depression (Taylor, 1990). Indeed, since its early description, catalepsy by itself has been considered a symptom to be encountered in "hysteria," epilepsy, delirium, melancholia, mania, hypochondria, and acute dementia.

Some forms of cataleptic behavior follow an emotional trauma or an episode where an unacceptable impulse is provoked. An exemplary case history is described by H. François in the *Dictionnaire encyclopédique des sciences médicales* (1874), where a soldier, sitting with friends around a table, suddenly grasps a bottle to hit a colleague with and remains in a "frozen" position for several hours. This type of episode has been considered more indicative of dissociative and conversion disorders than the more severe psychiatric syndromes.

Since the nineteenth century, there had been reports in the literature of a rare, life-threatening form of psychosis or mania, which, although explained and classified in several manners, usually referred to an acute lethal condition. In 1934 Stauder coined the term fatal or lethal catatonia. This disorder, after a short prodrome characterized by insomnia, anorexia, and excitation, gradually evolves into extreme agitation and destructive behavior, accompanied by somatic symptoms such as tachycardia, high blood pressure, acrocyanosis, diaphoresis and hyperpyrexia (up to 43.5 °C). In its end stage there is cardiovascular collapse, stupor, rigidity, and death. It is important to differentiate this entity from neuroleptic malignant syndrome (NMS) first described by

Table 7   Illnesses in which catatonic signs and symptoms have been reported at onset.

Psychiatric conditions

Schizophrenia
Affective disorders
Conversion disorders
Dissociative disorders
Reactive psychosis

Neurologic conditions

Basal ganglia disorders (arteriosclerotic Parkinsonism, focal lesions of the pallidum)
Disorders of the limbic system and temporal lobes (viral encephalitis, vascular lesions of the temporal lobes, tumors of the septum pellucidum)
Diencephalon disorders (tumors, hemorrhage in the third ventricle, focal thalamic lesions)
Other lesions and disturbances (frontal lobe tumors, anterior cerebral artery aneurysms, arteriovenous malformations, diffuse brain trauma, diffuse encephalomalacia, petit mal epilepsy, postictal states, tuberous sclerosis, Wernicke's encephalopathy, narcolepsy, intracranial hemorrhage, cerebral cortex infarctions, subdural hematomas)

Metabolic conditions

Diabetic ketoacidosis, hypercalcemia, intermittent acute porphyria, pellagra, homocystinuria, hepatic encephalopathy

Toxic agents

Organic fluorides, illuminating gases, mescaline, ethanol, phencyclidine (PCP), neuroleptics (neuroleptic malignant syndrome, neuroleptic-induced catatonia)

(After Stoudemire, 1982, with permission.)

Delay in 1960. The latter is an iatrogenic form of catatonia and is essentially a side effect of all neuroleptics, although initially described as occurring with chlorpromazine, which is a phenothiazine. The two clinical presentations are hard to differentiate because of the psychotic state, the muscular rigidity, and the clouding of consciousness present in both. However, some clinicians state that it is possible to differentiate by analyzing the timing of the hyperthermia, which is said to precede the rigidity and catatonic symptoms in lethal catatonia, but to be present only at the later stuporous stage of NMS. Both conditions can be fatal and obviously the treatment is radically different (Gabris & Miller, 1983; Mann et al., 1986; Castillo et al., 1989).

Although classically associated with psychiatric disorders, it is important to remember that the clinical signs of catatonia are present in several conditions of neurological, metabolic, infectious, and toxic origin.

Beyond the crucial elements of the diagnostic investigation, i.e. history, mental status, and examination, there are the obvious laboratory examinations. X-rays and particularly CAT scans can be helpful in detecting BASAL GANGLIA or frontal lobe abnormalities and calcifications, diffuse cortical atrophy, or ventricular enlargement. EEG can be helpful in diagnosing some seizure disorders, particularly of the temporal lobe. More specifically, it has been said that the ocular nystagmus response to caloric testing is helpful because it is normal in the functional psychoses. The standard lumbar puncture and interpretation of cerebrospinal fluid may reveal abnormal glucose levels, protein levels, etc. Of particular interest in the case of the neuroleptic malignant syndrome are creatine phosphokinase levels, which have proved to be most helpful in the diagnosis and monitoring of this condition. In essence, all these tests are done to exclude medical conditions and one is left with "idiopathic" cases of catatonia (Weinberger, 1984; Stoudemire, 1982).

There is considerable literature suggesting the use of amobarbital or lorazepam intravenously to release the more or less unconsciously defended thought content and affective components. Under medication, patients suffering from brain diseases usually demonstrate disorganization and simplification of verbalizations, as well as growing confusion. The schizophrenic or hysteric patients, on the other hand, become more communicative and able to describe the content of their delusions or fantasies. This is a temporary effect and, after several hours, the patient usually returns to the original state (Gelenberg, 1976; Salam & Kilzieh, 1988).

PREVALENCE

It is hard to determine why this psychosis, which in the past represented anywhere from 10 to 15 percent of patients in mental hospitals, has gradually diminished and become a rarity. Bleuler thought that half of his schizophrenic patients presented catatonic features at some time during their illness. A correlation with the incidence of viral encephalitis has been postulated by some authors. At present, the current edition of the American Diagnostic Manual questions whether it is worthwhile to include catatonia as a category. When discussing incidence, it is important to specify if we are referring to catatonic schizophrenia which, at the present time, represents a very rare disorder, or including the catatonic features seen more frequently in affective disorders. In the latter case, the percentage of prevalence may be as much as 15 to 20 percent in bipolar disorders (Abrams & Taylor, 1976; Magrinat et al., 1983; Taylor & Abrams, 1977).

ETIOLOGY AND CONCEPTUALIZATION

In the past 65 years, there have been two diametrically opposed sets of ideas to explain the clinical picture. Several investigators claimed that catatonia had a strictly organic etiology and argued that the clinical presentation was due to the impairment either of the basal ganglia or, secondly, to a more diffuse lesion. On the other hand, there were others who believed that catatonia was a manifestation of intense mental regression, a lower functioning of the mind due to unconscious emotional repression. They felt that mutism and AKINESIA were evidence of unwillingness to express conflict; in essence, a defense against unspeakable impulses. It would be to persist in a narrow analysis to conceptualize catatonia in this "either/or" perspective. It appears preferable to consider the behavior as a resultant and an adaptation to cerebral as well as psychic insults.

It is helpful to look at the historical experimental data concerning this pathological picture and review some of the psychoanalytic hypotheses to clarify current thinking.

191

Since 1921 (Dejong) bulbocapnine has been mentioned as a drug capable of provoking cataleptoid-like states in animals, including catalepsy, hyperkinesia, negativism, and flexion spasms. Following several studies both with this substance and others, Baruk concluded that catatonia was proportional to diffusion within the entire brain and not localized to any specific area. He also proposed that catatonia could be secondary to toxic colibacillus ENCEPHALITIS, to tuberculous allergic reactions, and severe hepatic and uraemic conditions.

The advent of modern psychopharmacology and the analysis of the role played by different amines and indoles, particularly the role of the basal ganglia in severe extrapyramidal side effects, helped clarify the pathophysiology of catatonia. In the 1960s, the investigation of drug-induced catatonia by Poirier and Sourkes, involving alphamethyltyrosine, alphamethyldopa, and reserpine, demonstrated that the tremor and akinesia could be reversed temporarily by L-dopa, as well as benztropine and other anticholinergic compounds. Indeed, catalepsy became a pharmacological behavioral test to screen for neuroleptics, because of the specific action that we now know to be a blocking of dopamine transmission in the basal ganglia and the nigrastriatal pathways.

Other authors considered catatonia to be associated with frontal lobe dysfunction because of the role of these structures in attention, emotional control, and motor regulation (Taylor, 1990). A parallel was drawn with frontal lobe patients described as presenting a dissociation between cognition and behavior, as if aware of their errors but incapable of modifying them. Mesulam considered that the brain stem also plays a role in the syndrome of akinetic mutism and stereotypy. There is CAT scan evidence of atrophy in the brain stem and the vermis of the cerebellum.

There continues to be some literature which shows that it is helpful to conceptualize catatonia as a psychological defensive reaction where the person is able to block verbal or motoric behavior provoked by an overwhelming affect or unconscious conflict. The clinical picture would result from a generalized form of disorganization with "active" immobility; in essence, an unconscious but positive attempt to stop the acting out of unacceptable impulses. It is hypothesized that the schizophrenic presents with an access, because of his or her psychosis, to unspeakable internal affects and cognitions which have to be behaviorally blocked by virtue of their nature. Both psychoanalysts and neurologists have pointed to the similarity of the dissociation in hysterical conversion reactions and catatonia (Juni, 1982).

TREATMENT

Obviously, because we are addressing a syndrome, it follows that after diagnosis the treatment should be directed to the primary condition. Electroconvulsive therapy (ECT) particularly the unilateral, nondominant type, has consistently been shown to be the therapy of choice for a catatonic state. There is often a dramatic reversal of the clinical picture after only 2 or 3 treatment sessions. In some cases where there is severe dehydration and cachexia, it becomes an urgent indication. Neuroleptics are too slow in onset of action and often have limited effect. The therapeutic results of ECT, although partially understood in the perspective of the prevalence of affective disorders presenting catatonic symptoms, are at present unexplained, despite a putative neurotransmitter and neuroendocrine augmentation accompanied by a lowering of the blood–brain barrier (Taylor, 1977).

It is best to be prudent with neuroleptics, although they are indicated in lethal catatonia, because of the differential diagnosis with neuroleptic malignant syndrome, where the treatment is obviously to stop those medications.

In the recent literature, benzodiazepines have been found to be helpful not only in the diagnosis, but also in the treatment of catatonia (Menza & Harris, 1989). Given their relative innocuousness, a therapeutic trial should be attempted, providing the condition is not overly serious. It may be interesting to ponder, in terms of theoretical psychopharmacological explanations, the effects of both benzodiazepines and barbiturates on catatonia. Both groups of medications interact at the GABA-chloride ionophore complex, inhibiting neuronal firing. At low doses GABA agonists reduce cholinergic activity in the basal ganglia. However, at higher doses they also reduce dopaminergic transmission, particularly in the basal ganglia as opposed to the limbic system. Obviously, both groups of medications are anticonvulsants as well and their effect on ictal activity may offer a partial explanation of this effect.

The psychotherapeutic approaches to treatment, in combination with medication, can help the subject reassess the internal conflicts and better integrate his or her affects and cognitions.

CONCLUSION

Catatonia is a rare heterogeneous disorder sometimes secondary to neurological, metabolic, or toxic insult. Diagnosis and treatment of the primary condition are crucial. Psychiatrically, it is important to consider the possibility of an affective rather than a schizophrenic condition. Present literature considers that, most likely, catatonia is a frontal lobe syndrome resulting either from damage to its motor regulatory systems or disruption of connections with the subcortical structures (basal ganglia, brain stem). At present, the treatments proposed are electroconvulsive therapy and benzodiazepines.

BIBLIOGRAPHY

Abrams, R., & Taylor, M. A. (1976). Catatonia, a prospective clinical study. *Archives of General Psychiatry, 33*, 579–81.

Baruk, H. (1970). La catatonie de Kahlbaum, la schizophrénie et la révision de la nosographie psychiatrique. *Semaine des Hôpitaux de Paris, 46*, 1697–729.

Castillo, E., Rubin, R. T., & Holsboer-Trachsler, E. (1989). Clinical differentiation between lethal catatonia and neuroleptic malignant syndrome. *American Journal of Psychiatry, 146*, 324–8.

Gabris, G., & Müller, C. (1983). La catatonie dite "pernicieuse" [The so-called "lethal catatonia"]. *L'Encéphale, IX*, 365–85.

Gelenberg, A. J. (1976). The catatonic syndrome. *The Lancet, June 19*, 1339–41.

Gjessing, L. R. (1974). A review of periodic catatonia. *Biological Psychiatry, 8*, 23–45.

Juni, S. (1982). On the conceptualization and treatment of catatonia. *American Journal of Psychoanalysis, 42*, 327–34.

Larochelle, L., Bédard, P., Poirier, L. J., & Sourkes, T. L. (1971). Correlative neuroanatomical and neuropharmacological study of tremor and catatonia in the monkey. *Neuropharmacology, 10*, 273–88.

Magrinat, G., Danziger, J. A., Lorenzo, I. C., & Flemenbaum, A. (1983). A reassessment of catatonia. *Comprehensive Psychiatry, 24*, 218–28.

Mann, S. C., Caroff, S. N., & Bleier, H. R. (1986). Lethal catatonia. *American Journal of Psychiatry, 143*, 1374–81.

Menza, M. A., & Harris, D. (1989). Benzodiazepines and catatonia: an overview. *Biological Psychiatry, 26*, 842–6.

Salam, S. A., & Kilzieh, N. (1988). Lorazepam treatment of psychogenic catatonia: an update. *Journal of Clinical Psychiatry, 49*: 12 (Suppl.), 16–21.

Stoudemire, A. (1982). The differential diagnosis of catatonic states. *Psychosomatics, 23*, 245–52.

Task Force on DSM-IV (1991). *DSM-IV options book: Work in progress (9/1/91)*. Washington, DC: American Psychiatric Association.

Taylor, M. A. (1990). Catatonia, a review of a behavioral neurologic syndrome. *Neuropsychiatry, Neuropsychology and Behavioral Neurology, 3*, 48–72.

Taylor, M. A., & Abrams, R. (1977). Catatonia, prevalence and importance in the manic phase of manic-depressive illness. *Archives of General Psychiatry, 34*, 1223–5.

Weinberger, D. R. (1984). Brain disease and psychiatric illness: when should a psychiatrist order a CAT scan? *American Journal of Psychiatry, 141*, 1521–7.

GILBERT D. PINARD

caudate nucleus   The caudate nucleus is one of the nuclei which form the BASAL GANGLIA. The body of the caudate nucleus lies lateral and slightly superior to the THALAMUS, from where its tail passes backward, down, and finally forward again to connect with the AMYGDALA. Anteriorly it passes down into the head of the caudate nucleus which is in turn at the anterior end of the PUTAMEN and GLOBUS PALLIDUS around which the caudate is arranged. The caudate nucleus has important connections to the dorsomedial nuclei of the thalamus, to the globus pallidus, and to motor areas of the cortex, and its primary function is normally regarded as contributing to motor abilities.

central aphasia   *See* APHASIA.

central epilepsy   *See* EPILEPSY.

cerebellum The cerebellum lies above the MEDULLA and the PONS and occupies the greater part of the posterior cranial fossa. It has generally been considered to be part of a feedback circuit governing the activity of the extrapyramidal motor system. Controlling tone and involuntary movement and providing coordination and integration of motor activities, the concept of possible nonmotor functions of the cerebellum was formulated theoretically in experimental animals by Watson (1978). Between 1960 and 1975, for the first time in the literature, the role of the cortico-subcortical loops in human behavior was elaborated (Botez & Barbeau, 1971). This basic principle, which was developed at the midbrain, diencephalic, and cortical levels of the central nervous system (CNS), can be summarized as follows (Botez & Barbeau, 1971): a subcortical lesion will induce a behavioral deficit that is similar to one determined by a lesion of the cortical structure on which the respective subcortical structure has its anatomical and physiological projections. This behavioral deficit evoked by the subcortical lesion is usually milder than that caused by the cortical lesion.

This principle has been confirmed in recent years, and there is an extensive literature on the subject.

In the 1960s "the starting mechanism of speech" or mechanism of speech initiation was defined (Botez & Barbeau, 1971). We held that it may be separated from the phylogenetic point of view into two parts: an older part (vocalization function) correlated mainly with facio-vocal and emotional expression (i.e. the central gray and cingulate gyrus); and a newer part primarily encompassing interactions between the various levels of a cortico-subcortical servo-mechanism, including the supplementary motor area, the ventrolateral thalamic area, the periaqueductal gray and, secondarily, the *cerebellum*, the cortico-striate projections, and the striatum itself. "Speech, as the output side of information processing and the vehicle of language, requires constant modulation and control from subcortical mechanisms."

The association between cerebellar damage and mental or neuropsychological disorders has been mentioned in the literature (as reviewed by

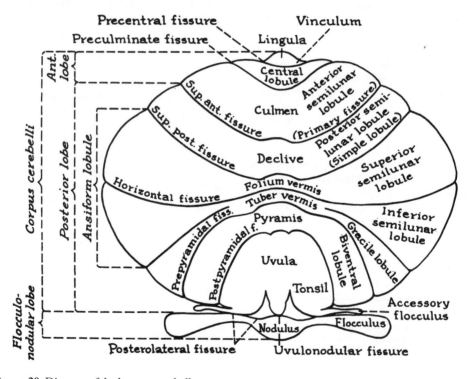

Figure 28 Diagram of the human cerebellum.

Schmahmann, 1991) but no firm clinical and physiopathological, i.e. cause and effect, relationships were documented in neurological patients before the 1985 report of Botez and colleagues. This paper clearly established the cause–effect relationship between neuropsychological disorders and bilateral cerebellar damage; that report and subsequent studies (Botez et al., 1989) emphasized the role of cerebello-frontal and cerebello-parietal pathways as anatomical substrata of the mild frontal- and parietal-like syndromes encountered in cerebellar patients. The clinical neuropsychological findings prompted the start of experimental studies in cerebellar mutant mice, which were initially published in the same year (Lalonde & Botez, 1985). These papers were followed by the tentative reviews of Leiner and others (1991) and since then a growing body of evidence has pointed towards a role of the cerebellum in cognitive functions.

ANATOMOPHYSIOLOGICAL BACKGROUND

Only some of the main aspects will be summarized, as details can be found in classical textbooks.

The cerebellum is a massive, organized accumulation of neurons located above the medulla oblongata and the pons. It is covered superiorly by the cerebellar hemispheres. The cerebellum is connected to the brain stem by three distinct bundles of nerve fibers, the inferior, middle, and superior cerebellar peduncles, also known as the restiform body, brachium pontis, and brachium conjunctivum respectively. The major subdivisions of the cerebellum are the median unpaired vermis and the paired lateral hemispheres. From Figure 28 it may be inferred that the corpus cerebelli include the anterior and posterior lobes; the flocculonodular lobe is separated from the corpus cerebelli by the posterolateral fissure. The flocculonodular lobe, also called the archicerebellum (denoting its early phylogenetic appearance), has predominantly vestibular connections. The anterior lobe, pyramis, and uvula comprise the paleocerebellum, which classically receives proprioceptive and exteroceptive information from the head and body. The posterior lobe, except for the pyramis and uvula, makes up the neocerebellum, which developed phylogenetically in conjunction with the cerebral cortex.

During phylogenetic evolution, the cerebellum and cerebral cortex were enlarged dramatically; within the enlarged cerebellum, the number of nerve cells exceeded the population in the cerebral cortex. At the cortical level, enlargement was striking in the association areas whereas, in the cerebellum, there was massive enlargement of the neocerebellum (lateral and posterior parts of the cerebellar hemispheres) and of the new phylogenetic part of its dentate (lateral) output nuc-

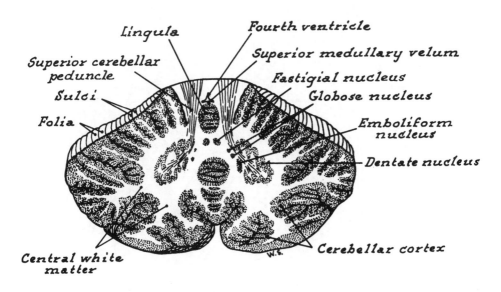

Figure 29 Horizontal section of the cerebellum.

cerebellum

leus. The pontine nuclei also underwent a
dramatic increase in size during mammalian
evolution and attained their largest development
in humans. As already observed (Leiner et al.,
1991), while we can ascribe well-known motor
functions to the anterior lobe of the cerebellum,
the functions of the lateral-posterior parts are less
known in classical neurology. Recent data provide
increasing evidence that these cerebellar regions
are concerned with cognitive functions.

Figure 29 represents a schematic section of the
cerebellum that is composed of three parts: the
cerebellar cortex, a core of white matter, and the
deep, i.e. dentate (or lateral) nuclei, the
emboliform, globose, and fastigial nuclei. The
emboliform and globose nuclei are collectively
known as the interpositus nucleus (especially in
lower mammals).

Histologically, the cerebellar cortex consists of
two layers: the outermost or molecular (basket,
stellate, and Golgi cells) and the innermost or
granular layers (Figure 30). The Purkinje cells
are large efferent neurons of the cerebellar

cortex, and their axons project to the cerebellar
nuclei. Afferent fibers to the cerebellum are of
two types: mossy and climbing fibers. Mossy
fibers originate from the pontine nuclei, whereas
climbing fibers originate from the inferior olive.
The intrinsic circuits of the cerebellum could be
summarized as follows: afferent mossy fibers
synapse with terminal granule cells which,
through their parallel fibers, make contact with
the dendritic terminals of Purkinje cells.
Through their axons, the Purkinje cells provide
output to the cerebellar nuclei.

In classical neurology, lesions of the archicerebellum and paleocerebellum usually result in
ataxia of gait. Lesions of the paleocerebellum
induce cerebellar hypotonia, whereas neocere-
bellar lesions evoke ataxic and dysmetric movements, intentional tremors, and asynergia.
Nystagmus could occur as a result of lesions of
vestibulocerebellar connections.

As demonstrated by Kemp and Powell (Wiesendanger et al., 1979), there are two main classic
cerebro-cerebellar loops underlying *motor control*

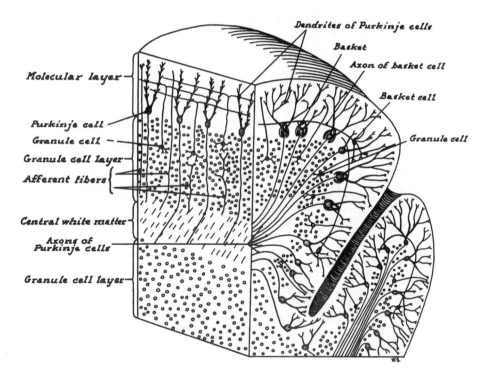

Figure 30 Diagrammatic representation of a longitudinal section of a cerebellar folium (left) and
cross-sections of two adjacent folia (right).

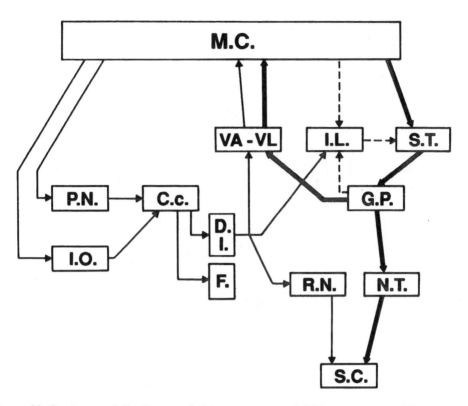

Figure 31 Cerebro-cerebellar loops underlying motor control. MC, motor cortex; VA, n. ventralis anterior thalami; VL, n. ventralis lateralis; IL, intralaminar nuclei; ST, striatum; GP, globus pallidus; Cc, corpus cerebelli; PN, pontine nuclei; IO, inferior olive; D, dentate n.; I, interpositus n.; F, fastigial n.; RN, red nucleus; NT, n. tegmenti; SC, spinal cord.

(Figure 31). The first neural circuit is the cortical → ponto (and olivary) → cerebellar → dentate (magnocellular part) → ventral anterior and ventral lateral thalamic nuclei → cortical pathway. From the dentate nucleus, motor control is exerted on the spinal cord via the red nucleus. The second loop involves the striatum, globus pallidus (external and internal parts) the ventrolateral thalamic nucleus and motor cortex (Figure 31).

The input and output systems of the cerebellum, which could be related to cognition, are illustrated in Figures 32 and 33. Frontal lobe connections to the pons originate from both motor and associative areas. Motor projections derive from primary, i.e. Rolandic 4 areas, as well as from the supplementary motor area (SMA) and area 6, whereas association projections come from premotor and prefrontal areas (8 through 12

and 44 through 47). Broca's area could be included in the association areas (Leiner et al., 1991).

The pontine nuclei receive heavy projections from association areas of the frontal neocortex, from the posterior parietal cortex, and the superior temporal sulcus. Paralimbic and autonomical projections to the pons derive from the limbic lobe (especially from the cingulate gyrus), the hypothalamus, and mammillary bodies (Figure 32).

Projections from the cerebellum back to the cerebral association areas are less known than the cortico-pontine projections. Dentate nucleus projections via the thalamus to the association cortices include medial dorsal, ventrolateral, and intralaminar thalamic nuclei (Figure 33). Parts of the ventrolateral and intralaminar nuclei (particularly the central lateral nucleus) have strong projections to the posterior parietal cortex and

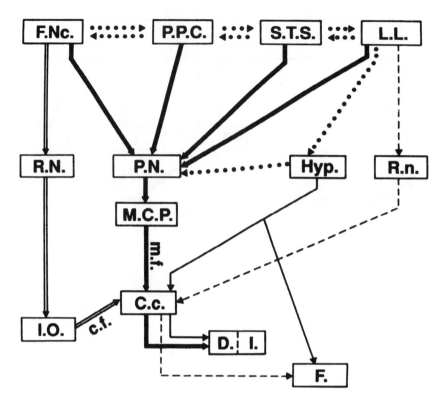

Figure 32 Cerebellar afferents. FNc, frontal neocortex; PPC, posterior parietal cortex; STS, superior temporal sulcus; LL, limbic lobe; RN, red nucleus; PN, pontine nuclei; Hyp., hypothalamus; Rn., reticular nuclei; MCP, middle cerebellar peduncle; Cc, corpus cerebelli; IO, inferior olive; c.f. climbing fibers; m.f. mossy fibers; D, dentate n.; I, interpositus n.; F, fastigial n.

superior temporal sulcus (Figure 33). On the other hand, reciprocal hypothalamic connections to the cerebellar cortex and fastigial nucleus have also been found.

The various cortico-cerebellar-cortical loops involving not only motor cortical areas but also associative areas provide the anatomical background for information-processing mechanisms. The cerebellum, like the basal ganglia and thalamus, receives information from the cerebral cortex for processing and sends the results of this processing back to the cortex, to both sensory motor and association areas. In turn, these areas can send information back to the cerebellum for further processing (Leiner et al., 1991a).

CHEMICAL NEUROANATOMY

Experiments and clinical studies indicate that behavioral disorders (motor or cognitive) caused by cerebellar lesions are not only related to classical anatomophysiological cerebellar loops but possibly also to neurochemical pathways (Botez et al., 1991a).

It should be remembered that the main sources of noradrenaline, serotonin, dopamine and acetylcholine are the locus ceruleus, raphé nuclei of the brain stem, substantia nigra, and nucleus basalis of Meynert respectively. Whereas the cerebellar sources of noradrenaline, serotonin and acetylcholine are well-established, the origin of cerebellar dopamine is not yet clear; dopaminergic innervation of the cerebellum was proved only recently in the rat. Table 8 provides a short summary of the localization of main neurotransmitters in the mammalian cerebellum. The relationship between some neurotransmitters and behavioral disorders will be discussed at the end of this entry.

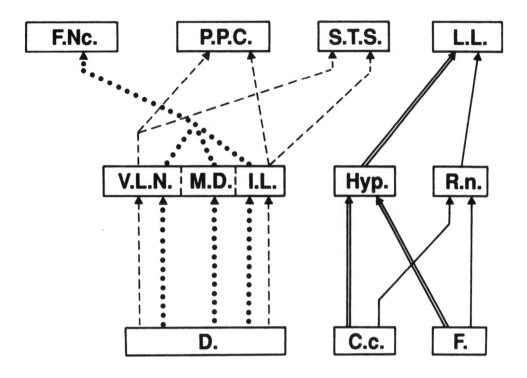

Figure 33 Cerebellar efferents. FNc, PPC, STS and LL, frontal neocortex, posterior parietal cortex, superior temporal sulcus, limbic lobe respectively. VLN, MD, IL, ventralis lateralis, medial dorsal, and intralaminar thalamic nuclei respectively. Hyp., hypothalamus; RN, reticular nuclei; D, dentate n.; Cc, corpus cerebelli; F, fastigial n.

Table 8　Proposed neurotransmitters and receptor subtypes in cerebellar structures of the mammalian brain.

Structures	Neurotransmitters
Granule cells	Glutamate, aspartate; extracerebellar afferents: ser-
Molecular layer of cerebellar cortex (basket, stellate and Golgi cells)	otonin, gamma aminobutyric acid (GABA), dopamine, noradrenaline; taurine and neuropeptides
Purkinje cells	GABA; extracerebellar afferents = noradrenaline, ser-otonin, dopamine
Inferior olive (climbing fibers)	Glutamate, aspartate; possibly serotonin
Pontine area, spinal cord, reticular nuclei (mossy fibers)	Acetylcholine, serotonin excitatory amino acids (gluta-mate aspartate a.s.o.)
Cerebellar cortex	Acetylcholine, noradrenaline, serotonin, dopamine
Dentate, interpositus and fastigial nuclei	Serotonin, glutamate, dopamine (afferents)

Receptor subtypes	
On granule cells	N-methyl-D-aspartate (NMDA)
On Purkinje cells	Non-NMDA

BEHAVIORAL AND NEUROPSYCHO-LOGICAL STUDIES IN HUMANS

The roles of the basal ganglia, cingulate gyrus, SMA, and cerebellum *in the initiation of movement*, as postulated since 1962 (see Botez & Barbeau, 1971), were confirmed more recently (Leiner et al., 1991). It is generally accepted that the cerebellum and its input and output pathways play a significant role in motor programming, which precedes motor acts, as well as in motor learning.

Studies on the role of the cerebellum in *motor learning* have focused on the acquisition and retention of simple reflexes or responses, adaptation of the vestibulo-ocular reflex and, in a few cases, more complex behavior involving visuo-motor adaptation by humans. Recently, motor learning in patients with cerebellar dysfunction was assessed by performance of two tasks (Sanes et al., 1990). The first consists of repetitive tracing of an irregular geometrical pattern with the hand under normal visual guidance, and the second involves repetitive tracing of a different geometrical pattern with mirror-reversed vision. Cerebellar patients are impaired in the skilled performance of movement in the normal vision task, probably because of a failure of motor adaptation.

Patients with combined cerebellar and brain-stem atrophy show a deficit in the mirror-reversed vision task, which can be considered as a failure in motor skill learning. The anatomical background of this phenomenon is probably altered information processing to the cerebellum via the climbing and mossy fibers. Sanes and colleagues (1990) concluded that: (i) the cerebellum contributes to the learning of movement skills; and (ii) structure inputs to the cerebellum "are critical in this process."

After our initial paper (Botez et al., 1985), where we documented the possible relationship between the *parietal-like* and *frontal-like* syndromes occurring in our first two patients, we published neuropsychological studies of 73 cases of bilateral and unilateral cerebellar damage compared to 71 control subjects.

The principles of this research were: (1) to use a comprehensive neuropsychological test battery with three objectives: (i) to assess general intellectual abilities; (ii) to examine in more detail specific cognitive functions, i.e. frontal- and parietal-like syndromes; and (iii) to evaluate the speed of information processing (SIP) by simple visual and auditory reaction time (RT); (2) to adapt neuropsychological testing to the degree of cerebellar motor involvement (epileptic patients with cerebellar atrophy on CT scans but without a clinically striking cerebellar syndrome underwent a different battery from those with epileptic olivopontocerebellar atrophies (OPCA) or Friedreich's ataxia (FA)); (3) to evaluate separately patients with bilateral cerebellar involvement versus those with unilateral cerebellar damage; (4) to rule out, by computed tomography (CT) scans and magnetic resonance imaging (MRI; see SCAN), all patients with supratentorial deficits, more specifically those with diffuse vascular disease of the brain, as well as those with hydrocephalus or cerebral atrophies (severe exclusion and inclusion criteria were therefore established before including patients in the study); (5) to conduct single-photon-emission computed tomography (SPECT) assessments in patients with unilateral cerebellar infarcts as well as in those with OPCA and FA; (6) to perform cerebrospinal fluid (CSF) determinations of 5-hydroxyindoleacetic acid (5HIAA), 3-methoxy-4-hydroxyphenyl ethylene glycol (MHPG) and homovanillic acid (HVA), which are the metabolites of serotonin, noradrenaline, and dopamine respectively, for correlation with neuropsychological findings.

Thirty-three outpatient epileptics with normal CT scans (Group 1) and 31 patients with cerebellar and brain-stem atrophy (Group 2) were randomly included in the second investigation (Botez et al., 1989). There were no statistically significant differences between groups with regard to age, education, and number of grand mal and other seizures. Neuropsychological assessment revealed lower performances by the atrophic group on the following measures: full IQ scale, verbal IQ scale, performance IQ scale, information, arithmetic, block design, object assembly, digit symbol, Stroop test forms I and II, and the B-M dexterity test. No significant differences were observed between the two groups for the remaining five subtests of the WAIS scale (comprehension, digit span, similarities, picture arrangement, picture completion), or for the immediate recall and delayed recall subtests belonging to the Wechsler Memory Scale. Visual and auditory RT and movement time (MT) were measured separately with a Lafayette apparatus, using the method of Hamsher and Benton.

Fifteen OPCA patients and 15 FA patients compared with pair-matched controls were evaluated neuropsychologically (Botez-Marquard & Botez, 1993). The OPCA cases had significantly lower performances on the Standard Progressive Matrices of Raven (SPMR), Rey's complex figure, Trail B, similarities and block design (timed and untimed version) with a tendency toward significant differences in the Hooper Visual Organization Test. No impairment was found in visual memory (copy of Rey's complex figure), digit span forward and backward, picture arrangement, and immediate memory learning. The FA patients were impaired on SPMR, Rey's complex figure, and block design (timed version). No impairment was found in FA patients on digit span forward and backward, similarities, picture arrangement, Hooper's visual organization, and immediate memory learning tests. Both visual and auditory RTs were lengthened in FA and OPCA patients. Multiple-choice task RTs were also measured in OPCA patients and revealed significant lengthening in comparison to their controls.

Analyses of the composite scores of neuropsychological performance in our studies showed that the cerebellum interfered with the following complex behavioral functions: (i) *visuospatial organization for a concrete task*, a function related to the cerebello-parietal loops, as demonstrated by deficient performances on the object assembly, digit symbol and block design subtests; (ii) *planning and programming of daily activity*, a function related to the cerebello-frontal loops; deficient performance on the Stroop test was relevant in this matter. The last function to be impaired was SIP: visual and auditory RT performances were deficient in the atrophic group whereas MT showed no significant differences between the two groups. These findings confirmed the fact that RT performances reflecting motor abilities are independent from RT performances reflecting SIP.

The mild frontal-like syndrome observed in cerebellar patients was found recently by some other research workers. In an elegant paper, El-Awar and colleagues (1991) reported deficits in delayed alternation tasks in OPCA patients. By using the tower of Hanoi, a nine-problem task, Grafman and others (1992) showed a cognitive planning deficit in 12 patients with bilateral cerebellar atrophies.

In another study we compared neuropsychological performances in 22 patients with cerebellar hereditary ataxias, i.e. with bilateral cerebellar damage (BCD), and 8 patients with chronic, well-delimited unilateral cerebellar infarcts (UCI) versus two respectively matched control groups. BCD patients scored lower performances on SPMR, Rey's complex figure, similarities, and the Hooper Visual Organization Test. No significant differences were found for the following tests: Rey's 15-word; visual recall memorization of Rey's complex figure; digit span forward and backward, and picture arrangement. Visual and auditory RT and MT were significantly lengthened in BCD patients versus their controls. Correlations between SPMR and visual and auditory RT in the control groups confirmed data from the literature: r fell to the range of $-.15$ to $-.49$. The correlation between SPMR and RT in BCD patients was definitely stronger and relatively homogeneous with r placed between $-.58$ and $-.68$. These findings reinforced previous psychological observations: speed of information processing (SIP) generalizes across experimental tasks and reliably indicates intellectual ability.

Neuropsychological assessments, including simple visual and auditory RT determinations, did not reveal any impairment in chronic UCI patients as compared to their controls.

In two *acute* unilateral cerebellar infarcts involving both posterior-inferior cerebellar and superior cerebellar arteries, we found – 5 and 10 days respectively after the stroke – markedly lengthened RTs and low performance on SPMR. After three months, performance was in the normal range compared with the controls.

SPECT and PET studies showed decreased metabolism in contralateral cerebellar structures following unilateral frontoparietal infarcts; this *cerebro-cerebellar diaschisis* is the result of remote transneuronal metabolic depression of the corticopontocerebellar pathways. Using SPECT, we demonstrated a reverse phenomenon, i.e. *cerebello-cerebral diaschisis*: reduced cerebellar hexamethylpropyleneamine oxime (HMPAO) uptake was invariably accompanied by a diminution of HMPAO in the contralateral basal ganglia and frontoparietal cortex. Diaschisis was observed even 15 years after the stroke (Botez et al., 1991).

In conclusion, despite the presence of cerebello-cerebral diaschisis in unilateral cerebellar infarcts, no impaired neuropsychological or RT performances were noted.

A series of experimental findings supports our data, showing an absence of RT or some other neuropsychological deficits in patients with chronic UCI. Unilateral experimental dentate lesions in monkeys lengthened auditory RT in the immediate post-lesion period; auditory RT gradually declined over about 20 days post-operatively, approaching normal values (Spidalieri et al., 1983).

Furthermore, unilateral lesions of the right dentate and interpositus nuclei in monkeys produced severe movement dysfunction of the ipsilateral limb which recovered in 10 to 15 days (Dr Yves Lamarre, personal communication). After recovery, left cerebellar nuclei were lesioned, which caused a deficit in the left arm and in the right contralateral arm that had recovered from the previous lesion inflicted on the right side. In a monkey in which the middle cerebellar peduncle was destroyed unintentionally by a stereotaxic lesion aimed at the dentate nucleus, Wiesendanger and others (1979) observed that, besides ataxia and dysmetria, the animal displayed marked inattention on the side of the lesion during the first postoperative days. The transient nature of this inattention was also characteristic of unilateral lesions of association areas of the cerebral cortex in monkeys. These experimental findings and our observations on humans converge to the same conclusion: there is some functional relationship between both sides of the cerebellum which could compensate for both motor and cognitive behavior.

Our bilateral cerebellar-damaged (epileptic, FA, and OPCA) patients presented slower RT and MT than their controls. Significant differences in MT reflected motor (i.e. coordination) deficits per se, whereas RT (a test of cognition) measured SIP. Reaction time, recognized as one of the best behavioral measures of central nervous system integrity (Jensen, 1993), primarily reflects cognitive processing speed. Although reaction time involves both central (premotor) and peripheral (muscle contraction) components, it has been demonstrated through electromyography that it is the central component that comprises the majority of the stimulus-response latency and is primarily related to behavioral slowing. Besides experimental studies on

monkeys showing RT lengthening after cerebellar lesions (Spidalieri et al., 1983), Ricklan and others (quoted by Watson, 1978) found that in human epileptics whose treatment included implantation of electrodes in the cerebellar cortex, stimulation increased RT to visual stimuli presented tachistoscopically.

In another study (Botez-Marquard et al., 1989), we analyzed SIP by measuring simple warned visual and auditory RT and its relationship to intelligence in patients with lesions at various levels of the CNS: cerebellar (CR), Parkinsonian, well-delimited chronic right cerebral hemisphere infarcts, and chronic left hemisphere infarcts. The CR group showed the most significant diminution of SIP as measured by RT with both hands ($p < 0.001$); a significant negative correlation between SIP and SPMR was noted. The Parkinsonian group registered a significant reduction of SIP only on auditory RT ($p < 0.03$) with a significant negative correlation for all RTs versus SPMR. Neither right nor left cerebral hemisphere infarcts, however, presented a significant decrease in SIP or a negative correlation with SPMR.

The role of subcortical structures in speed of information processing (SIP) has already been recognized. Our studies as well as more recent data from the literature suggest that the cerebellum is *directly* involved in SIP, thus showing that it is engaged in rapid motor and cognitive processing of information. Second, the cerebellar patients – as compared to the controls – generally had slower intellectual abilities as reflected by lower performance on SPMR. Third, mild frontal-like and parietal-like syndromes were observed in all groups of patients studied. The cerebellum and its pathways interfere with visuospatial organization for concrete tasks, as well as with the planning and programming of daily activities. The role of the cerebellum in these syndromes is mainly *indirect* through various cerebello-cortical, anatomophysiological and neurochemical pathways (see Figures 31–33). It has to be pointed out, however, that FA patients have milder frontal-like syndromes than OPCA patients and this could be due to the pathological background of these two diseases: whereas in OPCA all efferents and afferents as well as the cerebellum itself are impaired from the onset of the disease, in FA the cerebellum is moderately affected.

Bauman and Kemper (quoted by Courchesne et al., 1994) showed histoanatomic abnormalities, i.e. loss of Purkinje cells in the limbic areas and in the cerebellum *in autistic patients*. Using MR technology, Courchesne and others (1994) described vermian abnormalities but also parietal lobe abnormalities in patients with infantile autism. We believe that in our state of knowledge it is rather difficult to draw conclusions about a specific role of the cerebellum in autistic behavior because the lesions due to a possible maldevelopment are not confined only in the cerebellum. On the other hand, we did not observe in 104 patients with acquired well-delimited cerebellar disease (unilateral or bilateral lesions) a single patient with a tendency to display an autistic behavior.

IS REPLACEMENT THERAPY POSSIBLE IN CEREBELLAR NEUROBEHAVIORAL DISORDERS?

There were no beneficial results in cerebellar ataxias following the administration of cholinergic agents, such as physostigmine, lecithin, and choline chloride (Botez et al., 1991b). Although disturbed GABA metabolism could be supposed in patients with hereditary cerebellar ataxias, GABA agonists were also not helpful in improving their motor behavior.

Noradrenaline is reduced in the cerebellar cortex of postmortem OPCA patients (El-Awar et al., 1991). Low levels of CSF 3-methoxy-4-hydroxyphenylethylene glycol (MHPG), a noradrenaline metabolite, were detected by us (Botez & Young, unpublished paper) in FA patients. In Korsakoff's psychosis, diminished brain noradrenergic and dopaminergic activities are related to impairments on different psychometric tasks. Lengthened RT performances and some neuropsychological deficits in OPCA and FA patients could be the consequence of a noradrenaline deficiency. An impairment in learning patterned motor movements in rats with noradrenergic lesions was recently found.

Dopamine is considered to be a neurotransmitter underlying the *initiation* of action. Its depletion impairs RT in experimental animals (Amalric & Koob, quoted by Botez et al., 1991b). Sawaguchi (quoted by Botez et al., 1991b) described the sensitivities to noradrenaline and dopamine of neurons of the prefrontal cortex in a conscious monkey which showed changes in activity during a visual reaction task. Whereas the former mostly has an excitatory influence, the latter has an inhibitory impact.

Lesions of nucleus fastigii were associated with relatively low dopamine levels in the ipsilateral forebrain; in contrast, dopamine ipsilateral to the cerebellar cortical lesion was increased. This finding is interpreted to indicate the removal of cerebellar inhibitory influences on dopamine nuclei. Of particular interest is an efferent pathway described by Snider and others (quoted by Botez et al., 1991b), arising from cells in the nuclei interpositus, dentatus, and fastigius, and passing through the ventral two-thirds of the brachium conjunctivum in cats; the fibers cross the midline at the level of decussation, sending extensive degenerative terminals into the nucleus ruber. From there they enter the dorsal-ventral tegmental area, the substantia nigra, and nucleus interpeduncularis. Some projections originating from the fastigial nucleus to the substantia nigra are homolateral. Projections are sent from there to the neostriatum and neocortex. This is the dopaminergic pathway.

The reverse cerebello-cortical diaschisis described (Botez et al., 1991a) follows the neurochemical dopaminergic pathway, i.e. the cerebellum (interpositus-dentate) → substantia nigra (and red nucleus) → striatum → frontoparietal neocortex. It is interesting to note that this diaschisis does not follow the classical anatomophysiological cerebello-dento-thalamic-cortical pathway but rather the dopaminergic pathway.

Glutamate is an excitatory neurotransmitter of granule cells in the cerebellum; in OPCA cases and in experimental animals, the death of Purkinje cells is associated with glutamate toxicity by Plaitakis (see Botez et al., 1991a). Glutamate dysfunction, i.e. glutamate neurotoxicity, is mediated by N-methyl-D-aspartate (NMDA) receptors in rat cerebellar granule cells.

In an open clinical trial, the lengthened RT and MT in OPCA patients was improved by administration of amantadine hydrochloride. This action could be explained as follows (Botez et al., 1991b): (i) amantadine blocks NMDA receptors, diminishing glutamate neurotoxicity (see above); (ii) amantadine has a dopaminergic action, being a possible replacement therapy in OPCA patients in whom CSF homovanillic acid (HVA), the dopamine metabolite, was diminished.

Low CSF 5-hydroxyindoleacetic acid, the *serotonin* metabolite, was found in some ataxic patients. Serotonin has specific inhibitory effects on glutamate excitatory activity; the motor improvement observed in some ataxic patients after the administration of serotonin precursors may be due to its inhibitory action on glutamate excitotoxicity (Trouillas et al., 1988).

The neuroradiological correlates of RT and MT measurements in OPCA patients were recently studied. Those with severe versus mild-moderate atrophy as assessed by three neuroradiological measures, i.e. brain stem, brachium pontis, and fourth ventricle ratios, presented few significantly lengthened RT and MT performances. In contrast, patients with severe atrophy revealed by the midbrain ratio had significantly lengthened simple visual and auditory RT and MT performances for all eight measures. This could be explained by the fact that atrophy at the midbrain level is the only one which involves dopaminergic, noradrenergic, and glutamatergic structures and pathways.

There is some distinct evidence that dysfunction of glutamatergic, dopaminergic, noradrenergic, and perhaps serotonergic pathways underlies the motor deficit, as well as the impairment of SIP and probably of some other neuropsychological performances in cerebellar diseases. More neuropsychological studies related to CSF neurochemistry and pharmacology are needed.

THE CEREBELLUM AND LANGUAGE

Leiner and colleagues (1991) postulated a possible role for the cerebellum in *language* skills. We hypothesized about the role of the cerebellum in the initiation of speech more than 20 years ago (Botez & Barbeau, 1971). In children with William's syndrome who are proficient in language, the cerebellum is normal in size, but in Down's syndrome patients who are dysfunctional in language, the neocerebellum is smaller than normal (see Leiner et al., 1991). It is certain that the cerebellum participates in triggering or starting speech initiation, but there is no clinical evidence of language comprehension disorders or naming difficulties (i.e. word-finding difficulties) – except, of course, DYSARTHRIA – in adult cerebellar patients.

MEMORY AND LEARNING

We did not find disorders of immediate memory and learning in cerebellar patients. Some recent unpublished results from our laboratory have shown that cerebellar patients have, however, memory retrieval difficulties and also diminished performance when an interfering list of words is used. The global memory quotient is diminished in OPCA patients compared with their controls. The cerebello-hypothalamic and limbic loops (Figures 32 and 33), as well as the involvement of noradrenergic pathways, could be responsible for memory disorders and some minor learning difficulties.

TIMING SENSE AND SOMATOSENSORY DISCRIMINATION

Ivry and Keele (1989) employed two experimental tasks designed to test the role of the cerebellum in timing performance. They used: (1) a production task in which the subjects perform rhythmic tapping; and (2) a perception task in which their perceptual acuity at comparable temporal intervals is tested. They compared performances in Parkinsonian, cerebellar, and cortical damaged patients versus normal age-matched controls. On the tapping task, Parkinsonian patients performed as well as their age-matched controls whereas the cerebellar and cortical groups were: (1) much more variable in this task than the controls; and (2) significantly impaired in comparison to Parkinsonian patients.

Only the cerebellar group showed a deficit in perception of the duration task. Comparison with control subjects revealed a significant difference which only approached significance between cerebellar and Parkinsonian patients. Ivry and Keele (1989) concluded that only cerebellar patients are impaired in the ability to discriminate perceptually small differences in duration. They demonstrated that this perceptual deficit was specific to the perception of time because cerebellar patients were unaffected in some control tasks, for example, on a task measuring the perception of loudness. Cerebellar patients showed the greatest increase in variability of central time-keeper estimates (clock) whereas both the cortical and cerebellar groups presented impairments in the implementation system (motor delay).

The authors advanced the idea that the timing mechanism could be considered as a well-delimited component of the motor control system. However, it appears that "the domain of the cerebellar timing process is not limited to the motor system, but is employed by other perceptual and cognitive systems when temporally predictive computations are needed" (Ivry & Keele, 1989).

In patients with predominantly cerebellar median lesions, the implementation score was responsible for the increase in overall variability, while lesions in the lateral cerebellum produced large clock deviations.

The lateral part of the cerebellum seems to be involved in controlling *time sense* and *the programming of finger movements*. Inhoff and others (quoted by Leiner et al., 1991) instructed cerebellar patients to execute movement sequences in response to a simple reaction signal. Each sentence to be executed consisted of either a single, two, or three key-press components. The execution of programmed responses was evaluated in the pattern of response onset time and inter-key press time. Their findings supported the hypothesis that "the translation of a programmed sequence of responses into action involves cerebellar structures which schedule a sequence of ordered responses before the onset of movement."

PSYCHIATRIC DISEASES AND MOOD DISORDERS

Over a century ago, it was reported that patients with cerebellar agenesis are mentally subnormal (see the review by Schmahmann, 1991). On computed tomographic scans Heath and others (quoted by Schmahmann, 1991) observed pathological features in the cerebellar vermis in 40 percent of schizophrenic patients. The relationship remains unclear.

Heath et al. (quoted by Watson, 1978) correlated electrical responses in the fastigial nucleus of an emotionally disturbed woman with emotional states; fastigial activity increased when the patient experienced fear or anger.

Elliott (quoted by Leiner et al., 1991) reported a lack of behavioral self-control, including episodic rage, which was occasionally observed after removal of the midline (paleo)cerebellum. These findings could be correlated with modifications of aggressive behavior in adult rhesus monkeys following midline (vermal) lesions. Cerebellar-limbic pathways (cf. Figures 32, 33) might be the neural basis of this behavior.

EXPERIMENTAL STUDIES IN ANIMALS

Experimental analysis of cerebellar damage has mostly been limited to Pavlovian rather than instrumental learning.

Classical conditioning and the cerebellum Classical conditioning of the nictitating membrane (a third cartilaginous eyelid) response is impaired by lesions of the olivo-cerebellar system but not by injury to tissues above the thalamus (McCormick & Thompson, 1984). The basic paradigm is as follows: an unconditioned stimulus (US) (e.g. a corneal air puff or periorbital electric shock) is paired with a conditioned stimulus (CS) (e.g. a light or tone) until the CS alone elicits the conditioned response, i.e. a blink of the rabbit's external eyelid and a sweep of the nictitating membrane. This classical conditioning paradigm serves as a working model of the Marr/Albus motor learning test, in which US information to the cerebellum derives from the olive while CS information derives from the pons. In confirmation of this theory, Yeo and others (quoted by Lalonde & Botez, 1990) found that lesions of medial parts of the rostral dorsal accessory olive and principal olive abolished nictitating membrane conditioning in the rabbit. In further confirmation of this theory, the nictitating membrane response can be conditioned with corneal air puffs as US and electrical stimulation of the dorsolateral, lateral, and medial pontine nuclei as the CS (Steinmetz et al., quoted by Lalonde & Botez, 1990). Since the cerebellum contributes in associative learning in the classical conditioning paradigm, does it contribute to associative learning in other paradigms? Are the behavioral deficits following cerebellar damage more general than previously recognized? Are spatial tasks more sensitive to cerebellar lesions than nonspatial ones? These questions remain to be answered.

Spatial learning and the cerebellum In view of the motor difficulties encountered by animals with cerebellar damage in dry mazes, attempts have been made to circumvent this problem with the use of water mazes. Animals with cerebellar damage swim well. Thus there is hope that learning defects could be more easily dissociable from motor defects in such paradigms. Pellegrino and Altman (quoted by Lalonde & Botez, 1990) tested groups of rats that varied according to the time at which the cerebellum was X-irradiated during the first 15 postnatal days. Rats X-irradiated on days 4–15 were impaired on a spatial alternation task but not on acquisition and reversal of a left-right position habit in a water maze.

Moreover, rats X-irradiated on days 4–15 and 12–15 had deficits in a double alternation task in the same maze. There were no group differences in swimming times. These results are at variance with the conclusion that the cerebellum plays no part in maze learning.

Discrimination learning, emotion, and the cerebellum A few experiments have been reported concerning the effects of cerebellar lesions on shock avoidance with simultaneous discrimination learning. Rats with cerebellar lesions were impaired in performance under high but not low motivational conditions of shock avoidance. Differential impairments according to motivational conditions may be explained by cerebellar connections to brain centers critical in emotion, such as the hypothalamus, so that the adverse effect of cerebellar lesions may be due to excessive arousal. Watson (1978) has reviewed evidence on how the cerebellum acts on arousal mechanisms.

BEHAVIORAL EVALUATION OF CEREBELLAR MUTANT MICE

One goal of our experiments on cerebellar mutant mice was to measure motor activity and coordination on the one hand with visuospatial learning on the other. It is obvious from general observations that all five cerebellar mutants tested so far (nervous, lurcher, weaver, staggerer, Purkinje cell degeneration (pcd)) have deficits in motor coordination, have an ataxic gait, and fall frequently after rearing. However, mutants differ from each other in several respects. It has been found that, despite ataxia, nervous, lurcher, and pcd mutants have normal activity levels as measured in a T-maze. In contrast, weaver and staggerer mutants are less active than normal littermate controls (Lalonde & Botez, 1990).

Since nervous, lurcher, and pcd mutants had massive losses of Purkinje cells at the time they were tested (1 month old), these results indicate that Purkinje cell degeneration is not sufficient to cause a decrease in motor activity. It has been reported that, together with Purkinje cell loss, there is degeneration of cerebellar granule cells, of inferior olive neurons, and a decrease in deep nuclei weight in staggerer mutants. It is possible that these additional cell losses are the reason that staggerer mutants are less active. On the other hand, degeneration of the olivo-cerebellar system may cause biochemical alterations in extracerebellar regions (such as dopamine-containing neurons) important in motor activity. It is already known that weaver mutants have a deficiency of striatal dopamine concentrations because of nigral cell losses. Hypoactivity in this mutant may be caused by combined depletion of cerebellar granule cells and substantia nigra cells (Tables 9 and 10).

In addition to horizontal activity in a maze, vertical activity in the stem of the maze has also been evaluated, together with hole-poking exploration of a single hole in a steel cage. Weaver and staggerer mutants exhibited fewer rears and hole pokes than normal mice. Nervous and lurcher mutants showed no decrease in either test, whereas pcd mutants scored a lower number of rears but hole-poking was normal (Table 10). Taken together, various motor activity and exploration tests indicate that weaver and staggerer mutants are the least active whereas nervous and lurcher mutants are the most active and, in certain tests, even manifest patterns of hyperactivity (Table 10).

Visuospatial analysis in cerebellar mutants has been tested in an adaptation of the Morris water maze by a rectangular basin under both visible

Table 9 Neuropathological characteristics of cerebellar mutant mice.

Mutants	Predominant cell loss
Nervous	Purkinje cells
Lurcher	Purkinje cells, cerebellar granule cells, inferior olive cells
Weaver	Cerebellar granule cells, substantia nigra cells
Staggerer	Purkinje cells, cerebellar granule cells, inferior olive cells
Pcd	Purkinje cells, inferior olive cells

Table 10   Motor activity and exploration in cerebellar mutant mice.

Mutants	Behavioral tests			Spatial learning	
	Motor activity (T-maze)	Hole-poking (steel cage)	Rears	Invisible platform	Visible platform
Nervous	0	0	+	?	?
Lurcher	0	+	0	X	X
Weaver	X	X	X	X	X
Staggerer	X	X	X	X	0
Pcd	0	0	X	?	?

X Decreased;   0 Not different;   + Increased;   ? Not tested.

and invisible platform conditions (Lalonde & Botez, 1990). All three mutants tested (lurcher, weaver, staggerer) were impaired but in different ways. Staggerer mutants were slower to reach the invisible but not the visible platform, whereas lurchers and weavers were impaired in both (Table 10).

It must be remembered that in terms of motor activity the performance of staggerers is worse than that of lurchers. The reverse is the case in navigation. Thus, although the cerebellum is involved in motor coordination and navigational skills, these functions are not correlated in these mutants.

In general, the results of mutant mice studies are in agreement with emerging neuropsychological evidence of visuospatial deficits in patients with cerebellar disease. However, the severity of motor deficits may not be correlated to the severity of cognitive deficits.

PET AND SPECT STUDIES

Recent advanced activation techniques using positron emission tomographic (PET) measurements of cerebral blood flow have made it possible to address concerns relevant to clinical neuropsychology with a precision not previously available. PET enables the demonstration of activated neuronal populations in the human brain by measuring regional cerebellar blood flow (rCBF) and regional glucose and oxygen metabolic rates coupled to neuronal activity.

In 1977 Ingvar and associates introduced the term ideagraphy, which is the identification, by either metabolic or circulatory PET scan studies, of human brain activation caused by events that are simply ideational and are not coupled to any sensory input or motor output.

Decety and Ingvar (1990) defined mental simulation of movement (MSM) as "an imagined rehearsal of a motor act with the specific intent of learning and improving it, without any simultaneous sensory input or any overt input, i.e. any muscular movement. It constitutes a pure cognitive activity." These researchers investigated MSM as a cognitive model of a motor act which requires several components, such as motivation, attentional resources, visual and kinesthetic imagery. Various MSM tasks were used: the subjects were asked to imagine tennis movements, graphic movements, or to project visually that they were walking along a well-known route in their home town, silently counting.

By measuring ^{133}Xenon rCBF, Decety and Philippon (see Decety & Ingvar, 1990) studied normal subjects imaging a graphic movement either with the right or left hand. Regions corresponding to the prefrontal cortex, the supplementary motor area, and the cerebellum were activated significantly. SPECT revealed a significant bilateral rCBF increase in the cerebellum ($p < 0.001$) as well as in the basal ganglia ($p < 0.01$) during mental simulation of tennis training in normal volunteers. Similar forms of activation were noted during silent counting.

Petersen and others (quoted by Schmahmann, 1991) performed a PET study of single word processing. Of the tasks used the simplest was visual fixation alone on a color TV monitor. The inferior lateral occipital cortex striate, extrastriate, and left putamen were activated. The second task was passive observation of the word presented either visually or auditorily; different classical cortical areas were activated. The third task was to speak each presented word aloud; in this output task – besides cortical area activation – the superior anterior cerebellum was also activated. The fourth task was to generate a semantically appropriate verb aloud in response to each presented noun. Only cortical areas were activated. Two other association-monitoring tasks were used: (i) in a semantic monitoring task, the subjects noted members of a semantic category (dangerous animals); and (ii) in a rhyme-monitoring task, they judged whether visually presented pairs of words rhymed. On these two association tasks, in addition to specific cortical areas, the anterior, posterior, and inferior lateral cerebellum were activated. It therefore seems that word association activates the lateral and posterior lobules of the cerebellum.

Roland (1993) summarized PET data on tasks which produced changes in rCBF and regional cerebral metabolism (rCMR) in the cerebellum. The lateral part of the anterior lobe was activated by vibration, flexion, extension of the hand or fingers, and motor sequences, motor sequence learning, tactile learning, tactile recognition, somatosensory discrimination, preparation for reading repeating words, and spontaneous speech. Lateral and posterior lobe activation was observed during tactile learning, somatosensory discrimination, route finding, and word association. The dentate nucleus was activated mainly during somatosensory discrimination. It has to be emphasized that cerebellar activation is *always* accompanied by activation of classical (and even nonclassical) cortical elementary and associative areas.

What is the practical value of cerebellar activation during cognitive tasks? As mentioned earlier in this entry, reverse cerebello-cerebral diaschisis in patients with chronic unilateral cerebellar infarcts does not induce neuropsychological deficits. We believe that the findings of these fascinating studies have to be interpreted cautiously from the practical clinical point of view.

Our investigations have shown that bilateral cerebellar lesions induce mild frontal-like and parietal-like syndromes through anatomophysiological and neurochemical cerebello-cortical loops; the cerebellum is directly involved in the control of SIP. It acts as a learning machine, as emphasized by Ito, and contributes effectively to motor learning. The role of the cerebellum in the initiation of language skills is well-known, but its role in language comprehension, as postulated by Leiner and others (1991), remains to be proven (if it exists at all) in cerebellar patients. A slowing of general intellectual abilities has been documented in cerebellar patients. Some memory retrieval difficulties occurring with bilateral cerebellar lesions have been found. Unilateral cerebellar infarcts seem not to be followed by major neuropsychological deficits and are well compensated. Ivry and Keele (1989) documented the role of the cerebellum in the control of timing sense and considered it to be like "a clock."

A series of experimental animal studies in our laboratory and elsewhere have confirmed the role of the cerebellum in behavioral processes in the fields of classical conditioning, spatial learning, emotion, and motor coordination.

Fascinating SPECT and PET experiments have demonstrated cerebellar activation during various cognitive tasks; however, it must be indicated that cerebellar activation is always accompanied by activation of classical cortical areas. Clinical and PET investigations support the fact that posterior and lateral, new, phylogenetically developed cerebellar areas are especially related to cognition. The authors of this entry are strongly convinced that future research on cognitive functions of the cerebellum should not be confined only to anatomophysiological, clinical neuropsychological, or even PET and SPECT approaches, but should include neurochemical and pharmacological approaches in both humans and animals.

Note This work was supported by grants from the Canadian Association of Friedreich's Ataxia and from the Du Pont Merck Pharmaceutical Company, Wilmington, Delaware. Gratitude is expressed to Ovid Da Silva for his editorial input and to Michèle Mathieu for her secretarial assistance.

BIBLIOGRAPHY

Botez, M. I., & Barbeau, A. (1971). Role of subcortical structures, and particularly of the thalamus, in the mechanisms of speech and language. *International Journal of Neurology, 8,* 300–20.

Botez, M. I., Botez, T., Elie, R., & Attig, E. (1989). Role of the cerebellum in complex human behavior. *Italian Journal of Neurological Sciences, 10,* 291–300.

Botez, M. I., Gravel, J., Attig, E., & Vézina, J. L. (1985). Reversible chronic cerebellar ataxia after phenytoin intoxication: possible role of the cerebellum in cognitive thought. *Neurology (NY)*, *35*, 1152–7.

Botez, M. I., Léveillé, J., Lambert, R., & Botez, T. (1991a). Single photon emission computed tomography (SPECT) in cerebellar disease: cerebello-cerebral diaschisis. *European Neurology*, *31*, 405–12.

Botez, M. I., Young, S. N., Botez, T., & Pedraza, O. L. (1991b). Treatment of heredo-degenerative ataxias with amantadine hydrochloride. *Canadian Journal of Neurological Sciences*, *18*, 307–11.

Botez-Marquard, T., & Botez, M. I. (1993). Cognitive behavior in heredo-degenerative ataxias. *European Neurology*, *33*, 351–7.

Botez-Marquard, T., Botez, M. I., Cardu, B., & Léveillé, J. (1989). Speed of information processing and its relationship to intelligence at various levels of the central nervous system. *Neurology*, *39*, 318.

Courchesne, E., Saitoh, O., Young-Courchesne, R., & Press, G. A. (1994). Abnormality of cerebellar vermian lobules VI and VII in patients with infantile autism. *American Journal of Radiology*, *162*, 123–30.

Decety, J., & Ingvar, D. H. (1990). Brain structures participating in mental simulation of motor behavior: a neuropsychological interpretation. *Acta Psychologica*, *73*, 13–34.

El-Awar, M., Kish, S., Oscar-Berman, M., Robitaille, Y., Schut, L. S., & Freedman, M. (1991). Selective delayed alternation deficits in dominantly inherited olivopontocerebellar atrophy. *Brain and Cognition*, *16*, 121–9.

Grafman, J., Litvan, I., Massaquoi, S., Stewart, M., Sirigu, A., & Hallett, M. (1992). Cognitive planning deficit in patients with cerebellar atrophy. *Neurology*, *42*, 1493–6.

Ivry, R. B., & Keele, S. W. (1989). Timing functions of the cerebellum. *Journal of Cognitive Neurosciences*, *1*, 136–52.

Jensen, A. R. (1993). Spearman's *g*: link between psychometrics and biology. *Annals of the New York Academy of Sciences*, *702*, 103–29.

Lalonde, R., & Botez, M. I. (1985). Exploration and habituation in nervous mutant mice. *Behavioural Brain Research*, *17*, 83–6.

Lalonde, R., & Botez, M. I. (1990). The cerebellum and learning processes in animals. *Brain Research Reviews*, *15*, 325–32.

Leiner, H. C., Leiner, A. L., & Dow, R. S. (1991). The human cerebro-cerebellar system: its computing, cognitive and language skills. *Behavioral Brain Research*, *44*, 113–28.

McCormick, D. A., & Thompson, R. F. (1984). Cerebellum: essential involvement in the classically conditioned eyelid response. *Science*, *223*, 296–9.

Roland, P. E. (1993). Partition of human cerebellum in sensory-motor activities, learning and cognition. *Canadian Journal of Neurological Sciences*, *20 (supplement 3)*, S75.

Sanes, J. N., Dimitrov, B., & Hallet, M. (1990). Motor learning in patients with cerebellar dysfunction. *Brain*, *113*, 103–20.

Schmahmann, J. (1991). An emerging concept: the cerebellar contribution to higher function. *Archives of Neurology*, *48*, 1178–87.

Spidalieri, G., Busby, L., & Lamarre, Y. (1983). Fast ballistic arm movements triggered by visual, auditory and somesthetic stimuli in the monkey. II. Effects of unilateral dentate lesion on discharge of precentral cortical neurons and reaction time. *Journal of Neurophysiology*, *50*, 1359–79.

Trouillas, P., Brudon, F., & Adeleine, P. (1988). Improvement of cerebellar ataxia with levo-rotatory form of 5-hydroxytryptan. *Archives of Neurology*, *45*, 1217–22.

Watson, P. J. (1978). Nonmotor functions of the cerebellum. *Psychological Bulletin*, *85*, 944–67.

Wiesendanger, M., Ruegg, D. G., & Wiesendanger, R. (1979). The corticopontine system in primates: anatomical and functional considerations. In J. Massion and K. Sasaki (Eds), *Cerebro-cerebellar interactions* (pp. 45–64). Amsterdam: Elsevier/North Holland Biomedical Press.

M.I. BOTEZ, ROBERT LALONDE,
AND THÉRÈSE BOTEZ

cerebral dominance *See* LATERALIZATION.

cerebral palsy Cerebral palsy (CP) may be defined as a "persistent, but not unchanging, disorder of movement and posture due to non-progressive disorder of the immature brain" (Brett, 1991). The deficit may affect one or more parts of the nervous system and so the symptoms vary. This definition focuses on the main items in the etiology, namely: an early and fixed disorder of the brain and arbitrary age limits, such as the first 2 or 3 years of life.

The incidence of cerebral palsy varies according to different series from 1 to 3 cases per 1,000 live births. The prevalence is currently rated at 2 per 1,000 live births.

CLASSIFICATION AND MAIN CLINICAL FEATURES

Ingram's classification with the following categories – hemiplegia, bilateral hemiplegia, diplegia, ataxia, dyskinesia, and "other" – is adopted in this article (Ingram, 1984).

Hemiplegia In most children with the hemiplegic form the disorder is congenital.

Antenatal factors are important as predisposing conditions in about two-thirds of cases. In about half the cases detrimental antenatal events interact with perinatal risk factors (Hagberg et al., 1984). In many cases (42 percent) the etiology is unknown, although the cryptogenic forms have been reduced by improved imaging techniques. Indeed, CT scans often show an area of infarction confined to the corresponding hemisphere secondary to a perinatal stroke.

In congenital hemiplegia the motor handicap is usually associated with normal intelligence and behavior.

Acquired hemiplegia, which accounts for between a tenth and a third of most series of hemiplegic patients, is the outcome of many causes: vascular, traumatic, inflammatory, and epileptic.

Hemiplegia affects mainly the right side of the body and especially the arm, which is hypotonic in the first month of life to become spastic later. In addition to the dominant feature of motor impairment, several other disorders may be associated: sensory, visual field (HEMIANOPIA), speech, and mental development. Intellectual deficit, however, is less common than in double hemiplegia and diplegia.

Bilateral hemiplegia (tetraplegia) All four limbs are affected, the upper limbs being more severely spastic than the lower.

The most frequent causes are: perinatal distress, fetal malformation, infection or vascular trouble, less often postnatal cerebral insults. Mental retardation and epilepsy are very common, as are bulbar muscle involvement, ocular defects and microcephaly.

Spastic diplegia All four limbs are spastic, the upper less severely than the lower limbs.

The condition is almost always congenital (mainly among preterm infants), although in diplegic infants born at term antenatal and perinatal risk factors are often associated (Hagberg et al., 1984).

Intelligence is less severely affected than in tetraplegic cerebral palsy and is generally within normal limits or a little below, although the increased survival of patients with spastic diplegia among low birthweight infants, since the introduction of neonatal intensive care, has meant that there are now more children with more severe physical and mental handicap.

Other problems such as epilepsy, visual and ocular defects, or deafness may be associated.

Dyskinetic (athetoid) cerebral palsy The motor symptoms, typical extrapyramidal movements, dyskinetic or athetoid, become evident only many months after birth.

Perinatal risk factors (mainly birth asphyxia), often preceded by fetal disturbances, have become the commonest cause of dyskinetic CP, since the risk of neonatal hyperbilirubinemia has been reduced.

Speech is very often impaired in these children, while intelligence is within the normal range in most patients.

Ataxic cerebral palsy Motor impairment is of cerebellar origin and is associated in the pure form with marked hypotonia, which is the predominant clinical feature in the first months of life, together with delay in achieving the motor milestones.

Perinatal abnormalities (prolonged and difficult or precipitate delivery, fetal distress, and so on) or postnatal factors are at the origin of ataxic cerebral palsy in a few children, but in most cases the condition is congenital with no defined risk factors (Hagberg et al., 1984). Intellectual impairment, speech disorders, ocular problems, and epilepsy may also occur.

MENTAL DEVELOPMENT

The variety and extent of CNS lesions in children with cerebral palsy explain how it is that the motor, sensory, and communication disorders are so often compounded by psychological, especially cognitive, impairment. And yet the nexus between brain damage and psychic disorder is far from straightforward. A brain lesion does not always impinge, either generally or sectorially, on the higher functions. Even extensive brain damage is consistent with quite normal psychological development. Further, children with or without brain damage may develop quite similar psychological disorders, while children with similar brain damage may have disorders that differ both in severity and type.

On this subject, MRI scanning supplies information on ventricular dilatation and reduction of the white substance, which reflect the severity of the motor disability, but not on mental impairment (Yokochi et al., 1991). Further, the CT-determined extent of brain damage was found to correlate with the IQ only in children with lesions after age 5, there being no correlation in children with earlier damage. More specific information on the connection between functional and structural damage seems recently to have emerged from research into the regional uptake of glucose in different clinical forms of cerebral palsy. FDG-PET investigations seem to show that the distribution of metabolic changes almost always extends beyond the anatomically affected region. For example, in patients with spastic diplegia, PET reveals focal areas of decreased metabolism in the cortex without apparent structural abnormalities, whereas in patients with choreoathetosis the metabolism in the cortex is relatively normal but markedly reduced in the thalamus and in the nucleus lentiformis (Kerrigan et al., 1991).

Given the early onset of the disorders, it is hardly ever possible to attempt any syndromal classification (frontal, parietal, callosal, or other), as is possible with disorders of later onset. The cognitive disorder in cerebral palsy is rarely focal; more often it expresses global disorganization.

The mental deficit arises from an interaction between the effects of the structural deficit or lesion in the brain and those arising from the associated sensory and motor deficits. The cognitive processes in the early stages of development are accomplished via sensory channels, chiefly sight and hearing, and object manipulation.

The presence of multiple sensory and motor, as well as speech, disorders makes it exceedingly difficult as a rule to arrive at a score of intelligence (IQ) in a cerebral palsy child by means of routine psychometric tests. It is nonetheless considered possible to arrive at an all-round estimate of ability in at least 90 percent of cases. The

Wechsler Intelligence Scale for Children (WISC) is particularly helpful in detecting the cerebral dysfunction profile from a higher (10 points or more) mean verbal subtest score and a lower mean performance subtest score, since both verbal and performance tasks are included in the same scale. The detection of brain damage by means of the verbal higher than performance formula may be extended to progressively younger children, and this discrepancy between verbal and performance scores can be picked up even in preschool children.

Another test designed specifically for the individual testing of cerebral palsy children is the Columbia Mental Maturity Scale, which consists of 100 card drawings of likeness and differences.

Early studies by 13 teams combining 3,705 cases of cerebral palsy yield the following distribution of intelligence: IQ under 71: 45 percent; between 70 and 89: 23 percent; between 90 and 119: 26 percent; over 120: 6 percent (Denhoff & Pick-Robinault, 1960). A more recent survey from the USA (1979) of 1,000 cerebral palsy children, mostly under the age of 10, suggests that both the frequency and the severity of mental retardation associated with cerebral palsy are greater than previously reported. The mean IQ for the whole sample was found to be 52, and 85 percent of the children in the sample had IQs under 85. In that sample children with hemiplegia and monoplegia tended to attain borderline to low-average IQs, children with spastic quadriplegia a mean IQ of 46 and children with hypotonic cerebral palsy came off worst with a mean IQ of 16. In another epidemiological survey from Great Britain (1985), based on indirect data, 77 percent of 527 cerebral palsy subjects were said to have some mental disability.

SENSORY AND PERCEPTUAL-MOTOR DISORDERS

Neurosensory disorders are often hard to assess because of poor awareness and cooperation on the part of patients. They may be present in all forms of cerebral palsy but are most frequent among hemiplegics, in whom they become more marked with age.

The sensory impairment may be global but the abilities most commonly affected are stereognosia, two-point discrimination, GRAPHES-THESIA, and finger AGNOSIA, especially in spastic diplegics. Less affected are the response to touch and pain and the position sense of the fingers. Right/left discrimination may be affected too, and also somatognosia, though this only in hemiplegics.

The *ocular defects* found in cerebral palsy concern the extraocular muscles, visual acuity, object perception, and eye dominance. It is generally thought that over 50 percent of cerebral palsy children have oculomotor defects and 25 percent or more subnormal vision. Strabismus is one of the commoner disorders. Others are optic atrophy, congenital cataract, coloboma of the iris, and paresis of gaze. Such defects are commonly found in all types of cerebral palsy but mostly in the spastic varieties.

HEMIANOPIA is found in approximately 25 percent of spastic hemiplegic children.

These early developmental abnormalities, combined with oculomotor incoordination and atypical eye–hand patterns, may affect learning ability and the acquisition of fine skills.

Perceptual and perceptual-motor dysfunctions are so insidiously hidden among the gross neuromotor disabilities of cerebral palsy children that they are often overlooked.

One of the problems most frequently encountered is visual perception of form. The child has difficulty in recognizing the complete conformation of a design or picture. This has been described in connection with figure-background difficulties. Other disturbances may come to light through the faulty reproduction of figures or drawings.

The Marianne Frostig Developmental Test of Visual Perception seemed to be a convenient tool for the analysis of specific perceptual and visuomotor disorders. According to a study by Abercrombie and others (1964) of various cerebral palsy types, the athetoid group showed no specific perceptual or visuomotor disorder on this test while the diplegics, very variable in their performances, all showed signs of perceptual disorder on one or more subtests. Peritrigonal lesions, especially in the parietal lobe, revealed by MRI in diplegic children, may play a part in this impairment (Yokochi et al., 1991). The performances on the same test varied in hemiplegics but none was generally low as in some of the diplegics.

HEARING AND SPEECH PROBLEMS

The incidence of hearing loss among cerebral palsy children is calculated to be between 10 and 40 per cent. Spastics are less impaired than ataxic children and much less than athetoid patients.

Of the various types of deafness the *central* type (affecting the nervous system from the brain stem to the cortex) is more frequent among cerebral palsy patients than *perceptive* (nerve) or *conduction* deafness (affecting transmission of sound as far as the inner ear). The causes of central deafness include traumatic events and anoxia-ischemia responsible for the brain damage, and at one time very frequently kernicterus, which could cause simple nuclear deafness and also more complex forms of vestibular dysfunction. This explains the frequency of hearing loss in series of athetoid cerebral palsy.

Speech disorders may be in part related to hearing difficulties, though there may be other reasons too. Delay and poverty of language often depend on the degree of mental deficit. DYSARTHRIA, DYSPRAXIA and APHASIA are very common problems. Dysarthria is a speech disorder due to a disturbance in the muscular control of the speech mechanism, resulting from impairment of any of the basic motor processes involved in the execution of speech. Dyspraxia is a central disorder of motor speech programming affecting the complex sequence of muscle contractions involved in speaking. Aphasia is another frequent dysfunction in cerebral palsy children as a result of neurological impairment disrupting the normal language-learning process and affecting both expression and comprehension.

NEUROPSYCHOLOGICAL PROFILE IN HEMIPLEGIC CEREBRAL PALSY

The neuropsychological profile has been fairly extensively studied in hemiplegic cerebral palsy, partly because the relative sparing of intellectual function in these subjects has allowed a thorough evaluation of various higher functions, and partly because in the case of a unilateral localized cerebral lesion it is possible to study the influence both of the side on which the lesion occurred and the time of the lesion. This should throw light both on cerebral PLASTICITY and on LATERALIZATION.

PERCEPTUAL-MOTOR DYSFUNCTIONS

The principal sensory functions to be affected are stereognosia, two-point discrimination, graphesthesia, and tactile localization. Elementary sensibility is more often spared.

Raven's Progressive Matrices Test elicits no significant correlation between visuoperceptual abilities (see also VISUOPERCEPTUAL DISORDERS) and lesion side. There is some difference in the process of development of spatial and class relationships in that right-lesioned children generally fail to generate *next-to* relations (i.e. placing one object next to another) with the same frequency as normal or left-lesioned children, although they perceive *in* and *on* relations (i.e. one object containing another) correctly. Children with congenital right hemisphere lesions also seem to have a spatial cognitive deficit in drawing, revealed by a failure to integrate different elements into a coherent spatial configuration.

Further, some studies show impairment of visuomotor performance in both the affected and the "good" hand. So it seems that in children unilateral lesions, whether right- or left-sided, may result in bilateral visuomotor impairment.

Dyspraxia may also occur in children with hemiplegia, right or left, but this dysfunction might be a consequence of their difficulty in execution, secondary to distal weakness, rather than of impaired motor planning.

INTELLIGENCE AND ACADEMIC ACHIEVEMENT

The IQs of hemiplegic children have been the most extensively reported and they are on average 20 points below normal. The reliability of some of the data is highly questionable, however, because of the probable inclusion, in some groups, of patients with bilateral brain damage and of patients with seizure disorders.

The two problems that have received most attention in this area are the influence of lesion side and the influence of time of lesion onset. The latter point is crucial to the development of the higher functions, for cerebral plasticity, which allows extensive anatomicofunctional remodelling in cases of very early damage, is nonetheless limited. Even children with very early lesions do not seem able to develop their cognitive abilities in the same way as normal children after 6–8 years of age.

With regard to the influence of lesion side on cognitive abilities, some studies of children with very early, even congenital, brain damage argue for the presence of sectoral cognitive or language

deficits, such as to differentiate them from normal subjects. These data suggest that there are areas in the brain programmed for processing given functions and that damage to these areas causes irremediable loss of functional specialization. Thus, however early the damage, the scores on verbal tests are likely to be lower when the left side is affected and the scores on visuospatial tests are likely to be lower when the right side is affected.

The published data on this issue are somewhat discordant. Some studies have shown that lesions occurring before the age of 1 year, whether in the right or the left hemisphere, implied below-normal mean scores both on the verbal and on the performance IQ, whereas lesions occurring after that age induced side-related effects. In other words, left-sided lesions influenced both the VIQ and the PIQ whereas right-sided lesions affected only the PIQ.

According to others, the one-year watershed does not differentiate scores by time of lesion onset. Early and late lesions of the right hemisphere lower only the performance scores, while lesions of the left hemisphere lower both verbal and performance scores. The recent data of Vargha-Khadem and others (1992) on children with hemiplegia secondary to perinatal damage to right or left hemisphere, who presented lower IQ and Memory Quotient (MQ), show no side differences. In these children the frequency and degree of deficit correlated strongly only with the presence of seizures and/or the severity of the EEG abnormalities. These authors interpreted the lack of side difference as support for the hemisphere equipotentiality hypothesis and the theory of cognitive crowding.

Reading and spelling are more likely to be impaired by early damage to the left than to the right hemisphere. Some language measures, such as lexical comprehension and production, are equally affected by early lesions on either side, whereas others, such as syntactic production, show marked asymmetry of effect (early left-hemisphere lesions). Subjects with early left lesions produced syntactically simpler output with many more syntactic errors than did their controls or early right-lesioned subjects (Aram & Whitaker, 1988).

The data on mathematical abilities are few and contradictory. Some authors number acalculia among the major neuropsychological deficits associated with language disorder in subjects with

213

left lesions, while others failed to detect any side-related arithmetic disorder.

NEGLECT

The NEGLECT syndrome in adults has been associated with various cerebral lesions, mainly in the right hemisphere, and has been widely studied in its different behavioral manifestations: hemi-inattention, HEMIAKINESIA, ALLESTHESIA, hemi-spatial neglect, and EXTINCTION. Very few neuro-psychological data have been published on neglect following a unilateral hemisphere lesion in children, and the few that there are concern mostly acquired damage, in which neglect resembles that observed in adults with similarly localized lesions and is usually temporary.

Some data on DICHOTIC LISTENING in congenital hemiplegic subjects show poorer scores for the ear contralateral to the damaged hemisphere, but the pattern of deficit is opposite to that seen in adults. The congenital left-hemisphere-damaged group fared worse on pitch discrimination than either right-damaged subjects or controls, while the congenital right-hemisphere-damaged group fared significantly worse on syllable discrimination. These unexpected findings have been explained in terms of the crowding hypothesis.

Tactile extinction has been found in both congenital and acquired right and left hemiplegia. It is generally contralateral to the lesion side, although a few male patients with right hemiplegia have shown ipsilateral extinction. This deficit may be explained by either the sensory or the attentional hypothesis (Lenti et al., 1991).

Hemi-inattention and extinction in hemiplegic subjects shed light on some of the behavioral features often seen in clinical practice: the scant attention paid to the function of the paretic side, irrespective of the severity of the motor deficit, and body image disorder.

BIBLIOGRAPHY

Abercrombie, M. L. J., Gardiner, P. A., Hansen, E., Jonckheere, J., Lindon, R. L., Solomon, G., & Tyson, M. C. (1964). Visual, perceptual and visuomotor impairment in physically handicapped children. *Perceptual and Motor Skills, 18,* 561–625.

Aram, D. M., & Whitaker, H. A. (1988). Cognitive sequelae of unilateral lesions acquired in early childhood. In D. L. Molfese & S. J. Segalowitz (Eds), *Brain lateralization in children* (pp. 417–36). New York and London: Guilford.

Brett, E. M. (1991). Cerebral palsy, perinatal injury to the spinal cord and brachial plexus birth injury. In E. M. Brett (Ed.), *Pediatric neurology* (pp. 285–316). Edinburgh: Churchill Livingstone.

Denhoff, E., & Pick Robinault, I. (1960). *Cerebral palsy and related disorders.* New York: McGraw-Hill.

Hagberg, B., Hagberg, G., & Olow, I. (1984). The changing panorama of cerebral palsy in Sweden. IV. Epidemiological trends 1959–1978. *Acta Pediatrica Scandinavica, 73,* 433–40.

Ingram, T. T. S. (1984). A historical review of the definition and classification of cerebral palsies. In F. Stanley & E. Alberman (Eds), *The epidemiology of the cerebral palsies.* Clinics in Developmental Medicine No. 87, SIMP (pp. 1–11), Oxford: Blackwell Scientific; Philadelphia: J. B. Lippincott.

Kerrigan, J. F., Chugani, H. T., & Phelps, M. E. (1991). Regional cerebral glucose metabolism in clinical subtypes of cerebral palsy. *Pediatric Neurology, 7,* 415–25.

Lenti, C., Radice, L., Cerioli, M., & Musetti, L. (1991). Tactile extinction in childhood hemiplegia. *Developmental Medicine and Child Neurology, 33,* 789–94.

Vargha-Khadem, F., Isaacs, E., Van der Werf, S., Robb, S., & Wilson, J. (1992). Development of intelligence and memory in children with hemiplegic cerebral palsy. *Brain, 115,* 315–29.

Yokochi, K., Aiba, K., Horie, M., Inukai, K., Fujimoto, S., Kodama, M., & Kodama, K. (1991). Magnetic resonance imaging in children with spastic diplegia: correlation with the severity of their motor and mental abnormality. *Developmental Medicine and Child Neurology, 33,* 18–25.

CARLO LENTI

cerebrospinal fluid (CSF)   The cerebrospinal fluid (CSF) occupies the space within the skull and the outer MENINGES, between the arachnoid layer and the pia mater, and also the spaces within the brain (the VENTRICLES) and spinal cord (the central canal). The subarachnoid space and the ventricular system communicate through various holes, making these spaces continuous.

The CSF, which is partly secreted from the choroid plexus of the two lateral ventricles (other constituents diffuse directly across the limiting membranes), is of very constant composition, and differs in several important respects from plasma. It acts as both a fluid buffer for the mechanical protection of the brain and spinal cord and has metabolic functions, not fully understood. The fluid, after circulating around the ventricular spaces and around the spinal cord and subarachnoid space, is absorbed into the veins of the pia mater and subarachnoid space and some escapes into the venous sinuses and into the lymphatic system.

The CSF is under positive pressure in the ventricular system, which drives the circulation from the lateral ventricles through the chain of medial ventricles and out into the subarachnoid space. When this circulation is obstructed HYDROCEPHALUS occurs, the increasing pressure resulting in ventricular dilation and displacement of brain tissue. Cerebral edema may also result in an increase in pressure in the CSF as the swollen brain exerts increased pressure upon the ventricular system. For these reasons, the monitoring of the CSF pressure is important in managing a range of neurological conditions, and, in intensive care, the pressure of the CSF may now be continuously monitored. Abnormally low pressure in the CSF (low pressure hydrocephalus) may have as serious a consequence as abnormally raised pressure.

Examination of the constitution of the CSF, by a sample obtained through LUMBAR PUNCTURE, may reveal information which is diagnostic of a range of cerebral diseases. These include the organisms associated with cerebral infections, proteins indicative of certain diseases and neoplasms, and neoplastic cells may themselves be identifiable in the CSF. Blood may be detected in the CSF when a hemorrhage communicates with the subarachnoid space. Normal CSF is, however, consistent with a range of conditions including degenerative conditions associated with dementia, and it can never exclude a pathological process within the brain. Nevertheless, in certain conditions, particularly encephalitis and cerebral abscess, CSF examination may be critical in establishing a diagnosis.

J. GRAHAM BEAUMONT

cerebrovascular accident (CVA) A cerebrovascular accident (CVA) is a sudden failure of the blood supply to a part of the brain, and is more popularly known as a STROKE. It may result from an INFARCT or from an intracerebral hemorrhage. It is of sudden or rapid onset, in terms of minutes, and is accompanied by focal neurological signs: commonly hemiplegia on the contralateral side, sensory loss, homonymous HEMIANOPIA, and dysphasia (if the hemisphere subserving language is affected).

It is the most common neurological disease, affecting 1.5 per 1,000 overall and 1 per 100 over the age of 75. Males and females are almost equally affected. The primary causes are emboli originating in the arteries or the heart, hemorrhage resulting from the rupture of an aneurysm, hypotension (although hypertension is a risk factor) and other vascular diseases. The cause is unrelated to the nature of the ensuing stroke, except that in ischemic conditions there may have been previous TIAs, and there may be a stepwise progression of a series of minor strokes over a protracted period. Initial mortality is high, with 20 percent failing to survive beyond one month, while about 40 percent make a relatively full recovery.

The neuropsychological assessment and interventions are according to the demonstrated site of the lesion and the focal impairments which may be observed.

Charles Bonnet syndrome Charles Bonnet compiled the self-observations of his grandfather, who reported a range of visual hallucinatory disturbances associated with decreased visual acuity. The hallucinations may be continuous or almost continuous over prolonged periods of time (even years), and are commonly figured, multiple, and characterized by rich and brilliant colors. Lilliputian people, animals, and objects may be seen, and animation may be present. The visions more normally occupy the entire visual field and appear clearly located in space, although the patient retains awareness of the unreality of the hallucination. The hallucinations are clearly linked to reduced visual acuity, especially of acute onset.

chimeric figure Chimeric figures are composed of the left and right lateral halves of two different stimuli joined at the vertical meridian, which is the point of visual fixation when the stimulus is presented. These figures have been principally used in the DIVIDED VISUAL FIELD TECHNIQUE with COMMISSUROTOMY patients, and also with normal subjects. When used in this way the left half of the figure, for example, the left half of a picture of the face of a young woman, is presented to the right cerebral hemisphere and the right half of the figure, perhaps the right half of a picture of the face of an old man, is presented to the left hemisphere. Following brief exposure, the right hand will select the whole picture of the old man from among a set of test stimuli while the left hand will pick out the picture of the young woman. Verbal report will also identify the old man, and the unusual nature of the stimulus will not be apparent to the patient.

Chimeric stimuli have also been used with normal subjects with similar results, and reports have suggested that under certain conditions normal subjects may similarly be unaware of the chimeric nature of the stimulus.

chorea Chorea is a form of involuntary movement or dyskinesia, in which relatively gross movements of an apparently purposive nature follow one another in a disorderly and uncontrolled fashion. These movements arise, not in the pyramidal system of voluntary movement, but in the extrapyramidal system controlled by the BASAL GANGLIA.

Choreiform (or "choreic") movements of the face, which may include frowning, smiling, raising the eyebrows, pursing the lips, and movements of the mouth and tongue, are always bilateral. In the limbs, movements are more pronounced in the arms than in the legs. The choreiform movements interfere with normal intentional movements, making the patient ataxic and dysarthric and interfering with chewing and swallowing. The choreiform movements cease during sleep.

The typical pattern of the movements differs according to the associated condition, of which the principal examples are HUNTINGTON'S DISEASE (previously known as Huntington's chorea), Sydenham's chorea, and HEMIBALLISMUS. This is consonant with the differing pathology in these conditions: in Huntington's disease the corpus STRIATUM is affected together with ganglion cells in the forebrain, in Sydenham's chorea the corpus striatum and closely related structures, in hemi-

ballismus the contralateral subthalamic nuclei. In all forms of chorea there is a reduction in the neurotransmitter dopamine and certain of its metabolites in the caudate nucleus, and it is thought that the choreiform movements result from overstimulation of a damaged striatum by a relatively normal nigrostriatal pathway.

choreiform syndrome Choreiform syndrome (Prechtl's syndrome) is a disorder of involuntary movements in children, in which CHOREA is the principal feature.

Children with this disorder may be of normal, even above average, intelligence and possess normal motor coordination, except that their motor activity is interrupted repeatedly by irregular jerky choreiform movements. These children are also likely to exhibit TICS and cases have been reported which develop into GILLES DE LA TOURETTE SYNDROME. The syndrome was diagnosed in 3 percent of a consecutive series of admissions to a learning disabilities clinic over a two-year period.

If children with this syndrome are matched with normal children on the basis of age and intelligence, the affected children show poor coordination, impulsivity, clumsiness and a reduced attention span. When the disorder was first described, an associated reading difficulty was considered to be an important feature, but the significance of this has received less emphasis in more recent discussions.

cingulate gyrus The cingulate gyrus is a region of cortex on the medial surface of each cerebral hemisphere, lying superior to the CORPUS CALLOSUM. It is sometimes referred to as one of the layers of the "paralimbic cortex," being older than the neocortex in terms of its phylogenetic development. It receives projections from secondary neocortex, and thus provides an alternative to the secondary-tertiary projection route for sensory information. It has been linked with processes of visual ATTENTION and NEGLECT. With lateralized intracranial pressure, or displacement by a space-occupying lesion, the cingulate gyrus may become herniated under the falx with compression of the anterior cerebral arteries and consequent infarction.

cingulectomy Cingulectomy is a form of PSY-CHOSURGERY, alternatively referred to as *cingulotomy*, in which the surgical target is the anterior portion of the cingulum, a fiber tract which connects the CINGULATE GYRUS with the HIPPOCAMPUS (*see* LIMBIC SYSTEM). Destruction of this portion of the cingulum may alleviate severe emotional disorders which do not respond to pharmacotherapy.

circumlocution Circumlocution is generally taken to indicate an aphasic word-finding difficulty. Given their inability to access a word which they need in speech, patients may substitute a descriptive phrase in its place. If in producing the substitute phrase, there needs to be further substitution for an unavailable word, then the wordy, lengthy output becomes increasingly circumlocutory, and may be referred to as "empty speech." This may occur in a patient with good comprehension, accurate repetition, and otherwise fluent speech output without paraphasias, although it may also be a feature of all fluent aphasias.

cLEMs *See* LEMs.

clinical neuropsychology *See* NEUROPSY-CHOLOGY.

closed head injury A closed head injury results from a trauma to the head which does not penetrate the skull and MENINGES and enter the brain (as opposed to a *penetrating brain injury*). It may have two types of consequence: primary and secondary.

The primary effects are instantaneous, respond poorly to treatment, and are often the limiting factor in recovery. Most of these effects are due to acceleration which may be translational or angular (twisting). Translational forces produce differential movements of the skull and brain, which may produce surface lacerations from internal features of the skull and damage to the cortex as it is slammed against the skull. Internal pressures may also be built up within the brain itself and may result in cavitation as liquids within the brain rapidly vaporize and then condense, producing an effect similar to an explosion within the head. Angular forces produce shearing strains which result in multiple tearing of neural and microvascular elements throughout the deep portions of the brain.

The secondary effects of closed head injury are infarction (*see* INFARCT) and necrosis (death) of cells due to pressure. These effects come about by a range of mechanisms. The primary effects of the injury produce HEMATOMA, cerebral EDEMA, and vasospasm, and these changes in turn will result in an increase in intracranial pressure, with consequential effects upon brain perfusion and raising the possibility of brain herniation in which portions of the brain are squeezed through the more restricted apertures in the meninges and bony case surrounding the brain. These pathological changes, which may be temporary and treatable, nonetheless may produce irreversible changes through infarction and necrosis. Hematomas may also lead directly to cell necrosis. The effects of closed head injury are often so severe, even following relatively minor impacts, because the brain is contained within a relatively closed system and so cannot accommodate changes in volume following œdema, and because cells in the central nervous system are largely unable to regenerate after the effects of damage.

J. GRAHAM BEAUMONT

cluster headache Cluster headaches, normally caused by migraine, are acute recurrent attacks of headache, sometimes termed "migrainous neuralgia." The headaches are unilateral, always on the same side, and are commoner in men than women. The pain typically lasts up to an hour, but may recur several times a day over a period of weeks before there is a pain-free interval, often of many months.

colliculus, inferior The two inferior colliculi are a pair of rounded elevations on the dorsal surface of the upper part of the midbrain. Together with the superior colliculi, they form the *corpora quadragemina*, which are the main elements of the *tectum*. The inferior colliculi receive fibers from and transmit fibers to the spinal cord, and form an important element in the auditory system.

Certain fibres passing into the brain in the

auditory nerve are routed to and terminate in the inferior colliculus. By a further relay these fibers transmit information on to the medial GENICULATE BODY of the THALAMUS. Certain fibers pass directly through the inferior colliculus to the medial geniculate body. The inferior colliculus therefore acts not only as a relay station within the auditory system but permits the integration of auditory information with sensory and motor information passing up and down the spinal cord.

colliculus, superior   The two superior colliculi are a pair of rounded elevations on the dorsal surface of the upper part of the midbrain. Together with the inferior colliculi, they form the *corpora quadragemina*, which are the main elements of the *tectum*. The superior colliculi receive fibers from and transmit fibers to the spinal cord, and form an important element in the visual system.

The optic tract as it passes through the brain is routed to the lateral GENICULATE BODY of the THALAMUS from which most of the fibers continue posteriorly to the occipital visual cortex. Some fibers, however, continue from the lateral geniculate to terminate in the superior colliculus. In the superior colliculus, and the pretectal area adjacent to it, the light and accommodation reflexes which control pupillary size are organized. The superior colliculus also plays a role in the coordination of eye movements through reflex movements of the eyeballs, and head turning in response to visual stimuli.

Some have considered the superior colliculi to play a role greater than the reflex control of eye and head movements, being a sensory integration center. Animal studies have demonstrated that lesions of one superior colliculus may produce a multimodal unilateral neglect syndrome, and may also interfere with the capacity to acquire novel visual discriminations. The superior colliculi, as important elements in the secondary visual system (*see* BLINDSIGHT), may well play a wider and more important role in vision than is often assumed.

color agnosia   *See* AGNOSIA; VISUOPERCEPTUAL DISORDERS.

coma vigil   *See* MUTISM, AKINETIC.

commissurotomy   (Less commonly, commissurectomy; also called forebrain commissurotomy, corpus callosotomy, or split-brain operation.) Strictly speaking, a commissurotomy is any surgical interruption of commissural fiber tracts (commissures). Commissures consist of axons, which connect the right and left sides of the nervous system. The majority of these connections are homotopical, i.e. topographically identical areas on both sides are connected and they are reciprocal. However, some heterotopic connections exist. Commissural connections are found in the spinal cord as well as between many parts of the brain. In the context of clinical neuropsychology, commissurotomy refers almost always to the midline sectioning of the commissures connecting cerebral cortical regions. This forebrain commissurotomy, even though it may only involve sectioning of the corpus callosum (callosotomy), is frequently referred to as the "split-brain operation."

THE COMMISSURES OF THE BRAIN

The most prominent of the commissures is the CORPUS CALLOSUM. In a midsagittal section of a human brain (see Figure 34) its length from the rostral bend (genu) to the caudal end (splenium)

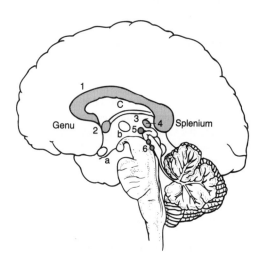

Figure 34 A midsagittal section of a human brain. **1,** corpus callosum; **2,** anterior commissure; **3,** hippocampal commissure; **4,** habenular commissure; **5,** posterior commissure; **6,** midbrain commissures; a, chiasma opticum; b, massa intermedia; c, fornix.

reaches approximately 10 cm. It is estimated to contain 200 million axons, which interconnect all major portions of the cerebral cortex. Most of the clinical and research data concerning human commissural functions are related to the callosum. Much less is known about the *anterior commissure* (commissura rostralis). It is a compact bundle of fibers approximately 2 to 3 mm in diameter. The anterior part of it is related to the olfactory system and the larger posterior portion connects the anterior temporal lobes of both hemispheres.

The right and left hippocampal formations are connected via the *hippocampal commissure* (commissura fornicis). There are further connections of the hippocampal cortices running through the rather small *habenular commissure* of the epithalamus. At the posterior end of the third ventricle, in the caudal wall of the pineal recess, we also find another small commissural bundle. This is the *posterior commissure*. The terminations of its fibers are not completely known, but they are thought to include several diencephalic nuclei. Finally, both inferior and superior colliculi are connected by commissures (*midbrain commissures*) that also contain ascending and descending decussating fibers.

COMMISSURAL FUNCTIONS

Often the commissures are referred to as the commissural system, and attempts have been made to find the specific unitary function of this system. Thus it has been considered a channel for the transmission of information between both sides of the nervous system. Due to the predominantly contralateral body–brain connections, the corpus callosum may provide the missing information from the respective ipsilateral side. One problem with this explanation is that the densest commissural connections exist between regions representing the midline visual field and the body trunk as well as the proximal extremities, which are already receiving ipsilateral in addition to contralateral inputs. Peripheral distal regions, with almost exclusively contralateral connections, on the other hand, appear to be devoid of commissural connections. Inhibitory functions have been postulated as well, permitting one hemisphere to function without interference from the other, or allowing for the exclusive application of specialized right or left hemisphere skills (*see* LATERALIZATION) to a particular task.

Commissural connections in a certain (physiological) sense may have a particular function, just as associative fibers or cells of a particular layer of the cortex may have a specific function. In neuropsychological terms, however, functions of the commissures are more safely considered in relation to the functions of the areas of which they are an integral part. Considering the variety of different, highly specialized brain areas connected by commissures, even within a single sensory modality, commissures interconnecting various specialized subfields subserving this modality may be involved in quite different functions. On an even larger scale, such differences have to be expected for commissures interconnecting brain areas of even greater functional diversity.

COMMISSUROTOMY (SPLIT-BRAIN OPERATION) FOR THE TREATMENT OF EPILEPSY

The most common indication for split-brain surgery is the treatment of epilepsies which have proved intractable to medication. Often only the anterior portion of the corpus callosum (i.e. the genu and the anterior part of the trunk) is sectioned (partial commissurotomy). If seizure activity is not sufficiently reduced, the commissurotomy may be extended to include all of the corpus callosum; sometimes the anterior commissure as well as the posterior, the habenular, and the hippocampal commissures are also cut. At times the so-called massa intermedia has also been sectioned. This structure, however, is not a commissure; rather, it arises from a merging of the midline nuclei of the thalamus in the third ventricle (hence this structure is also called connexus interthalamicus or adhaesio interthalamica). In humans it is highly variable in size and shape; it may also be absent, without any known functional consequences.

The rationale for the introduction of commissurotomy for the treatment of epilepsy was to contain the spread of seizures from an epileptic focus within one hemisphere. This was seen as a less destructive intervention than the often quite extensive excisions of tissue from which epileptic seizures may originate (see LOBECTOMY). Experiments with split-brain animals as early as 1890 had indicated that the procedure might be effective while causing few side effects. Bykoff's (1924) studies are an example of the split-brain operation's effectiveness to functionally separate both hemispheres in split-brain dogs. Bykoff demonstrated that generalizations of conditioned salivary reactions to tactile stimuli remained confined to stimulation of body parts controlled by one hemisphere. In normal animals a spread was observed to the other half of the body, such that stimulation of homotopical locations resulted in reactions of almost equal strength. It was also possible in the operated animals, but not in animals with intact commissures, to achieve differential conditioning using different stimuli at homotopical points on both sides of the body. Outside the experimental situation the split-brain animals appeared to be normal.

In the late 1930s Van Wagenen performed the first commissurotomies in humans for the treatment of epilepsy (Van Wagenen & Herren, 1940). The therapeutic results of these first operations, in which portions of the callosum were left intact to various degrees, thus amounting to partial commissurotomies, appear to have been less than had been hoped. Subsequently, with the exception of several operations in children, undocumented in the literature, the procedure appears to have been abandoned. Nevertheless, the study of these first split-brain patients had important repercussions. Some patients were reported to complain about left-sided muscular dyscoordination, but otherwise appeared to be basically unaffected by the operation in their everyday behavior. Neuropsychological investigations could not find any deficits in what were believed to be tests of interhemispheric transfer. In retrospect, these studies can be criticized for several methodological flaws. In some tasks there was insufficient control of lateralization; in others pretransfer learning did not extend far enough to reach steady performance levels. Thus comparisons between original learning, for example with one hand, and subsequent transfer learning with the other hand, did not result in any significant differences due to extreme variability in right- and left-hand performance. Also, a low level of performance in most tasks can very often be achieved by several alternative functional circuits, thus masking any deficit due to the loss of a specific function possibly subserved by callosal connections. Furthermore, since sizable portions of the corpus callosum had been left intact in these patients, alternative routes of information transmission may have been available. Despite the animal data already mentioned, or the disconnection syndromes due to lesions of the callosum which had been described in humans (e.g. Liepmann, 1908; Trescher & Ford, 1937), the fact that no disconnection syndrome could be demonstrated in these patients was taken to indicate that lesions of the callosum may perhaps cause degradation of functional capacities in general, but no specific defects.

Holistic ideas of brain functions, and particularly of callosal functions, came under attack when Sperry and his students in the 1950s demonstrated various specific disconnection deficits in split-brain cats and monkeys. Together with the very influential clinical research on war veterans demonstrating functional double DIS-SOCIATIONS in the effects of circumscribed lesions in young and otherwise healthy people, they pushed the pendulum again in the direction of a more localizationist view of brain functions.

These ideas also led to the reintroduction of split-brain surgery for the therapy of epilepsy (Bogen & Vogel, 1962). At first, complete transections of the forebrain commissures appeared to be necessary to guarantee a reduction in seizure activity. Some time later, partial anterior commissurotomies by the same neurosurgeons were shown to be effective as well. Since the animal research from Sperry's laboratory had demonstrated specific disconnection deficits with appropriate control of lateralization of stimuli and/or responses during testing, techniques of lateralized presentation of stimuli and attempts to control for cross-cueing characterized the testing program that Sperry, Bogen, and colleagues initiated for the study of the so-called Los Angeles series of split-brain patients in the sixties. At approximately the same time disconnection syndromes due to pathological lesions of the callosum were rediscovered (e.g. Geschwind & Kaplan, 1962), and in the following two decades observations on patients with partial and complete commissurotomies due to surgical lesions or pathological processes proliferated. Nevertheless, it is the early studies of Sperry and his colleagues and students which more or less defined what has become known as the disconnection syndrome or the split-brain syndrome (see below). It is mainly these studies, reinforced by the Nobel Prize awarded to Roger Sperry in 1981, which provided a major boost to clinical and experimental research into laterality. The study of lateral cerebral asymmetries in turn had and still has an enormous influence on many areas of brain research, as well as many other fields.

Despite the obvious success in the reduction of seizure activity in the patients operated on by Bogen and Vogel, only singular cases of split-brain surgery, mainly outside the United States, were reported for some time. It was not until several years later that split-brain operations for the treatment of epilepsy were performed elsewhere in the United States (Wilson et al., 1977). Meanwhile, interest in commissurotomy has steadily grown, and a number of epilepsy centers worldwide have taken up this procedure to treat a select group of patients. Most of these patients suffer from severe and potentially very damaging drop attacks and generalized motor seizures, as well as hemiatrophic processes or other lateralized brain damage and consequent hemiparetic seizures (Engel, 1987).

DISCONNECTION SYNDROMES FOLLOWING PARTIAL AND COMPLETE COMMISSUROTOMIES

Destruction of nerve fiber connections anywhere in the brain can result in a disconnection syndrome (*see* DISCONNECTION SYNDROME, and, for example, conduction APHASIA). As is the case with lesions thought to interrupt a direct connection between areas within a hemisphere, the sectioning of direct cortical interhemispheric connections does not really result in complete disconnection in the sense of isolation. There are potentially many alternative subcortical routes for interhemispheric interaction. The full range of these connections is not known; neither is their normal functional role nor the circumstances under which they can compensate for the loss of the forebrain commissures or the extent to which such compensation is possible.

As a probable consequence of these alternative routes, as well as differences in normal plastic changes with life-long experiences or adaptations following pathological disturbances, the resulting disconnection syndrome after commissurotomies can vary widely. There are also changes in the syndrome over time, again with large differences between individuals as to the rate and type of changes. The most important variables with regard to these individual differences appear to be etiology and the time course of epilepsy, the age of the patient at the time of surgery, the extent of extracallosal damage, the course of postoperative recovery, and presurgical neuropsychological status. The following pertains to right-handed patients. In view of the variability with regard to lateralized cerebral functions in left-handers, it appears impossible to draw conclusions from the very few left-handed split-brain patients studied so far.

ACUTE SYNDROME FOLLOWING COMPLETE COMMISSUROTOMY

One of the transient effects of a complete commissurotomy in many patients is MUTISM. In some patients it may be present for only a few days, while others may continue to make no effort to speak for weeks, although he or she may readily communicate in writing. The cause of mutism is not known; it is suspected to be related to the extent of extracallosal damage, especially of anterior cingulate and septal areas.

Another acute symptom is intermanual conflict. Patients report attempting to do something with one hand and then finding themselves struggling to do something else with the other hand. In some cases synkinetic movements may prevent one hand from letting go while an object is grasped with the other hand. Other instances involve successive conflicting acts. In one case it was reported that a patient buttoned his shirt with one hand while the other hand followed to unbutton it again. Or a newspaper was thrown on the table with one hand and then picked up again with the other. Many of these latter conflicts fit the description of an ALIEN HAND syndrome. Patients have the feeling that they cannot control the actions of one hand (almost always the left hand). For example, they pick a particular shirt from the closet with their right hand and then the left hand reaches for still another one. These problems appear to persist only in patients who at the time of the operation were older, or in patients in whom extracallosal damage cannot be excluded.

A further highly variable and mostly acute consequence of commissurotomy is left-sided limb kinetic DYSPRAXIA or APRAXIA. Patients cannot perform on verbal command particular movements with their left extremities, such as crossing themselves, giving a military salute, performing a movement as if hammering a nail or opening a door with a key, and similar gestures. The dyspraxia may also be seen in lower limb movements, such as showing how to kick a ball, stamping out a cigarette, or stamping the ground defiantly. The patients have no problems following the commands with their right limbs, and they may also perform the correct movement with their left limbs in the course of a naturally occurring situation. Often, as with other dyspraxias, the deficit is less marked when the patient is asked to perform a movement using an actual object.

CHRONIC SYNDROME FOLLOWING COMPLETE COMMISSUROTOMY

In the long term, the most impressive fact about the split-brain patients is their apparent normality. Relatives report that after the operation they observed no changes in personality or in general social behavior. Several months after the operation a routine medical examination would not pick up any abnormalities.

A possible exception may be some deficits in anterograde memory functions. However, there is no agreement on this issue. Since the patients described in these reports differ greatly, not only with regard to their pre- and postoperative history but also in the type of split-brain surgery they had, it cannot be stated with certainty that commissural lesions per se lead to memory deficits. It is possible that the destruction of the hippocampal commissures and the fornix in patients in whom the surgery extended below the corpus callosum is responsible for some of the problems observed. In others, accidental damage to anterior limbic structures may contribute indirectly to learning and memory deficits. A further possibility more closely related to anterior commissurotomies is that disconnection of the frontal cortical regions may produce such difficulties indirectly through changes in attentional mechanisms. Finally, it is possible that in some patients the commissurotomy eliminated a route which preoperatively had been used to compensate for unilateral deficiencies in medial temporal lobe memory mechanisms.

CHRONIC DISCONNECTION SYNDROME

Very clear-cut signs of disconnection with very little change over decades can be demonstrated in controlled laboratory experiments on split-brain patients. While in everyday behavior quite complex bimanual coordinations are performed without problems, even a relatively simple two-hand coordination test of which the patient has no preoperative experience may now present a problem. While moving one hand, the patient may be unable to move the other hand simultaneously in a controlled fashion. Again there are large individual differences, with younger patients after some time learning to alternate hand movements quickly, using visual feedback for control. Or they may use shoulder and whole-body motions on one side and hand movements on the other, apparently using one hemisphere to control both via ipsilateral and contralateral projections. All patients have difficulties with moving both hands such that each hand moves at a different rate. They always fall into symmetrical or parallel movement patterns against their will. However, in the same test, they are equally unable to voluntarily produce and maintain precisely synchronized bilateral symmetrical or parallel movements.

Disconnection effects can be demonstrated as well in all sensory modalities, as long as stimulus inputs can be lateralized to one hemisphere. Stimuli presented to the left visual half-field and objects to be felt only with the left hand are perceived only by the right hemisphere and vice versa. Thus patients are usually unable to retrieve an object felt or seen by the right hemisphere with their right hands, and since the right hemisphere lacks expressive language, they are unable to talk about what they are holding in their left hands or about what they have seen in their left visual half-fields. Cross-modal as well as intra-modal comparisons of stimuli are impossible, as long as they are presented such that each will be perceived by only one hemisphere. Postures imposed on the fingers of one hand out of sight cannot be copied with the opposite hand; neither can such finger postures be produced with the fingers of the right hand if pictures of the postures are presented to the right hemisphere, and vice versa.

In the auditory modality the so-called DICHOTIC LISTENING effect is dramatically enhanced. Patients can report words individually presented to each ear separately. If, however, two different words are presented simultaneously, one to each ear, only words heard with the right ear can be reliably reproduced.

If the anterior commissure is cut in addition to the corpus callosum and the nasal septum of the patient is intact, odors presented to one nostril will be perceived only by the ipsilateral hemisphere.

While one hemisphere is perceiving a sensory stimulus, the other cortical half appears to be oblivious to what is going on in its disconnected partner. When only the right hemisphere has been presented with a stimulus, the patient will even deny having seen or felt anything. Despite the verbal denial by the left hemisphere, the right hemisphere meanwhile may appropriately follow an instruction, for example, by correctly matching or manipulating an object with the left hand out of sight. If a stimulus to the right hemisphere results in a reaction, which can be perceived by the left hemisphere, the patient may try to explain this reaction. These explanations often indicate that the left hemisphere did not have sufficient knowledge of what it was that the patient experienced with the right cortical half. Thus, in the laboratory, the dominant impression is that each hemisphere has its own separate experiences, to such an extent that Sperry concluded that there existed two separate and independent streams of consciousness in these patients.

Over the years, with extensive testing experience, some patients appear to have been able to use subtle cues available to both hemispheres to solve some interhemispheric transfer problems. They may, for example, use sounds made by objects they are asked to compare, or they may rely on pain and temperature information which reaches both hemispheres via ipsilateral as well as contralateral projections from the periphery. Thus objects with sharp points or edges may be recognized interhemispherically or discriminations can be transferred if they can be made on the basis of similarity of material, due to differences in sensations of temperature with plastic, wooden, or metal objects. Other information used includes feedback from movements of the eyes, head, or arm. Thus left-handed writing with whole arm movements, although out of sight, can apparently be "read" by the left hemisphere, at least to the degree of making an intelligent guess about what it was that the right hemisphere responded to.

It must be kept in mind, however, that these latter observations were made with single exceptional patients with decades of experience in being tested. While they may provide some clues as to the alternative routes by which the surgically separated cortical halves can still communicate, the fact that the commissurotomy appears to have so little negative effect on everyday life activities does not need such elaborate explanations. Most of it can be explained by the fact that in daily life all the information is always available to both hemispheres anyway in one form or another. While in some modalities lateralization may occur, e.g. for tactile stereognostic information, this can be compensated by information from another modality. Vision is of great importance here; because of constant eye movements and bilateral representations of the foveal retina, lateralization of visual inputs appears to be all but impossible in daily life. As far as motor functions are concerned, a possible explanation of the lack of apparent deficits may come from the fact that the majority of our daily behavior is made up of highly overlearned routines. Where cortical involvement is necessary, reliance on exchange of kinesthetic, proprioceptive information via subcortical routes and visual control may lead to some slowing. But this will not show prominently in everyday behavior.

The issue of emotional and motivational processes is more complex. Such processes can be elicited through stimulation of either hemisphere. However, subsequently both hemispheres appear to be affected by these processes. Another aspect of great importance in this respect is the obvious dominance of the communicating left hemisphere. Although under laboratory conditions each hemisphere can initiate and control actions in the environment, even in this situation right hemisphere capacities cannot be tested adequately unless interference from the left hemisphere is prevented. Outside the laboratory, the left hemisphere clearly appears to be in control. With the exception of the previously mentioned alien hand syndrome, the patient never feels split. As can be inferred from laboratory observations, a major reason for this appears to be that, even if the right hemisphere is responsible for a certain behavior, the left hemisphere considers it to be its own, by fitting it into its own realm of consciousness. If explanations are requested, those provided by the left hemisphere are often clearly designed to avoid cognitive dissonance.

DISCONNECTION SYNDROME FOLLOWING PARTIAL COMMISSUROTOMY

Partial commissurotomies in epileptic patients have been performed mainly after it became clear that the most obvious disconnection effects resulted from lesions of the splenium and caudal portions of the trunk of the callosum. In particular, in cases with ictal activity involving the frontal cortex, a partial commissurotomy (of the anterior portions of the callosum) appeared to be able to provide the benefits of seizure reduction without the disconnection deficits. The same operation has also been proposed as a diagnostic option in cases with unclear lateralization of ictal activities.

Following partial anterior section of the callosum, the acute signs of a commissurotomy, such as mutism or left-sided dyspraxia, if present at all, are much less pronounced. No disconnection in the sensory domain has been described. There are subtle deficits in motor coordination, insofar as the exchange of feedforward or corollary motor information between the hemispheres is disrupted. The patients have to rely on proprioceptive and visual feedback. However, the patients may still perform quite well in less demanding tasks like doing an "Etch-a-Sketch" drawing. If such a task is made more demanding, for example, by requiring longer sequences of continuously coordinated movements, or by eliminating visual feedback, distinct deficits can be demonstrated.

As in the case of complete commissurotomies, there are isolated reports of memory deficits with partial commissurotomies. They appear to be more pronounced with concomitant lesions of the anterior commissure. As mentioned before, it is difficult to attribute these deficits solely to lesioning of the commissures. Brain damage due to a long history of epilepsy is a confounding factor, as is the possibility of extracallosal damage during the operation and the indirect effects of attentional deficits.

SPLIT-BRAIN RESEARCH IN HUMANS AND LATERALITY

The phenomenon of functional lateral cerebral asymmetry in humans had been known long before the split-brain studies. Almost all of what we know about left and right hemisphere specialization came from comparisons of groups of patients with unilateral left or right hemisphere lesions. This implied inferring functions from deficits and comparisons between groups of individuals who differ in many respects. The importance of human split-brain studies lies in the fact that they demonstrated functional differences between more or less intact right and left cerebral hemispheres within one and the same individual.

Another important contribution of this research, especially of the pioneering work of Sperry and his students and colleagues, is to have pointed out that the specialization is not absolute; each hemisphere may be able to solve a problem for which the other is thought to be specialized, such as, for example, facial recognition or language comprehension. Thus split-brain research through its spectacular findings not only helped to popularize the concept of LATERALIZATION, it also broadened the theoretical base for investigating and explaining hemispheric specialization.

SPLIT-BRAIN, RIGHT HEMISPHERE CAPACITIES, AND CONSCIOUSNESS

The right hemisphere in split-brain patients has been demonstrated not only to possess superior spatial perceptual skills, but also to be able to comprehend single words, distinguish words from non-words, follow verbal and written commands, perform object categorizations and simple number arithmetic, as well as other cognitive tasks. Others have taken the lack of propositional speech in the right hemisphere to deny language capacities, with consequent characterization of right hemisphere cognitive skills on or below the level of those of chimpanzees. Those who make not only cognitive skills but consciousness dependent on language functions have also denied consciousness to the right hemisphere. The dispute over right hemisphere capacities and consciousness, extending into the dualism versus monism debate, is mainly a dispute over definitions of language and consciousness which cannot be reviewed here. It should be noted that some language-related skills were also present in the right hemispheres of patients whose brain injury was postpubertal (Bogen, 1993), to counter the argument that the history of severe epilepsy in the split-brain patients led to abnormal lateralization not representative of normal brains. With regard to consciousness, while there is no absolute test of consciousness in all its possible definitions, the right hemisphere has been shown to possess recognition of self and self-identity (Preilowski, 1979).

COMMISSUROTOMY IN ANIMAL RESEARCH

In experiments with cats, dogs, and nonhuman primates, the same commissures that are involved in human commissurotomies have been cut to study the neuroanatomy and the functions of these commissures, as well as the brain regions which they interconnect. In experiments with lagomorphs and rodents, and especially in birds, fish, and reptiles, a number of additional, mostly midbrain commissures are of relevance. Most of the research, however, has concentrated on functions of the corpus callosum and was performed on mammals. Here, complete commissurotomies were also often used to create two more or less independently operating hemispheres. As in research on laterality, the performance of both hemispheres could then be compared within the same animal. The effects of various experimental manipulations on one hemisphere were also studied, using the other half as a control within the same organism. Thus the split-brain method has been applied to a wide range of questions concerning areas as diverse as perceptual or learning and memory functions, the dynamics of epileptic seizures, or those of minimal brain damage and recovery of function following brain lesions.

In recent years the use of split-brain methods has declined. The loss of split-brain investigations, especially in nonhuman primates, to parallel clinical studies is particularly problematic as, with a certain distance from the earlier work, it becomes apparent that some important questions remain unanswered. For example, there is the very basic issue of whether the functions of either half of the brain or the two halves of a brain without intact commissures can be compared in a meaningful way with those of an intact brain. It also appears more and more unlikely that the two halves of a split-brain animal really are functionally equivalent. As we have to make more and more adjustments in our neuroanatomical picture of the commissures (e.g. Innocenti, 1988; Killackey, 1985) as well as in our appreciation of plastic changes in brain functions (e.g. Merzenich et al., 1990), a re-evaluation of the functional properties of the commissures through animal research, as a possible corrective to some oversimplified models applied to human clinical and experimental neuropsychology, remains necessary (Preilowski, 1993).

BIBLIOGRAPHY

Bogen, J. E. (1993). The callosal syndromes. In K. M. Heilman & E. Valenstein (Eds), *Clinical neuropsychology* (3rd edn). New York: Oxford University Press.

Bogen, J. E., & Vogel, P. J. (1962). Cerebral commissurotomy in man. *Bulletin of the Los Angeles Neurological Society*, *27*, 169–72.

Bykoff, K. (1924). Versuche an Hunden mit Durchschneiden des Corpus Callosum. *Zentralblatt der gesamten Neurologie und Psychiatrie 1925*, *39*, 199.

Engel, J. J. (Ed.). (1987). *Surgical treatment of the epilepsies*. New York: Raven Press.

Geschwind, N., & Kaplan, E. (1962). A human disconnection syndrome. *Neurology*, *12*, 675–85.

Innocenti, G. M. (1986). General organization of callosal connections in the cerebral cortex. In E. G. Jones & A. Peters (Eds), *Cerebral cortex*, (Vol. 5): *Sensory-motor areas and aspects of cortical connectivity* (pp. 291–353). New York: Plenum.

Killackey, H. P. (1985). The organization of somatosensory callosal projections. A new interpretation. In A. G. Reeves (Ed.), *Epilepsy and the corpus callosum* (pp. 41–53). New York: Plenum.

Liepmann, H. (1908). *Drei Aufsätze aus dem Apraxiegebiet*. Berlin: Karger.

Merzenich, M. M., Recanzone, G. H., Jenkins, W. M., & Grajski, K. A. (1990). Adaptive mechanisms in cortical networks underlying cortical contributions to learning and non-declarative memory. In *Cold Spring Harbor Symposia on Quantitative Biology*, *LV* (pp. 873–87). Plainview, NY: Cold Spring Harbor Laboratory Press.

Preilowski, B. (1979). Consciousness after complete surgical section of the forebrain commissures in man. In I. Steele Russell, M. W. Van Hof, & G. Berlucchi (Eds), *Structure and function of cerebral commissures* (pp. 411–20). London: Macmillan.

Preilowski, B. (1987). Split-brain methods. In J. N. Hingtgen, D. Hellhammer, & G. Huppmann (Eds), *Advanced methods in psychobiology* (pp. 85–149). Toronto: C. J. Hogrefe.

Preilowski, B. (1993). Cerebral asymmetry, interhemispheric interaction and handedness: second thoughts about comparative laterality research with non-human primates, about a theory and some preliminary results. In J. P. Ward & W. D. Hopkins (Eds), *Primate laterality: Current behavioral evidence of primate asymmetries* (pp. 125–48). New York: Springer.

Reeves, A. G. (Ed.) (1985). *Epilepsy and the corpus callosum*. New York: Plenum.

Sperry, R. W. (1974). Lateral specialization in the surgically separated hemispheres. In F. O. Schmitt & F. G. Worden (Eds.), *The neurosciences: Third study program* (pp. 5–19). Cambridge, MA: MIT Press.

Trescher, J. H., & Ford, F. R. (1937). Colloid cyst of the third ventricle. *Archives of Neurology and Psychiatry, 37,* 939–73.

Trevarthen, C. (Ed.). (1990). *Brain circuits and functions of the mind: Essays in honor of Roger W. Sperry.* New York: Cambridge University Press.

Van Wagenen, W. P., & Herren, R. Y. (1940). Surgical division of commissural pathways in the corpus callosum. *Archives of Neurology and Psychiatry, 44,* 740–59.

Wilson, D. H., Reeves, A., Gazzaniga, M. S., & Culver, C. (1977). Cerebral commissurotomy for control of intractable seizures. *Neurology, 27,* 708–15.

BRUNO PREILOWSKI

completion   *See* VISUOPERCEPTUAL DISORDERS.

computerized tomography   *See* CAT SCAN.

conduction aphasia   *See* APHASIA.

confabulation   When amnesic patients give prompt, full, and detailed, but incorrect, responses to questions requiring the recall of information, this is referred to as confabulation. The recall is not only incorrect, but may often be bizarre. It is considered to be a prominent feature of the AMNESIC SYNDROME, but may occur in other patients, particularly those with global amnesias.

The classic description of KORSAKOFF'S SYNDROME includes confabulation as a frequent, though not essential, feature of the disorder. It is most marked during the acute stages of the disorder, and amnesic patients appear to be able to adjust to this aspect of their amnesic difficulties. Confabulation is more marked among those with the amnesic syndrome resulting from chronic alcoholism than in post-encephalitic states. Memory disorders which follow from nutritional deficiency (especially of thiamine: Wernicke–Korsakoff syndrome), from normal-pressure HYDROCEPHALUS, and from certain head injuries, may also be associated with confabulation.

Confabulation has been linked by some to lesions of the frontal lobes, and considered to result from a failure to monitor the accuracy of the report which is generated. Stuss and Benson (1984) obtained clear evidence for the link between confabulation and frontal pathology, whether the confabulation was severe and fantastic or only present in a milder form elicited by prompts given by the examiner. In their study, the extent of confabulation did not correlate with the severity of the associated memory disturbance, but did relate to the ability to self-correct.

While confabulation for recent events is relatively easy to identify, confabulation for more remote events may be more difficult to establish, unless the context is particularly bizarre or implausible. It is always incumbent upon the neuropsychologist accurately to verify the content of suspected confabulatory responses: bizarre reports are not necessarily inaccurate. Confabulation may also interfere with cognitive and gnostic performance during assessment, and if this is suspected the patient may be asked to undertake a verbal interference task (such as counting backwards) to assess whether performance improves under this condition. Comparisons with nonverbal response modes may also be made. It may, of course, be the case that if verbal intrusions associated with confabulation are demonstrated, then this may be the result of primary defective planning, monitoring or verbal mediation processes in the frontal lobe of which the confabulation is a secondary effect.

BIBLIOGRAPHY

Stuss, D. T., & Benson, D. F. (1984). Neuropsychological studies of the frontal lobes. *Psychological Bulletin, 95,* 3–28.

J. GRAHAM BEAUMONT

confusional state   A relatively common condition in which a disruption of the attentional *matrix* emerges as the most salient feature of the clinical picture.

The term "attention" is used to designate a family of hypothetical mechanisms for selecting the part of the stimulus space which is to capture the center of awareness while holding other distracting stimuli at bay. The overall process can be considered as a composite of two major operations: (1) A *matrix* or *state* function which regulates the information processing speed, detection efficiency, focusing power, vigilance level, resistance to interference, and signal-to-noise ratio. This component, also known as tonic attention, is generally associated with neural mechanisms in the reticular activating system. (2) A *vector* or *channel* function which regulates the direction and target of attention in any one of the behaviorally relevant spaces (e.g. extrapersonal, mnemonic, semantic, visceral, etc.). This component, also known as selective attention, is associated with more rostral elements of the neuraxis, especially the neocortex.

This *physiological* dichotomy is largely blurred at the psychological level since most attentional behaviors eventually represent an interaction between both components. Some behaviors, such as the detection of blips on a radar screen, are heavily dependent on the matrix aspect, whereas others, such as the ability to focus on one of many simultaneous conversations in the environment, would appear to place a greater premium on the vector aspect of attention.

Disturbances of the attentional matrix (as in a confusional state) are part of everyday experience. The behavior which follows a sudden awakening from sleep by an unexpected telephone call is a fairly common example. Although the individual may give the external appearance of being awake, it may be difficult to focus on the telephone conversation, to avoid distractibility, or to organize thought and speech coherently. It may even be difficult to recruit all the information necessary for proper orientation in time and space. What should have been simple actions, such as using a pen to write down a message, suddenly requires undue effort and may result in a great deal of fumbling and perhaps even a few attempts at writing with the wrong end of the pen. Finding the correct word or controlling immediate but inappropriate response tendencies may prove impossible. If such an individual were administered tests that place a premium on attention and vigilance, the performance could be quite unflattering. Such an individual can be said to be in an acute confusional state. Naturally, no medical intervention becomes necessary, since either voluntary mental effort or a few more hours of sleep will effectively reverse all these difficulties.

Acute confusional states, also known as delirium, organic psychoses, or acute organic brain syndromes, may also arise as pathological alterations of mental state, especially in patients with a wide variety of metabolic encephalopathies. It is fair to say that confusional states constitute the single most common species of mental state disturbance that most physicians and hospital-based neuropsychologists will see.

THE CLINICAL PICTURE OF CONFUSIONAL STATES

A confusional state can be defined as a change of mental state where the *most salient deficit* is a disruption of the attentional matrix. This does not mean that deficits of attention and vigilance necessarily emerge in isolation. Patients in acute confusional states may have additional cognitive and behavioral disturbances. Some of these are secondary to the attentional difficulties, while others may be independent. It is also important to realize that not all patients with attentional disturbances can automatically be described as being in a confusional state. For example, patients with the amnestic form of Alzheimer's disease commonly also have attentional difficulties. However, they cannot be said to be in a confusional state, since the salient feature is amnesia rather than inattention. It should also be stressed that while most acute confusional states occur in the context of a metabolic encephalopathy, the two conditions are not synonymous. For example, some metabolic-toxic encephalopathies may lead to paranoid, delusional, hallucinatory states, where the psychotic disturbance rather than inattention becomes the most salient feature of the clinical picture.

The central role of the attentional disorder in confusional states has been stressed in many clinical descriptions of this condition (Adams & Victor, 1974; Chedru and Geschwind, 1972; Mesulam & Geschwind, 1976). In lay usage, confusion often indicates disorientation. Many patients in confusional states are in fact also disoriented. However, this is not a necessary feature and it is possible to see patients in confusional states who maintain their orientation. It is the salience of the attentional deficit rather than the presence of disorientation which is the sine qua non for the diagnosis of a confusional state.

The clinical picture of a patient in an acute confusional state is familiar to most clinicians. There are usually no focal neurological signs of a motor or sensory nature with the possible exception of a coarse tremor, myoclonus, or asterixis. Attentional deficits arise at several levels of behavior. Vigilance is defective in intensity as well as in selectivity. Attention either wanders aimlessly or is suddenly focused with inappropriate intensity, even if for a fleeting moment, on an irrelevant stimulus which becomes the source of distractibility. Thought and skilled movement also become vulnerable to interference, impersistence, and perseveration. The patient may volunteer that "concentration" and "thinking straight" require great effort. The stream of thought loses its coherence because of frequent intrusions by competing thoughts and sensations. Skilled movement sequences, even those that are as automatic as using the telephone or eating utensils, lose their coherence and show signs of disintegration, perseveration, and impersistence.

Performance in attentional tasks such as the Digit Span, the Stroop Interference Test, and the Alternating Sequences Task is impaired (Weintraub & Mesulam, 1985). When asked to recite the months of the year in reverse order, the patient may say: "December, November, October, September ... October, November, December, January," showing the inability to withhold the more customary response tendencies. This clinical description highlights the three cardinal features of confusional states: (1) disturbance of vigilance and heightened distractibility; (2) inability to maintain a coherent stream of thought; (3) inability to carry out a sequence of goal-directed movements.

Difficulties in additional aspects of mental function are also common in confusional states. Perceptual distortions may lead to illusions and even hallucinations. The patient is often, but not always, disoriented and gives evidence for faulty memory. Mild anomia, dysgraphia, dyscalculia, and constructional deficits are common. Judgment may be faulty, insight appears blunted, and affect is quite labile, with a curious tendency for facetious witticism (Adams & Victor, 1974; Mesulam & Geschwind, 1976). Some of these deficits are probably secondary to attentional difficulties.

For example, if the patient is allowed sufficient drilling during the acquisition stage of a learning task, memory improves. Calculations that appear devastated when tested mentally may prove to be quite accurate when the patient is allowed the use of a pencil and paper. Other deficits of mental state, on the other hand (e.g. poor judgment and hallucinations), may be affected independently by the underlying pathogen. In confusional states these additional deficits are, by definition, of lesser importance than the attentional difficulties.

Some confusional states are characterized by apathy. Others, especially when related to alcohol, barbiturates, or opiate withdrawal, lead to extreme agitation. In their more severe forms, confusional states may lead to stupor and coma. This gives rise to the widely held opinion that confusional states are merely disorders of wakefulness and arousal. However, in the early stages of most confusional states attention and vigilance are impaired out of proportion to the drowsiness, suggesting that the mechanisms of wakefulness and attention need not overlap completely. One other characteristic feature of confusional states is the rapid fluctuation of mental state that may occur from one hour to the next, and the rather typical nocturnal exacerbation. The clinical picture of confusional states would easily lend itself to staging.

CAUSES AND MECHANISMS

The causes of confusional states can be divided into five major groups: (1) toxic–metabolic encephalopathies; (2) multifocal brain lesions; (3) head trauma; (4) seizures; (5) space-occupying processes; (6) focal brain lesions.

Confusional states are most commonly caused by *toxic-metabolic encephalopathies*. The adequate function of the central nervous system depends on the metabolic integrity of its constituent neurons and glia. Any condition which interferes with the nutritional requirements, acid–base balance, or electrolyte environment of these cells could interfere with nervous function. It is therefore not surprising that metabolic disturbances ranging from renal insufficiency to hepatic failure, anemia, endocrinopathies, hyperglycemia, anoxia, acidosis, alkalosis, etc. may each cause an encephalopathy. Withdrawal from alcohol, barbiturates, or opiates, as well as the intake of various psychoactive drugs including analgesics, hypnotics, sedatives, tranquillizers, neuroleptics, antidepressants, and even antihypertensives can also cause a toxic encephalopathy.

In some of the toxic and metabolic encephalopathies the common denominator appears to be an interference with neurotransmitter action (Faraj et al., 1976). Toxins and drugs which interfere with cholinergic transmission are particularly apt to produce confusional states. A variety of medications including neuroleptics, antidepressants and antihistamines also have marked anticholinergic activity. Since many elderly, psychiatric, or depressed patients receive combined treatment with antidepressants and neuroleptics, and since anticholinergic drugs may be added to the regimen to prevent the extrapyramidal effects of neuroleptics, it is easy to see how such patients may be subjected to considerable anticholinergic effects. In the setting of a surgical service of a general hospital, Tune et al. (1981) found that 7 of 8 patients who developed a post-operative confusional state had serum anticholinesterase activity higher than 1.5 picomolar atropine equivalents, whereas only 4 of the 17 patients who were not in a confusional state had levels in that range. Interference with central cholinergic pathways may therefore represent a major mechanism for the emergence of confusional states.

Multifocal brain diseases such as those seen in degenerative abiotrophies (e.g. Alzheimer's disease), meningitis, encephalitis (e.g. with the Human Immunodeficiency Virus in AIDS), anoxia, vasculitis, disseminated intravascular coagulation (Collins et al., 1975), and fat embolism (Dines et al., 1975) can result in confusional states, especially in the acute period. These conditions are characterized by a myriad of small lesions spread throughout the brain. A confusional state may be seen in relation to *head trauma* either as part of a concussion syndrome or even as a fixed and chronic sequel. *Epileptic* patients may develop confusional states either post-ictally or in the course of complex partial seizures (Markand et al., 1978). *Space-occupying lesions*, especially subdural hematoma, may present as a confusional state. Finally, there are a number of *focal lesions*, usually acquired as part of a cerebrovascular accident, which can also result in confusional states. These include unilateral lesions in the parahippocampal-fusiform-lingual gyri on either side of the brain and infarcts of posterior parietal and inferior prefrontal regions in the right hemisphere (Horenstein et al., 1967; Medina et al., 1974; Mesulam et al., 1976).

It is remarkable that so many different processes could lead to a similar clinical picture. In the case of seizures and head trauma, it is likely that the attentional difficulty results from a structural or electrical interference with ascending reticular pathways. A similar mechanism may well account for confusional states in subdural hematoma where the supratentorial mass effect may result in brain-stem compression. The question could be asked why there should be such a predilection for attentional disturbances in metabolic-toxic-multifocal brain diseases, in contrast, for example, to the relative rarity of salient aphasic and amnestic syndromes in this group of conditions. Perhaps attention has the least "safety factor" so that it emerges as the most salient cognitive difficulty whenever there is widespread disease of the nervous system. In other words, inattention could be the characteristic outcome of MINIMAL BRAIN DYSFUNCTION so long as this dysfunction is multifocal.

While the relationship between confusional states and metabolic-toxic-multifocal conditions implies that attention might be a widely distributed function, the cases of confusional states which follow focal infarctions suggest the presence of anatomical specialization for attentional processes, even at the level of the neocortical mantle. For example, lesions in the high-order (heteromodal) association cortex of the right frontal or parietal lobes can give rise to confusional states which may sometimes be indistinguishable from those that arise in the course of metabolic-toxic-encephalopathy (Mesulam et al., 1976). Even the toxic-metabolic encephalopathies may be affecting the brain quite selectively. For example, alcohol as well as anesthetic agents have their greatest depressant effect on the reticular formation and on high-order association cortex (Hyvarinen et al., 1978; Perrin et al., 1974).

One feature common to high-order association cortex as well as to the reticular formation is that each stands at the end of a polysynaptic chain of information processing. This may explain why functions such as attention, which depend on the most polysynaptic chains of information processing, are most vulnerable to toxic-metabolic encephalopathy. It may initially seem that this explanation cannot apply to the case of multifocal brain disease where the lesions are randomly distributed. However, one could argue that long polysynaptic chains of neurons are likely to experience a greater cumulative effect of randomly distributed lesions. Thus, randomly distributed brain disease as well as toxic-metabolic encephalopathies could both selectively influence the physiological function of high-order association areas. This explanation reconciles the apparent disparity of having focal infarcts in high-order association areas give rise to clinical deficits which are similar to those seen after toxic-metabolic encephalopathies and multifocal brain involvement.

BIOLOGY OF THE ATTENTIONAL MATRIX

Approximately a hundred years ago, Ferrier in 1880 and then Bianchi in 1895 observed that bilateral frontal lobe lesions in rhesus monkeys severely impaired attentiveness and curiosity. These reports generated considerable interest in the relationship between the cerebral cortex and the process of attention. However, the work of Dempsey and Morison (1942) on the recruiting response, and that of Moruzzi and Magoun (1949) on EEG desynchronization rapidly shifted the emphasis to the brain stem. Although vestiges of such subcortical theories of attention can occasionally be detected in the contemporary literature, there is now an emerging sense that neocortex, basal forebrain, thalamus, brain stem, and ascending cholinergic and monoaminergic pathways are all collectively involved in the modulation of the attentional matrix.

The pedunculopontine and laterodorsal tegmental nuclei of the rostral brain stem provide the principal cholinergic innervation for thalamic nuclei (Mesulam et al., 1983). The basal forebrain, on the other hand, contains the neurons which provide the major cholinergic input for the entire cerebral cortex. Acetylcholine acts as a neuromodulator which makes neurons more responsive to depolarizing inputs (Krnjevic, 1981). The ascending cholinergic pathways which originate in the brain stem and basal forebrain may thus provide a mechanism for modulating the excitability of the thalamus and cerebral cortex in a way that can influence the overall information processing capacity of the nervous system.

The rostral brain stem also provides noradrenergic and serotonergic innervation to the cortex and thalamus. The serotonergic pathways originate from the raphé nuclei. The nora-drenergic pathway originates from the nucleus locus coeruleus. The suggestion has been made that noradrenalin increases the postsynaptic evoked response relative to spontaneous activity, thus enhancing the signal-to-noise ratio in neural transmission (Morrison & Magistretti, 1983). Agents which increase central noradrenergic activity, such as dextroamphetamine and methylphenidate, have been shown to enhance attentiveness in cognitive tasks (Rapoport et al., 1978). In animals, the interruption of the noradrenergic pathways from the nucleus locus coeruleus to the neocortex impairs the ability to ignore irrelevant stimuli, thus increasing distractibility (Mason & Fibiger, 1979).

Unimodal association areas and even primary sensory areas participate in modality-specific attentional processes. The more generalized and complex aspects of attention, however, are coordinated at the level of heteromodal (polymodal) association cortex (Mesulam, 1981; Mesulam et al., 1976). Heteromodal association areas are regions which are not devoted to any single modality and which receive convergent input not only from several sensory association regions but also from limbic-paralimbic areas (Mesulam, 1985). These heteromodal areas are sensitive to the more abstract components of incoming information and also to its motivational relevance. There are at least three heteromodal association fields in the primate brain: the prefrontal cortex, the posterior parietal cortex, and the ventral temporal lobe (Mesulam et al., 1977; Seltzer & Pandya, 1976). It is interesting that acute infarcts, even when unilateral, in any one of these three heteromodal fields (but not elsewhere) give rise to generalized attentional deficits in the form of confusional states (Horenstein et al., 1967; Medina et al., 1974; Mesulam et al., 1976). In the case of the prefrontal and posterior parietal heteromodal fields, the confusional state almost always occurs after right-sided lesions, raising the possibility of a right hemisphere dominance for neural mechanisms that regulate the attentional matrix.

The prefrontal cortex is a heteromodal cortical region intimately related to the maintenance of the attentional matrix. In a series of experiments based on determinations of regional cerebral blood flow, subjects were given pairs of auditory, visual, and somatosensory stimuli (Roland, 1982). The subjects were simultaneously exposed to all three modalities in each trial, even though they were asked to ignore two of the channels while making a difficult sensory discrimination in only one of the modalities. Three conclusions emerged. First, the primary and unimodal areas for an individual channel were activated even in trials where information from that modality was to be ignored. Second, the activation in the modality-specific (primary and unimodal) cortical areas for the channel in which the discrimination was being made was greater than in the other modality-specific areas. Third, a part of the prefrontal heteromodal cortex showed preferential activation during these trimodal attention tasks, regardless of the modality in which the discrimination was being made. These observations show that attentional filtering occurs at a quite advanced stage of information processing, since unimodal areas in the unattended modalities continue to be active. This undoubtedly introduces much greater flexibility than if sensory influx were to be barred at a more peripheral level. Furthermore, there appears to be a region in the superomesial prefrontal cortex which may be essential for the differential tuning of the attentional matrix across the entire multimodal sensorial space (Roland, 1982).

Several additional lines of evidence highlight the importance of the frontal lobe to attention. Two attention-related components of the evoked potential, the P300 and the contingent negative variation, are closely related to frontal lobe mechanisms. The contingent negative variation is a surface negative potential which may reflect the readiness that a task-related warning stimulus elicits, and is most readily recorded over the frontal cortex (Boyd et al., 1982; Cohen, 1971; Rohrbaugh et al., 1976). Furthermore, the P300 component which is elicited in response to novel stimuli is markedly attenuated in patients with frontal lesions. These observations suggest that the frontal lobe may play a major role in attending to complex and novel stimuli. In keeping with these aspects of frontal lobe function, patients with lesions in the prefrontal cortex commonly show deficits in many tests sensitive to disruptions of the matrix. In fact, some species of the frontal lobe syndrome fit the description of a confusional state.

CONCLUSION

The attentional matrix is controlled by a large-scale distributed network whose major components include the brain-stem reticular formation, the basal forebrain, thalamic nuclei, and high-order association cortex, especially in the frontal lobes. Disease processes that interfere with the function of one or more components of this network cause a perturbation of the attentional tone (Mesulam, 1990). The diagnosis of confusional state is made when such a disruption leads to the clinical presentation of the patient. Patients with confusional states offer unique opportunities for investigating the cognitive and biological properties of attentional processes.

BIBLIOGRAPHY

Adams, R. D. & Victor, M. (1974). *Delirium and other confusional states*. In M. M. Wintrobe, G. W. Thorn, R. D. Adams, E. Braunwald, K. J. Isselbacher, & R. G. Petersdorf (Eds), *Principles of internal medicine* (pp. 149–56). New York: McGraw-Hill.

Boyd, E. H., Boyd, E. S., & Brown, L. E. (1982). Precentral cortex unit activity during the M-wave and contingent negative variation in behaving squirrel monkeys. *Experimental Neurology*, *75*, 535–54.

Chedru, F., & Geschwind, N. (1972). Disorders of higher cortical functions in acute confusional states. *Cortex*, *8*, 395–411.

Cohen, J. (1971). The contingent negative variation in visual attention. *EEG Clinical Neurophysiology*, *31*, 287–305.

Collins, R. C., Al-Monddhiry, H., Chernik, N. L., & Posner, J. B. (1975). Neurological manifestations of intravascular coagulation in patients with cancer. *Neurology*, *25*, 795–806.

Dines, D. E., Burgher, L. W., & Okazaki, H. (1975). The clinical and pathological correlation of fat embolism syndrome. *Mayo Clinic Proceedings*, *50*, 407–11.

Faraj, B. A., Bowen, P. A., Isaacs, J. W., & Rudman, D. (1976). Hypertyraminemia in cirrhotic patients. *New England Journal of Medicine*, *294*, 1360–4.

Horenstein, S. Chamberlin, W., & Conomy, J. (1967). Infarction of the fusiform and calcarine regions: agitated delirium and hemianopia. *Transactions of the American Neurology Association*, *92*, 85–9.

Hyvarinen, J., Laakso, M., Roine, R., Leinonen, L., & Sippel, H. (1978). Effect of ethanol on neuronal activity in the parietal association cortex of alert monkeys. *Brain*, *101*, 701–15.

Krnjevic, K. (1981). Cellular mechanisms of cholinergic arousal. *Behavioral Brain Science*, *4*, 484–5.

Markand, O. N., Wheeler, G. L., & Pollack, S. L. (1978). Complex partial status epilecticus (psychomotor status). *Neurology*, *28*, 189–96.

Mason, S. T., & Fibiger, H. C. (1979). Noradrenaline and selective attention. *Life Science*, *25*, 1949–56.

Medina, J. L., Rubino, F. A., & Ross, A. (1974). Agitated delirium caused by infarction of the hippocampal formation and fusiform and lingual gyri: a case report. *Neurology*, *24*, 1181–3.

Mesulam, M.-M. (1981). A cortical network for directed attention and unilateral neglect. *Annals of Neurology*, *10*, 309–25.

Mesulam, M.-M. (1985). Patterns in behavioral neuroanatomy. In M.-M. Mesulam (Ed.), *Principles of behavioral neurology (Contemporary Neurology Series)*, (pp. 1–70). Philadelphia: F. A. Davis.

Mesulam, M.-M. (1990). Large-scale neurocognitive network for distributed processing for attention, language and memory. *Annals of Neurology*, *28*, 597–613.

Mesulam, M.-M., & Geschwind, N. (1976). Disordered mental states in the post-operative period. *Urological Clinics of North America*, *3*, 199–216.

Mesulam, M.-M., Mufson, E. J., Wainer, B. H., & Levey A. I. (1983). Central cholinergic pathways in the rat: an overview based on an alternative nomenclature (Chl–Ch6). *Neuroscience*, *10*, 1185–201.

Mesulam, M.-M., Van Hoesen, G. W., Pandya, D. N., & Geschwind, N. (1977). Limbic and sensory connections of the inferior parietal lobule (area PG) in the rhesus monkey: a study with a new method for horseradish peroxidase histochemistry. *Brain Research*, *136*, 393–414.

Mesulam, M.-M., Waxman, S. G., Geschwind, N., & Sabin, T. D. (1976). Acute confusional states with right middle cerebral artery infarctions. *Journal of Neurology, Neurosurgery and Psychiatry*, *39*, 84–9.

Morrison, J. H., & Magistretti, P. J. (1983). Monamines and peptides in cerebral cortex. *Trends in Neuroscience*, *6*, 146–51.

Perrin, R. G., Hockman, C. H., Kalant, H., & Livingston, K. E. (1974). Acute effects of ethanol on spontaneous and auditory evoked electrical activity in cat brain. *EEG Clinical Neurophysiology*, *36*, 19–31.

Rapoport, J. L., Buchsbaum, M. S., Zahn, T. P., Weingartner, H., Ludlow, C., & Mikkelsen, E. J. (1978). Dextroamphetamine: cognitive and behavioral effects in normal prepubertal boys. *Science*, *199*, 560–3.

Rohrbaugh, J. W., Syndulko, K., & Lindsley, D. B. (1976). Brain wave components of the contingent negative variation in humans. *Science*, *191*, 1055–7.

Roland, P. E. (1982). Cortical regulation of selective attention in man. A regional cerebral blood flow study. *Journal of Neurophysiology*, *48*, 1059–78.

Seltzer, B., & Pandya, D. N. (1976). Some cortical projections to the hippocampal area in the rhesus monkey. *Experimental Neurology*, *50*, 146–60.

Tune, L. E., Damlouji, N. F., Holland, A., Gardner, T. J., Folstein, M. F., & Coyle, J. T. (1981). Association of postoperative delirium with raised serum levels of anticholinergic drugs. *Lancet*, Sept. 26, 651–3.

Weintraub, S., & Mesulam, M.-M. (1985). The examination of mental state. In M.-M. Mesulam (Ed.), *Principles of behavioral neurology (Contemporary Neurology Series)*, (pp. 71–123). Philadelphia: F. A. Davis.

M.-MARSEL MESULAM

congenital disorders "Congenital disorder" is a term used to classify an extremely wide variety of abnormalities in the structure or function of bodily parts or systems that are present at or from birth. In general, the term presupposes that the disorder in question developed during the prenatal phase of development and was evident at birth. Two related terms, *congenital anomaly* and *congenital malformation*, typically refer to aberrations, whether major or minor, in the structure of a body part (e.g. more than five fingers on a hand). When the term "congenital disorder" is used, however, it usually implies a functional impairment as opposed to a structural abnormality alone. Any organ, bodily structure, or system can be affected by a congenital disorder.

In some cases, it may be postulated that the cause of a disorder originated in the prenatal phase of development, even if the problem was not manifest at birth. In such cases, the term "congenital disorders" can be applied, it being assumed that the dysfunction was present at birth but was not detected until later in development, when the functioning of that organ or system became impaired.

The causes of some congenital disorders are well known. The basis for dysfunction may be related to chromosomal abnormalities, an inborn error of metabolism, maternal infections during pregnancy, or maternal substance abuse during that time. The causes of other congenital disorders are less well understood. There may be no significant family history of disease or impairment and no known complications of pregnancy or delivery.

Given the wide variety of conditions classified as congenital disorders, it is clearly not possible to discuss the entire range. The specific disorders reviewed in this entry have been selected, based on their frequency in the population, clinical severity, and particular relevance to the area of neuropsychology or psychiatry. This entry serves to highlight the main clinical features of each disorder and to outline the associated neuropsychological sequelae. For a more detailed review of congenital disorders, the reader is referred to Jones (1988).

CHROMOSOMAL ABNORMALITIES AND INHERITED DISORDERS

Several congenital disorders arise as a result of chromosomal abnormalities. To help in understanding the nature of their specific problems, a very basic overview of human genetics is presented below. Humans have 23 pairs of chromosomes; of these, 22 pairs are autosomes and are possessed equally by males and females. The other pair, being comprised of the sex chromosomes, are different in males and females: males have an X and Y pair of sex chromosomes (XY), whereas females have a pair of X sex chromosomes (XX). Twenty-three single chromosomes are inherited from each parent to form the 23 pairs of chromosomes in an offspring. The chromosomes contain the genetic material that dictates both hereditary transmission and individual development. The term "genotype" is used to describe the chromosomal make-up of an individual. The manner in which the genotype is expressed in observable or quantifiable characteristics is referred to as the "phenotype" of an individual. Chromosomal abnormalities can

occur in either the autosomes or the sex chromosomes. The abnormalities can arise from the partial or entire deletion of a chromosome, from the addition of an extra chromosome, or via "mosaicism," which occurs when there is a combination of normal and abnormal chromosomal material. When a chromosomal abnormality is transmitted on one of the sex chromosomes, it is considered a "sex-linked" abnormality.

In some cases, only a single gene or set of genes may be affected rather than the entire chromosome. The term "gene locus" refers to the location or position of a particular gene on a chromosome. At each gene locus, the actual genes can be present in two different forms, one of which is inherited from the mother and one from the father. These two different forms are called "alleles." In some cases, both alleles will be the same, in which case the person is considered to be homozygous for that gene. However, if the alleles inherited from each parent are different at that location, the person is considered to be heterozygous for that gene. The phenotypes of certain characteristics, such as eye color, are determined by a single gene (i.e. one pair of alleles). In such cases, when an individual is heterozygous for that gene, the phenotypic expression may vary if one allele is "dominant" over the other "recessive" allele.

The term "sex-linked recessive characteristic" refers to the fact that some characteristics, which are coded from genetic information carried on an X sex chromosome, are recessive. Females are less likely to express a recessive sex-linked characteristic because they have another X chromosome which may contain the dominant allele. A sex-linked recessive characteristic will only be expressed in a female if she inherits the recessive allele from both her mother and her father. In contrast, males will always phenotypically express a recessive, sex-linked characteristic because they only inherit one X chromosome. Their other sex chromosome (Y) may not contain an allele for that particular characteristic. Hemophilia, a congenital hereditary disorder of blood coagulation, is an example of a disorder that is transmitted by an X-linked recessive trait by a female carrier to her male child.

Down's syndrome (DS) is a congenital disorder caused by a chromosomal abnormality in which the twenty-first pair of chromosomes in an affected individual contains an extra third chromosome, or part of a third chromosome. It is one of the leading causes of mental retardation (MR), the severity of which varies considerably across individuals. Phenotypically, DS is characterized by specific physical and cognitive attributes. Affected individuals generally exhibit hypotonicity, slanting eyes with epicanthal eye folds, large tongues, fine hair, and possible growth failure. These children are at increased risk of exhibiting congenital heart defects and intestinal stenosis (i.e. blockage). The incidence of acute leukemia is also increased in these individuals. Early, prenatal detection of DS is possible through amniocentesis, a procedure which involves obtaining a sample of amniotic fluid for chromosomal analysis. The risk of DS is positively correlated with maternal age, although the reason for this association is not clear.

Cognitively, infants with DS may appear developmentally normal at birth and through the initial six months of life. After this period, there may be a deceleration in the rate of cognitive development, eventually resulting in MR. There is a wide variation in the level of cognitive impairment, but no well-established characteristic neuropsychological profile. Environmental factors have also been seen to impact severely on cognitive outcome. With regard to behavioral development, children with DS have been rated by their parents as exhibiting more behavioral problems, especially attentional difficulties, as compared to their unaffected siblings (Cuskelly & Dadds, 1992).

The risk of developing Alzheimer's disease as affected individuals reach their forties and fifties is substantially higher than in the general population. Haxby (1989), in a study of 29 young (< 35 years old) and old (> 35 years old) adults with DS found that all were developing neuropathological changes associated with Alzheimer's disease, yet only a small percentage (n = 4) were exhibiting clinically significant dementia. Those who evidenced dementia exhibited global deficits in all areas of functioning except simple language, whereas older, nondemented DS adults were deficient compared to younger DS adults in the areas of visuospatial construction and long-term memory. Carr (1994) provides an excellent review of long-term outcome associated with DS.

Turner's syndrome (TS) is a congenital disorder arising from an abnormality of the X sex chromosome. Females who are affected with TS are lacking some or all of the second X chromosome (XO rather than XX as in the normal female). The condition affects approximately 1 in 3,000 female births, but is not associated with mental retardation. Physically, the disorder is associated with infertility and other congenital malformations, including short stature, webbed neck, and short fingers. In adolescence, affected individuals do not develop secondary sex characteristics unless treated with female hormones. Turner's syndrome provides a unique opportunity to investigate the impact of hormonal influences on brain development and function, as affected individuals are not endogenously exposed to sex hormones.

Cognitive abilities in TS appear to vary according to the severity of the chromosomal abnormality. An estimated 50–55 percent of individuals with TS have total deletion of the second X chromosome (XO), whereas the rest exhibit only partial deletion or mosaicism. Overall, verbal abilities tend to be in the average range. Specific vulnerabilities are noted on visual-perceptual tasks and numerical reasoning (Rovet, 1993).

The deficits in performance skills as compared to verbal abilities led some investigators to hypothesize that the deficits may be lateralized in the right hemisphere. In a study designed to test this hypothesis, Pennington and others (1985) compared women with TS to three different groups of brain-injured women (those with right, left, or diffuse lesions). Lateralization of deficits associated with TS was not demonstrated in this study. The pattern of mild neuropsychological impairments noted in the women with TS was most similar to the women with diffuse, as opposed to right hemisphere, brain damage (Pennington et al., 1985).

Discrepancies between verbal and performance scale scores on the Wechsler IQ tests have been noted to range from 8 to 20 points. The cognitive deficits seen in individuals with total deletion are generally more severe than in those with partial deletions. In a cross-sectional study of pre-adolescent and adolescent girls with Turner's syndrome, Swillen and colleagues (1993) found that hormonal therapy was associated with improved visuospatial abilities.

Fragile X syndrome, which occurs much more frequently in males than females, is another example of a sex chromosome abnormality. It is a leading cause of mental retardation (MR). There is considerable variability in the phenotypic expression of fragile X syndrome, with many affected individuals manifesting autistic-type behaviors. Not all individuals who exhibit a fragile-X syndrome genotypically will express the characteristics phenotypically.

It is estimated that approximately 10 percent of boys with severe MR (i.e IQ > 40) have fragile X syndrome. In a recent, comprehensive review of the literature, Turk (1992) highlighted the wide variability in the level of cognitive functioning observed in these individuals. However, most studies found that performance skills are more affected than verbal abilities, and there may be a gradual deterioration in cognitive abilities, with intellectual functioning reaching a plateau in late childhood. Delays in speech and language abilities are common. There appears to be a link between fragile X syndrome and AUTISM, though there is no consensus regarding the percentage of autism cases caused by the fragile X syndrome.

Klinefelter's syndrome is another example of a congenital disorder involving the sex chromosomes. It affects only males and is characterized by an extra X chromosome (XXY rather than XY in normal males). In their review of the literature, Flint and Yule (1994) found that Klinefelter's syndrome is not associated with deficits in general intellectual functioning. However, a higher incidence of language difficulties has been noted, the specificity of which has not been consistently demonstrated.

INBORN ERRORS OF METABOLISM

Inborn errors of metabolism are examples of inherited disorders in which the body is unable to metabolize certain proteins or compounds present in normal diets as a result of an enzyme deficiency. There are many different types of metabolic disorders, most of which have profound neurological and neuropsychological consequences if left untreated. The symptoms of some inborn errors of metabolism are not manifest at birth and are not detected phenotypically until developmental delay or neurological damage have already occurred. Newborn screening programs have been developed to identify cases early and thus prevent irreversible neurological impairment. The inborn errors of metabolism commonly identified through newborn screening programs include phenylketonuria, galactosemia, congenital hypothyroidism, homocystinuria,

maple syrup urine disease, and biotinidase deficiency. Only three disorders are presented in this entry.

Phenylketonuria (PKU) is an autosomal, recessive, inborn error of phenylalanine (Phe) metabolism involving a deficiency of the enzyme phenylalanine hydroxylase. PKU affects about 1 in 14,000 live births and is much more prevalent in Caucasians than in African Americans or Asians. As a result of the enzyme deficiency, Phe, a protein present in many foods, cannot be metabolized into tyrosine. Subsequently, the levels of Phe, and its organic metabolites, become elevated. Children who are born with PKU will appear developmentally normal at birth. However, if left untreated, the chronically elevated levels of Phe will result in severe mental retardation and other neurological sequelae at about 6 months of age. Fortunately, the consequences of PKU can be prevented through early identification via newborn screening programs, and through prompt implementation of treatment.

The goal of treatment for PKU is to decrease the level of Phe in the body through dietary reduction of foods containing Phe. Unlike treatment for other inborn errors of metabolism (e.g. biotinidase deficiency), in which the primary enzyme deficiency can be targeted directly, the defect in phenylalanine hydroxylase cannot be altered. Rather, the treatment of PKU serves to correct the secondary and tertiary metabolic abnormalities caused by the enzyme deficiency. Although early identification and treatment will prevent severe mental retardation, those children receiving treatment at an early stage are still at risk of developing specific cognitive, academic, and behavior difficulties.

Cognitive functioning of children with early-treated PKU is related to the quality of their dietary treatment and subsequent metabolic control. Compared to age- and IQ-matched controls, even these children with early-treated PKU demonstrate relative weaknesses on tests of executive functioning – specifically tasks that assess verbal fluency, planning, and visual search skills (Walsh et al., 1990). Performance on executive functioning tasks has been associated with average lifetime metabolic control and blood Phe level at the time of testing. Deficits in sustained attention have been observed and appear to be influenced by current Phe levels as well (De Sonneville et al., 1989). Other neuropsychological impairments associated with early-treated PKU include expressive language difficulties, slower reaction times, and increased frequency of visual EVOKED POTENTIAL abnormalities. An increase in the prevalence of behavioral problems, especially HYPERACTIVITY, has also been noted.

Studies of adults with early-treated PKU suggest that performance on certain neuropsychological tests, such as those requiring problem-solving or sustained attention, is associated with current Phe levels. General intellectual functioning, on the other hand, while related to lifetime Phe levels, is particularly dependent on metabolic control during the first few years of life (see Ris et al., 1994). These findings would suggest optimal neuropsychological functioning is best obtained by continuation of treatment into adulthood (*see also* PHENYLKETONURIA).

Galactosemia is an inborn error of metabolism, typically caused by a deficiency in the enzyme galactose-1-phosphate uridyltransferase, which prevents the body from metabolizing galactose (a derivative of the lactose in milk) into glucose. Early identification through newborn screening programs is extremely critical; life-threatening illness will develop quickly in an affected newborn after the ingestion of milk. If left untreated, the consequences of galactosemia include hepatomegaly (enlargement of the liver), cataracts, severe growth retardation, and mental retardation. Although treatment, which includes a lactose-free diet, can prevent the severe neurological consequences, even early-treated children with galactosemia are at risk for speech and language deficits and visual-perceptual problems. Although receptive language skills appear to remain relatively intact, articulation, expressive language, and word retrieval are areas of vulnerability (Waisbren et al., 1983). In their study of 24 individuals with treated galactosemia, Nelson and colleagues (1991) found that over half (54 percent) exhibited verbal DYSPRAXIA. Areas of academic difficulty include arithmetic and handwriting.

Congenital hypothyroidism (CH), also known as "cretinism," is included under the category of an inborn error of metabolism, but can also occur as the result of a defect in the thyroid gland, hypothalamus, or pituitary gland.

Screening for CH is included in many newborn screening programs and treatment consists of thyroid hormone supplementation. If left un-

treated, the condition will result in mental and growth retardation. Cognitive abilities in individuals with early-treated CH tend to be in the average range, but slightly below that of their healthy siblings or peers. In general, affected children who are identified and treated early develop normally during the first two years of life. However, by the age of 3 years, children with CH, compared to their peers (matched for age, sex, and social class), are at risk for developing problems with quantitative abilities and on tasks requiring quick motor responses (Murphy et al., 1990). Language deficits have also been observed. Visual-spatial difficulties are often observed by the age of 5 years. There is a relationship between severity of the CH and cognitive outcome, although this association may not always be detected in the early years of life. It is not clear, however, whether the specific problems observed in early childhood persist as the child develops. A follow-up study of school-age children with CH did not find evidence for specific, residual learning difficulties associated with CH (New England Congenital Hypothyroidism Collaborative, 1990).

DEVELOPMENTAL DISORDERS

The term developmental disorder is used to classify a range of conditions in which the primary problems lie in the acquisition of cognitive, language, social, or motor abilities. Mental retardation, autism, and learning disorders are included in the category of "developmental disorders." Some developmental disorders involve a global delay in skill acquisition, such as mental retardation, whereas others involve a delay in only a very specific area of functioning, such as expressive language ability. Some developmental disorders involve a delay in a cluster of specific skills, as in autism, where there is a marked disturbance in communication skills, reciprocal social interaction, and a restricted repertoire of interests.

Only one developmental disorder, Rett's disorder, has been selected for review in this entry. However, the reader is referred to Lord and Rutter (1994) for a comprehensive review in the area of autism and to Bishop (1994) for an overview of communication disorders.

Rett's disorder is a recently recognized problem of unknown etiology that affects only girls. Though first described in the literature in the

1960s, the disorder did not become well-recognized until more recently, when Hagberg and others (1983) published a review of 35 cases who exhibited similar forms of encephalopathy. Children affected with Rett's disorder experience normal development until 7 to 18 months of age. After this time, a delay in the development of gross motor skills is typically noted, followed by a progressive deterioration in those motor skills already acquired (e.g. loss of ability to crawl) plus other higher cortical functions. Loss of purposeful hand movements, jerky truncal ATAXIA, abnormal breathing patterns and deceleration of head growth, resulting in MICROCEPHALY, become evident.

Stereotyped hand movements may develop, resembling hand-washing or hand-wringing. The progressive encephalopathy results in severe mental retardation, accompanied by deficits in expressive and receptive language, and eventually results in dementia. Seizures and spasticity may also develop in the later stages. Four clinical stages have been identified. The syndrome appears to affect 1 in approximately 15,000 live female births.

STRUCTURAL DISORDERS

As noted earlier, some congenital disorders arise as the result of a structural defect that impacts the function of a given organ or body system.

Agenesis of the corpus callosum is one example of a structural congenital disorder. The term "agenesis" means failure to develop. Affected individuals are born without a CORPUS CALLOSUM. The term "partial agenesis" describes a condition in which only a portion of the corpus callosum is missing. This disorder is particularly significant for neuropsychology, as it provides an unusual opportunity to explore the role of the corpus callosum in interhemispheric function and general cognitive development in a naturally occurring condition. Consequences of this disorder can be compared to the cognitive outcomes in cases of surgical removal of the corpus callosum (i.e. COMMISSUROTOMY).

Children with CALLOSAL AGENESIS have been noted to exhibit difficulties with the discrimination of phonemes and perform poorly on tasks that place a high demand on rhyming skills (Temple et al., 1989). Some researchers have argued that problems in phonemic discrimination and other phonological processing skills represent the fundamental deficits in developmental DYSLEXIA. Temple, Jeeves, and Vilarroya (1990) suggest that the development of phonological reading skills (i.e. learning to read by sounding out the phonemes that comprise a word) may be at risk in children with agenesis of the corpus callosum, despite average vocabulary skills.

Spina bifida is another example of a structural disorder. It is the most frequently occurring structural defect involving the central nervous system and arises as the result of a malformation of the spinal column caused by the incomplete closure of one or more vertebrae. Spina bifida occurs in approximately 1 in 1,000 live births. It is often associated with HYDROCEPHALUS, a condition in which a large volume of CEREBROSPINAL FLUID (CSF) collects within the skull as the result of obstruction of one of the normal routes through which CSF travels. The physical and cognitive outcome of spina bifida depends on the level of the lesion. Affected individuals can experience paralysis below the level of the lesion (including neurogenic incontinence). When hydrocephalus occurs in conjunction with spina bifida, attentional problems and language deficits, specifically difficulties in comprehension of abstract language and the production of irrelevant speech, have been observed.

In a follow-up of cases into young adulthood, Hunt (1990) found a range of impairments. Out of 117 cases enrolled in the study at birth, 69 survived to the age of 16 years. Of these survivors, the majority (n = 47) had an IQ in the normal range; a smaller percentage (n = 12) had IQ scores in the 60–79 range. Cognitive abilities were associated with level of sensory impairment.

MATERNAL INFECTIONS AND SUBSTANCE ABUSE

Certain congenital disorders can arise as the result of a mother's health status or behavior during pregnancy. Infections during pregnancy, including venereal disease, as well as the ingestion of certain substances during that time, can serve to introduce teratogenic agents into the uterine environment which can have a harmful impact on the developing fetus. Only a few infections are reviewed in this entry, with maternal alcohol abuse being discussed to illustrate the potential damage that can occur during the prenatal phase of development. In most cases, the type and degree of the damage caused to the fetus is associated with the time at which the teratogen is introduced into the uterine environment. Those systems and structures which are undergoing the most rapid stages of development at the time of exposure are the most vulnerable. The central nervous system is most at risk during the later stages of pregnancy and into the first few years of life.

Maternal infections

Congenital herpes is a condition in which an infant contracts the herpes simplex virus from its mother. Transmission of the virus from an infected mother to her offspring generally occurs during delivery, rather than during pregnancy. The risk of transmission of the herpes virus from mother to child can be reduced if the child is delivered by Cesarean section, particularly if the mother has an infection at the time of the birth. Congenital herpes can be fatal to the newborn or can result in encephalitis and subsequent mental retardation (MR), as well as damage to the eyes (including blindness) and other skin and oral infections (*see also* ENCEPHALITIS). *Congenital cytomegalovirus* (CMV), another form of herpes virus, is a major cause of congenital impairment, including MR and deafness.

Congenital human immunodeficiency virus (HIV), can be transmitted prenatally or perinatally from an infected woman to her unborn child. Encephalopathy and loss of previously acquired developmental milestones are part of the clinical course. Three stages of disease progression have been identified. The reader is referred to Thompson and others (1994) for an extensive and recent review of this area (*see also* AIDS).

Congenital rubella syndrome is an example of a congenital disorder that can arise if a woman contracts rubella during pregnancy. It may result in the death of an unborn fetus. Premature delivery, as well as several congenital defects, including mental retardation, deafness, eye problems, and heart defects are associated with this syndrome.

Maternal substance abuse

Fetal alcohol syndrome (FAS) arises as the result of prenatal exposure to alcohol. It is associated with slow physical growth, developmental delay, and distinctive craniofacial dysmorphic features. HYPERACTIVITY and behavioral problems as-

sociated with FAS, such as sleeping and eating difficulties, have been documented as well.

CONCLUSIONS

As is evident in this general overview, the term "congenital disorder" encompasses a wide variety of conditions in which structural and functional impairments arise in the prenatal phase of development. Congenital disorders are of interest to neuropsychologists as they provide the opportunity to investigate the relationships between abnormal brain development and the resulting cognitive and behavioral impairments. Furthermore, cases of naturally occurring structural defects (e.g. agenesis of the corpus callosum) can be compared to cases in which the structural defect was produced surgically (e.g. commissurotomy). Congenital disorders also provide the opportunity to explore the role of brain–behavior relationships within a developmental context, as the nature of cognitive strengths and vulnerabilities associated with particular conditions may change as a child matures.

The cognitive deficits associated with many of the congenital disorders have been investigated. Several disorders, such as PKU and Turner's syndrome, have been shown to be associated with specific behavioral and neuropsychological profiles or phenotypes. In some disorders, the general cognitive outcome (e.g. normal versus impaired functioning) has been well established, but investigators are now becoming more aware of particular areas of cognitive strengths and vulnerabilities associated with these disorders. Information provided by neuropsychological evaluations regarding possible specific deficits related to a disorder can be invaluable to parents and teachers involved in the education of a child with that disorder. Screening and early intervention may help ameliorate long-term difficulties in cognitive, academic, or psychological functioning.

It is important to note that the term "congenital" is not synonymous with "untreatable." Although certain treatments (e.g. gene replacement therapy) are not yet available, other environmental interventions, such as dietary therapy for inborn errors of metabolism, can have a significant impact on the physical, cognitive, and behavioral outcomes of affected individuals. In these cases, in which treatment can substantially impact the consequences of a congenital disorder, whether physical or cognitive, it is imperative that clinicians and researchers consider the extent to which individuals have been exposed to and are compliant with treatment regimens. In particular, studies that focus on populations at risk for poor adherence (e.g. adolescents) should take these issues into consideration when investigating neuropsychological abilities.

In the next few years, the inclusion of magnetic resonance imaging (MRI) technology in studies of individuals affected with congenital disorders will no doubt shed additional light onto the structural and functional deficits associated with particular disorders. Those conditions in which treatment produces modifications in outcome or transient effects on functioning (e.g. hormonal therapy in Turner's syndrome, current Phe levels in PKU) provide the opportunity to gain further insight into brain–behavior relationships. The behavioral phenotyping of various congenital disorders is another area of intense investigation, as researchers attempt to establish cognitive and behavioral profiles unique to various conditions. Research in all these areas will no doubt continue to make distinctive contributions to the field of neuropsychology.

BIBLIOGRAPHY

Bishop, D. V. M. (1994). Developmental disorders of speech and language. In M. Rutter, E. Taylor, and L. Hersov (Eds.), *Child and adolescent psychiatry: Modern approaches*, 3rd edn (pp. 546–68). Oxford: Blackwell Scientific.

Carr, J. (1994). Long-term outcome for people with Down's syndrome. *Journal of Child Psychology and Psychiatry, 35*, 425–39.

Cuskelly, M., & Dadds, M. (1992). Behavioral problems in children with Down's syndrome and their siblings. *Journal of Child Psychology and Psychiatry, 33*, 749–61.

De Sonneville, L. M. J., Schmidt, E., & Michel, U. (1989). Information processing in early-treated PKU. *Journal of Clinical and Experimental Neuropsychology, 11*, 362.

Flint, J., & Yule, W. (1994). Behavioral phenotypes. In M. Rutter, E. Taylor, & L. Hersov (Eds), *Child and adolescent psychiatry: Modern approaches*, 4th edn (pp. 666–87). Oxford: Blackwell Scientific.

Hagberg, B., Aicardi, J., Dias, K., & Ramos, O. (1983). A progressive syndrome of autism, dementia, ataxia, and loss of purposeful hand use in girls: Rett's syndrome: report of 35 cases. *Annals of Neurology, 14*, 471–9.

Haxby, J. V. (1989). Neuropsychological evaluation of adults with Down's syndrome: Patterns of selective impairment in nondemented old adults. *Journal of Mental Deficiency Research, 33*, 193–210.

Hunt, G. M. (1990). Open spina bifida: outcome for a complete cohort treated unselectively and followed into adulthood. *Developmental Medicine and Child Neurology, 32*, 108–18.

Jones, K. L. (Ed.). (1988). *Smith's recognizable patterns of human malformation*, 4th edn. Philadelphia: Saunders.

Lord, C., & Rutter, R. (1994). Autism and pervasive developmental disorders. In M. Rutter, E. Taylor, & L. Hersov (Eds), *Child and adolescent psychiatry: Modern approaches*, 3rd edn (pp. 569–93). Oxford: Blackwell Scientific.

Murphy, G. H., Hulse, J. A., Smith, I., & Grant, D. B. (1990). Congenital hypothyroidism: physiological and psychological factors in early development. *Journal of Child Psychology and Psychiatry, 31*, 711–25.

Nelson, C. D., Waggoner, D. D., Donnell, G. N., Tuerck, J. M., & Buist, N. R. (1991). Verbal dyspraxia in treated galactosemia. *Pediatrics, 88*, 346–50.

New England Congenital Hypothyroidism Collaborative. (1990). Elementary school performance of children with hypothyroidism. *Journal of Pediatrics, 116*, 27–32.

Pennington, B. F., Heaton, R. K., Karzmark, P., Pendelton, M. G., Lehman, R., & Shucard, D. W. (1985). The neuropsychological phenotype in Turner syndrome. *Cortex, 21*, 391–404.

Ris, M. D., Williams, S. E., Hunt, M. M., Berry, H. K., Leslie, N. (1994). Early treated PKU: adult neuropsychologic outcome. *Journal of Pediatrics, 124*, 388–92.

Rovet, J. F. (1993). The psychoeducational characteristics of children with Turner syndrome. *Journal of Learning Disabilities, 26*, 333–41.

Rutter, M., & Casaer, P. (1991). *Biological risk factors for psychosocial disorders*. Cambridge: Cambridge University Press.

Scriver, D. R., Beaudet, A. L., Sly, W. S., & Valle, D. (Eds), *The metabolic basis of inherited disease*, 6th edn New York: McGraw-Hill.

Swillen, A., Fyrns, J. P., Kleczkowska, A., Massa, G., Vanderschueren-Lodeweyckz, M., Vanden-Berge, H. (1993). Intelligence, behaviour and psychosocial development in Turner syndrome: a cross-sectional study of 50 preadolescent and adolescent girls (4–20). *Genetic Counselling, 4,* 7–18.

Temple, C. M., Jeeves, M. A., & Vilarroya, O. (1989). Ten pen men: rhyming skills in two children with callosal agenesis. *Brain and Language, 37,* 548–64.

Temple, C. M., Jeeves, M. A., Vilarroya, O. (1990). Reading in callosal agenesis. *Brain and Language, 39,* 235–53.

Thompson, D., Westwell, P., Viney, D. (1994). Psychiatric aspects of Human Immunodeficiency Virus in childhood and adolescence. In M. Rutter, E. Taylor, & L. Hersov (Eds), *Child and adolescent psychiatry: Modern approaches,* 3rd edn (pp. 711–19). Oxford: Blackwell Scientific.

Turk, J. (1992). The fragile-X syndrome: on the way to a behavioral phenotype. *British Journal of Psychiatry, 160,* 24–35.

Waisbren, S. E., Norman, T. R., Schnell, R. R., & Levy, H. (1983). Speech and language deficits in early-treated children with galactosemia. *Journal of Pediatrics, 102,* 75–7.

Walsh, M. C., Pennington, B. F., Ozonoff, S., Rouse, B., & McCabe, E. R. B. (1990). Neuropsychology of early-treated phenylketonuria: specific executive function deficits. *Child Development, 61,* 1697–713.

J. WARNER-ROGERS

conjugate lateral eye movements   *See* LEMs.

connectionism   *See* NEUROPSYCHOLOGY.

consciousness   As our level of consciousness varies, so can the level of cognitive processing received by environmental stimuli around us, and so also can our subjective experience of awareness. When we are aware of something – of an event in the world detected by our senses, or a memory of a past event – that event can be said to be represented in our conscious mind. Other events may be processed and even gain responses without our being aware of them: these events have received *preconscious processing.* Memories of past events belong to the unconscious mind until the very moment when we become aware of them. Observers have no direct access to the level of consciousness currently being experienced by another person, and must rely upon what the other person reports as their current awareness, and upon performance measures. Changes in our ability to give responses to new stimuli provide an indirect measure of the level of consciousness and provide a valuable correlate of subjective experience.

Variations in our state of awareness can come through changes in arousal, for instance, through sleepiness or induced by drugs, or through an intentional and momentary change in the focusing of ATTENTION. Focused attention gives rise to perceptual clarity, and is regarded here as processing at the highest available level of consciousness. Variations in awareness are associated with changes in the information that is processed and in the responses that we can make to the sensory input. We are maximally aware of the input when our attention is focused upon it, less aware when our attention is divided between inputs, and less aware still when our attention is directed towards a second source of information. At the extreme end of this continuum is processing without awareness – the recognition of stimuli without consciousness representation. Demonstrations that purport to show the semantic identification of inputs under conditions of *subliminal perception,* or in sleeping subjects, or in patients under ANESTHESIA, all come into this category of cognition without awareness.

The processing of an input provides us with an index of the perceiver's awareness, but there is not a perfect match between awareness and richness of processing. We have no direct access to an individual's level of consciousness, and the extent and richness of processing under different states of awareness provide our only means of assessing the level of consciousness currently enjoyed by the recipient of the input. Intuitively this is known by anyone who attempts to determine whether another person is awake or asleep by asking simply, "Can you hear me?" Assessment of the level of consciousness of a subject can be made more formally, but on the same basis. Empirical studies have observed the extent of cognitive processing gained by stimuli when the subject's attention is controlled by the demands of the task, or when the stimulus is presented in subthreshold conditions and is therefore not available for verbal report, or when the subject is not conscious (asleep or anesthetized).

CONSCIOUSNESS, ATTENTION, AND COGNITION

Laboratory studies (and our own intuitions) suggest that incoming stimuli that do not receive attention are less likely to be understood than are those that are attended to. When adult readers have to divide their attention between a shadowing task (repeating each spoken word as it is heard) and a reading task, performance is considerably worse than when full attention can be given to reading (Kleiman, 1975). In this experiment, sentence comprehension was damaged by attention being directed to the shadowing of a spoken list of words. Importantly, and in a second experimental condition, the recognition of individual printed words was less influenced by the division of attention between tasks.

Focusing our attention upon a spoken message enhances comprehension, and the effectiveness of focusing can be observed by comparison with word detection, when attention is divided. Johnston and Wilson (1980) compared the effects of focused attention against the effects of asking subjects to listen to two messages at once, using a DICHOTIC LISTENING task. The direction of attention was manipulated by either informing the listener as to which message would contain the target word (pre-cueing), or providing no information upon which selection of messages could be made.

Johnston and Wilson first established that, with attention divided between the two messages, performance is influenced by the word presented at the same time as the target. This effect disappeared when the subjects were pre-cued as to which message would contain the target, and could therefore focus upon an attended message. The comparison between the conditions which induced divided and focused attention provides us with a demonstration of the effects of inattention. Nontargets in an unattended message were unable to influence the detectability of simultaneous targets: the influence of their meaning might be said to have been "attenuated" by the listeners focusing upon the attended message.

Investigations of the effects of attention upon detection provide a straightforward conclusion: when a message is unattended there is poor detection of the targets contained in it. Failing to attend to a message results in a failure to respond to single words within that message, and the Johnston and Wilson (1980) experiment provides evidence to suggest that effects of nontarget words can be eliminated by directing attention away from them. These effects of attention are not confounded by attended and unattended messages competing for limited response systems, and are most easily interpreted as being due to unattended messages failing to gain the perceptual analysis required for target detection. Although unattended words are not readily detected (that is, they are not available for verbal report, nor available to awareness), they can continue to influence ongoing behavior, as has been demonstrated in the dichotic shadowing experiments reported by Lewis (1970) and Underwood (1977). This indicates that they have not been recognized at the level where a conscious representation has been formed, but that recognition can be independent of availability for report.

At this point a useful distinction can be made between *implicit* and *explicit* memories, a distinction which Schacter and his colleagues have found helpful in describing performance in amnesic, hypnotic, and anesthetized subjects (for example, see Schacter, 1987; Schacter et al., 1988; Kihlstrom & Schacter, 1990). Whereas we can reflect on some past events in personal experience and provide a verbal report on the context in which an event occurred, there are other forms of knowledge which may not be available for verbal report but which are available only in the sense that our behavior is changed. These are explicit and implicit forms of knowledge respectively, and there are now a number of demonstrations of evidence of implicit memory in the absence of explicit memory. A subject in a memory experiment may be unable to provide an item as a response in a recall task, but may offer the item in a word association task, or show an effect of priming from this "unavailable" item, or may know some obscure fact without knowing from where the knowledge originated. Memories which do not have a conscious representation are not necessarily dormant, and this can be demonstrated to exist by their indirect effects upon other activities. Eich (1984) used the distinction between implicit and explicit memories to demonstrate the semantic processing of unattended messages with a dichotic listening task. Recognition of unattended spoken words remained at chance level (i.e. no explicit influence), even when the words had influenced the interpretation of homophones (i.e. an implicit influence). Awareness of an event is neither a necessary consequence of cognition nor a necessary condition for cognition.

CONSCIOUSNESS AND SERIAL BEHAVIOR

It is clearly not the case that we need to attend to all inputs in order to respond appropriately to them. Although the data on the detection of unattended targets suggest that inattention can result in a deficit in the explicit perception of single items, we have experimental and everyday evidence to suggest that performance can sometimes proceed without attention, particularly in serial continuous tasks. Driving a car is a complex information processing task – the inputs include those from the engine, instruments, and traffic conditions, and the outputs involve changes to these conditions – and yet we can drive while holding a conversation with a passenger. In numerous everyday activities we make appropriate responses to environmental conditions while our attention seems to be directed elsewhere. These examples of dual-task performance could be considered as providing support for the view that perception of the environment does not require attention and that complex cognitive activities can proceed without conscious representation.

Three combinations of tasks have been cited as providing the best examples of dual-task performance, those reported by Allport, Antonis, and Reynolds (1972), who used musical performance plus shadowing, Shaffer (1975), who used typing plus shadowing, and Hirst and colleagues (1980), who used reading plus dictation. Each of the tasks required the subject to perform two transcription tasks, in which a continuous output was made to a continuous input. Why should practiced performers be able to perform a difficult task such as shadowing at the same time as performing another skilled activity? Broadbent's (1982) analysis of the three transcription experiments concluded first that there was evidence that the two tasks could not be performed without some interference between them, and second that the performers might have been skillfully sampling the messages one at a time. As the auditory tasks

used in these experiments did not require continuous sampling, Broadbent argued that there would have been sufficient time to share attention between the two tasks. It must remain an open question, therefore, as to whether claims for automatized behavior provide evidence of cognition with conscious representation.

Our responses to the visual world are influenced by events not currently receiving attention, and this can be demonstrated by a fine-grained analysis of eye fixations made during reading. The directions of our eyes are sometimes claimed to provide an index of the contents of our minds. The most discriminating part of the retina – the FOVEA – is a small area densely packed with cone receptors, which is usually brought into alignment when patterns are inspected. As an image's distance from the fovea increases, so our visual acuity for that image decreases, but the area of the fovea is not well defined, because there is a gradient of acuity. A safe working assumption is that the fovea has a diameter of about two degrees, and this gives maximum sensitivity to eight or ten printed letters when a book is read at a comfortable distance of, say 50 cm. It is this restriction upon the area of sensitivity which results in our saccadic eye movements during reading. Foveal scrutiny of a pattern will make the greatest detail available and it is this area which will be associated with the greatest perceptual clarity, but the contents of the viewer's mind are not restricted to that part of the world gaining the benefit of foveation (*see* EYE MOVEMENT).

Just and Carpenter's (1980) eye–mind assumption provides a strong statement of the relationship between attention and the direction of our eyes: "the eye remains fixated on a word as long as the word is being processed" (p. 330), that is, the direction of the reader's eyes provides us with a measure of what is going through the reader's mind. The eye–mind assumption considers that a fixation will continue until all of the cognitive processes activated by the fixated word have been completed. The assumption can be challenged with evidence that information ahead of fixation is also processed. If information from earlier fixations and from information not yet fixated can both influence the current fixation duration, then the measure of fixation duration will be an indication of the processing of past, present, and future information. If this is the case, then the time taken to process a newly fixated word will only be partly indicated by the duration of the gaze upon a word, because past and future information will also be contributing to the time taken by processing.

For the eye–mind assumption to hold, the evidence would need to demonstrate that all processing of an object is completed during its inspection. Carpenter and Just (1983) allow for the continued processing of previously encountered words, but words ahead of fixation also influence the current fixation behavior. The assumption requires that there are no influences of nonfixated words during reading, and this can be shown to be false. The most useful evidence concerns influences upon eye guidance. Readers do not fixate every word when comprehending text, and the words which are skipped tend to be uninformative in some way. They may be highly predictable from the context of the passage, or they may be from predictable syntactic classes. Words which are not fixated can nevertheless influence performance, both in natural reading tasks and in tachistoscopic recognition tasks. Furthermore, a reader's eyes move towards words which have been primed by associates, and towards parts of words which are most informative.

The assumption is supported by good evidence: the difficulty of encoding of a word is the best predictor of the duration of gaze, and the encoding of the words immediately preceding and following the word have little effect upon this duration. However, it is not supported by evidence of nonfixated events being processed, such as in tachistoscope studies of unattended words which influence the processing of fixated words and pictures (e.g. Dallas & Merikle, 1976; Underwood, 1976).

If we are to challenge the use of the eye–mind assumption then it is necessary to demonstrate that, during reading, some features of text can be processed when they are not gaining foveal inspection. One problem for the assumption would arise if it were possible to demonstrate that, under some circumstances, the eye is drawn to a feature of text, for this would be a demonstration of pre-fixational processing. Such a demonstration has been provided in experiments, in which a reader's eye movements were monitored during sentence comprehension tasks (Underwood et al., 1990). Readers made selective fixations upon the informative parts of words. These informationally complex words were associated with initial in-

spections which reflected their distributions of information. (For example, consider the words *moralistic*, which has more information in the first few letters than in the last few, and *supervisor*, which has an imbalance of information in the last few letters.) When the informative group of letters was at the beginning, then the very first fixation tended to be towards the beginning of the word. This result suggests that the information value of letters away from fixation, in the parafovea of vision, had been recognized to the extent that it could help determine the location of the next fixation.

SEMANTIC ACTIVATION WITHOUT CONSCIOUS IDENTIFICATION?

Can we recognize the meanings of messages of which we have no conscious representation? There is still some debate over the effectiveness of subliminal messages – messages presented at a stimulus intensity insufficient for the perceiver to gain awareness of them – and it is necessary to consider the means used to prevent awareness and the method of inquiring of the perceiver's state of awareness.

There are a number of means by which a stimulus can be presented so as to be out of conscious access: a spoken message may be presented too quietly and a visual message too briefly or too dimly for the perceiver to be able to give a report, or masking techniques can be employed. For example, in the case of visually presented words, the message may be followed immediately by a backwards mask in the form of a second stimulus. This masking stimulus is most effective when it is a random display of letter-like features (that is, a pattern mask), and other techniques involve the use of masking displays of randomly placed dots and other nonlinguistic features, and the use of dichoptic masking, in which the message is presented to one eye while relatively bright light is presented to the other.

Reviews of the large number of studies using these techniques have been provided by Dixon (1981) and Holender (1986), with opposing conclusions. The question of whether there are any convincing demonstrations of the semantic processing of subliminal messages hinges on the issue of whether the perceiver has been aware of the effective message. A priming word presented under subliminal conditions may have an effect upon a subsequent target word, for example, as in the experiments of Fowler and colleagues (1981), Balota (1983), and Marcel (1983), but the critics of these experiments query the measures taken to ensure that the "subliminal" prime was not available for conscious scrutiny. Part of the problem here is that the experimenter is obliged to rely upon verbal report as the only index of the level of conscious representation. If the subject can say what the word is, then it is a supraliminal presentation, otherwise it is subliminal, but this objective measure does not necessarily match with subjective impressions. The perceiver may be unable to identify a word well enough for verbal report while still knowing something of the presentation. While verbal reports are all or none the process of becoming aware of a stimulus may be more gradual. The moment immediately before we are able to give a verbal report extensive processing will have been completed, and it is this processing which may be responsible for the positive results obtained in studies of subliminal words.

In the case of subliminal demonstrations this dissociation between objective and subjective discrimination has the perceiver declaring that nothing can be seen, while being affected by the stimulus, or while otherwise being able to make forced-choice guesses better than chance. The BLINDSIGHT patients also demonstrate this dissociation.

Given that there are separate subjective and objective thresholds (see also Cheesman & Merikle, 1984), and given that perceivers are not often asked after each presentation whether they were able to report the subliminal word, the critics of the notion of "semantic activation without conscious identification" have good reason to be doubtful. We cannot be certain that the perceivers were unaware of the messages at the time of presentation. What is needed is a converging operation, whereby a secondary index of processing would give support to the claim that the effective message has not been available as a conscious representation.

Dixon (1981) suggested that this converging measure could be a qualitative difference in the effect of the message under subliminal and supraliminal conditions. When the perceiver can report the message its effect should be not only different in magnitude from when it cannot be reported, but the effect should also vary in type or direction. This would provide an independent

assessment of whether the perceiver was aware of the message. One example of this qualitative change is provided by Marcel (1980), in which the effect of an ambiguous word was observed under masking conditions. A set of three words terminated with a target, and it was the response to the target that was measured. The first word and the target were not related in meaning, but both were related to the second word, through its two meanings. For example, in the triplet *save – bank – river* the first word might prime the second, but once the second word is interpreted it should not prime the terminal word. This in fact was the pattern of results obtained when all three words were presented supraliminally, but when the second word was pattern-masked, and unavailable for verbal report, then a qualitative change was observed in the results. With a subliminal second word a priming effect was found. Other demonstrations of this qualitative change have been reported for auditory and visual investigations of subliminal presentations by, for example, Groeger (1984, 1986). Schacter's (1987) distinction between implicit and explicit memories may again be an appropriate framework for regarding these demonstrations, in that events which are prevented from achieving a conscious level of representation are recorded as having influences upon the processing of other events. Implicit representations are inferred by their effects, which can be observed even when the representations themselves are not available for verbal report.

COGNITION WITHOUT CONSCIOUSNESS: MEMORY UNDER ANESTHESIA?

The implicit/explicit memory distinction also provides a promising approach to the question of the extent that patients undergoing surgery under anesthesia can know of the events around them. Anecdotal stories apart, there are a number of cases reported in the literature of anesthetized patients who have been able to repeat comments made by surgeons, either in response to conventional enquiry or when subsequently hypnotized (e.g. Bennett, 1987; Cheek, 1959, 1964; Levinson, 1965). These reports from patients could arise from a number of possibilities:

● the anesthetic was inadequate and acted merely as an analgesic, that is, the patients did

not lose consciousness and were fully aware of the spoken comments made in their hearing at that time;
- the patients were anesthetized as intended, and full perceptual representations can be maintained without awareness, as explicit memories;
- the patients were anesthetized as intended, but only implicit memories are available in the absence of knowledge of the spatiotemporal context in which the events were experienced.

The absence of full verbal reports from all patients may, if either of the first two possibilities are valid, result from amnesia associated with the anesthetic. This amnesia may then be overcome by hypnosis and this would account for the availability of more detailed accounts from hypnotized patients. Obtaining evidence of clear perception during anesthetized surgery is difficult, and has not been demonstrated. This does not mean that clear perception followed by amnesia does not occur, but demonstrations may have to rely upon the use of physiological measures such as event-related potentials. Kihlstrom and Schacter (1990) favor the view of implicit memories being available after anesthetized surgery, and suggest that these memories could result from "implicit perceptions" which resemble the perceptual processing gained by subliminal and unattended stimuli and which are also demonstrated by blindsight patients. In support they offer a number of studies in which patients are presented with tape-recorded materials during anesthetized surgery, and who subsequently report no awareness of these materials. This establishes the absence of explicit memories, and to confirm the availability of implicit memories a number of techniques have been used. For example, Bennett, Davis, and Giannini (1985) observed 9 out of 11 patients making a specific manual gesture in response to a signal described in the tape recording. In another study, no recall (explicit memory) was found of a list of low frequency words, but greater familiarity with those words was reported when they were seen as part of a longer list. It is not well established that patients gain implicit memories of events during anesthetized surgery, and there are a number of reports of a failure to find changes in behavior as a result of these surgical events (see Millar, 1987). One problem here is the particular anesthetic mixture used during surgery. Different

mixtures have different influences on the central nervous system, and the perceptions, memories, and indeed, awareness of a patient may vary according to the anesthetic in use.

CONSCIOUSNESS AND COGNITION

From a number of studies in a range of investigations of the relationship between conscious experience and cognitive processing it is possible to come to a singular conclusion. Cognitive processing can proceed in the absence of conscious awareness, resulting in implicit memories of events of which the perceiver is unaware. This conclusion is supported by evidence from manipulations of the perceiver's attention in hearing and in vision, and from studies of the effects of stimuli presented below the threshold for verbal report. An implicit memory can be formed in the absence of knowledge of the spatiotemporal context of the event, is inferred on the basis of changes in behavior in the absence of conscious, reportable recollections of the event, and is more likely to involve the activation of existing knowledge structures than to involve the formation of new concepts and structures. The distinction between implicit memories, for which conscious processing does not appear to be necessary, and explicit memories, for which it is, may prove to be helpful in our eventual understanding of the role of consciousness in cognition. Understanding familiar stimuli may be possible without the perceiver's awareness, but it may be that only with conscious processing are we able to understand and develop the new concepts that can be described and discussed as explicit memories.

See also COMMISSUROTOMY; DISCONNECTION SYNDROME; VEGETATIVE STATE.

BIBLIOGRAPHY
Allport, D. A., Antonis, B., & Reynolds, P. (1972). On the division of attention: a disproof of the single channel hypothesis. *Quarterly Journal of Experimental Psychology, 24*, 225–35.
Balota, D. A. (1983). Automatic semantic activation and episodic memory encoding. *Journal of Verbal Learning and Verbal Behavior, 22*, 88–104.
Bennett, H. L. (1987). Learning and memory in anaesthesia. In M. Rosen & J. N. Lunn (Eds), *Consciousness, awareness and pain in general anaesthesia* (pp. 132–49). London: Butterworths.

Bennett, H. L., Davis, H. S., & Giannini, J. A. (1985). Non-verbal response to intraoperative conversation. *British Journal of Anaesthesia, 57,* 174–9.

Broadbent, D. E. (1982). Task combination and selective intake of information. *Acta Psychologica, 50,* 253–90.

Carpenter, P. A., & Just, M. A. (1983). What your eyes do while your mind is reading. In K. Rayner (Ed.), *Eye movements in reading: Perceptual and language processes* (pp. 275–307). New York: Academic Press.

Cheek, D. B. (1959). Unconscious perception of meaningful sounds during surgical anaesthesia as revealed under hypnosis. *American Journal of Clinical Hypnosis, 1,* 101–13.

Cheek, D. B. (1964). Surgical memory and reaction to careless conversation. *American Journal of Clinical Hypnosis, 6,* 237.

Cheesman, J., & Merikle, P. M. (1984). Priming with and without awareness. *Perception and Psychophysics, 36,* 387–95.

Dallas, M., & Merikle, P. M. (1976). Semantic processing of non-attended visual information. *Canadian Journal of Psychology, 30,* 15–21.

Dixon, N. F. (1981). *Preconscious processing.* Chichester: Wiley.

Eich, E. (1984). Memory for unattended events: remembering with and without awareness. *Memory and Cognition, 12,* 105–11.

Fowler, C. A., Wolford, G., Slade, R., & Tassinary, L. (1981). Lexical access with and without awareness. *Journal of Experimental Psychology: General, 110,* 341–62.

Groeger, J. A. (1984). Evidence of unconscious semantic processing from a forced error situation. *British Journal of Psychology, 75,* 304–14.

Groeger, J. A. (1986). Predominant and non-dominant analysis: effects of level of presentation. *British Journal of Psychology, 77,* 109–16.

Hirst, W., Spelke, E. S., Reaves, C. C., Caharack, G., & Neisser, U. (1980). Dividing attention without alternation or automaticity. *Journal of Experimental Psychology: General, 109,* 98–117.

Holender, D. (1986). Semantic activation without conscious identification in dichotic listening, parafoveal vision, and visual masking: a survey and appraisal. *Behavioural and Brain Sciences, 9,* 1–66.

Johnston, W. A., & Wilson, J. (1980). Perceptual processing of non-targets in an attention task. *Memory and Cognition, 8,* 372–7.

Just, M. A., & Carpenter, P. A. (1980). A theory of reading: from eye fixations to comprehension. *Psychological Review, 87,* 329–54.

Kihlstrom, J. F., & Schacter, D. L. (1990). Anaesthesia, amnesia, and the cognitive unconscious. In B. Bonke, W. Fitch, & K. Millar (Eds), *Memory and awareness in anaesthesia* (pp. 21–44). Amsterdam: Swets & Zeitlinger.

Kleiman, G. M. (1975). Speech recoding in reading. *Journal of Verbal Learning and Verbal Behaviour, 14,* 323–39.

Levinson, B. W. (1965). States of awareness during general anaesthesia: preliminary communication. *British Journal of Anaesthesia, 37,* 544–6.

Lewis, J. L. (1970). Semantic processing of unattended messages using dichotic listening. *Journal of Experimental Psychology, 85,* 225–8.

Marcel, A. J. (1980). Conscious and preconscious recognition of polysemous words: locating the selective effect of prior verbal context. In R. S. Nickerson (Ed.), *Attention and Performance,* Vol. VIII (pp. 435–57). Hillsdale, NJ: Erlbaum.

Marcel, A. J. (1983). Conscious and unconscious perception: experiments on visual masking and word recognition. *Cognitive Psychology, 15,* 197–237.

Millar, K. (1987). Assessment of memory for anaesthesia. In F. Guerra & J. A. Aldrete (Eds), *Emotional and psychological responses to anaesthesia and surgery* (pp. 1–8). New York: Grune & Stratton.

Schacter, D. L. (1987). Implicit memory: history and current status. *Journal of Experimental Psychology: Learning, Memory and Cognition, 13,* 501–18.

Schacter, D. L., McAndrews, M. P., & Moscovitch, M. (1988). Access to consciousness: dissociations between implicit and explicit knowledge in neurological syndromes. In L. Weiskrantz (Ed.), *Thought without language* (pp. 242–78). Oxford: Oxford University Press.

Shaffer, L. H. (1975). Multiple attention in continuous verbal tasks. In P. M. A. Rabbitt and S. Dornic (Eds), *Attention and performance,* Vol. V (pp. 157–67). London: Academic Press.

Underwood, G. (1976). Semantic interference from unattended printed words. *British Journal of Psychology, 67,* 327–38.

Underwood, G. (1977). Contextual facilitation

from attended and unattended messages. *Journal of Verbal Learning and Verbal Behavior, 16*, 99–106.

Underwood, G., Clews, S., & Everatt, J. (1990). How do readers know where to look next? Local information distributions influence eye fixations. *Quarterly Journal of Experimental Psychology, 42A*, 39–65.

GEOFFREY UNDERWOOD

constructional apraxia *See* APRAXIA; GERSTMANN SYNDROME; PARIETAL LOBE.

contiguity, disorders of In Jakobson's pioneering work on neurolinguistics, aphasia was regarded as reducible to either a disorder of similarity or a disorder of contiguity. Disorders of contiguity related to syntagmatic linguistic signs and were thought to be evident in impairments in the ability to form propositions and construct complex linguistic entities from simple linguistic units. The concept is of historical importance, but has little contemporary usage.

contre coup Contre coup is a form of CLOSED HEAD INJURY in which the main effects of the impact to the skull occur at a location opposite to the point of impact.

Contre coup injuries result from two processes. The first is the ability of the brain, being suspended within the CEREBROSPINAL FLUID, to move more freely than the skull within which it is contained. Acceleration forces generated by an impact will therefore produce greater motion in the brain than in the head as a whole, with the effect that the brain continues to move after the head has stopped moving, bringing it sharply into contact with the inside of the skull opposite to the point of impact. Secondly, theoretical models of the process of cavitation, by which the acceleration-deceleration forces produce rapid vaporization and then condensation of the liquids within the brain with violent results, demonstrate that these effects are more likely to occur in the negative pressure zone opposite to the point of impact.

conversion reaction *See* HYSTERIA.

coprolalia Forced vocalizations which commonly take the form of obscene words or phrases comprise coprolalic speech. It is most commonly seen to accompany multiple tics in the rare inherited disorder, GILLES DE LA TOURETTE's syndrome. This condition is commoner among boys than girls, and usually has an onset before the age of 11. Coprolalia may occur in the absence of tics, as in the *latah* reaction among Malays. The organic basis for coprolalia has not been clearly established, but it may respond to pharmacotherapy, and may be classified as a form of DYSTONIA.

corollary discharge Teuber hypothesized the existence of a corollary discharge to maintain the stability of the perceived external world. When a voluntary movement is initiated, two efferent signals are generated: one travels to the muscles involved in the voluntary action, the other (the corollary discharge) combines with the reafferent signals and is fed back into central processing mechanisms. More specifically, frontal lobe signals are sent to parietal and temporal association cortex which permits the relevant sensory systems to anticipate motor acts. The existence of the corollary discharge has not been unequivocally demonstrated, but it has proved a useful hypothesis.

corpus callosum The corpus callosum is the principal commissure in the cerebral hemispheres; the prominent broad band of fibers which links homolateral points in the cortex of the two hemispheres. It is easy to visualize in a medial sagittal section of the brain, and is named from the coarse and horny appearance of its surface. It forms a canopy over the thalamus, the fornix, and the head and body of the caudate nucleus at each side. At the anterior end it curves forwards and under forming the *rostrum* and behind that the *genu* of the corpus callosum; the posterior third is named the SPLENIUM. The corpus callosum interconnects homotopic points from all regions of the cortex, apart from certain areas of the temporal lobes (which are connected by the anterior commissure). Callosal fibers, being long corticocortical neurons, are relatively late to myelinate and the corpus callosum is not fully developed until around the age of puberty.

Until quite recent times the corpus callosum was thought by some to play no functional role beyond mechanical support within the forebrain, but its significance became evident with the influential studies of COMMISSUROTOMY (the split-brain patients) from about 1960. These studies conclusively demonstrated that the corpus callosum plays a major and crucial role in exchanging information between the cortices of the two hemispheres and so providing neuropsychological integration between the relatively independent left and right hemisphere systems. Section of the corpus callosum, for example, results in an inability to name objects (dependent on left hemisphere language systems) presented to the left hand, or in the left visual half field (as the relevant sensory information is projected to the right hemisphere).

Individual differences in the size of the corpus callosum, which by inference suggest differences in the number of callosal fibers, have been linked with sex, with handedness, and with various pathological conditions; for example, a reduced corpus callosum has been reported in both schizophrenia and in developmental dyslexia. However, not all these reports have been confirmed in the literature, and their precise significance is open to debate. The corpus callosum may vary not only in volume but also in fiber density, and it is difficult to disentangle primary causational factors from secondary results of medication or of abnormal psychological development or experience.

Tumors of the corpus callosum present a distinct clinical picture with mental changes being more pronounced than with tumors in almost any other location. These changes include apathy, drowsiness, and memory dysfunction although affective changes may also occur. Tumors affecting the genu or the rostrum may produce a GRASP REFLEX. Left-sided apraxia may also result from such a midline tumor by disconnection of the right corticospinal tracts (controlling the left hand) from the mechanisms controlling skilled performance located in the left hemisphere.

J. GRAHAM BEAUMONT

cortex The cortex (from the Latin for "rind" or "bark") is the outer layer of the human forebrain. Strictly, the term *cerebral cortex* should be used, as many organs within the body also possess a cortex,

and even within the head, the CEREBELLUM also has a cortex; nevertheless, in an unqualified form, "cortex" is used by neuropsychologists to refer to the cerebral cortex.

The human forebrain (the cerebral hemispheres) is entirely surrounded by a layer of grey matter on its outer surface, which is the cortex. The gray coloration results from the nuclei of the very considerable number of neural cells located in the cortex, cells which project downward to almost all structures within the central nervous system, as well as cells which communicate with other cortical cells (cortico-cortical connections). The cortex is a region of very dense interconnectivity. It varies in thickness from about 1.5 mm at the frontal poles to about 4.5 mm around the central fissure. The human brain, quite distinctively, is folded into a complex pattern of gyri and sulci, so that the total surface area of the cortex of about 2,500 sq cm can be contained within the skull. The cortex is divided into six anatomically distinct layers, which vary in their relative thickness in different areas of the cortex, but the distinctions among these layers are not normally of significance for the neuropsychologist.

The cortex, while appearing quite haphazard in its arrangement of gyri and sulci, has a number of fairly constant landmarks, as well as a regularity of pattern which is greater than might at first be apparent. The division of the cortex into the left and right cerebral hemispheres is obvious, and the subdivision of each of the hemispheres into four lobes (FRONTAL, TEMPORAL, PARIETAL, and OCCIPITAL) is readily identified by the landmarks of the two major fissures: the SYLVIAN FISSURE (or lateral sulcus) and the central or Rolandic fissure (*see* ROLANDIC AREA). (Other features of functional significance are noted in the context of the discussion of specific topics.)

cortical blindness Extensive bilateral damage to the striate cortex of the occipital lobe may result in cortical blindness. It is distinguished from peripheral causes of blindness by the normal appearance of the optic disk and retina within the eye and the preservation of pupillary reflexes on ophthalmological examination. The condition most commonly results from severe infarction of the posterior cerebral arteries or the basilar artery, but may also follow severe occipital trauma and certain other cerebral diseases. The onset may be sudden and total, or may be the final stage of steps of increasing HEMIANOPIA. Temporary periods of cortical blindness may be associated with epileptic phenomena, with migraine, or with TIAs.

Recovery from cortical blindness, more rapid following closed head injury and much slower following vascular lesions if any recovery occurs, follows a classic pattern: perception of light and dark, perception of movement, perception of colour and lastly perception of form. There is a gradient of increasing definition of contours as recovery progresses. In the late stages of recovery the difficulty with object perception may simulate a visual AGNOSIA, particularly if there is prolonged presentation of the object, a condition referred to as *cerebral asthenopia*.

Two unusual conditions may accompany cortical blindness. One is ANTON'S SYNDROME, where patients are blind but deny being blind and may confabulate concerning what they see; the other is BLINDSIGHT, where patients assert their blindness but may nevertheless preserve some visual functions due to the operation of the more primitive secondary visual system.

While patients who are cortically blind generally report that they continue to dream and experience visual images, cases have been described in which the recall of visual memories is impossible, or the visual image of colors cannot be formed. Visual hallucinations have frequently been reported to be associated with cortical blindness, and confusional states are also common, characterized by disorientation, attentional disorders, and memory defects.

cortical deafness   Patients who are regarded as suffering from cortical deafness show a severe lack of awareness of auditory stimuli during normal functional tasks and have abnormal pure tone thresholds as established by audiometry. Complete deafness rarely, if ever, results from cortical lesions alone. The condition is generally seen only with bilateral lesions of primary auditory cortex in the superior temporal cortex in the region of Heschl's gyrus. However, the term is sometimes used to indicate less severe disturbances of auditory function in the absence of gross audiometric changes, that is, partial deafness of cortical origin, which might more properly be termed auditory AGNOSIA. It may be difficult to distinguish between auditory agnosia and cortical deafness.

Cortical deafness is uncommon, as it is rare for traumatic lesions to occur simultaneously in the two primary auditory cortices in the lateral temporal lobes. The bilateral projection of the auditory pathways up to the temporal lobe preserves auditory sensation from the effects of unilateral auditory disorders by comparison with vision, for example, where the pathways are completely crossed from retina to cortex. Even when bilateral lesions of the two primary auditory cortices do occur, the evidence is that this does not invariably lead to a total loss of audiometric sensitivity. Indeed, some writers have doubted whether cortical deafness does, in fact, exist. Bilateral subcortical lesions in the region of the internal capsule may isolate the auditory cortex without directly affecting it, and so produce cortical deafness. Lesions of the medial geniculate bodies may also account for the deafness.

One situation where total deafness seems reliably to occur is when a lesion in one temporal lobe is followed after an intervening period by a second lesion, often of a vascular nature, in the homolateral position in the contralateral temporal lobe. Even in such cases, patients may retain a response to environmental sounds and show rather inconsistent response to auditory stimuli. This may lead to the suspicion of a psychogenic basis for the disorder, but is more likely to be due to varying levels of auditory attention. Deafness due to cortical lesions is commonly transient.

A phenomenon similar to ANTON'S SYNDROME in the visual modality has been described, in that a patient with cortical deafness may act as if unaware of the deficit.

See also AUDITORY PERCEPTUAL DISORDERS.

J. GRAHAM BEAUMONT

corticobulbar pathway   The corticobulbar motor pathway, between the cortex and the pontobulbar area of the brain stem, has been hypothesized to play a role in the generation of emotional facial expression. Bilateral lesions of this pathway may release reflex mechanisms for emotional expression from cortical control. The resulting syndrome may involve involuntary crying or laughing, but in a stereotypic form and without graded intensity. It may be triggered by various stimuli, but neither its initiation nor its termination are under voluntary control. This remains a hypothesis without clear empirical support (*see* PSEUDOBULBAR PALSY).

Cotard syndrome The Cotard syndrome is a form of nihilistic delusion in which patients believe that they are dead. The delusion may be accompanied by delusions of putrefaction or the absence of parts of the body, and the condition is also associated with tendencies to suicide and self-injury. Although rare, it is normally seen in a context of severe depression, although it has been reported to occur in cases of typhoid fever, and in those with frontal and temporal lobe epilepsy or with medial frontal cortical atrophy. The Cotard syndrome is also associated with delusional misidentification in the form of the CAPGRAS and FREGOLI SYNDROMES.

cranial nerves Peripheral nerves are of two kinds, cranial and spinal. These are attached to the brain and spinal cord respectively. In humans, there are twelve pairs of cranial nerves, numbered rostrocaudally: I olfactory, II optic, III oculomotor, IV trochlear, V trigeminal, VI abducent, VII facial (including the nervus intermedius), VIII vestibulocochlear, IX glossopharyngeal, X vagus, XI accessory, XII hypoglossal.

The cranial nerves contain motor and sensory nerve fibers. The former stem from neuronal cell bodies located in motor nuclei within the brain. Most of the latter arise from cell bodies in ganglia located on the cranial nerves themselves, close to their points of exit from the skull. These terminate by synapsing on sensory nuclei within the brain. Both types of fiber generally form roots which traverse the central nervous system surface through an *attachment zone* which is specific for each nerve. The transition from central to peripheral nervous tissue generally occurs at or a little outside the plane of the BRAIN STEM surface. As the roots cross the subarachnoid space (*see* MENINGES) they generally unite to form a single nerve trunk. This passes through the skull, outside which most branches arise. Through these, each nerve is distributed to a specific territory within the head and neck.

Cranial nerves vary much more in morphology and fiber composition than the relatively stereotyped spinal nerves. Unlike the latter they show little evidence of a repeating pattern corresponding to the segments of the body. This has been obscured during evolution in association with the extensive phylogenetic changes which have occurred in the morphology of the head region

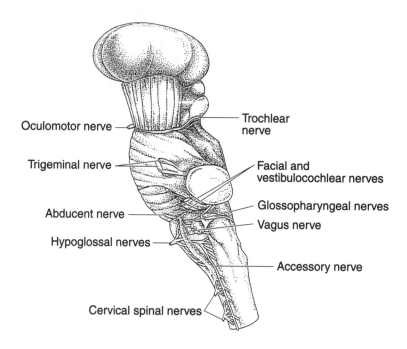

Figure 35 Roots of the cranial nerves: lateral view.

and especially of the brain, special senses, and pharyngeal (branchial) arch derivatives. Taken together, the cranial nerves include a wider variety of fiber types than the spinal nerves. Both may contain motor fibers innervating voluntary muscle, sensory fibers innervating skin and deeper tissues, as well as efferent (outgoing) autonomic fibers and afferent (incoming) fibers from viscera. In addition the cranial nerves include afferent fibers mediating the special senses and also taste fibers. Some cranial nerves consist almost exclusively of one type of motor or sensory fiber, while others consist of several, both motor and sensory.

I   OLFACTORY

This is the nerve of smell (OLFACTION). The bipolar olfactory neuron cell bodies lie in the epithelium lining the olfactory area in the upper part of the nose. Cilia from their peripheral processes lie in the overlying fluid and possess a variety of classes of receptor in their cell membranes. Individual receptors respond selectively to the three-dimensional configuration of odorant molecules, sometimes in extremely low concentrations. Their central processes are very thin nonmyelinated axons. On each side these run in 20 or so fascicles which comprise the nerve. Each

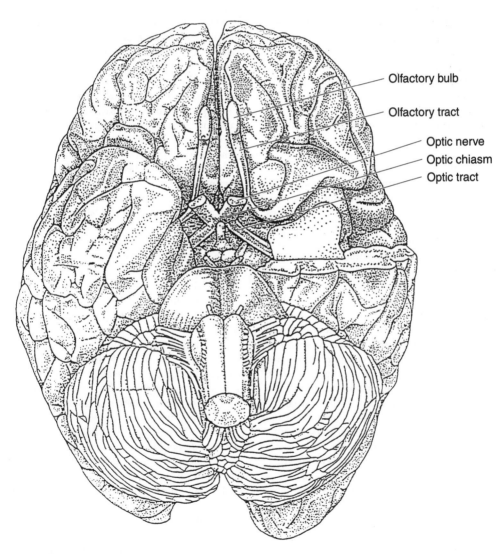

Olfactory bulb

Olfactory tract

Optic nerve
Optic chiasm
Optic tract

Figure 36 Roots of the cranial nerves: inferior view.

251

fascicle enters the skull through an individual opening and terminates separately in the olfactory bulb. This contains primitive (three-layered) cerebral cortex and is comparatively under-developed in humans. The olfactory tract connects it to the rest of the hemisphere. Destruction of an olfactory nerve due, for example, to head injury leads to ANOSMIA on that side. The human brain is capable of distinguishing between thousands of different odors. Moreover, olfaction and TASTE (see facial nerve) are closely integrated centrally in the appreciation of the flavors and tastes of foodstuffs. Olfactory neurons are unique among vertebrate nerve cells in that their cell bodies lie in the surface epithelium of the body – a topological relationship which they share with embryonic neuronal precursors. Furthermore, unlike the vast majority of types of neuron, their cell bodies undergo turnover at maturity. Also, a single neuron links the periphery to the cerebral cortex. In other sensory systems, such as the spinothalamic, it is commonly the third neuron of a series which does so.

II OPTIC

This is not a true peripheral nerve, but a brain tract. It consists of central nervous tissue surrounded by extensions of the MENINGES. It runs backwards from the eyeball through the orbit and enters the cranial cavity. Here the two nerves join below the hypothalamus at the OPTIC CHIASM. From each side of this an optic tract runs backwards to the lateral geniculate body, part of the thalamus. Optic nerve fibers are axons of retinal ganglion cells. In the retina they are normally nonmyelinated. They acquire myelin sheaths as they leave the eyeball. At the optic chiasm fibers from the medial half of each retina cross the midline to enter the opposite tract. Those of the lateral half remain uncrossed. Each optic tract therefore consists of fibers from the medial half of the contralateral retina and the lateral half of the ipsilateral retina. These terminate in two principal sites: in the lateral geniculate body, from where they are relayed to the visual cortex for conscious visual perception, and in the region of the upper midbrain, where they terminate in the pretectal nucleus and the superior COLLICULUS, centers for visual reflexes (see below). At all levels between the retina and the cortex, optic pathway fibers have a highly ordered (retinotopic) arrangement relative to their points

of origin in the retina. Variations in this arrangement along the pathway enable the sites of lesions producing VISUAL FIELD DEFECTS to be predicted.

III OCULOMOTOR, IV TROCHLEAR, AND VI ABDUCENT

These three nerves supply the extrinsic ocular muscles in the orbit. The *oculomotor* nucleus lies in the gray matter of the upper midbrain. It contains subdivisions corresponding to individual muscles and another, the Edinger–Westphal nucleus, which is parasympathetic. On leaving the midbrain the nerve passes forwards into the lateral wall of the cavernous venous sinus. Its branches enter the orbit. Here they supply the medial, superior, and inferior rectus muscles as well as the inferior oblique muscle and the voluntary part of the levator palpebrae superioris, which elevates the upper eyelid. The parasympathetic component relays in the ciliary ganglion. Its postganglionic fibers are involved in light and accommodation reflexes. They enter the eyeball and supply the smooth muscle of the constrictor of the pupil and the ciliary muscle. Contraction of the latter permits the lens to increase in convexity, thereby shortening its focal length for accommodation. These actions are opposed by sympathetic neurons. Pupillary size, shape, and reflex function may be abnormal in a variety of conditions, including SYPHILIS, which is associated with the ARGYLL ROBERTSON PUPIL.

The *trochlear* nucleus lies in the lower midbrain in line with that of the oculomotor. Its fibers follow a unique course. They leave the nucleus, curve backwards around the gray matter, cross the midline and emerge from the dorsal brain-stem surface on the side opposite to their origin. The nerve passes forwards beside the midbrain and its subsequent course resembles that of the oculomotor. It supplies the superior oblique muscle. Its dorsal emergence contravenes the general rule that motor nerves are attached ventrally and sensory nerves dorsally.

The *abducent* nucleus lies in the PONS and the nerve emerges ventrally at the pontomedullary junction. In its course to the orbit it runs in the medial wall of the cavernous sinus, close to the internal carotid artery. It supplies the lateral rectus muscle.

Where they leave the brain stem, the three nerves contain few, if any, sensory (proprioceptive) fibers carrying feedback from their muscles.

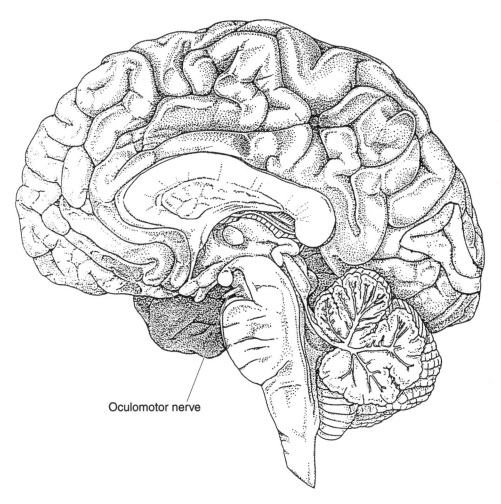

Figure 37 Root of the oculomotor nerve: sagittal view.

These are present in the nerves close to the muscles but leave them and pass to the brain stem via branches of the trigeminal nerve.

Activity of the motor nuclei of the three nerves is closely coordinated in producing EYE MOVE-MENTS. They are controlled by centers for vergence, in which the two visual axes converge, and for GAZE, in which the axes move in parallel (conjugate movement). The pons contains two lateral gaze centers, one for conjugate movement to each side. These are influenced by cortical and brain-stem centers such as the FRONTAL EYE FIELDS, the superior colliculi and the vestibular nuclei. The midbrain contains vertical gaze centers, two for upward and two for downward conjugate movement.

Oculomotor paralysis results in severe deficiency of eyeball movement. The visual axis tends to be deviated downwards and outwards due to unopposed action of the two non-paralyzed muscles and the eyelid droops (*ptosis*). Abducent paralysis results in a medial squint due to the unopposed medial rectus. Trochlear paralysis results in double vision on attempting to look down and outwards to the affected side.

V TRIGEMINAL

The trigeminal nerve subserves general sensation for most of the head, supplying the skin of the face and anterior scalp, and the linings of the nose and mouth. These fibers enter the pons in its sensory root. Peripherally, they are distributed through its three divisions, the ophthalmic, maxillary, and mandibular. These radiate from the trigeminal ganglion, in which most of the unipolar sensory cell bodies lie. The ophthalmic runs in the lateral wall of the cavernous sinus. Its branches traverse the orbit and supply the upper trigeminal territory, including the paranasal air sinuses and conjunctiva. The maxillary division supplies the middle part of the face, including the palate and the upper lip and teeth. The mandibular division supplies the lower face, the anterior part of the tongue, and the lower lip and teeth. In *trigeminal neuralgia*, the cause of which is unknown, excruciating pain is commonly experienced in the distribution of one or more of the divisions. The trigeminal motor root joins the mandibular division, and supplies the muscles of mastication, which produce jaw movements, and also muscles in the floor of the mouth, palate, and middle ear.

Trigeminal proprioceptive fibers carry feedback from the muscles to which it is motor. They also subserve proprioception from muscle groups which receive only motor innervation from other cranial nerves, for example, the muscles of facial expression, supplied by the facial nerve. Unusually, their cell bodies are in the midbrain. The trigeminal sensory nuclei extend along the pons, medulla, and upper cervical spinal cord. In addition to trigeminal afferents, general sensory fibers of the facial, glossopharyngeal, and vagus nerves also terminate in them.

No taste or autonomic fibers enter or leave the pons in the trigeminal nerve. However, both types, derived from other nerves, join trigeminal branches and are distributed with them. For example, the chorda tympani branch of the facial nerve, containing taste and parasympathetic fibers, joins the lingual branch of the trigeminal.

VII FACIAL

The facial and vestibulocochlear (VIII) nerves are attached to the brain stem near the pontomedullary junction. Between the two nerves is the *nervus intermedius* which joins the facial and is generally considered part of it. The facial follows a tortuous path through the skull, passing close to the internal and middle parts of the ear. It may be affected by disease of the latter. It leaves the skull and divides in the parotid salivary gland, diseases of which may also damage the nerve. Its branches radiate over the face and are motor to the muscles of facial expression, including those of the scalp

and forehead. Complete interruption of facial motoneuron function at or distal to its nucleus, for example in Bell's palsy, causes paralysis of all the muscles supplied. By contrast, in lesions of the facial upper motoneurons of the CORTICOBULBAR PATHWAY (e.g. in a STROKE), function of the upper facial muscles may be spared because of redundancy in their upper motoneuron supply.

The nervus intermedius contributes taste and parasympathetic fibers. Most taste fibers leave the facial in the skull through the chorda tympani nerve. This runs in the wall of the middle ear cavity, crossing the eardrum (hence its name) and eventually joins the lingual nerve to supply taste buds on the oral surface of the tongue. Other facial branches supply taste buds on the palate. Facial (and also glossopharyngeal and vagal) taste fibers terminate centrally in the nucleus solitarius in the medulla. It is widely accepted that a different class of taste receptor cell responds to each of the four basic modalities: sweet, salty, sour, and bitter.

The chorda tympani also contains parasympathetic fibers. These originate in the superior salivatory nucleus in the pons. Some relay in the submandibular ganglion to supply the sublingual and submandibular salivary glands. Others, relaying in the pterygopalatine ganglion ("the ganglion of hay fever") innervate the lacrimal and nasal glands.

VIII VESTIBULOCOCHLEAR

The cochlear and vestibular parts of this nerve innervate the cochlea and the membranous labyrinth respectively, parts of the internal ear, which lies in the temporal bone. From here the nerve runs centrally, first through the bone and then across the subarachnoid space. Most of the latter nerve segment consists of central nervous tissue. It joins the brain stem near the pontomedullary junction, where the cochlear and vestibular nuclei lie. The *cochlear* nerve subserves hearing. Its bipolar cell bodies lie in the spiral ganglion in the cochlea itself. They are myelinated, which promotes rapid impulse conduction along them. Their peripheral processes innervate the *spiral organ* of the cochlea. Their central processes terminate in the cochlear nuclei. Both the cochlea and its nuclei show a tonotopic arrangement whereby specific parts of each respond to individual sound frequencies. The nerve also contains efferent fibers, running from the brain stem to the spiral organ. These may facilitate or inhibit the initiation of impulses mediating specific sound frequencies. This may help to selectively focus attention on some sounds. In some forms of ear disease *tinnitus* may occur – the subjective perception of sound in the absence of a corresponding auditory stimulus.

The bipolar *vestibular* neurons lie close to the internal ear. Their peripheral processes innervate the *maculae* of the utricle and saccule, which monitor static head position, and the *cristae* of the three semicircular canals, which monitor head movements. Accordingly, vestibular disease is associated with vertigo and other disorders of balance. Most vestibular central processes terminate in the vestibular nuclei in the floor of the fourth ventricle of the brain. Some bypass these and terminate in the CEREBELLUM. Some of the vestibular nuclei are connected to the oculomotor, trochlear, and abducent nuclei through the medial longitudinal fasciculus. By means of these connections, they automatically control eyeball position, helping to keep the gaze fixed on a target during head movement. Disorders of this system may produce *nystagmus*, a type of involuntary oscillating eyeball movement. Because of their close proximity, the facial and vestibulocochlear nerves may be affected together by conditions such as *acoustic neuroma*, a tumor of the vestibulocochlear nerve, producing a combination of symptoms and signs of disease in both nerves.

IX GLOSSOPHARYNGEAL

This small nerve is attached to the upper medulla. After leaving the skull it becomes associated with the wall of the pharynx and its outgrowths. It is mainly sensory, and gives taste and other sensory supply to the tonsil and the back of the tongue. It also supplies the auditory (Eustachian) tube and middle ear. Because of these connections, pain due to pharyngeal disease may be perceived as originating in the middle ear. Its parasympathetic fibers from the inferior salivatory nucleus relay in the otic ganglion below the skull base. From here, fibers run to the parotid gland in the auriculotemporal branch of the trigeminal. Blood pressure and oxygen tension are monitored from the carotid sinus and body respectively, via the sinus branch.

X VAGUS AND XI ACCESSORY

The *vagus* has an extensive distribution, hence its name (Latin *vagus*, wandering). It arises in the medulla. Just outside the skull it is joined by the cranial part of the accessory (see below). It descends through the neck into the thorax and accompanies the esophagus through the diaphragm into the abdomen. It provides parasympathetic input to the enteric nervous system in the wall of the alimentary tract and its derivatives, which it influences as far distally as the transverse colon, and also to the thoracic viscera. The preganglionic cell bodies lie in the dorsal vagal nucleus. The ganglia lie in, on, or near the viscera supplied. The vagus contains a variety of sensory fibers from the thoracic viscera, conveying the afferent limbs of respiratory and cardiovascular reflexes. These, with corresponding fibers in the glossopharyngeal, end in the nucleus solitarius. It also carries conscious sensation from part of the external ear (see trigeminal nerve), the lower pharynx, and the larynx, and taste from the lowermost part of the pharyngeal surface of the tongue and the epiglottis (see facial nerve).

The *accessory* nerve has cranial and spinal parts. The former consists of motoneuron fibers arising in the nucleus ambiguus in the medulla. These join the vagus and are distributed with it, supplying the striated muscle of the larynx, most of the pharynx, and the upper esophagus. Movements of the pharynx, face, tongue, mandible, and soft palate are coordinated in the brain stem during speech, mastication, and swallowing, through integration of activity in the motor nuclei controlling them. Swallowing and vomiting centers are associated with the nucleus solitarius.

The *spinal* accessory is motor and arises in the upper cervical cord. The trunk enters the cranial cavity by ascending through the foramen magnum. It adheres to the cranial accessory over a short distance, without significant fiber exchange, near its exit from the skull. It descends in the neck to supply the sternocleidomastoid and trapezius muscles. These receive proprioceptive innervation from upper cervical spinal nerves.

XII HYPOGLOSSAL

The hypoglossal roots emerge from the medulla in line with the upper cervical ventral spinal roots. Like these they are purely motor. The trunk leaves the skull and descends in the neck. It then turns forwards to supply the extrinsic and intrinsic lingual muscles, which change tongue position and shape respectively. In hypoglossal paralysis, when the tongue is protruded it deviates to the opposite side under the action of the intact muscles.

BIBLIOGRAPHY

Brodal, A. (1981). *Neurological anatomy in relation to clinical medicine*, 3rd edn. Oxford: Oxford University Press.

Kandel, E. R., Schwartz, J. H., & Jessell, T. M. (Eds). (1991). *Principles of neural science*, 3rd edn. New York: Elsevier.

Williams, P. L., Warwick, R., Dyson, M., & Bannister, L. H. (Eds). (1989). *Gray's Anatomy*, 37th edn (pp. 1094–123). Edinburgh: Churchill Livingstone.

JOHN P. FRAHER

Creutzfeldt–Jakob disease (also **Jakob–Creutzfeldt disease**) Creutzfeldt–Jakob disease is a transmissible dementing illness which runs a rapid course due to neuronal degeneration and astrocyte proliferation, the brain becoming riddled with small cavities. The illness is accompanied by seizures, but otherwise with variable neurological signs. The cause has been attributed to a slow-acting virus and to other genetic transmissible material. Parallels have been explored with kuru in humans, and with scrapie and bovine spongiform encephalitis in animals. Cannibalism has been blamed for its transmission in certain societies where this is practiced, and there are reports of its medical transmission in both living and post-mortem brain tissue.

critical period The critical period is a concept employed in the study of development to indicate the period of time during which a psychological skill is best learned. The evidence is most clear for the skills of walking, language, and sensorimotor coordination for which critical periods have been identified. If for some reason there is no opportunity for the skill to be learnt during the appropriate critical period, perhaps as a result of environmental restriction or ill health, then it will be much more difficult for the skill subsequently to be gained, and the normal level of skill is unlikely to be attained.

Similar effects have been observed in the development of other animals, the development of the visual system in kittens being the classic example, and the concept may also be extended to include critical periods for the biochemical sensitivity of systems important to normal development of the nervous system. It is inferred that the nervous system is organized for development in a way that facilitates certain kinds of learning at a particular stage.

crossed aphasia *See* APHASIA.

CT scan (also **CAT scan**) Computerized tomography scan (computerized axial tomography scan). (*See* SCAN.)

D

deblocking One of the strategies employed in APHASIA therapy is the deblocking method. In this method a successful response in an intact channel is used to evoke a response in a previously blocked channel. For example, a printed word, which the patient is able to recognize, is presented immediately before the same spoken word, previously not comprehended, to facilitate its comprehension. This may be regarded as a form of intermodality facilitation.

deep dyslexia *See* DYSLEXIA.

degenerative diseases In degenerative diseases there is a loss of neural tissue, either as a result of pathology of the nerve cells, or of the supportive tissues. Gross degeneration may lead to ATROPHY of the brain.

Acute neurological disease states may be associated with degeneration when the cause is ANOXIA, or else a DEMENTIA which is complicated by a cerebral infection. However, degenerative states are more commonly associated with chronic disease states, of which the principal examples are dementia of the Alzheimer type, multi-infarct dementia, PICK'S DISEASE, CREUTZFELDT–JAKOB DISEASE, normal pressure HYDROCEPHALUS, MULTIPLE SCLEROSIS, PARKINSON'S DISEASE, Schilder's disease, Wilson's disease, progressive supranuclear palsy, various encephalopathies, and progressive myoclonic epilepsy. The precise pathology differs among these various diseases, and the neuropsychological concomitants are also dependent on the pattern and sites of the degeneration. However, most of these conditions produce a diffuse loss of neural function across the cortex and within multiple subcortical structures; therefore they are associated with general and progressive cognitive decline, accompanied in many cases by changes in personality and affect.

déjà vu An inappropriate sense of familiarity with respect to novel objects or places is known as déjà vu (literally "already seen").

The more common use of the term relates to an altered perceptual experience during the aura preceding a temporal lobe seizure, often accompanied by other distortions of perception or feelings of derealization or depersonalization. The phenomenon is simply a change in the quality of recognition, with strong feelings of familiarity for whatever is the current focus of attention. It is presumed that some dysfunction of the memory systems contained within the anterior temporal lobe results in the faulty attribution of familiarity to novel or unfamiliar stimuli.

An alternative use of the term refers to the sensation in relation to visual HALLUCINATIONS, where the scene is clear and detailed in the sense of a vivid visual memory, where the patient has the sense of living through an already experienced event, often accompanied by the affective state which applied on the previous (real) occasion. These hallucinations are so vivid as to be more vivid and real than a film or video image, yet the patient does not believe in the reality of the experience.

The term déjà vu is also used more loosely to refer to any sense of inappropriate familiarity which may be reported by neurotic patients or even by normal subjects. Many normal subjects will report occasional sensations of déjà vu with respect to either objects or places, and the phenomenon alone in the absence of other neurological signs is not indicative of pathology. The conditions which produce déjà vu are similar to those which result in its converse, JAMAIS VU.

257

dementia Dementia is a generic term used to characterize acquired, intellectual (cognitive) impairment, usually, but not exclusively, resulting from pathological degeneration of cortical and/or subcortical cerebral structures. Vascular, metabolic, demyelinating, and infectious disorders are also known to cause dementia. Although historically controversial, the distinction between subcortical and cortical dementia has become increasingly utilized, in large part due to research which suggests that cortical dementia may differ significantly from subcortical dementia in many respects. As is suggested by the cortical–subcortical distinction, the neuropathology of dementia varies considerably. Dementia also varies with respect to age of onset, pathophysiology, pattern of neuropsychological impairment, and progression. Dementia does not appear to be a consequence of normal aging, although many of the neuropathological changes in dementia, particularly in dementia of the Alzheimer type (DAT), occur in normal aging and the prevalence of DAT increases significantly with age. In contrast, many dementias become initially apparent in the presenium, particularly those classified as subcortical dementias.

Subcortical dementia (axial dementia) is a controversial diagnostic concept used to describe a broad range of degenerative, vascular, metabolic, and demyelinating disorders. While cortical dementias are reportedly characterized by AMNESIA, APHASIA, APRAXIA, and AGNOSIA, symptoms of axial dementia principally include bradyphrenia, BRADYKINESIA, impairments in memory, abstraction, and reasoning, as well as abnormalities in mood (Cummings, 1990). Reports by Albert, Feldman, and Willis (1974) ignited a contemporary debate on axial dementia, although dementias presumably resulting from subcortical disease were described in some detail decades earlier (Mandell & Albert, 1990).

Criticism of the cortical–axial dichotomy has been focused on the supposed lack of clinical and neuropsychological evidence to support different diagnostic entities. In addition, a classification system based on theoretical independence of brain regions (cortical–subcortical) known to have intimate neuronal connections is thought to be untenable (Whitehouse, 1986). Debate regarding the diagnostic validity and utility of a cortical–axial dementia framework is likely to continue for some time, but recognition that dementias vary with respect to clinical presentation, neuropathology, and pathophysiological processes seems undisputed. Classification systems other than cortical–axial dichotomy have yet to be derived, but dementia can be discussed with respect to neuropathology, clinical progression, neuropsychological dysfunction, and psychopathology without resorting to formal nosology.

ALZHEIMER'S DISEASE

Dementia of the Alzheimer type (DAT) is currently thought to be the leading cause of dementia. Current estimates of incidence vary considerably and appear to be dependent on sample characteristics. Problems in diagnosis and longitudinal monitoring influence empirical findings, but conservative estimates suggest an incidence of approximately 6 percent in persons over 65 years of age. Familial DAT may account for as much as 20 percent of the reported cases and genetic studies have implicated several modes of possible inheritance (autosomal dominant, and polygenic–multifactorial). Although some studies suggest that familial DAT differs in many respects from sporadic (presumably non-inherited) DAT, recent research efforts have not found consistently substantive differences between familial and sporadic DAT with respect to neuropsychological presentation or clinical progression. Research continues to address the relationship between heritability, onset, clinical presentation, and progression of DAT.

Although the etiology of DAT is unknown, symptoms of illness are known to result from degeneration in cortical and possibly subcortical neurons. The presence of neurofibulary tangles, neuritic plaques, and granulovacular degeneration is characteristic. Histological abnormalities may have patterns rather than being random. Primary motor and sensory cortices appear relatively spared while certain limbic structures, especially the hippocampus, amygdala, and basal forebrain, are more dramatically affected. Recent autopsy studies suggest differential presence of neuritic plaques and neurofibulary tangles in the entorhinal cortex and subiculum (input–output from hippocampus), which is thought to effectively disconnect memory systems and produce the profound mnestic dysfunction observed in DAT (Damasio & Van Hoesen, 1986). Whether similar patterns of histological changes are consistent across large numbers of patients is not yet known.

Clinical criteria for the diagnosis of probable DAT include onset between ages 40 and 90, dementia documented by clinical examination and confirmed by neuropsychological assessment, impairment in two or more areas of cognitive functioning without a disturbance in consciousness (delirium), progressive worsening of cognitive dysfunction, and an absence of other CNS disease known to produce dementia (McKahnn et al., 1984). DAT is usually diagnosed long after onset of the illness. Retrospective analysis by family members often identifies symptoms (typically memory problems), that were ignored or minimized at the time they occurred. When patients present for neurological examination, disturbance in memory and other cognitive–linguistic functions is often quite apparent.

DAT is described as having numerous stages of progressively worsening memory, language, and visual spatial skills, as well as changes in personality. DAT often progresses in a generally predictable fashion (stages), but in some cases generalizations (mild, moderate, severe) fail to characterize the illness adequately. Nevertheless, in the initial phase of the disorder, impairment in new learning and memory is most obvious, while routine, over-learned tasks may be performed adequately. Sustained concentration is usually difficult and patients may begin avoiding situations where cognitive demands are high. Typical problems include "forgetting" things to be done (plans), previously familiar and especially novel persons (faces and/or names), and even personally significant events (episodic memory). Significant retrograde memory loss is often less apparent than anterograde memory impairment, and studies have shown that patients with DAT begin to evidence rapid forgetting of unfamiliar information. Dysfunctional encoding and retrieval processes have been implicated in the memory disturbance in DAT.

As the disorder progresses, disorientation becomes increasingly apparent, retrograde memory loss increases, and anterograde memory is most often severely impaired. There may be material asymmetry in memory impairment, but research is unclear on factors predisposing to material specific deficits. Unlike declarative memory, procedural memory or memory for skills (motoric) and habits appears relatively spared, and priming has been shown to facilitate recall.

Initially, language impairment is somewhat less apparent than mnestic disturbance and may be relatively absent in some patients until later stages of the illness. Most often though, verbal fluency is noticeably impaired and dysnomia is commonly observed. The semantic and/or perceptual components of naming may be impaired and category fluency is reported to be more impaired than letter fluency, presumably because of a disintegration in lexical–semantic processing. Less common variants of DAT include disproportionate impairment in language or visuospatial skills, with relative sparing of cognitive abilities typically affected earlier in the illness. Progressive aphasia "without dementia" has been reported as a distinct clinical syndrome (Mesulam, 1987), although more recent evidence suggests that persons with progressive aphasia eventually develop dementia.

Visuospatial impairment is typically less apparent than memory and language deficits although a relatively rapid and disproportionate decline in visuospatial skills may occur. In addition, visuospatial dysfunction is often exacerbated by memory deficits. Failure to learn novel routes or faces is common, as is being lost in familiar places, but whether these deficits reflect primary visuospatial dysfunction is unclear. Impairment in perceptual discrimination, constructional skills, and visuospatial problem-solving abilities are common. Visuospatial abilities, like other skills dependent on heteromodal cortices, disintegrate as the disease progresses.

Personality change and psychiatric disturbance commonly occur in DAT, although the presence of symptoms varies considerably across patients, depending on premorbid personality as well as stage and progression of the illness. The Diagnostic and Statistical Manual of Mental Disorders (DSM IV) identifies four psychiatric subtypes of DAT including dementia with delirium, delusions, depression, and uncomplicated progression. The incidence of each subtype varies, but the frequency of depressive and delusional subtypes are reported to be most common.

Mood disturbance (dysphoria) may be present in the early stages of the illness, especially when awareness of cognitive deficits remains intact. In some cases disturbances in mood persists, but in many cases dysphoria is reported to be transitory. As the disease progresses, paranoid mentation and delusions commonly occur, possibly due to patients' attempts to organize extrapersonal stimuli without functional memory and cognitive systems. For example, patients commonly believe they are being stolen from, have unfaithful spouses, or are about to be abandoned. Misidentification syndromes are commonly observed. Hallucinations occur less frequently than delusions, but are observable in a number of patients.

As indicated by the National Institute of Neurologic and Communicative Disorders and Stroke (NINCDS) diagnostic criteria (McKahnn et al., 1984), neuropsychological assessment plays a significant role in diagnosis at present. Assessment strategies vary considerably, but the Consortium to Establish a Registry for Alzheimer's Disease (CERAD) has recommended a standardized assessment strategy which includes measures of various language, memory, and visuospatial skills (Morris et al., 1989). Existing research has demonstrated the diagnostic sensitivity of the CERAD protocol. Delayed recall and confrontation naming have been shown to be especially sensitive in detecting mild DAT, but due to the relatively early and severe impairment of memory in DAT, lexical–semantic and visuospatial measures are thought to be the most appropriate methods for assessing progression of the illness (Welsh et al., 1992).

Clinicians and researchers specializing in dementia recommend that, whenever possible, problem-solving, reasoning, attention, language, visuospatial and memory measures be included in dementia assessments. Recommended tests vary, but all tests used should be appropriate for elderly persons (length, required effort, age norms, education level), sensitive to changes in cognition, and reliable. Considering the consequences of false positive diagnoses, conservative interpretation of neuropsychological tests is recommended. Some authors provide strict interpretive guidelines or cutting scores, while others utilize pattern analysis or more qualitative interpretation of test data.

By design, most research endeavors rigorously select patients for inclusion, most often excluding patients with serious medical problems, psychiatric illnesses, or multiple dementing disorders. While selection in research is necessary for methodological reasons, most patients presenting for assessment in clinics and hospitals have complex medical psychiatric histories which complicate the diagnostic process. Therefore recommendations based on research with highly selected populations need to be applied judiciously in most clinical situations.

Efficacious treatment for dementia is unavailable at the present time. Drugs typically used to facilitate cholinergic systems (choline, lethicin) have not proved helpful in reducing cognitive –linguistic dysfunction in DAT. A number of potentially therapeutic drugs are being evaluated, and some patients have shown statistically significant changes on neuropsychological tests following drug therapy, but the clinical significance of these results has yet to be determined. In any case, early diagnosis, family education, environmental management, and proper follow-up are important. Documented variability in the rate of cognitive and behavioral decline in DAT suggests some patients may maintain a stable level of cognitive functioning for many years while others may show rather rapid deterioration requiring medical/psychiatric supervision and hospitalization. Structuring the environment to reduce cognitive demands while providing appropriate but not intrusive supervision can enable many persons who have DAT to function adequately outside an institution, at least until the later stages of the illness.

VASCULAR DEMENTIA

Multi-infarct dementia, now referred to as vascular dementia, is reported to be second only to DAT in incidence. Some researchers feel vascular dementia is underdiagnosed, while others suggest the incidence of vascular dementia is considerably overestimated. A number of researchers argue that patients with vascular dementia are more likely to experience sudden death due to cardiac disease, which may inflate estimates of DAT, particularly if epidemiological studies focus on elderly hospitalized populations. In addition, the relatively frequent occurrence of hypothesized etiological factors (cardiac disease, hypertension, stroke, systemic disease) suggests that vascular dementias may be more common than is documented at present, but debate regarding the incidence of vascular dementia alone and in combination with DAT continues (Joynt, 1988).

As with dementia in general, some researchers classify vascular dementia as cortical or axial disorders (Chui, 1989). Classification schemes may also consider pattern of infarcts, vessel size, infarcted structures, and supposed "principal features" of related dementia (Cummings & Benson, 1992). Using these criteria, several distinct types of vascular disorders have been identified, including lacunar dementia, Binswanger's disease, and cortical vascular dementia.

Lacunar dementia describes a condition characterized by ischemia in arterioles innervating subcortical structures, typically the striatum, thalamus and external capsule. Multiple ischemic events are necessary to qualify for a diagnosis of lacunar dementia. In contrast, Binswanger's disease is characterized by an apparent progressive demyelination and atrophy of subcortical white matter, as well as the presence of arteriosclerosis and the lacunae observed in lacunar dementia. Both disorders appear to be associated with hypertension and systemic vascular disease.

Cortical infarctions are also reported to produce dementia, although many persons suffer more than one cerebrovascular event (stroke) without developing dementia. Dominant hemisphere infarctions typically produce well-documented language disturbances which complicate cognitive assessment and documentation of the decline necessary for a diagnosis of dementia. Nondominant cerebrovascular events also result in characteristic impairment in attention (neglect), regulation, awareness (anosognosia), prosody, and visuospatial skills.

Neuropsychological sequelae of vascular dementia depend to a large extent on the type of disorder and findings which are for the most part quite variable. Impairment in intellectual, reasoning, attention, language (fluency naming) and memory skills has been documented (Almkvist et al., 1992). In some cases the neuropsychological sequelae of vascular dementia are indistinguishable from those found in DAT, but vascular dementia is reported to produce disproportionate motor and sensory deficits compared to DAT. Motor deficits may include extrapyramidal symptoms and specific disorders, such as thalamic vascular dementia, are reported to occur.

Psychiatric symptoms of vascular dementia have not been researched extensively. Abulia, dysphoria, labile affect (pseudobulbar), and anosognosia are common sequelae of vascular dementia. Depressive disorders are thought to be intimately related to cortical and subcortical cerebrovascular disease. In many cases, frontal subcortical lesions produce changes in arousal, attention, prosody, and awareness that are classified as affective disorder, but on closer examination they appear quantitatively and qualitatively distinct from typical affective illness.

Treatment for vascular dementia is primarily preventive in nature. Common risk factors may be addressed, but once dementia is apparent, intervention for hypertension, cardiac disease, or systemic disease may slow but not reverse the dementia process. Since the severity of dementia seems related to the volume of impaired brain tissue (Mielk et al., 1992) medical interventions to slow or minimize further vascular events are strongly recommended.

HIV

Unlike vascular dementia and DAT, dementia resulting from human immunodeficiency virus (HIV) is known to have an infectious etiology. HIV encephalopathy or AIDS dementia complex (ADC) usually becomes apparent at some point in the evolution of the disorder. HIV dementia progresses rapidly, possibly reflecting the momentum of the illness, but there also appears to be considerable variability in onset and progression. Autopsy studies have shown numerous pathological changes in subcortical white matter and nuclei, but the precise pathophysiological basis for dementia in ADC is yet to be determined.

Dementia is common in the later stages of the illness, but cognitive symptoms have been reported to be evident even prior to seroconversion. Bradyphrenia, impaired attention, decreased concentration, and impaired fine motor speed coordination may be observed early in the illness. Once the disease has progressed, more significant impairment in mental flexibility and speed, attention, sequential processing, visual motor skills, and memory functions becomes apparent.

Recent National Institute of Mental Health (NIMH) proposals regarding assessment strategies recommend test batteries which include measures of intelligence, attention, processing speed, memory, abstraction, language, visual/spatial skills, as well as construction and motor abilities (Butters et al., 1990). Recommended abbreviated versions of this battery emphasize assessment of vocabulary skills, verbal memory, visual memory, mood and anxiety. Since neuropsychological deficits may appear earlier than other symptoms of AIDS, the NIH workshop group concluded that early identification of cognitive impairment has the potential to provide valuable information for drug efficacy studies as well as treatment planning.

EXTRAPYRAMIDAL DISORDERS

Numerous degenerative disorders, such as Parkinson's disease, Huntington's disease, progressive supernuclear palsy (Steel–Richardson–Olszewski syndrome), Hallervorden–Spatz disease, Wilson's disease, and others are known to cause dementia. Except for Parkinson's disease, which is relatively common, these disorders are rare and they differ with respect to age of onset, pathophysiology, clinical presentation, and neuropsychological dysfunction.

Parkinson's disease is usually diagnosed in middle age (40–60 years) while progressive supernuclear palsy (PSP) becomes evident much later in life (60–70 years). In contrast, Hallervorden–Spatz and Wilson's disease most often manifest themselves in childhood to early adulthood. Parkinson's disease is by far the most common extrapyramidal disorder producing dementia. Huntington's disease, which results in psychiatric symptoms, profound chorea, and dementia, is much less common, as are PSP, Wilson's disease, and Hallervorden–Spatz.

The neuropathological process varies considerably in these diseases. Parkinson's disease is characterized by nigrostriatal degeneration, and the presence of Lewy bodies, but diverse changes in subcortical structures may also occur. Dopaminergic systems are severely depleted and the impact on motor functions is profound. In some cases of Parkinson's disease, cortical changes found in DAT (neurofibrillary tangles and senile plaques) are also observed. Huntington's disease affects the neostriatum (caudate, putamen, and globus pallidus) although histological changes in the thalamus and other structures may also be apparent. The cortex may or may not be involved, but the cerebellum and brain stem are reportedly spared. Hallervorden–Spatz characteristically affects the globus pallidus and substantia nigra, while Wilson's disease is known for progressive lenticular degeneration due to excessive unbound copper. Differences in neuropathology, pathophysiology, and onset progression make comparison of these disorders somewhat difficult, but there is reported to be similarity in neuropsychological impairment.

Consistent with the concept of subcortical dementia, a person suffering from these disorders tends to show bradyphrenia, bradykinesia, impairments in attention, concentration, and memory, with a general absence of significant language disturbance. Huntington's disease is somewhat atypical in the sense that changes in personality are reported to occur prior to obvious disturbance in cognition.

Symptoms in Parkinson's disease (PD) include bradykinesia, resting tremor, cogwheel rigidity, micrographia, hypophonia, and dysarthria. Although dementia commonly occurs in PD, prevalence estimates vary, and the neuropsychological characteristics are reported to be heterogeneous. In general though, bradyphrenia and memory dysfunction are prominent features of the illness, but unlike DAT, procedural memory appears impaired. Language skills (naming and fluency) are usually less affected in PD compared to DAT, but speech is clearly dysfunctional (dysarthria, dysprosody, decreased phrase length). Visuospatial, visual motor, and executive regulatory deficits are also observed.

Huntington's disease is also known to be characterized by impairments in attention and concentration early in the illness. Studies comparing memory dysfunction in Huntington's disease, Korsakoff's disease and DAT have found impaired retrieval and procedural learning, but generally spared recognition recall in Huntington's disease, at least on verbal tests. Like Parkinson's disease, Huntington's disease patients evidence impaired performance on most motor tests, therefore performance on constructional and visual-motor measures usually reveals considerable impairment.

At the present time, treatment of these disorders is palliative, although early intervention in Wilson's disease may result in reversal of the dementia process. Levodopa, combined with carbodopa, is common therapy for Parkinson's disease. Huntington's disease is usually treated with haloperidol, which reduces choreiform movements. Numerous other drugs have been applied to the treatment of these illnesses without success. Drug efficacy studies continue to search for agents which can slow or reverse the disease process in extrapyramidal disorders.

Neuropsychological evaluation strategies vary, but assessment of attention, concentration, memory, language, motor functions, as well as reasoning and abstraction, is recommended. Due to the common presence of anxiety dysphoria, psychosis, and suicidality, psychiatric measurement techniques are also included in most clinical and research trials (Huber & Shuttleworth, 1990).

PSEUDODEMENTIA

Pseudodementia is the term most often used to describe reversible cognitive impairment resulting from psychiatric illnesses, as opposed to a degenerative central nervous system disorder. Major affective disorder (depression) is the most common "pseudodementia" although other psychiatric disturbances such as mania or schizophrenia are considered to be capable of producing symptoms of dementia.

Recent theoretical models suggest pseudodementia, depression in particular, may be best classified as an axial dementia (Cummings & Benson, 1992). Severe depression is known to result in symptoms (bradyphrenia, bradykinesia, impaired attention, concentration, memory and vegetative disturbance) typically observed in axial dementia. In contrast, some theoretical models attempting to account for the diversity of symptoms in depressive disorders emphasize the interplay between cortical and subcortical systems.

Pseudodementia has been shown to exist independently of dementia, although the conditions often coexist. Pseudodementia has also been shown to be stable over time, suggesting that the illness is not a prelude to the development of a "genuine" dementing disorder. Finally, depressive disorders are commonly associated with neurological illness. Symptoms of depression, such as anhedonia, bradykinesia, bradyphrenia, dysphoria, and hypoarousal are frequently observed in patients with cerebrovascular, traumatic, and non-dementing degenerative disorders. In spite of symptoms of depression, many of these patients do not show signs of pseudodementia.

Neuropsychological assessment may be helpful in diagnosing pseudodementia. While memory tests may not adequately discriminate pseudodementias, recognition memory is usually better preserved. In addition, changes in language, gnosis, and praxis typically observed in dementia, particularly DAT, are typically not observed in pseudodementia.

Treatment is clearly available for pseudo-

dementia and the disorder may be completely reversible. Antidepressants, lithium, and under the right circumstances electroconvulsive therapy (ECT) may be used to treat this disorder. Response to intervention is limited by factors normally operative in psychiatric treatment of the elderly.

CONCLUSION

Many disorders of differing etiology may cause dementia. In addition to the degenerative, vascular, infectious, and other disorders discussed, dementia may be caused by numerous neuropathological processes not presented here. Various toxic-metabolic, neoplastic, traumatic, and genetic disorders may also cause dementia (Cummings & Benson, 1992). Increased understanding of the pattern and progression of neurobehavioral deficits in dementia has assisted development of diagnostic and classification criteria. In the future, neuropsychological assessment will continue to play a significant role in diagnosis, classification, and measurement of treatment outcome in dementia.

BIBLIOGRAPHY

Albert, M. L., Feldman, R. G., & Willis, A. L. (1974). The "subcortical dementia" of progressive supranuclear palsy. *Journal of Neurology, Neurosurgery and Psychiatry, 37*, 121–30.

Almkvist, O., Wahlund, L., Andersson-Lundman, G., Basun, H., & Backman, L. (1992). White matter hyperintensity and neuropsychological functions in dementia and health in aging, *Archives of Neurology, 49*, 626–32.

Butters, N., Grant, I., Haxby, J., Judd, L. L., Martin, A., McClelland, J., Peguegnate, W., Schacter, D., & Stover, E. (1990). Assessment of age-related cognitive changes: Recommendation of the NIMH Workshop on neuropsychological assessment approaches. *Journal of Clinical and Experimental Neuropsychology, 12*, 963–78.

Chui, H. C. (1989). Dementia: a review emphasizing clinical pathologic correlation and brain-behavioral relationships. *Archives of Neurology, 46*, 806–14.

Cummings, J. L. (1990). Subcortical dementia: Introduction. In J. L. Cummings (Ed.), *Subcortical dementia* (pp. 3–16). New York: Oxford University Press.

Cummings, J. L., & Benson, D. F. (1992). *Dementia: A clinical approach*. Boston: Butterworth-Heinemann.

Damasio, A. R., & Van Hoesen, G. W. (1986). Neuroanatomical correlates of amnesia in Alzheimer's disease. In A. B. Scheibel, A. F. Wechessler, & N. A. B. Bazier (Eds), *The biological substrates of Alzheimer's disease* (pp. 65–72). Orlando: Academic Press.

Huber, S. J., & Shuttleworth, E. C. (1990). Neuropsychological assessment of subcortical dementia. In J. L. Cummings (Ed.), *Subcortical dementia* (pp. 71–86). New York: Oxford University Press.

Joynt, R. J. (1988). Vascular dementia: Too much or too little? *Archives of Neurology, 45,* 801.

McKahnn, G., Drachman, D., Fostein, M., Katzman, R., & Price, D. (1984). Clinical diagnosis of Alzheimer's disease: Report of the NINCDS-ADRDA Workgroup under the auspices of the Department of Health and Human Services Task Force on Alzheimer's disease. *Neurology, 34,* 939–44.

Mandell, A. N., & Albert, M. K. (1990). History of subcortical dementia. In J. L. Cummings (Ed.), *Subcortical dementia* (pp. 17–30). New York: Oxford University Press.

Mesulam, M.-M. (1987). Primary progressive aphasia: differentiation from Alzheimer's disease. *Annals of Neurology, 37,* 448–53.

Mielke, R., Herholz, K., Gond, M., Kessler, J., & Heiss, W. D. (1992). Severity of vascular dementia is related to volume of metabolically impaired tissue. *Archives of Neurology, 49,* 909–15.

Morris, J. C., Heyman, A., Moh, R. C., Hughes, J. D. van Belle, G., Fillenbaum, E. D., Mellitis, E., Clark, C., & CERAD investigators. (1989). The Consortium to Establish a Registry for Alzheimer's Disease (CERAD). Part I. Clinical and neuropsychological assessment of Alzheimer's disease. *Neurology, 39,* 1159–65.

Welsh, K. A., Butters, N., Hughes, J. P., Moh, R. C., & Heyman, A. (1992). Detection and staging of dementia in Alzheimer's disease: use of the neuropsychological measures developed for the Consortium to Establish a Registry for Alzheimer's Disease. *Archives of Neurology, 49,* 448–52.

Whitehouse, P. J. (1986). The concept of subcortical and cortical dementia: another look. *Annals of Neurology, 19,* 1–6.

STEPHEN N. MACCIOCHI AND JEFFREY T. BARTH

denervation hypersensitivity Among the processes hypothesized to occur during recovery, central denervation hypersensitivity is one of the more controversial. The essential idea is that certain central structures become more responsive following damage as the remaining active fibers from the damaged region exert a greater effect on the region which has been denervated and promote recovery. Hypersensitivity has been most clearly observed in effector organs of the autonomic nervous system, but has also been observed in structures of the central nervous system. However, the opposite effect, that initial hypersensitivity could induce inhibition of function by DIASCHISIS, has also been argued.

denial Denial, the statement that some state of affairs does not exist, is a feature of a number of neuropsychological phenomena. It may alternatively be referred to as ANOSOGNOSIA.

Evidence of denial can be obtained not only from explicit statements which the patient may make, refusing to accept the presence of some disability, but also from the failure to spontaneously report the disability, a failure to make any complaint. The patient may recognize the disability, but yet have no emotional response to the difficulty. An affected limb may be disowned by the patient, or a hemiplegic limb described as tired, weak, or numb, and may be referred to in the third person ("it . . ." rather than "my . . .").

There are various explanations for denial, including the psychodynamic form of repression motivated by an instinctive urge to maintain the body's integrity. Denial may be a pre-existing personality characteristic which is employed as a defense mechanism in the face of the threat posed by the illness. Goldstein referred to denial as "a quite normal biological reaction to a very grave threat."

Other explanations of denial relate more specifically to the context in which it is expressed. Denial is not uncommonly seen in association with disorders of BODY SCHEMA so that the patient not only neglects one half of the body, but denies the existence of these defects, or alternatively disowns the relevant affected limbs. This phenomenon could be due to the psychodynamic explanation, to alterations in attention to the body parts, or to a defective body schema. The point has been raised that none of these explanations satisfactorily accounts for the preponderance of right (usually parietal) lesions leading to left-sided symptoms, and the counter-objection that left-sided lesions are likely to render the patient aphasic and so make the denial less apparent, is not entirely persuasive. It may be important to distinguish between denial associated with emotional flattening (ANOSODIAPHORIA), which might be associated with specific right hemisphere emotional systems, from explicit denial of illness (verbal anosognosia); interestingly, frank denial may abate to emotional flattening and a degree of indifference during the process of recovery. Disconnection between the cerebral hemispheres (*see* DISCONNECTION SYNDROME) has also been employed as an explanation of denial, in that the right hemisphere lesion may serve to disconnect the relevant somesthetic information received in the right hemisphere from its recognition and interpretation in the language-based left hemisphere. None of these explanations fully accounts for frank denial of illness.

Denial of CORTICAL BLINDNESS is known as ANTON'S SYNDROME, and may result from the destruction of both primary and secondary visual cortex together. Denial also occurs as a common feature in the AMNESIC SYNDROME following chronic alcoholism, although not following encephalitis. Patients with APRAXIA may also exhibit denial, and in this context it appears at least as frequently among dysphasic patients with right-sided hemiparesis.

The bizarre circumstances of the CAPGRAS SYNDROME may also involve some form of denial. The essential feature of this rare disorder is that the patient believes that individuals who appear familiar, usually close family members, are in fact imposters who have assumed an identical appearance. In the case originally described, the patient, as a result of a vivid hallucinatory experience, believed the relevant family members to be dead and had no memory of his head injury owing to his severe memory deficit. The resulting behavior can then be understood in terms of both denial and confabulation.

It may be mistaken to expect a single explanation for the variety of contexts in which denial of illness or denial of specific disability may be expressed. It occurs in association with a number of quite distinct neuropsychological states, and it may be that its origin in these various states is not dependent on the same dysfunctional process.

J. GRAHAM BEAUMONT

depersonalization Depersonalization is the loss of the sense of personal identity, coherence, or location and is an abnormality of the perception of self. It is common among all neuropsychological states, although it may be poorly expressed. It appears to result from a dissolution of the perceptual boundaries between inner conscious experience and the experience of the external environment, a failure to distinguish between self and non-self, and may be accompanied by an alarming sense of the imminent loss of bodily or personal integrity.

Depersonalization is particularly characteristic of certain temporal lobe lesions in the company of other psychotic schizophreniform disturbances and personality changes. In this context, the phenomenon may also be a feature of the aura preceding temporal lobe seizures in association with other perceptual disturbances such as DÉJÀ VU and JAMAIS VU.

depression In everyday use, the term "depression" denotes a transient lowering of mood, a mixture of sadness and inertia. Depression of clinical severity is far more complex, involving changes in mood, thought, activity, social behavior, and vegetative functions. Mood is sad or empty, and responses to pleasurable events are reduced or absent (anhedonia); thoughts center on themes of hopelessness, helplessness, worthlessness, and guilt; fatigue is prominent, normal levels of activity require great effort, and ability to concentrate is reduced; social interaction is diminished; sexual behavior, appetite, and weight are decreased; and sleep is poor. Frequently there are marked diurnal variations, usually with improvements toward the evening. No one symptom is invariably present; all symptoms may also occur in other conditions.

The central features of depression are a profound lowering of mood (described as depressed, sad, hopeless, not caring, or unable to experience pleasure), and/or a loss of interest or pleasure in usual activities or pastimes, which is often more obvious to observers than to the individual affected. Feelings of worthlessness and guilt can be so excessive and inappropriate as to reach delusional proportions ("psychotic depression") and thoughts of suicide (sometimes accompanied by suicide attempts) are common. Severe depressions are usually accompanied by a prominent psychomotor agitation or retardation (sometimes both): characteristic agitated behaviors include an inability to sit still, pacing, hand-wringing, pulling of hair or clothing, and outbursts of shouting, complaining, or crying; retardation refers to slowed body movements, a decrease in amount of speech, with protracted pauses, and a lack of facial animation.

The most important subclassification of depression is into two major subtypes, endogenous, also known as "melancholia," and reactive. The distinction between "endogenous" and "reactive" depressions is often thought to refer to whether the depression has an obvious precipitant (reactive) or not (endogenous); a corollary of this position is the belief that while reactive depressions are "psychological" in origin, endogenous depressions result from some form of spontaneous brain malfunction. These views are mistaken, and have been a source of much confusion. The endogenous/reactive distinction does not refer to causation, but rather to a crucial aspect of the clinical picture: a reactive patient is one whose mood "reacts" to psychosocial intervention. In other words, the reactive patient can be cheered up but the endogenous patient cannot. Endogenous depressions are usually, though not always, more severe than nonendogenous ones; the presence of pronounced psychomotor change almost invariably denotes an endogenous depression. Other "biological" symptoms, such as weight loss, also tend to be associated with the endogenous subtype, as do certain neuroendocrine and neurophysiological "markers," in particular increased activity in the hypothalamus-pituitary-adrenal (HPA) system and decreased latency to enter the first period of rapid eye movement (REM) sleep.

Another important distinction is between unipolar and bipolar depressions. Depression is a recurrent disorder, which is likely to reoccur 4–5 years after the first episode, and subsequently with a shorter and shorter period between episodes. In bipolar disorder, episodes of mania or hypomania are interspersed between the episodes of depression. The depressive pole of bipolar disorder tends to be of the endogenous type, and thus less variable than unipolar depression. Otherwise, unipolar and bipolar depressions do not differ in their symptomatology.

The great majority of neuropsychological studies of depressed patients have tended to use diagnostically heterogeneous groups, and there are relatively few unipolar/bipolar and endogenous/nonendogenous comparisons. On the basis of similarities and differences in depressive symptomatology, endogenous/nonendogenous differences might be expected in neuropsychological performance, while unipolar/bipolar differences might not. However, there are at present few indications that performance relates clearly to either classification. Furthermore, it is likely that neuropsychological performance differs between medicated (but nonrecovered) and unmedicated patients, but there are currently few data in this area. There are certainly instances of tests in which differences between endogenous/nonendogenous, unipolar/bipolar or medicated/nonmedicated patients have been reported, but little evidence that any of these results can be reliably replicated. For this reason, the following account of neuropsychological test performance in depressed patients makes no attempt to relate impairments to diagnostic subgroups or medication status. However, it must be recognized that the paucity of information on well-defined subgroups is far from ideal, since these factors are almost certainly responsible for at least some of the inconsistencies in the data.

THE CEREBRAL CORTEX AND DEPRESSION

Studies of the perception and expression of emotions in normal subjects provide a backdrop against which to consider the clinical evidence. Emotions are more readily perceived with left ear or left visual hemifield presentation, and are expressed more strongly on the left side of the face, implying a localization within the right hemisphere; these functions are correspondingly impaired by right hemispheric damage. However, there is also evidence that some aspects of the perception and expression of positive emotions are controlled by the left hemisphere. In depression there is a shift in the salience of emotionally negative material (increased) relative to that of emotionally positive material (decreased), and this would be consistent with an increase in activation of the right hemisphere relative to the left.

Evidence from a number of sources supports this concept. EEG studies of depressed patients have tended to find a relatively greater activation (EEG desynchronization) in right frontal regions relative to left frontal regions, and leftward eye movements tend to be increased in depressed patients (presumably, reflecting a relatively greater activation of the right FRONTAL EYE FIELDS). Further evidence for a decrease in left hemispheric activation is provided by observations of decreased energy metabolism in the left frontal cortex of depressed patients, as revealed by PET scanning studies, as well as abnormalities of cerebral blood flow in the same region. Another line of evidence, difficult to interpret but supportive of the concept of a differential involvement of the two hemispheres, comes from studies demonstrating that unilateral electroconvulsive therapy (ECT) applied to the nondominant (right) hemisphere is as effective in the treatment of depression as bilateral ECT, and in some studies superior to bilateral ECT, but unilateral ECT applied to the dominant (left) hemisphere is clearly inferior to bilateral ECT.

On the basis of these data, it might be expected that damage to the dominant hemisphere might cause depression, but damage to the nondominant hemisphere would not. However, the clinical picture is far more complex. As predicted, there are many reports of depressive CATASTROPHIC REACTIONS following left hemispheric damage, and of INDIFFERENCE or euphoria following right hemispheric damage. However, some studies, including the largest (Lishman, 1973), have reported a high frequency of depression in patients with right hemisphere lesions. The picture becomes clearer when the location of the damage is considered. Within the left hemisphere, the severity of depression increases with proximity to the frontal pole. However, within the right hemisphere, indifference/euphoric reactions are associated with anterior lesions, while depressions tend to result from more posterior lesions; consistent with a posterior locus are studies reporting abnormalities of right posterior cerebral blood flow in depressed patients (Jeste et al., 1988). It must be emphasized that, while the concept of a left anterior-right posterior axis is a useful heuristic device, many cases of depression have been reported following cortical damage outside these areas. However, the significance of these cases remains to be determined. There are numerous pitfalls in the way of a clear interpretation of depressive reactions in brain-damaged patients; for example, few studies have used appropriate intact or physically impaired control groups, and psychiatric histories are rarely provided.

NEUROPSYCHOLOGICAL TEST PERFORMANCE

A recent comprehensive review of studies of neuropsychological test performance in depressed patients (Cassens et al., 1990) confirms the initial report of Flor-Henry (1976) of a pervasive impairment in nonverbal functions traditionally ascribed to the nondominant hemisphere. Although the data are not wholly consistent, impairments are usually reported in a wide variety of tests of visual or tactile memory, and in tests of visuospatial or visuomotor skill. An impairment of right hemisphere function is also indicated by perceptual asymmetries in depressed patients, such as a poor left-ear performance in DICHOTIC LISTENING tasks. Consistent with these findings, and in particular, with impairment on visuospatial tasks such as the Categories Test, depression is frequently associated with low WAIS-R performance IQ scores.

Impairments are also seen in verbal tasks, but these are less comprehensive and, in most cases, less consistent. It is also unclear whether the impairments are related to verbal test content as such, rather than other task-related features, such as task complexity or test duration. Thus, depressed patients usually have a normal WAIS verbal IQ, and six studies out of seven found no impairment of auditory verbal short-term memory (digit span); paired associate learning was impaired in only two studies out of five, while six studies out of seven found impaired list recall and seven studies out of nine found impairments of story recall (Cassens et al., 1990). A similar pattern may be discerned in tests of receptive verbal skills; for example, depressed patients show impaired story comprehension, but no impairment of ability to repeat sentences.

Interpretation of the verbal test performance data is complicated by the presence in depressed patients of a general mental slowing, as revealed, for example, in finger-tapping, pegboard and trail-making tasks, or increased speech pause time. It is likely that nonspecific factors of this kind, related to motivational or motor impairments, are responsible for at least some of the verbal impairments. This seems a plausible way to account for a decrease in verbal fluency, and could in principle explain impairments of, for example, story comprehension and recall. However, the possibility of genuine verbal performance deficits, either across the board or in

267

subgroups of patients, cannot at present be discounted.

Some of the deficits discussed, such as verbal fluency, motor speed, and verbal memory, are consistent with a functional impairment of the left frontal cortex, as expected on the basis of the PET scanning studies, and depressive reactions following left frontal damage. Impairments are also sometimes observed in other tests of frontal function, such as the Stroop Test and proverb interpretation. However, deficits on "frontal" tests are observed less reliably than impairments of nonverbal performance. For example, a group of depressed patients studied by Hart and others (1987) showed impaired performance on the WAIS Block Design and Digit-Symbol subtests, but performed normally in a right-left discrimination test and in the Wisconsin Card Sorting Test. This discrepancy might reflect a lesser sensitivity of "frontal" tests or a lesser degree of frontal impairment in depressed patients, relative to their right posterior deficits. However, it is clear that the between-groups design of these studies is at least partly responsible, since individual depressed patients may perform as poorly in the Wisconsin Card Sorting Test as patients with known frontal lobe damage (Cassens et al., 1990).

To summarize, the neuropsychological test performance of depressed patients is consistent with pronounced deficits of right posterior cortical functioning and with less pervasive, but sometimes equally severe, left frontal dysfunction. However, at the level of the individual patient, a wide variety of patterns of impairment are observed, ranging from patients in whom neuropsychological performance is relatively intact, through patients with predominantly visuospatial deficits, to patients with a global pseudodementia. Crucially, the degree of neuropsychological impairment is not correlated with the severity of depression (Cassens et al., 1990).

The functional significance of neuropsychological impairments in depression is currently unknown. However, these deficits, when present, are markers of the depressed state; neuropsychological test performance improves when the depression is successfully treated with antidepressant drugs or ECT, and there is no evidence of neuropsychological deficits following recovery.

POSSIBLE RELATIONSHIP TO NEUROCHEMICAL CHANGES

The lack of correlation between severity of depression and performance deficits in tests of cortical functioning serves to redirect attention to subcortical mechanisms in the control of mood. For example, there has been considerable recent interest in the finding of CT scanning studies that the cerebral ventricles are enlarged in a subgroup of schizophrenic patients, characterized by predominantly negative symptoms: it is less well known that exactly the same pathology, of a similar magnitude, is seen in a similar proportion (around 20 percent) of depressed patients (Jeste et al., 1988). However, the primary focus of interest in relation to depression has for many years been the monoamine NEUROTRANSMITTERS, serotonin (5-HT), noradrenaline (NA), and more recently, dopamine (DA). For most practical purposes, direct methods are not available to study the neurochemistry of the living human brain. The evidence of neurochemical abnormalities therefore derives largely from post-mortem studies and from indirect sources, such as measurement of the levels of neurotransmitter metabolites in the blood or CEREBROSPINAL FLUID (CSF).

It is outside the scope of this entry to discuss in detail the evidence that depression is associated with alterations of neurotransmitter function, but some aspects of the organization of the monoaminergic systems and their functioning in mood disorders are germane to an understanding of the neuropsychology of depression. The cell bodies of the major pathways in all systems are located in a small number of compact nuclei in the hindbrain and midbrain. Their axons run forward in well-defined pathways, but then diverge to terminate in wide areas of the forebrain. The postsynaptic actions of monoamine transmitters are relatively long-lasting, and although there is some topographical organization within each system, the cells within each nucleus tend to fire synchronously, resulting in the simultaneous release of transmitter throughout the area of innervation. This mode of functioning suggests that the monoamine systems act to bias or modulate activity states in the forebrain, rather than to carry precise information.

The best-established neurochemical abnormality in depression is a decrease in CSF concentrations of the DA metabolite homovanillic acid in a group of patients who display pronounced psychomotor retardation, suggesting a reduction in the release of DA in these patients. DA neurons are an important component of the motor output system of the brain, and it remains unclear whether decreased DA activity is causal in depression, or simply reflects the decreased motor output of retarded patients. However, the high incidence of depression associated with PARKINSON'S DISEASE (which results from the degeneration of DA neurons) suggests a causal role for DA depletion. A decrease in DA function could explain the mental slowing of depressed patients, as revealed in tests such as verbal fluency. Interestingly, the dorsolateral prefrontal cortex is the only area of the cerebral cortex that is significantly innervated by DA neurons. Furthermore, there is evidence that, in humans, DA is preferentially involved in left hemisphere functions (Tucker & Williamson, 1984); for example, a significant correlation has been reported between CSF HVA and EVOKED POTENTIALS recorded from the left hemisphere, but not the right. These observations make it plausible that the left frontal deactivation observed in depressed patients, and the associated "frontal" performance deficits, may be related to a decrease in DA release within the frontal cortex.

A second major abnormality is a decrease in CSF concentrations of the 5HT metabolite 5-hydroxyindoleacetic acid (5HIAA). This abnormality is associated more closely with suicide and personality disorder than with depression as such, and is also seen in other disorders, such as bulimia nervosa; it is thought that this marker relates to poor impulse control, rather than depression per se. In general, studies that have identified a decrease in CSF 5HIAA in depressed patients have also reported the same abnormality in mania and following recovery; low CSF 5HIAA appears to be a trait marker rather than a marker for the depressed state. If this is correct, then changes in 5HT function are unlikely to be implicated in the neuropsychological deficits, which are absent following recovery.

Studies of NA metabolism in depression are conflicting and difficult to interpret, for technical reasons that are not discussed here. However, some of the hormonal (increased HPA activity) and EEG (decreased REM sleep latency) markers of depression are consistent with a reduced level of NA function, which accords with some of the

biochemical data. While the precise nature of the NA abnormality remains controversial, what is clear is that the various markers of NA activity normalize on recovery. The functions of NA in the forebrain have also proved difficult to elucidate, but a consensus has developed around the view that the NA innervation of the cerebral cortex is involved primarily in attention and the efficient processing of information. There is also some evidence that NA may be preferentially involved in right hemisphere function. Lesions to the right, but not the left, frontal cortex have been reported to cause an antidepressant-reversible hyperactivity in rats, as well as a depletion of cortical NA; and these effects were also seen in animals subjected to a neurotoxic lesion that selectively destroyed NA (and DA) neurons in the right (but not the left) frontal lobe (Robinson & Stitt, 1981). NA neurons enter the cortex at the anterior pole, but diverge to provide a relatively uniform distribution of terminals throughout the cortex. Abnormal levels of activity in these neurons could cause a decrease in information processing throughout the hemisphere, and it is conceivable that this might be the mechanism underlying the impairments of right hemisphere function in depression.

It is important to emphasize the speculative nature of these hypotheses relating neuropsychological deficits to neurochemical dysfunctions. They do, however, illustrate the important principle that at some point it will be necessary to achieve a conceptual integration between neuropsychological and neuropharmacological approaches to depression (and other functional disorders).

BIBLIOGRAPHY

Cassens, G., Wolfe, L., & Zola, M. (1990). The neuropsychology of depressions. *Journal of Neuropsychiatry, 2,* 202–13.

Flor-Henry, P. (1976). Lateralized temporal-limbic dysfunction and psychopathology. *Annals of the New York Academy of Science, 280,* 777–97.

Hart, R. P., Quentus, J. A., Taylor, R. J., & Harkus, S. W. (1987). Rate of forgetting in dementia and depression. *Journal of Consulting and Clinical Psychology, 55,* 101–5.

Jeste, D. V., Lohr, J. B., & Goodwin, F. K. (1988). Neuroanatomical studies of major affective disorders. A review and suggestions for future research. *British Journal of Psychiatry*, *153*, 444–59.

Kinsbourne, M. (Ed.). (1988). *Cerebral hemisphere function in depression*. Washington: American Psychiatric Press.

Lishman, W. A. (1973). The psychiatric sequelae of head injury: a review. *Psychosomatic Medicine*, *3*, 304–18.

Robinson, R. G., & Stitt, T. G. (1981). Intracortical 6-hydroxydopamine induces an asymmetrical behavioral response in the rat. *Brain Research*, *213*, 387–95.

Tucker, D. M., & Williamson, P. A. (1984). Asymmetric neural control systems in human self-regulation. *Psychological Review*, *91*, 185–215.

Willner, P. (1985). *Depression: A psychobiological synthesis*. New York: John Wiley.

PAUL WILLNER

development *See* MATURATION.

developmental dyslexia *See* DYSLEXIA.

diaschisis Diaschisis is the principle that recent lesions may have effects at a distance from the site of the lesion within the brain. An acute lesion may therefore have widespread consequences, due to the interruption of patterns of excitation and inhibition across mutually interacting neural systems, which may diminish with the passage of time. Diaschisis will affect those aspects of a functional system which are most recently developed, least fixed in structure, and most voluntary. Diaschisis is one element in the range of explanations for RECOVERY OF FUNCTION.

dichhaptic technique Dichhaptic presentation of stimuli refers to the procedure whereby different haptic (or tactile) stimuli are presented simultaneously to the two hands. The dichhaptic procedure is one of several lateral perceptual techniques used to study hemispheric functional specialization or LATERALIZATION. Various methods exist to study lateralization: (1) study of cognitive deficits in patients having unilateral brain damage – the approach which first revealed hemispheric specialization in the human brain; (2) ELECTRICAL STIMULATION mapping; (3) INTRACAROTID SODIUM AMYTAL testing; (4) lateral perceptual techniques including DICHOTIC LISTENING and the DIVIDED VISUAL FIELD TECHNIQUE; (5) study of split-brain patients (those having COMMISSUROTOMY); (6) electrophysiological studies of EEG and EVOKED POTENTIALS; and (7) brain imaging revealing LOCALIZATION of function using xenon inhalation and PET SCAN techniques. Functional MAGNETIC RESONANCE IMAGING studies (fMRI) will probably be a key approach in the near future.

One of the advantages of lateral perceptual techniques such as dichhaptic stimulation is that they can provide information on hemispheric specialization in neurologically intact people and in groups readily selected for specific characteristics, such as hand preference, reading ability, or age.

Dichotic listening and divided visual field tasks were developed in the 1950s and their use as possible indices of the pattern of brain lateralization was recognized by the early 1960s. The anatomy between sense organs and the brain for the SOMESTHETIC SYSTEM is similar to that for the auditory system. There are both contralateral (crossed) and ipsilateral (same-side) connections between sense organs and the brain, with the contralateral connections being structurally or physiologically predominant. Thus, in the tactual modality, the input from the right hand initially goes predominantly to the left somatosensory cortex, whereas that from the left hand goes to the right side. Haptic presentation involves stimulation of the surface of the skin under conditions in which a person is permitted to actively explore or palpate the object. Tactile stimulation refers to passive touch. The dichhaptic technique was developed to be analogous to the dichotic procedure and was first described by Witelson (1974) who coined the term "dichhaptic" (Witelson, 1976) (replacing the laboratory term of "double feelies") to refer to an experimental situation in which subjects were asked to palpate (haptic) out of view different objects in the two hands simultaneously. Figure 38 schematically describes the procedure. Since then, the term has sometimes been used to refer to any form of bilaterally simultaneous tactile stimulation, whether or not active exploration is involved (e.g. Oscar-Berman et al., 1978), and has sometimes been spelled with a single h (e.g. Yandell & Elias, 1983) rather than two. Here we shall use the broader definition (but the original spelling) and comment on all forms of simultaneous tactile stimulation that have been employed to assess hemispheric specialization.

The task was first used with children. The impetus was to develop a task to probe right-hemisphere specialization for form perception in neurologically intact children in a study of lateralization in children with developmental DYSLEXIA compared to children with normal reading ability.

Witelson (1974) created a number of novel and unnameable two-dimensional shapes from thin styrofoam sheets. The children were presented with a different shape to each hand and permitted to palpate them for ten seconds. The children

were then asked to select the two objects they had felt by pointing to the matching stimuli, which were presented along with four distractors in a visual display. In a linguistic dichhaptic task, Witelson used pairs of styrofoam letters. A pair of letters was presented for a two-second period and then one second later a second pair was presented for two seconds. The subjects then named the four letters they had felt. As predicted, the children (normal, strongly right-handed, school-age boys aged 6–14 years) showed greater accuracy in the recognition of nonsense shapes felt by the left rather than the right hand, but a trend for right-hand superiority for the letters. In contrast, a small group of six left-handers failed to show any difference between hands. In a subsequent study (Witelson, 1976), a SEX DIFFERENCE in lateralization was observed. No asymmetry was noted for the young girls, although by early

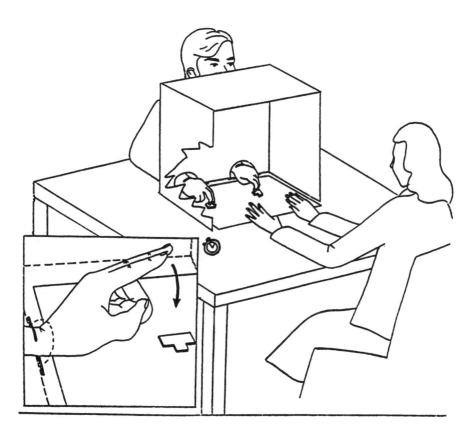

Figure 38 Schematic representation of dichhaptic stimulation set-up. The subject simultaneously palpates two different items, out of view, one with each hand for a limited time period. (Adapted from Witelson, 1974, with permission.)

adolescence a tendency toward perceptual asymmetry appeared. These results indicated right-hemisphere specialization for form perception in boys as early as age 6 years and less lateralization in girls than boys for this aspect of cognition. Boys with developmental dyslexia failed to show the typical pattern of better left-hand accuracy for form perception although they did show greater right-ear accuracy on a verbal dichotic listening task (Witelson, 1977). These results led to the hypothesis of bihemispheric lateralization of form perception and left-hemisphere processing of both spatial and verbal material in developmental dyslexia, that is, "Two right hemispheres and none left."

Several studies soon followed, using dichhaptic tasks with similar stimuli in children and adults. For example, Cioffi and Kandel (1979) found a left-hand superiority on a similar nonsense shapes test for boys, but also for young girls. Etaugh and Levy (1981) reported a left-hand superiority for shapes in children as young as 4 years of age. On a letters task similar to Witelson's (1974), Cioffi and Kandel observed a sex difference; but on a more demanding linguistic task, a right-hand superiority overall was found. Gibson and Bryden (1983) also found a tendency for right-hand superiority for the perception of letters.

Gottfried and Rose (1978) developed a modification of the dichhaptic task for use with infants. One-year-olds were familiarized with an object tactually in one hand, and visual recognition memory for the item was assessed by a paired-comparison technique that indicates degree of preference for a novel stimulus. Left-hand superiority was observed in the male infants, suggesting evidence of right-hemisphere specialization for form perception by 1 year of age. Females showed no difference.

Dozens of studies now exist in the literature, using some variation of the dichhaptic technique. Although the majority show the typical pattern, there is some inconsistency in the results regarding lateralization and the presence of sex differences. In general the findings have conformed to the general view that the right hemisphere is more specialized for spatial tasks and the left for linguistic, sequential tasks (e.g. Bradshaw & Nettleton, 1981).

These studies have also contributed to the issue of the onset or developmental course of hemispheric specialization and to the possibility of a sex difference in lateralization. Several reviews exist and the reader is referred to these (Hiscock, 1988, Table 5.3; Minami et al., 1994; Summers & Lederman, 1990; Witelson, 1987).

METHODOLOGICAL CONSIDERATIONS AND VARIATIONS

The exposure time of 10 seconds used by Witelson (1974) for exploration of the stimuli creates a potential problem, in that a subject could potentially alternate palpation or attention to the exploration between the hands, thus reducing the simultaneity or competing aspect of the task and making it into more of a serial unimanual task. As a consequence of such considerations, other experimenters have attempted to develop procedures that permitted closer control over stimulus parameters. For example, Lassonde and others (1986) attached their stimuli to moving belts with velcro and drove two belts along with a motor that moved them in discrete steps. This allowed the experimenters to control the time subjects could explore a stimulus fairly accurately, as well as the interval between successive pairs. In another approach, Oscar-Berman and others (1978) had two experimenters simultaneously trace out separate patterns on the hands of their subjects. Nachshon and Carmon (1975) constructed a device that employed solenoids to present punctate stimuli to the fingertips at controlled time intervals.

The task of identifying letters by touch allows some ambiguity in the cognitive task involved – a feature not recognized at the outset of the research (Witelson, 1974). The naming of a letter clearly has to be preceded by form recognition of the shape of the letter, thus possibly eliciting right-hemisphere as well as left-hemisphere processing. This hypothesis was supported by subsequent studies which increased the linguistic demands of the task (e.g. Cioffi & Kandel, 1979). This feature of two types of processing in one task adds complexity in the interpretation of results but also adds an interesting possibility of assessing a preferred cognitive strategy in different people.

The use of multiple pairs of stimuli opens the way for subjects to adopt a variety of different strategies that may determine the specific patterns of results obtained (Bryden, 1978). For example, when two stimuli are presented sequentially to each hand, as in Witelson's (1974) letters task, the subject has the choice of identifying the first pair of stimuli followed by the second pair, or of identifying those items presented to one hand followed by those presented to the other. A bias to report the left hand first could lead to an artificial left-hand advantage for such a condition. Identifying the items pair by pair could reduce the magnitude of any lateral asymmetry by reducing the asymmetry in the time difference of report between one hand and the other.

Several investigators have attempted to control for order of recall by instructing subjects to report the items in a specific order (e.g. Gibson & Bryden, 1983; Oscar-Berman et al., 1978; Koenig, 1987). In the study by Oscar-Berman and others (1978), lateral asymmetries were seen only for the second hand reported, while Koenig (1987) found them only with the first hand reported.

A wide variety of different types of stimuli have been employed in dichhaptic studies. In addition to the two-dimensional nonsense shapes and letters employed by Witelson (1974), researchers have also used three-dimensional nonsense shapes (Summers & Lederman, 1990), textures varying in roughness (Koenig, 1987), and patterns of punctate stimuli (Minami et al., 1994), to name but a few.

In some studies, for example, the one by Gardner and colleagues (1977), left–right differences in reaction time as well as in accuracy were recorded in studies with adults. In other studies, the tactual-visual integration required for the response mode based on visual examination was eliminated, and response by tactual recognition was used (Flanery & Balling, 1979).

The technique of studying lateralization with the use of two concurrent tasks (interference paradigm or DUAL TASK technique) has been used with dichhaptic tasks. For example, the subject can be requested to count backwards while engaged in a tactual task.

DICHHAPTIC VERSUS UNIMANUAL STIMULATION

The dichhaptic task was designed theoretically with the idea that, as in dichotic listening, competing stimulation would yield greater asymmetries than would unimanual stimulation. In a minority of studies, monaural stimulation yielded some perceptual asymmetry (e.g. Bradshaw et al., 1981). In the somesthetic system, Dodds (1978) and Hatta (1978) observed a left-hand advantage for unimanual tactile form perception. Left-hand superiority has been reported for an alternative spatial task, the tactile determination of direction

(e.g. Benton et al., 1973). In contrast, Nachshon and Carmon (1975) and Minami and colleagues (1994) found a fairly strong right-hand advantage for a putatively unimanual spatial task.

The examples of tasks used in the experimental studies described present a sampling of the diversity possible, and demonstrate how perceptual techniques may make use of the anatomy of the nervous system in order to study localization of function in the brain.

BIBLIOGRAPHY

Benton, A. L., Levin, H. S., & Varney, N. R. (1973). Tactile perception of direction in normal subjects. *Neurology, 23*, 1248–50.

Bradshaw, J. L., Farrelly, J., & Taylor, M. J. (1981). Synonym and antonym pairs in the detection of dichotically and monaurally presented targets: competing monaural stimulation can generate a REA. *Acta Psychologica, 47*, 189–205.

Bradshaw, J. L., & Nettleton, N. C. (1981). The nature of hemispheric specialization in man. *Behavioral and Brain Sciences, 4*, 51–92.

Bryden, M. P. (1978). Strategy effects in the assessment of hemispheric asymmetry. In G. Underwood (Ed.), *Strategies of information processing* (pp. 117–49), London: Academic Press.

Cioffi, J., & Kandel, G. L. (1979). Laterality of stereognostic accuracy of children for words, shapes and bigrams: a sex difference for bigrams. *Science, 204*, 1432–4.

Dodds, A. G. (1978). Hemispheric differences in tactuo-spatial processing. *Neuropsychologia, 16*, 247–54.

Etaugh, C., & Levy, R. B. (1981). Hemispheric specialization for tactile-spatial processing in preschool children. *Perceptual and Motor Skills, 53*, 621–2.

Flanery, R. C., & Balling, J. D. (1979). Developmental changes in hemisphere specialization for tactile spatial ability. *Developmental Psychology, 15*, 364–72.

Gardner, E. B., English, A. G., Flannery, B. M., Hartnett, M. B., McCormick, J. K., & Wilhelmy, B. B. (1977). Shape-recognition accuracy and response latency in a bilateral tactile task. *Neuropsychologia, 15*, 607–16.

Gibson, C., & Bryden, M. P. (1983). Dichhaptic recognition of words and letters in children. *Canadian Journal of Psychology, 37*, 132–43.

Gottfried, A. W., & Rose, S. A. (1978).

Developmental tactile-visual cross-modal functioning in infancy: issues and future directions. Paper presented at the International Conference on Infant Studies, Providence, RI (March).

Hatta, T. (1978). The functional asymmetry of tactile pattern learning in normal subjects. *Psychologia*, *21*, 83–9.

Hiscock, M. (1988). Behavioral asymmetries in normal children. In D. L. Molfese & S. J. Segalowitz (Eds), *Brain lateralization in children* (pp. 85–169). New York: Guilford.

Koenig, O. (1987). Dichhaptic recognition of textures in normal adults. *Neuropsychologia*, *25*, 295–8.

Lassonde, M., Sauerwein, H., Geoffroy, G., & Décarie, M. (1986). Effects of early and late transection of the corpus callosum in children: a study of tactile and tactuomotor transfer and integration. *Brain*, *109*, 953–67.

Minami, K., Hay, V., Bryden, M. P., & Free, T. (1994). Laterality effects for tactile patterns. *International Journal of Neuroscience*, *74*, 55–69.

Nachshon, I., & Carmon, A. (1975). Hand preference in sequential and spatial discrimination tasks. *Cortex*, *11*, 121–31.

Oscar-Berman, M., Rehbein, L., Porfert, A., & Goodglass, H. (1978). Dichhaptic hand-order effects with verbal and nonverbal tactile stimulation. *Brain and Language*, *6*, 323–33.

Summers, D. C., & Lederman, S. J. (1990). Perceptual asymmetries in the somatosensory system: a dichhaptic experiment and critical review of the literature from 1929 to 1986. *Cortex*, *26*, 201–26.

Witelson, S. F. (1974). Hemispheric specialization for linguistic and nonlinguistic tactual perception using a dichotomous stimulation technique. *Cortex*, *10*, 3–17.

Witelson, S. F. (1976). Sex and the single hemisphere: specialization of the right hemisphere for spatial processing. *Science*, *193*, 425–7.

Witelson, S. F. (1977). Developmental dyslexia: two right hemispheres and none left. *Science*, *195*, 309–11.

Witelson, S. F. (1987). Neurobiological aspects of language in children. *Child Development*, *58*, 653–88.

Yandell, L., & Elias, J. W. (1983). Left hemispheric advantage for a visuospatial-dichaptic matching task. *Cortex*, *19*, 69–77.

SANDRA F. WITELSON AND M. P. BRYDEN

dichotic listening In dichotic listening, subjects are asked to listen to two different auditory messages presented simultaneously, one to each ear, and to indicate what they have heard. In her seminal study, Kimura (1961) presented two short lists of numbers, one to each ear, and found that normal subjects were more accurate in reporting the numbers presented to the right ear than those presented to the left ear. Furthermore, by studying patients with known language lateralization as determined by the sodium amytal technique (INTRACAROTID SODIUM AMYTAL), she found that this right-ear advantage (REA) was related to the lateralization of language to the left cerebral hemisphere. Thus the dichotic listening technique was seen to provide a noninvasive means of testing normal subjects for the lateralization of cerebral function.

Subsequent research has consistently verified the REA in normal subjects (Bryden, 1988b) and the link to cerebral lateralization (Zatorre, 1989). Furthermore, a left-ear advantage (LEA) has been found for numerous types of nonverbal stimuli, including musical passages, tone sequences, and the affective tone of speech. Much of the research on dichotic listening and its relevance to both clinical and normal populations has been reviewed in the volume edited by Hugdahl (1988).

EXPERIMENTAL PROCEDURES

In the early studies of the REA for verbal material (e.g. Kimura, 1961), subjects were presented with short lists of words or numbers in each ear. Such procedures introduced problems of short-term memory and opened the task to various subject-controlled strategies, such as preferentially attending to one ear. Subsequently, Studdert-Kennedy and Shankweiler (1970) showed that the REA was most robust for the initial stop consonants (/b/, /d/, /g/, /p/, /t/, /k/) in consonant–vowel–consonant (CVC) syllables, rather weaker for the terminal consonants, and weakest of all for the vowels. On the basis of this work, simple consonant–vowel (CV) stimulus pairs, employing the stop consonants paired with some constant vowel (e.g. /a/) became a popular stimulus set. Subjects were simply asked to indicate which of the six possible stimuli they heard on any given trial. Such a procedure grossly reduced the memory load involved with dichotic lists, and limited the different strategies subjects could use. Bryden, Munhall, and Allard (1983) subsequently recommended using CV pairs with instructions to attend specifically to one ear in a further attempt to reduce subject-generated attentional strategies. They recommended comparing performance on the left ear when it was the attended ear to performance on the right ear when it was the attended ear, and showed that this procedure reduced intersubject variability.

More recently, three other verbal procedures have enjoyed some success. The first is dichotic monitoring (Geffen & Caudrey, 1981), in which long lists of words are presented rapidly to the two ears, and the subject is asked to indicate whenever a prespecified target word appears. Since subjects sometimes indicate that the target was heard when it was not presented (a "false alarm"), this procedure has the advantage of making possible a signal detection analysis of hits and false alarms. Performance has been shown to relate to cerebral speech lateralization (Geffen & Caudrey, 1981).

In another approach, Halwes and his colleagues (Wexler & Halwes, 1983) have refined the usual CV task by using meaningful words and selecting only those contrasts that give reliable ear effects. They have produced a fused dichotic words test, in which rhyming words differing only in the initial phoneme are paired. By splicing the initial phoneme onto a constant ending, the two dichotic sounds fuse so that subjects normally profess to hear only a single word. Again, this leads to a robust REA in normal subjects, and has been shown to accurately classify individuals with known cerebral speech lateralization (Zatorre, 1989).

Graves, Morley, and Marcopulos (1987) have developed a technique for titrating interaural intensity differences, and have used the difference in intensity between the two ears when performance is equated as a measure of the ear advantage. They report an average REA, in right-handers, of about 3 db for phoneme discrimination, and a similar LEA for intonation discrimination.

For nonverbal material, where subjects cannot report the items verbally, other procedures have been required. Kimura (1964), for example, provided four binaural forced-choice alternatives following dichotic presentation of two short musical passages. As with the list procedure, this procedure placed heavy demands on short-term memory, as it was some 20 sec after the dichotic

presentation before all the alternatives had been presented. Others have used a target detection procedure, in which the subject is to respond "yes" if a particular target sound is present and "no" if it is not.

The specific procedures used in dichotic presentation are limited only by the ingenuity of the experimenter. However, when devising new procedures, one should keep in mind potential problems arising from subject-controlled strategy effects, short-term memory effects, and attentional biases. The best advice is to keep the task and response requirements simple.

MODELS OF DICHOTIC LISTENING

One of the earliest models of dichotic performance was the structural model of Kimura (1967). She postulated three effects. First, transmission along the contralateral pathways was faster and more efficient than transmission along the ipsilateral pathways, so that information from one ear was better transmitted to the opposite hemisphere. Second, the functional specialization of the two hemispheres determined where the input was analyzed, so that verbal information had to reach the left (speech) hemisphere and nonverbal information had to reach the right hemisphere. Thus verbal information input to the left ear transmitted to the right hemisphere had to be further transmitted by way of the corpus callosum to the left hemisphere prior to final analysis. This extra step resulted in left-ear verbal information being degraded by the time it was analyzed, and produced the REA. Finally, Kimura also suggested that activity along the ascending contralateral pathways blocked the ipsilateral signals, thus preventing them from reaching the cortex. This occlusion effect was proposed to account for the large REA observed with dichotic presentation as opposed to monaural presentation.

An alternative view, emphasizing the attentional aspect of dichotic listening, was proposed by Kinsbourne (1975). He argued that the expectation of dealing with verbal material served to activate the left hemisphere and make it more prepared to accept new input. Conversely, when nonverbal material was expected, the right hemisphere would be activated. This selective activation of one cerebral hemisphere would then provide the basis for the observed laterality effects.

A somewhat more complex model has been proposed by Efron and his colleagues (Efron et al., 1983). They consider verbal and nonverbal stimuli to represent a continuum from an REA for the most complex verbal stimuli involving rapid temporal transitions to an LEA for simple tone patterns. Because of asymmetries in the ascending auditory pathways, the performance of individual subjects may be shifted to the right or left along this continuum. Then they propose a "temporal lobe enhancement mechanism" (TLEM) in each hemisphere that enhances the perceptual salience of acoustic signals presented to the contralateral ear. They see the efficacy of the TLEM as being related to the relative size of the temporal planum and primary auditory cortex in the two hemispheres. They argue that simpler sounds are analyzed in the auditory cortex, which is larger on the right, while more complex signals are dependent upon the temporal planum, which is larger on the left.

A good general review of the various models of dichotic performance has been provided by Geffen and Quinn (1984). They propose a modified structural model, patterned after that of Kimura (1967) but with no provision for suppression of the ipsilateral pathway by activity in the contralateral pathway. Geffen and Quinn suggest that sounds in one half of space are qualitatively better processed in the contralateral hemisphere. Therefore, the REA occurs because the left hemisphere is specialized for language, the ipsilateral pathway is weak and the callosal pathway is indirect. Geffen and Quinn suggest that the REA can be overcome by voluntary attention to the left ear and that an REA will be observed for monaural tasks when the processing demands are heavy.

VERBAL LATERALITY EFFECTS

The REA for verbal material is one of the most robust findings of experimental neuropsychology; it can be observed with virtually any experimental procedure, and with meaningful words, nonsense syllables, or even backwards speech. As would be expected from the literature on the relation of handedness to aphasia, the REA is more evident in right-handed subjects than in left-handed people, with about 81 percent of right-handers and only 64 percent of left-handers demonstrating an REA (Bryden, 1988b). Some studies have claimed a relation between the dichotic REA and

other subject variables, such as the subjects' familial history of left-handedness, the posture employed in handwriting, and the presence of indicators of "latent left-handedness" such as left-eye dominance or folding the arms with the left arm superior, although none of these has been consistently documented (Bryden, 1988b). In general, there is also an increased likelihood of obtaining an REA in male subjects as opposed to female subjects (Bryden, 1988b), but the effect is small and there are numerous exceptions to this rule.

Developmental studies have indicated that the verbal REA can be obtained with conventional procedures in children of kindergarten age and, using dishabituation techniques, can be seen in infants as young as 3 and 4 months of age. The probability of observing an REA does not appear to change substantially with age, thus suggesting that lateralization of speech is present soon after birth and does not develop gradually.

NONVERBAL LATERALITY EFFECTS

In addition to the verbal studies, many investigators have demonstrated laterality effects, usually favoring the left ear, for diverse types of nonverbal material. Thus, in one early study Kimura (1964) found an LEA for dichotically presented musical passages. The early work with musical stimuli has been throughly reviewed by Gates and Bradshaw (1977), and the more recent work by Peretz and Morais (1988). In general, when the spectral characteristics of the music are more important to the task, as with paired chords, an LEA is seen; when temporal characteristics are more important, as with rhythms, an REA is often obtained. Furthermore, there is evidence that professional musicians will show an REA for material that reveals an LEA in nonmusicians.

LEAs can also be observed for vocal nonverbal sounds such as laughing or crying. Likewise, LEAs are found for dichotically presented environmental sounds, sonar signals, and Morse code signals.

Finally, an LEA is observed for emotional sounds, such as the tone in which various utterances are spoken. In one example of such a task, Bryden and MacRae (1988) paired two-syllable rhyming words were spoken with different emotional expressions. When subjects were asked to detect the presence of a specific affect, such as "anger," they showed an LEA, but produced an

REA when asked to detect a specific target word.

As with the verbal laterality effects, nonverbal LEAs are seen in very young infants and in older children.

EFFECTS OF NEUROLOGICAL DAMAGE

When neurological patients with temporal lobe damage are studied, it is typical to find impaired performance on the ear contralateral to the damaged hemisphere, in what has been termed a "lesion effect." Under certain circumstances, however, neurological patients show a decrement on the ipsilateral ear rather than the contralateral one, a "paradoxical extinction effect." Impaired performance on the ipsilateral ear normally follows deep lesions that destroy callosal connections, thus disrupting transmission of ipsilateral ear information via the stronger contralateral pathway (Eslinger & Damasio, 1988).

As would be expected from a model such as that of Kimura (1967), performance on the left ear is reduced to near zero following section of the corpus callosum (Sparks & Geschwind, 1968). Sparks and Geschwind also found that performance on the left ear was enhanced when the competing right-ear material was distorted or when speech noise was employed, thus indicating that interference with incoming left-ear information was maximal when the signals reaching the left temporal lobe from the two ears were most similar. Such findings are in agreement with Kimura's (1967) structural model, and indicate the importance of callosal transfer in dichotic listening. Sidtis and colleagues (1981), investigating staged section of the corpus callosum, found that section of the posterior 3 to 4 cm of the callosum was sufficient to produce almost complete loss of the ipsilateral information. The implications of the findings from callosal section have been reviewed by Sidtis (1988).

In addition, there are reports of enhanced verbal REAs following frontal lobe damage and damage to the basal ganglia. Eslinger and Damasio (1988) suggest that these may result from damage to higher-order attentional mechanisms.

ALTERATIONS IN DICHOTIC LATERALITY

Because dichotic procedures are relatively easy to administer, there have been numerous studies of dichotic performance in various pathological groups. One of the most commonly studied groups are children with developmental dyslexia or reading disability. Bryden's (1988a) review concludes that the majority of such studies support the view that the verbal REA is somewhat reduced in such children, indicating weaker language lateralization. However, the effects are not large, and many studies fail to show differences between normal and reading-disabled children. Kershner and Morton (1990) have considered a number of alternatives, and prefer an explanation in terms of excessive bilateral activation, making it more difficult to allocate attention to a specific ear.

In addition, reduced REAs for verbal material have been reported for people with Down's syndrome (Pipe, 1983). Pipe also found normal REAs in severely retarded children without Down's syndrome. Despite some evidence that autistic children show a smaller REA than do normal controls (Prior & Bradshaw, 1979), the evidence concerning shifts in laterality in autism is inconsistent.

Dichotic laterality effects have also been found to be altered in various psychopathologies (see Hugdahl, 1988). Thus, for example, schizophrenic patients have been found to show a very large REA for lists of numbers, but virtually no REA for nonsense syllable pairs. With both types of material, the recovery pattern is one of returning to a normal REA. Such findings have been interpreted as indicating left-hemisphere over-activation in schizophrenia. In contrast, depressed patients show a reduced REA for verbal material, and fail to show an LEA for nonverbal material.

CONCLUSIONS

Dichotic listening procedures have fascinated researchers for many years and have taught us many things, both about normal individuals and about clinical populations. The correlation between dichotic ear effects and functional lateralization is not perfect, with the consequence that one cannot infer speech lateralization from observing dichotic listening performance. Nevertheless, different populations do vary in their patterns of dichotic laterality, and these variations may not only give us important clues about cerebral mechanisms, but also lead to a better understanding of mechanisms of attention and memory. As is so often the case with behavioral procedures, the important task is to understand the procedure thoroughly and to know how different factors may affect the observed performance.

BIBLIOGRAPHY

Bryden, M. P. (1988a). Does laterality make any difference? Thoughts on the relation between cerebral asymmetry and reading. In D. L. Molfese & S. J. Segalowitz (Eds), *Brain lateralization in children: Developmental implications* (pp. 509–25). New York: Guilford.

Bryden, M. P. (1988b). An overview of the dichotic listening procedure and its relation to cerebral organization. In K. Hugdahl (Ed.), *Handbook of dichotic listening: Theory, methods, and research* (pp. 1–44). Chichester: John Wiley.

Bryden, M. P., & MacRae, L. (1988). Dichotic laterality effects obtained with emotional words. *Neuropsychiatry, Neuropsychology, and Behavioral Neurology, 1*, 171–6.

Bryden, M. P., Munhall, K., & Allard, F. (1983). Attentional biases and the right-ear effect in dichotic listening. *Brain and Language, 18*, 236–48.

Efron, R., Koss, B., & Yund, E. W. (1983). Central auditory processing. IV. Ear dominance – spatial and temporal complexity. *Brain and Language, 19*, 264–82.

Eslinger, P. J., & Damasio, H. (1988). Anatomical correlates of paradoxic ear extinction. In K. Hugdahl (Ed.), *Handbook of dichotic listening: Theory, methods, and research* (pp. 139–60). Chichester: John Wiley.

Gates, A., & Bradshaw, J. L. (1977). The role of the cerebral hemispheres in music. *Brain and Language, 4*, 403–31.

Geffen, G., & Caudrey, D. (1981). Reliability and validity of the dichotic monitoring test for language laterality. *Neuropsychologia, 19*, 413–24.

Geffen, G., & Quinn, K. (1984). Hemispheric specialization and ear advantages in processing speech. *Psychological Bulletin, 96*, 273–91.

Graves, R. E., Morley, S., & Marcopulos, B. A. (1987). Measurement of the dichotic listening ear advantage for intersubject and interstimulus comparisons. *Journal of Clinical and Experimental Neuropsychology, 9*, 511–26.

Hugdahl, K. (Ed.). (1988). *Handbook of dichotic listening: Theory, methods, and research*. Chichester: John Wiley.

Kershner, J. R., & Morton, L. L. (1990).

Directed attention dichotic listening in reading disabled children: a test of four models of maladaptive lateralization. *Neuropsychologia, 28*, 181–98.

Kimura, D. (1961). Cerebral dominance and the perception of verbal stimuli. *Canadian Journal of Psychology, 15*, 166–71.

Kimura, D. (1964). Left-right differences in the perception of melodies. *Quarterly Journal of Experimental Psychology, 16*, 355–8.

Kimura, D. (1967). Functional asymmetry of the brain in dichotic listening. *Cortex, 3*, 163–78.

Kinsbourne, M. (1975). The mechanism of hemispheric control of the lateral gradient of attention. In P. M. A. Rabbitt & S. Dornic (Eds), *Attention and Performance V* (pp. 81–97). New York: Academic Press.

Peretz, I., & Morais, J. (1988). Determinants of laterality for music: towards an information processing account. In K. Hugdahl (Ed.), *Handbook of dichotic listening: Theory, methods, and research* (pp. 323–58). Chichester: John Wiley.

Pipe, M.-E. (1983). Dichotic-listening performance following auditory discrimination training in Down's syndrome and developmentally retarded children. *Cortex, 19*, 481–91.

Prior, M. R., & Bradshaw, J. L. (1979). Hemispheric functioning in autistic children. *Cortex, 15*, 73–81.

Sidtis, J. J., Volpe, B. T., Holtzman, J. D., Wilson, D. H., & Gazzaniga, M. S. (1981). Cognitive interaction after staged callosal section: Evidence for transfer of semantic activation. *Science, 212*, 344–6.

Sparks, R., & Geschwind, N. (1968). Dichotic listening in man after section of neocortical commissures. *Cortex, 4*, 3–16.

Studdert-Kennedy, M., & Shankweiler, D. (1970). Hemispheric specialization for speech perception. *Journal of the Acoustical Society of America, 48*, 479–94.

Wexler, B. E., & Halwes, T. (1983). Increasing the power of dichotic methods: The fused rhymed words test. *Neuropsychologia, 21*, 59–66.

Zatorre, R. J. (1989). Perceptual asymmetry on the dichotic fused words tests and cerebral speech lateralization determined by the carotid sodium amytal test. *Neuropsychologia, 27*, 1207–19.

M. P. BRYDEN

diencephalon The diencephalon is one of the regions of the BRAIN STEM. It includes three structures: the epithalamus, the THALAMUS, and the HYPOTHALAMUS. It is also sometimes referred to as the interbrain, and is an important way station between the forebrain and the lower regions of the brain stem. Although the functions of the epithalamus in humans are not understood, the functions of the other structures may be summarized as motivation and affect.

differentiation   *See* MATURATION.

diplegia Diplegia is a movement disorder due to bilateral weakness or spasticity of the limbs in which the legs are more severely affected than the arms. It is closely related to HEMIPLEGIA. It is most commonly a congenital disorder and a form of CEREBRAL PALSY. The associated lesion principally involves the corticospinal tracts in association with symmetrical cortical atrophy, which may also result in mental retardation, involuntary movements, and ataxia.

diplopia Diplopia is the medical term for double vision, in which two images of a single object are perceived. It results from paralysis, or partial paralysis, of the movements of one of the eyes so that the image no longer falls on corresponding points of the two retinae. The apparent displacement occurs in the plane of action of the affected muscle; and the displacement of the images increases as the eyes are moved further in the normal diection of pull of the affected muscle. Not all causes of diplopia are neurological, but when they are the diseases most commonly diagnosed are multiple sclerosis, myasthenia gravis, and cerebral atheroma in the elderly.

disconnection syndrome A set of deficits following interruption of large tracts of cerebral nerve fibers is called a disconnection syndrome. The clearest example is the syndrome following complete cerebral COMMISSUROTOMY wherein all of the neocortical commissure, including the CORPUS CALLOSUM, anterior commissures, and hippocampal commissure, are sectioned (severed). This results in loss of normal communica-

tion between the two cerebral hemispheres. Partial callosal disconnections occur with various diseases as well as being produced surgically. This entry focuses on surgical disconnection to alleviate intractable multifocal epilepsy.

Following complete cerebral commissurotomy, it is customary to distinguish an acute syndrome, lasting weeks to a few months after operation, from a chronic syndrome. The chronic syndrome typically persists in a stable condition for many years, although with some progressive compensation as time goes by.

COMPLETE DISCONNECTION
Acute disconnection   When the corpus callosum (as well as the anterior and hippocampal commissures) of a right-handed, left-hemisphere dominant patient is sectioned by retraction of the right hemisphere, there often follow mild AKINESIA, imperviousness, and MUTISM, as well as competitive movements between the two hands. There are severe left-hand APRAXIA to verbal command, left-arm HYPOTONIA, well coordinated but repetitive reaching, groping or grasping with the left hand, and bilateral BABINSKI RESPONSES. Symptoms vary across patients and reflect edema from retraction as well as DIASCHISTIC shock to both hemispheres from the radical disconnection. It is suggested by some that complete callosotomy (section of the corpus callosum alone; *see* COMMISSUROTOMY) in cases where speech and manual dominance are in opposite hemispheres may result in loss of the ability to initiate spontaneous speech (Sussmann, McKeever; the names of scientists associated with specific results are added in parentheses to allow their publications to be traced).

Commonly, in the early postoperative period there are episodes of intermanual conflict, in which the hands act at cross purposes. Patients sometimes complain that their left hand behaves in a "foreign" or "alien" manner, and they routinely express surprise at apparently purposeful left hand actions (autocriticism).

Largely absent from the acute disconnection syndrome are florid symptoms associated with unilateral lesions, including APHASIA, AGNOSIA, PROSOPAGNOSIA, and DENIAL, as may occur with NEGLECT.
Chronic disconnection   Within a few months after the operation, patients appear normal on routine neurological examination and in social situations.

279

Long-term personal interaction with the patients reveals a few persisting cognitive lacunae. Most noticeably, the patients have a moderate memory deficit, demonstrating lower memory than intelligence quotients, particular difficulty with uncommon paired word associates, story passages and topographical memory, and selective difficulty in acquisition of new information (D. W. Zaidel). It is believed that these deficits are mainly due to callosal rather than fornix damage (D. W. Zaidel). Patients often get lost in a familiar lab, tell the same stories, and cannot recall episodic information about the relative recency and chronological ordering of recent events (D. W. Zaidel and Sperry). Also, the patients tend to demonstrate some pragmatic deficits in conversation, inappropriate or exaggerated politeness, and a slight tendency to confabulate. They show impoverished verbal description of emotional personal experiences (ALEXITHYMIA). The patients fail to sustain simultaneous reading of extended texts and rarely read for enjoyment.

In contrast to everyday interactions, lateralized testing in which the stimuli and/or responses are restricted to one hemisphere reveals lack of communication between the two disconnected hemispheres, each of which appears to have its own perceptual, learning and memory systems. Thus, a typical right-handed commissurotomy patient with left hemisphere (LH) speech cannot name stimuli in the left sensory field, whether the left visual hemifield (LVF) or the left hand (Lh), and such a patient cannot make reliable same–different judgments about stimuli in opposite sensory fields, usually the two visual hemifields or the two hands.

When different but acoustically similar auditory linguistic stimuli are presented simultaneously to the two ears (DICHOTIC LISTENING), patients do not name the left-ear stimuli, which normally reach the LH via the isthmus of the corpus callosum (Milner and Taylor). This is due to suppression of the ipsilateral auditory pathways. Suppression can be maximized by precise acoustic overlap of the dichotic signals and is then resistant to manipulation of attention or experience. There is a corresponding suppression of the right ear for nonverbal identification of auditory stimuli specialized in the RH, such as complex pitch discrimination (Sidtis). There is no interhemispheric transfer for touch, pressure, and proprioception. Hand postures impressed on one

(unseen) hand by the examiner cannot be mimicked in the opposite hand, and a brief flash of a hand form to one visual hemifield cannot be copied by the contralateral hand (Sperry). After complete cerebral commissurotomy there is a substantial loss of intermanual point localization, that is, loss of the ability to identify exact points stimulated on the other side of the body, especially distal parts such as the fingertips. In all these cases intrahemispheric comparisons are intact.

One would expect bimanual coordination to suffer following commissurotomy but this does not appear to be the case. Motor skills learned prior to surgery, such as swimming, riding a bicycle, piano-playing, cooking, tying shoe laces, bead-stringing, and similar skills all appear intact. New bimanual tasks consisting of fine finger movements or parallel hand movements are normally executed. However, bimanual interdependent control, such as required in an "Etch-a-Sketch"-type task, is severely impaired (D. W. Zaidel). Even patients with partial commissurotomy (intact splenium with divided anterior and hippocampal commissures) are severely limited in such bimanual coordination. Further, the chronic disconnection syndrome shows persisting mild to moderate left-hand apraxia to verbal command in spite of good imitation and adequate auditory language comprehension in the disconnected RH (D. W. Zaidel). Finally, following complete commissurotomy the patient is unable to name but can signal with the left hand odors presented to the right nostril (Gordon).

Interhemispheric transfer With time, patients acquire a variety of noncallosal transfer mechanisms. This includes cross-cueing, ipsilateral sensory/motor projections, especially on the left side, and a number of routes for subcallosal communication. Transfer of high-level semantic information can occur (Cronin-Golomb and Myers) although its extent is as yet uncertain. For example, Sergent found that complete commissurotomy patients in the Los Angeles series could assess the alignment of arrows in the two VFs, the parity of a bilateral dot pattern, the larger of two digits in opposite fields, or the lexicality of a word straddling the midline. Corballis could not replicate this on the same patients and Gazzaniga and his associates failed to find similar transfer in callosotomy patients from the Dartmouth series.

Some results remain unexplained. For example, it is known that patient LB in the Los Angeles series can often name LVF stimuli although he has never been able to compare stimuli across the midline (Johnson). Comparable tests on patient NG showed that she could not name LVF stimuli but she could compare (meaningful or nonsense) shapes across the midline (Clarke).

Implicit transfer We may say that implicit interhemispheric transfer (priming) occurs in the split-brain if both naming of LVF stimuli and cross-matching fail, but there is nonetheless some influence of an unattended stimulus in one VF on a decision about an attended target in the other. No account of interhemispheric priming in the split-brain literature to date is fully satisfactory, although each demonstrates some significant interhemispheric effects. This includes spatial attentional priming (Holzmann and Passarotti), negative priming in lexical categorizations or digit parity decisions (Lambert), lexicality priming in lateralized lexical decision (Iacoboni), and bilateral Stroop (Weekes). In most cases where interhemispheric priming effects do occur (with the exception of spatial attention), they may be attributable to a unification late in the development of the motor plans (response programming) in the two hemispheres.

What accounts for the normally unified everyday behavior of the patients? First, there are bihemispherically appreciated visual and manual explorations of space, including conjugate eye movements. Second, there is some bilateral representation of sensory information. Third, there is ongoing hormonal communication via blood and cerebrospinal fluid. Fourth, and perhaps most important, there are a variety of connecting subcallosal pathways in the cerebellum, midbrain, pons, and both hypo- and subthalamus.

PARTIAL DISCONNECTION

Callosal channels Anatomical, physiological, and behavioral observations in clinical and normal populations converge on the view that the corpus callosum contains function-specific channels that interconnect cortical regions in the two cerebral hemispheres. The anteroposterior arrangement of these channels generally respects the anteroposterior arrangement of corresponding cortical regions. As a result, different partial sections produce different elements of the complete disconnection syndrome.

The evidence from partial commissurotomy for regional functional specialization is limited by the small number of cases, extracallosal pathology, lack of pre- and post-operative comparisons, and apparent individual differences in callosal organization. Complete division of the SPLENIUM, including the tip, is necessary and sufficient for visual disconnection. Two dramatic syndromes usually associated with posterior callosal disconnection are pure ALEXIA and optic APHASIA, where visual and sometimes semantic disconnection are invoked in addition to right homonymous HEMIANOPIA to help explain selective failure of reading or naming of visual stimuli respectively. If only the tip of the splenium is spared, there is good visual transfer but persisting unilateral left hemifield ANOMIA, unilateral left-hand apraxia, deficits in both tactile and kinesthetic transfer, and a large right-ear advantage in dichotic listening.

Surgical section of the anterior two-thirds of the corpus callosum, sparing the splenium, can result in little or no disconnection symptoms. There may be some relatively subtle deficits in bimanual coordination and in tactile or motor transfer, and memory for new events is also impaired. Nonepileptic patients with surgical removal of parts of the trunk of the corpus callosum sometimes have more or less subtle tactile or motor disconnection symptoms. Division of the isthmus usually but not always results in auditory disconnection. One possible cause of differences across patients is the extent of extracallosal damage, which may interrupt some callosal conduction or disable a region that usually suppresses inhibition of transfer through some callosal channels.

Complete callosotomy, but sparing the anterior commissure, appears to result in the complete disconnection syndrome (Gazzaniga).

HEMISPHERIC SPECIALIZATION AND INDEPENDENCE

The full disconnection syndrome has supported the doctrine of complementary hemispheric specialization: LH specialization for language and analytic processing, RH specialization for visuospatial and Gestalt processing. But more important, it has advanced the concept of hemispheric independence: that each hemisphere can constitute a separate cognitive system operating independently of and in parallel with the other (Sperry).

Attention There is some controversy over whether the disconnected RH is more vigilant than the disconnected LH (Dimond) or not (Ellenberg and I. Sperry). Experiments on covert orienting of spatial attention using the Posner paradigm confirm the existence of two different attentional systems in the two hemispheres (E. Zaidel). Both disconnected hemispheres show benefits from valid cues but the RH is more likely to show costs from invalid cues (Passarotti). There are also suggestions that the attentional system in the LH is more object-based and that in the RH it is more location-based (Driver). A visual search task has suggested independent allocation of attention in the two disconnected hemispheres (Luck).

Perception and space The disconnected RH was superior to the disconnected LH on modified versions of spatial relations tests (Levy and Kumar), on part-whole and Gestalt completion tests (Nebes), on the use of perspective cues (Cronin-Golomb), and on tests of geometric invariance (Franco). The disconnected RH was also superior for complex pitch discrimination (Sidtis) and for harmonic progression (Tramo and Barucha). The disconnected LH was superior in figure-ground disembedding (E. Zaidel). The components of mental imagery are differentially specialized: the RH was found superior for mental rotation (Corballis and Sergent), the LH superior for image generation (Farah). But there are no hemispheric differences for image scaling and scanning (Mattison), and both hemispheres are capable of performing all these component operations. Other tests, such as the Mooney Faces or face recognition tests, failed to show the expected RH superiority (E. Zaidel). Experiments on hierarchic perception showed only an inconsistent RH specialization for global decisions and LH specialization for local decisions (Robertson and Weekes).

Nonverbal Piagetian tests for spatial development (stereognosis, localization of topographical positions) at the pre-operational and concrete operational stages showed mixed hemispheric superiorities across tests and patients and did not succeed in characterizing each hemisphere as performing at some consistent developmental stage (E. Zaidel).

Memory The disconnected RH was superior for memory of tactile nonsense shapes either when the responses were signaled by touch (Milner and Taylor) or by drawing (Kumar), and the disconnected LH was superior for tactile or visual memory for ordered sequences of figures, both common objects and nonsense shapes (D. W.

Zaidel). The multiple-choice version of Benton's Visual Retention Test showed an RH advantage at short (15 sec) delays but no hemisphere difference at 60 sec delays (E. Zaidel). Finally, concept decision tests of long-term semantic memory with pictorial exemplars showed an advantage for atypical exemplars in the LH and for typical exemplars in the RH. There was a typicality effect only in the RH (D. W. Zaidel). In all of these tests, memory in either disconnected hemisphere is generally lower than normal, though better than in patients with AMNESIA, suggesting that the forebrain commissures are important for the formation of some kinds of memory.

Language The disconnected LH has a generally normal clinical language profile. Its subtle psychometric deficit may be attributed to lack of normal RH contribution. In the Los Angeles series the disconnected RH has no speech, little writing, a substantial visual vocabulary (Sperry and Gazzinaga), and a larger and surprisingly rich auditory vocabulary. Visual word recognition in the RH proceeds ideographically, without grapheme–phoneme translation. Both disconnected hemispheres show sensitivity to word frequency, concreteness, emotionality, and length. The disconnected RH has a rich if diffusely organized lexical semantic system but a poor phonology and an impoverished syntax. It has a very limited short-term verbal memory capacity of 2 ± 1 items. The RH understands the meaning of verbs but has difficulty initiating action to printed or pictured commands. It has special paralinguistic competence in appreciating the communicative significance of prosody, facial expression and bodily postures (Borowitz). The mental age profile of RH language abilities is very irregular, showing no correspondence to any single stage in first language acquisition.

Reasoning The disconnected RH was superior on a tactile version of a concept formation test (Kumar) and it can process abstract concepts (Cronin-Golomb). The RH was superior on both a tactile (D. W. Zaidel and Sperry) and a visual (E. Zaidel) version of the Raven Colored Progressive Matrices, which requires the coordination of abstract rules. The LH was superior on the more difficult Raven Standard Progressive Matrices. A form board version of the test which permits a trial and error strategy showed that only the LH benefited from error correction (E. Zaidel).

Learning This important area has been neglected and deserves further study. The disconnected RH can be superior in tactile concept classification tests by sensory cue (size, shape, roughness; Kumar). The LH was superior on reversal learning of letter sequences (Lee-Teng). The RH may be competent to detect certain linguistic errors, such as spelling violations in words, but it fails to take advantage of external error correction (E. Zaidel). Training with feedback improves lateralized lexical decision in both hemispheres but especially in the LH. Rotation of mental images shows an initial RH superiority but greater learning from experience in the LH (Corballis). It is likely that the two hemispheres use different learning strategies. RH performance is more variable from session to session than the LH. The RH has not been shown to possess one-trial learning nor to benefit from feedback during trial and error but has responded better with redundant, complete, and concrete models.

CONTROL

In general, not only partially but also fully split-brain patients behave in a coordinated, purposeful, and consistent manner, belying the independent, parallel, usually different and occasionally conflicting processing of the same information from the environment by the two disconnected hemispheres. Free field performance often resembles that of the superior hemisphere (horse race), especially when the task is linguistic and performed better in the disconnected LH. Occasionally the LH dominates free field responses even when it is inferior to the RH. On rare occasions the RH dominates in spite of being inferior, particularly when the task has prominent visuospatial components. Thus, hemispheric dominance in responding is not always the same as the superior unilateral competence (Levy and Trevarthen).

When the two hemispheres receive competing stimuli at the same time, the response mode tends to determine which hemisphere controls behavior: Lh responses reflect RH decisions and Rh responses reflect LH decisions, even when these decisions are in mutual conflict. A variant of this technique presents brief chimeras consisting of competing half stimuli around fixation, divided along the vertical meridian (Levy and Trevarthen). In this case, both the nature of the task and the response mode interact to select a behaviorally dominant hemisphere.

Bimanual responses facilitate interhemispheric cooperation for compatible stimuli in the two VFs even in the split brain. It seems that motor responses tend to be unified so that in the chronic condition the two hands do not respond in conflict with each other even when the two hemispheres make conflicting decisions.

The disconnected LH can be said to be generally dominant for several reasons. First, it is more likely than the RH to assume control over behavior in free field situations. Second, it has better ipsilateral visual and tactile-kinesthetic sensory-motor control than the RH. Third, LH performance is more stable and less sensitive to small task differences. Fourth, the split-brain patient routinely neglects and denies RH experiences.

CONSCIOUSNESS

Each disconnected hemisphere possesses not only a separate sensory-motor interface with the environment, its own perceptual, mnestic, cognitive and linguistic repertoire, but also a distinct personality, as well as characteristic preferences and dislikes. The two hemispheres have similar, but not identical, concepts of self, past and future, family, social culture and history (Sperry). After some testing experience with the patients, examiners spontaneously refer to the two hemispheres as if they were distinct people, e.g. "the LH was upset at the RH responses today." While such references may be regarded as shorthand for patterns of behavior with specific lateralized stimuli and responses, they nonetheless express a strong phenomenological sense of two coexisting streams of consciousness. But while both sides can most probably be simultaneously and independently conscious, it is not clear that they both simultaneously possess free wills and thus that the split-brain includes two distinct, and possibly incompatible, loci of moral responsibility (Mackay).

Recognizing that the disconnected RH is conscious provides additional evidence that language is not necessary for human consciousness. Using the split brain as a model for the normal mind, an individual's consciousness can then be viewed as the net result of an interaction among at least two distinct states of consciousness. The question then arises why the normal person with an intact brain experiences consciousness as unified rather than dual. Sperry reasoned that normal consciousness is a higher emergent entity that transcends the separate awareness in the connected left and right hemispheres, supersedes them in controlling thought and action, and integrates their activity. Alternatively, Bogen and many others argue that normal consciousness is also dual, with partially separate parallel processing in the two hemispheres which sometimes does result in subjective feelings of conflict. Moreover, some normal subjects behave like split-brain patients during lateralized tests, thus demonstrating spontaneous or dynamic functional disconnection (Landio and Iacoboni).

It is noteworthy that the two chronically disconnected hemispheres generally do not engage in overt conflict. This is partly explained by characteristic RH passivity, LH dominance, and a unified system of motor control, as well as shared subcortical structures. Such conflict has usually been observed in the acute stage following disconnection and in partial disconnection due to natural lesions, as in cases of the ALIEN HAND syndrome. However, even in the chronic stage we routinely encounter LH autocriticism and denial of RH experiences.

GENERALIZABILITY

The Los Angeles series of commissurotomy patients is unique because (1) the patients were relatively high functioning; (2) they suffered from relatively minor extracallosal damage rather than from massive early lesions causing hemispheric functional reorganization; indeed, few of the patients had any history of early functional deficits; (3) these patients have diverse neurological histories yet show similar functional hemispheric profiles; (4) in general, the predominant hemisphericity of extracallosal damage in these patients does not correlate with behavioral laterality effects. Thus, it is unlikely that the disconnection syndrome observed in these patients represents an abnormal state of cerebral dominance.

The chronically disconnected LH does not show neglect of the left half of space or PROSOPAGNOSIA and the disconnected RH is neither word deaf nor WORD BLIND. The linguistic profiles of the disconnected RH do resemble those of patients with dominant HEMISPHERECTOMY or with amytal anesthesia of the LH, as well as the pattern observed in large heterogeneous aphasic populations. Indeed, RH language is now often used to reinterpret perplexing symptoms of some paradoxical syndromes, such as covert reading in pure alexia, semantic errors in deep DYSLEXIA or misnaming with good miming in optic aphasia.

Overall, the disconnected hemispheres are generally free of the dramatic deficits that sometimes follow focal hemispheric damage. It seems that certain focal lesions involve both diaschisis and pathological inhibition of residual competence in the healthy hemisphere. As a result, the disconnected hemispheres often suggest greater hemispheric capabilities than inferred from lesion studies. At the same time, even when the hemispheres of normal subjects demonstrate independent strategies or apparently different representations, their competence and range of abilities is greater than seen in the disconnected hemispheres. It is likely that the normal hemispheres can borrow resources from each other and affect each other by more or less subtle automatic priming/interference effects. Even the split brain permits some interhemispheric exchange through multiple subcortical pathways, so that the competence of the disconnected hemispheres in turn may overestimate the overall competence of residual hemispheres following hemispherectomy for lesions of late onset. Some normal cognitive effects, such as the consistency effect in hierarchic perception (global interference with local decisions), the Stroop effect, discourse processing, or verbal access to emotions may be necessarily interhemispheric, hence reduced in the split brain.

The split brain remains a model system for behavioral laterality effects in the normal brain. It operationalizes the concept of "degree of hemispheric specialization" by demonstrating independent processing of the same task in each hemisphere and interpreting the expressions "hemisphere X performed better than hemisphere Y on test A by amount d" or "hemisphere X performed task A better than task B by amount d." Further, the split brain has motivated the useful distinction for behavioral laterality effects in normal subjects between "callosal relay" tasks that are exclusively specialized in one hemisphere, "direct access" tasks that can be processed independently in each hemisphere, and "interhemispheric" tasks that routinely require hemispheric integration.

The disconnection syndrome has been adduced as a useful model for other conditions of congenital cognitive deficits. Thus, schizophrenia is sometimes believed to involve symmetrically hyperactive callosal function (David) (as well as frontal LH dysfunction), ALEXITHYMIA is said to involve asymmetrically hypoactive callosal function (Hoppe) (selective deficit in RH to LH callosal transfer), and developmental dyslexia may involve impaired interhemispheric control (as well as LH language dysfunction) (Bloch).

BIBLIOGRAPHY

Bogen, J. E. (1990). Partial hemispheric independence with the neocommissures intact. In C. Trevarthen (Ed.), *Brain circuits and functions of the mind* (pp. 215–30). Cambridge: Cambridge University Press.

Bogen, J. E. (1993). The callosal syndrome. In K. M. Heilman & E. Valenstein (Eds), *Clinical neuropsychology*, 3rd edn (pp. 337–407). New York: Oxford University Press.

Nebes, R. D. (Ed.). (1990). The commissurotomized brain. In F. Boller & J. Grafman (Eds), *Handbook of neuropsychology*, Vol. 4, section 7 (pp. 3–168). Amsterdam: Elsevier.

Sperry, R. W. (1968). Mental unity following surgical disconnection of the cerebral hemispheres. In *The Harvey Lectures*, series 62 (pp. 293–323). New York: Academic Press.

Sperry, R. W. (1974). Lateral specialization in the surgically separated hemispheres. In F. O. Schmitt & F. G. Worden (Eds), *Neuroscience 3rd Study Program* (pp. 5–19). Cambridge, MA: MIT Press.

Trevarthen, C. (Ed.). (1990). *Brain circuits and functions of the mind; Essays in honor of R. W. Sperry*. Part III. *Cerebral hemispheres and human consciousness* (pp. 211–388). Cambridge: Cambridge University Press.

Zaidel, D. W. (1990). Memory and spatial cognition following commissurotomy. In R. D. Nebes (Ed.), The commissurotomized brain (see above) (pp. 151–66). Amsterdam: Elsevier.

Zaidel, D. W. (1994). A view of the world from a split brain perspective. In E. M. R. Critchley (Ed.), *The neurological boundaries of reality* (pp. 161–74). London: Farrand Press.

Zaidel, E. (1978). Concepts of cerebral dominance in the split brain. In P. Buser & A. Rougeul Buser (Eds), *Cerebral correlates of conscious experience* (pp. 263–84). Amsterdam: Elsevier.

Zaidel, E., Zaidel, D. W., & Bogen, J. E. (1990). Testing the commissurotomy patient. In A. A. Boulton, G. B. Baker, & M. Hiscock (Eds), *Neuromethods*. Vol. 15: *Methods in human neuropsychology* (pp. 147–201). Clifton, NJ: Humana Press.

ERAN ZAIDEL, DAHLIA W. ZAIDEL,
AND JOSEPH E. BOGEN

disinhibition Disinhibition may refer to the removal of inhibition in any neural system. However, the term is more commonly applied to a behavioral change of a social or sexual nature. Socially, there is over-familiarity, tactlessness, over-talkativeness, silly joking and punning, often accompanied by childish excitement. Breaches of normal manners are common, with errors of judgment, lack of concern and insight. Sexually, indiscretions may occur which may extend to sexual touching or public masturbation; lack of control of anger may also result in verbal or physical aggression. These behavioral changes are commonly associated with lesions of the FRONTAL LOBE, but also occur with lesions of the BRAIN STEM.

dissociation Dissociation is the demonstration that a specific function may be impaired while another related function remains unimpaired; the two functions are then said to be dissociated. The inference drawn from a dissociation is that the two functions are supported by different neural structures. A simple example would be in disorders of reading (ALEXIA) and writing (AGRAPHIA). These disorders commonly occur together. However, as cases may be seen in which alexia occurs without agraphia, and agraphia without alexia, they are said to be dissociable; a dissociation has been demonstrated. The conclusion is that while the functions may be spatially contiguous in the brain, and therefore both are likely to be affected by a single lesion, or they may rely upon common functional elements which, if impaired, result in a deficit in both functions, there are elements to each function which are dissociated, which are specific to the particular function (reading or writing), and which may be impaired and lead to a deficit in that function alone.

A special case of dissociation which is of importance among the research strategies available to clinical neuropsychologists is *double dissociation*. This principle states that it is insufficient to associate a particular function to a specific cerebral region on the basis of dissociation evidence alone. In terms of the logic of the double dissociation analysis it is necessary to consider two locations and two functions. If lesions of area A affect function X but not function Y, and lesions of area B affect function Y but not function X, then double dissociation has been demonstrated. An even stronger position is sometimes adopted: that lesions of area A should affect function X and no other function, while lesions of area B should affect function Y and no other function; but this strong demonstration of double dissociation is difficult to achieve in practice.

The double dissociation principle is an undoubted contribution to the conceptual analysis of lesion effects, but it does rely upon a model of relatively strict and stable localization. It may also be difficult to apply in a complex clinical situation with varied and interacting behavioral deficits resulting from a complex pattern of cerebral lesions. An additional problem with the double dissociation strategy, as well as with less elegant research designs, is that the investigator may be trying to establish that a particular ability is not affected by a particular lesion. This is the problem of affirming the null hypothesis and is beset by methodological and statistical difficulties. The investigator can never be sure that no effect is present and that sufficiently sensitive tests and an adequate research design have been employed. The general sensitivity of standard psychometric procedures when applied in neuropsychology is a particular problem within this context (*see* ASSESSMENT; METHODOLOGICAL ISSUES).

J. GRAHAM BEAUMONT

divided visual field technique The divided visual field technique refers to a variety of experimental paradigms that involve flashing visual stimuli briefly to one side or the other of a fixation point and recording measures of response accuracy and reaction time. The technique has become popular as a noninvasive, inexpensive way to study hemispheric asymmetry or laterality. This is done by comparing performance when a stimulus is flashed to the left side of the observer's fixation point (left visual field or LVF) with performance when the same stimulus is flashed to the right side of the observer's fixation point (right visual field or RVF). Like many experimental procedures, the divided visual field technique has advantages and disadvantages. When used properly, it can provide an important means of testing hypotheses about hemispheric asymmetry. At the same time, the direction and magnitude of visual field differences can be influenced by many factors in addition to hemispheric asymmetry, therefore appropriate control procedures are essential when the technique is used to study hemispheric asymmetry.

When both eyes are fixated on the same point in space, information from each visual half-field projects directly to the visual cortex of the contralateral hemisphere, that is, there is a direct connection from the LVF to the right hemisphere and from the RVF to the left hemisphere. This comes about because of the anatomy of the primate visual system. Specifically, those portions of the optic nerve that carry information from the temporal halves of the two retinas project to the hemisphere ipsilateral to each eye. At the same time, those portions of the optic nerve that carry information from the nasal halves of the two retinas cross at the OPTIC CHIASM so as to project to the hemisphere contralateral to each eye. Given this anatomical arrangement, it is possible to present a visual stimulus so that it projects directly to only one cerebral hemisphere by presenting it to only one side of an individual's fixation point. Of course, this presupposes that the individual maintains the same eye fixation for as long as the visual stimulus is present. For this reason, stimulus duration is typically below the latency required for a voluntary shift in eye position in response to the onset of a visual stimulus (approximately 200 msec).

Examination of the ability of humans to identify visual stimuli such as letters as a function of where they occur in the visual field has a long history. The earliest studies of this sort were not conducted with hemispheric asymmetry in mind. Instead, much of the interest was on whether individuals scanned some post-exposure trace of a multi-element display in a systematic order (e.g. left to right) and whether the direction of the scan was related to such things as the scanning order used for reading. In fact, the order of post-exposure scanning contributes to visual half-field asymmetries. This creates potential problems in using visual half-field asymmetries to make inferences about hemispheric asymmetry unless steps are taken to control for asymmetric scanning biases.

DIVIDED VISUAL FIELD STUDIES OF SPLIT-BRAIN PATIENTS

Growth in the use of visual half-field asymmetry to study information processing differences between the hemispheres can be traced to studies with patients who have had the left and right hemispheres surgically disconnected in order to control the spread of epileptic seizures. Such COMMISSUROTOMY (or split-brain) patients provide the opportunity to investigate the competence of each hemisphere, assuming that ways can be found to test each hemisphere separately from its partner. Beginning in the early 1960s, the divided visual field technique was adapted for this purpose and the results were quite striking. For example, when single words or pictures of familiar objects were flashed to the RVF (left hemisphere), split-brain patients had no trouble naming them. However, when the same stimuli were flashed to the LVF (right hemisphere), the stimuli could not be named. Such results are consistent with the well-established dominance of the left hemisphere for a number of linguistic processes and with the fact that the right hemisphere is virtually unable to generate speech in most people. These dramatic findings obtained with split-brain patients reinforced the idea that hemispheric asymmetry can influence visual half-field asymmetries and helped create the *Zeitgeist* that has led to an explosion of divided visual field studies with neurologically intact individuals.

DIVIDED VISUAL FIELD STUDIES OF NEUROLOGICALLY INTACT INDIVIDUALS

Early studies with neurologically intact individuals produced visual half-field asymmetries that were generally consistent with those obtained from split-brain patients and with hemispheric asymmetries inferred from the study of neurological patients. For example, in right-handed individuals there is typically an RVF advantage for identifying words and pronounceable nonsense syllables. To be sure, this perceptual asymmetry is smaller than in split-brain patients. Nevertheless, in view of the many connections between the two hemispheres in the intact brain, the presence of reliable asymmetries at all is remarkable. Furthermore, when stimulus duration is sufficiently short to prevent eye movements that bring the stimulus into central vision, and when only a single stimulus is presented on each trial, the RVF

advantage for word recognition is obtained for both languages like English that are processed from left to right and for languages like Hebrew that are processed from right to left. Thus the effects are not easily attributed to biases in the order of post-exposure scanning. In addition, LVF advantages are often obtained for tasks for which the right hemisphere seems dominant, based on studies with neurological patients. Included are certain tasks involving photographs of faces and tasks involving certain judgments of spatial location (for review, see Bradshaw, 1989; articles in J. Sergent, 1986; Hellige, 1993; Davidson & Hugdahl, 1995).

Given that the divided visual field technique has both convergent and face validity as a way of investigating hemispheric asymmetry, it is important to consider how it is that hemispheric asymmetry might produce perceptual asymmetry in neurologically intact individuals. One possibility is that, despite connections between the two hemispheres, whichever hemisphere receives the stimulus information directly (i.e. the hemisphere contralateral to the stimulated visual field) performs all of the information processing required by the task. According to this *direct access* view, visual half-field asymmetries occur for the same reason in both split-brain patients and in neurologically intact individuals. A second possibility is that, when there is hemispheric asymmetry for the task being performed, the dominant hemisphere eventually processes stimulus information from both visual fields. On this *callosal relay* view, performance is better when the stimulus reaches the dominant hemisphere directly (from the visual field that projects to that hemisphere) than when the stimulus projects first to the nondominant hemisphere and information about that stimulus is transferred via the CORPUS CALLOSUM to the dominant hemisphere. An important assumption of this view is that information is degraded by traversing a less direct pathway to the dominant hemisphere. A third possibility is that performing a task for which one hemisphere is dominant creates an *arousal asymmetry* in favor of the dominant hemisphere. On this view, attention is directed more quickly and more easily to the side of space contralateral to the more aroused hemisphere. Rather than identifying one of these mechanisms as correct and the others as incorrect, research over the last 30 years suggests that all three may contribute to visual half-field asymmetries (see the chapters by Hellige and Zaidel in Hellige, 1983; also Hellige, 1993).

POTENTIAL ARTIFACTS AND METHODOLOGICAL CONSIDERATIONS

Although hemispheric asymmetry can (and often does) influence visual half-field asymmetry, there are a host of other factors that also influence perceptual asymmetry. When the goal is the study of hemispheric asymmetry, it is critical that the studies be designed to minimize the contribution of these other factors or to rule them out completely. Biases in the direction of post-exposure scanning have already been noted as contributing to visual half-field asymmetries when visual displays contain more than one item, especially if some items on each trial are in the LVF and others are in the RVF. As ways of minimizing the effects of left-right scanning biases, investigators typically present only a single item on each trial and, when more than one item is necessary (e.g. having observers indicate whether two simultaneously presented letters are identical or not), arranging the items vertically rather than horizontally. It is for this reason that words in visual half-field studies are frequently presented with the letters arranged vertically.

Other factors that can influence visual half-field asymmetry include such things as the dominance of one eye over the other in combination with the dominance of either nasal or temporal hemiretinal pathways and systematic biases in covert visual attention. Several of these factors and ways to control for them are discussed in Beaumont (1982), Bryden (1982), Hellige (1983, 1993), and J. Sergent (1986). Although there are many factors that contribute to any single visual field asymmetry, it should be noted that most of the unwanted factors do not predict changes in visual field advantage as a function of the manipulation of task-related variables. For example, if some combination of peripheral pathway asymmetries biases an individual in favor of the RVF, then this will be true regardless of the stimuli or of the specific information processing requirements of the task being performed. However, this sort of bias could not account for the fact that opposite visual field advantages are obtained for different tasks or for different conditions within the same experiment. That is, Visual Field by Task interactions are usually more difficult to dismiss as

artifacts of these other factors than are the main effects of visual field or the simple effects of visual field at any one level of some task variable (for discussion see Hellige, 1983). For this reason, more emphasis should be placed on Visual Field by Task interactions than on the simple effects of visual field.

An interesting question concerns the effect of perceptual reference frames on visual half-field asymmetry. It is usually assumed that what is important is whether a stimulus is to the left or right of the center of the fovea. This is not always the case. For example, Robertson and Lamb (1988) required observers to indicate whether a set of identical letters (e.g. four uppercase R's) was normal in orientation or mirror-image reversed. With the stimulus display frame upright, they found that reaction time was faster when the letters were presented to the RVF than when the letters were presented to the LVF. When the stimulus display frame was rotated 90 degrees clockwise or counterclockwise, the "RVF" and "LVF" stimuli actually appeared in the upper or lower visual field. However, relative to the "top" of the rotated display, the stimuli continued to appear in the *relative LVF* or *relative RVF* location. In these rotated conditions, reaction time was faster for the relative RVF condition than for the relative LVF condition, with the difference being equal to the magnitude of the RVF advantage in the upright display condition; that is, the entire visual half-field difference in the upright condition can be attributed to the relative position of stimuli within a perceptual, object-centered frame of reference rather than to left/right location with respect to the fovea. These results underscore the fact that some visual half-field differences may have nothing to do with hemispheric asymmetry. However, such strong effects of an object-centered frame of reference may be restricted to judgments of mirror-image reflection of stimuli. For example, in a task that required identification of consonant-vowel-consonant nonsense syllables, Hellige and colleagues (1991) found the expected RVF advantage when stimulus displays were upright and no effects of relative visual field in rotated displays. In addition, differences between the types of errors found on LVF and RVF trials were also restricted to the upright condition, consistent with an explanation in terms of left-hemisphere dominance for phonetic processing.

THE ROLE OF INPUT FACTORS IN VISUAL HALF-FIELD ASYMMETRY

A necessary requirement of visual half-field studies is that stimuli be presented very briefly and to off-center areas of the retina that are not the most effective for identifying visual stimuli. In this sense, the visual half-field technique may be particularly susceptible to hemispheric asymmetries that occur relatively early in visual processing. It is important to remember this when the goal is to study hemispheric asymmetries for more abstract aspects of cognitive processing. Furthermore, in any visual half-field experiment, stimuli must be presented at some specific stimulus duration, luminance, size, distance from the fovea and so forth. The specific combination of perceptual parameters chosen for an experiment can influence the pattern of visual half-field asymmetry. This should be kept in mind in both the design and interpretation of experiments using the visual half-field technique. The fact that input factors can have such effects is almost certainly one cause of variation in the results of experiments that differ in the perceptual parameters that were used but that are otherwise very similar. In addition to being important for methodological reasons, understanding the role of input factors is important for understanding some of the mechanisms that underlie hemispheric differences for processing visual information.

It is generally the case that manipulations that degrade the quality of visual input disrupt performance more when stimuli are presented to the RVF than when stimuli are presented to the LVF (for reviews see articles in J. Sergent, 1986; Kitterle et al., 1990; Hellige, 1993). This is particularly true when the quality of visual input is reduced in a manner that selectively impairs the processing of local details that must be carried by visual channels tuned to relatively high visual spatial frequencies. This has led to the hypothesis that, at some level of processing beyond the sensory cortex, the two cerebral hemispheres are preferentially sensitive to different spatial-frequency outputs from the visual channels (see the articles by J. Sergent and Hellige in Sergent, 1986). Visual half-field studies with sine-wave gratings (which contain only a single, well-specified, spatial frequency) are consistent with this hypothesis. Specifically, these experiments and others suggest that, for the identification (but not the detection) of visual stimuli, the left and right hemispheres make most efficient use of relatively high and relatively low spatial frequencies respectively. In view of the support for the spatial frequency hypothesis, it is instructive to consider in less technical terms the kinds of visual information that must be conveyed by lower versus higher ranges of spatial frequency. If relatively high spatial frequencies are removed from a complex stimulus (e.g. a face), the stimulus looks blurred. You can see this for yourself by looking at things through a set of strong reading glasses (assuming that you do not ordinarily use them). If your vision is ordinarily normal, wearing these glasses produces what is known as dioptric blur – an effective means of selectively removing relatively high spatial frequencies. The more powerful the lenses, the greater the range of high frequencies removed. In such a blurred world, you can still make out the larger characteristics of objects (e.g. the outer contour of faces) because this information is carried by the moderate to low spatial frequency channels, which are not influenced much by dioptric blur. Unfortunately, there is no easy way to illustrate for yourself what the visual world looks like when relatively low frequencies are selectively removed and relatively high frequencies remain. In general, however, the high spatial frequencies are most useful for processing small details (e.g. the inner features of a face) and are not particularly useful for extracting the larger configural properties.

The fact that input factors can exert a powerful influence on visual half-field asymmetries does not mean that other factors are unimportant. For example, the RVF (left-hemisphere) advantage for tasks demanding linguistic/phonetic analysis (e.g. word recognition, lexical decisions) occurs across a very wide range of input parameters. Indeed, it is questionable whether asymmetry for such tasks is influenced at all by input factors. This suggests that the effects of input parameters become less important when hemispheric asymmetry for more abstract cognitive aspects of a task becomes greater.

INTERHEMISPHERIC INTERACTION

The predominant focus of visual half-field experiments has been on investigating hemispheric differences. It is also important to understand how the hemispheres interact with each other to produce unified information processing. The following modification of the visual half-field technique has proved useful for doing this. In addition to LVF and RVF trials, the same stimulus is sometimes presented simultaneously to both LVF and RVF locations (redundant bilateral trials). The quantitative and qualitative nature of performance on redundant bilateral trials is then compared to performance on LVF and RVF trials to determine whether modes of processing favored by one hemisphere or the other tend to dominate when the viewing conditions allow both hemispheres to have equal access to the stimulus (see Hellige et al., 1989). So far, such studies have identified interesting dissociations between the mode of processing preferred on redundant bilateral trials and the mode of processing associated with superior performance on unilateral trials.

BIBLIOGRAPHY

Bradshaw, J. L. (1989). *Hemispheric specialization and psychological function*. New York: Wiley.

Davidson, R. J., & Hugdahl, K. (Eds). (1995). *Brain asymmetry*. Cambridge, MA: MIT Press.

Hellige, J. B. (Ed.). (1983). *Cerebral hemisphere asymmetry: Method, theory, and application*. New York: Praeger.

Hellige, J. B. (1993). *Hemispheric asymmetry: What's right and what's left*. Cambridge, MA: Harvard University Press.

Hellige, J. B., Cowin, E. L., Eng, T., & Sergent, J. (1991). Perceptual reference frames and visual field asymmetry for verbal processing. *Neuropsychologia, 29*, 929–39.

Hellige, J. B., Taylor, A. K., & Eng, T. L. (1989). Interhemispheric interaction when both hemispheres have access to the same stimulus information. *Journal of Experimental Psychology: Human Perception and Performance, 15*, 711–22.

Kitterle, F. L., Christman, S., & Hellige, J. B. (1990). Hemispheric differences are found in the identification, but not the detection, of low versus high spatial frequencies. *Perception and Psychophysics, 48*, 297–306.

Robertson, L. C., & Lamb, M. R. (1988). The role of perceptual reference frames in visual field asymmetries. *Neuropsychologia, 26*, 145–52.

Sergent, J. (Ed.). (1986). Methodological issues concerning the use of the tachistoscope in neuropsychological research. Special issue of *Brain and Cognition, 5*, 127–252.

JOSEPH B. HELLIGE

dominance *See* LATERALIZATION.

dorsal column   The dorsal columns are important fibers tracts within the spinal cord. Their principal functional significance is in carrying somatic sensory information from the dorsal nerve roots in the cord up to the level of the brain stem (*see* SOMESTHETIC SYSTEM).

dreamy state   Dreamy states are an aptly named alteration of consciousness in which a sense of unreality envelops the subject. They are important because they are associated with both auditory and visual hallucinations, although more commonly with auditory hallucinations. They have been elicited by cortical stimulation of the superior and lateral surface of the temporal lobes, when a hallucination of recognizable voices most commonly accompanies the dreamy state. The parallel with imagery experienced while awaking from or falling into sleep is obvious.

dressing apraxia   *See* APRAXIA.

drug intoxication   *See* TOXICOLOGY.

dual task paradigm   In the dual task situation subjects are asked to perform a primary task while at the same time performing a second task. Three relevant measures are usually employed: performance on each of the two tasks separately and on the dual task condition. This paradigm usually entails a manual task and a second task that may be either motor or cognitive. The aim is to study the effect of cognitive activity upon manual performance and vice versa. The manual task might be unimanual or one performed by both hands with one hand leading the sequence.

This method was first shown to be relevant to neuropsychology by Kinsbourne and Cook (1971) and was followed by a number of other studies whose main conclusion is that verbal and nonverbal tasks have differential effects on concurrent manual performance. Verbal activity has been shown to be more disrupting for right-hand than left-hand performance, while nonverbal activity impairs the activity of both hands equally (or the left more than the right in a minority of cases). Concurrent verbal activity has also been shown to interfere with the strategy used in the task rather than just with the level of motor performance (Semenza, 1983).

The dual task methodology is also thought to be informative about skills putatively mediated by modular cognitive architecture. Its application is usually predicated on the argument that two tasks will interfere heavily if they both require the involvement of the same cognitive module(s); that is, if they both compete for the same cognitive resources (Shallice, 1988). If they can be mediated by separate modules (and pathways), then it should be possible to combine the two tasks with little interference (a limited decrement could be expected, however, even when the tasks concerned do not compete for cognitive resources, due to things such as greater neural noise when the two tasks are being performed, greater stimulus uncertainty, or the need to keep multiple goals active). With this logic the dual task paradigm is viewed as being able to provide an analogue of the DISSOCIATIONS (*see also* METHODOLOGICAL ISSUES) in neuropsychology. The prerequisite for being able to combine two tasks is that they utilize separate functional subsystems; they should, therefore, be dissociated in neurological patients.

A variation of the paradigm is the concurrent memory load technique in which subjects are first given a set of items to retain in their memory. A primary task is then performed, after which recall or recognition of the memory load items is tested. Interference would result from the need to devote certain resources to retaining the memory load items while the primary task is being performed. The conditions that cause interference seem to involve items which subjects may rehearse between presentation and test.

BIBLIOGRAPHY

Kinsbourne, M., & Cook, J. (1971). Generalized and lateralized effects of concurrent verbalization on a unimanual skill. *Quarterly Journal of Experimental Psychology, 23*, 341–5.

Semenza, C. (1983). Effect of concurrent activity on strategies in copying designs. *Perceptual and Motor Skills, 43*, 1003–7.

Shallice, T. (1988). *From neuropsychology to mental structure*. Cambridge: Cambridge University Press.

T. M. SGARAMELLA AND C. SEMENZA

dualism *See* MIND–BODY PROBLEM.

dysarthria Dysarthria is a difficulty in speech production resulting from incoordination of the speech apparatus. It is therefore not an APHASIA, but a disorder of articulation resulting from a defect in the mechanisms of the larynx, pharynx, or tongue. Among the disorders of articulation it may be distinguished from problems of sound selection and central motor deficits in speech control, which are aphasic in nature.

dyschromatopsia The central or acquired defect in the discrimination of colors is known as dyschromatopsia; although it may also be known as acquired achromatopsia, color blindness or color imperception. Bilateral lesions of the occipitotemporal border regions are thought to be critical in the production of this deficit, which is commonly also associated with visual field defects, and possibly with facial agnosia.

dysdiadochokinesis Dysdiadochokinesis refers to the inability to perform alternating movements rapidly and regularly. It is commonly demonstrated by requiring the patient to alternately form a fist and open the hand, or to alternately pronate and supinate the forearm. It is a symptom of cerebellar dysfunction.

dyseidetic A dyseidetic patient has difficulty in recognizing words by their visual configuration. Within current dual-route models of DYSLEXIA it refers to a dysfunction of the whole-word reading route, while the phonological route remains intact. The patient may therefore succesfully employ phonic skills in reading regular words (to which phoneme-to-grapheme conversion rules correctly apply), or to spell a word with a regular form. Dyseidetic individuals have difficulty in building a sight vocabulary and produce regularization errors in reading and spelling.

dyslexia As a class of acquired disorders of reading, dyslexia may be highly selective, in that the difficulty coping with written language may occur in the absence of any other impairments, or it may be accompanied by other deficits of language, perception, or memory that are causally related to the reading disturbance. Consequently, there is a variety of major dyslexic subtypes, with a different functional explanation required for each of them.

The fact that human beings can use an orthographic code as a substitute for spoken language, and that this kind of representation allows us to fluently derive the sound and meaning of written words and sentences, has been crucial to the development and proliferation of knowledge. It is hard to imagine how a technologically advanced culture could evolve without first discovering a way of coding language in a medium that allows the information to be permanently stored and widely accessible, and that is easily compatible with the normal mechanisms for sentence comprehension and production. In general terms, reading is possible because the brain, exposed to a period of appropriate learning conditions, can fashion out of its existing machinery for processing linguistic and visual representations a set of *additional* routines that can rapidly take squiggles on the page and convert them into meaningful words and sentences.

What do we currently know about the nature and organization of these routines? One source of evidence that has played a very crucial role in our attempts to answer this question has been the performance of individuals with acquired reading disorders. From detailed analyses of such cases, we have begun to arrive at an initial understanding of the specialized functional components that allow us to rapidly and automatically translate written word forms into other linguistic representations.

THE MAPPING OF ORTHOGRAPHY TO MEANING: THE SEMANTIC ROUTINE

There was little clear progress in our understanding of the specialized mechanisms that can be disrupted to produce reading disorders until the recent convergence of methods in cognitive and neuropsychology. Earlier work by neurologists was based on the assumption that written words were transcoded immediately into an auditory form, based on the sounds of their constituent letters. Most reading disorders were simply considered to be the outcome of an underlying core language deficit, aside from a more peripheral

subtype that was thought of as a disconnection between letter percepts and auditory word forms (see De Bleser & Luzatti, 1989, for an excellent review of nineteenth-century work on reading and writing disorders). There were dissenting viewpoints along the way, of course: Beringer and Stein (1930) reported a case that they were forced to classify as "pure alexia," using the impoverished nomenclature of the period, showing apparently unimpaired spontaneous speech, language comprehension, and written production, but whose errors in reading words were frequently semantic approximations to the targets (e.g. "fox" was read as "hare" and "India" as "elephant"). The claim by Beringer and Stein that the reading disorder occurred without any concomitant disturbance in auditory language implied, of course, that a great deal of complexity and specialization must underlie the procedures that map print to sound and meaning, despite earlier views. Many years went by, however, before this notion gained acceptance.

The existence of a form of dyslexia in which semantic errors (e.g. "colonel" read as "uniform") were a dominant feature, continued to be reported sporadically in the literature (Low, 1931; Goldstein, 1948; Simmel & Goldshmidt, 1953) and was eventually fully validated by Marshall and Newcombe (1973), who drew attention to its theoretical import. They described evidence from a patient GR who, before sustaining a left hemisphere injury, was clearly an intelligent and literate adult. In addition to producing numerous *semantic* errors when asked to read individual words in free vision (examples include "play" for act, "shut" for close, "cousin" for uncle, and "long" for tall) GR would sometimes make *derivational* errors (thus "entertainment" for entertain, "born" for birth, and "wisdom" for wise), as well as *visual* errors ("shock" for stock, "sausage" for saucer, and "crocodile" for crocus). His performance was very sensitive to the grammatical category of the words he was required to read. *Concrete* nouns were read much more accurately than other words; *adjectives, adverbs*, and *abstract* nouns were of intermediate difficulty, and *function* words (e.g. for, his, the, in, and some) were seldom read correctly, his most frequent response to these items being a complete omission. Finally, the patient could not read *any* pronounceable nonsense words, regardless of how elementary their spelling pattern, and would either resort to producing a visually similar word in an attempt to cope with the task demands (e.g. "wet" for wep, "damp" for dup) or would be completely unable to generate any response.

This complicated set of features – now termed *deep dyslexia* – has been documented by many investigators since the original description by Marshall and Newcombe. Coltheart (1980) reviewed 15 cases, Kremlin (1982) described a further 8 patients with the same combination of symptoms or *symptom complex*, and an additional 10 were summarized by Coltheart and colleagues (1987).

To arrive at a preliminary interpretation of deep dyslexia, Marshall and Newcombe began by emphasizing the fact that the patient they first observed could *not* be relying on any procedure that *first* assembled the pronunciation of a spelling sequence *before* the meaning of the word was contacted. It must be that the orthography of the *whole word* was being used for access to meaning and pronunciation – how else could the patient

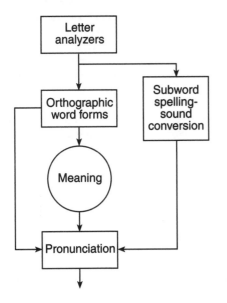

Figure 39 The general processing framework initially used to interpret the fact that deep dyslexic patients are forced to read by directly mapping the visual form of the word to meaning. For these patients the route from orthographic forms to meaning is still partially available, but the remaining transcoding options that bypass meaning are not.

read a word like "moon" (concrete) but not "soon" (an adverb) or "yoon" (a spelling pattern without any premorbidly stored orthographic representation) if not by using the entire spelling pattern as the means of gaining access to a semantic description? Words *without* meaning (i.e. pronounceable nonsense words) would find no address in the system and so could only yield a null response. In addition, access to meaning for some visual word forms may be partial or incomplete; e.g. the activation for the sequence "lion" may be something like < large, dangerous, feline >, leading to a semantically related but incorrect response such as "tiger."

FURTHER REFINEMENTS

The conceptualization of deep dyslexia was based on the inference that the patients must be reading by mapping each word in terms of the spelling pattern *as a whole* onto meaning, and then deriving a pronunciation for the word as a concept. Notice that this claim does *not* imply that reading in deep dyslexics occurs without analysis of the individual letters; the explanation does not require that the patients are reading via a kind of holistic extraction of features that directly activate the word, only that access to meaning relies on first contacting a stored, abstract, orthographic representation corresponding to the exact sequence of letters on the page (e.g. FLOWER, flower, or for that matter FloWeR, all have precisely the same orthographic form and therefore map onto *one* entry in this system), without first deriving a pronunciation.

This idea seems surprising – our intuitions tell us that we arrive at the sound of a written word *before* we understand what the word denotes, yet the performance of deep dyslexics clearly indicates that they are forced to derive a pronunciation *from* the meaning, presumably by using a purely visual routine that directly interprets the word's orthographic pattern. One question immediately arises from this account of the disorder: Is reading in deep dyslexia a property of the normal system, damaged in such a way that only a subset of its components can now operate on written words, or has there been a *qualitative* change in the system, radically altering its habitual mode of operation? Related to this question is the coherence of the full set of symptoms – *the symptom complex* – that constitutes the reading disorder: What underlies the fact that patients

293

who produce semantic errors in reading also show a complicated profile that invariably includes visual errors, greater difficulty reading low imageable (abstract) words than high imageable (concrete) words, additional word-class effects (nouns better than function words, for example), derivational errors, etc?

The most prosaic explanation is that the pattern is simply due to a set of independent, co-occurring deficits that are associated because their neuroanatomical substrates are physically close. The difficulty with this account is that the phenomenon of semantic errors appears to virtually guarantee the additional presence of all the remaining symptoms that characterize deep dyslexia (Coltheart et al., 1987). Given the fact that the patient fails to arrive at the correct semantic interpretation of written words and produces semantic paralexias, all the other symptoms follow routinely. How could this be if the explanation for the syndrome is simply due to the neuroanatomical proximity of a number of functionally separate processing components?

Another hypothesis is based on the idea that deep dyslexia is the outcome of an alternative form of reading that does not normally occur, mediated by the *right* instead of the left hemisphere. Some evidence for this claim derives from the similarity between the performance of deep dyslexic patients and right hemisphere reading in a small group of patients who have undergone resection of the corpus callosum and anterior commissure for intractable epilepsy. These patients will make semantic errors in a word –picture matching task when the words are presented only to the right hemisphere (Zaidel & Peters, 1981), analogous to the errors observed in deep dyslexia. In addition, *normal* readers engaged in word recognition tasks for items flashed briefly in the left visual field (projecting to the right hemisphere) have been reported to show an advantage for concrete or high imagery words relative to abstract (low imagery) words (Ellis & Shepherd, 1974; Hines, 1976; Day, 1979), again evoking a comparison with the performance of deep dyslexics.

Unfortunately, despite its intuitive appeal, the right hemisphere hypothesis remains unsatisfactory. Detailed critiques have been formulated by Patterson and Besner (1984) and Shallice (1988), and the main points of their arguments can be summarized as follows: the

effect of concreteness on visual word recognition in the left visual field of normal readers has not been widely replicated and Patterson and Besner have identified a host of methodological problems in the original studies. The force of the analogy between the reading performance of deep dyslexics and that of the disconnected right hemisphere of commissurotomized patients has also been questioned; indeed, the fact that the right hemisphere in a few such neurosurgical cases (many of whom may have undergone substantial cortical reorganization because of early-onset epilepsy) demonstrates partial knowledge of the meaning of some words, hardly provides clear support for the much more sweeping claim that deep dyslexia is a manifestation of normal right hemisphere reading mechanisms. Finally, at least one patient has been described, with many of the characteristics of deep dyslexia, whose reading was abolished after a second *left* hemisphere stroke (Roeltgen, 1987).

A more promising approach to an integrated account of deep dyslexia as a symptom complex has emerged recently in the form of computational models incorporating a large number of relatively simple neuron-like elements that interact in parallel by means of weighted connections. These "connectionist" architectures (see Quinlan, 1991, for an excellent review) typically make use of representations that are distributed over numerous weighted associations between processing units. There has been wide interest among cognitive and neuroscientists in such models because their structure embodies the massive parallelism that is understood to characterize the hardware of the brain.

In a current application of this methodology to deep dyslexia, Hinton and Shallice (1991; see also Plaut and Shallice, 1993) have productively utilized the idea of "attractors" in meaning space, corresponding to bounded regions that delineate each familiar, nameable concept. If the input to these semantic representations from visual (orthographic) words is inherently a bit noisy, the attractor basins will nevertheless continue to move the activation of the word into the correct part of semantic space. When the system is damaged though (by randomly turning off a portion of the weighted connections, for example, or removing some of the processing units), the word may sometimes move to a nearby attractor, one that in fact may correspond to the meaning of a related word. Thus the network will map the word "peach" to the meaning of "apricot," say, because the activation projects into a region of semantic space that is close to but does not actually match the basin of the target. The account proposed by Hinton and Shallice could in principle extend to morphologically related words, clarifying the source of errors like "restless" for restful.

There is a further and rather unexpected consequence that emerges directly from this type of interactive architecture, given appropriate damage to the system. As Hinton and Shallice (1991) point out: "In a connectionist network, similar inputs tend to cause similar outputs, and generally a lot of training and large weights are required to make very similar inputs give very different outputs. Now, if each meaning has a large basin of attraction, the network is free to make the visual form of the word point to any location within this basin, so the network will, if it can, choose to make visually similar words point to nearby points in semantic space. Damage that moves the boundaries of the basins of attraction in semantic space will then have a tendency to cause mixed errors or even visual ones" (p. 75). Surprisingly, then, a change that interferes with the mapping from written words to regions in semantic space can produce a pure visual error like "rat" for mat, or alternatively, "rat" for cat, a type of mixed error (both visual and semantic) that is relatively common in deep dyslexia, occurring much more frequently than the proportion predicted by chance alone.

Additional work based on this approach to the modelling of deep dyslexia has also yielded some success in capturing the effect of word imageability on reading performance. Plaut and Shallice (1993) rely on the idea that words vary substantially in the number of semantic predicates or features they evoke, and that abstract or low imagery words have fewer predicates than concrete words (Jones, 1985). They note that the implemented account developed by Hinton and Shallice included both direct pairwise connections between semantic units or *sememes* (to ensure that activated features are locally consistent by developing lateral inhibitory interactions between the activation of rival units) and a group of "clean-up" units that send connections to and receive connections from many individual feature units. This device allowed *combinations* of sememes to influence each other from different sub-

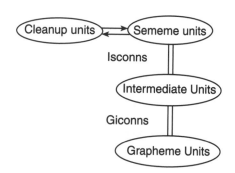

Figure 40 A more recent network architecture for modelling semantic errors in deep dyslexia. Graphemes are mapped to intermediate units and then to sememe units (semantic features). The interactive links between sememes and clean-up units allow combinations of sememes to influence each other, and ensures global consistency among semantic features. (*Giconns* refer to grapheme-to-intermediate connections, *isconns* to intermediate-to-sememe connections.)

sets, and enforced more global consistency among them.

Damage to the network will result in abstract words being less effective than concrete words at engaging the semantic clean-up mechanism, because they intrinsically have fewer features that make up their representation, so abstract words (and words from other grammatical classes as well, like function words) must depend more heavily on unmodulated mapping from words into semantic space. Concrete words, however, have many more features in their representation, both unique and shared, and therefore benefit from stronger clean-up during activation. It is interesting that severe damage to the clean-up units will yield a *reversed* concreteness effect (abstract words read much better than concrete words), because abstract words can still rely on direct connection from words to sememe units, but concrete words, having more extensive semantic features, depend more heavily on the activity of clean-up units, and so yield more errors. This unusual dissociation has indeed been documented in a case of *concrete word dyslexia* by Warrington (1981).

THE NON-SEMANTIC ROUTINE FROM SPELLING TO SOUND

Apparently, in defiance of our intuitions, the normal reading mechanisms can map written words onto a stored representation of the orthographic form, and from this representation can gain direct entry to meaning. Of course, such a *direct* reading routine cannot be the only or even the primary mode of access: we can easily derive the pronunciation of spelling patterns with no meaning that we have never seen before (e.g. nonsense words like "snark" and "boojum"), and we can also use the pronunciation we obtain from a written string to *indirectly* contact a meaning. So patterns like "yot" or "brane" do not match the stored orthographic forms "yacht" and "brain," but nevertheless we can easily determine the sound of these "pseudohomophones," and we realize immediately that they correspond to the sound (and hence the meaning) of known words in our vocabulary.

The presence of two parallel and independent routines from spelling to sound, one activating the stored orthographic form of a given word and the other assembling a pronunciation based on the phonemic values of subword units, has been clearly revealed by the detailed analysis of individual cases of acquired dyslexia. Marshall and Newcombe (1973), who emphasized the dichotomy at the outset, described a form of dyslexia in which the patient can read nonsense words (in marked contrast to deep dyslexics) but has great difficulty reading aloud and comprehending written words that do not conform to the usual correspondences between spelling and sound of the language. Thus the nonsense word "grint" is correctly read, as are the words "hint, stint, flint etc.," but the exception word "pint" is misread using the conventional pronunciation of the segment INT (i.e., a shortened vowel). Given the error, the patient will then also fail to understand the meaning of the word and, based on the incorrect pronunciation, will in fact consider the word to be nonsensical. Comprehension of auditory words is by contrast quite normal.

The explanation of this kind of reading, known as *surface dyslexia*, is that the orthographic representation of many words has been lost or can no longer be reliably accessed after brain damage. The patient is forced to use a routine that assigns a pronunciation to the orthography determined by the regular (i.e. predictable) correspondences of the subword spelling units, and then to rely on this representation to contact the meaning. So the patient will have trouble reading words like "pint" that violate the conventional relationships between spelling and sound (i.e. orthographically irregular or exceptional words, of which there are many examples in English), but will cope much better with regular words like "hint, flint, print," because the pronunciation of these words can be assembled without consulting orthographic knowledge specific to their entire form. Even regular words, however, are not dealt with normally, given the patient's reliance on pronunciation. Homophones like "fare" and "fair" will inevitably remain ambiguous, the patient opting for a definition that is governed by intrinsic bias or context rather than the particular orthography of the word.

FURTHER REFINEMENTS

The initial descriptions of surface dyslexia (Marshall & Newcombe, 1973; Coltheart et al., 1983), though clearly pointing to a reading disorder that was qualitatively distinct from deep dyslexia, were not entirely consistent with the view that the two types were *complementary*. If surface dyslexia was just the reverse of the dissociation responsible for deep dyslexia, patients should be relying on a relatively *intact* mechanism that treats words analytically by assembling a pronunciation from subword orthographic units. Unfortunately, the error patterns were a good deal more complex than the one dictated by this simple viewpoint. First, many responses of modal surface dyslexics tend to be real words, even when they are confronted with a word like "steak." The response based on conventional pronunciation of the EAK segment should be the nonword "steek" (given the correspondence in freak, leak, beak, etc.) but it is not unusual to see errors like "stack" or "stuck" among the expected (and unproblematic) regularizations. Perhaps more troublesome is the fact that many misreadings are obviously not just due to the routinized application of principles of spelling to sound, even if we are willing to assume that these principles are operating somewhat unreliably in the patients. For example, the patient documented by Marshall and Newcombe (1973) produced "increase" for "incense" and "bargain" for "barge," errors that indicate an attempt to reconstruct whole words from a partial analysis of the orthography rather than a veridical application of spelling to sound translation. Marcel (1980) drew an analogy between this kind of strategy and the errors one sees in beginning readers; he disputed the inference that a separate functional mechanism exists for reading independent of a whole-word (lexical) procedure. At the very least, spelling-to-sound relationships must be embedded in a lexical framework.

The question of the precise nature of the procedures that allow a normal reader to quickly assign a pronunciation to familiar words, as well as to words that have never been viewed before, remains a focus of much research. A number of recent developments have led to a deeper understanding of the problem. First, the mixed (and confusing) pattern of errors originally documented in surface dyslexic readers no longer appears to require an explanation based only on the operation of the impaired system operating under essentially normal strategic control. Shallice (1988), following arguments by Henderson (1982), provides cogent reasons for the assumption that the numerous complications in the error patterns must be due to a compensatory procedure mustered by the patients to cope with damaged activation in the visual word form system. A second point is that there is now very good evidence that *nonsemantic* readers – patients who have suffered damage to the representation of word and object meaning – indeed show precisely the pattern expected from an account based on the distinction between word and subword translation of spelling to sound. These cases (e.g. Schwartz et al., 1980; Bub et al, 1985; McCarthy & Warrington, 1986) fail to understand many words (both written and spoken), and reading aloud indicates that (i) some words, especially more common ones (e.g. "break"), are read via *word-specific* mapping from spelling to sound, because despite the comprehension failure, the patient will read many irregular words correctly; (ii) other words, particularly less common ones (e.g. "steak"), are misread and almost all the errors indicate correct application of spelling to sound correspondences at the subword level (i.e. the response to "steak" would be "steek," conforming to the pronunciation of words like freak, creak, sneak).

These results clearly support the existence of two functionally separate routines operating in parallel for the translation of print into sound, one that involves the mapping of visual word forms to meaning, followed by a naming response, and the other based on the transcoding of visual words directly to a pronunciation (the "nonsemantic" procedure).

But what of the normal ability to read nonsense words aloud? These items have no meaning, so they cannot be transcoded by activating semantic representations, and they also do not correspond to any individual whole-word orthographic forms that would be available for directly mapping items within the stored vocabulary of the reader to a spoken response. There are basically two approaches to this question. One tack is to assume that both words and nonsense words are served by a unitary nonsemantic routine. The system must then hold orthographic representations that allow for *word-specific* as well as more *general* correspondences between spelling and sound. For example, Shallice and McCarthy (1985) argue for a range of segments for mapping orthography to a pronunciation, including single graphemes (the smallest unit, like "oo," that can be assigned a response), subsyllables, syllables, and words. Correspondences based on the larger units are assumed to be more vulnerable to the effects of neurological disease. Seidenberg and McClelland (1989) take a different position, opting for an orthographic mechanism that has no explicit representation for whole words, but instead contains numerous triplets of letter combinations (1,000 in their implemented model), plus an explicit marker (denoted by #) for word boundaries. A given sequence of letters will activate an orthographic unit if the string contains a sequence of three consecutive characters that matches one of the triplets; for example, "made" will activate *#ma, ad, ade*, or *de#*. A similar kind of representation was adopted for assigning a pronunciation to the orthographic pattern. The model makes a number of predictions about normal reading that yield an encouraging match with initial experimental evidence.

An alternative to the idea that a *unitary* system of orthographic correspondences is all that is needed for reading both familiar and unfamiliar words is that the brain must in fact have *dual* routines available that are to some extent functionally independent. One mechanism assigns a pronunciation to visual words on the basis of the sequence of letters as a whole, the other functions by having a set of more general correspondences derived from subword units. In a recent defense of this notion, Coltheart and colleagues (1993) point out that certain dyslexic patients have completely lost the ability to read nonsense words but continue to read legitimate words at a high

297

level of accuracy. These patients (referred to as phonological dyslexics), according to any unitary model, must be relying on access to meaning from orthography to obtain a pronunciation of the word. Yet there is good reason to argue that, in certain cases, this cannot be the mechanism by which a response has been generated. Funnell (1983) described a patient whose reading of nonsense words was completely abolished but who correctly read many words aloud, despite the fact that his comprehension of them was severely impaired. A similar case has been reported by Coslett (1991) – an acquired phonological dyslexic whose reading of words (including abstract words) proved to be excellent but who no longer understood many of these same items. It is difficult to avoid the inference that, in such cases, a procedure normally responsible for mapping subword units to a pronunciation has been damaged, and that a separate mechanism remains available for reading whole words aloud, *without* first gaining access to meaning. Coltheart and his collaborators develop an implemented model that extracts systematic and extensive principles of the relationships between spelling and sound, given a corpus of words to learn from, and hold to the view that "our ability to deal with linguistic stimuli we have not previously encountered . . . can only be explained by postulating that we have learned systems of general linguistic rules, and our ability at the same time to deal correctly with exceptions to these rules . . . can only be explained by postulating the existence of systems of word-specific lexical representations" (p. 606).

Obviously, the debate on the nature of the routines for mapping visual words to sound hinges on some fundamental issues. Does the brain explicitly maintain rules for coping with generalities, in addition to whole word units, when embodying a linguistic system like orthography, or is there another kind of representational system that is being used, one that derives regularities implicitly, out of the activation pattern associated with more primitive elements? Doubtless, significant future progress will depend in large part on a successful resolution of this issue.

FROM LETTERS TO VISUAL WORDS

The dyslexias described thus far may be termed "central," in that the disturbance occurs *after* letters have been perceptually synthesized into higher-level visual units. Additional subtypes are

clearly the result of damage to mechanisms that prevent normal access to orthographic forms. *Pure* alexia is a disorder in which the patient has no language deficits and retains the ability to spell words; but reading, when attempted, is limited to an extremely laborious process yielding massive effects of array length on the time taken to identify a word (hence the modern term "letter-by-letter reading"). In general, the patient will need 3 or 4 seconds to read (name or classify) even common three-letter words and, for every increase in word length by one additional letter, performance may be correspondingly slowed by 2 or 3 seconds.

A complete interpretation of this striking dyslexia has remained elusive. One account holds that the impairment is due to a generalized disturbance in the perception of multiple visual forms (Rapp & Caramazza, 1991; Kinsbourne & Warrington, 1962), or is the outcome of inefficiency in the processing of a single visual element that becomes magnified when many elements (i.e. strings of letters) must be identified at once (Farah, 1990; Friedman & Alexander, 1984). A weakness suffered by all current versions of this kind of explanation is that the evidence has been based essentially on the co-occurrence of a perceptual disturbance (say, abnormal effects on a letter matching task) with the characteristic profile of letter-by-letter reading. This type of observed association leaves unproven the claim that the peripheral disturbance is directly responsible for the dyslexia.

Some recent observations may prove relevant in formulating a more precise account. It is now clear that at least some patients are capable of deriving fast, though incomplete access to the identity of a written word. Thus, Shallice and Saffran (1986) have described a letter-by-letter reader who appeared capable of reasonably accurate word/nonsense word decisions and semantic classification, even when the targets were displayed too briefly for him to report. This kind of "tacit or covert" reading has been documented in a number of other cases (Coslett & Saffran, 1989; Coslett et al., 1993). Presumably, word activation must still be rapidly occurring in certain pure alexics, but not in such a way as to yield a fully identified, conscious percept. How the interaction between letters and words has been altered to produce this kind of striking dissociation remains a question for future research.

Finally, and still more peripherally, a number of dyslexic cases have been documented that reflect a disruption in attentional systems that filter information from regions outside the intended focus (Shallice & Warrington, 1977). This failure results in numerous intrusion errors ("win fed" may be read as "fin fed"). Similar mistakes have been observed in normal readers attempting to report one of a set of words under limited viewing conditions (Mozer, 1983). Neglect dyslexia, an additional form of disorder that is the outcome of a general attentional deficit, is characterized by errors at the beginning or end of words ("enigma" reads as "stigma"). Recent accounts (e.g. Ellis et al., 1987; Costello & Warrington, 1987) distinguish between letter position and identity, suggesting that, in neglect dyslexia, attentional focus is limited to a subset of the letter identities.

BIBLIOGRAPHY

Bub, D., Cancelliere, A., & Kertesz, A. (1985). Whole-word and analytic translation of spelling to sound in a nonsemantic reader. In K. E. Patterson, J. C. Marshall, & M. Coltheart (Eds), *Surface dyslexia: Neuropsychological and cognitive studies of phonological reading* (pp. 15–34). Hillsdale, NJ: Erlbaum.

Coltheart, M. (1980). Deep dyslexia: a review of the syndrome. In M. Coltheart, K. E. Patterson, & J. C. Marshall (Eds), *Deep dyslexia* (pp. 22–48). London: Routledge.

Coltheart, M., Masterson, J., Byng, S., Prior., M., & Riddoch, J. (1983). Surface dyslexia. *Quarterly Journal of Experimental Psychology*, *35A*, 469–95.

Coltheart, M., Patterson, K., & Marshall, J. C. (1987). Deep dyslexia since 1980. In M. Coltheart, K. E. Patterson, & J. C. Marshall (Eds), *Deep dyslexia* (pp. 407–51). London: Routledge.

Coltheart, M., Curtis, B., Atkins, P., & Haller, M. (1993). Models of reading aloud: dual-route and parallel distributed processing approaches. *Psychological Review, 100*, 589–608.

Coslett, H. B. (1991). Read but not write "idea": evidence for a third reading mechanism. *Brain and Language, 40*, 425–33.

Coslett, H. B., & Saffran, E. M. (1989). Evidence for preserved reading in "pure alexia." *Brain, 112*, 327–59.

Coslett, H. B., Saffran, E. M., Greenbaum, S., & Schwartz, H. (1993). Reading in pure alexia. *Brain, 116*, 21–37.

Costello, A. de L., & Warrington, E. K. (1987). Dissociation of visuospatial neglect and neglect dyslexia. *Journal of Neurology, Neurosurgery and Psychiatry, 50*, 1110–16.

Day, J. L. (1979). Visual half-field recognition as a function of syntactic class and imageability. *Neuropsychologia, 17*, 515–19.

De Bleser, R., & Luzzatti, C. (1989). Models of reading and writing and their disorders in classical German aphasiology. *Cognitive Neuropsychology, 6*, 501–14.

Ellis, H. D., & Shepherd, J. W. (1974). Recognition of abstract and concrete words presented in the left and right visual fields. *Journal of Experimental Psychology, 103*, 1035–6.

Ellis, A. W., Flude, B. M., & Young, A. W. (1987). "Neglect dyslexia" and the early visual processing of letters in words and nonwords. *Cognitive Neuropsychology, 4*, 439–64.

Farah, M. (1990). *Visual agnosia: Disorders of object recognition and what they tell us about normal vision*. Cambridge, MA: MIT Press.

Friedman, R. B., & Alexander, M. P. (1984). Pictures, images and pure alexia: a case study. *Cognitive Neuropsychology, 1*, 9–23.

Funnell, E. (1983). Phonological processes in reading: new evidence from acquired dyslexia. *British Journal of Psychology, 74*, 159–80.

Henderson, L. (1982). *Orthography and word recognition in reading*. London: Academic Press.

Hines, D. (1976). Recognition of verbs, abstract nouns and concrete nouns from left and right visual fields. *Neuropsychologia, 14*, 211–16.

Hinton, G. E., & Shallice, T. (1991). Lesioning an attractor network: investigations of acquired dyslexia. *Psychological Review, 98*, 74–95.

Jones, G. V. (1985). Deep dyslexia, imageability and the ease of predication. *Brain and Language, 24*, 1–19.

Kinsbourne, M., & Warrington, K. E. (1962). A disorder of simultaneous form perception. *Brain, 85*, 461–86.

Kremin, H. (1982). Alexia: theory and research. In R. N. Malatesha & P. G. Aaron (Eds), *Reading disorders: Varieties and treatments*. New York: Academic Press.

McCarthy, R. A., & Warrington, E. K. (1986). Phonological reading: phenomena and paradoxes. *Cortex, 22*, 359–80.

Marcel, A. (1980). Surface dyslexia and beginning reading: a revised hypothesis of the pronunciation of print and its impairments. In M.

Coltheart, K. E. Patterson, & J. C. Marshall (Eds), *Deep dyslexia* (pp. 227–58). London: Routledge.

Marshall, J. C., & Newcombe, F. (1973). Patterns of paralexia: a psycholinguistic approach. *Journal of Psycholinguistic Research, 2*, 175–99.

Mozer, M. C. (1983). Letter migration in word perception. *Journal of Experimental Psychology: Human Perception and Performance, 9*, 531–46.

Patterson, K. E., & Besner, D. (1984). Is the right hemisphere literate? *Cognitive Neuropsychology, 1*, 315–42.

Plaut, D. C., & Shallice, T. (1993). Deep dyslexia: a case study of connectionist neuropsychology. *Cognitive Neuropsychology, 10*, 377–500.

Quinlan, P. T. (1991). *Connectionism and psychology: A psychological perspective on new connectionist research*. Chicago: University of Chicago Press.

Rapp, B. C., & Caramazza, A. (1991). Spatially determined deficits in letter and word processing. *Cognitive Neuropsychology, 8*, 275–311.

Roeltgen, D. P. (1987). Loss of deep dyslexic reading ability from a second left hemisphere lesion. *Archives of Neurology, 44*, 346–8.

Schwartz, M. F., Saffran, E. M., & Marin, O. S. M. (1980). Fractionating the reading process in dementia: evidence for word-specific print-to-sound associations. In M. Coltheart, K. E. Patterson, & J. C. Marshall (Eds), *Deep dyslexia* (pp. 259–69). London: Routledge.

Seidenberg, M. S., & McClelland, J. L. (1989). A distributed, developmental model of word recognition and naming. *Psychological Review, 96*, 523–68.

Shallice, T. (1988). *From neuropsychology to mental structure*. New York: Cambridge University Press.

Shallice, T., & McCarthy, R. (1985). Phonological reading: from patterns of impairment to possible procedures. In K. E. Patterson, M. Coltheart, & J. C. Marshall (Eds), *Surface dyslexia* (pp. 361–97). Hillsdale, NJ: Erlbaum.

Shallice, T., & Saffran, E. M. (1986). Lexical processing in the absence of explicit word identification: evidence from a letter-by-letter reader. *Cognitive Neuropsychology, 3*, 429–58.

Shallice, T., & Warrington, E. K. (1977). The possible role of selctive attention in acquired dyslexia. *Neuropsychologia, 15*, 31–41.

Simmel, M. L., & Goldshmidt, K. H. (1953). Prolonged posteclamptic aphasia: report of a case. *AMA Archives of Neurology and Psychiatry, 69*, 80–3.

Warrington, E. K. (1981). Concrete word dyslexia. *British Journal of Psychology, 72*, 175–96.

Zaidel, E., & Peters, A. M. (1981). Phonological encoding and ideographic reading by the disconnected right hemisphere: two case studies. *Brain and Language, 14*, 205–34.

DANIEL N. BUB

dysorthographia   Dysorthographia may refer to any disorder of production in writing, but is generally taken to refer to those associated with AGRAPHIA in nonfluent APHASIA. Although classic descriptions of motor (nonfluent) aphasia describe its occurrence in the absence of a disorder of writing, clinical evidence has shown that most disorders of oral language are accompanied by disorders of writing. Although the presentation of these dysorthographias is highly variable, the effects are generally seen at the word level, while writing of individual graphemes is preserved. The disorder affects writing to dictation more than copying, the writing of real words rather than nonwords, and words more than symbols and numbers.

dyspraxia   Dyspraxia is the relative inability to carry out purposeful movements in the absence of paralysis of the relevant musculature (APRAXIA). In neuropsychology the prefixes *a-* and *dys-*, although they should strictly indicate a total loss of a function and a partial loss of a function respectively, are used rather loosely. However, a dyspraxic deficit can generally be assumed to be less severe than an apraxic deficit.

dysprosody   Dysprosody is the loss of expressive intonation, rhythm, or accent in spoken language. It is therefore a disorder of phonemic production as an aspect of motor or nonfluent APHASIA, and may be the only residual feature of this disorder as recovery progresses. It has been suggested that dysprosody may result from an overcorrection of the difficulties of phonemic production through auditory or kinesthetic feedback, and may be conceived as a disorder of phonemic programming.

dystonia Dystonia is a disorder of movement characterized by distorted postures of the limbs and trunk associated with excessive muscular tone, which may be interrupted by frequent involuntary repetitive twisting movements. It is therefore closely related to CHOREA and ATHETOSIS. Dystonia results from lesions of the basal ganglia, the putamen, and their connections, and may be general or, more commonly, localized as in TORTICOLLIS, BLETHAROSPASM, spastic DYSARTHRIA, and writer's cramp. There is a strong genetic basis to the disorder.

E

echolalia Echolalia is the automatic repetition of a word or phrase. The term is more commonly used when the patient repeats the last word or phrase used by an examiner, but may also refer to repetitions occurring during the course of speech. A single repetition is usual, but further repetitions may occur. Strictly speaking, echolalia refers to repetition of phrases, and *pallilalia* to the repetition of single words (*logoclonia* for the repetition of final syllables), but the term is generally used more loosely.

The condition is most commonly seen in adults with nominal aphasia (*see* ANOMIA), where the speech is normally fluent (and repetition is unaffected) and the echolalia may be understood as a strategy to reduce the difficulties of word-finding by employing the words supplied by the examiner. This strategy may not necessarily be at a high cognitive level; it may be the case that the words most recently heard have a high valency which makes them more likely to be selected for the speech production systems.

When repetition is preserved, but fluent speech output is filled with phonemic and verbal paraphasias, as in transcortical sensory APHASIA, there may be a strong tendency to echolalia. Alternatively, particularly when repetition occurs during the course of the patient's speech, echolalia may be understood as a perseverative phenomenon which may be a result of attentional disorganization.

In the general breakdown of language accompanying DEMENTIA, in which incoherence of language output may be seen, echolalia may also occur and in this case is understood as a relatively automatic, reflex form of verbal response, but others have suggested that the phenomenon is due to disinhibition of language control mechanisms, or the presence of a mixed form of transcortical aphasia. When echolalia is observed in dementia, then automatic sentence completion may also be seen.

Echolalia is also a prominent feature of infantile autism, and the overlap between this symptom and the symptom as it appears in receptive language disorders in children has encouraged hypotheses of the neurological or neuropsychological basis of autism.

J. GRAHAM BEAUMONT

echopraxia Echopraxia is the automatic repetition of a movement, analogous to ECHOLALIA. It is normally seen as the compulsive imitation of actions or movements, and a distinction is sometimes made between the actions (*echopraxia*) and movements (*echokinesis*) being repeated. Echopraxia may occur, but rarely, in GILLES DE LA TOURETTE SYNDROME.

ECT ECT (electroconvulsive therapy) or *ECS (electroconvulsive shock)* is a psychiatric treatment for depression administered when there is a poor response to antidepressant medication, or where a more rapid response to treatment is desirable, for example, when there is a high risk of suicide or self-harm. ECT is administered by placing two electrodes over the temporal regions and applying an alternating current of between 70 and 120 volts for a duration of about 500 msec, thereby inducing a convulsion. As protection for the patient, muscle relaxants and tranquillizers are given prior to the shock, and the treatment is repeated on about 10 occasions over two to three weeks. There is still debate about its appropriate role as a treatment within psychiatry.

The neuropsychological significance of ECT, apart from interest in the ways in which the treatment has its effect, lies in the side effects which occur in memory, being a clinical parallel with the controlled experimental work on ECS carried out with animals. Bilateral ECT (the form usually administered, with one electrode over each hemisphere) normally induces memory changes, even with the limited number of treatments normally given, although these changes appear reversible and return to pretreatment levels within about six months. The effects are cumulative, with increasing effects as more treatments are given. Certain effects may persist beyond six months, especially in personal and autobiographical memory, although these are not regarded as being seriously disabling.

There is some evidence that unilateral administration of ECT (both electrodes being over the same hemisphere) may reduce the effects of ECT on memory without diminishing the primary response to the treatment. Further, left-sided treatment may have its effects on verbal memory, while right-sided treatment may affect nonverbal memory, right-sided unilateral ECT being therefore less disturbing for the patient. However, these conclusions are not universally accepted and both bilateral and unilateral ECT continue to be administered.

There is an obvious parallel between the effects of ECT and the effects of temporal lobe lesions on memory, both of which are a form of anterograde amnesia. Given that the HIPPOCAMPUS and the AMYGDALA, within the temporal lobe, are significant sources of epileptic activity, it seems reasonable to conclude that the involvement of these medial temporal structures is important both in the temporal lobe lesion effects and in the effects on memory of ECT. It is known that repeated seizure activity in the hippocampus may lead to chronic changes in this structure, which include the loss of cells, and the concern has therefore been raised that repeated ECT may also produce similar pathological changes. For this reason, among others, it is considered good practice to limit the course of ECT to about 10 sessions and to give only a single course. Nonetheless, the clinical neuro-psychologist may encounter patients who have in the past received many more ECT treatments (some over 100) and in such patients chronic deficits in both memory and general cognitive function may be observed, which may well be attributable to treatment by ECT.

J. GRAHAM BEAUMONT

ectopia Ectopia is a general medical term which refers to abnormal development of some structure at an inappropriate location. Within the nervous system, application of the term arises in two principal contexts.

Extracerebral ectopias are a heterogeneous group of cerebral malformations by which neural masses are located within the meningeal space, but external to the cerebral hemispheres, and consequently they are a form of HETEROTOPIA. This abnormality of early development has been associated with fetal exposure to alcohol, but may not be linked only with early exposure to toxic agents. Traumatic processes, particularly between 8 and 20 weeks of gestation, may also cause abnormal neural cell migration and development.

Ectopia lentis is an abnormality in the development of the eye, and presents as glaucoma with poor vision. It is a rare genetically determined condition and is linked with a number of other developmental abnormalities.

edema (also **oedema**)   More correctly *cerebral edema*, edema is any swelling of the brain substance or surrounding tissues. It is an extremely common response to any cerebral insult in the acute phase, often associated with raised intracranial pressure, and may be accompanied by displacement of regions of the brain if localized. There are three types of cerebral edema: *vasogenic*, which results from increased membrane permeability caused by trauma or tumor; *cytotoxic*, associated with cell death, commonly from an anoxic episode; and *interstitial*, accompanying HYDROCEPHALUS. The effects of edema associated with significantly increased intracranial pressure may be relieved by neurosurgical or drug treatment, but less severe forms will resolve spontaneously in the course of the acute phase.

EEG   *See* ELECTROENCEPHALOGRAPHY.

electrical stimulation   Electrical stimulation of the brain involves the application of low physiological levels of electrical current to the brain substance through electrodes placed on the cortex or implanted more deeply into brain tissue. As the brain itself contains no sensory receptors, this can be achieved without awareness on the part of the patient of the stimulation itself.

Electrocortical stimulation, stimulation by electrodes placed over the cortex, has proved a valuable tool for the neurosurgeon and has, at the same time, yielded important information about the functions of the cortex. Stimulation of the cortex exposed at surgery may evoke behavioral responses, which can include the subjective reports of the patient who is brought out of deep anesthesia for the period of stimulation. This permits the surgeon to assess the functional significance of a particular cortical area prior to making an incision, so informing decisions about the extent of any surgical removal being considered. However, at the same time this procedure generates case knowledge about cortical functions which has, for example, been collated by Penfield and his colleagues for the regions which lie in the ROLANDIC AREA.

The conclusions of these studies are broadly consonant with the division of the cortex into three levels: primary, secondary, and tertiary. The primary level of the cortex is concerned with sensory reception or the discrete individual movements of voluntary motor output. Stimulation of these primary sensory areas produces a sensation: a PHOSPHENE in the visual cortex, a pure tone in the primary auditory cortex, a touch localized to a part of the body in somatosensory cortex, or movement of a single body part in the case of primary motor cortex. Stimulation of the surrounding secondary cortex evokes a perception in the relevant modality, so an integrated visual percept, an image, may be experienced on stimulation of secondary visual cortex, a melody or identifiable environmental sound from secondary auditory cortex, a touch perception which might, for example, be the forearm being gently stroked by velvet, from secondary somatosensory cortex. If the secondary motor cortex is stimulated, then a more complex integrated and potentially purposive movement may result. The tertiary or association cortex has been much less studied by means of electrical stimulation, and the effects of stimulation of these areas are harder to interpret. Direct stimulation of the primary cortex has also been attempted as a prosthesis for cases in which the sensory apparatus or pathways leading to the cortex are dysfunctional, but while the technique may be feasible in principle, no effective system has yet been developed.

Electrical stimulation of the subcortical regions of the brain is also undertaken in *stereotactic* neurosurgery, where the position of the inserted probe, which is directed according to three-dimensional coordinates under X-ray guidance, may be assessed by stimulation of the site which has been reached. The procedure of PSYCHOSURGERY may use electrical stimulation through electrodes implanted in this way either to gain the therapeutic effect, or by using supraphysiological currents to achieve the destruction of tissue. Recent interest has also developed in the use of electrical stimulation of the BRAIN STEM in the treatment of VEGETATIVE STATES, but adequate controlled trials have yet to demonstrate the validity of the apparent outcome.
See also SENSORIMOTOR CORTEX.

J. GRAHAM BEAUMONT

electroconvulsive therapy *See* ECT.

electroencephalography The electrical changes associated with neuronal activity in the brain can be measured via a technique known as electroencephalography (EEG). The techniques of EEG recording are well established and well documented and will be outlined here only briefly. More detailed technical information can be acquired from Fisch (1991).

MEASUREMENT OF EEG ACTIVITY

EEG measurement generally entails the attachment of metal electrodes of a fixed size to the scalp at standard locations. These electrodes pick up the activity associated with the changes in interneuronal electrical potentials and the potential difference between pairs of electrodes can then be measured. The comparison between two active recording sites is known as the *bipolar derivation*. Single active electrodes may be compared to common inactive *reference* electrodes for comparison; these may be noncephalic sites, such as the earlobes or mastoid. Different combinations of electrode pairs can be selected to examine different cortical areas of particular interest. These combinations are known as *montages*.

Each of these signals is then amplified. As the medium frequencies are those of interest to the electroencephalographer, the signal is also fed through high and low frequency filters. Signal artifacts, which may comprise noncerebral activity from eye movements, muscle activity, or heartbeats have to be screened out. These are sometimes obvious by visual inspection, such as the slow frontal activity associated with eye movements; the identification and removal of such artifacts from the data is of crucial importance in ensuring the validity of the EEG data. Originally the amplified signals were used to move ink pens over a moving paper chart with the resultant record providing a visual display of the changes between pairs of electrodes, each pair providing one channel of recording. Such analogue recordings were then visually inspected (see below). The arrival of computer technology now allows the input of digitized signals into a range of analytical and statistical packages, sometimes incorporating automatic artifact rejection procedures.

For standard clinical EEGs, electrodes are attached at locations determined by an internationally agreed system. This standardized placement is known as the *10/20 system*. The distance from the patient's nasion to inion and between the preauricular points is measured. Each electrode is placed at 10/20 percent intersections of these lines. This results in a montage combining 21 recording and 1 reference electrodes. Electrodes are referred to by an initial letter indicating their location (F = frontal, P = parietal, T = temporal, O = occipital) and a number, with odd numbers referring to left hemisphere electrodes and even numbers to right hemisphere electrodes, or the letter z indicating a vertex site. Currently, research techniques are moving towards an increasing density of electrodes to provide data for sophisticated mathematical analyses of EEG data – several workers report data from more than 100 channels. The technical aspects of wiring a patient/participant up with 128 electrodes should not be underestimated, even when using a cap with preset electrode placements.

DESCRIPTIONS OF EEG ACTIVITY

The best-known level of description is in terms of different *frequencies*. The first to be described, by Hans Berger in 1929, was the *alpha rhythm*, referring to activity between 8 and 13 cycles per second. Other frequencies commonly referred to are the slow *delta* waves (< 4 cycles per

second), *theta* waves (4– < 8 cycles per second) and *beta* waves. This latter term originally referred to activity above 13 cycles, but now reference can be found to beta 1 (> 13–16), beta 2 (> 16–20), and beta 3 (> 20 cycles and above).

In addition, EEG activity may be referred to in terms of *amplitude*. Different frequencies have characteristic ranges of amplitude (alpha is generally less than 50 μv, beta less than 35 μv) and sometimes inter-frequency variations in amplitude are associated with specific experimental variations. Variations in amplitude are hypothesized to arise from variations in the synchronization of the neuronal activity being measured; increasing activation is associated with *desynchronization* of the populations of nerve cells, with the resultant activity measured as low-voltage fast responses, whereas reduction in activation is associated with *synchronization* and high-voltage slow responses.

Particular patterns of activity may also be referred to in the description of an EEG record, for example, *spike and wave activity*. This comprises a spike of high amplitude immediately followed by a slow wave of similar amplitude. This complex repeats itself at frequencies of about 3 Hz. The presence of this pattern is indicative of convulsive disorders (*see also* EPILEPSY).

Finally, reference can be found to slow DC shifts occurring over several seconds. The best-known is the *contingent negative variation* (CNV) described by a pioneer of EEG, W. Grey Walter. This can be observed in subjects preparing to make a response (e.g. in a reaction time test) and has therefore been described as related to anticipatory decision making.

NORMAL EEG ACTIVITY

In the normal waking adult, a standardized EEG procedure should generate a record of predominantly alpha rhythm posteriorly distributed, with an absence of slow wave and of paroxysmal activity. Within the alpha waveband the frequency is relatively constant for an individual, with the two hemispheres showing the same frequency. The alpha rhythm should be emphasized by closing the eyes and blocked on eyes opening, or by requiring the subject to pay attention to a particular task. Asymmetrical alpha blocking may indicate that the two hemispheres are differentially engaged in the task concerned. With task demands, the faster, lower amplitude beta activity should become evident.

In the sleeping adult EEG is used to characterize four stages, ranging from drowsiness to deep sleep. Stage 1 sleep shows beta-like activity, stage 2 shows slower background activity with intermittent sharply pointed waveforms or *sleep spindles*, stages 3 and 4 display increasing proportions of delta wave activity. An additional stage is accompanied by rapid eye movements (REM) and hence is referred to as REM sleep. The sleep is apparently deepest at this point, but the EEG shows the fast low-amplitude pattern characteristic of early sleep stages. It is during this stage that dreaming occurs (*see* SLEEP).

It should be noted that there are marked age-related changes in EEG. Developmental changes are evident up to the age of about 20 years. These can be characterized by changes in characteristic frequencies from the slower theta-type activity, which is relatively common in a child's EEG, to the faster alpha and beta wavebands. Over about 60 years of age, the EEG may be characterized more by beta than by alpha activity, which becomes slower and less reactive.

ABNORMAL EEG ACTIVITY

This is rather more difficult to define. Inter- and intra-individual differences in EEG signals are quite considerable, so it is difficult to establish criteria for what is normal and what is abnormal in an EEG record, with the possible exception of the paroxysmal EEG signals characteristic of epilepsy, or the presence of delta waves indicative of tumors. The presence of theta activity in the adult EEG is statistically abnormal and has been associated with psychopathic disorders.

Any review of the literature will uncover rather vague reference to an "excess of abnormal EEG" or "diffuse EEG abnormalities." The physiological significance of such observations is rarely discussed although such abnormalities may be reported in conjunction with other observations, such as enlarged cerebral ventricles in some schizophrenics (Weinberger et al., 1980). Non-specific EEG abnormalities can comprise EEG slowing, referring to a greater preponderance of EEG activity in the lower frequency range, or a shift to the lower end of a given frequency range, particularly alpha. Similarly, low amplitude variability within an EEG record may be reported. Although this has been hypothesized to reflect a lack of plasticity in neural functioning, there is no supporting evidence for this.

Additional abnormalities may refer to lack of alpha blocking with task demands, either unilaterally or bilaterally. This is a measure of the EEG's usefulness in monitoring implicit processes, such as attention. These data can be correlated with behavioral measures such as task performance to indicate the validity of such inferences. An extension of this is in the investigation of conditions where attentional disorders are possibly central, such as schizophrenia.

In deciding on the abnormality or otherwise of EEG records, it is suggested that much more extensive normative data bases are required before the criteria for abnormality can be established. It is also the case that more research is needed on the physiological significance of EEG changes to strengthen its role as a clinical tool.

ANALYSIS OF EEG ACTIVITY

Originally, analysis of EEG records was by visual inspection of the analogue records, with different channels identifying the location of particular patterns or anomalies. Some variations in frequency can be seen by the trained eye, such as the appearance and disappearance of alpha activity as a function of eyes open or closed. It is possible to observe the presence of anomalous delta activity, generally present during certain stages of sleep but evident in the waking EEG of cerebral tumors. The presence of spike and wave patterns is a crucial diagnostic indicator of epileptiform problems.

With contemporary computerized data collection, analysis is carried out on digitized signals. Again, for more detailed technical information of the procedures involved the reader is referred to Fisch (1991) or Gevins and Remond (1987).

One early outcome of more sophisticated analysis was the use of averaging techniques which combined the signals from large numbers of stimulus repetitions to produce an average evoked response (*see also* EVOKED POTENTIALS). A consequence of this averaging technique is the removal of background "noise" and the enhancement of any recurring characteristic. The resultant waveform can then be described in terms of its latency and amplitude. Such data can then be investigated as a function of the particular eliciting stimulus situation. The advantage of this technique is its temporal resolution, allowing analysis of changes occurring within milliseconds of the stimulus event. A disadvantage is the paradigm required, involving the use of simple stimuli to be repeated many times, as it is not always possible to operationalize the process of interest in this way. However, this use of EEG has become one of its key research roles, particularly with respect to specific psychological processes.

For analysis of the raw EEG signal one commonly used technique is that of *spectral analysis*, whereby amplitude characteristics of the frequency domain of the EEG signal can be assessed. The particular mathematical technique involved is known as *fast Fourier transform (FFT)* – this technique divides the complex EEG waveform into the simpler waveforms of specific frequency bands, generally the traditional ones of alpha, beta, delta, theta, and calculates the signal amplitude within each of these bands. A subsequent stage involves the creation of the *power spectrum*, using the squared coefficients of the FFT. This gives a measure of frequency vs intensity, and can be crudely viewed as a measure of the "amount" of a particular frequency to be found in the EEG signal at the time under analysis. With a power spectrum it is possible to consider, for example, the *absolute band values* (the amount of activity within a specific frequency) or the *relative band value* (comparing amounts of different frequencies). These spectra can be graphically plotted to give a visual display of the signal. A *compressed spectral array* stacks successive spectral plots and gives a measure of changes over time. *Spectral edge frequency* gives a measure of the frequency below which a set percentage of the signal is found and can be used to plot the changes in EEG activity over time.

These measures can then be used to provide more detailed descriptors of cortical activity as a function of particular events. For example, one can compare the amount of alpha activity over a given time or during a specific task or compare changes within a given frequency band, e.g. 8 Hz activity shifting to 12 Hz activity with task onset. Similarly one can compare power spectra within and between subject groups to provide a measure of individual differences.

An additional statistical technique that has received some attention is *coherence analysis*. This draws on the observation of increasing desynchronization in cortical areas that become activated. Changes in the correlation between

EEG from different areas could therefore be interpreted as changes in the synchronization of activity from these areas. Coherence analysis computes the correlation between pairs of areas (i.e. electrodes) as a function of frequency. It is claimed that this allows an insight into the functional organization of the brain by providing indices of the changing areas of activity during any given process. For example, changes in interhemispheric coherence could provide a measure of the relative contributions of the hemispheres. It has thus proved popular in the study of conditions where anomalies of hemispheric balance are suggested. Various methodological issues, particularly the use of inappropriate reference electrodes, have led to criticism of the utility of this measure (French & Beaumont, 1984). However, it has the advantage of being a statistical technique related to specific physiological characteristics of cortical activity. Many of the more sophisticated EEG analytical batteries include coherence analysis and it may yet prove a useful descriptor of EEG changes, anomalous or otherwise.

Also of interest are the *spatial* characteristics of the EEG signal, its distribution across the cortex, and the changes in this distribution as a function of e.g. time, task demands, and subject characteristics. Commonly used comparisons are those of right and left hemisphere activity, as a whole or as a function of the different lobes. Similarly, anterior–posterior comparisons can be made.

A contemporary technique which allows an inspection of spatial characteristics of the EEG signal is *topographic mapping*. The simplest form provides amplitude maps for each of the classical frequencies, with either color-coded or grayscale maps depicting the variations in amplitude of the given frequency over the cortex at a particular point in time. Power maps indicate the intensity of the signal in given frequencies at different locations. In addition, statistical maps can be produced with the values from statistical comparisons mapped at the relevant points on the cortex, providing an "instant snapshot" of areas where statistically significant changes have occurred.

Topographic maps have provided the kind of instantaneous visibility missing from the early chart-gazing approach and the more contemporary statistical quantification techniques. It is important to realize, however, that they must be viewed with considerable caution (Kahn et al., 1988). The statistical technique by which the maps are produced involves an interpolation procedure where the values lying between the electrodes are statistically estimated or approximated to produce a sort of "value of best fit." These values, which are depicted as part of the final map, do not reflect real EEG data. This particular problem can be overcome by increasing the density of electrodes over the surface of the scalp, but this can have consequences for ease of recording. It also has consequences for the validity of statistically significant findings when they are based on a large number of comparisons. Perhaps the best use of the maps is as a heuristic device to guide subsequent statistical analysis of the raw data.

A more sophisticated analysis arises from the application of electromagnetic field theory (Fender, 1987). The changes in polarization of nerve cells produce electrical potentials and magnetic fields which are directly related to the activation patterns of the underlying nerve cell populations. If neurons are conceived of as *dipoles*, electrical sources which project positive and negative fields in opposite directions, EEG signals can be modelled as arising from specific dipole current sources. The orientation of these dipoles with respect to the surface of the cortex where recording is taking place will determine the negativity or positivity of the signal measured. Mathematical modelling techniques can be applied to the raw EEG signal to calculate the origin of the signal and any changes occurring. These are known as dipole localization methods or *dipole approximation techniques* (Lehmann et al., 1991). The use of such techniques is at a relatively early stage and methodological issues, such as allowances for the shape of the head within which the signals are generated and the conductivity of the tissue through which the signals pass, are still under consideration.

Also related to the analysis of the magnetic fields generated by electrical potential gradients is the use of the *magnetoencephalogram (MEG)*. This is still a methodologically complex procedure and involves multichannel recording. However, reliable estimates of the distribution of electrical activity throughout the brain have been claimed and this could well be an additional way forward for EEG techniques.

In any consideration of the utility of EEG as a spatial measure it is important to remember that the origin of these signals is still under discussion (see below), therefore care must be taken in extrapolating from patterns of activity observed at the cortex, however sophisticated the statistical techniques used to generate and describe such patterns.

Recent discussion of EEG has suggested that the linear techniques employed by statisticians are, in fact, inappropriate for the analysis of this form of signal and that nonlinear methods, such as *chaos* analysis, would be more beneficial. This complicated mathematical process is claimed to model more closely the nonrandom periodicity characteristic of EEG. Additionally it is possible to describe signal characteristics and signal changes in terms of so-called chaotic attractors which model the action of the signal generators which are hypothesized to underlie EEG activity (see below). Use of this form of analysis imposes some methodological constraints in terms of the length of EEG epochs required for analysis, but it is viewed by many as a promising way forward in EEG analysis (Skarda & Freeman, 1987).

Further, whatever the form of analysis selected, it should be noted that with each stage of any form of analysis we get further from the original raw signal; it is therefore important to be sure that the analysis employed is providing the information in the best form to answer the question posed.

ORIGINS OF EEG ACTIVITY

From early on, the presence of rhythmicity in the EEG suggested the presence of some form of *generators* or pacemakers, driving groups of neurons in varying patterns of activity. The location of such pacemakers is of importance if EEG is to have any utility in the identification of sites of normal or abnormal activity.

Modelling such generators as electrical dipoles (see above), researchers applying dipole approximation techniques to FFT data have concluded that different EEG frequency bands are generated by neural populations in different brain locations. Michel and colleagues (1992) suggest a deep anterior source for delta, a shallower more posterior source for alpha, with beta activity generated from a deeper and more anterior source than alpha.

It must be remembered that researchers are applying complex mathematical models of signal generation which it is *assumed* have fairly close parallels to the reality of EEG generation. However, dipole approximation techniques have been shown to have some success in identifying epileptic foci, for example. This would appear to be a promising way forward in the use of a signal whose use for spatial analysis has lagged some way behind the sophistication of its temporal resolution.

APPLICATIONS OF EEG MEASURES

It is sometimes possible to get so involved in the minutiae of the acquisition and analysis of EEG data that its role as a research tool is forgotten.

As a psychophysiological measure, one can consider both its physiological significance, i.e. its role in identifying the organic bases of normal and abnormal processes, and its psychological significance, i.e the light it sheds on the different stages of specific psychological functions.

Clinical applications of EEG measures

The physiological role almost invariably interacts with the clinical role of EEG. There are several questions which one can ask of the use of EEG, the answers to which can determine its effectiveness. Does it provide a unique index of the condition under consideration? Does it provide evidence of the organic basis of the condition? Could it provide useful clinical information in addition to that provided by other clinical measures? Could it identify previously unsuspected organic dysfunction or, alternatively, could it rule out organic dysfunction?

The answer to these questions is mainly positive. EEG measures clearly have an important role in the localization of spike foci in epileptiform disorders and, as such, can be said to provide a unique physiological signature. EEG's role in the identification and classification of epileptiform disorders could therefore be claimed as its *raison d'être*. Similarly, the characterization of sleep stages could be considered under this heading. The finding of EEG spiking in the temporal areas in some schizophrenic patients supports hypotheses concerning limbic system involvement in schizophrenia. The consistent finding of abnormal EEGs in children with attentional deficit disorder suggests an organic basis to the condition, although the reported "diffuse generalized slowing" does not take this suggestion beyond the descriptive level. Abnormal EEG

features in childhood autism again provide support for evidence that this is an organic disorder; the tendency for these features to be found more often in the right hemisphere narrows the focus of further investigations. EEG can be important in identifying the presence of organic disorder which was not otherwise suspected, e.g. in cases of depression in the elderly associated with degenerative disorders, or it can rule out organic disorder, e.g. in distinguishing between temporal lobe epilepsy and schizophrenia.

On the whole, the clinical utility of EEG has to be acknowledged as limited. This is related to the current weakness in spatial resolution and a consequent uncertainty concerning the physiological significance of observed abnormalities. EEG data can at best be viewed as providing rather indirect clues in the identification of the biological bases of different states and conditions. One example is the relatively consistent finding of lower mean alpha frequencies in schizophrenia, and also greater incidences of beta activity. It is possible that this might index abnormal levels of arousal, but such an interpretation is rather speculative. A more detailed review of the current clinical applications of the EEG is to be found in Binnie and Prior (1994).

EEG measures in the study of normal and abnormal cognition

A rather stronger role is provided by linking observations of localized changes in EEG to particular kinds of psychological processes. This role for EEG illustrates its greatest strength, its utility in assessing functional (or dysfunctional) activity. If we wish to monitor the changes in cortical activity associated with a particular process *while that process is occurring*, then currently EEG is one of the best methods. It is true that positron emission tomography (PET) and MAGNETIC RESONANCE IMAGING (MRI) scans allow much more sophisticated *spatial* resolution and are potentially much more powerful localizing tools. However, these techniques can be variously described as invasive, potentially dangerous, time-consuming, labor-intensive, and extremely costly. Even allowing for this, they cannot as yet provide the *temporal* resolution possible with the more subtle EEG analysis or AEP techniques, providing data on changes in activity in terms of milliseconds.

An early example of the use of EEG in

assessing the psychological state of an individual and the role of cortical activation in a psychological process is the use of alpha activity in the assessment of attentional state. As described above, alpha is usually found over the posterior regions of the brain, particularly the occipital areas. It is generally present when the subject is in a relaxed but alert state. It is generally most pronounced when subjects are asked to close their eyes; it attenuates on eye opening or with light flashes or with requests to carry out specific tasks (e.g. mental arithmetic). This phenomenon is known as *alpha blocking* and the amount and timing of such blocking is often used as an index of attention. It has been demonstrated that the topography of alpha blocking can vary as a function of task demands, e.g. mental arithmetic producing more blocking in the left parietal regions, thus suggesting the usefulness of this measure as an index of specific cognitive processing.

Ray and Cole (1985) suggest that, whereas alpha activity is an appropriate measure of attentional stance, beta activity is more responsive to specific task demands and therefore provides a useful index of variations in cortical activity with the nature of the task. It is clear that multifrequency analysis is necessary to try and get as full a picture as possible. The sophisticated analytical techniques now available mean that it is relatively easy to compare power spectra in all the traditional wavebands over the whole cortex and to report findings as a function of differential hemispheric engagement and/or differential involvement of the classical cortical areas. One measure of cortical changes as a function of cognitive processing considers *event related desynchronization* (Pfurtscheller & Aranibar, 1977). This considers amplitude attenuation in both alpha and beta bands as a function of different kinds of processing demands, and can be used to localize regional differences in cortical activation as a function of task demands. Topographic mapping techniques (described above) are similarly employed (Duffy, 1988).

Measures ranging from simple alpha blocking to power spectral analysis and ERD coherence have been applied to the study of *hemispheric specialization*, the concept that, in humans, the two hemispheres are differently specialized for particular types of cognitive processing. A crude dichotomy describes the left hemisphere as generally responsible for linguistic functions, with the right hemisphere associated with spatial processing (*see also* LATERALIZATION). EEG clearly lends itself to such research, allowing continuous analysis of functional processing taking place over fairly long periods of time. Such research has provided evidence of, for example, right parietal involvement in imaging, left temporal involvement in mnemonic processes.

With respect to a dysfunctioning organism, if the difficulty is associated with a functional rather than a structural problem, then psychophysiological techniques such as EEG provide the best data. A useful analogy might be to think of such problems as software rather than hardware disorders. This is not to deny that structural and functional problems must be inextricably linked but to note that, with the occurrence of specific dysfunctions in the apparent absence of any organic problem, EEG techniques provide invaluable research tools. It may also be that, if the structural disorder is at the level of interneuronal connectivity, then techniques such as EEG are the best we currently have available to assess this, given the present constraints of techniques such as PET and MRI.

The techniques applied to the study of normal cognition can also be applied to the study of abnormal cognition, e.g. investigations of cortical activity in children with developmental dyslexia whose reading difficulties are characterized by phonological processing weaknesses, or EEG correlates of face processing in autistic children.

With all such studies (as indeed with any psychophysiological measure) it should be remembered that one is dealing with a signal which is constantly changing anyway as a function of the intrinsic activity of neuronal cells. In addition, many such tasks show variations in motor activity or sensory processing demands, which are just as likely to influence EEG activity as the more subtle cognitive variations (Gevins et al., 1979).

EEG measures in the study of sleep

As described above, it is through the use of EEG techniques that we have gained some insight into the processes of sleep, if not its function. Behavioral observation had suggested that there were different stages in sleep, ranging from very heavy sleep, from which it is most difficult to rouse the sleeper, to restless "shallow" sleep. Once techniques required for assessing EEG throughout a night's sleep were perfected, it became clear that these stages were physiologically different as well. One observation where the EEG findings were of particular significance was of so-called paradoxical sleep, where the EEG indicates a relatively high state of alertness but muscle tension measures indicate the deepest stage of relaxation. As this stage is most frequently accompanied by dreaming, it is possible that the EEG is indexing some form of processing related to this, but no findings have confirmed this.

It cannot be said that EEG has taken sleep researchers much beyond the descriptive level. It allowed insight into sleep as an active process and, combined with organic research techniques, provided some information on the location of various key structures. It provides descriptive data for the study of some sleep abnormalities and can be used to monitor the effectiveness and consequences of narcoleptics.

CONCLUSION

It should be remembered that EEG's status as a provider of information is very much a function of the way in which this information is acquired, the procedural, analytical, and interpretative decisions made *en route*. Questions such as the number of electrodes to use, the analytical techniques to be employed, the methodological controls to be used, must be carefully considered. The increasing sophistication of measurement, analysis, and mapping techniques should not disguise the fact that EEG is a crude measure obtained at some distance from its source. Even though EEG electrodes are small in size, they are recording activity from many thousands of neurons. More particularly they are recording activity at the surface of the brain, whereas the generators of such activity may be located certainly below the surface of the brain and potentially some distance from the recording site.

To assess the importance of EEG measures in contemporary neuropsychological research we need to consider how much it can add to the other research techniques available. A measure of the activity of the brain should clearly be a central feature in the understanding of the function or dysfunction of this organ. It is clear that currently we do not know enough about the physiological significance of the measures we can obtain to make other than descriptive use of EEG data, with notable exceptions, as in epilepsy. However, this situation could be improved by the combination of EEG techniques with the more powerful localizing techniques of PET and MRI and the application of sophisticated mathematical models to EEG data. The spatial resolution of EEG may improve with the application of highly sophisticated mathematical techniques (e.g. dipole localization) to data from large numbers of electrodes, or with the application of techniques such as MEG. This could allow researchers to make many more meaningful inferences from EEG data.

As a psychophysiological measure it provides an important index in the assessment of particular behavioral states. Its temporal resolution can allow the "tracking" of activity across the cortex while the process of interest is occurring. This is clearly more applicable to evoked potential measures, but it should be remembered that the paradigms appropriate for the measurement of EPs are not always appropriate for the task of interest, for example, it is difficult to model the reading process solely via the use of EP paradigms.

Given the role of EEG in assessing the functional aspects of cortical activity, it clearly has a central role in research into areas where particular functions are of interest, such as various stages of the reading process. If we consider the deconstruction of various processes into particular modules along the lines of contemporary cognitive neuropsychology, then researchers who are interested in the possible differential involvement of different parts of the cortex (or even subcortex) need a technique which may allow the measurement of this involvement. It is possible to envisage the use of EEG techniques to map the brain activity involved in, for example, face recognition or movement planning, and to confirm the independence or interdependence of different subprocesses of such activities. Early EEG research was allied to rather crude localizationist theories; contemporary techniques might earn it a place in the sophisticated modelling approach currently employed by the cognitive neuropsychology school.

Although EEG research has clearly come a long way since Berger's work in 1929, much more sophistication is required if this important technique is to retain its central role in our understanding of the role of the brain in human behavior.

BIBLIOGRAPHY

Binnie, C. D., & Prior, P. F. (1994). Electro-encephalography. *Journal of Neurology, Neurosurgery and Psychiatry, 57*, 1308–19.

Duffy, F. (Ed.). (1988). *Topographic mapping of brain electrical activity*. Boston: Butterworths.

Fender, D. H. (1987). Source localization of brain electrical activity. In A. S. Gevins & A. Remond (Eds), *Handbook of electroencephalography and clinical neurophysiology: Methods of analysis of brain electrical and magnetic signals*, Vol. 1 (pp. 355–99). Amsterdam, Elsevier.

Fisch, B. J. (1991). *Spehlmann's EEG primer*, 2nd rev. edn. Amsterdam: Elsevier.

French, C. C., & Beaumont, J. G. (1984). A critical review of EEG coherence studies of hemispheric function. *International Journal of Psychophysiology, 1*, 241–54.

Gevins, A. S., & Remond, A. (Eds). (1987). *Handbook of electroencephalography and clinical neurophysiology: Methods of analysis of brain electrical and magnetic signals*, Vol. 1. Amsterdam: Elsevier.

Gevins, A. S., Zeitlin, G. M., Doyle, J. C., Yingling, C. D., Schafer, R. E., Callaway, E., & Yeager, C. (1979). EEG patterns during "cognitive" tasks. I. Methodology and analysis of complex behaviours. *Electroencephalography and Clinical Neurophysiology, 47*, 693–703.

Kahn, E. M., Weiner, R. D., Brenner, R. P., & Coppola, R. (1988). Topographic maps of brain electrical activity: pitfalls and precautions. *Biological Psychiatry, 23*, 628–36.

Lehmann, D., Michel, C. M., Henggeler, B., & Brandeis, D. (1991). Source localisation of spontaneous EEG using the FFT dipole approximation: different frequency bands, and differences with classes of thoughts. In I. D. Dvorak & A. V. Holden (Eds), *Mathematical approaches to brain functioning diagnostics* (pp. 159–69). Manchester: Manchester University Press.

Michel, C. M., Lehmann, B., Henggler, B., & Brandeis, D. (1992). Localization of the sources of EEG delta, theta, alpha and beta frequency bands using the FFT dipole approximation. *Electroencephalography and Clinical Neurophysiology, 82*, 38–44.

Neidermeyer, E., & Lopes da Silva, F. (Eds). (1987). *Electroencephalogaphy: Basic principles, clinical applications and related fields*, 2nd edn. Baltimore: Urban and Schwartzenberg.

Pfurtscheller, G., & Aranibar, A. (1977). Event-related cortical desynchronisation detected by power measurements of scalp EEG. *Electroencephalography and Clinical Neurophysiology, 42*, 817–26.

Pfurtscheller, G., & Lopes da Silva, F. H. (Eds). (1988). *Functional brain imaging*. Hans Huber.

Ray, W. J., & Cole, H. W. (1985). EEG alpha activity reflects attentional demands and beta activity reflects emotional and cognitive processes. *Science, 228*, 750–2.

Skarda, C. A., & Freeman, W. J. (1987). How brains make chaos in order to make sense of the world. *Behavioural and Brain Sciences, 10*, 161–95.

Weinberger, D. R., Bigelow, L. B., Kleinman, J. E., Klein, S. T., Rosenblatt, J., & Wyatt, R. J. (1980). Cerebral ventricular enlargement in chronic schizophrenia: an association with poor response to treatment. *Archives of General Psychiatry, 37*, 11–13.

GEORGINA M. J. RIPPON

emotional disorders (emotion) The term "emotion" here denotes reactions to an appropriately evocative stimulus involving cognitive appraisal (or perception), expressive behavior, physiological arousal, subjective experience ("feelings"), and goal-directed activity (Plutchik, 1984). Emotion is to be distinguished from affect (i.e. a relatively brief episodic event) and mood (i.e. pervasive, sustained feeling).

There are two general classes of theory about emotion: (a) theories in which stress is placed on the role of cognitive processes (e.g. evaluation, attribution) in mediating emotional experience, and (b) more biologically oriented theories which postulate separate systems for cognition and emotion, with reciprocity and interaction between them. Such theories consider emotional experience to be mediated by motoric and neurophysiological feedback, and are particularly relevant to the neuropsychological study of emotion. In this paper a neuropsychological perspective is assumed; see Buck (1988) for a more general psychological and physiological approach.

In studying emotion from a neuropsychological perspective, a number of parameters are critical. *First* are interhemispheric factors, that is, whether emotion is controlled by the right or left cerebral hemisphere. *Second*, a related parameter involves intrahemispheric factors. In this domain, one distinction relates to caudality – whether control within a hemisphere depends on anterior (i.e. frontal lobe) or posterior (i.e. temporal, parietal, occipital) structures. Another distinction relates to the vertical dimension of neuroanatomical control; inputs from limbic system and subcortical structures, in addition to neocortical structures, have also been implicated. The term neocortex refers to the gray matter covering the cerebral hemisphere (or "pallium"), showing stratification and organization of the most highly evolved type. The *third* parameter pertains to the actual mode of processing the emotion, whether via perception, expression, physiological arousal, or experience. The term perception is used to refer to the processing or "comprehension" of the emotional aspect of a stimulus. It is important to learn how these modes function individually as well as how they are related to each other. The *fourth* parameter is the communication channel, that is, the modality or way in which an emotion is processed, including facial, prosodic/intonational, lexical, gestural, and postural channels. The term lexical refers to verbal and speech content. It is important to ascertain whether there is a single central brain mechanism for these various channels and whether the channels are interrelated. The *fifth* parameter refers to the notion of discrete emotions (e.g. happiness, disgust) versus the superordinate level of emotional dimension (e.g. pleasantness/unpleasantness, approach/avoidance).

The neuropsychological literature is beginning to address the issue of whether there is a single system (i.e. a central mechanism) or multiple systems in the human brain for aspects of emotional processing. For neurologically normal adults, one wonders whether aspects of emotion are correlated, and, for neurological populations, whether deficits in various aspects of emotion occur together. In this vein, a componential approach to emotional processing has been proposed (Borod, 1993b) that applies to the five parameters described above. By assuming the componential approach, it is possible to ascertain whether components (e.g. face, prosody, and gesture) within a particular parameter or level of processing (e.g. communication channel) are overlapping or independent from each other.

HISTORY

Studies of unilateral brain-damaged patients and normal adult subjects have provided most of our knowledge base regarding brain/behavior relationships for emotional processing.

Brain damage One of the earliest discussions of emotion and the brain was in 1880 by Hughlings Jackson, who observed that emotional words (i.e. curses) could be selectively spared in aphasics with left hemisphere lesions. In 1912 Mills observed that right hemisphere pathology was associated with deficits in emotional expression. In the past two decades systematic studies of brain-damaged patients have provided experimental data about emotion, expanding on earlier anecdotal evidence and case studies.

Most studies have used patients with well-defined lesions of the right or left cerebral hemisphere and have typically examined level of performance on tasks involving emotional processing. Using this design, impaired performance is associated with the compromised hemisphere, and preserved performance is ascribed to the intact hemisphere.

In 1972 Gainotti examined emotional behavior in brain-damaged patients during a standard neuropsychological evaluation. He observed indifference reactions (inappropriate joking, euphoria, denial, minimization of deficits) in patients with right-hemisphere brain damage (RBD), and catastrophic reactions and depression in patients with left-hemisphere brain damage (LBD). These findings were corroborated by a series of studies in the 1960s using the INTRACAROTID SODIUM AMYTAL (ISA) or Wada test procedure. Intracarotid injections of sodium amytal result in temporary inactivation of the hemisphere ipsilateral to the injection site. In some but not all ISA studies, indifference/euphoric/laughter reactions occur with right-hemisphere injections and catastrophic/dysphoric/crying responses with left-hemisphere injections.

Whereas one interpretation of these data supports the right hemisphere's unique specialization for emotion, another view is that the right hemisphere is specialized for negative emotions and the left hemisphere for positive emotions. In the former view, the indifference reaction is taken as a lack of emotional responsivity; in the latter view, the euphoria that sometimes accompanies right-hemisphere damage is attributed to the intact left hemisphere.

While the research just described dealt with

313

inferences about destructive lesions or inactive hemispheres, another line of research has focused on hemispheric activity and so-called "irritative lesions." For example, Bear and Fedio in the mid-1970s examined personality characteristics of temporal lobe epileptics (TLE). During the interictal phases, patients with right-sided TLE were characterized as extremely emotive, whereas patients with left-sided TLE showed ruminative intellectual tendencies and were obsessive and humorless. Such descriptions were not inconsistent with Flor-Henry's report of a relationship between a right TLE focus and affective disorders (i.e. manic-depressive reactions) and between a left TLE focus and thought disorder (i.e. schizophrenic-like reactions). It was hypothesized that irritative lesions of TLE were actually exacerbating the characteristics of a particular hemisphere, and this theory was compatible with the hypothesis that the right hemisphere has a special role in emotional processing.

Psychiatric disorders One of the earliest observations in the psychiatric domain was the association between a preponderance of left-sided bodily complaints and the following disorders: conversion reactions (*see* HYSTERIA), hypochondriasis, phobias, psychoses, and PAIN syndromes. Given contralateral connectivity of sensorimotor pathways, these findings were interpreted as implicating the right hemisphere in emotional disorders.

During the same period (1970s and 1980s), neuropsychological mechanisms underlying psychiatric disorders were being investigated. (See reviews by Borod and Koff (1989) and Cutting (1992) for a direct treatment of this literature.) Briefly, a wide range of procedures (e.g. EEG, dichotic listening, neuropsychological testing) initially implicated right-hemisphere dysfunction in unipolar depression and left-hemisphere dysfunction in schizophrenia. The data for schizophrenia have been further refined, such that negative-symptom Type II schizophrenia with flat affect is more likely to have right-hemisphere dysfunction than is positive-symptom Type I schizophrenia. Affective behavioral similarities between Type II schizophrenics and RBDs (e.g. Borod et al., 1990) have been recently corroborated to some degree by Wolkin and colleagues' (1992) PET findings of right frontal hypometabolism in flat-affect chronic schizophrenics. On the other hand, Flor-Henry's original emphasis on left temporal lobe dysfunction in schizophrenic thought disorder has recently been underscored by a finding by Shenton and colleagues (1992) of volumetric reductions of the left superior temporal gyrus in schizophrenics with predominantly positive symptoms. In studies of depression, right-hemisphere mediation has been most frequently reported, with both increased right frontal activity and right posterior dysfunction in unipolar depression.

Normal adults Neuropsychological research on emotion in normal adult subjects has focused on laterality. Darwin appears to have made the first observations about laterality and emotion in his 1872 description of facial asymmetry during emotional expression (i.e. "snarling"). Darwin pointed out that the muscles on one side of the face may be incapable of movement, but he did not make any neuroanatomical speculations. In 1902, using the composite photograph technique, Hallervorden described the normal resting right hemiface (presumably controlled by the left hemisphere) as "apperceptive," sensible, and active, and the left hemiface (controlled by the right hemisphere) as "perceptive," affective, and directionless. This work was continued by Wolff in the 1930s but has not been corroborated by more recent studies. In the late 1930s and early 1940s, Lynn and Lynn used a movie camera to measure facial asymmetry ("facedness") during spontaneous smiling and laughter, and correlated measures of facial asymmetry with measures of lateral dominance and personality traits.

It was not until the 1970s that emotional perception began to be studied. The development of the DICHOTIC LISTENING procedure made it possible to study LATERALIZATION for auditory perceptual stimuli, followed by the tachistoscope and free-field viewing within the visual perceptual domain. Given the typical contralateral innervation of the central nervous system, superiority of the left side (e.g. left ear, left visual field, left hemispace) implies greater right-hemisphere involvement. Conjugate lateral eye movements (LEMs) have also been used as an index of underlying hemispheric activity.

The most recent research on emotion has utilized new electrophysiological and neuroradiological techniques (e.g. Davidson's (1984) work on frontal lobe EEG asymmetries and emotion). It is hoped that studies using procedures such as event-related potentials, regional cerebral blood flow, and metabolic imaging

(SPECT, PET, MRI) will enable the on-line study of all components of emotion in real time, thus providing a clearer window into brain–behavior relationships.

NEUROPSYCHOLOGICAL THEORIES OF EMOTION

A number of neuropsychological theories have emerged to explain hemispheric mechanisms underlying emotion. Three separate hypotheses are described below.

Hemispheric asymmetries for emotion have been much less clear-cut than those for cognitive functions. "Hemispheric specialization" refers to differential representation of functions in the two hemispheres. In right-handed individuals, the left hemisphere is thought to be the primary mediator of verbal and linguistic functions, the numerical symbol system, and complex voluntary movement, whereas the right hemisphere has a primary role in nonverbal and spatial functions, attention, and melody. Left- versus right-hemisphere strategies are described respectively as analytic vs synthetic, linear vs configurational, serial vs simultaneous, detailed vs holistic, and temporal vs spatial. Left-hemisphere processing involves abstract, logical, and sequential reasoning, whereas right-hemisphere processing involves concrete, perceptual insight.

Right hemisphere hypothesis The right hemisphere hypothesis maintains that the right hemisphere is specialized for emotion, regardless of the pleasantness level or "valence" of the emotion. On a psychological level, support for this hypothesis is based on the notion that emotional processing involves strategies (e.g. integrative, holistic) and functions (e.g. nonverbal, visuospatial) for which the right hemisphere is dominant. On a neuroanatomical level, the structure of the right hemisphere is consistent with the strategies and functions associated with emotional processing. In particular, the right hemisphere has been described as having greater capacity for multimodal integration, greater interlobular organization, and a greater degree of neural interconnectivity among regions than the left hemisphere.

Valence hypothesis There are two versions of the valence hypothesis. One version postulates that the right hemisphere is specialized for unpleasant/negative emotions and the left hemisphere for pleasant/positive emotions, regardless of processing mode. The other version of this hypothesis contends that this pattern of differential hemispheric specialization occurs for the *expression* and *experience* of emotion, whereas the right hemisphere is dominant for the *perception* of emotions of both valences. One can only speculate about how differential effects of valence may have evolved. Because negative emotions are linked with survival (e.g. removing oneself from danger), a system would be required that is sensitive to multimodal inputs and able to quickly scan and evaluate the entire situation. Such behaviors seem more linked to Gestalt, synthetic processing (a right hemisphere function) than to discrete, focused analysis (a left hemisphere function). Positive emotions, on the other hand, may be more dominated by left hemisphere processing, being perhaps more linguistic and communicative than emotional and reactive.

Approach/avoidance hypothesis The third hypothesis postulates that the left hemisphere is specialized for "approach" emotions and the right hemisphere for "avoidance" emotions (Davidson, 1984; Kinsbourne, 1982). In this formulation, withdrawal/avoidance emotions are linked with the right hemisphere's involvement in arousal, habituation, and undifferentiated automatic movements. Approach behaviors, on the other hand, are linked with the left hemisphere because of its specialization for activation and focal attention; further, the left hemisphere is considered superior for motor behavior, fine manual control, and sequentially executed movement, processes which would seem more critical in approach than avoidance behaviors. Conceptual overlap clearly exists between the valence and approach/avoidance hypotheses, as most pleasant emotions (e.g. happiness) have an approach component, whereas most unpleasant emotions (e.g. disgust) have an avoidance component. Anger may be an exception, being both negative and related to approach.

LITERATURE REVIEW

The neuropsychological literature on emotion will be summarized below. This summary will be organized around four components of emotional processing: perception, expression, arousal, and experience. Evidence will be limited to data from normal and brain-damaged subjects, and interhemispheric, intrahemispheric, and valence factors will be considered. The data for percep-

315

tion and expression will be organized according to the communication channels of face, voice, and speech content.

Perception In *normal adults*, for the *prosodic channel*, the dichotic listening paradigm is used with response measures of identification, discrimination, or reaction time. Subjects are typically required to identify the emotion conveyed in the stimulus. Prosody refers to features in speech (e.g. melody, intonation, stresses, pauses) that convey the emotional attitude of the speaker. Dichotic listening experiments have demonstrated a left-ear (right hemisphere) advantage for processing the emotional tone of natural speech, nonsense syllables, and nonverbal vocalizations (e.g. laughter, shrieks).

For the *facial channel*, the tachistoscopic paradigm is typically used and requires a discrimination or identification response with speed and accuracy as dependent variables. A left visual-field advantage (right hemisphere) has been obtained for the perception of emotional facial expressions, with photographic, chimeric, cartoon, and line-drawing stimuli. This advantage appears to be independent of the left visual-field superiority for neutral facial recognition and visuospatial perception. In addition, the neuropsychological literature has demonstrated a left hemispace bias for processing emotional CHIMERIC FIGURES (i.e. faces) during free-field viewing.

For the *lexical channel*, the tachistoscopic procedure has been used to examine speed and accuracy of processing emotional versus nonemotional words. While some studies have found a left visual-field advantage, others have failed to find a difference.

In general, the perception findings for normal adults are consistent across individual emotions and across dimensions (pleasant vs unpleasant emotions).

In *brain-damaged adults*, subjects typically are required to identify the emotion expressed in a stimulus or to discriminate between two emotionally toned stimuli. For the *prosodic channel*, in most studies, right brain-damaged subjects (RBDs) relative to left brain-damaged subjects (LBDs) and normal controls (NCs) have been shown to be impaired in making judgments about the emotional tone of spoken sentences. For the facial channel, deficits in perceiving facial emotion are associated more frequently with pathology of the

right rather than the left hemisphere. For the lexical channel, RBDs have shown impairment (compared to LBDs and NCs) in processing emotional vs nonemotional words and sentences.

For the most part, these findings are consistent across individual emotions (e.g. disgust) and specific dimensions (e.g. unpleasantness). When intrahemispheric site of lesion is considered, for facial and prosodic channels, posterior (e.g. parietal, temporal) structures appear to be the most critical.

In conclusion, findings from studies with normal subjects suggest that the right hemisphere is generally dominant for emotional perception for both facial and prosodic channels, irrespective of valence. Further research is required for the lexical channel. Among brain-damaged subjects, RBDs typically are more impaired than LBDs and NCs across all three channels, regardless of valence. When intrahemispheric site of lesion is examined, posterior regions are important for facial and prosodic perception, but of unclear relevance in lexical perception studies.

Expression To study facial expression in normal adults, the facial channel most lends itself to laterality paradigms. Because the lower two-thirds of the face are predominantly innervated by the contralateral cerebral hemisphere, activity on one side of the face (or "hemiface") has been interpreted to reflect mediation by the contralateral cerebral hemisphere.

One of the main distinctions in the study of emotional expression is that between posed and spontaneous expression. Posed or voluntary movements are behaviors which are deliberately intended by or requested of an individual; spontaneous or involuntary movements are those unintended movements which are part of an instinctual reaction to an appropriately evocative emotional stimulus. A major concern regarding the two modes of facial expression is whether innervation is ipsilateral, contralateral, or bilateral. This issue has important implications for the study of hemispheric specialization. Neuroanatomical evidence suggests that voluntary (posed) expression (in the lower face) is contralaterally innervated by cortical structures through the pyramidal system. Although involuntary (spontaneous) expression is presumed to be innervated by subcortical structures through the extrapyramidal system, there is a lack of consensus about whether its pathways are contra- or ipsilateral and just how they are distributed to the lower versus the upper face.

In a recent review of the facial asymmetry literature in normals (Borod, 1993a), 24 studies of posed expression and 23 studies of spontaneous expression were examined. Overall, a significant majority of studies reported that the left hemiface moves more extensively and appears more intense than the right hemiface. Furthermore, these findings are not confounded by nonemotional factors (i.e. hemiface mobility, hemiface size, and resting face asymmetries). In general, this left-sided finding occurred for both posed and spontaneous conditions and for both positive and negative emotions. It should be noted, however, that there was a slight tendency for left-hemiface expressivity to be more frequent for negative emotions and for right-hemiface expressivity to be more frequent for positive emotions. In general, the preponderance of left-sided findings appears to implicate the right cerebral hemisphere as dominant for the facial expression of emotion. From a neuropsychological perspective, these data provide stronger support for the right hemisphere hypothesis than for the valence hypothesis.

To study emotional expression in *brain-damaged adults*, patients with well-defined lesions of the right or left hemisphere serve as subjects. Lesions in this population are due to cerebrovascular accidents (CVAs) and sometimes to tumor or surgical excision of pathological tissue. Level of performance on tasks designed to elicit posed and spontaneous emotional expression is evaluated via measures of accuracy (or appropriateness), frequency (or expressivity), and intensity (or emotionality). These measurements typically are made by carefully trained raters, among whom interrater reliability has been established using Likert-type scales, although more objective techniques (e.g. measurement of facial action units, acoustical/spectral analysis, discourse analysis) have also been used.

For the *prosodic channel*, the majority of studies have shown that RBDs are impaired relative to LBDs and NCs in their ability to produce prosody with accuracy, intensity, and appropriate acoustical modulation, irrespective of the emotion type or expression elicitation condition. For the most part, there has been no specific intrahemispheric localization with respect to the rostral/caudal dimension, and subcortical, as well as cortical, structures have been implicated.

The *lexical channel* has received relatively less attention in the neuropsychological literature. Although the left hemisphere is clearly responsible for most linguistic functions, the right hemisphere is also involved in some aspects of language functioning (Joannette et al., 1990). Recently a few studies have been conducted to examine lexical emotional expression, using an immediate or recollected memory paradigm. In these studies RBDs were more impaired than LBDs and NCs, irrespective of emotional valence and intrahemispheric lesion site.

For the *facial channel* the findings have been less consistent than those for prosodic and lexical expression with respect to side of lesion (right vs left). In a review by Borod (1993a) one set of studies (I) reports that RBDs are significantly impaired in expressing facial emotion relative to LBDs and/or NCs. The other set (II) reports that both RBDs and LBDs show deficits or do not differ from normal adult control subjects. The differences between the two sets are of interest. Subjects in set I were more likely to be older males, to have cerebrovascular pathology, and to have been evaluated at a longer time post stroke onset; further, they were requested to produce approximately equal numbers of positive and negative emotions, and their expressions were evaluated by raters. Subjects in set II, by contrast, were younger and of both genders, had brain tumors or surgical excisions, and were tested more acutely; they were requested to produce mostly negative emotions, and their expressions were evaluated via facial action unit analytic techniques. Overall, when emotional valence was considered for the facial channel, there were no systematic differences; in a handful of studies where RBDs showed selective deficits for positive or negative emotions, findings were equally divided between the two valences. When intrahemispheric site of lesion was a factor, patients with anterior lesions (i.e. those involving frontal structures) were more impaired than those with posterior lesions.

In conclusion, for normals, the majority of studies suggest that the right hemisphere is dominant for posed and spontaneous expression of facial emotion. For brain-damaged subjects, findings differed as a function of communication channel. For prosodic and lexical channels, RBDs were generally more impaired than LBDs and NCs, regardless of intrahemispheric lesion site or valence. For the facial channel, findings for lesion side were less consistent; although the majority of studies found RBDs to be the most impaired, other studies found that both RBDs and LBDs were impaired or not different from NCs. When lesion site was considered, anterior structures appeared to be more critical for facial expression than posterior ones. Of interest was the fact that emotional valence occasionally made a difference for RBDs, but studies were about evenly divided as to whether deficits were more prominent for positive or negative emotions.

Arousal The idea has been advanced that the right hemisphere (and in particular parietal regions) has a special role in arousal. This notion is supported, in part, by observations of unilateral spatial neglect following damage to the right more than to the left hemisphere. In addition, a number of studies have examined hemispheric specialization for physiological arousal, using measures of autonomic nervous system (ANS) responding (e.g. skin conductance, heart rate, skin temperature). Research with normals has reported that emotional stimuli presented with lateralized procedures produce a greater ANS response when presented to the right than to the left hemisphere. Studies with unilateral lesion patients have found that RBDs, relative to LBDs, show abnormal patterns of ANS responding.

These findings are of interest in light of the suggestion (e.g. Heilman & Bowers, 1990) that the right versus the left hemisphere is more in touch with subcortical systems important for arousal and intention. Although there is ample documentation that limbic system structures are involved in emotion, there is currently little evidence of more substantial or more direct anatomical connections between subcortical/limbic structures and right- versus left-hemisphere cortical structures (e.g. Borod, 1992; Tucker, 1991). Although many levels of the nervous system appear to be involved in emotion, few studies have addressed how "higher" levels are coordinated with "lower" ones. One such attempt (Eidelberg & Galaburda, 1984) postulated a specialized neural network connecting area PEG of the inferior parietal lobe with both cortical association areas and limbic afferents. Interestingly, a right-hemisphere bias has been shown for this particular system, suggesting a link between neocortical arousal and attention, right-hemisphere parietal structures, and the limbic system.

Experience In the study of emotional experience in normals, mood induction or imagery procedures are typically used, and responding has been indexed with EEG recordings or more on-line procedures (e.g. BLOOD FLOW, PET). The EEG studies generally report frontal asymmetries, with greater right-hemisphere activation for negative experience and left-hemisphere for positive. Another technique used is the LEM procedure. LEMs in response to questions requiring reflective thinking or imagery have been hypothesized to indicate activation of the hemisphere contralateral to the direction of eye movement. While some studies have found support for the right-hemisphere hypothesis (more left LEMs), others have supported the valence hypothesis (more left LEMs for negative emotion and right LEMs for positive emotion). Others failed to find directional differences as a function of emotion. Further, a preponderance of left-sided LEMs has been reported under conditions involving arousal.

In brain-damaged patients experience is typically indexed with self-report measures of feelings. To date, a handful of studies has suggested that both RBDs and LBDs are capable of accurately assessing their emotional experience, in spite of simultaneous deficits in emotional expression.

EMOTIONAL DISTURBANCES IN NEUROLOGICAL DISORDERS

In addition to studying brain mechanisms underlying emotion, there has been considerable work on emotional disorders associated with neurological diseases.

Work in this area began with observations about emotional sequelae to stroke. Observations in the early 1970s documented catastrophic reactions in LBDs and indifference/euphoric reactions in RBDs. Among LBD aphasics, anterior patients (with relatively intact comprehension) were described as displaying illness-appropriate depressive reactions and posterior aphasics (with impaired comprehension) as appearing unconcerned or unaware of their illnesses. These behaviors were interpreted as reactions to the comprehension component of the patients' aphasia. More recently the focus has been on affective disorders associated with stroke (Starkstein & Robinson, 1988). Originally research demonstrated that depression occurs closer to the frontal pole in LBDs and further from the frontal pole in RBDs. Currently the literature is divided, with some studies reporting that depression occurs more frequently with LBD, others with RBD, and others with equal frequency in LBD and RBD (with estimates as high as 60 percent).

Depression has also been frequently described in PARKINSON'S DISEASE (PD), with estimates ranging from 12 percent to 90 percent (Raskin et al., 1990). One theory claims that depression reflects biochemical and neuroanatomical changes that are intrinsic to PD, another that depression is a reaction to the illness. The second theory has been challenged due to the lack of correlation in PDs between the severity of depression and the duration of the motoric impairment or level of functional disability. Other aspects of emotional processing have been studied in PD. A few studies have shown deficits in PDs relative to NCs for the perception and expression of facial and prosodic emotion (reviewed in Borod et al. (1990)). In another subcortical dementia, HUNTINGTON'S DISEASE (HD), a wide range of emotional disorders has been reported, including depression, apathy, mania, and psychosis. Both paranoid states and schizophrenic reactions have been described, and suicidal ideation (be it reactive or organic) is common. Mayeux (1983) has suggested that emotional disorders in PD and HD are caused by neuropathological changes within the basal ganglia and associated neurotransmitter alterations.

MULTIPLE SCLEROSIS (MS), a demyelinating white-matter disease, has also been associated with emotional disorders (Rao et al., 1992). Depression is most common, with estimates ranging from 27 percent to 54 percent. Also noted are euphoria and pathological crying and laughter.

Moving from the subcortical to the cortical level, there are dementias that also have associated emotional disorders. In Alzheimer's disease approximately 30 per cent of patients meet criteria for clinical depression. In PICK'S DISEASE frontal-lobe personality changes are common (e.g. inappropriate behavior, apathy). Finally, Cummings has described disinhibition, apathy, and mood alterations in FRONTAL LOBE degeneration.

Traumatic brain injury is another disorder that can produce emotional changes. In that condition, depending on trauma type and damage extent, a range of personality disturbances has been described by Prigatano – both active (e.g. irritability,

anger, anxiety, paranoia) and passive (e.g. aspontaneity, depression, denial). It is conjectured that damage to frontal, temporal, and limbic structures in head trauma plays a role in the development of personality changes. Similarly, exposure to solvents, many of which have affinities for limbic structures, often leads to personality and affective alterations. Finally, long-term exposure to alcohol can produce a KORSAKOFF'S PSYCHOSIS with associated frontal lobe pathology and personality changes (e.g. confabulation, apathy, passivity/withdrawal).

IMPLICATIONS

Research Obviously, more research is needed to pinpoint the nature and prevalence of emotional disorders associated with neurological disorders. Specific emotional processing deficits in such disorders have yet to be described, due in part to the lack of valid and reliable assessment techniques.

Clinical Neuropsychological research on emotion has a number of clinical applications. For example, emotional context has been shown to facilitate the performance of LBD aphasics on tasks involving comprehension, discourse production, reading, writing, and praxis. Further, this research may have implications for speech therapy. There are therapeutic techniques (e.g. MELODIC INTONATION THERAPY (MIT)) which presumably utilize preserved right hemisphere functions to improve speech/language production among aphasics.

Finally, this work has implications for the assessment of affect in neurological disorders. Compared to the many instruments available for evaluating cognitive deficits in brain damage, there are relatively few for affective deficits. In the last few years a number of batteries have emerged in the clinical literature (for a review see Borod, 1992). In our own research program on emotion, we have developed a battery of tests (Borod et al., 1990) to assess a wide range of neuropsychological parameters of emotional processing (e.g. expression, perception). Through the development of such batteries neuropsychologists can make further advances in the diagnosis and remediation of emotional processing deficits.

BIBLIOGRAPHY

Borod, J. (1992). Interhemispheric and intrahemispheric control of emotion: a focus on unilateral brain damage. *Journal of Consulting and Clinical Psychology, 60*, 339–48.

Borod, J. (1993a). Cerebral mechanisms underlying facial, prosodic, and lexical emotional expression: a review of neuropsychological studies and methodological issues. *Neuropsychology, 7*, 445–63.

Borod, J. (1993b). Emotion and the brain – anatomy and theory: an introduction to the Special Section. *Neuropsychology, 7*, 427–32.

Borod, J., & Koff, E. (1989). The neuropsychology of emotion: evidence from normal, neurological, and psychiatric populations. In E. Perecman (Ed.), *Integrating theory and practice in clinical neuropsychology* (pp. 175–215). Hillsdale, NJ: Erlbaum.

Borod, J., Welkowitz, J., Alpert, M., Brozgold, A., Martin, C., Peselow, E., & Diller, L. (1990). Parameters of emotional processing in neuropsychiatric disorders: conceptual issues and a battery of tests. *Journal of Communication Disorders, 23*, 247–71.

Buck, R. (1988). *Human motivation and emotion*. New York: John Wiley.

Cutting, J. (1992). The role of right hemisphere dysfunction in psychiatric disorders. *British Journal of Psychiatry, 160*, 583–8.

Davidson, R. (1984). Affect, cognition, and hemispheric specialization. In C. Izard, J. Kagan, & R. Zajonc (Eds), *Emotions, cognition, and behavior* (pp. 320–65). Cambridge: Cambridge University Press.

Eidelberg, D., & Galaburda, A. (1984). Divergent architectonic asymmetries in the human brain. *Archives of Neurology, 41*, 843–52.

Heilman, K., & Bowers, D. (1990). Neuropsychological studies of emotional changes induced by right and left hemispheric studies. In N. Stein, B. Leventhal, & T. Trabasso (Eds), *Psychological and biological approaches to emotion* (pp. 97–113). Hillsdale, NJ: Erlbaum.

Joannette, Y., Goulet, P., & Hannequin, D. (1990). *Right hemisphere and verbal communication*. New York: Springer Verlag.

Kinsbourne, M. (1982). Hemispheric specialization and the growth of human understanding. *American Psychologist, 37*, 411–420.

Mayeux, R. (1983). Emotional changes associated with basal ganglia disorders. In K. Heilman & P. Satz (Eds), *Neuropsychology of human emotion* (pp. 141–64). New York: Guilford.

Plutchik, R. (1984). Emotions: a general psychoevolutionary theory. In K. Scherer & P. Ekman (Eds), *Approaches to emotion* (pp. 197–219). Hillsdale, NJ: Erlbaum.

Rao, S., Huber, S., & Bornstein, R. (1992). Emotional changes with multiple sclerosis and Parkinson's disease. *Journal of Consulting and Clinical Psychology, 60*, 369–78.

Raskin, S., Borod, J., & Tweedy, J. (1990). Neuropsychological aspects of Parkinson's disease. *Neuropsychology Review, 1*, 185–221.

Shenton, M., Kikinis, R., Jolesz, F., Pollak, S., Le May, M., Wible, C., Hokama, H., Martin, J., Metcalf, D., Coleman, M., & McCarley, R. (1992). Abnormalities of the left temporal lobe and thought disorder in schizophrenia: a quantitative magnetic resonance imaging study. *New England Journal of Medicine, 327*, 604–12.

Starkstein, S., & Robinson, R. (1988). Lateralized emotional response following stroke. In M. Kinsbourne (Ed), *Cerebral hemisphere function in depression* (pp. 25–47). Washington: American Psychiatric Press.

Tucker, D. (1991). Developing emotions and cortical networks. In M. Gunnar & C. Nelson (Eds), *Minnesota symposium on child psychology*, Vol. 24: *Developmental behavioral neuroscience* (pp. 75–128). Hillsdale, NJ: Erlbaum.

Wolkin, A., Sanfilipo, M., Wolf, A., Angrist, B., Brodie, J., & Rotrosen, J. (1992). Negative symptoms and hypofrontality in chronic schizophrenia. *Archives of General Psychiatry, 49*, 959–65.

JOAN C. BOROD

encephalitis Encephalitis is inflammation of the brain. This is a pathological definition and inflammation is one of the principal pathological changes associated with disease. It is characterized by cells from the immune system moving out of blood vessels into tissues, with accompanying fluid and proteins. Most cases of encephalitis recover, so post-mortem material is not obtained, and there is no indication for biopsy. Thus the disease has to be diagnosed clinically, and clinical definitions have been developed by known associations between clinical and pathological features. Most cases are acute, and many are associated with a virus infection, proven or presumed. There is a conceptual overlap between virus encephalitis and the so-called spongiform encephalopathies, which are due to infection with a sub-viral particle but in which inflammation is not prominent.

TERMINOLOGY

This is confusing. Historically, the term encephalitis appeared around 1800. Previously the condition had been known as brain fever, phrenitis, or cerebritis. The first two terms are now obsolete, and cerebritis is reserved for inflammation of the brain associated with a bacterial infection, for example, around an abscess or in the brain surface adjacent to the inflamed meninges in bacterial meningitis. When there is similar brain involvement in virus meningitis it is called meningo-encephalitis. Encephalitis associated with inflammation of the spinal cord, or myelitis, is called encephalomyelitis.

Polioencephalitis can mean any encephalitis involving the gray matter of the brain, or specifically that variety due to the poliovirus. These cases are due to virus invasion of the brain; hence they are called primary viral encephalitis. Leucoencephalitis means that it is the white matter which is involved. The usual term for this is now acute disseminated encephalomyelitis, or ADEM. This is commonly preceded by a systemic virus infection or a vaccination, and is therefore known as secondary, or post viral, or post vaccinal encephalitis. *Multiple sclerosis* is regarded as a separate entity, even though it does consist of recurrent foci of inflammation in the white matter, some apparently triggered by virus infections.

Myalgic encephalomyelitis, or ME, is an unfortunate term which has crept into public usage to describe a fatigue state. It is a misnomer, and has led to much misunderstanding. The existence of fatigue states is not disputed, and some begin after a virus infection, but there is no evidence that the brain is inflamed. The term should be abandoned for reasons advanced by the neurologist William Gowers in 1888, when he deplored the use of the term encephalitis "as a convenient designation for obscure cases, the exact nature of which is unknown."

THE CLINICAL PICTURE

The typical presentation of encephalitis is with a febrile illness, impairment of consciousness, neurological signs, and fits. The neurological deficits may be in cognitive, motor, sensory, or visual function, and are usually diffuse and of only mild to moderate severity, rather than focal and severe. They may indicate disorders of the hemispheres, brain stem, or spinal cord. There may be a history of preceding infection, either specific, like measles, mumps, or chickenpox, or nonspecific, in the form of a flu-like illness. There may have been a recent vaccination. In some cases the diagnosis cannot be made until other conditions have been excluded, such as tumor, stroke, intracranial hemorrhage, abscess, tuberculous meningitis, and venous thrombosis. Others will show such distinctive features that there is little risk of confusion. Some of these more specific syndromes will now be described. These are clinical entities, easily recognized, each of them illustrating some underlying factors in etiology. However, they do not fall neatly into subgroups.

A patient may present with a febrile illness and neck stiffness, due to an acute lymphocytic meningitis of virus origin. If they then develop impairment of consciousness or other evidence of brain disorder, the diagnosis of virus meningo-encephalitis will be clear-cut. Brain-stem encephalitis is usually part of a more diffuse picture, but can occur rarely in isolation. It then needs to be distinguished from a brain-stem tumor, which typically differs by producing raised intracranial pressure. An acute disorder of cerebellar function, known as acute cerebellar ataxia, can also occur in isolation, and indeed is the form taken by some 50 percent of cases of encephalitis which follow chickenpox. Herpes simplex virus affects predominantly the FRONTAL and TEMPORAL LOBES, and may begin asymmetrically. The presentation is typically with a personality change, focal epileptic fits, and focal signs suggestive of a unilateral lesion, such as a visual field defect or a hemiplegia. Such a picture strongly suggests an abscess or tumor, necessitating a CAT SCAN of the head. This may reveal the correct diagnosis, by showing the patchy hemorrhage typical of this form of encephalitis.

Encephalitis lethargica was an epidemic disease which spread to much of the world between 1916 and 1930, but which is now seen rarely, if at all. It produced a characteristic picture of sleepiness or reversal of sleep rhythm, coupled with eye movement disorders, and with other brain-stem and more diffuse signs. It sometimes caused an acute transient Parkinsonian syndrome, or a chronic one as a long-term sequel. Another specific condition, now rare, is subacute sclerosing panencephalitis, associated with a chronic measles infection. This is a disease of very gradual onset in children and young people, beginning with intellectual decline and proceeding to problems with motor control and unusual repetitive jerking movements, accompanied by a characteristic EEG. In Russian spring-summer encephalitis, a tick-borne disease caused by an arbovirus, involvement of the cervical cord is common, producing neurological signs in both arms. Herpes zoster, or shingles, is a segmental rash produced by the proliferation of latent varicella/zoster virus in a dorsal root ganglion. This can be complicated by focal paralysis produced by spread of the primary virus infection within the adjacent central nervous system, whether the spinal cord or the brain stem. It can also be complicated by a diffuse encephalomyelitis, of secondary or post-viral type.

Some viruses can not only initiate a range of central nervous syndromes, including diffuse encephalitis and isolated transverse myelitis, but also give rise to the Guillain–Barré syndrome, an inflammatory demyelinating disorder of the peripheral nerves. Cytomegalovirus (CMV) is one example.

Rabies is unusual in being transmitted almost invariably by a bite from an infected animal, and wild reservoirs of infection reside in various species, including wolves and bats. Apart from the bite itself, the first symptoms are non-specific, with malaise or headache, followed by fear and agitation, disturbed sleep, hallucination, and fits. The specific feature of hydrophobia is due to spasm of the throat muscles provoked by attempts to swallow. The untreated disease is universally fatal.

Lastly, encephalitis can be associated with AIDS, which predisposes to various infections. The AIDS virus itself is responsible for most cases, which have a subacute or chronic onset. There is an increased predisposition to CMV infections, but the incidence of herpes simplex encephalitis is not increased. Most of the associated brain infections are not due to viruses.

INVESTIGATIONS

Some of these will be carried out to exclude other disorders, and the commonest is a CAT scan, which will detect most of the alternative diagnoses, as well as herpes simplex encephalitis. In other cases the scan may be normal or show evidence of brain swelling. The EEG may show positive features favoring a diagnosis of encephalitis, with slowing or deficiency of the normal rhythm and an increased quantity of slow activity in either the theta or the delta range. There may be focal or generalized discharges typical of epilepsy. The cerebrospinal fluid typically contains an increased white cell count, and a slightly raised protein level. There may be oligoclonal bands, typical of local synthesis of immunoglobulin within the nervous system. If there is no increase in the cell count the diagnosis is probably a metabolic encephalopathy. MAGNETIC RESONANCE IMAGING (MRI) can show multiple areas of demyelination in cases of ADEM, which may be difficult to distinguish from a first episode of multiple sclerosis. The continuing appearance of new lesions on repeated scanning favors the latter diagnosis.

Investigations need to be performed to diagnose the responsible virus. These include cultures from body fluids, including a throat swab and a rectal swab. A virus can rarely be cultured from the cerebrospinal fluid, unless the cell count is very high, but virus antigen or nucleic acid may be found. Virus isolation from a brain biopsy is definitive, but is rarely available. Tests on paired specimens of serum, one early and one late, may show a diagnostic rise in an antibody to a specific virus.

CAUSES AND EPIDEMIOLOGY

In the UK most cases are sporadic. However, a preceding infection, such as influenza, may be epidemic and there may be a rush of cases of encephalitis associated with this, but the actual prevalence of the complication is low, less than one case in a thousand. No factor has yet been identified which tells us why these individuals develop encephalitis when most people do not. Cases of ADEM without apparent preceding infection may still prove on careful virological investigation to be associated with a specific virus. Minor epidemics of virus meningitis may occur, in association with widespread infection with an enterovirus, and a small proportion of these may have an associated encephalitis or myelitis. The commonest single virus to be incriminated as the cause of sporadic cases is herpes simplex.

In other countries all of these can occur, and

also other sporadic disorders such as rabies. There are also epidemic forms of encephalitis, caused by arboviruses. These constitute a large group, variously subdivided, with a complex nomenclature. Some are carried by insects and some by ticks. There are specific varieties occurring in many countries, and they may infect other members of the animal kingdom, such as birds, small rodents, or horses.

PATHOLOGY AND PATHOGENESIS

In primary viral encephalitis the virus directly invades brain tissue. In rabies it enters a peripheral nerve and travels centripetally up this nerve to the spinal cord and brain, and herpes simplex may do something similar through the olfactory nerves. In most diseases the virus reaches the brain via the bloodstream, crosses the blood-brain barrier, perhaps by infecting endothelial cells on the way, and typically damages neurons by entering them and causing cytolysis or cell death. Other cell types, such as astrocytes, and also blood vessels, may be damaged as well, and in addition there is an inflammatory reaction with infiltration of white cells and microglia, the immune cells specific to the nervous system. There will also be macrophages, which mop up debris. Although the cells come from the blood vessels, and may appear to be clustered around them, they diffuse rapidly into the areas of greatest damage. The viruses causing this picture have been called the neurotropic viruses, because of their affinity for nerve cells. They include herpes simplex, varicella-zoster, polio, other enteroviruses, and arboviruses.

In secondary or post-viral encephalitis it is the myelin sheaths in the white matter of the brain which are damaged. The earliest change is swelling of the sheaths, which progresses to destruction, and there are inflammatory infiltrates of white cells, particularly around venules, sometimes with some hemorrhage. The macrophages often contain myelin fragments. In theory such appearances could be caused by direct virus cytolysis of oligodendrocytes, the cells which support the myelin sheath. However, such a mechanism has never been proved, and the damage is almost certainly caused by an autoimmune reaction against myelin itself. The changes are identical in human cases of encephalitis following a virus infection, in those following vaccination, and in experimental animal disease

produced by inoculation with myelin antigens. The mechanisms producing the immune reaction are not known in the case of the virus infections. With regard to vaccination, encephalitis was much commoner after the early rabies vaccine, prepared in rabbit brain, than in preparations made in duck eggs or, later still, tissue culture.

Although these two forms of pathology have been described separately they can occur to some extent in combination. It has already been mentioned that the varicella-zoster virus is capable of damaging nerve cells by direct invasion, and also of producing ADEM, by a putative immune mechanism. Measles virus may be capable of causing both forms of damage as well, but the changes are predominantly those of ADEM and neuronal damage is hard to find. Dead nerve cells cannot recover, so the prognosis for the primary viral form of disease is worse than that for ADEM, which in mild cases may involve only temporary swelling of myelin sheaths with very little destruction.

The spongiform encephalopathies, or prion diseases, are rare neurological disorders due to an infectious agent, but they are not strictly encephalitic because there is no inflammation. They include CREUTZFELDT–JAKOB DISEASE, a rare form of human dementia, and bovine spongiform encephalopathy (BSE), as well as eight other human and animal syndromes. They are characterized pathologically by accumulation of an abnormal form of a normal cell membrane protein, called prion protein, which is also the transmissible agent. Creutzfeldt–Jakob disease has not become more frequent since the outbreak of bovine spongiform encephalopathy.

TREATMENT

Prevention is ideal. Treatment of a bite from a rabid animal is one example, and another is vaccination against a dangerous virus. In the case of rabies, vaccination after the bite is highly effective, and since the disease is 100 per cent fatal even those vaccines with a high chance of producing an encephalitis on their own account were worth using. Current vaccines are much safer. Post-infectious encephalomyelitis due to measles and other types of illnesses has certainly been reduced by vaccination. The incidence of encephalitis after measles was about one in a thousand cases, but the risk after vaccination is a hundred times less. As a result of widespread vaccination against smallpox in the UK, a situation eventually developed in which more illness was being caused by vaccination than by the disease itself. In fact, there were no cases at all of the disease, but an incidence of about one in a hundred thousand for post-vaccine encephalomyelitis. Nevertheless it was not feasible to discontinue vaccination until the worldwide WHO campaign to stamp out smallpox had been successful. There was an unfortunate time when an ill-advised media campaign against the use of vaccine to protect from whooping cough, in the mistaken idea that vaccination did more harm than good, led to widespread concern among parents who thus refused their children the vaccine. Many unnecessary deaths were caused as a result.

Once a case of encephalitis has developed the management consists of general medical care, including when necessary the care of the unconscious patient. Corticosteroid drugs may be beneficial if the brain is significantly swollen, but are not given routinely. Antibiotics are not indicated except for complications such as chest infections. Antiviral drugs are effective against DNA viruses such as herpes and varicella-zoster. Anticonvulsants may be needed for epilepsy. In cases with residual disability a rehabilitation program may be needed, as after any disease damaging the nervous system.

OUTCOME

In the UK there is probably an overall mortality rate of some 30 percent for all cases of encephalitis, and a risk of permanent sequelae in another 30 percent. The figures vary according to the original illness. Those for mild cases of ADEM are much better, and those for herpes simplex encephalitis much worse, with a mortality of some 50 percent even in treated cases. In arbovirus epidemics there is generally a 10 percent mortality, and the prevalence of sequelae varies from virus to virus but can be as high as 50 percent. Residual problems include specific neurological deficits, continuing epilepsy, disturbances of memory or cognition, and personality change. Neurological deficits are especially likely after damage to the spinal cord. Serious focal neurological deficits are typical of cases of herpes simplex encephalitis which recover, and many of these have memory disturbance, associated with the predilection of this disease to

affect the inferior frontal and mesial temporal structures. The commonest personality change after other forms of encephalitis is a mild frontal lobe syndrome.

BIBLIOGRAPHY

Brew, B. J. (1994). The clinical spectrum and pathogenesis of HIV encephalopathy, myelopathy, and peripheral neuropathy. *Current Opinion in Neurology, 7,* 209–16.

Davis, L. E. (1987). Acute viral meningitis and encephalitis. In P. G. E. Kennedy & R. T. Johnson (Eds), *Infections of the nervous system* (pp.156–76). London: Butterworth.

Pruisner, S. B. (1994). *Prion diseases of humans and animals. Journal of the Royal College of Physicians, 28/2,* supplement.

Tselis, A. C., & Lisak, R. P. (1995). Acute disseminated encephalomyelitis and isolated central nervous system demyelinative syndromes. *Current Opinion in Neurology, 8,* 227–9.

NIGEL LEGG

encephalopathy   Encephalopathy refers to an inflammation of the central nervous system resulting from a reaction to chemical, allergic, toxic, or physical factors. It can produce significant motor, cognitive, and behavioral changes and can lead to coma and death in more severe cases. It should be distinguished from encephalitis, which refers to inflammation of the central nervous system resulting from viral infection. Neither term refers to a specific condition but rather to the effects of that condition. Given the large number of different factors that can result in an encephalopathy, only a few examples will be mentioned here.

Boxers can suffer from a chronic progressive traumatic encephalopathy resulting from the cumulative effects of frequent but mild head injuries received during the course of their sport. In more severe cases there are pyramidal, extrapyramidal, and cerebellar signs along with evidence of a dementing process. The sufferers are often described as being "punch drunk."

Encephalopathy is the most serious manifestation of lead poisoning. Adults may present with delirium along with poor concentration and memory, headaches, personality changes, and abdominal pain. Encephalopathy resulting from lead intoxication is rare in adults. In children, on the other hand, it is more common and can result in forceful vomiting, ataxia, and seizures.

Other specific conditions that can lead to encephalopathy are chronic liver disease, severe hypertension, radiation injuries, and the presence of carcinoma, as well as reaction to certain chemical agents and allergens. Perhaps the most well known encephalopathy is that resulting from a thiamine deficiency and known as WERNICKE'S ENCEPHALOPATHY.

MARCUS J. C. ROGERS

endorphin Endorphins (together with encephalins) are naturally occurring opiate-like polypeptide NEUROTRANSMITTERS. Their discovery followed the identification of receptors sensitive to opiates and the inference that similar substances must be produced naturally in the brain. Their principal interest lies in their function as modulators of the PAIN pathways; but it is also thought that a release of these neuropeptides during trauma may also result in the complex hallucinations of the "near-death experience." The endorphin system is highly complex and research continues to identify new endorphins and novel mechanisms of their action.

entorhinal cortex The entorhinal cortex is an area of the cortex which lies on the medial surface of the temporal lobe, in the superior part and towards the anterior end of the lobe. Its significance is that it forms part of the LIMBIC SYSTEM and the loop of connections known as the Papez circuit. The entorhinal cortex is a part of the parahippocampal gyrus. Functionally, the entorhinal cortex is part of the dopaminergic system arising from the midbrain and targeted upon the STRIATUM, particularly the AMYGDALA, the SEPTUM and the entorhinal cortex. The entorhinal cortex also receives input from the inferior temporal cortex (PYRIFORM CORTEX), and in turn provides the HIPPOCAMPUS with its single most massive input.

epicritic innervation Two anatomically distinct systems innervate the skin: PROTOPATHIC and epicritic. The epicritic system is considered to serve receptors that support light touch and temperature, and to be characterized by limited radiation and referral of sensation. Although originally considered to be distinguished at a peripheral level, these two systems are now thought to be associated with independent mechanisms at a more central level, in the thalamus and central transmission pathways. The concept is now little used as interest has focused on more specific functions and neural pathways.

epilepsy Epilepsy is a condition characterized by recurrent fits, or seizures. Single grand mal seizures are very common – one person in 20 will have a fit during their lives. But for a diagnosis of epilepsy to be considered two fits must occur with no obvious cause within two years. Many people outgrow their epilepsy; anyone who has had a two-year period free from fits will be regarded as no longer suffering from the condition.

At least one person in 200, and perhaps as many as one in 100, suffers from epilepsy. It is, on the whole, a disease of the young. About one-quarter of people with epilepsy will have developed the condition by the age of 5; half will have done so by 11, and three-quarters by the age of 18. A tendency to epilepsy can be inherited. For someone with one parent with the disease the chances of developing it increase to one in 40.

Epilepsy developing in adulthood may be due to a brain tumor, but this is rare and occurs only in about 10 percent of cases. Even in the 50–55 age group, when brain tumors are most common, about 85 percent of people who develop epilepsy do so from some other cause – perhaps the blockage of a small blood vessel within the brain. Research shows that the epilepsy of 80 percent of people whose fits start after the age of 25 can be successfully controlled by drugs.

SEIZURES

A seizure is a paroxysmal burst of abnormal electrical activity within the gray matter of the brain. Information is transferred within the brain as electrical impulses are passed from cell to cell by chemical messengers. As each brain cell "fires," it stimulates a neighboring cell and this in turn fires and excites the next cell along the pathway. How excitable the brain is depends on the balance of those chemical messengers which excite and those which inhibit cell firing. If the brain cells are more excitable than is normal, they will fire more easily and, instead of the orderly passage of electrical messages from cell to cell along a specific path, there is a sudden burst of electrical activity within a group or groups of cells – a seizure.

The main inhibitory neurotransmitter is gamma-amino butyric acid (GABA). GABAergic cells damp down the excitatory activity of neural transmission. The main excitatory neurotransmitter is glutamate. Neural transmission is, however, carried out by over 50 other known types of neurotransmitter.

During a seizure the abnormal electrical discharge may be limited to one part of the brain (a partial seizure) or it may spread rapidly to affect a much larger area, perhaps even the whole brain (a generalized seizure).

In a few people the whole brain is so highly excitable that seizures may develop spontaneously within it. The effects of the seizure will depend on which part and how much of the brain is affected.

Anyone can have a seizure under certain conditions. Drug or alcohol withdrawal, for example, a high temperature in some infants, extreme sleep deprivation or prolonged hunger, may all occasionally produce the sudden burst of electrical firing that leads to a seizure. But if the seizure threshold of the brain is low (i.e. the brain is more excitable than normal) many other factors, for example, drowsiness, low blood sugar, flickering lights, or, in some people, sleep, will trigger off the abnormal electrical discharge of a seizure. Women are usually more likely to have seizures during a menstrual period (*catamenial epilepsy*). Seizures are also often spontaneously triggered, with no apparent precipitating factor.

Brain excitability is probably partly inherited and is determined by genes which have their strongest effect in childhood and thereafter become progressively weaker. This kind of inherited epilepsy, developing without apparent cause, used to be called *idiopathic epilepsy* or *primary generalized epilepsy*.

Often, even though there is an inherited tendency to seizures, epilepsy will not always develop unless there is some additional "insult" to the brain – perhaps damage at birth or later, through injury, infection, or lack of oxygen.

Damage to the frontal and temporal lobes is more likely to cause seizures than damage to the back of the brain (the occipital and parietal lobes).

FOCAL SEIZURE GENESIS

One model of seizure genesis defines two populations of epileptogenic cells in the damaged area, group 1 and group 2. Group 1 cells are partially damaged neurons at the center of the focus. These cells are pacemaker cells, which fire *continuously* in an abnormal, bursting mode. Their activity is not modified to any significant extent by surrounding brain activity.

Group 2 cells are partially damaged neurons surrounding the focus. They can fire in both the bursting, epileptic mode, and in a normal mode, and can be modified by surrounding brain activity. When a seizure occurs, the continuously discharging group 1 cells recruit group 2 cells, spreading abnormal discharges to produce a focal seizure. Secondarily generalized seizures occur when normal neurons are recruited into the seizure discharge. Thus the activity of the neurons surrounding the focus determines the likelihood of a seizure occurring and spreading. This model also carries the implication that alteration in the level of excitation in the area of an epileptic focus can *prevent* seizure activity from arising and spreading.

EVOKED SEIZURES

In susceptible individuals, any form of appropriate (usually rhythmic) peripheral stimulation may evoke a seizure. Evoked seizures are said to occur in about 5 percent of people with epilepsy, though in hospital populations the rate may be nearer 25 percent. Flickering or strobe lights are a common cause of evoked seizures – the so-called *photosensitive epilepsy*. Reading, eating, stimulation of the skin, movement, sounds, smells can all trigger seizures by altering the level of activity within a damaged area of the cortex.

Seizures can be generated by an action of mind, either by a deliberate act of will (usually the manipulation of attention) or by the ongoing activity of mind, as in the *thinking epilepsies* which result from excitation of the seizure focus by mental activity, such as multiplication or addition.

TYPES OF SEIZURE

The international classification of seizures defines three types: partial seizures, generalized seizures, and unclassifiable seizures. What form a seizure takes depends on the part of the brain in which it arises, and how widely and rapidly it fans out from its point of origin.

Generalized seizures affect both sides of the body equally, and may arise over a wide area of the brain. The best known and most common of these is the *grand mal* attack. During a grand mal attack the person falls to the ground unconscious. The muscles of the body contract, the arms and legs go straight and rigid, the mouth clenches tight and the whole body is taut. The seizure may end with this "tonic" phase, or it may continue with a second, "clonic" phase during which the muscles of the body jerk in unison, starting at a rate of once a second, slowing to a rate of once every 4 to 6 seconds, and then stopping. Sometimes a convulsion consists only of the clonic phase. At the end of the seizure the muscles relax. Bowel and bladder control may be lost during the fit. The extent of the tonic and clonic phases of the fit will vary from time to time.

Another generalized seizure is the *absence* (what used to be called the *petit mal*) seizure. During an absence the person – nearly always a child – has a "blank" period from seconds up to half a minute or so, during which he or she is unaware of anything that is happening to him or her and looks as though he or she is day-dreaming or inattentive; the attacks may even pass unnoticed. However, an EEG recording made during one of these absences will reveal a characteristic pattern of spike and wave.

Other generalized seizures are *drop attacks*, which affect all ages and consist of a sudden loss of consciousness or muscle tone, so that the person does, literally, drop to the ground, and *myoclonic attacks*, which take the form of uncontrollable jerks or jerking of the muscles on one or both sides of the body, without necessarily causing any alteration of consciousness.

Infantile spasms (salaam attacks) are a rare (1 in 7,000) form of generalized epilepsy which develops between the ages of three months and a year, and which often results in permanent brain damage.

Partial (or focal) seizures are always caused by damage to some part of the brain. There are two types of partial seizures: *simple partial seizures*, in which consciousness is *not* affected, and *complex partial seizures*, in which there *is* a disturbance of consciousness.

Partial seizures begin in the localized, damaged area of the brain, though they may later spread. Partial seizures usually begin with a recognizable aura, often called the "warning," caused by the start of the electrical discharge within the brain. The characteristics of the aura will depend on the part of the brain involved. Seizures starting in the motor cortex (*Jacksonian epilepsy*), for example, usually begin with some body movement, usually a thumb or the face, perhaps an arm, hand, or foot. If the seizure arises in the sensory cortex, the aura may be a sensation, for example, an itching or tingling, or some feeling that is quite indescribable, though instantly recognizable to the sufferer. Seizures that arise in the occipital cortex give rise to auras that take the form of simple flashes or speckles of light, or more complex visual images.

Seizures caused by damage to the temporal lobe (usually complex partial seizures) often begin with a feeling arising in the stomach and moving up to the throat, usually accompanied by a sensation of fear, which can be so intense that the person fears they are going to die. Less often there may be an aura of taste or smell, usually unpleasant, or of some simple sound such as hummings or clicks. There may be feelings of déjà vu or precognition. Some people describe a feeling of reincarnation, or a sensation that the world is quite unrecognizable (jamais vu). Memories may be triggered off as part of the aura and – very rarely – intensely pleasant sexual or even mystical feelings can arise.

A few people have partial seizures that consist only of an aura, and some people manage to develop various techniques to abort their seizures at this stage, so that there is no loss of consciousness. However, more usually the seizure spreads, and results in more complex disturbances of sensation or bizarre behavior (called *automatism*) with some impairment of consciousness or confusion.

Sometimes a partial seizure may spread so rapidly through a wide area of the brain that it becomes generalized and there is a grand mal convulsion.

Seizure occurrence

The period before a seizure is often characterized by feelings of restlessness or irritability, or a change in mood or behavior. This "prodromal" phase may occur between one and 72 hours before the actual fit begins.

Tiredness or confusion are common after a seizure. After a grand mal seizure consciousness returns slowly, and the person may feel confused, disturbed, sleepy, and perhaps have a headache. They will usually sleep for about two hours, and wake up feeling better. However, for some people the after-effects last longer – occasionally for a week or more. After a temporal lobe seizure, return to normality begins with small repetitive movements, which become more complex and gradually fade into normal behavior.

Rarely there may be a prolonged state of confusion after a generalized or complex partial seizure, during which quite complex actions, perhaps dressing or undressing, may be performed, without the sufferer realizing what he or she is doing. This state of AUTOMATISM seldom lasts longer than a few minutes, but can rarely continue for as much as an hour. There is no subsequent memory for the events. Very occasionally the grand mal fit may be followed by a short mental illness or paranoid psychosis, lasting for up to 72 hours, in which patients feel that people around them are trying to harm them and so they may act impulsively and run away into danger.

DIAGNOSING EPILEPSY

A diagnosis of epilepsy is not one to be made lightly. Once it is made, the person concerned is given a "label" that may affect his or her chances of employment or lose them various privileges – their driving license, for example. It also means that they will have to start a regime of drug-taking that may continue for months or even years.

Many doctors advise a "wait and see" policy after a first fit. But, if there have been one or more previous attacks, referral to a neurologist is usual for tests to discover abnormalities in the structure or function of the brain.

Electroencephalogram (EEG)

Abnormalities of electrical activity show up on the EEG recording in about 75 percent of people with epilepsy. But an abnormal EEG is not necessarily proof of epilepsy, and neither does a normal EEG prove that no seizures are arising. Discharges in the depth do not always show up on a scalp EEG. The EEG pattern varies with the type of epilepsy: paroxysmal activity and spike and wave are both suggestive of generalized epilepsy. Focal spikes or sharp waveforms in the EEG are indicative of abnormal activity in one part of the brain, suggesting partial epilepsy.

During the recording the patient is asked to do various things which may provoke epileptic activity, including opening and closing the eyes, overbreathing, and sitting in front of a strobe (a flickering lamp).

Because sleep enhances epileptic activity in some people, a further recording may be made while the patient is asleep. In special circumstances (for example, to locate a possible area of damage in the temporal lobe if an operation to remove it is planned) a sphenoidal EEG recording may be made. This involves the insertion of electrodes just above the angle of the jaws, so that they lie outside the skull but as close as possible to the deeper part of the temporal lobes. A general anesthetic is then given in an attempt to induce abnormal EEG activity. Nowadays it is becoming more common for these electrodes to be placed within the skull, either by putting them through a hole in the base of the skull (the foramen ovale) out of which the fifth nerve comes, or by placing them stereotactically through a hole made in the skull.

Other investigations

CT SCAN (computerized axial tomography) is a special X-ray which shows up any areas of disease or evidence of a tumor within the brain.

Psychometric testing determines whether any particular area of the brain is functioning less well than another (see ASSESSMENT). Sometimes abnormality of brain functioning can be detected in this way even though nothing has shown up in the EEG or CT scan. Partial complex seizures often arise from the temporal lobes. In these patients there is often a disorder of memory, a poor memory for words if the damage is in the left temporal lobe, and a poor spatial memory if damage is on the right.

MRI scan (MAGNETIC RESONANCE IMAGING) builds up an image of the brain which can make it easier, in certain cases, to detect tumors or areas of injury within the brain.

Blood tests are used to see whether there is any medical reason for the seizures.

RISKS FROM SEIZURES

The observation of a grand mal convulsion is a frightening experience. However, the person is likely to have had many convulsions before and to have recovered satisfactorily from them. Heroic intervention is only very rarely, if ever, necessary.

All that is needed is to make sure that the patient does not harm her- or himself by hitting her or his head on the floor or nearby furniture while jerking. It is impossible to put anything into a patient's mouth during a fit, as the jaw muscles are clenched and any attempt to do so will break the patient's teeth. If there is blood or froth around the patient's mouth, wipe this away gently with a soft cloth and then, when the patient has stopped jerking, turn him or her onto his or her side in the recovery position. This will allow any fluid in his or her mouth to drain out quite naturally, and the airway will automatically be kept open. The patient will return to full consciousness within ten minutes.

The danger signs are seizures which do not stop after three to four minutes (*status epilepticus*). This is an emergency and medical help should be summoned immediately. Status epilepticus is extremely rare; more common are serial seizures, in which the patient does not regain consciousness between attacks. This too is an emergency but it is not as life-threatening as true status epilepticus.

Occasionally, after a grand mal seizure, quite often at night, patients may develop a severe psychiatric illness over the next two to three days. They will become suspicious, anxious, and fearful, feel people are against them, and may have auditory hallucinations. In response to these voices the patient may act precipitately by jumping out of windows or dashing into the road. This is also a medical emergency and help should be summoned immediately.

FEBRILE CONVULSIONS

Children's brains are more excitable, and therefore more "seizure prone" than adults. Between 3 percent and 6 percent of children tend to have convulsions when running a high temperature. They usually last only a few seconds or at the most a minute or two, and take the form of a grand mal seizure – the child becomes unconscious, the muscles go into spasm, with involuntary jerking and twitching, and then finally relax. Febrile convulsions often run in families. They are most common between the ages of 6 months and 3 years, and most children outgrow the tendency by about the age of 5. Only about 5 percent of

children who have febrile convulsions fail to outgrow them and develop true epilepsy.

Children run a greater risk than adults of developing status epilepticus (prolonged or repeated convulsions) during a fit, which is dangerous, and may cause permanent brain damage and even, occasionally, be fatal. Most doctors believe that children who have a tendency to febrile convulsions should be given regular anticonvulsant medication (usually sodium valproate) to prevent fits during their most susceptible years.

TREATMENT OF EPILEPSY

One hundred years ago about a third of sufferers lost their fits altogether with drug treatment, a third were improved, and a third were no better or worse after treatment. These figures are much the same today, but there are three important differences. The first is that there is a wider armory of drugs, and they have less damaging side effects. Second, a clearer understanding of the brain processes underlying the disease means that new drugs can be directed at more specific targets. Third, it is now widely recognized that there is a close relationship between the person, their seizures, their thought processes, and their lifestyle. Although drugs are still the first line of treatment, many people with epilepsy can be taught to exert at least some control over their own seizures.

Drugs

Drugs are the main treatment for epilepsy, and in almost every case have a beneficial effect on the frequency and severity of seizures. Unfortunately, all anticonvulsants also have side effects which must be weighed against the advantages of improved seizure control. The dilemma for the physician has always been how to damp down seizure activity without producing cognitive impairment in the sufferer. The often quoted words of Lennox (1942) are as true today as they were then: "Many physicians, in attempting to extinguish seizures, only succeed in drowning the finer intellectual processes of their patients."

The first drugs, such as the bromides, phenobarbitone, and phenytoin, all to some extent slowed thinking and motor behavior. Bromides are now seldom used and phenobarbitone is used only when other drugs fail, although it is an important drug in the third world because of its

epilepsy

Table 11 Drugs used to treat epilepsy.

Drugs	Uses	Common side effects
First-line drugs		
Carbamezapine (Tegretol)	Partial seizures Generalized tonic clonic seizures During pregnancy Brightening of mood in depressed people	Poor balance; double vision; blood diseases; water retention; thyroid abnormalities
Sodium valproate (Epilim)	Generalized seizures Absences (petit mal) To prevent febrile convulsions in susceptible children Myoclonic epilepsy Partial epilepsy	Hair loss and change in color; weight increase; tremor
Phenytoin (Epanutin)	Generalized tonic clonic seizures Focal epilepsy	Deterioration of balance; swollen gums; excessive hairiness; tingling in fingers and toes (peripheral neuritis)
Ethosuximide (Zarontin)	Absences (petit mal)	
Second-line drugs		
Diazepam (Valium)	Given intravenously (or as suppositories in children) to terminate status epilepticus or febrile convulsions Sometimes helpful in temporal lobe epilepsy	
Clonazepam (Rivotril)	Generalized tonic clonic seizures Partial seizures Myoclonic epilepsy	Marked drowsiness; personality changes
Clobazam (Frisium)	Partial and generalized tonic clonic seizures	Drowsiness with large doses
Phenobarbitone (Luminal)	Generalized tonic clonic seizures Partial seizures	Drowsiness; personality change; overactivity in children
New drugs		
Lamotogine (Lamictal)	Partial complex seizures	
Vigabatrine (Sabril)	Partial complex seizures	

low cost. Carbamazepine, sodium valproate, and phenytoin are the current first-line anticonvulsant drugs. In severe epilepsy a combination of drugs may be needed to establish control. However, the adding of different drugs to obtain seizure control is likely to produce significant toxic side effects.

State-of-the-art anticonvulsants are those specifically developed to decrease brain excitability. One such drug is Vigabatrine, which works by boosting GABA, a substance which decreases the excitability of the brain by inhibiting the transmission of electrical impulses within it. Another is

Lamotrogine, a drug which acts in part by decreasing brain excitability via glutamate.

Anticonvulsants may interfere with the action of other drugs, particularly alcohol, sedative drugs, anticoagulants, and oral contraceptives. Although epilepsy is no bar to pregnancy, because of the teratogenic effects of some anticonvulsant drugs, a woman who has epilepsy should always consult her doctor before embarking on a pregnancy. The rate of fetal malformation is increased by only one or two percentage points. The commonest malformations are cleft palate, heart defects, and spina bifida. All anticonvulsant drugs have some teratogenic risk, but Tegretol is thought to produce the fewest effects on the developing fetus.

When an individual has been free of fits for two to three years, the decision may be made to gradually reduce their drugs and perhaps eventually tail them off completely. However, when anticonvulsant drugs are stopped there is always a small risk that seizures may recur, and if they do, control will be harder to re-establish. There is also a risk that withdrawal of the drug may itself cause a seizure.

Surgery

Focal epilepsy can sometimes be successfully treated surgically. The operation is most often carried out to remove lesions in the temporal lobe. Provided the cases are carefully chosen, about 80 percent are much improved and approximately 50 percent lose their seizures altogether.

Stereotactic surgery, a method being developed to limit the spread of seizures by making a very small lesion within the brain, by means of an electrode, may prove helpful for a few people who have very severe or frequent seizures.

Behavioral treatment

The medical view of epilepsy is that seizures arise as a result of abnormal brain discharges, usually caused by a damaged area of brain tissue. However, it is becoming increasingly recognized that there is a close relationship between ongoing cerebral activity and the capacity of those cells involved in that activity to be diverted into a seizure process. There is evidence that children can both inhibit and generate their own seizures spontaneously. Many adult patients have behavioral strategies which they use either to inhibit seizures or to stop them spreading. In patients who have difficulties in coping with the stresses in their life the voluntary generation of seizures may come to form a response to difficult situations.

In focal epilepsy, the position of the focus will determine the relationship between individuals and their epilepsy, and those aspects of their psychic life and behavior which will both trigger and inhibit seizure activity. A complete treatment of epilepsy involves not just the giving of drugs, but also teaching patients how their feelings, thinking, and behavior can all be used in the control of their seizures.

Because of the close relationship between seizure activity and the ongoing patterns of excitation and inhibition in the neuronal pools which surround the epileptogenic focus, standard methods of behavior modification and psychophysiological treatments can be used to alter seizure activity. Most epileptic patients use cognitive strategies to inhibit seizure activity, both by avoiding circumstances likely to cause seizures, and attempting to abort seizures once they have begun. Reward management, relaxation, psychotherapy, and biofeedback have all been used with some success as treatment methods. However, more than one therapeutic factor in a conditioning program may lead to change. For example, the program's success will improve the patient's self-image and enhance self-esteem. Any consequent drug reduction will improve his or her alertness, well-being, and chances of employment.

LIVING WITH EPILEPSY

Driving

In the United Kingdom, no one who has had a fit after the age of 5 may hold a heavy goods vehicle or public transport driving license. However, people with epilepsy may reapply for an ordinary driving license when they have been fit-free (with or without medication) for two years. Some people only have seizures while asleep: in this case, if they have had no seizures which started when they were awake for three years, they may reapply for a driving license.

In other countries the regulations are different – in America there need only be a six-month fit-free period before a license is regained; in Japan the laws are draconian: anyone who has had one seizure is barred from driving for life.

There is no reason why people who have epilepsy should not take part in most sports, such as football or running. Where there is a greater element of risk common-sense precautions should be taken. A lifeguard should be present during swimming, for example, and mountaineers should be roped. Patients with epilepsy may have an occasional drink, but unfortunately the depressant effect of alcohol is enhanced by anticonvulsant drugs, so the patient rapidly becomes inebriated. Of more importance, as the alcohol is wearing off, about 8 hours after ingestion, the brain becomes much more excitable, and seizures are more likely to occur. A safe rule of thumb is to avoid drinking, or to limit drinking to no more than one pint (2 units) in an evening.

Most people who have epilepsy, or who have a family member with the disease, find it helpful to join a support group, such as the British Association for Epilepsy. It is always helpful to realize that other sufferers meet the same problems and have the same fear.

Children with epilepsy
Perhaps the greatest danger of childhood epilepsy is that it will permanently lower the child's self-esteem. There is a risk that both parents and teachers may become so over-concerned and over-protective that the child's social development and personality are restricted and he or she becomes isolated from other children. Difficult or bad behavior is often assumed to be an inevitable consequence of the child's epilepsy. Although those children whose epilepsy is due to brain damage, particularly to lesions in the temporal lobe (especially the left temporal lobe), do seem to be more prone to behavior disorders, it is worth remembering that all children are sometimes aggressive, inattentive, badly behaved, or restless. There is no good evidence to suggest that such behavior is more marked in children with uncomplicated epilepsy.

Some children who have epilepsy do, unfortunately, fail to achieve what they should be capable of at school, sometimes because of frequent absences, more often because of the effect of some anticonvulsant drugs (especially phenobarbitone and related drugs) on the child's behavior and concentration. However, often another major factor is the attitude of parents and school towards him or her. Once children are labelled "epileptic" there is a real danger that their teachers may underestimate their academic potential and give them neither stimulation nor encouragement.

Parents should make it clear to the school that they want the child to take part in the whole range of the school's activities, and that the staff should treat him or her just like the other children, in terms of punishment as well as reward. Psychometric testing is advisable, to establish what the child should be capable of and where his or her skills or difficulties lie.

OUTLOOK
Approximately one-third of all those people who develop epilepsy will eventually grow out of the condition and become fit-free. A further third will find that their seizures become less frequent and less severe with treatment, and the final third will remain unchanged. The outlook in any particular case depends on the cause of the epilepsy, the age of onset, and whether or not there is a family history of the disease. Temporal lobe epilepsy, for example, is one of the most difficult types to treat successfully. Where the epilepsy is the result of severe brain damage or of some degenerative brain disease, seizure control may be more difficult. But for those people who have straightforward epilepsy, uncomplicated by brain damage, the outlook is good.

Patients with epilepsy do have a reduced life expectancy and unfortunately some patients do die in a seizure. A grand mal seizure in a bath is one common situation; showers are safer for patients with grand mal seizures. Occasionally a patient with epilepsy will be found dead in the morning, having died in a seizure during the night. This sudden death syndrome is mainly confined to young adult males. Frequently these young men reject the diagnosis of epilepsy, are unhappy about taking their tablets, and play about with the dosage. Many of them also drink (see above).

There is considerable prejudice among the general public and also, unfortunately, among some doctors, which suggests that patients with epilepsy are aggressive, emotional, and have a high rate of psychiatric illness. There is now a large body of evidence which shows that patients with epilepsy but without significant brain damage are normally intelligent and show no evidence of a greater tendency to psychiatric illness than the general population. Those patients who do have brain damage have the deficits that would be expected, due to the brain damage rather than the epilepsy. However, some patients with epilepsy do have multiple fits and may acquire large numbers of anticonvulsant drugs. These patients are clearly at greater risk of developing psychiatric syndromes.

BIBLIOGRAPHY

Brown, S. B., & Fenwick, P. B. C. (1989). Evoked and psychogenic seizures: 2. Inhibition. *Acta Neurologica Scandinavica, 80*, 535–40.

Chadwick, D. (1994). Epilepsy. *Journal of Neurology, Neurosurgery and Psychiatry, 57*, 264–77.

Devinsky, O., & Bear, D. (1984). Varieties of aggressive behavior in temporal lobe epilepsy. *American Journal of Psychiatry, 141*, 651–6.

Fenwick, P. B. C., & Brown, S. B. (1989). Evoked and psychogenic seizures: 1. Precipitation. *Acta Neurologica Scandinavica, 80*, 541–7.

Goldstein, L. H. (1990). Behavioural and cognitive-behavioural treatments for epilepsy: a progress review. *British Journal of Clinical Psychology, 29*, 257–69.

Hermann, B. P., & Whitman, S. (1984). Behavioural and personality correlates of epilepsy: a review, methodological critique and conceptual model. *Psychological Bulletin, 95*, 451–97.

Malafosse, A., Genton, P., Hirsch, E., Marescaux, C., Broglin, D., & Bernasconi, R. (Eds). (1994). *Idiopathic generalized epilepsies: Clinical, experimental and genetic aspects*. London: John Libbey.

Trimble, M. R., & Thompson, P. (1986). Neuropsychological aspects of epilepsy. In I. Grant & K. M. Adams (Eds), *Neuropsychological aspects of neuropsychiatric disorders* (pp. 321–46). New York: Oxford University Press.

Wolf, P. (Ed.). (1994). *Epileptic seizures and syndromes*. London: John Libbey.

P. B. C. FENWICK

episodic dyscontrol syndrome The term "episodic dyscontrol syndrome" relates to a disorder characterized by uncontrollable bouts of aggression, but it is used rather differently depending on whether the affected individual is an adult or a child.

In adults the term is applied to phenomena of a quasi-epileptic nature in which violent aggressive outbursts occur with no or absolutely minimal provocation. The attacks are similar to true epileptic events in a number of ways: there is commonly an aura, and headache and drowsiness following the attacks. At other times the affected individual may have brief absences or other altered states of consciousness. Soft neurological signs are frequently observed, and there may be nonspecific abnormalities of the EEG in the temporal lobe, even when clinical temporal lobe epilepsy has been excluded. Opinion is divided as to whether these attacks of episodic dyscontrol are true epileptic phenomena or whether psychogenic factors are the principal cause.

In children a similar phenomenon may occur, but it is considered to be a subtype of hyperactivity. The explosions of violent behavior occur in children who habitually display attentional and organizational problems. There is a strong similarity to the episodic dyscontrol syndrome described in adults, in that these children similarly have mildly abnormal EEGs and symptoms which are suggestive of temporal lobe epilepsy.

equipotentiality The principle of equipotentiality states that, while sensory input to the brain is localized, perception involves the whole brain and the effects of brain lesions depend upon their extent, not upon their location.

Equipotential theory, developed around the principle of equipotentiality, was originally proposed by Flourens in the 1840s, but was actively supported by Goldstein, Head, and Lashley, among others, about a century later. Lashley's demonstration in rats that the behavioral effects of lesions depended upon their mass and not their location (the principle of mass action) was seen as powerful support for the theory. Subsequently the strict equipotential theory was moderated by the acceptance that some degree of LOCALIZATION was demonstrable in clinical studies of the human brain, with the resulting compromise of "relative localization" expressing the idea that both the mass and location of a lesion may be important in determining its behavioral effects.

Equipotentiality has, however, undergone a recent revival with the contemporary interest in connectionist models of the brain. The parallel distributed processing (PDP) models of cerebral function incorporate the concept of undifferentiated matrices of neural elements supporting a given function, which is consonant with the principle of equipotentiality. Speculation suggests that the connectionist matrices may be equipotential, while the whole matrix is to some degree localized, providing an explanatory basis for the rather pragmatic idea of relative localization.

erythropsia Erythropsia is a visual disorder similar to METAMORPHOPSIA, in which a modification of object color occurs. In erythropsia objects, irrespective of their nature or number, become tinged with a reddish hue; this is the most common form of the modifications by a monochromatic tint. As with all metamorphopsias, the disorder is associated with occipital and occipital-temporal cortical lesions, and is more common following right rather than left hemisphere lesions.

evoked potentials Evoked potentials are the electrical activity recorded from the nervous system in response to a stimulus. They are generally recorded from small electrodes fixed to the scalp, although it is also possible to use electrodes fixed to other parts of the body or electrodes implanted in the brain. Evoked potentials describe the time-course of electrical activity following a stimulus such as a flash of light, a shock to the median nerve, or an auditory tone pip. Unlike the random electrical activity of the electroencephalogram (EEG), the activity represented in an evoked potential is consistent and time-locked to the stimulus. This feature provides the basis of averaging which is the most commonly used method of extracting an evoked potential from the background EEG. Evoked potentials vary in amplitude from fractions of a microvolt for the potentials produced in the BRAIN STEM following a tone pip to tens of microvolts for potentials associated with cognitive tasks. The EEG activity is much larger and, following a single stimulus, the evoked potential is hidden in the EEG activity. By adding together the responses to a number of successive stimuli it is possible to extract the evoked potential because the consistent activity sums together, whereas the random activity in the EEG cancels out. The smaller the response the greater the number of stimuli that need to be added together to obtain the evoked potential. Averaging was introduced to the study

of evoked potentials by George Dawson towards the end of the 1940s. The original equipment was built especially for the purpose of averaging but, since the late 1960s, the general-purpose computer has formed the basis of averaging systems in research laboratories and clinical neurophysiology departments worldwide.

Although the equipment with which recordings are made is changing, the general principles of electrode placement are not. Extraneous electrical activity (e.g. from laboratory equipment and communication systems) is picked up by the body and has a much higher amplitude than the electrical activity in an evoked potential. In addition, other electrical activity produced by the body, such as that associated with muscle activity and the heart, is larger than that of the evoked potentials generated in the brain. The electric fields associated with this extraneous activity tend to be constant across the scalp, so that subtracting the activity at one scalp electrode from that recorded at another will cancel the common electrical potentials and leave those that differ between the two electrode placements. This is achieved by recording from "active" sites with respect to a common reference electrode located in a position (preferably on the scalp) at which little brain activity associated with the stimulus being studied is thought to occur; the ear-lobes or mastoids are used frequently. The electrical activity from the brain is in the order of a few microvolts and so the potential recorded from pairs of electrodes (active reference) is amplified by up to a million times before the analogue output from the amplifier is converted to a digital input for the averaging computer. The rate at which this conversion, or sampling, is done determines the fidelity with which the brain activity is represented in the computer; brain waves with higher frequency components, such as those from the brain stem, need faster sampling rates than the low-frequency potentials associated with cognitive tasks.

Evoked potentials are plotted as changes in amplitude over time with individual peaks being identified by their polarity (positive- or negative-going (P or N)) and either their latency with respect to stimulus onset or the sequential order of their occurrence. Thus, the second positive-going potential occurring 100 msec after a stimulus would be named either P2 or P100. The amplitude of peaks is measured with respect to either the preceding or following peak of opposite polarity or with reference to a pre-stimulus baseline.

Evoked potentials are generally separated into those generated in the primary sensory areas of the brain and those associated with cognitive function. The former are termed sensory or exogenous evoked potentials, whereas the latter are referred to as event-related or endogenous potentials. The terms evoked potential (EP) and event-related potential (ERP) will be used here to refer to sensory and cognitive potentials respectively. The division between cognitive and sensory potentials has become less distinct in recent years, with clear evidence that sensory potentials can be modulated by cognitive factors such as attention. These effects can occur as early as 40 msec following stimulus delivery.

The sensory evoked potentials provide an indication of the integrity of the sensory pathway being stimulated. The pattern-reversal visual evoked potential (VEP), for example, introduced into clinical neurophysiology by Halliday in the early 1970s, proved to be a sensitive indicator of visual dysfunction by identifying abnormally prolonged potentials in patients suspected of having multiple sclerosis but in whom there was no history of visual problems. The VEP is also capable of identifying the site of a lesion in the optic pathway from the distribution of potentials across the scalp overlying the OCCIPITAL LOBES in response to separate stimulation of the visual half-fields.

Somatosensory evoked potentials (SEP) in response to stimulation of the median nerve at the wrist can be recorded from electrodes on the neck and scalp. The first activity is the N9 which reflects the passage of the nerve volley as it approaches the spinal cord. Subsequent small amplitude potentials, probably generated in subcortical structures, are followed by the N20 component, which is generated in the primary somatosensory cortex. SEPs can also be recorded to stimulation of the lower limb and other nerves. The clinical utility of SEPs has been established in a variety of disorders including MULTIPLE SCLEROSIS and myoclonic EPILEPSY.

Auditory evoked potentials (AEP) occur following either a tone pip or click stimulus. The earliest potentials are a sequence of six or seven small wavelets arising from the BRAIN STEM during the first 12 msec following a stimulus

(brain stem auditory evoked potentials (BAEP)). These potentials are followed by a series of waves known as the middle-latency auditory evoked potentials, which end at about 60 msec following a stimulus, after which point the responses are referred to as long-latency evoked potentials. BAEPs have proved useful clinically in identifying demyelinating or neoplastic lesions of the auditory pathway.

A comprehensive review of the characteristics of sensory evoked potentials in healthy individuals and associated clinical applications can be found in Halliday (1993).

Evoked potentials associated with cognition (ERPs) are recorded whenever a delivered stimulus has some significance for the subject. In general, the potentials recorded are independent of stimulus modality. There are two well-established experimental procedures which result in the recording of ERPs. The first, originally described by Walter and colleagues (1964), is known as the contingent negative variation (CNV) and occurs in the interval between the presentation of a warning stimulus (S1) and an imperative stimulus (S2) which requires an action on the part of the subject, such as pressing a button to extinguish a flashing light. The electrical brain activity between S1 and S2 follows a slowly increasing negative course which terminates abruptly as soon as S2 is delivered. The time interval separating S1 and S2 is typically in the order of 1 to 2 seconds. The CNV has been separated into early and late phases, with the early phase being associated with orientation to the initial stimulus and the later phase being associated with the preparation to make a motor response. The second established procedure is known as the "oddball" paradigm in which the subject has to respond to a rare target stimulus occurring randomly in a sequence of frequent stimuli. Target stimuli typically have a probability of occurrence of 0.1 to 0.2 with frequent stimuli having the complementary probability. In the auditory modality, for example, the target stimulus might be a high pitch tone with a probability of 0.15 presented in random order with a low pitch tone. The early waveform of the ERP to both target and frequent stimuli (up to about 100 msec) is largely indistinguishable, but the potentials after this latency are different for the two stimulus categories. The response to the target includes an N2 (N250) and a P3 (P300), which do not generally occur in the response to the frequent stimulus.

Research involving the CNV has been largely hampered by the uncertainty concerning its relationship with a similar slow negative shift of electrical activity preceding voluntary movement. The requirement of a motor response to S2 in the CNV paradigm makes it difficult to separate cognitive from motor processes when interpreting the results of CNV studies. It is now clear, however, that it is possible to record a CNV potential in situations where S2 provides the subject with information, such as feedback about an earlier response, but a motor response is not required.

The oddball P300 has received a considerable amount of attention in studies of healthy individuals and in the investigation of disorders of intellect. The latency of P300 increases by between 1 and 2 msec each year of the adult lifespan and this change provides the basis for using the oddball P300 as a diagnostic test for DEMENTIA. If the latency of P300 recorded from an individual is prolonged beyond what would be expected from the regression line relating P300 latency to age in healthy people, then, because P300 is recorded in a cognitive task, it may be concluded that the individual is cognitively abnormal. The original study by Goodin and others (1978) demonstrating this technique found abnormal P300 potentials in 80 percent of the demented patients tested. Subsequent studies have reported success rates of between 100 percent and 0 percent. There is a variety of reasons for this unacceptably wide range of success. The first is that the clinical status of patients in different studies has varied from definitely to possibly demented. A second reason is that the inter-subject variability of P300 latency in healthy people tends to be high so that the confidence limits around the regression line relating P300 latency to age are too distant to be sensitive. A third reason is that it is difficult to identify a single psychological factor underlying the generation of P300 in the oddball test, although it is likely that attention, memory, and response selection all play a part. All or none of these factors could be affected in any demented individual.

Event-related potential tests involving auditory selective ATTENTION have demonstrated a negative-going potential between about 120 and 300 msec which reflects the ability of an individual to attend to one sound source rather than another. This potential, known as the processing negativity, is best observed in the difference waveform created by subtracting the evoked response from stimuli presented in the unattended ear from that recorded from stimuli presented in the attended ear. A typical procedure would be one in which high or low pitch tones are presented to one ear or the other in random order, with one of the 4 pitch/ear combinations being designated as a target on each run of the experiment. If the target on a particular run was the high tone in the left ear, then the processing negativity would be obtained by subtracting the response to the high tone presented in the unattended right ear from that recorded in the left ear. The greater the amplitude of the processing negativity, the better the ability to attend to the target ear.

A number of different evoked potential tests of memory function have been investigated. A general finding is that ERPs are larger for presented items that are recalled or recognized correctly on subsequent testing. In continuous recognition memory tests the ERPs to the second and subsequent presentations of a stimulus are larger than to the first presentation. ERPs recorded to the probe stimulus in modified versions of Sternberg's memory scanning task have established systematic changes in waveform associated with increasing memory load. Starr and Barrett (1987) demonstrated abnormal ERPs to probe stimuli in this task in conduction APHASIA. Some evidence for implicit memory function in PROSOPAGNOSIA has been provided by a report of larger ERPs to "unrecognized" faces of family members compared with ERPs to unknown faces. A potential occurring to a change in sequence of auditory stimuli soon after stimulus onset and known as the mismatch negativity (MMN) has been studied extensively by Näätänen and colleagues. The MMN is thought to occur because of a mismatch between the neuronal trace of the incoming stimulus and a template representing the current memory of recently presented stimuli. The MMN increases in amplitude and decreases in latency as the deviance between stimulus and template increases. Näätänen (1986) has suggested a parallel between the mechanism underlying generation of the MMN and echoic memory.

Evoked potentials have been shown to be sensitive to the congruence between an anticipated stimulus and that actually delivered. This was demonstrated for language by Kutas and Hillyard (1980), who presented subjects with sentences ending with an incongruous word (e.g. "He spread the warm bread with socks") and compared the ERPs to the final word with those obtained to congruous final words or final words which were semantically congruous but physically different from the preceding words in the sentence. The ERPs to the semantically incongruous words contain a negative potential occurring around 400 msec after stimulus onset (N400) which does not appear to the other words. Similar effects have *not* been observed for non-language stimuli, such as incongruent endings to melodies, and the current view is that N400 reflects post-lexical processes involved in semantic integration.

There is a widespread increase in the electrical activity of the brain recorded from the scalp preceding a self-paced voluntary movement (such as the extension of a finger). This activity, which was named the Bereitschaftspotential (BP) by Kornhuber and Deecke (1965), begins as a bilaterally symmetrical negative-going change some 1 to 1.5 seconds before movement onset. The gradient of the change increases over the central areas of the scalp contralateral to the moving hand at about 500 msec before movement and the potential continues until movement onset itself, after which it reverses in polarity. Recording of these potentials is different from that for stimulus-locked activity because the time of movement onset is not known before it occurs. The technique involves continuous recording of approximately 2 seconds of EEG activity, until the averaging computer is triggered by a signal linked to movement onset. This signal is derived ideally from the muscle activity associated with movement of the finger, but closing or opening of a response key or interruption of a light beam can also be used. There is some debate about the normality of this potential in PARKINSON'S DISEASE although Dick and his colleagues (1987) showed that the state of medication of patients seems to play the most important role in determining the amplitude of the BP and that the amplitude in healthy individuals can be modulated by dopaminergic drugs. In a task requiring a response with either hand it is possible to determine which hand a subject is likely to move before the movement is made by comparing the activity recorded from over central areas on one side of the head with that recorded over a similar position on the other side (Gratton et al., 1988). Using this information it is possible to establish the expectancies induced in subjects during the presentation of a series of stimuli, as well as the speed and accuracy with which they can correct performance associated with guesses that would have led to erroneous responses.

The technique described above for recording brain potentials preceding voluntary movement can also be used to study patients with involuntary movements such as MYOCLONIC JERKS or TICS (Barrett, 1992). This method, known as jerk-locked averaging, can identify whether there is abnormal activity in the brain preceding a myoclonic jerk and, together with the somatosensory evoked potential described earlier, can distinguish between cortical, subcortical, or spinal origins for the myoclonus. If the brain activity preceding a tic includes a potential similar to the BP, then it may be possible to conclude that the abnormal movement is voluntary rather than involuntary.

The field of application for evoked potentials is widespread and there have been some outstanding successes for sensory evoked potentials as an aid to neurological diagnosis. The event-related potentials have not proved so successful in terms of diagnosis, although significant group differences in terms of cognitive function have been established. Results from ERP tests derived from models of cognition suggest a bright future for this method of studying brain activity, particularly if it is used in conjunction with psychometric assessment and visualization of active structures using functional MAGNETIC RESONANCE IMAGING and positron emission tomography (PET).

BIBLIOGRAPHY

Barrett, G. (1992). Jerk-locked averaging: technique and application. *Journal of Clinical Neurophysiology*, 9, 495–508.

Barrett, G. (1993). Clinical applications of event-related potentials. In Halliday, A. M. (Ed.), *Evoked potentials in clinical testing*, 2nd edn (pp. 589–633). Edinburgh: Churchill Livingstone.

Dick, J. P. R., Cantello, R., Buruma, O., Gioux, M., Benecke, R., Day, B. L., Rothwell, J. C., Thompson, P. D., & Marsden, C. D. (1987). The Bereitschaftspotential, L-DOPA and Parkinson's disease. *Electroencephalography and Clinical Neurophysiology*, 66, 263–74.

Goodin, D. S., Squires, K. C., & Starr, A. (1978). Long latency event-related components of the auditory evoked potential in dementia. *Brain*, *101*, 635–48.

Gratton, G., Coles, M. G. H., Sirevaag, E. J., Eriksen, C. W., & Donchin, E. (1988). Pre- and poststimulus activation of response channels: a psychophysiological analysis. *Journal of Experimental Psychology: Human Perception and Performance*, *14*, 331–44.

Halliday, A. M. (Ed.). (1993). *Evoked potentials in clinical testing*, 2nd edn. Edinburgh: Churchill Livingstone.

Kornhuber, H. H., & Deecke, L. (1965). Hirnpotentialänderungen bei Willkürbewegungen und passiven Bewegungen des Menschen: Bereitschaftspotential und reafferente Potentiale. *Pflügers Archiv für die gesammte Physiologie*, *248*, 1–17.

Näätänen, R. (1986). Neurophysiological basis of the echoic memory as suggested by event-related potentials and magnetoencephalogram. In F. Klix & H. Hagendorf (Eds), *Human memory and cognitive capabilities* (pp. 615–28). Amsterdam: Elsevier/North-Holland.

Starr, A., & Barrett, G. (1987). Disordered auditory short-term memory in man and event-related potentials. *Brain*, *110*, 935–59.

Walter, W. G., Cooper, R., Aldridge, V. J., McCallum, W. C., & Winter, A. L. (1964). Contingent negative variation: an electric sign of sensorimotor association and expectancy in the human brain. *Nature (London)*, *203*, 380–4.

GEOFF BARRETT

experimental neuropsychology *See* NEUROPSYCHOLOGY.

expressive aphasia *See* APHASIA.

extinction Besides its uses in psychology as a term for the decline in the frequency of a conditioned behavior following the withdrawal of reinforcement, the reduction in response following regular and repeated presentation of a stimulus, "extinction" has a specific application in neuropsychology. Neuropsychologically, extinction occurs in the somatosensory modality under conditions of double simultaneous stimulation. In double simultaneous stimulation, two identical tactual stimuli are presented simultaneously either on opposite (homologous) positions on the body surface or in close proximity (heterologous positions). Extinction occurs when only one of the two stimuli is reported, although each would be reported if presented alone. The extinction is considered to follow from an inability simultaneously to perceive sensory stimuli arriving at different loci and is associated principally, but not exclusively, with lesions of the secondary somatosensory cortex in the parietal lobe, especially if the lesion is on the right. Of the two stimuli presented, it is normally the stimulus contralateral to the lesion which is subject to extinction.

extrapyramidal tract The extrapyramidal tract is alternatively, and more accurately, also known as the *extrapyramidal motor system*. It is often referred to as a "tract" by analogy with the pyramidal tract (or motor system) but, unlike the much simpler pyramidal tract, involves a complex set of neural centers and pathways. The extrapyramidal motor system is that which is controlled by the BASAL GANGLIA, but appears to control tone rather than movement in normal individuals. The system is termed "extrapyramidal" as it is that aspect of the motor system which is apart from the direct pyramidal system of voluntary movement.

Within the basal ganglia, the CAUDATE and the PUTAMEN receive input from most areas of the cerebral cortex, most of which input is inhibitory, and from specific nuclei of the THALAMUS (the intralaminar nuclei), most of which is excitatory. The caudate and the putamen then send fibers to the GLOBUS PALLIDUS, which has a two-way connection with the subthalamus, and also receives input from the SUBSTANTIA NIGRA. Both the subthalamus and the substantia nigra then project to reticular motor centers in the MEDULLA and, via the reticulospinal tract and the interneurons in the spinal cord, to control skeletal muscles via the anterior horn cells in the cord. The red nucleus is also considered to be part of the extrapyramidal system, as is the lateral vestibular nucleus, but each projects by separate tracts to the spinal interneurons. In addition, there is a feedback control mechanism which receives input quite widely from the extrapyramidal system and through the CEREBELLUM and the ventrolateral nucleus of the thalamus passes back to the cortex and on to re-enter the extrapyramidal system. This can be conceptualized as a feedback mechanism by which the thalamus and cortex regulate the extrapyramidal system, or by which the extrapyramidal system and the thalamus regulate the motor cortex. There are other interconnections which this simplified account does not include.

Disorders of the extrapyramidal system are characterized by changes in muscle tone, but also by various "spontaneous" disorders of movement which range from tremor to ATHETOSIS, CHOREA, and HEMIBALLISMUS, all of which are presumably due to the release of the inhibition normally exerted by the extrapyramidal centers.

See also PYRAMIDAL TRACT.

J. GRAHAM BEAUMONT

eye movement Movements of the eyes, which are normally *conjugate* in that the two eyes move together in an integrated manner, are controlled by an extremely complex neural system which involves the simultaneous control of twelve muscles through six CRANIAL NERVES. The system, principally located in the BRAIN STEM, receives input from both frontal and occipital cortical areas and from the vestibular apparatus.

In the brain stem, the medial longitudinal fasciculus which connects the superior COLLICULUS with the relevant cranial nerve nuclei and the center for lateral gaze, as well as the spinal anterior horn cells concerned with head movements, acts as the center of a complex which maintains normally functional conjugate eye movements. Disruption of any part of this system may result in a failure of conjugate gaze so that the patient complains of DIPLOPIA or double vision.

The next higher level of control over this system comes from centers in the PONS which are involved in the RETICULAR FORMATION, which can induce sudden saccadic movements to the left or right. Structures around the superior colliculus relate to point-to-point movement in the contralateral visual field, and also include a center which directs vertical eye movements, so that this is sometimes termed the "vertical gaze center." At this level vestibular information also enters the system so that eye movements may be adjusted in response to head movements, saccades following

head turning being mediated through the pontine gaze center, while smooth pursuit movements are achieved directly by connection into the medial longitudinal fasciculus. The CEREBELLUM also exerts an overall degree of control and coordination at this level of the system.

The highest level of control over eye movements involves the cerebral cortex. In the frontal lobe, the *frontal eye fields* (area 8; anterior to the premotor cortex in the superior anterior region of the frontal lobe) control contralateral saccadic movements, and lesions of this area may render the patient unable to move the eyes volitionally to the opposite side of visual space. The secondary visual cortex in the occipital lobe also contributes to the control of eye movements by a pathway which descends to the region around the superior colliculus, although these projections are bilateral. This pathway appears to mediate smooth pursuit movements, and patients with a lesion in this occipital area may be unable to execute smooth pursuit tracking of a visual object, even though saccadic visual jumps in fixation following the object may be retained. These frontal and occipital cortical regions involved in eye movements are themselves connected through the corticocortical fibers of the superior longitudinal fasciculus, which enables coordination between these two principal cortical centers. Given the complexity of the system which controls eye movements, the existence of a specialty of *neuro-ophthalmology* is no surprise.

Neuropsychologically, disorders of eye movement, besides being taken account of in the overall clinical functional state, have been of interest in the context of frontal lobe lesions, although there is still dispute about the relative role of orientational attentional mechanisms and of eye-movement defects in the reduced spontaneous head turning and eye movement in patients with frontal lobe lesions. Deficits in the ability to normally scan and inspect a stimulus have been shown to be associated with frontal lobe lesions and this may be a relevant factor in the decline of a number of more general higher-level functions which accompany frontal lobe pathology: motor skill disorders, executive deficits, and general intellectual functions which involve more than a semantic verbal response to an auditory stimulus. Impairments of gaze and visual tracking may also be of clinical significance in dementia and in states of low arousal (*see also* LATERAL EYE MOVE-MENTS).

J. GRAHAM BEAUMONT

eyedness Eyedness is an individual character-istic analogous to handedness. In situations of interocular conflict one eye will be dominant over the other; and in situations of monocular viewing, one eye will be preferred.

If two images are presented, one to each eye, so that the two images cannot be integrated into a single percept (the images falling on the two eyes are always slightly different due to binocular disparity) then one image will dominate over the other, and the eye to which this image is projected may be considered to be the dominant eye. In situations of monocular viewing, such as looking through a camera or telescope, or peering through a small aperture, an individual will habitually prefer to make use of a given eye. There is also an asymmetry in pointing; this is easily demonstrated by pointing at a distant object and then closing each eye in turn, on which it will be discovered that there is an alignment between the object, the fingertip, and one of the eyes which is the dominant one.

Unfortunately, the dominant or preferred eye for particular tasks is not always the same eye in any given individual, and in considering eyedness care must be taken to note the method of testing by which the eyedness has been established. While there is a preponderance of right eyedness in the population whatever the means of assess-ment, once this has been allowed for correlations across the different forms of eyedness within individuals are not strong. While there is a general correlation between handedness and eyedness, once the effect produced by there being a right preponderance of both in the population has been accounted for, the relationship in the normal population is not a strong one.

F

face recognition Species that depend heavily on social interaction must develop sophisticated recognition and memory systems to underpin the need to be able to interact differently with different individuals, according to what one knows about them. For humans, the face plays a key role in the recognition of other people.

The most extensively investigated impairment of face recognition is PROSOPAGNOSIA. This was identified as a distinct neuropsychological problem by Bodamer, whose seminal paper was published in 1947 (Ellis & Florence, 1990). Prosopagnosic patients are unable to recognize familiar faces, and rely on voice, context, name, or sometimes clothing or gait to achieve recognition of people they know. The problem in face recognition is not due to blindness (the patient can still see, and in many published cases can see quite well) or general intellectual impairment (people are still recognized from nonfacial cues). Yet even the most familiar faces may go unrecognized: famous people, friends, family, and the patient's own face when seen in a mirror.

This failure to recognize faces is indeed a social handicap. Newcombe, Mehta, and de Haan (1994) described some of the problems experienced by a retired mathematician who had been prosopagnosic all his life:

At the age of 16 years, while on holiday, he stood in a queue for 30 min next to a family friend whom he had known all his life, without any experience of familiarity. The friend complained – mildly – to his parents and his father reacted strongly to this apparent discourtesy. Soon after, cycling from the village to his home, he saw a man walking toward him. In his own words: "Mindful of my father's recent forceful comments, I decided to play it safe. As we passed, I said "Good morning, Sir." My father said later that I had never addressed him as politely before or since." (p. 108)

Although generally considered a rare deficit, there are now several hundred such case descriptions in the literature. These include cases where brain injury early or late in life has led to inability to recognize previously familiar faces, and developmental cases where the disorder is present from birth. The patients know when they are looking at a face, and can describe its features, but the loss of any sense of overt recognition is often complete, with no feeling of familiarity. In contrast, other aspects of face processing, such as the ability to interpret facial expressions, or to match views of unfamiliar faces, can remain remarkably intact in some (though by no means all) cases. The ability to recognize everyday objects other than faces may also remain good, and many prosopagnosic patients are able to read without difficulty. In one of the cases of early acquired deficit, a child who had remained unable to recognize any faces since suffering meningitis and subsequent complications in infancy was nonetheless able to learn to read (Young & Ellis, 1989); this underlines the implication that reading and face recognition depend on different types of visual analysis.

Deficits that are commonly associated with prosopagnosia include a VISUAL FIELD DEFECT in the left upper quadrant, ACHROMATOPSIA, and TOPOGRAPHICAL DISORDERS. These are useful clinical pointers, but they are thought to be due to anatomical proximity of otherwise unrelated processes rather than having any direct functional significance; cases of prosopagnosia without each of these associated deficits have been described, and they have also each been reported in the absence of prosopagnosia.

Studies of prosopagnosia have mostly concentrated on three separable issues: the location of the lesions responsible, to what extent the problem is specific to face recognition, and whether there exist different underlying forms of deficit.

LESIONS CAUSING PROSOPAGNOSIA

The underlying pathology involves lesions affecting ventro-medial regions of occipito-temporal cortex; these include the lingual, fusiform, and parahippocampal gyri, and more anterior parts of the temporal lobes. PET studies of normal observers have confirmed the importance of these regions to face perception (Sergent & Signoret, 1992). Bilateral lesions are usually present in the relatively small number of cases which have come to autopsy (Damasio et al., 1982), but cases involving unilateral lesions of the right cerebral hemisphere have been reported in several CT and MRI studies, and the PET findings with normal people also emphasize the importance of the right hemisphere.

A FACE-SPECIFIC DEFICIT?

Prosopagnosia involves a very severe impairment of face recognition, yet a number of prosopagnosic patients can read and recognize many everyday objects, so the deficit does not compromise all aspects of visual recognition. But is it only face recognition which is impaired?

In most cases, the answer is clearly "no." So, for example, recognition of familiar buildings, flowers, types of car, or animal species may all pose difficulties. Like faces, these are all visual categories with a high degree of inter-item similarity.

This has led to the hypothesis that what is lost in prosopagnosia is the ability to recognize the individual members of categories that contain several items of similar appearance. Ability to identify the general category to which the items belong (face, building, flower, etc.) is preserved, but within-category recognition is defective. Although this is an attractive idea, it no longer fits all the evidence. Instead of being consistently present, deficits for visual categories other than faces tend to vary from case to case. Moreover, there are also a few reports of highly circumscribed impairments. One of De Renzi's (1986) cases could find his own belongings when they were mixed in with similar objects, identify his own handwriting, pick out a Siamese cat among photographs of other cats, recognize his own car without reading the number plate, and sort domestic coins from foreign coins. In all of these tasks he was therefore able to identify individual members of visual categories with high inter-item similarity, yet he could not recognize the faces of

relatives and close friends. Just as strikingly, the deficit can affect mainly *human* faces; when McNeil and Warrington's (1993) prosopagnosic patient took up farming, he was able to learn to recognize his sheep, and correctly identified several of them from photographs of their faces!

Although they are exceptionally rare, the fact that such cases exist means that the possibility of face-specific deficits must be taken seriously.

DIFFERENT FORMS OF PROSOPAGNOSIA

There has been much discussion as to whether prosopagnosia can have more than one different underlying cause. Often a distinction is made between perceptual and mnestic forms.

For some patients prosopagnosia does seem to reflect defective face perception. For instance, one of Bodamer's cases maintained that people's faces all looked the same. They were like strangely flat, white oval plates, with emphatically dark eyes (Ellis & Florence, 1990). He was also unable to determine the age or sex of seen faces except by inferring these from the hairstyle, and his ability to interpret facial expressions was defective. He said that he could see the movements involved when people made angry or smiling facial expressions, but that these had no meaning for him.

Such cases contrast with other patients who have relatively intact perceptual abilities, but still cannot recognize the faces they perceive satisfactorily. Consider Mr W (Bruyer et al., 1983), one of the most thoroughly documented in the literature. Mr W could make accurate copies of drawings of faces, identify the sex of a face even when a hood covered the hair, correctly interpret facial expressions, and decide whether photographs of unfamiliar faces showed the same or different people. For all these tasks Mr W performed as well as normal control subjects, so when he looked at a face we have no grounds for thinking his perception was abnormal. Yet Mr W often had no sense of who the person might be. Since this problem could not be readily attributed to any defect of face perception, it seems reasonable that it might reflect defective ability to access previously stored representations of the appearances of familiar people.

This interpretation of some cases of prosopagnosia as a domain-specific impairment of face memory is strengthened by findings of covert recognition, which show clear parallels to priming effects found more generally in AMNESIA. Prosopagnosic patients usually fail all tests of overt recognition of familiar faces. They cannot name the face, give the person's occupation or other biographical details, or even state whether or not a face is that of a familiar person (all faces seem unfamiliar). Surprisingly, though, there is substantial evidence of covert recognition from physiological and behavioral measures (Bruyer, 1991).

In a path-breaking study, Bauer (1984) measured skin conductance while a prosopagnosic patient, LF, viewed a familiar face and listened to a list of five names. When the name belonged to the face LF was looking at, there was a greater skin conductance change than when someone else's name was read out. Yet if LF was asked to choose which name in the list was correct for the face, his performance was at chance level. Hence, there was a marked discrepancy between LF's inability to identify the face overtly and the relatively good recognition shown using the indirect skin conductance measure.

A number of other indices of nonconscious, covert recognition in prosopagnosia have also been developed. Matching of familiar faces is better than for unfamiliar faces, priming has been found from familiar faces onto the recognition of name targets, and learning of correct face-name pairings is better than learning of incorrect pairings (Bruyer, 1991). All these effects can be demonstrated when overt recognition of the faces is at chance level.

By no means all prosopagnosic patients show covert recognition, however. As might be expected, when there is evidence of substantial impairment of face perception, covert as well as overt performance can fall to chance level.

There is a parallel between preserved covert recognition abilities and those aspects of recognition that operate automatically for normal people. We cannot look at a familiar face and decide not to recognize it; the mechanisms responsible for visual recognition are not open to conscious control in this way. It seems that some of these automatic aspects of recognition continue to function in some cases of prosopagnosia. A simulation of this pattern can be made by halving some of the connection strengths in a computer model of the architecture of the recognition system (Burton et al., 1991). The network is then

no longer able to classify face inputs as familiar, yet it continues to display priming effects. This helps us to understand how covert responses can be preserved when there is no overt discrimination, but it does not solve the more difficult issue of what is involved in being aware of recognizing a face.

Despite the extensive range of covert effects demonstrated in the laboratory, prosopagnosic patients do not act as if they recognize faces in everyday life. Instead, most are acutely conscious of their problems in face recognition. However, some patients lack insight into their disability and show unawareness of impairment (ANOSO-GNOSIA). Case SP was very poor at recognizing familiar faces, yet she maintained that she recognized faces "as well as before" even when directly confronted with her failure to recognize photographs of familiar faces (Young et al., 1990a). In contrast, SP showed adequate insight into other physical and cognitive problems produced by her illness; her lack of insight into her face recognition impairment involved a deficit-specific anosognosia. Such deficit-specific anosognosias may reflect impairment to mechanisms used for monitoring performance in everyday life; we can all make occasional errors of recognition, so we constantly monitor our own performance to correct these errors quickly and avoid embarrassment whenever possible.

OTHER TYPES OF FACE AND PERSON RECOGNITION IMPAIRMENT

As well as prosopagnosia, there are other types of impairment that can compromise face recognition. These have been reviewed by Young (1992). Some correspond to breakdown at different levels of recognition. Cases of inability to recognize people from face, voice, or name have been described; these seem to reflect loss of semantic information about the identities of individuals. There are also reports of problems of name retrieval (ANOMIA), in which familiar people are successfully recognized and appropriate semantic information is accessed, but their names cannot be recalled.

Taken together, these different types of problem fit the view that recognition of others is a multistage process. This is consistent with studies of everyday difficulties and errors, which can also reflect breakdown at different levels of recognition. For example:

343

1 We may completely fail to recognize a familiar face, and mistakenly think that the person is unfamiliar.

2 We may recognize the face as familiar, but be unable to bring to mind any other details about the person, such as her or his occupation or name.

3 We may recognize the face as familiar and remember appropriate semantic information about the person, while failing to remember her or his name.

Each of these types of everyday error can also arise after neuropsychological impairment; a brain-injured patient will then make her or his characteristic error to many or almost all seen faces.

A different type of problem reflects inability to learn new faces. Case ELD (Hanley et al., 1990) was severely impaired on tests of unfamiliar face memory, and showed poor recognition of faces of people who had become famous since her illness in 1985. Yet her ability to recognize people who had been familiar to her before her illness was normal, and she could also recognize people who had only become familiar since 1985 from their names, and perform normally on tests of verbal memory. This makes an interesting contrast with the mnestic form of prosopagnosia, in which impaired retrograde memory for premorbidly known faces is usually accompanied by a severe anterograde impairment (i.e. an inability to learn new faces). Cases such as ELD, who only suffer anterograde impairment, suggest that these anterograde and retrograde components of mnestic prosopagnosia may be dissociable.

Problems may also affect one side of the seen face. KL (Young et al., 1990b) experienced difficulty in recognizing the left sides of faces (i.e. the side falling to *his* left) but was able to recognize the left sides of objects. Young and colleagues (1990b) considered that this reflected impairment of an attentional mechanism for faces, producing a domain-specific form of unilateral neglect.

Exactly how all these different types of impairment relate to each other remains to be worked out. The main point, though, is clear: face recognition impairments reflect damage to a complex underlying system, which can break down in different ways. This point is already well-established in other areas, such as language deficits, but it has only been appreciated relatively recently for face recognition.

WHAT HELP CAN BE GIVEN?

Although face recognition impairments are socially disabling, there has been little work on remediation. Most patients simply develop their own strategies for tackling the problem. They may note carefully what clothes someone is wearing, ask relatives always to wear a particular distinctive item, or become adept at initiating or maintaining a conversation while they work out who they are talking to. These strategies are never completely effective and occasionally go seriously wrong; one patient lost a legal action when he discussed his case with his opponent's lawyer, under the misapprehension it was his own advocate because he was wearing similar court clothes.

The few attempts at direct remediation by training in face-processing skills have given no grounds for optimism (Ellis & Young, 1988). However, more promising approaches may derive from recent observations that deficits of overt recognition need not be absolute. Sergent and Poncet (1990) found that their patient, PV, could achieve overt recognition of some faces if several members of the same semantic category were presented together. This only happened when PV could determine the category herself; otherwise she continued to fail to recognize the faces overtly even when the occupational category was pointed out to her.

Sergent and Poncet (1990, p. 1000) suggested that this shows that "neither the facial representations nor the semantic information were critically disturbed in PV, and her prosopagnosia may thus reflect faulty connections between faces and their memories." They thought that the simultaneous presentation of several members of the same category may have temporarily raised the activation level above the appropriate threshold.

Such findings in prosopagnosia show that the boundary between awareness and lack of awareness is not as completely impassable as it seems to the patients' everyday experience. However, the circumstances under which this has been found to happen are at present very limited, and it remains to be seen whether they can be translated into anything which would give significant remedial assistance in real life.

BIBLIOGRAPHY

Bauer, R. M. (1984). Autonomic recognition of names and faces in prosopagnosia: a neuropsychological application of the guilty knowledge test. *Neuropsychologia, 22,* 457–69.

Bruyer, R. (1991). Covert face recognition in prosopagnosia: a review. *Brain and Cognition, 15,* 223–35.

Bruyer, R., Laterre, C., Seron, X., Feyereisen, P., Strypstein, E., Pierrard, E., & Rectem, D. (1983). A case of prosopagnosia with some preserved covert remembrance of familiar faces. *Brain and Cognition, 2,* 257–84.

Burton, A. M., Young, A. W., Bruce, V., Johnston, R., & Ellis, A. W. (1991). Understanding covert recognition. *Cognition, 39,* 129–66.

Damasio, A. R., Damasio, H., & Van Hoesen, G. W. (1982). Prosopagnosia: anatomic basis and behavioral mechanisms. *Neurology, 32,* 331–41.

De Renzi, E. (1986). Current issues in prosopagnosia. In H. D. Ellis, M. A. Jeeves, F. Newcombe, & A. Young (Eds), *Aspects of face processing* (pp. 243–52). Dordrecht: Martinus Nijhoff.

Ellis, H. D., & Florence, M. (1990). Bodamer's (1947) paper on prosopagnosia. *Cognitive Neuropsychology, 7,* 81–105.

Ellis, H. D., & Young, A. W. (1988). Training in face-processing skills for a child with acquired prosopagnosia. *Developmental Neuropsychology, 4,* 283–94.

Hanley, J. R., Pearson, N., & Young, A. W. (1990). Impaired memory for new visual forms. *Brain, 113,* 1131–48.

McNeil, J. E., & Warrington, E. K. (1993). Prosopagnosia: a face specific disorder. *Quarterly Journal of Experimental Psychology, 46A,* 1–10.

Newcombe, F., Mehta, Z., & de Haan, E. H. F. (1994). Category specificity in visual recognition. In M. J. Farah & G. Ratcliff (Eds), *The neuropsychology of high-level vision: collected tutorial essays* (pp. 103–32). Hillsdale, NJ: Erlbaum.

Sergent, J., & Poncet, M. (1990). From covert to overt recognition of faces in a prosopagnosic patient. *Brain, 113,* 989–1004.

Sergent, J., & Signoret, J.-L. (1992). Functional and anatomical decomposition of face processing: evidence from prosopagnosia and PET study of normal subjects. *Philosophical Transactions of the Royal Society, London, B 335,* 55–62.

Young, A. W. (1992). Face recognition impairments. *Philosophical Transactions of the Royal Society, London, B 335,* 47–54.

Young, A. W., de Haan, E. H. F., & Newcombe, F. (1990a). Unawareness of impaired face recognition. *Brain and Cognition, 14,* 1–18.

Young, A. W., de Haan, E. H. F., Newcombe, F., & Hay, D. C. (1990b). Facial neglect. *Neuropsychologia, 28,* 391–415.

Young, A. W., & Ellis, H. D. (1989). Childhood prosopagnosia. *Brain and Cognition, 9,* 16–47.

ANDREW W. YOUNG

facial agnosia *See* AGNOSIA.

facial diplegia Facial diplegia is a general and bilateral disorder of movements of the face as a result of a cortical lesion of the motor area for the face. Its importance is in being distinguished from buccofacial APRAXIA. In principle the two disorders are distinct in that facial diplegia affects all movements including reflex and automatic movements, while buccofacial apraxia affects only voluntary movements. In the latter the patient will be unable to carry out verbal commands to protrude the tongue, blow, suck, and smile while able to perform these activities spontaneously; in facial diplegia all these activities will be defective. However, in practice, the two conditions can be difficult to distinguish as the automatic movements preserved in buccofacial apraxia may be limited to swallowing and chewing (with primarily facial movements therefore affected).

fear Fear is an emotion which is normally associated with the functions of the LIMBIC SYSTEM and the HYPOTHALAMUS. It may also be of significance as an aspect of the aura preceding complex partial seizures (*see* EPILEPSY), which may be presumed to result from the involvement of temporal lobe limbic structures in the genesis of the seizures. There has been some suggestion that involvement of emotional aspects in the complex partial seizure aura may be associated more with right-sided foci than with left-sided foci, the right hemisphere being presumed to be the hemisphere supporting emotional behavior, but the available evidence cannot be said to support this conclusion.

finger agnosia *See* AGNOSIA; GERSTMANN SYNDROME.

fluent aphasia *See* APHASIA.

fornix The fornix is one of the elements of the LIMBIC SYSTEM. Each fornix runs between the mammillary body, anteriorly, from which it rises up through the columns of the fornix, passing around the THALAMUS where, passing back above the thalamus and below the CORPUS CALLOSUM, it becomes the body of the fornix before turning down and moving anterior again where it runs into the HIPPOCAMPUS. As with other limbic structures, lesions of the fornix result in severe memory deficits: difficulty in learning new material and in recalling remote events.

fovea The fovea is a small depression in the centre of the retina which is filled with closely packed cones which each project to a single ganglion cell, therefore producing a high degree of visual resolution. The fovea is set within a small area known as the *macular region* (more properly the *macula lutea*) and corresponds to the point of visual fixation.

Although only a small portion of the retina, the fovea and macular region, because of their role in supporting high-resolution vision, project to fibers making up a large portion of the optic nerve and to about two-thirds of the primary visual cortex. The area of the calcarine fissure closest to the occipital pole is devoted to foveal and macular vision; the more anterior portions support peripheral vision.

As the fovea and macula occupy such a large portion of the visual projection, a large lesion is required to destroy this portion completely. As a slightly paradoxical result, HEMIANOPIA affecting the complete peripheral field is more common than it is in the foveal field, and it is therefore not uncommon to observe a hemianopia in which central vision is preserved; a condition referred to as *macular sparing*.

Fregoli syndrome The Fregoli syndrome is a rare form of delusional misidentification in which the patient believes that the physical identity of others has dramatically changed, while their minds remain as before the physical change. It is therefore a delusion complementary to the CAPGRAS SYNDROME and a form of mental REDUPLICATION.

Friedreich's ataxia *See* ATAXIA.

frontal eye field *See* EYE MOVEMENT.

frontal lobectomy, lobotomy *See* LOBECTOMY.

frontal lobes The frontal lobes refer to the rostral cerebral region superior to the Sylvian fissure and anterior to the Rolandic fissure, and encompass approximately 24–33 percent of the adult human brain. The two roughly symmetrical left and right frontal lobes are descriptively divided into three areas defined by the surface location: basilar-orbital, dorsolateral, and medial (see Figure 41). Another commonly used anatomical definition and subdivision is based on Brodmann area numbers: area 4 (the precentral gyrus) – primary motor area; area 6, posterior part of area 8 (frontal eyefields), and areas 44 and 45 (Broca's area) – premotor region; the remainder is labelled prefrontal cortex, frequently divided into basal-medial (areas 9–13, 24, 32), dorsolateral (9–12, 46, 47), mesial (9–12), and orbital (10–15, 47) sections. Two other ways of defining the frontal lobes anatomically are based on cytoarchitectural divisions and thalamocortical connections.

Confusion in the understanding of the terms "frontal lobes" and "frontal lobe functions" or "dysfunctions" frequently arises, as the operational definitions of their anatomy and cognitive processes vary in different publications. The brain region described by the term "frontal lobes" may range from the more limited prefrontal cortex to a much greater area, including such regions as the anterior cingulate. The label "frontal functions" may denote those cognitive abilities observed to be altered after focal pathology to the frontal lobes. The same label has also been used to identify those processes impaired after pathology in other brain regions, such as the basal

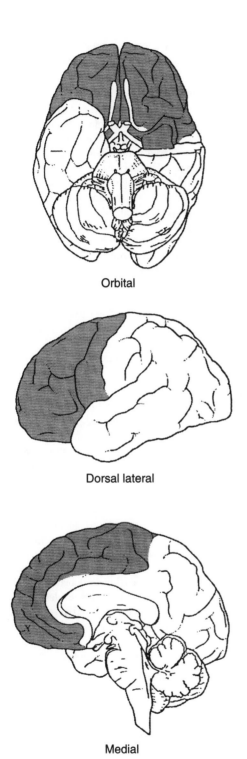

Orbital

Dorsal lateral

Medial

Figure 41 The three areas of the frontal lobes.

ganglia or dorsomedial nucleus, which are intimately connected with the frontal lobes, or after more diffuse pathology. In these instances a general term such as frontal systems, or more specific terms such as frontal-thalamic functional systems, have also been used. Cognitive neuropsychologists stress psychological function rather than anatomical localization. Executive control functions, supervisory system, or dysexecutive syndrome are general terms that have been used to describe these functions and dysfunctions that have been considered "frontal," but their anatomical basis has been of secondary concern. It is important to define operationally the psychological processes, to understand how these processes fit within a theoretical framework and, if brain–behavior relations are a focus of research, to identify clearly the associated structural anatomical regions.

The emphasis in this review is on the functions associated with the anatomical region known as the frontal lobes. While most frequently the descriptions relate to the prefrontal cortex, the term "frontal lobes" will be used. Certain functions will be described, however, even if localization is uncertain or not definitely limited to the frontal lobes, if common usage labels these as frontal lobe functions.

The types of neuropathology recognized as sources of frontal behavioral symptomatology can be divided into two. The first are those that produce relatively well localized frontal damage, such as that caused by vascular pathology, neoplasms, trauma, and postsurgical states. All of these still have limitations for brain–behavior research in that the etiology of pathology that affects one frontal lobe may affect the other frontal lobe, may have more distant effects such as those caused by tumor pressure, or may even produce wide-ranging disturbances in addition to the more focal disturbance, as is frequent with traumatic brain injury. The second type of nervous system alterations or disorders considered "frontal" includes multiple sclerosis, certain movement disorders, various degenerative dementias, some infectious disorders, and aging, each of which may produce behavioral changes which have been interpreted as similar to those found after focal frontal lesions. Whether the behavioral changes observed in the second group of disorders truly reflect focal frontal lobe dysfunction, frontal system disturbance, or whether they should be considered as cognitive changes independent of any brain localization is controversial. In addition to these neurological disorders, many psychiatric disorders have been considered to have executive disturbances as a primary symptom, and actual frontal lobe dysfunction in these disorders has been hypothesized. Involvement of the frontal lobes in psychiatric disorders must still be interpreted with caution.

METHODOLOGICAL AND THEORETICAL ISSUES

The awareness of possible methodological questions in frontal lobe research serves as a context for the interpretation of published findings. There is often confusion as to whether the term frontal lobe function refers to an anatomical localized behavior or to a cognitive process independent of brain localization. In many studies, locus of pathology is often inadequately described. Localization of the lesion to one hemisphere and within a particular lobe is frequently not considered, even though the animal literature suggests the importance of localization. The number of subjects included in specific studies is frequently small, and findings are often not replicated.

The experimental tasks are often complex in order to fulfill the criteria required of a frontal lobe test. Such tests unfortunately are by definition multifactorial, tapping many abilities and making it difficult to differentiate which specific processes are impaired. There is an increasing awareness of the need to identify and isolate component processes if specific knowledge of the functions of the frontal lobe is to be obtained. An important allied theoretical issue is the question of homogeneity versus heterogeneity of function within the frontal lobes. Some have argued that most if not all frontal functions can be explained by one construct (homogeneity of function) such as working memory or inhibition. Other researchers provide evidence that suggests possible fractionation or separation of processes. This theoretical problem may represent a problem of semantics and/or incomplete functional analysis rather than an unresolvable dichotomy. It may be that certain frontal processes are distinct, elicited by specific task demands. At the same time, other functions may be a necessary substrate for any frontal process. Depending on what is being experimentally assessed, homogeneous or heterogeneous processes may be identified.

EARLY STUDIES

Early writings on the functions of the frontal lobes revealed many diverse opinions. Some authors labelled this brain region the seat of wisdom; others considered it the silent brain area. Case studies reported significant alterations in behavior after frontal lobe damage. In other studies, objective identification of dysfunction after frontal pathology was not identified. This apparent paradox has led to increasing research and gradual identification of more defined cognitive processes associated with the frontal lobes. Animal researchers and anatomists such as Fuster, Goldman-Rakic, Mishkin, Pandya, Petrides, and Nauta and their colleagues have contributed significantly to the increasing knowledge of frontal lobe anatomy and functional abilities. The emphasis in this synopsis, however, is on the psychological functions associated with the frontal lobes in humans.

FRONTAL LOBE FUNCTIONS

It is generally accepted that the prefrontal cortex does not play a significant role in behaviors that are routine, simple and/or over-learned even if these behaviors are relatively complex. Because of this, patients with even significant prefrontal lobe damage may perform within normal limits on many tasks, including perceptual, memory, and certain cognitive tasks. Since many items in general tests of intelligence also reflect previous learning, an overall IQ score may appear unaffected after damage to the frontal lobes. What is important are the cognitive demands of the particular task. This becomes evident in an outline of major findings observed in studies and observations of frontal lobe patients.

Sensory, perceptual-constructive, and motor functions

Basic sensory functions are primarily located in nonfrontal brain regions. While the frontal lobes have been suggested to contribute to certain visual syndromes such as BÁLINT'S, the relationships are not well established. Olfaction may be significantly diminished or altered. The olfactory bulb and tract lie on the orbital surface of the frontal lobes, and are frequently involved when the frontal lobes are damaged. However, impaired olfactory discrimination can also reflect pathology in a neural system involving the dorsomedial nucleus of the thalamus and the lateral posterior orbitofrontal region. The frontal lobes do not play an essential role at the level of simple perceptual abilities or when basic perceptual-constructive responses are required, as in reproducing a simple design. When planning and synthesis/integration processes are required in such tasks, however, the frontal lobes appear involved. Patients with frontal lesions are impaired on certain maze tests, tasks requiring integration of fragmented pictures, and measures of personal orientation.

Motor functions related to the motor and premotor regions are described in neuroanatomy texts, and will not be discussed here. An anatomical dissociation of two very general alterations in motor behavior has been suggested for more prefrontal regions: hypokinetic and slow – associated with lesions to dorsolateral/medial frontal regions; hyperkinetic and impulsive – associated with orbitofrontal area damage. Difficulties in performing sequences of motor movements may be observed in patients with frontal pathology. Perseveration of previous responses may occur. Some patients may not be able to inhibit motor responses when the context does not require a response or even in the face of commands that no response be made.

The frontal lobes participate in some praxis functions, although the definition of praxis is frequently used in a broad sense. Bucco-linguo-facial and limb APRAXIAS have been reported after left frontal lesions (although a right frontal white matter lesion involving the corpus callosum could theoretically also result in a unilateral left apraxia). Magnetic apraxia, in which the patient compulsively explores the immediate environment and, once contact is achieved, appears to be unable to release the movement, has also been described after frontal lobe damage. This general disorder subsumes several descriptions of motor deficits, in which there appears to be an excessive and erroneous dependence on environmental cues. In some patients with unilateral medial frontal lesions, an "alien hand" syndrome has been described whereby the hand contralateral to the lesion appears dissociated from conscious control. Lhermitte and colleagues have described utilization and imitation behaviors. In utilization be-

havior disorder, the patient uses objects in the environment, even when not required to do so. This disorder may be context-dependent, in that the use of objects may occur spontaneously, or be "induced" when objects are given directly to the patient. In imitation behavior disorder, the patient imitates the examiner's gestures even when instructed not to do so. Many of these described motor disorders can be subsumed under the general concept of a disturbance in intentional motor acts.

Attention

Attentional deficits are a prominent feature in patients with frontal lobe damage. In recent years, there has been an increase in the specificity of knowledge of the type of attentional problem in such patients. Disorders of general arousal and alertness are not common with chronic frontal lobe lesions, particularly if the lesion is limited to the prefrontal region and is unilateral. These functions, however, may be depressed if frontal pathology such as a tumor extends beyond frontal regions. There frequently is a deficit in directing attention in visual space, particularly if the lesion encroaches upon the frontal eye fields. In its most extreme form, frontal lobe patients, particularly those with right frontal damage, may exhibit NEGLECT or hemi-inattention. In contrast to the neglect deficit found in patients with lesions elsewhere, the disorder caused by frontal pathology can be interpreted as a primary deficit in exploratory motor behavior. In some studies, the deficit has been even further dissociated into separate components, such as difficulty suppressing a reflexive glance to a nontarget stimulus, and impairment in performing volitional eye movements.

Other attentional deficits reported after frontal lobe damage include an impairment in inhibition of responses to irrelevant stimuli, diminished reaction to novel stimuli, possible impaired habituation to repetitive novel stimuli, and a deficit in sustaining attention. These impairments in specific processes are described clinically by such terms as distractibility, neglect, and impulsivity. Some components of attentional processes may be related to specific regions within the frontal cortex. The right frontal region has been implicated in sustained and directed attention.

From a clinical perspective, it is important to

note that patients with even significant frontal lobe damage can perform normally on many neuropsychological tests of attention, and their level of performance may vary. Sources of variability in performance include the cognitive processing demands of the test and the extent and locus of the lesion.

Language

It has been speculated that the frontal lobes, particularly the prefrontal cortices, have a unique role in language and communication. The role of the frontal lobes in some instances has been established. DYSARTHRIA, defined as a disturbance of the complex speech musculature system, often reflects peripheral motor dysfunction but can be caused by damage to frontal motor regions. Some authors have described cortical dysarthria or apraxia of speech, defined as intact motor articulation but impaired smooth flow of speech patterns, occurring after left frontal damage. The classic syndrome of Broca's APHASIA does involve Broca's area in the frontal lobes, but extends to regions significantly beyond this defined area. A syndrome sometimes described as minor or little Broca, or aphemia, characterized by initial acute mutism followed by hypophonic slow speech with no real lasting aphasia, has been described, with some authors even differentiating patients characterized more by the output disorder (aphemia) from those having some language deficits (little Broca). On a continuum with these disorders is transcortical motor aphasia, which is similar in certain respects to Broca's aphasia, but differentiated from it by intact repetition abilities. This disorder has been related to smaller lesions somewhat anterior to Broca's area. Lesions in the supplementary motor area can impair spontaneous initiation of speech. Finally, the right frontal regions appear to mediate the affective components of communication. For example, patients with right frontal lesions analogous to Broca's area understand and recognize emotion, but show little spontaneous affective quality in speech, and are impaired in imitating the affective tone. The more speculative functions of prefrontal regions in communication remain to be investigated experimentally.

Memory/Learning

Focal frontal lesions do not result in a global or severe amnesia as traditionally defined. Patients with frontal lobe damage, for example, frequently perform normally on measures of long-term memory, particularly when tested in a recognition procedure. Frontal lobe damage, however, can affect successful memory functioning, particularly if task demands are such that planning and/or organizational abilities are required to establish encoding strategies or direction of memory search. Patients with frontal lobe pathology appear extremely susceptible to the effects of interference even in the absence of amnesia. Faulty retrieval strategies have been hypothesized as the primary deficit underlying CONFABULATION. Perhaps the most consistent deficit found in patients with frontal lobe damage has been on conditional associative learning tasks where the learning of associations between arbitrary cues and matched responses is required. This deficit has been interpreted as a general defect in the patients' use of external cues to guide behaviors.

Other concepts of memory function have been proposed as being related to the frontal lobes. One such is working memory, described as a series of short-term memory processes, coordinated by a central executive system related to the frontal lobes, which function to hold information temporarily while it is being processed. The operational definitions of working memory and consensus on what are working memory tasks, however, remain controversial. A second area of investigation has examined the involvement of the frontal lobes in remembering the contexts related to specific information. Patients with frontal lobe damage typically have difficulty remembering or judging the temporal order (when) of information, even though they remember the information itself. While memory for spatial (where) context has also been suggested as being impaired after frontal lobe damage, this may be a methodological confound of temporal discrimination with spatial context tasks. A specific type of memory for context is recall of the source of learned information. Source forgetting occurs when the targeted information is remembered, but the source of that information is not recalled. While this deficit has been related to frontal lobe damage, the effect is not striking. Patients with frontal lobe damage have also been described as having a deficit in metamemory, which can be defined as knowledge of the capacity of one's memory processes and of strategies which can improve memory performance. Additional research is required to substantiate and elaborate these findings.

Cognitive/executive functions

At times it has been difficult to classify the type of processes impaired after frontal lobe damage and a general label such as higher-order cognitive or executive functions has frequently been used. Many of these concepts are similar to those already discussed.

In general, many tasks labelled cognitive are minimally affected by frontal lobe lesions, at least after the more acute stages of recovery. As mentioned above, scores on general tests of intelligence may be unaffected by frontal lesions; however, verbal IQ may be diminished after left frontal lesions, although the influence of lesion size and extent of aphasia have not been clearly documented. Specific task demands can elicit impairment in patients with frontal lobe damage. Generation and fluency of output for many types of tasks including word and gesture fluency are frequently diminished after frontal lobe pathology. Patients with frontal lobe lesions may be impulsive in responses, have difficulty in formulating hypotheses, be impaired in shifting strategies of established responses, take more moves to achieve correct solutions on problem-solving tasks such as the Tower of Hanoi, and have problems in programming and selecting subgoals of responses. In recent years there have been attempts to use tasks borrowed from cognitive psychology and artificial intelligence, such as the Tower of Hanoi. Tasks have also been devised to assess the effects of frontal lobe pathology in making decisions in real life situations.

Significant questions have been raised about frontal lobe involvement in such tasks, and the theoretical concepts that have evolved. In many reports, the abilities ascribed to the frontal lobes have been proposed as a general executive or supervisory ability. In other cases, there has been an attempt to suggest that these processes are indeed separable and distinct components, and that the executive supervisory system can be fractionated. How the processes identified in the "cognitive" tasks compare to those identified in "memory" or "attentional" tasks also remains to be experimentally investigated. Whether these executive processes are somehow distinct, or whether the divisions are arbitrary and artificial are significant theoretical questions.

Personality, emotions, and self-awareness

Personality changes have been considered a hallmark of frontal lobe pathology, with the classic example being Phineas Gage. As a consequence of severe focal frontal lobe injury in a work-related accident, Phineas' personality was so dramatically altered that friends considered him a different person – "No longer Gage." The descriptions of the altered behavior in the many published reports, however, are heterogeneous and often contradictory, including extremes such as apathy and restlessness, depression and euphoria. The incongruities can be at least partially understood by the use of terms which may relate to specific and possibly independent processes. Using labels such as altered drive or initiation (apathy or restlessness, depending on direction of alteration), mood (the subjective feeling tone), affect (the overt expression of emotion), and differentiating these functions from their superordinate control provides a base to understand observations such as the ability to experience emotion dissociated from or incongruent with the ability to control the expression of emotion. Knowledge of the relationship of lesion location and behavior also clarifies previous ambiguities. For example, pathology in the anterior convexity and/or medial frontal regions results in apparent apathy and difficulty in initiating behaviors. Orbitofrontal damage, on the other hand, results in disinhibition. Recent studies have attempted to link depression with focal left frontal damage and hypomania with right frontal damage, but this association remains tenuous and requires further investigation.

These distinctions still do not address the overall complex of disorders of social behavior that have been described. What appears to be impaired in such cases are additional disturbances most apparent in a social context. These include the ability to establish appropriate goals or responses; to organize and integrate behaviors in time and space; to monitor and verify the veracity and appropriateness of a percept or action; to show adequate concern about the implications of actions; and to alter behaviors after feedback. Disturbed self-reflectiveness or self-awareness appears to be an essential component of the frontal personality disturbance. This disturbed self-awareness and self-monitoring does not necessarily imply absence of knowledge since these patients may demonstrate awareness of errors but be unable to use this information to alter their behavior. Specific behavioral syndromes associated with this basic disorder of self-monitoring are confabulation (production of incorrect even bizarre responses or behaviors in routine situations), reduplicative paramnesia (a delusional condition in which the patient believes two or more locations with similar attributes exist), and the Capgras syndrome (a delusional belief that an individual has been replaced by a substitute who resembles the original individual).

CLINICAL IMPLICATIONS

Assessment

There are several important considerations in the clinical assessment of frontal lobe dysfunction. If the pathology is confined to the prefrontal cortex, overt neurological deficits are unlikely to be observed. When the pathology involves premotor and motor regions, or includes frontal systems, the neurological deficits may provide evidence as to the etiology of the disorder and/or localization of pathology.

The neuropsychological/behavioral examination of frontal lobe or executive abilities can be difficult for many reasons. The clinician must be aware that commonly used clinical frontal lobe tests are in reality multifactorial and assess many abilities. The specificity of the tests must therefore be questioned. For example, performance on the Wisconsin Card Sorting Test (WCST), perhaps the most widely used frontal lobe test, may be impaired after damage in many brain regions. While the number of perseverative errors on this test provides a good index of focal frontal pathology, the data also suggest that no single test can be used to diagnose frontal lobe dysfunction. In addition to test specificity, the question of the sensitivity of the test must be asked. Still using the WCST as an example, a review of the literature demonstrated that, even though group differences identifying a significant frontal lobe impairment were present, the probability of individual patients with proven frontal lobe damage being classified as impaired on the frontal lobe tests varied notably.

The examiner may encounter the incongruous situation of a patient who descriptively has a "frontal syndrome" but performs perfectly on supposed frontal lobe tests. There are several possible explanations for this apparent incongruity. First, the test used may be specific for a particular region of the frontal lobes which is not damaged in the identified patient. This possibility is suggested by the idea of separate processes within the frontal lobes, and published results suggestive of specific localization. Second, each patient may differ in what was premorbidly routine for her or him, possibly invalidating the frontal lobe test used. Third, the testing situation may provide the external routine control that the patient lacks, with the examiner "becoming the frontal lobes" of the patient. The examiner may therefore need to rely on observations made in natural settings or tests designed to examine ongoing demands within a limited time setting to evaluate capacity for executive functioning in everyday life.

Rehabilitation

Rehabilitation in patients with frontal lobe damage has either been neglected or directed at recovery of general functions, as the essential impairments were often not identified. The rehabilitative approach for frontal dysfunction should be specific to each patient. In some patients with very severe executive dysfunction, the rehabilitation specialist works bottom-up, focusing on the intact abilities and re-instituting basic and routine lower-level processes. In some cases the therapist even restructures the patient's environment to control input and output as a means of improving overall functioning. At this level, the emphasis is on increasing knowledge and skills. If the patient has a rudimentary attentional capacity, then the rehabilitation focus might be on executive subfunctions such as imitating and sequencing of action programs, and higher level attentional skills such as selecting and sustaining attention. Another method is first to establish external control of executive functions, which through practice become gradually internalized. The third form of training attempted in patients who are capable emphasizes generalization and metacognitive, reflective abilities. Many persons with frontal lobe damage have limited insight into the implications of their problems (even though their factual knowledge may be correct), and awareness and self-regulating training such as self-instructional procedures may be attempted.

In general, the rehabilitation approach moves from simple structured activities with significant external support, to more complex activities with gradual reduction of external support, to the establishment of self-direction. It is important to realize that the validity and success of these techniques, and whether all proposed steps are possible in all patients, are still open to continuing experimental verification and replication.

THE IMPORTANCE OF THE FRONTAL LOBES

In some respects, the frontal lobes represent the utmost challenge of the understanding to the functional significance of the human brain. Concepts like self-awareness, planning, and supervisory control suggest the highest functional levels of cognitive processing.

Studies of the effects of frontal lobe damage have provided a significant advance in the domain of brain–behavior relationships. The questions asked have assisted the integration of modern cognitive psychology concepts into neuropsychology. The study of miscellaneous neurological conditions and various psychiatric disorders has been assisted by the growing knowledge of executive functions.

At the same time, the difficulties in procurement of subjects with focal frontal lesions and in operationally defining the functions of the frontal lobes have led to diverse methodological and theoretical problems, even in the best studies. For example, the patients studied may often have a complex neurological history and/or poorly defined anatomical localization. The experimental protocols may still not sufficiently isolate the processes in question.

Research into frontal lobe functioning is still in its infancy. The next decade will see significant advancements in knowledge of the anatomy, connections, and functions of the anterior region of the brain, in the delineation of the psychological constructs of supervisory or executive functions, and in the understanding of changes in executive functions in psychiatric disorders and with normal aging.

BIBLIOGRAPHY

Alexander, M. P., Benson, D. F., & Stuss, D. T. (1989). Frontal lobes and language. *Brain and Language*, *37*, 656–91.

Fuster, J. M. (1989). *The prefrontal cortex: Anatomy, physiology, and neuropsychology of the frontal lobe*, 2nd edn. New York: Raven.

Hebb, D. O. (1945). Man's frontal lobes: a critical review. *Archives of Neurology and Psychiatry*, *44*, 421–38.

Lhermitte, F. (1986). Human autonomy and the frontal lobes. Part II: Patient behavior in complex and social situations: The "Environmental Dependency Syndrome." *Annals of Neurology*, *19*, 335–43.

Luria, A. R. (1973). *The working brain: An introduction to neuropsychology*. New York: Basic Books.

Milner, B., & Petrides, M. (1984). Behavioural effects of frontal-lobe lesions in man. *Trends in Neuroscience*, *7*, 403–7.

Pandya, D. N., & Barnes, C. L. (1987). Architecture and connections of the frontal lobe. In E. Perecman (Ed.), *The frontal lobes revisited* (pp. 41–72). New York: IRBN Press.

Shallice, T. (1988). *From neuropsychology to mental structure*. Cambridge: Cambridge University Press.

Sohlberg, M. M., & Mateer, C. A. (1989). *Introduction to cognitive rehabilitation: Theory and practice*. New York: Guilford.

Stuss, D. T., & Benson, D. F. (1986). *The frontal lobes*. New York: Raven.

DONALD T. STUSS

fugue state   Fugue states are dissociative states which involve a clouding of consciousness and, while control of posture and muscle tone is preserved, the performance of actions without awareness of what is happening over a protracted period. The patient in a fugue state may wander, without apparent awareness of who they are, or what they are doing. The state may last for hours or even days, and the patient may be incoherent and perplexed while in the state, yet carry out apparently purposive yet not always sensible actions. Amnesia for the period of the fugue is common on recovery. Fugue states are generally considered to be either epileptic in origin, or to be hysterical, and the differentiation between the two may be diagnostically difficult and may commonly be a matter of dispute. The differences among fugues, *automatisms*, and other *twilight states* are largely a matter of context and degree.

Epileptic fugues, which are associated with temporal lobe seizures, may or may not be accompanied by cerebral dysrhythmia in the EEG, as continuous monitoring is rarely possible throughout the episode. The diagnosis of epileptic fugue is considered to be more likely if the period of the fugue is relatively brief (although cases with documented pathology have been reported with fugues up to at least 10 hours), where there is independent evidence of epileptic activity, where the behavior during the fugue is less orderly and purposeful, and where there is a lack of self-care on the part of the patient.

Fugues may also occur as a hysterical condition in which the patient wanders about with claimed loss of identity and memory, also with amnesia for the period of the fugue on recovery, which is often sudden. Such hysterical fugues are often considered to be associated with current life stresses and times of personal crisis, particularly where some gain for the patient from the behavior can be seen. In hysterical fugues the patient is less likely to demonstrate evident clouding of consciousness and other cognitive disturbances, will continue with essentially rational actions in a context of maintained awareness of the environment, and may maintain a good standard of self-care. A previous history of a related form of epileptic activity is usually absent. However, it should be emphasized that the existence of these two forms of fugue is a matter of dispute, and that even where the two forms are accepted, the distinction in individual cases may never be resolved (*see* EPILEPSY, HYSTERIA).

J. GRAHAM BEAUMONT

Funktionswandel　Funktionswandel refers to one aspect of apperceptive visual AGNOSIA, a condition in which patients fail to recognize objects because they cannot perceive adequately. The condition, while rare, is often a stage in the recovery from CORTICAL BLINDNESS, and affects all aspects of perception involving shape or pattern perception. Patients typically complain that the environment appears to change as they try to survey it, and that objects are only visible as they are moved. Funktionswandel refers to the time-dependent aspects of this disorder: local adaptation time (the time taken for a stimulus to fade from a portion of the visual field) and sensation time (the exposure duration necessary for recognition of some element within the visual field). The result is that stimuli tend either not to enter awareness, or else fall out from awareness, because of these temporal abnormalities. In itself a rare disorder; it usually occurs in the company of other visual and perceptual disturbances, and is therefore difficult to both recognize and to analyze.

fusiform gyrus　The fusiform gyrus lies on the medial surface of the TEMPORAL LOBE. It is separated from the adjacent hippocampal gyrus and at its anterior end the uncus by the *collateral sulcus* which in its anterior portion is termed the *rhinal fissure*. The functional significance of the fusiform gyrus is its implication in disorders of FACE RECOGNITION, although a lesion in this region alone may not be sufficient to produce the disorder.

G

gait Gait is one of several types of locomotion used by animals with legs. Under guidance of the senses the legs carry – translocate – the body from one place to another by reciprocal movements in a rhythmic change between phases of flexion (swing) and extension (support). In the bipedal gait which is typical for humans, one leg must by definition always be in contact with the ground. The mobility of the joints in different planes as connected to postural control of the body gives considerable adaptability for walking on uneven ground and for changes in direction and speed. The basal gait pattern is common to all but there are obvious individual differences. They depend in part upon differences in physical structure but there are evident superposed elements of learned behavior, easily observed and often described in works of fiction.

The earliest observed instance of human-like gait is the footprints of hominids 3.7 million years old, which were found in Laetoli in Tanzania in petrified volcano ash. The heels were put down before the toes, which is characteristic for the plantigrade gait of adult humans. Most four-legged animals and small children are toe-walkers, that is, they put down the toes before the heels.

Bipedal locomotion is essentially unstable and therefore dependent upon the postural control of the body. The relation between the swinging leg and the supporting one is an unavoidable part of the gait. Without this relationship the stepping movements are not gait but merely successive flexion and extension. Far from being a task only for the stepping mechanism of the legs, gait is also dependent upon our ability to stand, to counteract gravitation, and to maintain equilibrium.

For postural control all parts of the body participate with synchronous movements adapted to optimal balance and effectiveness. The body is functionally divided, approximately at the waist, into two parts physically balancing each other at each step. For instance, with increasing stride length the amplitude of the arm-swing also increases and deliberate changes of arm-swing will result in corresponding changes of stride length. The control of this balance is effected by appropriately programmed postural reflexes which engage all parts of the nervous system. The adequate stimuli for a large part of these reflexes are changes of the center of gravity. The center of gravity of the standing human is approximately in the middle of the pelvis. In level walking it describes smooth sinusoidal curves with an amplitude of approximately 5 cm in both horizontal and vertical directions. It results from an interplay in different planes of movements, principally those of the pelvis, hip joints, knees, and ankles. A good summary of this interplay is given in Rose and Gamble (1993).

The stepping mechanism's basal pattern of flexion and extension and also postural control in part is organized in the spinal cord. In cats whose spinal cord has been severed in the thoracic region it is possible to provoke not only gait but also gallop in the hindlegs, provided that the hindquarters are supported. It has been shown by Grillner and colleagues (1979) that a few segments of deafferented spinal cord in the cat are able to generate reciprocally alternating rhythmical discharges in motor nerves to flexors and extensors, so-called "fictive locomotion." In the intact individual this pattern generator is under the influence of segmental afferent inflow and descending motor pathways. A special role is played by the descending pathways in the ventral columns of the spinal cord and it is probably significant that it is here that the pathways are found which serve total limb movements, erect posture, and direction of progression. In primates, including Man, the spinal pattern generator will not function without this connection (Eidelberg et al., 1981).

Although the spinal cord contains an elementary control system for the stepping mechanism, which other areas are needed for natural gait is a fundamental question. It is obvious that for full adaptability of gait all sensory and motor abilities of the central nervous system are necessary. It has been shown in experiments with cats that animals lacking cortex, basal ganglia, and thalamus are still able to walk spontaneously even if there are defects in footfall and direction. They can therefore still accomplish three essential elements of walking – stepping, postural tonus, and equilibration.

It is also possible to control the gait of decerebrated animals through tonic electrical stimulation of certain areas in the brain stem, the so-called hypothalamic and mesencephalic locomotor regions respectively. For example, a decerebrate cat supported on a treadmill with stimulation electrodes in the mesencephalic locomotor region will start and stop walking as the stimulus is turned on and off.

The function of the brain stem preparations described indicates which structures are necessary for walking in Man too, even if in the latter still more encephalization has to be expected.

External stimulation may be used to activate the stepping mechanism in humans. Newborn babies may take steps if they are held with their feet against a support. In Parkinsonism and spasticity, disorders which are both characterized by bad gait, suitable external stimulation may sometimes be therapeutically useful in activating the stepping mechanism. Patients with Parkinson's disease not only take short strides but sometimes have a tendency to "stick to the floor" as though they have lost the ability to start walking. By slightly rocking them from side to side it is possible to help them not only to start but also, in cases where they are still walking, to increase their stride length. The same effect may be obtained by visual objects positioned with an extension at right angles to the walking direction. In patients with spasticity in their legs the stepping mechanism may be activated by stimuli provoking a flexor reflex. The last effect has been used with the peroneal stimulator, a device that not only contracts the dorsiflexor muscles of the foot via the peroneal nerve but also provokes a flexor reflex through afferent stimulation.

The observation that stimuli which provoke the flexor reflex facilitate the stepping mechanism should not be unexpected, remembering the obvious similarity between swing and stance on one side and the flexor reflex and the crossed extensor reflex on the other. A subject treading on a sharp object will lift the foot to avoid the pain. At the same time the contralateral leg extends to support the body. It is possible to identify two different spinal systems through which afferent stimulation will result in flexion and crossed extension. In the classical pattern, which is evoked by pain, the latency to movement is short. In the other pattern, which is released if the afferent stimulus occurs simultaneously with influence from supraspinal tracts, the latency is longer. It dominates over the short latency system and is released not only by painful but also by other afferent stimuli from skin, joints, and muscles commonly named flexor reflex afferents (FRA). It is probably this superior system for flexion and extension which constitutes the central pattern generator for gait. The term FRA does not mean that stimuli via these afferents necessarily result in flexion. The slight rocking which may be used to facilitate gait in Parkinson patients in fact provokes a stretch reflex in the leg towards which the rocking is done.

GAIT ANALYSIS

An important reason for gait studies is the handicap experienced by subjects with gait disorders. Many methods of studying them have been developed. Kinematic methods describe the movement pattern, kinetic methods the forces in connection with movement, electromyography the activity pattern of muscles, and measurements of oxygen consumption the energy expenditure. A review of the findings obtained by these methods is given in Rose and Gamble (1993). Notwithstanding their scientific value, many of these methods are time-consuming and of limited value in everyday practice, where visual inspection has a dominant role. In addition, visual inspection helps the observer to integrate the results of technical measurements into a functional totality.

The strength of visual inspection is substantially increased if measurements of velocity, stride length, and stride frequency are added. A stopwatch and a measuring tape are the only aids needed. The walkway should be at least 10 m long and the patient should be asked to walk at several speeds, including a comfortable pace and a very fast one.

Velocity, together with endurance, expresses the sum of all functions necessary for gait. If any of them fail, velocity will decrease. This is true if the subject is asked to walk at both maximum and ordinary velocity. A patient with a gait disorder will have a restricted range of possible speeds, often being able to walk with only one velocity. Comfortable gait velocity has been investigated in pedestrians unknowingly passing a measured distance. The results depend upon circumstances. For men they range between 1.24 m/s and 1.54 m/s, the lower velocities obtaining in parks and shopping areas. In these circumstances women tend to walk more slowly, but in a hospital corridor young nurses walk faster than medical students, and factory workers walk faster from work than to work. It is obvious that in studies of gait velocity it is necessary to provide a thorough description of existing circumstances. Regardless of all the varying influences which may be important for the outcome of its measurement, gait velocity gives a good idea of a patient's gait ability, especially if the recording is made under standardized laboratory conditions, and if the patient is compared to him- or herself at different stages of a gait disorder.

The whole gait cycle is called the stride. The stride length is the distance covered from "heel on" of one leg to "next heel on" of the same leg. The step length is the distance from "heel on" of one leg to "heel on" of the other leg. Right step is from left "heel on" to right "heel on" and vice versa. In walking in a straight line the right and the left stride are always the same length. The right and the left step lengths may, however, be different in pathological cases.

Gait velocity is the product of stride length (SL) and stride frequency (SF). The relation between stride length and stride frequency is linear if extreme values are excluded. If a subject is asked to walk at several freely chosen velocities from very slow to maximum a linear regression is easily determined:

$$SF = B0 + B1* SL$$

Its slope (B0) and intercept (B1) help to describe how velocity is increased, whether by primarily increasing stride length or stride frequency. For a given velocity women and children, for instance, take shorter strides than men, but the difference is less at slow than at faster velocities. The difference is primarily due to their shorter legs and also to the pelvic structure in the case of women. Except for anatomical factors, the relation between stride length and stride frequency is dependent upon psychological and pathological circumstances.

The equation for linear regression is very useful in describing how a subject changes his or her walking ability between two different test occasions. Patients with an above-knee prosthesis and patients with weak muscles around the hip tend to show increased or at least unchanged stride length relative to stride frequency, dependent upon an increased pendulousness of the leg during swing, but otherwise gait disorders almost always result in shorter strides in relation to stride frequency. This is not because of low velocity but is connected to impaired postural control due to paresis or pain, among other things.

The duration of the stride (S) is the inverse of stride frequency. Since the stride duration is the sum of the phases it is possible to describe the time relations between the phases with a few simple equations. The time relations indicate changes in the contact forces with the ground and are therefore of practical importance in gait analysis.

The stride has two main phases, the extension or support phase, stance (ST), and the flexion phase, swing (SW). Like most gait parameters, they change with walking speed. One of the legs must always be in the support phase. When both legs are on the ground it is called double support (DS). It decreases successively with velocity and becomes double swing when gait passes over to run. In this instant the stance and the swing phases have equal durations.

The part of support with only one foot against the ground is called single support (SS). Its duration will be short if the leg is weak or the support is painful. Since single support corresponds to swing on the contralateral side, a weak or painful leg will tend to manifest itself as a fast swing of the healthy leg.

Double support has two parts, one on each side of single support, corresponding to when body weight is transferred from right to left (DS_{rl}) or from left to right (DS_{lr}) respectively. They have the same duration but in a gait disorder, where the weight transference from one leg to the other is disturbed because of pain or weakness, the relation will be changed.

The duration of stance is the sum of single support and the two phases of double support. Since the duration of single support is the same as contralateral swing (SW$_{cl}$) it is possible to describe this as:

$$ST = DS_{rl} + SW_{cl} + DS_{lr}$$

This equation describes the time relations between the two legs and is therefore of importance in characterizing a limp. It also demonstrates the fact that dysfunction of one leg inevitably affects the function of the other.

The objective of gait analysis is to identify deviations from normal and their causes. The existence of a deviation from normal is usually easy to observe, but the identification of its cause may be more difficult. This is due to the fact that the primary gait disturbance is mixed with the effect of compensatory reactions which are evoked to maintain propulsion and postural control. The effect of a compensatory postural change is a change of the loads on bones and muscles, a change which will diminish pain, or the adverse effects of weakness and bad coordination. This compensatory change of the gait pattern may be considerable and the part mainly observed in a gait disturbance.

The primary effects can strike the peripheral movement apparatus, including muscles and peripheral nerves as well as the central nervous system. In the first case the compensation is effected by a normal central nervous system. In the second case the compensation has to be effected by an already damaged central organization.

An example of compensation of a primary peripheral affect is the so-called cock gait of a patient with damage to the peroneal nerve with resulting paresis of muscles which dorsiflex the ankle. To achieve toe clearance the patient must increase the flexion of hip and knee during swing.

When the inability to dorsiflex the foot is due to damage of the central nervous system, as in hemiparesis, the compensatory movement is quite different. In this case the leg tends to be spastically extended during swing and therefore has to be moved outwards in a circular movement, so-called *circumduction*.

It is useful to divide the compensatory reactions into three stages, *acute*, *subacute* and *chronic*, each with different significance. The *acute* compensation is seen in the stumbling corrective reaction (Forssberg, 1979). The disturbing factor is unexpected, and if balance is retained the normal pattern of movement is regained after a few strides. The correction is unconditioned; it is dependent upon genetically determined postural reflexes. In the *subacute* compensatory reaction the primary defect is already established. The pattern of movement is conditioned to the defect, it is well adapted and consistent. The gait following an injury of the ankle may serve as an example. The compensatory change disappears with healing of the injury. If the healing takes a long time the changed movement pattern may remain as a "bad" habit and need physiotherapy to remove it. In the *chronic* compensatory change there are structural changes in muscles, bones, and joints. They will not disappear if the primary defect is healed and, if reconstructive surgery is considered, the origin and present state of the defect must be thoroughly evaluated if lasting benefit is to be obtained.

The main objective of compensation is to maintain propulsion in spite of pain, paresis, or risk of falling. Except for the specific changes in movement patterns already mentioned, there are general reactions, such as decreased velocity and shorter strides on a wide base. In a gait disorder the velocity is always decreased. This is to some degree an expression of the primary affect. A patient with a paresis cannot manage to move the body weight as fast as a healthy subject, but equally important is the fact that the patient may not be sufficiently strong to parry the forces arising at foot strike when the body decelerates. The deceleration forces become less when velocity is low and the obvious compensation is therefore to decrease velocity.

Another general method of compensation is to decrease stride length. Short strides are less risky, the duration of swing is shorter, and the period of double support is longer. The effect is to lessen postural strain. Simultaneously, short strides may be an expression of the paretic leg's inability to carry the body weight more than a short distance. Low velocity and short strides therefore express both the primary affect and how it is compensated.

The compensatory reactions imply an increased tax on available resources, which can be measured as an increase of EMG activity in relevant muscles and increased metabolism per stride.

BIBLIOGRAPHY

Eidelberg, E., Walden, J. G., & Nguyen, L. H.

(1981). Locomotor control in macaque monkeys. *Brain, 104,* 647–63.

Forssberg, H. (1979). Stumbling corrective reaction: a phasedependent compensatory reaction during locomotion. *Journal of Neurophysiology, 42,* 936–53.

Grillner, S. B., Zanger, P. (1979). On the central generation of locomotion in the low spinal cat. *Experimental Brain Research, 34,* 241–61.

Larsson, L.-E. (1985). Gait analysis: an introduction. In M. Swash & C. Kennard (Eds), *The scientific basis of clinical neurology* (pp. 98–107). Edinburgh: Churchill Livingstone.

Patla, A. E. (Ed.). (1991). *Advances in psychology.* Vol. 78: *Adaptability of human gait.* Amsterdam: North Holland.

Rose, J., & Gamble, J. G. (Eds) (1993). *Human walking,* 2nd edn. Baltimore, MD: Williams & Wilkins.

LARS-ERIK LARSSON

Ganser syndrome The Ganser syndrome is a neuropsychiatric syndrome in which the most striking symptom is the giving of approximate answers, also referred to as "answering past the point" or *vorbeireden*. It is generally regarded as a pseudodementia and of psychogenic origin, although it may be seen in association with a primary neurological illness.

The giving of approximate answers is an intriguing and bizarre behavior. In response to simple factual questions, the patient gives the incorrect answer, yet an answer which seems to demonstrate that the patient understands the purpose of the question and in some way knows the correct answer yet does not give it; the answer is wrong, but always close to the correct answer. Typical "Ganser responses" might be: "How many legs does a dog have? Five. How many states in the USA? 51. What is the color of the sky? Red." The patient may also give a common but incorrect name as his or her own and unusual circumlocutory definitions of common objects. It has been proposed that numerical answers are often incorrect by one integer, but this is not invariably the case, and may indeed be uncommon. The responses may also resemble those given in CONFABULATION.

Other symptoms are present in the Ganser syndrome: disorientation, fluctuations of consciousness, mood disturbances, hallucinations, and hysterical stigmata. The whole constellation of symptoms has a sudden offset, followed by complete amnesia for the period during which the symptoms prevailed. The patient is not incapacitated in the tasks of everyday life in the way that a dementing patient with similar cognitive disturbances would be affected. The condition has been explained in a variety of ways: as a hysterical reaction (*see* HYSTERIA), as a psychotic thought disorder (note the similarity with BUFFOONERY), as malingering (the impression that the patient is consciously and deliberately giving the incorrect answer is difficult to escape), and as organic confusion. However, a clear neurological basis for the disorder has never been established, and the presence of other psychiatric and particularly hysterical symptoms, and a context which would suggest psychogenesis, have resulted in the current view that the Ganser syndrome is not a true dementia but a pseudodementia. Nevertheless, reported cases have often followed head injury or other organic conditions, but these may have served to precipitate the disorder rather than representing the primary cause. It may be that the neurological disturbance interacts with the functional processes, giving an apparently neuropsychological expression to what are essentially psychogenic symptoms.

J. GRAHAM BEAUMONT

gaze Gaze is the current direction of eye fixation, and the control of gaze involves volitional control of the appropriate eye movements (*see* EYE MOVEMENT).

Gaze has also been associated with attentional mechanisms and in this context with selective activation of one of the two cerebral hemispheres. Kinsbourne's attentional hypothesis of hemispheric activation in the explanation of lateral cerebral asymmetries (*see* LATERALIZATION) involves lateral deviation of gaze, so that gaze is directed towards the side of visual space opposite to the hemisphere of greater activation (*see* LATERAL EYE MOVEMENTS). This lateral deviation of gaze is associated with the concurrent mental activity, and may be used as an index of relative hemispheric activation.

Psychic paralysis of gaze is an alternative term for BÁLINT'S SYNDROME and emphasizes the importance of control of gaze in the exploration of visual space. Bálint's syndrome involves a failure of voluntary gaze orientation, but only when higher-order mental tasks are involved, together with optic ataxia, a failure of conjugate eye movements under visual control as in grasping, which are both linked with a failure of visual attention so that peripheral visual stimuli fail to be perceived. In this syndrome gaze is normally spontaneously deviated to the right.

J. GRAHAM BEAUMONT

Gegenhalten   *Gegenhalten* or "counterpull" is a form of increased muscle tone in which the patient increasingly offers semivoluntary resistance to passive movement of a limb. For example, if the patient's elbow is extended the patient will resist, and the resistance will increase as the elbow is further extended. This motor sign is associated with frontal lobe disease, in particular with the involvement of areas 4 and 6 or their rich subcortical connections, when it is also likely to accompany motor paralysis.

gelastic epilepsy   *See* EPILEPSY; LAUGHING.

gender difference   *See* SEX DIFFERENCES.

general paralysis of the insane (GPI)   General paralysis of the insane (GPI), also known as *general paresis*, is a form of neurosyphilis, a cerebral infection.

First described in the early nineteenth century, the disease rapidly spread by venereal infection until it was pandemic throughout Europe, America, and beyond. Its historical importance, besides its significant social effects, is in its being the first psychiatric illness for which a clear neuropathological mechanism was demonstrated, followed by a test (the Wassermann reaction) and an effective treatment (penicillin). Following the introduction of penicillin, the prevalence of the disease declined to a point at which it became uncommon, but there have been recent increases, notably in North America.

While there are other forms of syphilitic disease, GPI is the only form in which the infecting spirochetes actually invade the brain and directly produce the ensuing lesions. Behaviorally, the result is a dementing process with an insidious onset, in which changes in affect or personality more commonly precede the deterioration in cognitive function. Males are more commonly affected than females, with an onset from infection of anything between 5 and 25 years. The age of onset is highly variable, modally between 30 and 50, and congenital cases occur in childhood.

The early symptoms are the insidious changes in temperament associated with many organic reactions: moodiness, irritability, apathy, and reduced emotional control. There may also be egocentricity and some degree of social disinhibition; the early cognitive changes are reduced concentration, mental slowing, and episodic forgetfulness. The course may then follow a variety of identified forms. The classic form is a grandiose type in which the patient is bombastic, euphoric, and good-humored with delusions of power, wealth, or status. However, other forms in which the course is a generalized dementia (simple dementing form), or strongly resembles a major depressive illness (depressive form), comprise a substantial proportion of cases. There is also a taboparetic form which resembles the condition tabes dorsalis (another form of syphilis of the nervous system characterized by pain and motor disorders in the lower limbs with a characteristic abnormal gait; GPI and tabes dorsalis are the two forms of parenchymatous neurosyphilis), as well as other rarer forms. In all forms there may be coarse tremor of the hands and face, which results in the majority of cases in a degree of DYSARTHRIA, a characteristic mask-like expression, reflex abnormalities, and ATAXIA.

Various serological tests are critical in the diagnosis of GPI and a good outcome can be obtained with early diagnosis and treatment, for which penicillin is still the agent of choice. Untreated, the infection runs a progressive course to death.

J. GRAHAM BEAUMONT

geniculate body   The geniculate bodies form two paired nuclei which are located in the THALAMUS. The *lateral* geniculate bodies are an important relay station in the visual system, receiving information from the optic nerves via the OPTIC CHIASM and passing information to the striate cortex of the occipital lobe, so forming the geniculostriate visual system. Topographic representation of the visual fields is preserved in the lateral geniculate bodies. The *medial* geniculate bodies form similar thalamic nuclei for the auditory system. Information from the auditory nerve via the inferior COLLICULUS passes to both the ventral and dorsal portions of the medial geniculate. From the ventral medial geniculate it passes to primary auditory cortex in the superior TEMPORAL LOBE, while the dorsal portion projects to secondary auditory cortex, providing multiple ascending pathways to the cortex.

J. GRAHAM BEAUMONT

Gerstmann syndrome   The Gerstmann syndrome refers to a constellation of deficits that frequently appear to cluster together. It consists of finger AGNOSIA, RIGHT–LEFT DISORIENTATION, AGRAPHIA, and ACALCULIA. This pattern of deficits was first observed by Josef Gerstmann in the 1930s. The syndrome now carries his name. It was suggested that this combination of deficits resulted from dominant hemisphere pathology. Later work appeared to highlight the parietal-occipital junction or angular gyrus, a finding which appeared to give the syndrome significant value in localizing lesions.

Later work brought into question the strength of the interrelationship between the four components of the syndrome. The main issue concerned whether these were the only symptoms and whether they did indeed invariably cluster together. Studies revealed that the four components of the Gerstmann syndrome frequently occur with other disorders of cognitive function such as constructional apraxia, dysphasia, or general intellectual impairment. Indeed, it has been observed that the strength of the concordance between the four entities of the syndrome is no stronger than between other combinations of functions related to the parietal lobe. Other researchers found that, in those instances where the defects did cluster together, they were usually accompanied by significant impairments in other areas, bringing into question the validity of the term "syndrome" in the pure sense of the word.

With regards to the value of the syndrome in localizing pathology, it is useful when looking for evidence of lesions in the dominant hemisphere and possibly within the parietal lobe itself. The certainty of such placement increases with the number of symptoms present; however, more recent research has brought into question the value of the syndrome in localizing any more specifically.

In support of the concept it has been suggested that the presence of a pure form of the Gerstmann syndrome is rarely observed simply because lesions confined to the critical area are rare. In addition, further research may reveal a common disturbance underlying each of the pertinent deficits, which may serve to strengthen the concept.

MARCUS J. C. ROGERS

gestural behavior   From a neuropsychological perspective, the term gestural behavior encompasses a broad range of abilities including "natural" gesture (e.g. the pantomimed use of objects), learned meaningful gestures (e.g. saluting) and structured gestural languages (e.g. American Sign Language for the Deaf). Both expression and comprehension of each aspect of this complex arena can be compromised by brain lesions.

The specific topic to be covered here is the comprehension of "natural" gestural language, which sometimes goes under the heading of *pantomime recognition*, that is, this entry will be dealing with a specific aspect of the gestural behavioral repertoire, comprehension of *meaningful gestural communications*, such as the pretended use of common objects. In particular, the discussion will concentrate on the nature and significance of deficits in this ability, its anatomic correlates, and its importance for APHASIA. While defective gestural comprehension has no specific name, it was at one time referred to as being symptomatic of a generalized deficit called ASYMBOLIA. As an operational definition, it may also be viewed as being the receptive side of ideomotor APRAXIA. It is important to note, as Critchley (1953) among others has demonstrated, that understanding of natural gestural communication can be well preserved in deaf signers who have lost the gestural language skills they had been taught, and is thus quite distinct from this type of "artificial" gestural language.

BACKGROUND

Comprehension of natural gestures (i.e. pantomime recognition) denotes the ability to understand a type of gestural communication in which an object's pretended use is depicted and the "receiver" accurately deciphers the movements to identify what object was being used. It is, in a simultaneously simple and complex way, a means of naming objects by gesture. As being part of the human, or more precisely, prehuman behavioral repertoire, meaningful natural gestural communication is an antecedent to spoken language dating back at least 2 million years. Indeed, it has been speculated that the rapid evolution of spoken language was made possible by the fact that hominids were already able to communicate by meaningful gestures (Hewes, 1973).

EARLY SPECULATIONS AND OBSERVATIONS

A number of nineteenth-century aphasiologists and behavioral neurologists noted that aphasic patients were often impaired in the comprehension of gestural as well as verbal *language symbols*. This conceptualization (i.e. "language symbols") led to the formulation of the concept of asymbolia. Put simply, this defined aphasia not as a disorder of language, but as a disorder of symbolization and symbol recognition. This concept, often associated with the otherwise undistinguished name of Finkelnburg, reached its most sophisticated conceptualization in the works of Hughlings Jackson (1878) and Henry Head (1920). That aphasics were impaired in gestural understanding was often used as proof that aphasia was indeed a symbolization disorder, or even a disability of dementia-like severity. However, as Hughlings Jackson noted, not all aphasics were impaired in use and comprehension of gestures and thus not all suffered a loss of what he termed *propositional thinking*. It remained possible that the determinants of impaired pantomime recognition were more specific, and that comprehension of natural gestures was a primary mental ability.

MODERN NEUROPSYCHOLOGICAL STUDIES

A series of studies have been performed since 1969, concerned with pantomime recognition defect (and whether it reflects asymbolia). While one could conceptualize pantomime recognition as being a non-verbal ability, multiple studies have demonstrated that defects in pantomime recognition occur almost exclusively in association with left hemisphere damage, the defect being highly uncommon except among aphasics (and patients with NEGLECT who fail because of visuoperceptual impairment having nothing specific to do with the gestural stimuli). Thus, impaired pantomime recognition is as essentially an aphasic deficit as more traditional language symptoms such as anomia or agraphia (Duffy et al., 1975).

Varney and Benton, in a series of studies (see Varney, 1982), were able to discard the notion that impaired pantomime recognition was evidence of a generalized asymbolia or loss of the ABSTRACT ATTITUDE, but gave impaired pantomime recognition a different significance for aphasia. Specifically, they employed a testing technique in which pantomimes were recorded on videotape and subjects identified the object whose use was pantomimed from among four choices. Borrowing from related work on sound recognition by De Renzi, Vignolo and associates, each test trial, besides the correct response (e.g. an axe), included a number of foils, an item belonging to the same semantic class (e.g. a saw), another test item not related to the stimulus (e.g. a fork), and an "odd" item, being an object whose use could not be pantomimed (e.g. an anvil). Thus, not only could subjects be evaluated in terms of number, but also the nature of correct vs incorrect responses could be seen (Varney & Benton, 1983).

In a series of studies, Varney and Benton (e.g. 1983) were able to demonstrate the following specific findings: (1) All aphasics with defects in pantomime recognition were also at least as severely impaired in reading comprehension. (2) Pantomime recognition had no other predictable relationships with aural comprehension or any other aspect of language functioning. (3) Some left brain-injured patients, including Wernicke and global aphasics, performed normally in pantomime recognition despite being grossly impaired in reading comprehension. (4) Errors in pantomime recognition very strongly favored the semantic foils (i.e. more than 70 percent of errors involved this foil when "chance" would predict 33 percent), suggesting that the patients had a rough but not exact understanding of the stimulus. (5) Severe defects in pantomime recognition could coexist with quite good performances on tests of non-verbal reasoning, such as WAIS Block Design or Raven's Progressive Matrices. (6)

Despite the close relationship between pantomime recognition and reading comprehension, no such relationship was found between pantomime recognition and letter recognition (Varney, 1982).

Overall, these findings suggested that the old concept of asymbolia might have elements worth saving, but it was not the explanation of the relationship between impaired gestural understanding (i.e. pantomime recognition) and aphasia. Specifically, it appeared that failure to understand gestures was part of a mental disability in which the patient was not impaired in auditory comprehension and not necessarily impaired in other visually mediated abilities except reading comprehension, but the disability involved at least some approximate understanding (partial misunderstanding) of the gestures' meaning. In another way, it could be said that impaired pantomime recognition or impaired gestural comprehension was part of a specific disturbance in the understanding of meaningful visual stimuli. While reading comprehension and gestural comprehension involve visually mediated and meaningful stimuli (and are closely related), letters of the alphabet were not meaningful in a semantic sense, aural comprehension was not visual, and non-verbal reasoning tasks were not communicative, much less semantically meaningful. Thus, impaired pantomime recognition lacked one or more important common elements with each of the abilities mentioned except reading. Even here, however, reading has properties not shared with gestural comprehension and can be impaired while pantomime recognition remains well within normal limits.

ANTHROPOLOGICAL CONSIDERATIONS

Gestural communication has been part of the hominid behavioral repertoire for a decidedly longer period than spoken language, and doubtless as the complexity of gestural communication increased there were corresponding changes in the brain for interpretation of these gestural communications as part of the evolutionary process (Hewes, 1973). Indeed, without better "decoders" more sophisticated gestural communications would have been pointless. Reading, by contrast, is a cultural development without the possibility of corresponding neuroanatomic adaptation, that is, written language was invented

only 6,000 years ago, literacy did not become common in Western culture until this century, and individuals from cultures with no written language tradition can learn to read. Thus, no part of the brain has been evolved for the specific purpose of decoding written words. Rather, the CNS processing which underlies the reading process involves structures and connections evolved for other purposes. In physical anthropology, this type of phenomenon is called preadaptation. In these circumstances, it could be said that the close association between impaired comprehension of gestures and impaired reading comprehension suggests that CNS tissue originally evolved for the interpretation of meaningful gestures is employed for at least part of the reading process (see Varney & Vilenski, 1980). It is interesting to note in this regard that pantomime recognition matures very rapidly in children and is at essentially adult levels between the ages of 4 and 6, the years when word reading is usually first taught successfully (i.e. it may be a developmental milestone necessary as a precursor for successful reading acquisition).

NEUROANATOMICAL CONSIDERATIONS

As impaired pantomime recognition is so closely associated with left hemisphere damage and impaired reading comprehension, one would suspect that the intrahemispheric lesions responsible for defective pantomime recognition would closely parallel those associated with the various lesion loci causing ALEXIA. This is indeed the case. Lesions in most areas of the posterior peri-Sylvian region (e.g. Wernicke's area, the angular gyrus) and lesions of the basal ganglia appear to be the primary responsible lesion sites. Specifically, the lesion sites associated with impaired pantomime recognition were Brodmann areas 40, 39, 41, 42, 22, and 37 (as well as the basal ganglia). The possible implication of the thalamus and occipital lobe has also been suggested.

Interestingly, the studies which reported the data mentioned above, Varney and Damasio (1987, 1989), found that patients could have lesions involving multiple areas on the posterior peri-Sylvian horseshoe without being impaired in pantomime recognition (though they were still impaired in reading comprehension). It was suggested that, while the majority of right-handed individuals showed left hemisphere dominance

363

for gestural comprehension, about 30 percent showed bilateral hemispheric involvement in the task (right dominance being highly unlikely, given that impaired pantomime recognition from right-sided lesions in patients without neglect is very rare). An alternative view, placing far more specific emphasis on lesions of Wernicke's area, has been expressed by Ferro et al. (1983).

CONCLUSION

The understanding of meaningful, natural, gestural communications, and the loss of that ability as a result of brain damage, have multiple and important implications for human brain function, particularly for how language processing evolved and how it can become impaired. The material presented above outlines a number of different facets of this process. However, further illumination of the issues raised above is necessary for a number of areas, and may eventually be resolved by new technologies like PET scanning and the improvement of cerebral blood flow technology.

BIBLIOGRAPHY

Critchley, M. (1953). *The parietal lobes*. London: Edward Arnold.
Duffy, R., Duffy, J., & Pearson, K. (1975). Pantomime recognition in aphasic patients. *Journal of Speech and Hearing Research, 18*, 115–32.
Ferro, J., Martens, I., Mariano, G., & Castro-Caldas, J. (1983). CT scan correlates of gesture recognition. *Journal of Neurology, Neurosurgery and Psychiatry, 46*, 943–52.
Head, H. (1920). *Aphasia and kindred disorders of speech*. London: Hafner.
Hewes, G. (1973). Primate communication and the gestural origin of language. *Current Anthropology, 14*, 5–24.
Jackson, H. (1878). On afflictions of speech from disease of the brain. *Brain, 1*, 304–30.
Varney, N. R. (1982). Pantomime recognition defect in aphasia: implications for the concept of asymbolia. *Brain and Language, 15*, 32–9.
Varney, N. R., & Benton, A. L. (1983). Qualitative aspects of pantomime recognition defect in aphasia. *Brain and Cognition, 1*, 132–9.
Varney, N. R., & Damasio, H. (1987). Locus of lesion in impaired pantomime recognition. *Cortex, 23*, 699–703.
Varney, N. R., & Damasio, H. (1989). The role of individual difference in determining the nature of comprehension defects in aphasia. *Cortex, 25*, 47–55.
Varney, N. R., & Vilenski, J. (1980). Neuropsychological implications for preadaptation and language evolution. *Journal of Human Evolution, 9*, 223–6.

NILS R. VARNEY

Gilles de La Tourette syndrome The syndrome of Gilles de la Tourette is a rare genetic disorder with an onset during childhood, characterized by facial TICS, with a minority of children also compelled to utter forced vocalizations and profanities (COPRALALIA). The genetic defect has been located on chromosome 18.

The syndrome is commoner among boys than girls in a ratio of about 3 to 1 (like so many developmental abnormalities). Onset in most cases is between the ages of 5 and 8 and is rare after 11. Although the facial tics are the most prominent, multiple tics occur and are different from other abnormal movements in showing a repeated stereotyped pattern. The tics may be of considerable force and severity and whole body movements may be involved, resulting in involuntary jumping, skipping, or hopping.

The compulsive vocalizations usually develop subsequent to the tics; initially grunts, barks, or coughing noises linked to the tics which may later develop into single words and then into expletives, oaths, and brief obscene phrases, often at around the time of puberty. Reviews suggest that this stage is reached in about half of all cases. There may also be a compulsion to think obscenities and this may be commoner than overt coprolalia. The symptoms are exacerbated by emotional arousal, but diminish with the ingestion of alcohol, during sexual arousal, and during periods of intense concentration. ECHOLALIA, ECHOPRAXIA, and echokinesis may also be present. The course is variable and the outcome uncertain, although there is a tendency to remission during adolescence.

There have been a variety of theories about the origins of this bizarre and intriguing syndrome, including psychogenic disturbances, psychoanalytic disorders, and early brain damage or infection. The debate among these explanations has largely been resolved by the identification of the associated genetic abnormality, although the precise nature of the mechanism which precipitates the disorder has not. Psychogenic factors, including childhood experiences, may well play a role in the expression of the disorder. The prominence of the abnormal movements naturally suggests an abnormality within the BASAL GANGLIA.

Although sufferers from Gilles de La Tourette syndrome are usually of normal and may be of superior intelligence, various neuropsychological deficits have been reported. The deficits noted have included drawing and memory for complex geometric figures (the Rey figure), together with reduced word fluency and memory for semantic verbal material. These findings naturally suggest deficits in the frontal and temporal lobes which might, in turn, be linked to deficiencies in the inhibition of, and perseveration of, complex motor movements, and the inhibition of socially unacceptable utterances, but this is speculative.

J. GRAHAM BEAUMONT

glioma   Gliomas (gliomata) are the commonest form of intracranial neoplasm, and grow from the glia or supporting tissue of the nervous system. All gliomas are infiltrative tumors and are therefore extremely difficult to remove and are likely to recur. The classification of gliomas is still a matter of debate, but the forms include: *astrocytomas*, which grow slowly and are relatively benign; *glioblastomas* (glioblastoma multiforme), which grow more rapidly and are extremely malignant; a form of glioma more commonly arising in childhood and in the cerebellum, *medulloblastoma*; and *oligodendroglioma*, a rare and relatively benign slow-growing tumor occurring more commonly in young adults.

global amnesia   *See* AMNESIA; AMNESIC SYNDROME.

global aphasia   *See* APHASIA.

globalists   The globalist school, active at the end of the nineteenth century, adopted a position counter to the associationists and localizationists (*see* ASSOCIATIONISM, LOCALIZATION). The globalists did not accept that higher-level func-

tions could be assigned to cortical areas, but asserted that such functions emerged as a dynamic process out of the integrated action of the entire brain. The debate between globalists and associationists/localizationists, centered principally around the cerebral representation of language function, continued well into the current century and has never been finally resolved. It is possible to see the influence of these two general approaches in the discussion of the effects of the COMMISSUROTOMY operation in the 1960s, and the issue has again been raised in considering the potential validity of connectionist models of neuropsychological function (*see* NEUROPSYCHOLOGY).

globus pallidus   The globus pallidus is a part of the BASAL GANGLIA which receives input from the CAUDATE NUCLEUS and sends projections to the ventral lateral nucleus of the THALAMUS. It lies medial to the PUTAMEN and below the thalamus. As part of the basal ganglia it is involved in motor function, and lesions may be associated with changes in posture, muscle tone, or abnormal movements, although certain disorders of the basal ganglia, such as PARKINSON'S DISEASE or HUNTINGTON'S DISEASE, also have behavioral and emotional aspects.

grand mal epilepsy   *See* EPILEPSY.

graphesthesia   Graphesthesia is the ability to identify symbolic material, normally numbers or letters, traced on the skin with a blunt instrument, and out of vision. Graphesthesia is therefore the loss of this ability, and is a somesthetic disturbance.

grasp reflex   The grasp reflex is normal in infants, but is an abnormal sign in adults and may follow focal or diffuse brain damage. The grasp reflex of the hand may be elicited by a moving tactile stimulus passing across the palm between the thumb and index finger, when the patient's thumb and fingers grasp in tonic flexion; attempts to withdraw the stimulating object result in strengthening of the grasp. A similar reflex may be observed in the foot on stimulation of the plantar aspect of the toes, so that the toes remain in tonic flexion. The hand grasp reflex is indicative of a lesion in the prefrontal cortex of the frontal lobe, and when it is unilateral is most commonly on the side contralateral to the lesion. The foot grasp reflex only occurs with lesions in the superior part of the prefrontal cortex.

groping reflex   The groping reflex is one of the primitive reflexes, that is, it is normal in infants but abnormal in children and adults. It is less common than the GRASP REFLEX with which it frequently occurs. The hand, and often the eyes, of the patient tend to follow an object (under examination, typically the fingers of the examiner) in a magnetic fashion. As with other primitive reflexes, it is generally regarded as a sign of the release of these reflexes from normal frontal lobe inhibition and is therefore indicative of a frontal lobe lesion.

H

hallucination A hallucination is a sensory perception without external stimulation of the relevant sensory organ. Hallucinations are therefore contrasted with *illusions*, which involve the misperception of real physical stimuli. In some cases the individual may believe the hallucination to be an event in the real world; at other times the hallucination may be embedded in a delusional context; and in still other cases the hallucination, while vivid, may be recognized as a purely subjective experience.

Hallucinations may occur with all types of cerebral pathology, most commonly in the context of confusion, dementia, delusions, or paroxysmal activity. There is, of course, debate about whether the hallucinations which characterize certain functional disorders, notably SCHIZOPHRENIA, have some form of organic basis, but there is a general observation that the hallucinations in functional states are more commonly auditory and somesthetic in character, while the hallucinations which accompany gross organic pathology are more likely to be visual or olfactory; but this is not universally the case. There may well be a bias towards the reporting of certain types of hallucination, in relation to given pathological states, in the literature.

Hallucinations may also occur in a relatively pure form in association with localized damage to elements of the visual system and this may be true for other sensory modalities; the visual system has been subject to more study in this respect. Visual hallucinations are reported to occur in around 2 to 3 per cent of patients with occipital lesions. Damage to the secondary visual cortex and to areas of the occipito- parietal region may result in hallucinations of objects, people, and animals which may be perceived as engaged in specific activities. While there is a tendency for unformed images to be reported with damage to the visual pathways and primary visual cortex, and for full percepts to follow damage to secondary visual association areas, this is not invariably the pattern and there are reports of well-formed visual hallucinations following eye disease. Other visual impairments may contribute to the occurrence of visual hallucinations, as may a high-level deficit in the ability to distinguish between veridical and hallucinatory percepts and the confidence in determining true percepts. One current hypothesis suggests that some hallucinations may arise from the faulty momentary reconstruction of the feature fragments of images, a result which is more likely to occur when defects in the system of visual perception result in the distortion of features, which makes the correct perception of the stimulus events less likely.

Hallucinations are also important in association with the aura preceding certain partial epilepsy phenomena, where they may be not only visual or auditory, but are also commonly hallucinations of smell (*see* EPILEPSY, temporal lobe epilepsy). Hallucinations also occur in NARCOLEPSY and in HYPNAGOGIC PHENOMENA, although they may commonly occur in any acute organic reaction.

J. GRAHAM BEAUMONT

handedness Humans differ from other animals in that nine out of ten of them prefer their *right* hand for skilled tasks. That alone is sufficiently surprising to merit detailed study. However, its association with cerebral language lateralization also makes handedness a useful surrogate for studying the far less tractable phenomenon of cerebral dominance. Research on handedness, and particularly its genetics, often therefore supposes that appropriate models for handedness may well also be appropriate models for language dominance.

Handedness is essentially very simple, and is probably best assessed, in the absence of known

367

social pressure, by the hand used for writing. Its measurement has sometimes been rendered overly complex while yet missing its full subtlety. Three principal problems arise: the distinction between *skill* and *preference*; the nature of the *distribution* of laterality scores; and the different *laterality measures* that can be derived.

A person can be right-handed in two distinct senses: given a moderately skilled unimanual task they *prefer* to use the right hand; and when tested in turn with right and left hands they are more *skilled* with the right hand. Handedness/skill and handedness/preference are generally highly correlated, although that is not always the case.

MEASUREMENT OF HANDEDNESS

Measurement of handedness/skill

Many tasks have been used for assessing skill in the two hands. One of the most frequently used is the Annett pegboard task which measures the time for each hand to move ten pegs in a board as quickly as possible from one row of holes to another. Although originally scored as $Time_{Left} - Time_{Right}$, a common form of scoring computes $100x(Time_{Left} - Time_{Right})/(Time_{Left} + Time_{Right})$ which assesses proportional hand differences independently of overall ability. Although popular, in part because it requires few instructions and can be used even at age 3 or 4, the test cannot be administered in groups and shows only small between-hand differences of about 4 percent, with a large overlap in distribution of right- and left-handers. Group testing is better carried out using the Tapley and Bryden task, in which a pencil is used in each hand in turn to place dots in as many circles as possible in 20 seconds. The laterality index is calculated as $100x(N_{Right} - N_{Left})/(N_{Right} + N_{Left})$. The test is quick and reliable, and produces larger hand differences (about 10–12 percent) with little overlap in performance of right- and left-hand writers. Nevertheless there is still substantial variation within right- and left-handers. Other useful tasks include Bishop's square-tracing task (Bishop, 1990), and the dot-making task of the National Child Development Study. Finger-tapping speed also differentiates right and left hands, but is not as useful for routine testing. Strength differences do not relate to handedness and do not assess skill. Practice affects overall performance on skill tests but even when intense has minimal impact on left–right differences; likewise extensive practice on asymmetric skilled tasks transfers little to other tasks.

Measurement of handedness/preference in adults

Hand preference in adults can be assessed using questionnaires, of which there are many in the literature, typically having 4 to 60 questions, asking about the preferred hand for a particular task on a three-, five-, or seven-point scale (e.g. always right, usually right, either, usually left, or always left). Questionnaires differ principally in length and appropriateness of items. The Edinburgh Handedness Inventory with 10 items is popular, although its original response method is eccentric, and is better used with the five-point scale described earlier (when perhaps it could be the standard questionnaire method for handedness research). The Annett questionnaire is similar in format but with 12 items on a three-point response scale. In recent years longer questionnaires have become popular, such as the Waterloo Handedness Questionnaire with 60 separate questions, a few of which are inappropriate outside North America. A laterality index from questionnaires is typically derived by scoring +2 for a response of "always right," +1 for "usually right," 0 for "either," −1 for "usually left," and −2 for "always left," summing responses across items (after reversing scores on questions for which right-handers normally use the left hand), and standardizing so that persons answering "always right" or "always left" to all items score +100 and −100 respectively; a complete lack of preference then scores as zero.

Questionnaires with less than 12 or so items typically show a J-shaped distribution of scores, with many right-handers in particular scoring at maximum (e.g. Figure 42e). Such floor and ceiling effects invalidate many statistical analyses. Questionnaires with more than about 25 items show distributions closer to a mixture of two normal distributions, with less censoring at the top and bottom ends of the scale. The distribution of left-handers is typically shifted somewhat more towards zero than is the distribution of right-handers, usually due to items with cultural biases (e.g. using a screwdriver, winding a clock, holding a knife when eating with a knife and fork); exclusion of such items restores symmetry.

Measurement of handedness/preference in children

Hand preference in children from the age of 10

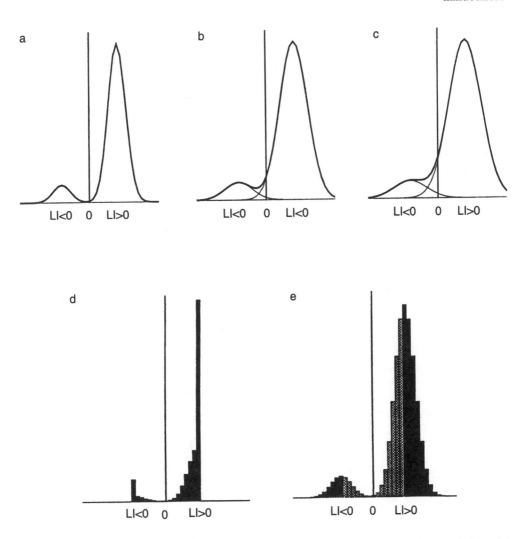

Figure 42 Laterality index distributions found for measures of handedness. a–c. Symmetric bimodal distributions with (a) almost no overlap, (b) mild overlap, and (c) moderate overlap, showing how the distribution can be bimodal or unimodal, according to the spread of the distributions. d. A typical J-shaped distribution of the type seen in handedness questionnaires, obtained by censoring the distribution of Figure 42a at the mean of each distribution. e. Arbitrary division of handedness into Left (left-hand distribution), Right (right-hand distribution), and "Mixed" (center distribution) showing how the "mixed" category confounds weak right-handers and weak left-handers.

can be assessed using questionnaires (Bryden & Steenhuis, 1991). With younger children, preference is usually assessed by performance measures in which it is observed which hand is used when the child carries out a number of simple tasks (such as drawing, hammering, taking a sweet). A laterality index can be derived by summing across measures as for questionnaires.

There are no standardized assessments of preference in infants, although many different measures show asymmetries.

Factorial structure of questionnaires

Several attempts have been made in recent years to use conventional methods of factor analysis for isolating different components of handedness.

Commonly two or more factors emerge, one of which appears to be "fine skill," involving the fingers in complex coordinated tasks, of which writing is the exemplar, and the other of which is "unskilled actions," often involving grosser, less subtle, more axial movements, as in carrying objects. The fine movement factor contains highly lateralized items and the unskilled factor the less lateralized items. These factors are probably artifacts due to violating the assumption in factor analysis that measures are multivariate normal. Item scores tend to be bimodal, with different proportions of right and left responses; factor analysis of such binomial measures results in artifactual "difficulty factors," and the factor structure should not therefore be trusted. Other multivariate techniques such as cluster analysis and association analysis may also produce artifacts with laterality data, and should not be relied on. At present handedness/preference is probably best conceptualized as unifactorial.

The distribution of laterality scores

Most measures of handedness/skill and handedness/preference consist of *mixture distributions*, usually of two normal distributions, one containing about 90 percent of the population and the other about 10 percent, placed approximately symmetrically about zero, and often censored at top and bottom ends (see Figure 42) – the *symmetric bimodal model*. The symmetry of such distributions makes it inappropriate to divide the distribution anywhere other than at zero.

Annett has claimed that her pegboard task is intrinsically unimodal, with the minor distribution centered at zero. Such a distribution is necessary in the right shift theory of the genetics of handedness (Annett, 1985), but is probably not supported by using appropriate statistical analysis (McManus, 1983) of empirical data, which finds a symmetric bimodal distribution even for the pegboard task. The apparent unimodal distribution is probably a result of the pegboard's particular task requirements (see Figures 42 a–c), and is not found for other tasks, even by Annett herself.

The four types of laterality measure

Bimodality of laterality scores has profound implications for the analysis of handedness and lateralization. Laterality scores should not be analyzed by statistical tests such as analysis of variance, t-tests, or correlations, both because they are far from normal, and because they seriously confound variation *within* component distributions with variation in proportions of subjects *between* component distributions. If the component distributions do not overlap substantially then two separate scores can readily be calculated: *direction of lateralization*, which is a binary variable, "right" if the laterality index is greater than zero, and "left" if the laterality index is less than or equal to zero (zero usually being included as left-handed); and *degree of lateralization*, the absolute value of the laterality index (i.e. ignoring its sign), approximately normal in distribution, and interpreted as strength of lateralization. If the components of the mixture overlap substantially then advanced statistical techniques can separate effects of direction and degree (McManus, 1983).

Some studies divide subjects into three classes: *right, left,* and *mixed*. This practice has little justification. If measurement is to "carve nature at its joints," then Figure 42 e shows that "mixed" handedness corresponds to no natural category; instead mixed handers are actually a mixture of weak right-handers and weak left-handers. If subjects are to be further subdivided then four groups are preferable (strong right, weak right, weak left, and strong left); alternatively the mean and SD of degree of lateralization should be reported separately for right- and left-handers. The problem is particularly serious in developmental studies if degree of lateralization increases with age, since the proportion of non-right-handers (i.e. mixed and left) will seemingly decrease with age, even though direction of lateralization is not truly changing.

In recent years the importance of distinguishing direction and degree of lateralization has been accepted. However, two other measures are as yet little used, despite one undoubtedly being important in understanding handedness. Consider a group of right-handers; their degree of lateralization is the mean lateralization score on individual questionnaire or performance items. Two different right-handers may have the same degree of lateralization and yet differ in *variance of lateralization* – one being moderately lateralized for all items, and the other showing strong lateralization for some items and no lateralization for other items. Although as yet hardly studied, variance of lateralization may be empirically important in distinguishing individuals.

The fourth measure, *ambiguous handedness*, requires that a set of items be administered twice to a subject. Two right-handed subjects may have an identical degree and variance of lateralization and yet one subject can be entirely consistent in hand usage *within tasks*, giving the same score *on both occasions*, whereas the other subject may be strongly right-handed on one occasion and subsequently weakly right-handed or even left-handed *at the same task*. This measure, of within-subject between-task unreliability, is called *ambiguous handedness* by Satz and his colleagues and differentiates children with autism from controls. In principle ambiguous handedness can be subdivided into *ambiguous direction of lateralization* and *ambiguous degree of lateralization*, although nothing has been published on that distinction. It should be noted that ambiguous handedness and degree of lateralization are inevitably partially confounded, although effects can be separated by analysis of covariance.

The interrelationship of handedness/preference and handedness/skill

For most subjects handedness/skill and handedness/preference are highly correlated, the preferred hand being more skilled on most tasks. An important exception finds a substantial minority of left-handers who, although more skilled at fine motor skills with the left hand, are more skilled at throwing with the *right* hand, are right-footed, and have stronger right hands. The origin of such *inconsistent left-handers* is not clear; neither is it clear if *inconsistent right-handers* exist in substantial numbers.

The association of skill and preference raises a causal question: Do right-handers prefer their right hand because it is more skillful, or is the right hand more skillful because of more practice due to being preferred? Cross-sectional studies in adults cannot answer that question. However, the finding that children with autism show population dominance for handedness/preference without the preferred hand being more skillful, implies that preference is causally prior to skill.

THE NEUROLOGICAL LOCUS OF HANDEDNESS

The anatomical locus of hand preference is not clear. The approximate, although not exact, bilateral symmetry of the bones, muscles, and nerves of right and left arms points to handedness originating in the central nervous system. A cortical origin is often assumed, partly because of skill asymmetries between hands, and partly because of the existence of other large functional asymmetries, as in Broca's area. However, if preference is prior to skill then handedness may result from subcortical mechanisms. Anatomical studies of the basal ganglia find asymmetries correlated with hand preference in the globus pallidus, an area functionally active in skilled motor learning. Lower in the hierarchy, handedness may be best construed as a "turning tendency," which in rats is mediated via small asymmetries in nigrostriatal dopamine and modified by injection into the substantia nigra.

THE FUNCTIONAL LOCUS OF HANDEDNESS

In right-handers the right hand is more skilled even on simple tasks such as repetitive tapping, at which it is faster and less variable. Peters has suggested that the superiority is due to more precise force modulation, due principally to more precise timing. Suggestions that handedness relates to superior visual-manual coordination are probably falsified by the normal incidence of right-handedness in congenitally blind subjects. It is interesting that handedness means precisely that, rather than a more general "sidedness," measures of asymmetry being greatest for distal movements and less for proximal, axial movements; this probably reflects two motor control systems, one pyramidal, contralateral, and distal, and the other non-pyramidal, bilateral, and proximal.

THE INCIDENCE OF LEFT-HANDEDNESS

Studies have claimed widely different incidences of left-handedness, from 1 percent to 35 percent. A recent meta-analysis of 284,665 individuals in 100 populations found an overall incidence of 7.78 percent, with a higher incidence in younger populations. No evidence was found for geographical differences; nevertheless questionnaire measures find differences between cultures, with lower incidences in Muslim and Far Eastern societies where cultural taboos prohibit left-hand use for activities such as eating. That right-handedness does not originate in cultural asymmetries due to writing is seen in a preliterate tribe of the Central Highlands of New Guinea of whom 10.3 percent were left-handed, a similar proportion to that elsewhere. Although anecdotes occasionally report populations with a majority of left-handers, none has been verified scientifically, and they are best viewed as modern myths.

Secular and age trends

Cross-sectional studies often find a lower incidence of left-handedness in older people. Interpretation is difficult because individual cross-sectional studies inevitably confound age effects and secular trends; thus, in a 1990 study, 30-year-olds were born in 1960 whereas 70-year-olds were born in 1920. Left-handedness has long been subject to social manipulation (Harris, 1990), particularly in the late nineteenth and early twentieth centuries, when schools forcibly prevented left-handed writing by children. Not surprisingly, that resulted in a lower manifest incidence of left-handedness. However, whether age trends can entirely explain secular trends is unclear, the effects not being disambiguated in a large meta-analysis. A study of 1,177,507 Americans showed no age effect in those aged under 41 (of whom 11.7 percent were left-handed writers), whereas above that age the incidence declined linearly. A far smaller age effect on throwing supported the existence of social pressure and secular trends. The point of inflection of the curve suggests that social pressures against left-handedness had ceased in the USA for cohorts born after 1945. Data on Victorian cricketers suggests that social pressure against left-handedness was absent in the early 1800s but present in the latter half of the century, only being lifted in the twentieth century.

Coren and Halpern (1991) interpreted age trends as evidence that left-handers have a reduced life expectancy. Their original data do not support that, since mean ages at death of right- and left-handers are not significantly different, and subsequent data relating age at death to handedness made serious epidemiological errors which ignored secular trends; neither have their data been replicated. Three causes for an increased mortality in left-handers were proposed: increased birth complications, auto-immune disorders, and accidents. The first two are considered below and rejected as unsupported by evidence. That accidents could be more common

in left-handers is very possible since in a complex, mechanical world their ergonomic needs are considered by few designers. Nevertheless, data claiming increased accidents in left-handers have yet to be replicated.

Sex differences

Sex differences in left-handedness have been controversial, although a meta-analysis shows clear evidence for left-handedness being more common in males than females, by about 27 percent; that is, for every five left-handed men there are four left-handed women. This ratio showed no secular or other changes, and in the recent very large US study is present at all ages; of those under age 41, 13.0 percent of males and 10.4 percent of females were left-handed writers.

The ontogeny of handedness

Handedness in young children is usually established between 18 months and 2 years of age. After that age, although direction seems fixed, degree of lateralization increases, probably throughout childhood and possibly throughout adulthood as well. Young infants show some evidence of predominant right-handedness, for instance, in how long they hold a rattle, although other asymmetries, the so-called turning tendencies such as the tonic neck reflex, do not seem to be obviously related to subsequent handedness. From 6 to 18 months infants pass through a "chaotic" phase of handedness, with direction of preference changing erratically, even from day to day, a phenomenon often causing confusion to parents. Despite such variability in infancy, ultrasonic observation of fetal behavior *in utero* suggests that even by 15 weeks of gestation about 90 percent of fetuses preferentially and consistently suck the right rather than the left thumb, with the direction related to subsequent head turning as neonates.

The phylogeny of handedness

That only a few people are left-handed has been recorded since ancient times, most notably in the Bible (Judges, 20: 15–16); and the associated symbolic differentiation of right and left into "good" and "bad" is prevalent in many geographically and temporally distinct cultures. Evidence for ancient handedness is necessarily indirect: during the past five millennia works of art portraying unimanual actions consistently show the left hand use in about 7.4 percent of cases; Neolithic bone tools of 7,000 years ago show evidence of being right-handed, as do Upper Paleolithic bone scrapers of 8,000 to 35,000 years ago, and stone tool flakes from 150,000–200,000 years ago. Wear patterns on teeth which are at least 250,000 years old are compatible with right-handedness, as also are flake patterns on Lower Pleistocene stone tools of 1.5–2 million years ago. Since hominids first clearly appear in the fossil record at that time, the implication is that right-handedness is an ancient trait whose evolution is tightly linked to human evolution itself.

Handedness, footedness, pawedness, and clawedness in nonhuman species

Individual animals in many species, including rats, mice, dogs, cats, rhesus monkeys, chimpanzees, and gorillas, show hand, foot, paw, or claw preference in the sense of repeatedly using one side rather than the other for skilled actions. However, in almost all species precisely 50 percent of individuals prefer the right side and 50 percent the left side; that is, they show *individual handedness* but not *population handedness*. Although primate species have been claimed to show population handedness, the studies suffer from methodological and statistical problems; careful studies have found no evidence for population handedness in gorillas or chimpanzees. An exception to the general rule seems to be the parrot, in which there may be population footedness, as was noted by Broca; the association of left-claw preference for holding objects, vocal mimicry, and asymmetric control of the syrinx in vocalization in some birds has provoked suggestions of a causal link, although the mechanism is unclear.

THEORIES OF LEFT-HANDEDNESS

Explanations of left-handedness suggest either a genetic or an environmental origin. Environmental theories come in weak and strong forms, with the strong forms assuming that right-handedness is universally the natural form, with environmental insults or pressures reversing that situation (Harris & Carlson, 1988).

Pathological left-handedness

The concept that left-handers are neurologically damaged is a recurrent one in the twentieth century, principally originating in the study of Gordon (1920). A particularly prevalent variant derives from the studies of Bakan, who suggested that left-handers showed an increased incidence of obstetric complications which caused minimal brain damage. Following the mathematical arguments of Satz, even if asymmetric damage randomly occurs in the right or left hemisphere, the consequence is necessarily increased left-handedness. Although mathematically correct the model fails empirically, a large number of studies failing to find increased obstetric complications in left-handers. An important exception is in extremely premature infants, weighing under 1 kilogram, in whom left-handedness is undoubtedly more common; however, that cannot be explained by Satz's model since laterality of lesions is unrelated to handedness. It is more likely that prematurity and left-handedness both result from developmental instability and fluctuating asymmetry caused by earlier developmental abnormalities. A similar explanation is necessary to explain the increased sinistrality found in much mental retardation, particularly in conditions such as trisomy 21 (Down's syndrome) with symmetric neurological damage: the implication in these cases is that individuals are not right-handers who have become pathologically left-handed, but rather that lateralization was never set up properly in the first place (primary rather than secondary pathological left-handedness). Bishop has assessed pathological left-handedness by measuring motor skill in the *nonpreferred* hand. Brain damage causing transfer of hand dominance from right to left should result in the right hand of such pathological left-handers being substantially impaired compared with the right hand of "natural" left-handers; Bishop estimates that only 1 in 20 left-handers has secondary pathological sinistrality. That pathological left-handedness undoubtedly occurs is seen in children with a history of severe, acute, neurological illness in the first three years of life; twice as many are left-handed as in matched controls, although the differences are mostly explained by concomitant sensory, motor, and intellectual deficits.

The Geschwind–Behan–Galaburda model of lateralization

Geschwind and Behan (1982) published an influential and much cited theory, subsequently extensively elaborated; the complex ramifications (McManus & Bryden, 1991) can only be summarized here. Essentially the theory is a strong pathological one, individuals normally being right-handed unless increased fetal testosterone levels retard left hemispheric development and cause left-handedness, atypical language lateralization, and a range of other conditions, of which the most surprising are immune disorders. The theory's most substantial evidence when first published was the highly counter-intuitive suggestion that immune deficits such as allergies, arthritis, asthma, diabetes, eczema, hay fever, migraine, myasthenia gravis, psoriasis, systemic lupus erythematosus, thyroid disorders, ulcerative colitis, and urticaria, were more common in left-handers. Many subsequent studies since have failed to replicate that suggestion, although a meta-analysis finds that although left- and right-handers are equally affected in most conditions, left-handers may be *more* vulnerable to ulcerative colitis, allergies and asthma, and *less* vulnerable to arthritis and myasthenia gravis. Such a pattern of results cannot be explained by the theory, and with a host of other failed predictions (Bryden et al., 1993) means that the Geschwind model does not provide the theoretical integration of disparate phenomena that was originally hoped.

GENETIC MODELS OF HANDEDNESS

The antiquity of human handedness, its seeming presence *in utero*, and the lack of major environmental correlates of handedness have suggested a genetic basis, a hypothesis supported by the undoubted tendency for handedness to run in families: in published data left-handedness occurred in 9.5 percent of children of two right-handed parents, 19.5 percent of children of one right- and one left-handed parent, and 26.1 percent of children of two left-handed parents (McManus & Bryden, 1992). The absence of an effect in adopted children makes a strong *prima facie* case for genetic causation. Nevertheless conventional Mendelian models have problems since neither right-handers nor left-handers "breed true." The difficulty is seemingly compounded by many studies showing substantial discordance in handedness of identical (monozygotic) twin pairs (McManus & Bryden, 1992), an effect which is not due to mirror-imaging, a phenomenon with no embryological foundation.

Discordance is not the problem it seems at first sight, since monozygotic discordance is more frequent among dizygotic twins, and discordance is predicted by some genetic models.

There have been a number of genetic models of handedness since Ramaley's first model in 1910. Most have failed because of not taking into account the biological basis of asymmetry (McManus & Bryden, 1992). In particular, models have ignored the phenomenon known in biology as *fluctuating asymmetry*, and results from developmental instability and hence random fluctuations in characteristics not under genetic control. Its role is undisputed in the genetics of *situs inversus*, the anatomical variant in which heart, lungs, and all viscera are mirror-reversals of their normal structures. This occurs in mice, due to the well-characterized *iv* mutation, and in humans, where it is also inherited. Handedness is not simply a further consequence of the same gene since humans with *situs inversus* have the same rate of left-handedness as do individuals with *situs solitus*, the normal anatomy.

Annett's Right-Shift (RS) model (Annett, 1985), and McManus' DC (Dextral-Chance) model have both integrated fluctuating asymmetry into their models. In each case there is one genotype (RS++ or DD) in which almost all individuals are right-handed, and a second genotype (RS−− or CC) in which 50 percent of individuals are right-handed and 50 percent left-handed. In both models heterozygotes (RS+− or DC) show additive inheritance, manifesting midway between the homozygotes. Both models predict that neither right- nor left-handers "breed true," and that monozygotic twins should show substantial discordance, since chance determination of handedness due to fluctuating asymmetry is independent in each twin.

Although superficially similar, the RS and DC models differ in many important respects. Phenotypically, the DC model argues that handedness/preference is primary, with handedness/skill differences being secondary, whereas the RS model invokes a primary role for handedness/skill differences (which are assumed to be normally distributed in genotypes), with handedness/preference being secondary and essentially arbitrary in incidence, depending on where a threshold is set in the continuous distribution of skill differences. The models differ in their predictions about the distribution of between-hand skill differences (see above), and insofar as the symmetric bimodal model is a better account of those distributions, then the DC genetic model is also superior.

The models also differ in explaining two separate phenomena concerning sex differences: the increased incidence of left-handedness in males, and the maternal effect, whereby left-handed females have more left-handed offspring (of either sex) than do left-handed males (McManus & Bryden, 1992). The RS model explains the increased incidence of left-handedness in males by a single additional parameter, whereby males are shifted more to the right than females. Although that parameter explains the difference in incidence it cannot explain the maternal effect adequately. The DC model explains the sex differences by invoking a second modifier gene located on the X-chromosome. Since the modifier manifests differently in males and females it explains the sex difference, and its different transmission by mothers and fathers also explains the maternal effect. This latter advantage argues in favour of the DC rather than the RS model.

A final difference between the RS and DC models is that, although the DC model argues that twins and singletons are equivalent in their inheritance of handedness, the RS model can only explain twin data by invoking a reduced right shift in twins (Annett, 1985), a biologically surprising effect without validatory support. Once more this should be taken as evidence in favor of the DC model.

Familial sinistrality

Familial sinistrality (FS) is a common measure in neuropsychology. *Broad FS*, having *any* left-handed relative, is a flawed measure, confounded with family size, not least since in the limit all humans are related to one another. *Narrow FS*, having first-degree left-handed relatives (parents, siblings, or children), is a more defined measure. It is theoretically sounder not solely to assess the phenotypes of relatives, but to use a specific genetic model to calculate exact genotype probabilities for probands based on the entire family tree. Data on calculated genotype probabilities show narrow FS to be a better predictor of genotypes than broad FS, although each measure leaves much true genetic variance unexplained. Familial sinistrality has been suggested as a criterion for distinguishing *natural* or inherited left-handedness from *pathological* or acquired left-handedness, only left-handers with sinistral relatives being assumed to be genetically left-handed. The argument is invalid since both RS and DC models predict that about 50 percent of genetic left-handers will show no FS. Similarly, although FS has been used to predict right hemisphere language dominance in left-handers, genetic modelling shows that it has minimal predictive power. However, FS *is* predictive of right hemisphere dominance in *right*-handers.

THE EVOLUTION OF HANDEDNESS

The reasons *why* handedness should have evolved, and why *right*-handedness in particular, are controversial. The latter can parsimoniously be explained by the gene for handedness being evolved from the gene for *situs*, affecting cerebral rather than cardiac tissue, and making the developing brain rather than the developing heart grow slightly more on the left side. The reasons for handedness at all are more contentious, and are complicated by being deeply intertwined with cerebral dominance, the causal interrelations being very unclear. Theorists have concentrated on the advantages of handedness for early humans for throwing or for feeding or on the cerebral dominance of generative grammars; and lateralization itself has been justified in terms of competition for limited neural space, and the need to prevent coordination problems between hemispheres. A final evolutionary problem concerns why some people are *left*-handed. If there are selective advantages to right-handedness then all individuals should be right-handed. The continued existence of left-handedness over many millennia suggests it must be advantageous; or to be more precise genetically, that there must be an overall heterozygote advantage. The precise advantage is unknown at present; but Annett's suggestion of an intellectual advantage for heterozygotes has severe theoretical and empirical problems.

HAND-CLASPING, ARM-FOLDING, LEG-CROSSING, EAR DOMINANCE, AND EYE DOMINANCE

Right- and left-handedness are sometimes confused with other related phenomena. When the hands are clasped with the fingers interlocked, either the right or left thumb is on top; similarly, when the arms are folded together one wrist is on top, and when the legs are crossed while sitting in a chair one knee is on top. All three behaviors are stable within individuals, show evidence of running in families, and are uncorrelated with one another or with handedness. In contrast, footedness for skilled actions is partly although not entirely correlated with handedness. Ear and eye dominance are sensory preferences. Ear dominance is little studied, typically being seen only in telephone usage. Eye dominance, which in many studies is uncorrelated with handedness, has been much studied, mainly because of theories which are not well supported, which relate crossed eye–hand dominance to reading difficulties. It can be subdivided into three uncorrelated components: sighting dominance (the usual meaning of eye dominance), sensory dominance, and acuity dominance. Eye dominance, like hand-clasping, arm-folding, and leg-crossing, runs in families and its inheritance can be modelled by the DC genetic model.

BIBLIOGRAPHY

Annett, M. (1985). *Left, right, hand and brain: The right shift theory*. Hillsdale, NJ: Erlbaum.

Bishop, D. V. M. (1990). *Handedness and developmental disorder*. Oxford: Blackwell.

Bryden, M. P., McManus, I. C., & Bulman-Fleming, M. B. (1994). Evaluating the empirical support for the Geschwind-Behan-Galaburda model of cerebral lateralization. *Brain and Cognition, 26*, 103–67.

Bryden, M. P., & Steenhuis, R. E. (1991). The assessment of handedness in children. In *Neuropsychological foundations of learning disabilities* (pp. 411–36). New York: Academic Press.

Harris, L. J. (1990). Cultural influences on handedness: historical and contemporary theory and evidence. In S. Coren (Ed.), *Left-handedness: Behavioral implications and anomalies* (pp. 195–258). Amsterdam: North-Holland.

Harris, L. J. (1992). Left-handedness. In I. Rapin & S. J. Segalowitz (Eds), *Handbook of neuropsychology*, Vol. 6, Section 10: *Child Neuropsychology (Part 1)* (pp. 145–208). Amsterdam: Elsevier.

Harris, L. J., & Carlson, D. F. (1988). Pathological left-handedness: an analysis of theories and evidence. In D. L. Molfese & S. J.

segalowitz (Eds), *Brain lateralization in children* (pp. 289–372). New York: Guilford.

McManus, I. C. (1983). The interpretation of laterality. *Cortex, 19*, 187–214.

McManus, I. C., & Bryden, M. P. (1991). Geschwind's theory of cerebral lateralization: developing a formal causal model. *Psychological Bulletin, 110*, 237–53.

McManus, I. C., & Bryden, M. P. (1992). The genetics of handedness, cerebral dominance and lateralization. In I. Rapin & S. J. Segalowitz (Eds), *Handbook of neuropsychology*, Vol. 6, Section 10: *Child neuropsychology (Part 1)* (pp. 115–44). Amsterdam: Elsevier.

CHRIS MCMANUS

hematoma A hematoma is a local swelling or tumor filled with effused blood. Besides being a consequence of bleeding within the brain, it may result from a subdural hemorrhage (*see also* SUBARACHNOID HEMORRHAGE) of the veins between the cortex and the venous sinuses, often a consequence of increased vulnerability following shrinkage of the brain in the elderly, or from an extradural hemorrhage of the arteries between the bone and the dura following head injury.

hemiagnosia Literally, hemiagnosia is an agnosia which applies to only one lateral half of sensory space. An example would be a disturbance of body image (ASOMATOGNOSIA) in which the disturbance was restricted to one side of the body. Nevertheless, it would be more common to term this a unilateral asomatognosia. The term "hemiagnosia" is, however, used for a particular syndrome: hemiagnosia for pain. This is seen only in patients with a significant reduction in the level of consciousness, and consists of an apparent inability to detect the nature or location of a painful stimulus, even though appropriate facial gestures or even verbal responses indicate perception of the pain; the patient makes no effort to drive away the painful stimulus with the functional hand.

hemiakinesia Patients with unilateral NEGLECT may fail to orient their eyes or head to stimuli appearing on the side contralateral to the lesion, to command, or when in pursuit of a moving object. This can be shown not to be attributable to a failure of the control of extraocular movements. Similarly, these patients may fail to use a limb opposite to the lesion, so that when instructed to raise both arms, they raise only the arm ipsilateral to the lesion, even when there is no weakness or paralysis of the arm which fails to move.

hemialexia Hemialexia is the inability to read words presented in one of the visual half-fields, normally the left visual right of right-handed subjects. It is a feature of COMMISSUROTOMY, but may also occur following natural lesions of the SPLENIUM of the CORPUS CALLOSUM even when there is no left HEMIANOPIA. It is inferred that the relevant visual information is projected to the right hemisphere, but is disconnected from the centers of the left hemisphere associated with language and particularly reading. Cases have been reported of patients who can name objects presented in the left half-field, while remaining hemialexic on the left and reading normally on the right.

hemianopia A hemianopia (also, less commonly, a *hemianopsia*) is a VISUAL FIELD DEFECT in which vision is lost in one lateral half of each visual field.

Lesions in the visual system produce clear effects which may be diagnostic. A lesion in the optic nerve results in blindness in one eye (monocular blindness), but more posterior lesions produce various forms of hemianopia. A lesion in the central part of the optic chiasm, most commonly produced by a pituitary tumor, will result in *bitemporal hemianopia* with the outer half of both visual fields affected. A lateral lesion of the optic chiasm will produce *nasal hemianopia* in one eye and will affect the inner (nasal) half of the visual field in the eye on the same side as the lesion.

Cerebral lesions more commonly disturb the optic tract and optic radiation (which extends from the lateral geniculate to the STRIATE CORTEX) by extending below the cortex into the underlying matter. Such lesions produce *homonymous hemianopia* affecting the visual half-field of both eyes contralateral to the side of the lesion. If the lesion is on the right side, then the nasal half of the right eye and the temporal half of the left eye will be affected. The result will be that all vision to the left of the current point of fixation will be lost. The area of visual field defect is not always identical on the two sides, and such incongruous hemianopias are more commonly seen after optic tract lesions.

If the lesion extends only partly into the optic radiation, then only the upper or the lower part of the visual fields will be affected, producing a *quadrantanopia*. Lesions of the temporal cortex are associated with loss in the upper part of the relevant visual fields, and lesions of the parietal lobe in the lower part. These quadrantanopias are also known as *upper (lower) quadrant hemianopias*.

When the lesion is in the visual cortex of the occipital lobe the result will be a homonymous hemianopia, but sight in the macular region, the area of high acuity in central vision, may be spared (*macular sparing*).

Assessment of visual field defects is normally carried out by confrontational testing and standard perimetry. Surprisingly, it is not uncommon to find patients with a hemianopia who are quite unaware of the extensive visual loss which they have suffered.

J. GRAHAM BEAUMONT

hemiasomatognosia An ASOMATOGNOSIA for one side of the body, more usually termed *unilateral asomatognosia*. (*See also* HEMIAGNOSIA.)

hemiballismus Hemiballismus is a form of CHOREA which affects only one side of the body, but in an unusually violent form. It most commonly occurs following stroke in elderly diabetic patients, involving the subthalamus nucleus on the side opposite to that affected. Unlike other forms of chorea, the proximal parts of the limb are more affected, resulting in wider and more dramatic movements.

hemi-inattention *See* ATTENTION; NEGLECT.

hemiparesis Hemiparesis is a muscular weakness affecting one side of the body. It may result from lesions at a variety of sites in the motor system, both within the brain and spinal cord (upper motor neuron lesions; extrapyramidal lesions; cerebellar lesions), as well as from lesions in the lower motor neurons, from muscular disorders, and hysteria. Hemiparesis affecting a substantial portion of one side of the body is most likely to have a cerebral origin. The pattern of weakness and associated features will naturally depend on the site and nature of the lesion.

hemiplegia Hemiplegia is the most frequent form of paralysis, which unilaterally involves an arm, a leg, and usually the face. Paralysis means complete or partial loss of voluntary movement due to interruption of the motor pathways. The term "paresis" is often used for a lesser degree of paralysis. However, the terms hemiplegia, hemiparalysis, and hemiparesis are often used interchangeably, but generally hemiparesis is used for slight and hemiplegia or hemiparalysis for severe unilateral loss of motor function (Adams & Victor, 1989).

NEUROANATOMICAL AND NEURO-PHYSIOLOGICAL CONSIDERATIONS

Hemiplegia is in most cases connected with the central motor pathways, also called the PYRAMIDAL TRACT or corticospinal pathway. The terminology is somewhat confusing.

Anatomically the pyramidal tract consists of those fibers which course longitudinally in the pyramid of the medulla oblongata (hence its name). The fibers arise from the cerebral cortex, and most of them continue in the spinal cord as the corticospinal tract. The fibers ending in the motor cranial nerve nuclei in the brain stem are called the CORTICOBULBAR TRACT. Thus, strictly speaking, the pyramidal tract contains the corticospinal and corticobulbar projections. The term "pyramidal tract" can therefore be used as a common name for these two components (Brodal, 1981).

The pyramidal tract was the first recognized fiber tract in the brain, described by Türck in 1851. Traditionally it was stated that the pyramidal tract fibers originate from the giant cells of Betz located in the fifth layer of the precentral gyrus or BRODMANN'S area 4. However, later studies demonstrated that the number of pyramidal tract fibers (about a million fibers in each

pyramid) far exceeds the number of Betz cells in Brodmann's area 4 (about 25,000 to 35,000 cells), and therefore the majority of pyramidal tract fibers come from cells other than the Betz cells in area 4 (Brodal, 1981). In many studies (some in Man but most in various animal species like the monkey and the cat) pyramidal tract fibers have been traced, besides area 4, from Brodmann's area 6 ("supplementary motor cortex"), areas 3, 1, and 2 ("primary sensory cortex"), and areas 5 and 7 (parietal cortex). These cortical areas represent the motor cortex, or rather the SENSORIMOTOR CORTEX: it was demonstrated that the classical precentral "motor" cortex receives sensory information, whereas motor functions are also located in the classical postcentral "sensory" cortex. It is therefore better to speak of the sensorimotor cortex, the precentral part being predominantly motor and the postcentral part being predominantly sensory (Brodal, 1981).

Studies with weak electrical stimuli have demonstrated a somatotopical arrangement of the sensorimotor cortex. The contralateral face, arm, trunk, and leg are represented on the cortex, with face and tongue on the inferior part of the lateral cortical surface, and the leg on the medial cortical surface of the hemisphere, often depicted as a homunculus. However, recent studies showed that the somatotopical arrangement is fairly flexible and that the body parts are often represented in more than one location.

The pyramidal tract fibers descend and converge from the sensorimotor cortex, via the posterior part of the corona radiata to the posterior limb of the internal capsule. The tract progressively shifts from the anterior half of the posterior limb into the posterior half of the posterior limb in the more caudal part of the internal capsule (Boiten & Lodder, 1991). From here, the tract further descends through the cerebral peduncle and pons to the pyramid of medulla oblongata where most fibers cross the midline and enter the spinal cord as the corticospinal tract. The corticospinal tract fibers end directly on the alpha motor neurons, which supply the muscle fibers, on the gamma motor neurons, which supply the muscle spindles, and on different kinds of interneurons, in the gray matter of the spinal cord. Stimulation of the sensorimotor cortex leads, via the pyramidal tract, to activation of the motor neurons, which causes contraction of the muscle fibers, leading to contralateral movements of the extremities. Clinical and experimental studies showed that the primary sensorimotor cortex, and hence the pyramidal tract, is important in initiating and controlling voluntary and fine and skilled movements, also being influenced by other brain regions and by somatosensory impulses.

LOCALIZATION AND ETIOLOGY OF THE LESIONS CAUSING HEMIPLEGIA

Hemiplegia can be caused by lesions anywhere along the course of the pyramidal tract from the sensorimotor cortex to the medullary pyramid: sensorimotor cortex, corona radiata (cerebral white matter), internal capsule, cerebral peduncle, pons, and medullary pyramid. The localization of the lesion can often be deduced from associated neurological symptoms and signs. Signs of cortical dysfunction (e.g. epileptic seizures, APHASIA, AGNOSIA, APRAXIA, VISUAL FIELD DEFECT, VISUOSPATIAL DISORDERS, ASTEREOGNOSIA) suggest in general a lesion involving the cortex. The pyramidal tract converges from a rather extensive sensorimotor cortex into a small tract running through the internal capsule. Therefore only large cortical lesions will cause a hemiplegia, which will in most cases be associated with these cortical signs. Isolated or pure hemiplegia (without signs of cortical dysfunction) is likely to be caused by a small lesion involving the posterior limb of the internal capsule (Fisher, 1982; Boiten & Lodder, 1991). In BRAIN-STEM lesions, the additional neurological signs permit a specific topical diagnosis: crossed signs with ipsilateral CRANIAL NERVE palsies and contralateral hemiplegia. For instance, a lesion of the cerebral peduncle goes with ipsilateral oculomotor nerve palsy and contralateral hemiplegia (Weber's syndrome); a lesion of the caudal pontine base with ipsilateral abducens or facial nerve palsy (or both) and contralateral hemiplegia (Millard–Gubler or Foville's syndrome); and a lesion of the medial or dorsolateral part of the medulla oblongata with ipsilateral hypoglossal nerve or glossopharyngeus-vagal nerve palsies and contralateral hemiplegia (Déjerine's and Wallenberg's syndrome respectively).

The lesions can also be localized by means of ancillary investigations, especially with modern neuroradiological techniques like CAT and MAGNETIC RESONANCE IMAGING.

The causes of the lesions resulting in hemiplegia are diverse. In most cases hemiplegia is caused by CEREBROVASCULAR diseases, like hemorrhage or infarction. Isolated or pure hemiplegia, also called pure motor stroke, is usually caused by small, deep infarcts, the so-called lacunar infarcts, usually in the internal capsule, corona radiata, or pons (Fisher, 1982; Boiten & Lodder, 1991). Therefore the syndrome of pure hemiplegia or pure motor stroke is called a lacunar syndrome. Other important causes of hemiplegia are trauma (cerebral contusion, epidural and subdural hemorrhage), TUMOR, infectious diseases (abscess, focal cerebritis complicating MENINGITIS, ENCEPHALITIS) and demyelinating diseases (like multiple sclerosis). These diseases can be diagnosed by their clinical presentation and mode of evolution, and by ancillary investigations like laboratory investigations, lumbar puncture, computerized axial tomography, and magnetic resonance imaging.

SYMPTOMS AND SIGNS OF HEMIPLEGIA

One should realize that spastic hemiplegia is not caused by a pure pyramidal tract lesion. Experimental studies in primates and some human cases demonstrated that a pure pyramidal tract lesion causes only slight impairment of voluntary movements and no spasticity (Davidoff, 1990). The notion that the syndrome of spastic hemiplegia with impairment of skilled voluntary movements, increased deep tendon reflexes, and a BABINSKI sign is called a pyramidal tract syndrome is therefore not quite right. The lesions causing spastic hemiplegia obviously damage, besides the pyramidal tract fibers, other corticofugal fibers, like corticothalamic and corticopontine fibers. The term "pyramidal tract syndrome" should therefore be discarded (Brodal, 1981).

In hemiplegia there is a complete or partial loss of voluntary movements of the arm, leg, and usually face on one side of the body. Symptoms and signs in the acute stage can differ from those in the subacute and chronic stage. In the arm and leg the fine and skilled movements, like those of fingers and toes, are more impaired than the gross, proximal movements. Generally, movements most recently acquired during evolution are the first to be lost after a pyramidal tract lesion (Walton, 1981). In the acute stage the paralyzed limbs are usually flaccid, whereas in the subacute and chronic stage (starting after some weeks) muscle tone gradually increases and becomes hypertonic or spastic. In SPASTICITY there is an increased resistance to passive movements. Hypertonia varies between different muscle groups of the limbs in hemiplegia (Walton, 1981). In the arm the adductors and internal rotators of the shoulder, the pronators of the forearm, and the flexors of elbow, wrist, and fingers are most affected. This distribution of most hypertonic muscle groups determines the position of the arm in hemiplegia, that is, adducted and internally rotated at the shoulder, and flexed at the elbow (with slight pronation), wrist, and fingers. In the leg adductors and extensors of the hip, extensors of the knee and plantar-flexors of the foot are most affected, yielding an adducted and extended leg with plantar flexion of the foot. This variation in hypertonia between different muscle groups leads to a typical GAIT disorder, the hemiplegic (spastic) gait. During walking the patient circumducts his or her spastic leg due to the inability to flex the hip, knee, and ankle, that is, the leg is moved and rotated outward at the hip describing a semicircle. The foot scrapes the floor because it is plantar flexed. The arm is flexed and does not swing naturally. In the chronic stage contractures (permanent contraction) usually develop in the spastic muscles.

The tendon reflexes are diminished or lost in the acute stage of hemiplegia due to the "neural shock." In the subacute and chronic stage the tendon reflexes become exaggerated, and clonus may develop. The superficial reflexes (e.g. abdominal reflexes) are diminished or lost. The plantar reflex becomes extensor, the so-called Babinski sign. Since the peripheral motor neuron is not damaged, there will be no marked muscle atrophy.

Especially in the acute stage of hemiplegia, the pyramidal tract lesion also causes other symptoms and signs. If the lesion is located in the cerebral HEMISPHERE, there may be an impairment of conjugate deviation of the eyes to the contralateral side or, in severe cases, the eyes are even deviated ipsilateral to the lesion ("the patient looks to his brain lesion"). If the lesion is located in the PONS the opposite occurs, being an impairment of conjugate deviation of the eyes ipsilateral to the lesion. These conjugate GAZE abnormalities usually disappear after a few hours or days. The abnormalities are due to dysfunction of the horizontal conjugate gaze centers in the hemisphere and pons respectively. Movements of the head may be impaired in the same way as the conjugate deviation of the eyes.

There may also be a facial weakness, e.g. weakness of retraction of the angle of the mouth. In pyramidal tract lesions, movements of the lower part of the face are more severely affected than those of the upper, because upper facial movements are innervated by both cerebral hemispheres, whereas the lower facial movements are innervated only by the contralateral hemisphere. Although pharyngeal and tongue movements are also largely innervated by both cerebral hemispheres, there may be a slight weakness of these movements to the contralateral side, especially in the acute stage. Other possible associated neurological signs are described in the section on localization of the lesions causing hemiplegia.

Functional recovery of the paralysis varies between patients. In most cases functional recovery of the arm is more unfavorable than that of the leg. Fine and skilled movements are generally impossible and only the gross and stereotyped movements return. Due to the extended position of the leg, most patients are able to walk again, even if functional recovery is incomplete.

INFANTILE HEMIPLEGIA

Infantile hemiplegia, also called *hemiplegia spastica infantilis*, is a hemiplegia which is already present at birth (so-called congenital hemiplegia), or which develops during the first years of life. Infantile hemiplegia is one of the forms of cerebral palsy. Cerebral palsy was for the first time associated with "abnormal parturition, difficult labor, premature birth, and asphyxia neonatorum" by Little in 1862 (Menkes, 1990). However, recent studies indicate that antenatal pathological factors are probably as important as perinatal problems in the pathogenesis of cerebral palsy. Although many causes of infantile hemiplegia are known, the pathogenesis is still not completely understood. Moreover, the cause in an individual infant is often obscure. The form of cerebral palsy is partially determined by the gestational age of the fetus. Premature infants more often have (spastic) DIPLEGIA, whereas term infants more often have (spastic) hemiplegia.

Infantile hemiplegia can be caused by a developmental anomaly of the brain or by an insult (e.g. trauma, ischemia, or hemorrhage) of antenatal, perinatal, postnatal, or infantile onset, to a previously normal developed brain, or by both (Menkes, 1990). Mechanical trauma to the neonatal brain during delivery can cause lacerations of the falx cerebri, tentorium, cerebral veins, and dural sinuses, with subsequent subdural hemorrhage.

More frequently the infantile hemiplegia is the result of (perinatal) asphyxia. During asphyxia the fetal brain is subjected to hypoxia and ischemia, leading to circulatory lesions and tissue necrosis. The location of the cerebral circulatory (ischemic) lesions are in part determined by the gestational age of the fetus at the time of the asphyxia (Menkes, 1990). Periventricular leukomalacia occurs particularly in premature infants, and it is the principal ischemic lesion of the premature infant. It consists of bilateral, fairly symmetrical necrosis, located periventricularly, in fact reflecting the vascular immaturity of this region. In the term newborn the ischemic lesions are located principally in the cortex, especially in the border zone or watershed areas between the large cerebral arteries. Both gray and white matter can be injured. Lesions involving damage to the deeper portions of the gyri, with consequently deepened and widened sulci producing a "mushroom" gyrus, have been called ulegyria (Menkes, 1990).

Besides subdural hemorrhage (caused by mechanical trauma), another type of intracranial hemorrhage causing infantile hemiplegia can occur in the newborn, the periventricular-intraventricular hemorrhage (PVH-IVH). This is the most common form of neonatal intracranial hemorrhage (Menkes, 1990). The site of the bleeding is determined by the maturity of the infant. In the premature infant hemorrhage originates in the capillaries of the germinal matrix, usually over the caudate nucleus, whereas in the term infant the choroid plexus becomes the principal site of the hemorrhage. The pathogenesis of PVH-IVH is not completely understood. Contributing factors are prematurity, perinatal asphyxia, dysmaturity, and forcipal extraction. PVH-IVH can be preceded by periventricular leukomalacia.

Developmental anomalies like aplasia of a cerebral hemisphere, porencephaly, micro- or agyria, and ectopic gray matter can also cause hemiplegia. Moreover, infants with a developmental anomaly are more prone to perinatal asphyxia.

In infancy and early childhood, usually during the first three years of life and prior to 6 years of age, acute hemiplegia can develop. The arterial occlusion in acute infantile hemiplegia can result from cardioembolism, Moyamoya disease, fibromuscular dysplasia, arterial dissection, vasculitis, or from infectious arteritis. Often the cause is unknown and in this group of patients the hemiparesis is preceded by fever, depressed consciousness, and seizures.

Clinically infantile hemiplegia is characterized by a unilateral spastic paralysis of arm and leg. Hemiplegia is usually detected during the first months of life, but only rarely at birth. Initial symptoms can be fisting (exaggeration of the palmar grasp reflex), hand dominance in the first year of life, which is unusual, and developmental retardation (e.g. long persistence of head lag) (Menkes, 1990). These are followed by disuse of extremities and gait disturbances. Most affected are fine movements of the hand, like the pincer grasp (thumb–forefinger). The increased muscle tone (spasticity) leads to typical posture, with the arm flexed and the leg extended with an equinus position of the foot. The infant circumducts the spastic leg during walking. The tendon reflexes are increased and the plantar reflex becomes extensor (Babinski sign). Many children have choreoathetotic movements of the affected limbs. Sensory abnormalities, homonymous hemianopia, neglect, and seizures can also occur. The unilateral hypertonia can lead to deformities of the thorax, to scoliosis, to luxation of the hip, etc. Many children have mental retardation. Patients with infantile hemiplegia need multidisciplinary support with a child neurologist, orthopedist, and rehabilitation specialist.

BIBLIOGRAPHY

Adams, R. D., & Victor, M. (1989). *Principles of neurology*. New York: McGraw-Hill.

Boiten, J., & Lodder, J. (1991). Discrete lesions in the sensorimotor control system: a clinical-topographical study of lacunar infarcts. *Journal of the Neurological Sciences, 105,* 150–4.

Brodal, A. (1981). *Neurological anatomy in relation to clinical medicine*. New York: Oxford University Press.

Davidoff, R. A. (1990). Pyramidal tract. *Neurology, 40,* 332–9.

Fisher, C. M. (1982). Lacunar strokes and infarcts: a review. *Neurology, 32,* 871–6.

Menkes, J. H. (1990). *Textbook of child neurology*. Philadelphia: Lea and Febiger.

Walton, J. N. (1981). *Brain's diseases of the nervous system*. Oxford: Oxford University Press.

JELIS BOITEN

hemisphere   The two hemispheres, more correctly the *cerebral hemispheres*, for other organs possess hemispheres, including the CEREBELLUM, are the two regions of the CORTEX of the forebrain. In Man they are the most prominent objects within the skull, being so large as to hide the subcortical structures and the brain stem. The two essentially independent hemispheres are separated by the median longitudinal fissure (in which runs the meningeal structure known as the *falx*) below which runs the CORPUS CALLOSUM which, together with the minor commissures, interconnects the two cortical hemispheres. Each hemisphere has a surface area of about 1,000 square centimetres. The cortex of each hemisphere is conventionally divided into four lobes (FRONTAL LOBE, OCCIPITAL LOBE, PARIETAL LOBE, TEMPORAL LOBE). There are a range of significant anatomical asymmetries between the two cerebral hemispheres which may be of functional significance (see, for example, PLANUM TEMPORALE).

Since the explosion of interest in the COMMISSUROTOMY or "split-brain" operation from about 1960, there has been a period of great interest in the differential neuropsychological functions of the two hemispheres (*see* LATERALIZATION), by both experimental laboratory studies and by clinical observation, although recognition of lateral differences in the effects of focal cortical lesions has been a feature of clinical neuropsychology throughout its modern history. Since the demonstration of the lateralization of language in the 1860s, it has been known that different effects may follow similar lesions at homologous sites in the two hemispheres.

It is virtually impossible to summarize the enormous literature on hemispheric laterality, but it is generally accepted that the left cerebral hemisphere is preferentially organized for linguistic, semantic, abstract, and symbolic processing while the right hemisphere is specialized for nonverbal, spatial, and holistic processing. Differences in the pattern of hemispheric lateralization have been associated with HANDEDNESS and,

less clearly, with sex and with psychiatric disorders.

J. GRAHAM BEAUMONT

hemispherectomy   Hemispherectomy is the surgical procedure which consists of removal of one cerebral hemisphere. The term is so descriptive that it has been used with qualifications to name other related surgical procedures.

Hemispherectomy was introduced in humans by Walter Dandy (1923) to treat extensive glioma of the nondominant hemisphere. From 1923 to 1928 Dandy used this operation in 5 patients with right hemispheric glioma. Hemispherectomy for the indication of tumor was used by some neurosurgeons but abandoned in the 1950s after the failure of the operation to prevent tumor progression.

The first hemispherectomy for control of seizures was performed by K. G. McKenzie in Toronto in 1938 on a child suffering from intractable seizures and infantile hemiplegia. Only following Krynaw's report on 12 such patients, published in 1950, did hemispherectomy become popular as the procedure of choice for control of epilepsy in patients with infantile hemiplegia.

INDICATIONS

Conditions responsible for seizures in patients who are candidates for hemispherectomy include: infantile hemiplegia (perinatal encephalopathy), chronic encephalitis, HHE (hemiplegia, hemiatrophy, epilepsy), head trauma, cerebrovascular accident, Sturge-Weber, hemimegalencephaly, infantile spasms (Villemure, 1992a).

Hemispherectomy is indicated for control of pharmacologically refractory seizures in patients harboring a unilateral hemiplegia and hemianopsia. The preoperative evaluation of the neurological function is very important to ensure that the hemispherectomy will not aggravate the patient's neurological condition. Patients presenting a hemiplegia with inability to perform individual finger movements or foot tapping should not have their motor function aggravated by the operation. Electroencephalographic demonstration of the unlateral epileptic activity responsible for the clinical seizures is essential. The radiological investigation usually demonstrates unilateral cerebral atrophy of a different degree.

In the majority of patients the psychological evaluation demonstrates pre-operatively an IQ below average and declining intellectual functions. The behavior observed in these patients is characterized by aggressiveness, outbursts of rage, and anti-social attitudes (Beardsworth & Adams, 1988; Lindsay et al., 1987).

In those patients who are candidates for hemispherectomy, the underlying pathology responsible for the severe brain damage has already created a severe neurological deficit that the hemispherectomy does not aggravate. In some instances of progressive neurological conditions due to severe hemispheric or diffuse brain damage, such as chronic encephalitis, hemispherectomy may be advisable prior to the presence of maximal hemispheric dysfunction. Controlling the seizures early allows better psychosocial development of the patients, especially when done early in life.

SURGICAL TECHNIQUES

The hemispherectomy technique used by Dandy (1928) consisted of removal of the cerebral cortex and white matter of one hemisphere, with excision of the caudate nucleus and basal ganglia; the most superficial structure which was spared was the thalamus. Some modifications to Dandy's original technique, proposed early on by Gardner (1933), preserved the caudate nucleus and basal ganglia as well as their vascularization, following the hypothesis that the motor recovery would be better in these instances. Two small series of patients were reported by Laine and others (1964) in France and French and others (1955) in the United States, comparing the effect of removing or sparing the caudate nucleus and basal ganglia at the time of hemispherectomy. Neither found any long-term difference in the motor recovery. Laine coined the terms "inter-thalamo-caudate" hemispherectomy when the caudate nucleus and basal ganglia were excised and "extra-thalamo-caudate" hemispherectomy when these structures were preserved.

The hemispherectomy technique used from the 1920s to the 1960s was characterized by anatomical removal of most of the hemisphere and thus named "anatomical hemispherectomy," where the end result is the creation of a large intracranial cavity.

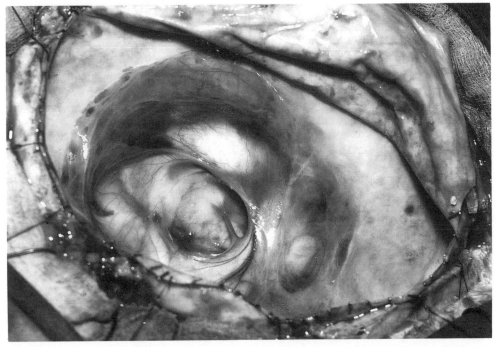

Figure 43 Pre-operative photograph demonstrating the large cavity resulting from "anatomical hemispherectomy." (Reproduced from *Epilepsy Research*, supplement 5, 1992, 209–15, with the permission of Elsevier Science Publishers.)

hemispherectomy

In the mid-1960s anatomical hemispherectomy was found to be associated with a late and often fatal complication called "superficial cerebral hemosiderosis" (SCH). This complication, which occurred from 4 to 25 years post-operatively (median 8 years) was seen in 15 to 33 percent (average 25 percent) of patients who had undergone neurological deterioration and hydrocephalus, leading to death in up to 30 percent of them. This complication, first described by Oppenheimer and Griffith (1966), was recognized universally (Falconer & Wilson, 1969; Ransohoff & Hess, 1973; Rasmussen, 1973) and so frequently that anatomical hemispherectomy was abandoned in the late 1960s for less extensive surgical procedures. Smaller surgical excisions was not associated with SCH but they had the disadvantage of not providing seizure control as good as hemispherectomy.

"Hemi-hemispherectomy," consisting of excision of half the hemisphere, either anterior (fronto-temporal lobectomies) or posterior (temporo-parieto-occipital lobectomies), which had been used in certain instances before, became popular as replacements for hemispherectomy. The surgical procedure "subtotal hemispherectomy," where only a third to a quarter of the hemisphere is preserved, was also used instead of hemispherectomy to avoid the severe late complication of SCH; in these procedures, the least epileptogenic portions of the hemisphere was preserved. The subtotal removal of the hemisphere was not associated with SCH, but was less successful in controlling seizures (Rasmussen, 1973).

Modifications of anatomical hemispherectomy have been proposed in the last three decades to protect patients against SCH, while still provid-

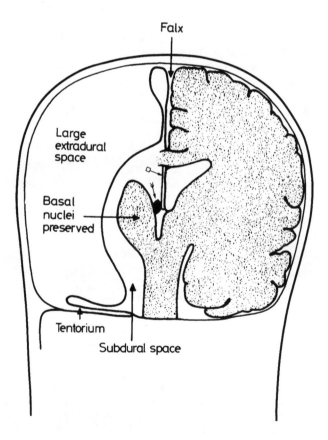

Figure 44 Schematic representation of "modified hemispherectomy." (Reproduced from *Journal of Neurology, Neurosurgery and Psychiatry, 46*, 1983, 617–19, with permission of the *British Medical Journal*.)

ing them with the best seizure control. These hemispherectomy techniques differ in their surgical principles and method but, in theory, for a given indication, they should have the same results in seizure control.

"Modified hemispherectomy" was first reported by P. J. E. Wilson in 1970 and popularized in the 1980s by C. B. T. Adams (1983). The surgical procedure consists of anatomical hemispherectomy, followed by occlusion of the ipsilateral foramen of Monroe and stitching of the dura so as to reduce the volume of the subdural cavity. This procedure aims at diminishing bleeding and membrane formation, as well as eliminating communication between the hemispherectomy cavity and the cerebrospinal fluid. This type of hemispherectomy has been used in Oxford on 25 patients with no incidence of SCH.

Hemidecortication, described by Ignelzi and

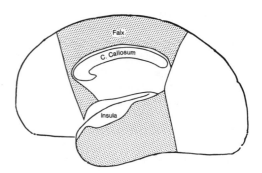

Figure 46 Schematic representation of functional hemispherectomy. (Reproduced from Grune & Stratton, *Operative neurosurgical techniques*, 1988, 1235–41, with permission of W. B. Saunders.)

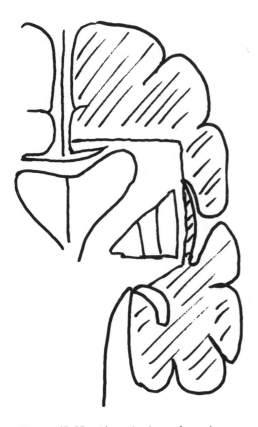

Figure 45 Hemidecortication: schematic representation (author's drawing, adapted from Ignelzi and Bucy, 1968).

Bucy in 1968, consists of excision of the gray matter of the diseased hemisphere, sparing the white matter and avoiding an opening in the ventricle. Hoffman advocates this technique in children suffering from Sturge-Weber or hemimegalencephaly, who would be candidates for hemispherectomy (Villemure et al., 1993). This procedure has also been widely used at Johns Hopkins (Vining et al., 1993). Winston and colleagues (1992) have proposed a variation in the hemidecortication technique; they named their technique hemicorticectomy. In this latter type of hemispherectomy, the cortex is removed in slabs rather than piecemeal.

"Functional hemispherectomy" was first carried out by Rasmussen (1973). Rasmussen and Villemure promoted this technique of hemispherectomy, which consists of subtotal anatomical excision of the hemisphere, but complete physiological disconnection. It provides protection against SCH as subtotal hemispherectomy did, and gives the patient maximum benefit toward seizure control, as did complete anatomical hemispherectomy.

The procedure consists of excision of the central region, including the parasagittal tissue, and temporal lobectomy; the residual frontal and parieto-occipital lobes are then disconnected from the ipsilateral and contralateral hemisphere by complete callosotomy and isolation from the ipsilateral deep structures (Villemure & Rasmussen, 1990).

The necessity to remove the insular cortex

during hemispherectomy has caused concern; in a retrospective analysis of a group of 55 hemispherectomy patients where half had the insular cortex resected and the other half had it spared, Villemure and colleagues (1989) found that there were more seizure-free patients when the insular cortex was spared, suggesting that its removal was not essential. At the Montreal Neurological Hospital, insulectomy at the time of hemispherectomy is now carried out routinely, following the observation of residual insular seizures in one patient who underwent functional hemispherectomy with sparing of the insula.

While there are different sizes of the parts of the central region and temporal lobe removed in functional hemispherectomy, usually depending on the underlying pathology and degree of atrophy, we believe that the smallest possible brain excision that will create an isolated hemisphere should be termed "hemispherotomy." This term was coined by Delalande to describe a type of functional hemispherectomy done through a frontal vertex approach (Delelande et al., 1992). The technique of hemispherotomy which we have utilized, "the peri-insular hemispherotomy," consists first in exposing the lateral ventricle (Villemure & Mascott, 1993, 1995). This is accomplished by removal of the frontal, parietal, and temporal operculum, and a section of the corona radiata in a plane perpendicular and through the circular sulcus of the insula. The disconnection above the fissure is carried out as

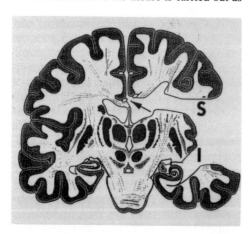

Figure 47 Schematic representation of "peri-insular hemispherectomy." Note the supra- (S) and infra-insular (I) windows and the parasagittal callosotomy (arrow).

outlined in functional hemispherectomy by using only a small suprasylvian window to enter the dilated ventricle, through which the parasagittal callosotomy as well as the frontal and parieto-occipital disconnections are completed. The hippocampus is excised by subpial aspiration, all the way back to the trigone level, or is amputated at the fimbria-fornix; the amygdala is also excised by subpial aspiration.

Hemispherotomy represents the technical variant of functional hemispherectomy where the ratio of disconnection versus excision is the greatest. This procedure requires minimal brain exposure, thus necessitating only a small skin incision and bone flap with subsequently reduced blood loss and operating time.

RESULTS

Though for the lay person it is difficult to conceive that a person may benefit from the influence of only one cerebral hemisphere, the results of hemispherectomy are very convincing.

The impact of hemispherectomy toward seizure control and psychosocial development, as well as the complications associated with this operation, will be discussed briefly. Hemispherectomy provides complete seizure control in 70 to 80 percent of patients and major improvement (more than 80 percent reduction of seizures) in another 15 to 20 percent of patients. Some patients continue to experience seizures, probably originating from the residual, good hemisphere (Villemure et al., 1993). Controlling or improving the seizure is associated with improved intellectual abilities (improved IQ, capacity to learn) and improved social integration (Beardsworth & Adams, 1988; Lindsay et al., 1987).

Hemispherectomy remains a major surgical procedure; no cases of SCH have been reported associated with the different new hemispherectomy techniques. Infection, hydrocephalus, and peri-operative hemodynamic instability represent the complications most frequently encountered (Brian et al., 1990; Cabiese et al., 1957; Falconer & Wilson, 1969).

CONCLUSION

The term hemispherectomy remains so descriptive of the extent of the surgical procedure that, in general, it has continued to be used and preferred by most surgeons, despite the different surgical techniques.

Hemispherectomy for control of pharmacologically resistant epilepsy in patients with unilateral hemisperic deficit secondary to unilateral brain damage resulting from diverse etiologies provides complete or almost complete seizure control in the great majority of patients. Furthermore, it allows the patient who becomes seizure-free to improve in intellectual development and social integration. Surgical methods developed over the past 30 years as substitutes for anatomical hemispherectomy appear to have eliminated the complication of SCH. Further development in surgical techniques of hemispherectomy, where disconnection of the hemisphere predominates over excision, appears to be associated with the lowest rate of complications.

Note This entry is dedicated to the memory of Justine Sergent in recognition of our friendship.

BIBLIOGRAPHY

Adams, C. B. T. (1983). Hemispherectomy: a modification. *Journal of Neurology, Neurosurgery and Psychiatry, 46*, 617–19.

Beardsworth, E. D., & Adams, C. B. T. (1988). Modified hemispherectomy for epilepsy: early results in 10 cases. *British Journal of Neurosurgery, 2*, 73–84.

Brian, J. E., Deshpande, J. K., & McPherson, R. W. (1990). Management of cerebral hemispherectomy in children. *Journal of Clinical Anesthesia, 2*, 91–5.

Cabiese, F., Jeni, R., & Landa, R. (1957). Fatal brain-stem shift following hemispherectomy. *Journal of Neurosurgery, 14*, 74–91.

Dandy, W. (1928). Removal of right cerebral hemisphere for certain tumors with hemiplegia. *Journal of the American Medical Association, 90*, 823–5.

Davies, K. G., Maxwell, R. E., & French, L. A. (1993). Hemispherectomy for intractable seizures: long-term results in 17 patients followed for up to 38 years. *Journal of Neurosurgery, 78*, 733–40.

Delalande, O., Pinard, J. M., Basdevant, C., Gauthe, M., Plouin, P., & Dulac, O. (1992). Hemispherotomy: a new procedure for central disconnection. *Epilepsia, 33*, suppl. 3, 99–100.

Falconer, M. A., & Wilson, P. J. E. (1969). Complications related to delayed hemorrhage after hemispherectomy. *Journal of Neurosurgery, 30*, 413–14.

French, L. A., Johnson, D. R., Brown, I. A., & Van Bergen, F. B. (1955), Cerebral hemispherectomy for control of intractable convulsive seizures. *Journal of Neurosurgery, 12*, 154–64.

Gardner, W. J. (1933). Removal of the right cerebral hemisphere for infiltrating glioma. *Journal of the American Medical Association, 12*, 154–164.

Griffith, H. B. (1967). Cerebral hemispherectomy for infantile hemiplegia in the light of late results. *Annals of the Royal College of Surgeons of England, 41*, 183–201.

Ignelzi, R. J., & Bucy, P. C. (1968). Cerebral hemidecortication in the treatment of infantile cerebral hemiatrophy. *Journal of Nervous and Mental Disease, 147*, 14–30.

Krynauw, R. A. (1950). Infantile hemiplegia treated by removing one cerebral hemisphere. *Journal of Neurology, Neurosurgery and Psychiatry, 13*, 243–67.

Laine, E., Pruvot, P., & Osson, D. (1964). Résultats éloignés de l'hémisphérectomie dans les cas d'hémiatrophie cérébrale infantile génératrice d'épilepsie. *Neurochirurgie, 10*, 507–22.

Lindsay, J., Ounsted, C., & Richards, P. (1987). Hemispherectomy for childhood epilepsy: a 36 years study. *Developmental and Medical Child Neurology, 29*, 592–600.

McKenzie, K. G. (1938). The present status of a patient who had the right cerebral hemisphere removed. *Journal of the American Medical Association, 111*, 168.

Obrador, A. (1952). About the surgical technique of hemispherectomy in cases of cerebral hemiatrophy. *Acta Neurochirurgica, 3*, 57–63.

Oppenheimer, D. R., & Griffith, H.B. (1966). Persistent intracranial bleeding as a complication of hemispherectomy. *Journal of Neurology, Neurosurgery and Psychiatry, 9*, 229–40.

Ransohoff, J., & Hess, W. (1973). Discussion in T. Rasmussen Post-operative superficial hemosiderosis of the brain, its diagnosis, treatment and prevention. *American Neurological Association, 98*, 133–7.

Rasmussen, T. (1973). Post-operative superficial hemosiderosis of the brain, its diagnosis, treatment and prevention. *American Neurological Association, 98*, 133–7.

Rasmussen, T. (1983). Hemispherectomy for seizures revisited. *Canadian Journal of Neurological Science, 10*, 7.

Villemure, J. G. (1992a). Hemispherectomy. In S. R. Resor & H. Kutt (Eds), *The medical treatment of epilepsy* (pp. 243–9). New York: Marcel Dekker.

Villemure, J. G. (1992b). Hemispherectomy techniques. In H. O. Luders (Ed.), *Epilepsy surgery* (pp. 569–78). New York: Raven.

Villemure, J. G. (1993) Hemispherectomy: techniques and complications. In E. Wyllie (Ed.), *The treatment of epilepsy: Principles and practice* (pp. 1116–19). Philadelphia: Lea and Febiger.

Villemure, J. G., Adams, C. B. T., Hoffman, H. J., & Peacock, W. J. (1993). Hemispherectomy. In J. Engel (Ed.), *Surgical treatment of the epilepsies* (pp. 511–18). New York: Raven.

Villemure, J. G., & Mascott, C. (1993). Hemispherotomy: the peri-insular approach. Technical aspects. *Epilepsia 34*, suppl. 6, 48.

Villemure, J. G., & Mascott, C. (1995). Peri-insular hemispherotomy: surgical principles and anatomy. *Neurosurgery* (in press).

Villemure, J. G., Mascott, C., Andermann, F., & Rasmussen, T. (1989). Hemispherectomy and the insula. *Epilepsia, 30*, 5.

Villemure, J. G., & Rasmussen, T. (1990). Functional hemispherectomy: methodology. *Journal of Epilepsy*, Supplement 3, 177–82.

Vining, E. P. G., Freeman, J. M., Brandt, J., Carson, B. S., & Uematsu, S. (1993). Progressive unilateral encephalopathy of childhood (Rasmussen's syndrome): a reappraisal. *Epilepsia, 34*, 639–50.

Wilson, P. J. E. (1970). Cerebral hemispherectomy for infantile hemiplegia. *Brain, 93*, 147–80.

Winston, K. R., Welch, K., Adler, J. R., & Erba, G. (1992). Cerebral hemicorticectomy for epilepsy. *Journal of Neurosurgery, 77*, 889–95.

JEAN-GUY VILLEMURE

hemisphericity Originally, the tendency to rely more on the left or right cerebral hemisphere for performing tasks, solving problems, or engaging in thought (Bogen et al., 1972). Later, subtypes of hemisphericity were distinguished (Bogen & Bogen, 1983): (1) *task* hemisphericity referred to greater activation of one hemisphere due to its specialization for the inherent nature of stimuli or of task requirements, (2) *individual* hemisphericity referred to an individual's greater reliance on a particular hemisphere for performance of a task. Individual hemisphericity implies hemispheric participation due to the characteristics of the individual, and may not always match hemispheric involvement that would be expected from the nature of the task. Task hemisphericity is dependent upon hemispheric specialization, which could change as a process of development. In some cases, such as speech, task hemisphericity mitigates expression of individual hemisphericity. By contrast, individual hemisphericity may vary more readily from time to time, and from situation to situation. A third concept, *cultural* hemisphericity, was defined by extending individual hemisphericity to a group of individuals characteristically homogeneous in some way, or to a cultural group with concordant thinking styles. Cultural hemisphericity would describe how a cultural group may jointly approach a problem, perceive a type of stimulus, or perform a task in a style more characteristic of the cognitive processing associated with the right or left hemisphere.

THE ORIGINAL CONCEPT
Terminology: task vs individual hemisphericity

The concept of task hemisphericity was based on a dichotomy of specialized brain functions emerging from research in the 1960s. (Hemispheric specialization was later recognized by the Nobel Committee by awarding the 1981 Prize in Physiology and Medicine to Roger W. Sperry.) Specialized functions were demonstrated by cognitive tests whose stimuli or task performance was better handled by one cerebral hemisphere relative to the other. While debate continues as to what constitutes the "purest" stimuli attributed to one hemisphere, or the most unique motor activity to be unilaterally controlled, the phenomenon of hemispheric specialization itself is not in dispute. There is a generally understood class of tasks – verbal or verbosequential – better performed by the left hemisphere, and another class – spatial or visuospatial – better performed by the right. It is also understood that this classification is dichotomous for convenience. There may be more than one ability or factor dominantly associated with a single hemisphere. The word dominant is meant to imply that the other hemisphere – in fact, the whole integrated brain – also participates in the task performance, but less so. Validity is derived empirically and accordingly defines the "average" brain, or the collective brain of a group of randomly selected, neurologically intact individuals.

The concept of individual hemisphericity has, by contrast to task hemisphericity, invoked considerable controversy, not only in definition, but also in validation, implication, and most important, in usefulness for scientific inquiry (Beaumont et al., 1984; Ehrlichman & Weinberger, 1978). Historically, individual hemisphericity meant that an individual tended to use one hemisphere more than the other to perceive stimuli, perform tasks, and solve problems (Bogen et al., 1972). Such reliance was not necessarily inherent, but could be learned; and not necessarily fixed, but could vary in time and across circumstances. Such variation notwithstanding, it was also believed that an individual's hemisphericity was characteristic of that person's behavior. Those who tended to rely on their right hemisphere, or who had a net bias in favor of performance by the right hemisphere, tended to do so most of the time. They would be expected to perform better on "right hemisphere" tasks than they would on "left hemisphere" tasks.

It is this original concept that has potentially the greatest utility in neuropsychological research. Individual hemisphericity describes cognitive behavior in terms of validated brain function. Brain function, by definition, is the end result of neuroanatomic structure, neuron-neuron interaction, and mechanisms of associated neurotransmitters, receptors, and metabolic processes. For example, if individual hemisphericity shifts as a result of an experimental manipulation (e.g. ingestion of a drug) or natural phenomenon (e.g. cerebral vascular accident), the underlying cerebral changes are of significant heuristic value.

Validation

Individual hemisphericity is a continuous variable whose value is based on behavioral measures which presumably reflect underlying neurophysiological processes. The strength of the behavioral/neurophysiological association requires that the behavioral measures (1) are valid, and (2) reflect the underlying neurophysiological activation of one cerebral hemisphere relative to the other. Criticism of the behavioral measures immediately arose (Beaumont et al., 1984) because of inadequate validation. Whereas task hemisphericity was established by emerging evidence from studies on unilateral lesion and com-

missurotomy patients, and on normal subjects, individual hemisphericity was mostly confused with cognitive laterality and, with a few exceptions, was never validated according to the original intent. Cognitive laterality indicated a hemispheric specialization in performance of a type of task, but *laterality* implies location. It does not address the relative contribution of the two hemispheres for a person's thinking or problem-solving approach. Another notion of individual hemisphericity was that it meant relative *activation* of the neurons in the left and right hemispheres. This led to the assumption that noncognitive measures, such as eye movements, hemispheric blood flow or glucose metabolism, could measure individual hemisphericity. Thus a number of studies estimated the relative right/left contribution to problem-solving merely by assessing the percentage of lateral eye movements in one direction or the other. The validity of this assumption was virtually never proven.

ALTERNATIVE MEASURES OF HEMISPHERICITY

Lateral eye movements

It was first observed (Day, 1964) that individuals tended to avert their eyes when asked a reflective question. Early speculation suggested that asymmetry in the direction of gaze might reflect hemispheric differences in function (Bakan, 1969). The idea was validated in a study (Kinsbourne, 1972) where 85 percent of the lateral eye movements were rightward for questions requiring verbal reflection or thought, while 77 percent were to the left for questions requiring spatial imagination. The study had an elegant experimental condition whereby eye movements, as dependent variables, were more to the left for spatial thought and more to the right for verbal thought, even when the stimulus question was exactly the same in both cases. (The question, "The ―― is above the ――, etc." was either to be repeated or sketched.) These results made eye movements a good indicator of *task* hemisphericity, that is, hemispheric specialization for verbal and spatial tasks influenced the direction of movement. Accordingly, eye movements assessed measures of cognitive LATERALITY (as did DICHOTIC LISTENING and tachistoscopic viewing), but not *individual* hemisphericity.

For lateral eye movement to be an index for individual hemisphericity, it must first be shown that the movements reflect increased hemisphere activation. Secondly, it must be shown that when there is a greater activation of one hemisphere, there will be better performance on tasks associated with that hemisphere. Data for either condition are sparse. In a study of BLOOD FLOW (Gur & Reivich, 1980), there was a significant increase in the right hemisphere for people who tended to avert their eyes to the left, but only a trend for a left hemisphere increase for right movers. Other evidence accrued from visually evoked electrocortical potentials (Shevrin et al., 1980). A relatively larger electrical response was observed in the left visual cortex for right movers and in the right cortex for left movers. While these results were in the predicted direction, the stimulus was not "cognitive" (a reversing checkerboard), the latency was relatively early (90 msec), and the relationship between the amplitude of an evoked response and its validity to reflect hemispheric activation had not been shown.

One study attempted to validate the second required condition, namely that a "left mover" would demonstrate better performance on tasks associated with the right hemisphere, and vice versa (Tucker & Suib, 1978). Information and vocabulary subtests of a standard IQ test were chosen to assess left hemispheric function; block design and object assembly assessed right hemisphere function. The validity of these choices was based on several studies of patients with unilateral left or right brain lesions. In support of the hypothesis, there was a modest correlation between direction of eye movement and the difference in performance between the "left" and "right" hemisphere tests.

In spite of the weak support for the assumption that lateral eye movements reflected individual hemisphericity, the measure was used repeatedly in published studies. Typically, subjects were classified into "left movers" or "right movers" on the basis of a few questions requiring reflective thought (e.g. Gur & Gur, 1974; Sackeim et al., 1977). Such groups were then compared to each other on a panoply of dependent measures including psychopathology (Sandel & Alcorn, 1980), expressivity (Newlin, 1981), and ALEXITHYMIA (Cole & Bakan, 1985). If the groups differed on the dependent measures, it was concluded that the differences reflected relative activation and contribution to the observed behavior by differential functioning of the cerebral hemispheres. (*See also* LATERAL EYE MOVEMENTS.)

Self-report surveys and questionnaires

The self-report method of estimating hemisphericity has the least validity. Typically, assessment instruments were constructed of seemingly face-valid statements about what might constitute "right hemisphere" or "left hemisphere" behavior. As an example, an examinee would be requested to endorse statements that might suggest a tendency to be organized, creative, or to think "spatially." A hemisphericity score would be derived according to the number of endorsed statements associated with the author's concept of right or left hemisphere behavior. When used as an independent measure, the hemisphericity measure, like lateral eye movements, would be compared to other variables from emotionality (Zenhausern et al., 1981) to business management skills.

The self-report measure of hemisphericity has no validity with respect to brain function. Endorsement of "left hemisphere" or "right hemisphere" self-report items is not associated with performance on verbal or spatial tasks; in fact, a slightly negative correlation has been reported (Knolle et al., 1987).

COGNITIVE ASSESSMENTS OF HEMISPHERICITY

Relative performance

The original intention in coining "hemisphericity" was to have a term to distinguish among people who tended to think and function more "spatially," as might be attributed to the right hemisphere, compared to those who performed more "verbally," as might be attributed to the left. The methods of assessment including lateral activation (e.g. eye movements) obscured the most direct measurement, and the one first applied to hemisphericity (Bogen et al., 1972): individual hemisphericity was estimated by the relative performance between a closure task (associated with the right hemisphere) and a word similarities test (associated with the left). This original estimate was based on raw scores on tests available at the time. But by the most straightforward application of the term, individual hemisphericity should be reflected by differences in performance between the *best examples* of standardized tests most associated with, or likely to be performed in, the right hemisphere as compared to tasks performed by the left. A person who performs better on tests associated with the right hemisphere would have "right hemisphericity," by definition. If several examples of right and left hemisphere tests are used, the tests for one hemisphere should be factor-related, and different from factor-related tests for the other hemisphere. The magnitude of hemisphericity estimated in this way is directly related to the degree of functional dominance in performance between the two factors of tests. It is important that hemisphericity should be independent of overall performance.

Validity is implicit in the methodology. Hemisphere-related tasks are chosen from a now vast literature. Both neurological patients and normal subjects demonstrate relative performance on several tasks which reflect relative dominance of hemispheric function. The better the choice of tests that assess the function of one hemisphere, the more closely they will cluster in factor scores. Hemisphericity would be independent of overall performance if standard scores are calculated and if the hemisphericity estimate is a difference between the "right hemisphere" composite and the "left hemisphere" composite.

Selection of tests of hemisphericity is not unlike selection of tests to measure any cognitive or behavioral entity. HANDEDNESS is a good example. The first question is: Does one want to measure relative hand "preference" or hand "performance"? For preference, subjects are asked to indicate which hand they use (or prefer) for a number of face valid items of unimanual hand use. For performance, skilled maneuvers are required, such as moving pegs or cutting patterns. Perhaps handedness would be best measured by more physiological measures, such as reflex or strength. All of these HANDEDNESS measures are intercorrelated, but selection of the most valid measure is, in some sense, dependent on the definition, and on the behavioral, as well as neurophysiological, significance of the entity called "handedness" (Annett, 1985).

Hemisphericity as a dichotomy

The one qualitative difficulty with the original concept of hemisphericity is the seemingly absolute dichotomy of hemispheric function. No single task or cluster of tasks is the province of only one hemisphere. The second hemisphere, as well as subcortical systems, are also involved in the cognitive ideation needed to complete complex tasks. Since there is a contribution by both hemispheres to any one task, what does it mean to link a test to the right or left hemisphere? Take the example of a verbal task that is, say, performed 90 percent by the left hemisphere but a spatial task that is performed 60 percent by the right. Equal performances on both (relative to a standard) would be interpreted as having no hemisphericity while, in fact, there was greater left hemisphere involvement. The situation is worse for measures of hemispheric activation because asymmetries of blood flow, eye movements, or glucose metabolism may reflect excitatory, inhibitory, or nonspecific functional differences. In other words, all "best" measures of hemispheric function assume equal asymmetry of dominance between the hemispheres. And, like handedness measures, all tasks associated with one hemisphere are assumed to be equal to each other, at least in terms of their asymmetrical engagement of hemispheric processing.

The empirical response to this dilemma is to determine whether the formulation of hemisphericity is heuristically useful, that is, does the variable hemisphericity predict meaningful relationships? If so, how can the dependent variables be explained in terms of the formulation of hemisphericity? When meaningful interpretations are demanded, estimates of hemisphericity by such techniques as lateral activation (e.g. eye movements) or self-report inventories fail to be useful. It is not that eye movements or inventories fail to relate to dependent variables, such as emotion or business skill, but rather the meaning of this relationship is obscure in terms of brain function. By contrast, when hemisphericity is defined in terms of relative performance between previously validated tasks of hemispheric function, interpretation of the dependent variables in terms of right and left brain processing is a good first-order approximation to the underlying situation.

A modified view of hemisphericity

In order to refine the original concept of hemisphericity in particular, and individual hemisphericity in general, it is necessary to refocus the concept that right and left hemispheric tasks are associated with the right and left hemicortical masses. At the same time, the well-established differences in cognitive processing attributed to the right and left hemispheres (most ideally, in the strongly familial right-handed, normally intelligent, neurologically intact male) must be recognized and preserved. The modified concept of hemisphericity replaces the anatomical dichotomy – right and left cerebral cortices – with non-localized entities – neurosystems. A neurosystem would include anatomical connections, as well as the associated neurotransmitters, receptors, and metabolites. These systems are extra-hemispheric and therefore are meant to include the possibility of functional contribution from both hemispheres. A "right" neurosystem would subserve tasks empirically chosen for their association with the right hemisphere. These tasks would be expected to invoke processing by neuroanatomical structures and neurotransmitter systems primarily in the right brain, but would invoke, as a matter of fact, processing by the part of the *same* neurosystem also located in the left hemisphere. Therefore, when "verbal" or "verbosequential" is compared to "spatial" or "visuospatial," the resultant hemisphericity reflects the relative performance of these neurosystems associated with the two hemispheres, wherever they actually may be anatomically located in an individual. If individuals differ in their hemisphericity, it would not be interpreted as a relative difference in efficiency or activation of their right and left hemispheres, but rather as a relative difference in efficiency or activation of the two (different) neurosystems.

This modified concept also precludes the expectation that laterality be correlated with hemisphericity. There is no theoretical reason why degree of ear dominance in dichotic listening, field dominance in tachistoscopic viewing, or lateral eye movements should be correlated with differences in levels of performance on visuospatial and verbosequential tests. In fact, they are not.

SAMPLE TESTS AND IMPLEMENTATION

A test battery

A battery of tests under development since the mid-1970s was designed to assess hemisphericity by comparing performance on tests chosen from the literature to be best measures of right and left

hemisphere function. (The end result, called the Cognitive Laterality Battery (Gordon, 1986), had an unfortunate misnomer in the title in light of the current confusion of "laterality" with "hemisphericity.") The tests were not intended to be presented laterally (i.e. exclusively to one hemisphere) because it is assumed that performance on the tests reflects efficiency of the hemisphere or, in the modified conceptualization, the neurosystem. Nevertheless, the tests fulfill the requirements of (1) initial selection to be associated with right or left hemispheric function, (2) factor loading on two orthogonal factors in several samples of normal subjects, and (3) availability of standardized norms. The factor structure is stable between the sexes and across age groups; the difference score – the hemisphericity measure – is stable over time (Gordon & Kravetz, 1991). There are significant differences in performance levels between males and females on some tests; but these are neutralized by calculating norms appropriate to each sex.

Tests associated with the left hemisphere include serial processing or temporal ordering. Subjects hear two-, three-, ... seven-item sequences of well-known environmental sounds and are required to write them down in the correct order. Another test uses numbers instead of sounds. Two tests of verbal output require writing as many words as possible in a minute that begin with a given letter or that fall within a given category. Tests associated with right hemisphere processing include locating points in (two-dimensional) space, mentally rotating pictured images of two- or three-dimensional geometric figures, and recognizing objects from silhouette forms (closure).

Hemisphericity scores (cognitive profiles) are calculated from the difference between the averaged standard scores for each cluster (factor) of tests. If an individual receives a difference score of zero, this means there is no greater ability to perform tests from one factor relative to the other. A score that signifies relatively better performance on the cluster of tests associated with the right hemisphere defines the person as having a right hemisphericity. In the modified concept, it would mean, first of all, that there is a neurosystem that is more involved in performing such tasks, and secondly, that this neurosystem is more efficient than the "verbosequential" neurosystem in this individual.

Application of the cognitive profile

One example where the cognitive profile has been contributory to scientific understanding is in individuals with specific learning disability. Deficits in verbal ability and sequencing skills are well-known correlates to learning difficulties, especially in reading. Theories have attributed this disorder to left hemisphere dysfunction (among other things). However, an application of cognitive tests to learning-disabled individuals not only confirmed the reduced verbosequential performance, but highlighted an *increased* visuospatial performance (Harness et al., 1984), that is, the cognitive profile reflected strong performance relying on functions associated with the right cerebral hemisphere, on a neurosystem associated with the right hemisphere. This conceptualization would suggest that understanding of learning disabilities should focus at least as much on a supra-efficient "right" neurosystem as on a sub-efficient "left" neurosystem.

Another example demonstrates a shift in cognitive profile in normal individuals as a function of sleep states (Gordon et al., 1982). Individuals were awakened twice during the night, once during Rapid Eye Movement sleep and once in Stage II sleep. Cognitive tests were given immediately at both times with the result that all subjects shifted, with respect to themselves, toward relatively better performance on visuospatial-type tests upon waking from Rapid Eye Movement sleep and relatively better verbosequential performance upon waking from Stage II sleep. Since it is unlikely to expect these shifts to be based on neuroanatomical changes, cognitive profile shifting reflects cycling of the neurochemical efficiency in the "right" or "left" neurosystems. Ultradian cycles of cognitive performance were also seen throughout the day (Gordon et al., 1995; Klein & Armitage, 1979), again suggesting the neurochemical nature of neurosystems underlying specialized cognitive function.

CULTURAL HEMISPHERICITY

The concept of cultural hemisphericity is an expansion of the individual hemisphericity idea to groups of ethnographically similar individuals. In the first description, the culture groups were urban and rural Americans of European descent, of African descent, and of descent from North American indigenous people. A test associated with right hemisphere function and a test of left

hemisphere function were administered with the result that the rural, the African Americans, and especially the Native Americans tended to perform relatively better on the "right hemisphere" test (Bogen et al., 1972). This finding was corroborated later in Americans of European and African descent (Thompson et al., 1979), in Aboriginal children compared to White Australian urban children (TenHouten, 1985), and individuals with subdominant social status in American societies (TenHouten, 1980). The results were interpreted to mean that these cultural or social groups tended to rely more on their right hemispheres. In the modified view this would be interpreted as relying more on neurosystems associated with right hemisphere function. Unfortunately, these findings have been limited in the variety of measures of assessment, leaving open the possibility that an unknown cultural bias in the tests themselves yielded unwarranted conclusions. However, the concept is worthy for heuristic reasons. If it were true that a particular culture group, especially one that was largely inbred and isolated, exhibited cognitive skills that were associated with one neurosystem more than the other, it would be reasonable to pursue investigations into the underlying genetic control, selective mating, and neurobiological factors.

SUMMARY

Hemisphericity is a concept that was initiated by observation of major differences in processing by the right and left cerebral hemispheres. Three levels of hemisphericity are distinguished. The simplest is task hemisphericity that refers to the hemisphere conducive to, or specialized for, processing or performing a task. Individual hemisphericity refers to the cerebral hemisphere that an individual is more likely to rely upon for performance of a task, *independent of the nature of the task itself*. For some individuals this might lead to performance of an inherently "right hemisphere" task with the "wrong" processing by the left hemisphere. An example would be to systematically analyze a three-dimensional object, instead of imagining its whole. It may also be the case that individual hemisphericity may not override task hemisphericity where there is strong specialization, as in the example of speech. Finally, cultural hemisphericity refers to the hemisphere relatively favored by people of an ethnographically homogeneous cultural group as compared to another cultural group.

A modified view of hemisphericity would not restrict the dichotomy of function to the anatomical entities – the right and left hemispheres per se – but rather to a neurosystem that, in the ideal case, would be most strongly associated with the right and left hemispheres. It should also be recalled that hemisphericity is a dichotomy because of the historical observation that there are qualitatively two different modes of cognitive thought. A broader concept of hemisphericity – better named, perhaps, "cognitive profile" – would be empirically defined as a vector including more than these two dimensions. However, the dichotomy has practical application in trying to understand the cerebral processes underlying cognitive function, and to understand how individuals come to differ in the manifestation of these processes.

BIBLIOGRAPHY

Annett, M. (1985). *Left, right, hand and brain: The right shift theory*. London: Lawrence Erlbaum.

Bakan, P. (1969). Hypnotizability, laterality of eye movements, and functional brain asymmetry. *Perceptual and Motor Skills, 28*, 927–32.

Beaumont, J. G., Young, A. W., & McManus, I. C. (1984). Hemisphericity: a critical review. *Cognitive Neuropsychology, 1*, 191–212.

Bogen, J. E., & Bogen, G. M. (1983). Hemispheric specialization and cerebral laterality. *Behavioral and Brain Sciences, 3*, 517–20.

Bogen, J. E., DeZure, R., TenHouten, W. D., & Marsh, J. F. (1972). The other side of the brain IV. The A/P ratio. *Bulletin of the Los Angeles Neurological Societies, 37*, 49–61.

Cole, G., & Bakan, P. (1985). Alexithymia, hemisphericity, and conjugate lateral eye movements. *Psychotherapy and Psychosomatics, 44*, 139–43.

Day, M. E. (1964). An eye movement phenomenon relating to attention, thought and anxiety. *Perceptual and Motor Skills, 19*, 443–6.

Ehrlichman, H., & Weinberger, A. (1978). Lateral eye movements and hemispheric asymmetry: a critical review. *Psychological Bulletin, 85*, 1080–101.

Gordon, H. W. (1986). The Cognitive Laterality Battery: tests of specialized cognitive function. *International Journal of Neuroscience, 29*, 223–44.

Gordon, H. W., Frooman, B., & Lavie, P. (1982). Shift in cognitive asymmetries between wakenings from REM and NREM sleep. *Neuropsychologia, 20*, 99–103.

Gordon, H. W., & Kravetz, S. (1991). The influence of gender, handedness, and performance level on specialized cognitive functioning. *Brain and Cognition, 15*, 37–61.

Gordon, H. W., Stoffer, D. S., & Lee, P. A. (1995). Ultradian rhythms in performance on tests of specialized cognitive function. *International Journal of Neuroscience* (in press).

Gur, R. C., & Gur, R. E. (1974). Handedness, sex, and eyedness as moderating variables in the relation between hypnotic susceptibility and functional brain asymmetry. *Journal of Abnormal Psychology, 83*, 635–43.

Gur, R. C., & Reivich, M. (1980). Cognitive task effects on hemispheric blood flow in humans: Evidence for individual differences in hemispheric activation. *Brain and Language, 9*, 78–92.

Harness, B. Z., Epstein, R., & Gordon, H. W. (1984). Cognitive profile of children referred to a clinic for learning disabilities. *Journal of Learning Disabilities, 17*, 346–52.

Kinsbourne, M. (1972). Eye and head turning indicates cerebral lateralization. *Science, 176*, 539–41.

Klein, R., & Armitage, R. (1979). Rhythms in human performance: 1½-hour oscillations in cognitive style. *Science, 204*, 1326–7.

Knolle, L., Gordon, H. W., & Gwany, D. (1987). Relationship between performance and preference measures of cognitive laterality. *Psychological Reports, 61*, 215–23.

Newlin, D. B. (1981). Hemisphericity, expressivity and autonomic arousal. *Biological Psychology, 12*, 13–23.

Sackheim, H. A., Packer, I. K., & Gur, R. C. (1977). Hemisphericity, cognitive set, and susceptibility to subliminal perception. *Journal of Abnormal Psychology, 86*, 624–30.

Sandel, A., & Alcorn, J. D. (1980). Individual hemisphericity and maladaptive behaviors. *Journal of Abnormal Psychology, 89*, 514–17.

Shevrin, H., Smokler, I., & Kooi, K. A. (1980). An empirical link between lateral eye movements and lateralized event-related brain potentials. *Biological Psychiatry, 15*, 691–7.

TenHouten, W. D. (1980). Social dominance and cerebral hemisphericity: discriminating race, socioeconomic status, and sex groups by performance on two lateralized tests. *International Journal of Neuroscience, 10*, 223–32.

TenHouten, W. D. (1985). Right hemisphericity of Australian Aboriginal children: effects of culture, sex, and age on performances of closure and similarities tests. *International Journal of Neuroscience, 28*, 125–46.

Thompson, A. L., Bogen, J. E., & Marsh, J. F., Jr. (1979). Cultural hemisphericity: evidence from cognitive tests. *International Journal of Neuroscience, 9*, 37–43.

Tucker, G. H., & Suib, M. R. (1978). Conjugate lateral eye movements (CLEM) direction and its relationship to performance on verbal and visuospatial tasks. *Neuropsychologia, 16*, 251–4.

Zenhausern, R., Notaro, J., Grosso, J., & Schiano, P. (1981). The interaction of hemispheric preference, laterality, and sex in the perception of emotional tone and verbal content. *International Journal of Neuroscience, 13*, 121–6.

HAROLD W. GORDON

Henschen's axiom Henschen's axiom states that restitution of speech in recovery from global aphasia is due to the activity of the hemisphere opposite to that premorbidly serving speech. Although it is associated with Henschen (1922), he gave credit to Wernicke and other contemporaries for this principle.

Heschl's gyrus Heschl's gyrus is close to the posterior end of the superior TEMPORAL LOBE, within the SYLVIAN FISSURE. Only the PLANUM TEMPORALE lies between it and the posterior termination of the fissure. Heschl's gyrus is the primary auditory cortex, and is one of the sites of lateral cortical asymmetry in humans. The area of Heschl's gyrus in the right hemisphere (in right-handed individuals) may be up to twice the extent of that in the left hemisphere; in this regard it complements the adjacent planum temporale, which is larger in the left hemisphere.

heterotopia A form of abnormal development of the nervous system, heterotopia is characterized by the appearance of displaced islands of gray matter within the subcortical white matter or in the walls of the ventricles. Heterotopia results from a failure in the normal process of cell migration, following differentiation, from inner layers of the lining of the brain through to the outer layers of the cortex.

Heubner's artery Heubner's artery is in the proximal territory of the anterior cerebral artery. It is noteworthy because of the distinctive vascular syndrome described by Critchley of unilateral and predominantly motor dysfunction, associated with vascular lesion of the anterior cerebral artery adjacent to the origin of Heubner's artery.

hippocampus Evidence implicates this brain region in memory. The finding that bilateral damage to the TEMPORAL LOBE which included hippocampal damage led to anterograde AMNESIA (originally studied in HM) has been extensively investigated (Scoville & Milner, 1957; Milner et al., 1968; Squire & Knowlton, 1994). Learning about new events (episodic memory) and facts (semantic memory) is severely impaired after the damage. The type of learning impaired has been characterized as declarative, or knowing that, as contrasted with procedural, or knowing how, which is spared in amnesia. Declarative memory includes what can be declared or brought to mind as a proposition or an image. It also includes episodic memory, that is, memory for particular episodes, and semantic memory, that is, memory for facts (Squire & Knowlton, 1994). There is also evidence in humans that damage to the FORNIX, one of the major afferent and efferent pathways of the hippocampus, produces anterograde amnesia (Gaffan, 1991). The memory of events which occurred up to some months before the brain damage may be relatively intact, so that permanent long-term memories are not stored in the hippocampus. Memories for a period of perhaps months before the brain damage may be impaired, and the relatively greater loss of recent rather than old memories has been referred to as the temporal gradient of retrograde amnesia (Squire, 1992).

There are left–right differences in the function of the hippocampus in humans. Left temporal lobe and hippocampal damage tends to impair verbal memory tasks, such as word-paired associate learning (Kolb & Whishaw, 1990), while damage to the right temporal lobe impairs conditional spatial response learning (Petrides, 1985). (In this task, arbitrary spatial responses must be learned to different stimuli, so that it is a type of episodic spatial memory task.)

Because it is not clear from the human evidence exactly which parts of the temporal lobe (the hippocampus, the entorhinal cortex, the parahippocampal gyrus, etc.) are crucial for this memory function, studies to investigate these regions, and the contribution each makes to memory, have been performed on animals.

FUNCTIONS OF THE HIPPOCAMPUS IN ANIMALS

In rats, damage to the hippocampus produces spatial learning deficits in tasks which require a cognitive map of allocentric space, that is, space defined as relations between objects and their places in the world. The deficits are not in processing egocentric space, that is, space defined relative to the body. An example of such a learning deficit is seen in a task in which the rat must learn to use room cues to swim through cloudy milk to find a hidden submerged platform (the Morris water maze; Morris, 1989). There may also be deficits in some nonspatial tasks (Jarrard, 1993).

In monkeys, which have a temporal lobe much more like that of humans, spatial learning and memory deficits are also evident after damage to the hippocampus or to one of its major connecting pathways, the fornix. Deficits in learning about the places of responses and about the places of stimuli are produced (see Gaffan & Harrison, 1989). All these tasks can be thought of as examples of spatial episodic memory, in that rapid learning of the task with one set of stimuli and responses is required, and later new stimuli and responses must be learned, so that on each occasion a particular memory of the stimulus response conditions currently used must be formed. For example, fornix lesions impair conditional left–right discrimination learning, in which the visual appearance of an object specifies whether a response is to be made to the left or the right. Fornix-sectioned monkeys are also impaired in learning on the basis of a spatial cue which object to choose (e.g. if two objects are on the left, choose object A, but if the two objects are on the right, choose object B). Similarly, macaques and humans with damage to the hip-

pocampus or fornix are impaired in object-place memory tasks in which not only the objects seen, but where they were seen, must be remembered (Angeli et al., 1993; Smith & Milner, 1981). Such object-place tasks require a whole scene or a snapshot-like memory in which spatial relations in a scene must be remembered in an episodic way.

Monkeys with fornix damage are also impaired in using information about their place in an environment. For example, Gaffan and Harrison (1989) found learning impairments when which of two or more objects the monkey had to choose depended on the position of the monkey in the room.

It now appears that the deficits in recognition memory produced by temporal lobe damage may be due not to damage to the hippocampus proper, but to the adjacent and connected entorhinal cortex and parahippocampal gyrus. The evidence for this is that tests of whether an object can be remembered in a delayed match-to-sample task are impaired by parahippocampal damage, but not much by damage to the hippocampus itself (Zola-Morgan et al., 1994). In a delayed match-to-sample task, an object or picture is shown, there is then a delay (of 10 seconds to several minutes) and then the object is shown again; if recognized, it must be selected.

SPATIAL AND NON-SPATIAL ASPECTS OF HIPPOCAMPAL FUNCTION

One way of relating the impairment of spatial processing to other aspects of hippocampal function is to note that this spatial processing involves a snapshot type of memory, in which one whole scene must be remembered (Gaffan & Harrison, 1989; Gaffan, 1994). This memory may then be a special case of episodic memory, which involves an arbitrary association of a set of events which describe a past episode. Further, the nonspatial tasks impaired by damage to the hippocampal system may be impaired because they are tasks in which a memory of a particular episode rather than of a general rule is involved. Thus the learning of tasks with non-general rules, such as choosing the object not previously rewarded (i.e. win shift, lose stay) may be impaired because to solve them the particular pairing in the particular context (of performing with this special rule) must be remembered in order to choose the correct object later. The natural rule, which will in the natural environment usually lead to reward, is to choose the object previously associated with reward. Another example is that choosing familiar rather than novel objects in a recognition memory task may be particularly difficult for monkeys with damage to the hippocampal system because it involves a special rule, choosing the familiar object in this task, rather than what may be a more general tendency, that is, to choose the novel rather than the familiar object. The latter rule is what normally guides behavior, as this rule is more likely to lead to reward for objects without an explicit reward association already in the natural environment. Further, recognition memory may be particularly impaired when this involves the memory of particular and arbitrary associations between parts of the image, especially when the same elements may occur in different combinations in other images. Also, the deficit in paired associate learning in humans may be especially evident when this involves arbitrary associations between words, for example, "window" and "take."

THE STRUCTURE AND CONNECTIONS OF THE HIPPOCAMPUS

Inputs converge into the hippocampus, via the parahippocampal gyrus and perirhinal cortex, which in turn feed into the entorhinal cortex and thus into the hippocampus, from virtually all association areas in the neocortex, including areas in the parietal cortex concerned with spatial function, temporal areas concerned with vision and hearing, and the frontal lobes (Figure 48). An extensively divergent system of output projections enables the hippocampus to feed back into most of the cortical areas from which it receives inputs.

INFORMATION IN THE HIPPOCAMPUS

In order to understand the role of the hippocampus in memory, it is necessary to know what information is represented in the hippocampus. Whole series of findings have shown that hippocampal pyramidal cells (e.g. CA3 and CA1 neurons) in rats respond when the rat is in a particular place in a spatial environment. In monkeys, it has been shown that there is a rich representation of space outside the monkey, in that (10 per cent of hippocampal) neurons in monkeys respond to particular positions in space

(see Rolls & O'Mara, 1993). In many cases this spatial encoding has been shown to be allocentric, that is, coded in world coordinates, not in egocentric coordinates relative to the body axis (Feigenbaum & Rolls, 1991). Moreover, 1 percent of hippocampal neurons combine information about the object shown and the place where it is shown, in that they respond in an object-place memory task differentially to the novel and familiar presentations of an object shown in a particular place (Rolls et al., 1989). Consistent with this, in a cue-controlled environment, some hippocampal neurons in primates respond to views of particular parts of the environment, irrespective of where the monkey is. These findings together show that there is a representation of space outside the organism in primates. This may be important, in that primates can explore space by moving the eyes to look at different places in the environment, and they can remember the location of what they see there. In contrast, the hippocampal spatial cells found so far in rats respond when the rat is in a particular place, perhaps related to the fact that rats normally need to visit places in order to explore and store information about them, consistent with their use of olfactory cues and their relatively poor vision compared to primates (O'Keefe, 1984; O'Keefe & Speakman, 1987). Another type of spatial information that has been found in primates is information about whole body motion (O'Mara et al., 1994). Such cells, for example, respond to clockwise but not counter-clockwise whole-body motion, or to forward but not backward linear translation. In some cases these neurons appear to be driven by vestibular information (in that they respond when the monkey is moved on a robot without performing the movement in the dark), while others are driven by the optic flow that is induced by whole-body motion (O'Mara et al., 1994). These cells may be important in short-range navigation, for which a memory of recent movements is needed. In addition, in monkeys, when conditional spatial response tasks are being performed, some hippocampal neurons respond to combinations of the visual image and the spatial response which must be linked by memory for the task to be performed correctly, and during the learning of such visual to spatial response associations, the responses of some hippocampal neurons become modified (Cahusac et al., 1993).

On the basis of these findings about neuronal activity in the hippocampus, and the effects of

397

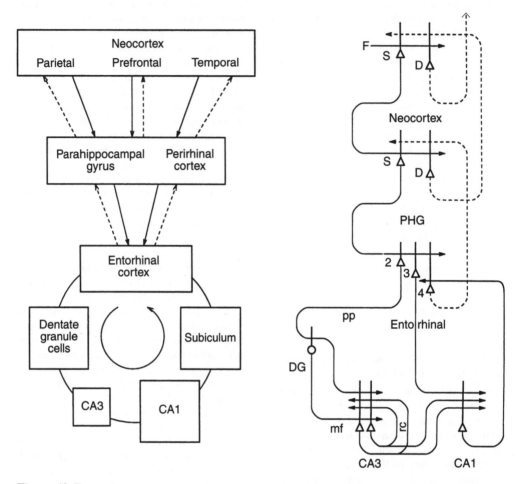

Figure 48 Forward connections (solid lines) from areas of cerebral association neocortex via the parahippocampal gyrus and perihinal cortex, and entorhinal cortex, to the hippocampus; and back-projections (dashed lines) via the hippocampal CA1 pyramidal cells, subiculum, and parahippocampal gyrus to the neocortex. There is great convergence in the forward connections down to the single network implemented in the CA3 pyramidal cells, and great divergence again in the back-projections. Left: block diagram. Right: more detailed representation of some of the principal excitatory neurons in the pathways. D, deep pyramidal cells; DG, dentate granule cells; F, forward inputs to areas of the association cortex from preceding cortical areas in the hierarchy; mf, mossy fibers; PHG, parahippocampal gyrus and perirhinal cortex; pp, perforant path; rc, recurrent collateral of the CA3 hippocampal pyramidal cells; S, superficial pyramidal cells; 2, pyramidal cells in layer 2 of the entorhinal cortex; 3, pyramidal cells in layer 3 of the entorhinal cortex. The thick lines above the cell bodies represent the dendrites.

damage to the hippocampus, the hypothesis is suggested that the importance of the hippocampus in spatial and other memories is that it can rapidly form "episodic" representations of information originating from many areas of the cerebral cortex, and act as an intermediate term buffer store.

Given that memories do not appear to be stored in the long term in the hippocampus, there must be a way to recall the information from the buffer store, and utilize it to help build long-term memories in the cerebral cortex. Ways in which the recall could operate are considered below.

In order to understand how the hippocampus could store the information it receives from the cerebral neocortex, and form, for example, episodic memories which link spatial information with information about objects which originate from different regions of the cerebral cortex, the internal circuitry of the hippocampus and how it could operate should be considered (see Rolls, 1989a, b; Treves & Rolls, 1994; see also Marr, 1971).

HIPPOCAMPAL CA3 CIRCUITRY

Projections from the entorhinal cortex reach the granule cells (of which there are 10^6 in the rat) in the dentate gyrus (DG) via the perforant path (pp). The granule cells project to CA3 cells via the mossy fibers (MF), which provide a *sparse* but possibly powerful connection to the $3 \cdot 10^5$ CA3 pyramidal cells in the rat. Each CA3 cell receives approximately 50 mossy fiber inputs, so that the sparseness of this connectivity is thus 0.005 per cent. By contrast, there are many more – possibly weaker – direct perforant path inputs onto each CA3 cell in the rat of the order of $4 \cdot 10^3$. The largest number of synapses (about $1.2 \cdot 10^4$ in the rat) on the dendrites of CA3 pyramidal cells is, however, provided by the (recurrent) axon collaterals of CA3 cells themselves (rc). It is remarkable that the recurrent collaterals are distributed to other CA3 cells throughout the hippocampus (see Treves & Rolls, 1994), so that effectively the CA3 system provides a single network, with a connectivity of approximately 4 percent between the different CA3 neurons (see Figure 48).

HIPPOCAMPAL LONG-TERM POTENTIATION

When the presynaptic terminals and the postsynaptic dendrites are conjunctively strongly activated for a short period (e.g. 100 ms), an increase in the synaptic connection strength occurs, as shown by the fact that subsequent stimulation of those terminals produces a larger effect on the postsynaptic cell. The effect is synapse-specific, and in most parts of the hippocampus (but not at the mossy fiber synapses) is associative, in that it requires conjunctive pre- and post-synaptic activity. Long-term potentiation (LTP) requires strong post-synaptic activation as one of the conditions for its induction, because the NMDA (N-methyl-D-aspartate)

channels which allow calcium to enter the post-synaptic cell are voltage-gated (depolarization) (Bliss & Collingridge, 1993). With its associativity, synapse specificity, and long duration (it has been demonstrated to last for as much as several weeks), it is an attractive candidate for one of the types of synaptic modification that underlie learning. Consistent with this, there is some evidence that blockade of LTP using blockers of the NMDA receptors prevents the formation of new hippocampal-dependent memories (Morris, 1989).

CA3 AS AN AUTOASSOCIATION MEMORY

On the basis of the evidence summarized above, Rolls (1989, 1990) has suggested that the CA3 stage acts as an autoassociation memory which enables episodic memories to be formed and stored for an intermediate term in the CA3 network, and that subsequently the extensive recurrent collateral connectivity between the CA3 cells allows for the retrieval of a whole representation to be initiated by the activation of some small part of the same representation (the cue). A quantitative model of how this could occur has been developed (Treves & Rolls, 1991, 1992, 1994). The model shows, for example, how it would be possible to store in the order of 36,000 memories in the rat hippocampus.

It is suggested that the systems level function of this autoassociation memory is to enable events occurring conjunctively in quite different parts of the association areas of the cerebral cortex to be associated together to form a memory which could well be described as episodic. Each episode would be defined by a conjunction of a set of events, and each episodic memory would consist of the association of one set of events (such as where, with whom, and what one ate at lunch on the preceding day). Once recalled in CA3, the recent episodic memory can, via the CA1 cells (which recode the representation into a more appropriate form), trigger recall via the back-projection pathways (dashed lines in Figure 48) of the activity that was originally present in the neocortex during learning. A quantitative theory of this recall function of the back-projection pathways has been developed (Treves & Rolls, 1994), and tested by simulation (Rolls, 1995). Once the neocortical representation that was present during the original episode has been reinstated from the hippocampus as a result of a recall cue, the neocortex is then able to utilize this information to build or add to structured long-term representations. The way in which these long-term neocortical memories are formed is not the subject of this entry, but the expectation is that this has to be very different from the rapid, one-shot, on-line, type of learning in which the hippocampus is involved. Setting up properly structured, often semantic, long-term memories may require a more gradual and organized approach (Treves & Rolls, 1994).

HIPPOCAMPAL FUNCTION AND ALZHEIMER'S DISEASE

The cortical pathological changes such as plaques and tangles that are associated with Alzheimer's disease are found in great density, and early on, in the entorhinal cortex and adjacent parahippocampal areas, which provide the major gateway from the cerebral cortex to the hippocampus (Van Hoesen, 1987). This damage may impair memory not only by deafferenting the hippocampus, but also by impairing neocortical recall of recent memories stored in the hippocampus via the hippocampal back-projection pathways.

See also AMNESIA, AMNESIC SYNDROME.

BIBLIOGRAPHY

Aigner, T. G., Mitchell, S. J., Aggleton, J. P., DeLong, M. R., Struble, R. G., Price, D. L., Wenk, G. L., Pettigrew, K. D., & Mishkin, M. (1991). Transient impairment of recognition memory following ibotenic acid lesions of the basal forebrain in macaques. *Experimental Brain Research, 86,* 18–26.

Angeli, S. J., Murray, E. A., & Mishkin, M. (1993). Hippocampectomized monkeys can remember one place but not two. *Neuropsychologia, 31,* 1021–30.

Bliss, T. V. P., & Collingridge, G. L. (1993). A synaptic model of memory: long-term potentiation in the hippocampus. *Nature, 361,* 31–9.

Cahusac, P. M. B., Rolls, E. T., Miyashita, Y., & Niki, H. (1993). Modification of the responses of hippocampal neurons in the monkey during the learning of a conditional spatial response task. *Hippocampus, 3,* 29–42.

Feigenbaum, J. D., & Rolls, E. T. (1991). Allocentric and egocentric spatial information processing in the hippocampal formation of the behaving primate. *Psychobiology, 19,* 21–40.

Gaffan, D. (1994). Scene-specific memory for objects: a model of episodic memory impairment in monkeys with fornix transection. *Journal of Cognitive Neuroscience, 6,* 305–20.

Gaffan, D., & Gaffan, E. A. (1991). Amnesia in man following transection of the fornix. *Brain, 114,* 2611–18.

Gaffan, D., & Harrison, S. (1989). Place memory and scene memory: effects of fornix transection in the monkey. *Experimental Brain Research, 74,* 202–12.

Jarrard, E. L. (1993). On the role of the hippocampus in learning and memory in the rat. *Behavioral and Neural Biology, 60,* 9–26.

Kolb, B., & Whishaw, I. Q. (1990). *Fundamentals of human neuropsychology,* 3rd edn. New York: Freeman.

Marr, D. (1971). Simple memory: a theory for archicortex. *Philosophical Transactions of the Royal Society London B, 262,* 24–81.

Morris, R. G. M. (1989). Does synaptic plasticity play a role in information storage in the vertebrate brain? In R. G. M. Morris (Ed.), *Parallel distributed processing: Implications for psychology and neurobiology* (pp. 248–85). Oxford: Oxford University Press.

O'Mara, S. M., Rolls, E. T., Berthoz, A., & Kesner, R. P. (1994). Neurons responding to whole-body motion in the primate hippocampus. *Journal of Neuroscience, 14,* 6511–23.

Parkinson, J. K., Murray, E. A., & Mishkin, M. (1988). A selective mnemonic role for the hippocampus in monkeys: memory for the location of objects. *Journal of Neuroscience, 8,* 4059–167.

Petrides, M. (1985). Deficits on conditional associative-learning tasks after frontal- and temporal-lobe lesions in man. *Neuropsychologia, 23,* 601–14.

Rolls, E. T. (1989). Functions of neuronal networks in the hippocampus and neocortex in memory. In J. H. Byrne & W. O. Berry (Eds), *Neural models of plasticity: Experimental and theoretical approaches* (pp. 240–65). San Diego: Academic Press.

Rolls, E. T. (1990). Functions of the primate hippocampus in spatial processing and memory. In D. S. Olton & R. P. Kesner (Eds), *Neurobiology of comparative cognition* (pp. 339–62). Hillsdale, NJ: Erlbaum.

Rolls, E. T., Miyashita, Y., Cahusac, P. M. B., Kesner, R. P., Niki, H., Feigenbaum, J., & Bach, L. (1989). Hippocampal neurons in the monkey with activity related to the place in which a stimulus is shown. *Journal of Neuroscience, 9*, 1835–45.

Rolls, E. T., & O'Mara, S. (1993). Neurophysiological and theoretical analysis of how the hippocampus functions in memory. In T. Ono, L. R. Squire, M. E. Raichle, D. I. Perrett, & M. Fukuda (Eds), *Brain mechanisms of perception and memory: From neuron to behavior* (pp. 276–300). New York: Oxford University Press.

Scoville, W. B., & Milner, B. (1957). Loss of recent memory after bilateral hippocampal lesions. *Journal of Neurology, Neurosurgery and Psychiatry, 20*, 11–21.

Smith, M. L., & Milner, B. (1981). The role of the right hippocampus in the recall of spatial location. *Neuropsychologia, 19*, 781–93.

Squire, L. R. (1992). Memory and the hippocampus: a synthesis from findings with rats, monkeys and humans. *Psychological Reviews, 99*, 195–231.

Squire, L. R., & Knowlton, B. J. (1994). Memory, hippocampus, and brain systems. In M. S. Gazzaniga (Ed.), *The cognitive neurosciences* (pp. 825–37). Cambridge, MA: MIT Press.

Treves, A., & Rolls, E. T. (1991). What determines the capacity of autoassociative memories in the brain? *Network, 2*, 371–97.

Treves, A., & Rolls, E. T. (1992) Computational constraints suggest the need for two distinct input systems to the hippocampal CA3 network. *Hippocampus, 2*, 189–99.

Treves, A., & Rolls, E. T. (1994). A computational analysis of the role of the hippocampus in memory. *Hippocampus, 4*, 374–91.

Van Hoesen, G. W. (1987). Neural correlates of cognitive impairment in Alzheimer's disease. In *Handbook of physiology, Section 1: The Nervous System. Vol. V. Higher functions of the brain.* Part 2 (pp. 87–100). Bethesda, MD: American Physiological Society.

Zola-Morgan, S., Squire, L. R., & Ramus, S. J. (1994). Severity of memory impairment in monkeys as a function of locus and extent of damage within the medial temporal lobe memory system. *Hippocampus, 4*, 483–95.

E. T. ROLLS

holoprosencephaly Holoprosencephaly is an abnormality of development in which the cerebral cortex forms as a single undifferentiated hemisphere, rather than developing normally into the grossly symmetrical left and right cortical hemispheres.

Huntington's disease or **chorea** First described by George Huntington in 1872, Huntington's disease, also known as Huntington's chorea, is a chronically progressive neurodegenerative disorder commonly characterized by a movement disorder, dementia, and psychiatric disturbances. Huntington's disease is genetically transmitted as an autosomal dominant trait with complete penetrance. The expression of Huntington's disease is related to a marked expansion of a trinucleotide repeat at a gene on chromosome 4, IT-15 (interesting transcript 15), and its novel protein product, "huntingtin" (The Huntington's Disease Collaborative Research Group, 1993). The availability of a preclinical test for Huntington's disease has added to the ethical controversy concerning genetic counselling, a relatively underdeveloped field with profound future implications.

Huntington's disease typically presents clinically between the ages of 35 and 40 and has a prevalence of approximately 5 to 10 per 100,000. The interval between symptom onset and severe disability or death is approximately 15 to 20 years. The disease is equally prevalent among males and females, but is less common in blacks and orientals than among whites. Age of onset shows less variation within than between affected families and tends to be earlier with paternal transmission. Progression rates tend to be inversely related to the age of onset and may be accelerated for females, as well as for people with low alcohol consumption or low body weight.

CLINICAL FEATURES

Movement

Huntington's disease is associated with a disorder of both voluntary and involuntary movements. The abnormal involuntary movements are usually choreoathetoid in type and may involve almost any part of the body. The most conspicuous involuntary movements often appear in the upper limbs and face, and patients may attempt to mask their disorder by integrating the abnormal movements into voluntary actions. Early in the course of the disease, the chorea may be exacerbated by stress and diminished by conscious control, but as the disease progresses the chorea may be more pronounced when voluntary movements are attempted (Folstein, 1989).

Although involuntary movements are ordinarily the initial and most salient feature of Huntington's disease, numerous more subtle deficits in voluntary movement also become apparent with progression. Patients may exhibit slowing, as well as deficits in the ability to initiate, sustain, or coordinate movements. These difficulties are apparent in gait, fine motor speed, manual dexterity, and reaching. Voluntary movements of the eyes also show impairment which may be evident in diminished velocity and marked jerkiness on ocular pursuit. Choreoathetotic movements in the oral-bucco-facial regions eventually result in a marked dysarthria that generally compromises all aspects of speech production until late in the disease, when a state of mutism is reached. Chorea also interferes with transport of food to the mouth, as well as chewing and swallowing, thus posing a distinct threat to the patient's life from choking (Folstein, 1989).

BEHAVIOR

Psychiatric disorders, including affective disturbance, psychotic processes, and disinhibition, are relatively common and may even appear before the onset of motor impairment. Affective disturbances are the most common psychiatric difficulty, with some reports documenting the incidence of major depression as high as 50 percent and hypomanic episodes as high as 10 percent. Suicide occurs with higher than base-rate likelihood. Apathy is prevalent but often situational, and the patient can be stimulated into action with explicit direction. Psychotic symptoms may also be present, with a schizophrenia-like syndrome including hallucinations, delusions, and a paranoid state in as many as one-third of cases, and a full-spectrum schizophrenia with thought disorder in as many as 12 percent of cases (Garron, 1973). Disinhibitory symptoms are also evident, with marked irritability evident in as many as 50 percent of cases and often the most proximal cause of hospitalization. Impulsivity is also manifest in abnormal sexual behavior, with a relatively high incidence of hypersexuality in males, as well as a relatively high rate of legal difficulties, arrests, and incarcerations.

COGNITION

Cognitive deficits may proceed or follow onset of motor anomalies and ordinarily progress at a similar rate. Although some language abilities remain relatively preserved until very late in the course of the disease, early impairments are evident in diminished information processing speed (bradyphrenia), and deficits in attention, executive functions, expressive language, visuo-spatial perception, and memory. Attention deficits are most evident with demands for sustained attention in the face of distraction. Disabilities in executive functions, including behavioral regulation and conceptual processing, are particularly evident in a diminished capacity to plan, organize, initiate, execute, and sustain behavioral sequences, as well as in the capacity to acquire, maintain, and shift among conceptual categories. With disease progression, there is a continuous deterioration of all cognitive faculties until the patient is rendered mute and intellectually devastated.

Language comprehension and basic skills including vocabulary and general knowledge are relatively preserved until late in the course of the illness. Comprehension difficulties may initially manifest in problems understanding complex directions or following the gist of conversations. Anomia and aphasia are relatively rare until the latter disease stages, but patients may exhibit early and subtle confrontation naming deficits secondary to visual misperceptions.

The expression of language, however, is often affected in the early stages of the disorder. The initial impairment may be a diminished verbal fluency marked by slowed verbal production, loss of conversational initiation, frequent hesitations, and an impoverished syntax. The progressive exacerbation of choreic movements of the muscles necessary for speech interfere with respiration, phonation, resonance, articulation, and prosody, resulting in a reduced ability to control volume, rate, timing, and spacing, thus producing speech that is erratic, explosive, and barely intelligible. Eventually, the dysarthria becomes so severe that patients lose voluntary control of their vocal apparatus and are rendered mute.

Visuospatial perception is also impaired in the early stages of the disease. Impairment is evident in a marked deficiency on the performance relative to the verbal scales of general intelligence tests. It is also apparent on a range of tests of visuospatial search and discrimination, as well as in an unusual compromise in the perception of egocentric spatial localization in the absence of a deficit in manipulation of spatial orientation of external objects. In general the limitations in visuospatial abilities are most evident under demands for visuomotor tracking, directional sense, or visuospatial integration.

Memory deficits are another early feature of Huntington's disease, with difficulties apparent for both verbal and nonverbal materials over relatively brief delays. As the disease progresses, memory deficits become more robust and appear on very simple tasks such as reciting strings of digits. Remote memory becomes increasingly compromised, and eventually a flat temporal gradient of retrograde amnesia may emerge in which the recall of highly familiar materials, such as the names of famous people or geographical locations, is equally impaired across all past decades. Motor skill learning or procedural memory may also show progressive deterioration. There has been considerable debate as to whether the memory problems represent deficits in the encoding or retrieval of information. A retrieval deficit is favored by a relative sparing of recognition memory over recall in the early stages of the disease. However, recognition memory also becomes impaired as the disease progresses.

VARIANTS

In addition to the typical expression of Huntington's disease described above, two variants distinguished by the age of symptom onset are generally recognized. Juvenile onset Huntington's disease, with onset before the age of 20, is more often characterized by paternal transmission, rigidity rather than chorea, rapid progression, a more severe clinical expression, and a higher risk of seizures. The longest segments of the aberrant trinucleotide repeat expansion at the Huntington's disease gene have been observed in juvenile onset cases. Late onset Huntington's disease appears after the age of 50 and is typically associated with maternal transmission, a slower rate of progression, and milder symptoms of motor and cognitive impairment. Psychiatric complications, such as depression, apathy, and anxiety, are often less severe and more responsive to pharmacotherapy, and a full-spectrum schizophrenia is rare. Although the late onset variant tends to have less robust neuropathological alterations relative to the juvenile variant, no qualitative differences have been documented to support distinct pathogenetic mechanisms. Theoretical mechanisms postulated to underlie the different variants have included maternally transmitted factors or "aging gene" modifiers, paternally transmitted gene "imprinting," and paternal and maternal transmission of differential propensities for methylation of DNA.

STRUCTURAL AND FUNCTIONAL CHANGES

Neuroradiology

In the late stages of Huntington's disease, a marked atrophy of the caudate and putamen is readily detectable with computed axial tomography (CT) and MAGNETIC RESONANCE IMAGING (MRI). Current research, however, has called into question the utility of these methods in detecting damage prior to the overt expression of cognitive and functional pathology. In contrast, aberrant glucose metabolism in the striatum has been reported very early in the disease with positron emission tomography (PET) before there is evidence of structural damage on CT, cognitive decline, or definite clinical signs of the disease.

In contrast to the reliable documentation of striatal damage, neuroradiology has not contributed unequivocal evidence of cortical damage. Slow wave activity and diminished alpha activity that correlate with caudate atrophy have been demonstrated with electroencephalography, but the diagnostic relevance of this finding is unclear. Cortical regional cerebral blood flow studies have documented a mild to moderate slowing at rest, and an unexplained hyperfrontality during a frontal activation task that correlates with the degree of caudate atrophy (Weinberger et al., 1988). Data from computed tomography have supported the notion of atrophy in the frontal cortex, but this damage has so far not been correlated with dementia or performance on neuropsychological tests of frontal function. Positron emission tomography has not provided evidence of aberrant glucose metabolism in the cerebral cortex, even in patients with relatively advanced disease.

Huntington's disease

Neuropathology

Neuropathological studies have consistently documented a severe atrophy, loss of neurons, and gliosis in the striatal nucleus, beginning in the caudate and spreading to the putamen and pallidum (Vonsattel et al., 1985). In later stages of the disease, neuron loss and gliosis may also be evident in the neocortex, particularly the frontal and occipital regions, but this deterioration has not been consistently observed. More moderate cell loss has been documented in the claustrum and subthalamic nuclei (i.e. ventrobasal thalamus), and the hippocampus, but there is an apparent sparing of the nucleus basalis, the brain stem, and spinal cord. The cerebellum was also believed to be spared, but recent evidence of cell loss in this area has been reported.

Neurochemistry

Although a specific neurochemical abnormality has not been directly linked to the pathogenesis of Huntington's disease, a number of anomalies have been observed. The most salient is a marked selectivity of the neuropathology, with early and prominent damage evident in the small to medium-sized spiny neurons, and a relative sparing of the medium to large aspiny neurons (Ferrante et al., 1985). The small to medium-sized spiny neurons comprise approximately 90 percent of striatal neurons which provide output projections from the striatum. These neurons appear to contain gamma amino butyric acid (GABA), along with various peptide cotransmitters, including substance P and enkephalin, all of which reportedly show marked reductions in Huntington's disease. In contrast, the medium to large aspiny neurons, which comprise approximately 10 percent of the striatal neurons, provide input from other cortical structures to the striatum, as well as connections within the striatum. Some of these neurons contain somatostatin, and elevations in striatal and cortical somatostatin have been observed.

The significant reduction in spiny neurons has focused attention on GABA as potentially the most critical neurotransmitter in Huntington's disease. Its relevance is underscored by the 70 to 90 percent reduction of GABA and its synthesizing enzyme, glutamic acid decarboxylase, in the striatum, pallidum, and substantia nigra, as well as from evidence of a 50 percent reduction in GABA receptor binding sites in the striatum, and a striatal reduction in glutamate. GABA reductions in Huntington's disease have also been documented in the nucleus accumbens, lateral pallidum, subthalamic nucleus, substantia nigra, and ventrolateral thalamic nucleus.

The activity of GABA-containing striatal efferents is modulated by dopaminergic and cholinergic inputs which also show a marked disruption in Huntington's disease. These irregularities are particularly significant because dopamine agonists have been shown to increase spontaneous involuntary movements, whereas cholinergic and GABA-ergics tend to reduce such movements. Neurons containing acetylcholine are diminished in the striatum, as are concentrations of the synthesizing enzyme choline acetyltransferase. There does not appear to be a reduction in terminals containing dopamine in the striatum or an abnormal concentration of tyrosine hydroxylase.

The relatively selective degeneration of striatal spiny neurons accompanied by sparing of the aspiny neurons has provided an important parameter for any biochemical model for the pathogenesis of Huntington's disease. A model that appears to meet this requirement has emerged from the discovery that local overactivity of excitatory amino acids could result in selective neuronal death after sustained depolarization, which is similar to the selective damage apparent in Huntington's disease (DiFiglia, 1990). This model has spawned considerable attention to the NMDA (N-methyl-D-aspartate) subtype of the glutamate receptor and its mediation of the excitotoxic effects of quinolinic acid. As yet, however, the excitatory neurotoxin model has not provided an acceptable account for why Huntington's disease has a delayed onset; nor does it account for the progressive deterioration within the neostriatum. Recent theoretical formulations have postulated an age-related decline in energy metabolism as an interactive mechanism that may overcome these theoretical limitations.

Functional relevance of structural damage

The relation between the basal ganglia and the frontocortical areas has been specified in terms of a series of segregated "loops" (Alexander et al., 1986). The putamen has connections to motor-related cortical structures, particularly the supplementary motor cortex. The caudate nucleus has no fiber connections with the motor cortex, except for the frontal eye fields and substantia nigra pars reticulata. Its major cortical connections are with the frontocortical regions, particularly the dorsolateral and orbital frontal cortex, and the limbic system. Given the relative selectivity of damage in Huntington's disease to the spiny projection neurons, these connections suggest functional anatomic relations in which movement abnormalities could relate to putamenal damage, whereas the cognitive and emotional changes might be most closely related to damage to the caudate.

A disruption of the efferent tracts between the striatum and substantia nigra has suggested to some that the progressive cognitive impairment associated with Huntington's disease could be a result of this "downstream" disconnection, with secondary effects on cortical functions (Weinberger et al., 1988). The sparing of gnosis and language functions until very late in the disease is consistent with this view, as are the similarities in cognitive function observed between Huntington's disease and other cortical "disconnection" syndromes, including PARKINSON'S DISEASE and progressive supranuclear palsy (PSP).

The anatomical correlate of emotional disregulation may also result from a "downstream" cortical disconnection. The limbic cortex is involved in emotional function and projects to the medial anterior caudate nucleus, a region that shows some of the earliest structural damage in Huntington's disease. The affective disorder in Huntington's disease may appear very early, providing temporal evidence of an association between the anterior caudate and emotional dysfunction. The similarities in emotional dysfunction among other "disconnection" symptoms such as Parkinson's disease and PSP, lend some support to the "disconnection" hypothesis of emotional dysfunction in Huntington's disease.

TREATMENT

There is currently no effective treatment available to stop the progression of Huntington's disease. Present therapeutic interventions are limited to symptom reduction and palliative care. Pharmaco-therapeutics have some utility in the reduction of movement disorders and psychiatric symptoms. In particular, low dose dopamine antagonists such as haloperidol or fluphenazine have proved useful in the attenuation of chorea,

irritability, hallucinations, and delusions. Tricyclic antidepressants, monoamine oxidase inhibitors, or ECT tend to ameliorate depression in Huntington's disease, though the beneficial effects appear specific to somatic signs of depression, with relatively minimal effects on the ruminative components, such as low self-esteem and hopelessness (Caine & Shoulson, 1983).

A number of behavioral treatment strategies have been proposed to reduce some of the more disabling aspects of certain symptoms (Folstein, 1989; White et al., 1992). Given the potentially lethal consequences of dysphagia, monitoring of meals may be important and patients may profit from training in effective eating strategies. The disabling effects of the progressive speech impairment may be reduced by limiting the demands placed on the patient, particularly with respect to speed and clarity. Speech therapy may also be indicated to provide alternative communication strategies, an approach that may be most effectively entrenched early in the disease while the patient retains a high capacity of language abilities.

Research into experimental therapeutics is ongoing, with many of the documented biochemical anomalies providing a guide to potentially effective intercession. The observed depletion of GABA has prompted several attempts to treat the disease by increasing the available GABA. These have included the use of the GABA-mimetic muscinol, Isoniazid, alpha-acetylenic GABA which inhibits GABA-transaminase, and THIP which is a GABA receptor agonist. None of these, however, has yet functionally significant efficacy.

The excitatory neurotoxin model has stimulated a number of attempts to limit excess glutamate in the striatum. One such attempt with Baclofen was successful in diminishing the amount of glutamate available, but the progressive deterioration was not attenuated and no symptomatic improvement was evident.

The role of somatostatin in the mediation of neurotransmitter regulation, particularly dopaminergic, along with the observed excess of somatostatin in the basal ganglia of Huntington's disease patients, prompted an efficacy evaluation of a somatostatin antagonist (Cysteamine) in the treatment of motor and cognitive dysfunction. The efficacy of this intervention could not be established.

In the preclinical domain, experimental investigations of fetal cell grafts in rodents have provided more encouraging results. Fetal cells transplanted from the striatum to a lesioned caudate nucleus have shown development of neostriatal neurons, and may form appropriate efferent and afferent connections (DiFiglia et al., 1988). Further, some of the movement deficits induced by excitotoxic lesions have been reversed by such grafts in rodents (Giordano et al., 1990). This area may hold considerable promise for the future development of effective treatments in Huntington's disease.

CONCLUSION

Huntington's disease is the model for an auto-somal dominant genetic disorder with multimodal degenerative consequences spanning personality, cognition, and motility. A convergence of psychi-atry, neuropsychology, and neurology has con-tributed to remarkable gains in the understanding of etiology and pathogenesis, but a considerable array of unknown features remain to be specified (Purdon et al., 1994). Moreover, although direct treatments for the pathology of Huntington's disease have yet to be discovered, a sizable literature exists in support of multidisciplinary treatment programs for palliative care (White et al., 1992). With the recent discovery of the pathological gene, advances in our understanding of the etiology, pathogenesis, and treatment of Huntington's disease are probably close at hand.

BIBLIOGRAPHY

Alexander, G. E., Delong, M. R., & Strick, P. L. (1986). Parallel organisation of functionally segregated circuits linking basal ganglia and cortex. *Annual Review of Neuroscience, 9,* 357–81.

Caine, E. D., & Shoulson, I. (1983). Psychiatric syndromes in Huntington's disease. *American Journal of Psychiatry, 140,* 728–33.

DiFiglia, M. (1990). Excitotoxic injury of the neostriatum: a model for Huntington's disease. *Trends in Neuroscience, 13,* 286–9.

DiFiglia, M., Schiff, L., & Deckel, A. W. (1988). Neuronal organization of fetal striatal grafts in kainate- and sham-lesioned rat caudate nuc-leus: light- and electron-microscopic obser-vations. *Journal of Neuroscience, 8,* 1112–30.

Ferrante, R. J., Kowall, N. W., Beal, M. F., Richardson, E. P., Bird, E. D., & Martin, J. B.

(1985). Selective sparing of a class of striatal neurons in Huntington's disease. *Science, 230,* 561–3.

Folstein, S. E. (1989). *Huntington's disease: A disorder of families.* Baltimore, MD: Johns Hopkins University Press.

Garron, D. C. (1973). Huntington's chorea and schizophrenia. In A. Barbeau, T. Chase, & G. Paulson (Eds), *Advances in neurology.* Vol. 1: *Huntington's chorea* (pp. 729–34). New York: Raven.

Giordano, M., Ford, L. M., Shipley, M. T., & Sandberg, P. R. (1990). Neural grafts and pharmacological intervention in a model of Huntington's disease. *Brain Research Bulletin, 25,* 453–65.

Huntington, G. (1872). On chorea. *Medical Surg-ical Report, 26,* 317–21.

Huntington's Disease Collaborative Research Group (1993). A novel gene containing a trinucleotide repeat that is expanded and un-stable on Huntington's disease chromosomes. *Cell, 72,* 971–83.

Purdon, S. E., Mohr, E., Ilivitsky, V., & Jones, B. D. W. (1994). Huntington's disease: etiology, pathogenesis, and treatment. *Journal of Psychi-atry and Neuroscience, 19,* 359–67.

Vonsattel, J. P., Meyers, R. H., Stevens, T. J., Ferrante, R. J., Bird, E. D., & Richardson, E. P. Jr. (1985). Neuropathological classification of Huntington's disease. *Journal of Neuropatho-logical and Experimental Neurology, 44,* 559–77.

Weinberger, D. R., Berman, K., Iadarola, M., Driesen, N., & Zec, R. F. (1988). Prefrontal cortical blood flow and cognitive function in Huntington's disease. *Journal of Neurology, Neurosurgery, and Psychiatry, 51,* 94–104.

White, R. F., Vasterling, J. J., Koroshetz, W. J., & Myers, R. (1992). Neuropsychology of Hun-tington's disease. In R. F. White (Ed.), *Clinical syndromes in adult neuropsychology: The practitioner's handbook* (pp. 213–51). London: Elsevier.

SCOT E. PURDON, THOMAS CHASE,
AND ERICH MOHR

hydrocephalus A dynamic pathological condi-tion of the brain VENTRICLES, hydrocephalus involves a progressive increase in volume of the ventricles due to a variety of pathological proces-ses that cause over-production of CEREBROSPINAL

FLUID (CSF), or obstruction of the passage of CSF between its sites of origin and absorption within the ventricles, subarachnoid space, or arachnoid villi. Whatever the anomaly of CSF flow dynamics, dilatation of the cerebral ventricles (ventriculomegaly) is the common result. As used currently, the term hydrocephalus refers to disorders involving excess cerebrospinal fluid accumulation and ventriculomegaly, whether or not the head is enlarged.

Hydrocephalus is usually accompanied by an increase in CSF pressure. The normal brain is bioelastic because of the venous capillaries, the extracellular space, and the lipids and proteins in the white matter. The effective CSF pressure (the gradient between the CSF pressure within the ventricles and venous blood) controls the degree to which fluid is displaced and brain tissue compressed. Normal CSF pressure is lower than the bioelastic limits of brain tissue, so stress is distributed within brain tissue. This intrinsic CSF regulatory-compensatory mechanism is upset by hydrocephalus, which increases intraventricular pressure and raises the effective CSF pressure, and this additional stress moves fluid out of the cells. The periventricular region receives the greatest stress, and as it yields the ventricles enlarge, which increases the pressure exerted on the brain tissue.

ETIOLOGIES OF HYDROCEPHALUS IN ADULTS vs CHILDREN

Hydrocephalus is a disorder that affects both children and adults, and it may be acquired at any age as a result of neoplasm, trauma, or brain infection. Childhood and adult hydrocephalus, however, have different characteristic etiologies. In adults, hydrocephalus normally arises from cerebrovascular anomalies of the deep white matter. In children, hydrocephalus is the common factor in a group of conditions that affect early brain development and that have in common raised CSF pressure and ventriculomegaly.

Normal pressure hydrocephalus in adults

Normal pressure hydrocephalus (NPH) is a form of chronic hydrocephalus occurring in adults and characterized by normal mean CSF pressure (but note that the CSF pulse pressure can be six times normal) and enlarged lateral ventricles. NPH reduces cerebral blood flow, alters oxidative

metabolism in cortical and subcortical regions, and reduces the density of capillaries in the corpus callosum, white matter, and periventricular gray matter. Prolonged NPH produces Alzheimer-like changes that include plaques, neurofibrillary tangles, basal ganglia atrophy, and degeneration in the cortex and hippocampus.

The classical symptom triad of NPH (gait apraxia, incontinence, and dementia) is thought to arise because of shearing forces on fibers within regions of the deep white matter. These fibers are also affected in deep white matter infarctions that occur as a result of decreased cerebral perfusion with age. Because deep white matter infarction and NPH co-occur, a common mechanism has been suggested whereby deep white matter infarction leads to decreased periventricular tensile strength and NPH. Current neuropsychological studies of adult hydrocephalus are concerned with comparing NPH to various forms of deep white matter infarct dementia, especially with respect to impairments in attention, memory, logical thinking, and speed and flexibility of cognitive processes.

Congenital and perinatal forms of hydrocephalus

Many CONGENITAL DISORDERS of early onset hydrocephalus are associated with abnormalities of neuroembryogenesis. Spina bifida, a defect in closure of the neural tube, is accompanied by a dysraphic spinal cord, by the Arnold–Chiari malformation involving a hindbrain deformity, agenesis of the cerebellum, and herniation of the cerebellum through the exits of the IV ventricle, as well as by other brain anomalies such as interdigitation of the hemispheres. Aqueduct stenosis is a congenital narrowing of the cerebral aqueduct by growth pressures from adjacent midbrain structures. The Dandy–Walker syndrome is a congenital malformation involving an enlarged posterior fossa, agenesis of the cerebellar vermis, and cystic dilatation of the IV ventricle.

Hydrocephalus often follows perinatal brain insults that involve periventricular leukomalacia, whereby the periventricular white matter is destroyed and then reabsorbed as a result of ischemia or hemorrhage; and infantile infections and adhesions that affect the ventricular system. Some form of hydrocephalus develops in 4 of every 1,000 infants from birth to 3 months of age.

EFFECTS OF HYDROCEPHALUS ON THE BRAIN

Investigations of how hydrocephalus affects the brain have included human tissue autopsy or biopsy and experimental animal models. Hydrocephalus has been induced in animals by inflammatory obstruction of subarachnoid spaces around the brain stem after injection of aluminum silicate, which obstructs CSF flow; by mechanical obstruction of CSF flow from the IV ventricle, as a result of injection of silicone oil into the cisterns; by obstruction of cerebral venous outflow; by inoculation of viruses; and by exposure to teratogenic or toxic agents.

Human and animal investigations have shown that hydrocephalus alters the development, structure, and function of the brain, both directly and as an indirect result of ventricular enlargement. The neuropathological effects of hydrocephalus depend on several factors, including the extent of hydrocephalus and ventriculomegaly, the level and duration of abnormal CSF pressure, the etiology of the hydrocephalus, and the age of the individual at onset of hydrocephalus. While some effects of hydrocephalus on the brain seem to occur regardless of age and etiology, others are somewhat different in adult and childhood forms of hydrocephalus.

Neuropathological studies of animals with infantile hydrocephalus show changes related to impaired neuronal maturation. These include loss of dendritic spines, decreased branching, and abnormal pyramidal dendrites.

Hydrocephalus produces changes in the ependyma, the epithelium lining the ventricles and central canal of the spinal cord. It flattens, stretches, tears or totally destroys the ependyma, these changes beginning within 12 hours after CSF obstruction. As the ventricles dilate, ependymal cells flatten to increase their surface area, but, because the ependyma cannot stretch indefinitely, focal loss of cilia and microvilli occurs in regions over the white matter along the roof and dorsolateral angle of the lateral ventricles.

Hydrocephalus creates changes in the cerebral vasculature. It reduces cerebral blood flow, alters oxidative metabolism in cortical and subcortical regions, and reduces the density of capillaries in the corpus callosum and white and periventricular gray matter. Cerebral blood vessels and capillaries become distorted or dysfunctional.

Hydrocephalus alters the constitution of the cerebral water and extracellular spaces. It creates periventricular edema for several mm from the ventricular surface, and enlarges the extracellular space in the white matter adjacent to the ventricles. Extracellular fluid normally flows into CSF spaces. It has been suggested that periventricular fluid collections are actually stagnant extracellular fluid, an abnormal microenvironment for neurons.

Hydrocephalus changes the concentration of NEUROTRANSMITTERS. Substances related to energy metabolism and information transfer (neurotransmitters and their metabolites) are found in the extracellular space, and these move around, depending on the volume and tortuosity of the extracellular space. Assays of human and animal CSF show that hydrocephalus alters the concentration of various neurotransmitters and neuropeptides. To the extent that hydrocephalus alters the tortuosity of the extracellular space, the flow of energy and information substances (and hence neuronal function) will be impaired.

Hydrocephalus and the white matter

The white matter of the brain is composed primarily of myelinated and unmyelinated axons, which transmit chemically mediated electrical signals, and oligodendrocytes, the cells that form myelin. White matter is affected by the biomechanism of hydrocephalus, as well as by particular etiologies that disturb white matter integrity.

Myelin basic protein has been identified in the CSF of hydrocephalic humans, which suggests that ventriculomegaly damages axons and myelin in the periventricular white matter. Biopsies of children with hydrocephalus show tissue damage in the periventricular white matter (axon degeneration and myelin breakdown in the acute stage, gliosis and atrophy in the chronic stage).

The CORPUS CALLOSUM is one white matter tract significantly affected by hydrocephalus. The corpus callosum is formed between gestational weeks 8 and 12, and AGENESIS is usually attributed to early disruption in neuroembryogenesis. Complete agenesis is rare, and is usually associated with gross midline or other abnormalities. Partial agenesis of the corpus callosum often occurs with aqueduct stenosis or spina bifida. Hydrocephalus can stretch or destroy an already formed corpus callosum, causing thinned or hypoplastic callosal structures.

Hydrocephalus affects other white matter tracts, particularly the projection fibres near the midline, which connect the hemispheres to the diencephalon and caudal regions. Lateral white matter tracts that connect cortical regions within each hemisphere are usually spared. Although infants with hydrocephalus have redundant cortical gyration in consequence of the cortex between the sulci becoming exposed to the brain surface, biopsies of hydrocephalic children show little change in cortical neurons.

TREATMENT

Hydrocephalus may improve spontaneously (drainage pathways may open up, CSF production may be decreased, or the absorption mechanism may become more efficient). More typically, shunt treatment (diversion of CSF from the ventricles into another body space by means of a tube and valve system) is required to reverse the abnormal CSF pressure. Even after treatment, however, the ventricles may not return to normal size because of continuing force exerted on the walls, a force that is directly proportional to the ventricular wall area and intraventricular pressure. And even with lowered CSF pressure, there may be enlarged ventricular surface area. Continuing symptoms are related to persisting abnormal stress on the brain tissue. Shunt treatment in children only partially reverses the neuropathological changes, and it need not fully restore cognitive function.

NEUROPSYCHOLOGICAL STUDIES OF CHILDREN WITH HYDROCEPHALUS

Hydrocephalus is a dynamic disorder. Although some of its effects on the brain may be permanent (white matter gliosis has been suggested to effect a permanent change in the extracellular space), at least some symptoms appear only when the condition attains a certain degree of severity. How the dynamics of the disorder relate to neuropsychological function is at present unclear. Also unclear is the role of associated complications such as shunt infections and ventriculitis. For both adults and children with hydrocephalus, the severity of ventriculomegaly remains to be fully understood in relation to cognitive function.

Nevertheless, research studies over the last 30 years have explored the neuropsychological abilities (intelligence, sensory-motor function,

visuospatial skill, language, memory, attention, and the like) of children with hydrocephalus. During this time, the focus of research investigations has changed. In an earlier treatment era, children with hydrocephalus were at risk for global mental retardation, and studies at that time monitored the incidence of mental retardation as a function of whether or not the hydrocephalus had been treated with a shunt. With improved treatment modalities, fewer children were mentally retarded, so the emphasis shifted to describing more specific cognitive impairments that limit school attainments and achievement. More recently, research has adopted a developmental perspective that considers the nature of the cognitive deficit, its characteristics over age, and its relationship to the particular forms and manifestations of early onset hydrocephalus. Neuropsychological studies at the present time concern: (i) the cognitive characteristics of hydrocephalic children successfully treated with shunts; (ii) the correlation of neuropathology and specific cognitive functions; (iii) the cognitive underpinnings of a particular language syndrome thought to characterize children with hydrocephalus; and (iv) the use of hydrocephalic populations to explore theory-driven questions in psychology and linguistics.

Children with hydrocephalus have long been observed to have a higher level of verbal than of nonverbal (or perceptual-motor) intelligence. Research investigations have explored specific psychomotor and cognitive skills related to this cognitive imbalance: sensory, motor, and spatial organization, eye–hand coordination, and problems with reading, handwriting, and number work.

Hydrocephalus stems from diverse etiologies and has a range of physical symptoms and manifestations. Some physical sequelae of childhood hydrocephalus (e.g. abnormal EYE MOVEMENTS; poor fine motor coordination) are associated with poorer performance on nonverbal, perceptual-motor tasks involving time constraints, as well as with VISUOPERCEPTUAL DISORDERS and VISUOSPATIAL DISORDERS. For these forms of nonverbal cognitive deficit, the connection between the symptoms of hydrocephalus and the type of impairment seems fairly transparent.

Anomalies of white matter development have consequences for cognitive function. In children with hydrocephalus, neither the overall thickness of the cortical mantle (visualized from AIR ENCEPH-ALOGRAMS or VENTRICULOGRAPHY) nor CSF volume (visualized from MAGNETIC RESONANCE IMAGING or MRI predicts cognitive function; however, extensive astrocytosis of the white matter is associated with mental retardation, and there is a correlation between state of myelination on MRI and psychomotor development. Recent research has extended the correlation of neuropathology with cognitive disorder. MRI studies of the brain in children with hydrocephalus have revealed changes in cerebral white matter tracts, problems in myelination, and atrophy of midline commissural structures like the corpus callosum, and related these neurodevelopmental anomalies to standardized measures of cognitive function.

Hydrocephalus also affects language, and here the connection between pathology and cognitive impairment is less obvious. Language was traditionally considered an area of strength for children with hydrocephalus, in that their speech and language appeared to be readily acquired, fluent (or even hyperfluent) and relatively well-structured. The seeming paradox, however, was that this fluent language seemed impoverished in content. The term "Cocktail Party Syndrome" was first applied 34 years ago to a pattern of aberrant speech, language, and behavior in children with hydrocephalus that involved fluent speech marked by verbal perseveration, excessive use of stereotyped social utterances, irrelevant verbosity, and over-familiarity of manner. For children with hydrocephalus, language was described as being an effective vehicle for social contact but an unsuccessful way of conveying meaning.

Research studies of the use and understanding of language in texts and in discourse contexts have confirmed the idea of content-poor language. Children with hydrocephalus tell fluent, fairly well-structured stories, but their narratives are verbose and lack core semantic content. Children with hydrocephalus also have difficulty deriving the full meaning of utterances within discourse contexts; specifically, understanding ambiguous statements, grasping common figurative expressions such as idioms; inferring what happened, given a particular situation; and making inferences that facilitate textual coherence. Children with hydrocephalus acquire fair word-decoding skills, but they have difficulty understanding what they read. Thus, even though they under-stand and produce many words, children with hydrocephalus miss much of the implicit and explicit message that words convey in discourse and in texts.

The language skills of children with hydrocephalus have also been used to address more theoretical questions. The fact that these children decode and understand single words better than written texts bears on models of reading comprehension. Their poor development of textual rhetoric (which involves the clarity, economy, and fullness with which text content can be understood or communicated) and well-preserved interpersonal rhetoric (which involves social aspects of discourse such as turn-taking) bear on the question of the dissociability of two classes of pragmatic linguistic constraints.

In the past, conditions like hydrocephalus held only moderate interest for neuropsychologists: cognitive skills in individuals with hydrocephalus were poorly delineated, and relatively little was known about how hydrocephalus affected the brain. Now a clearer picture is emerging of the cognitive profiles associated with the various forms of hydrocephalus, and MRI and other types of neuroimaging are providing a better visualization of the patterns of associated neurodevelopmental anomalies and structural white matter damage. The study of hydrocephalus now appears to provide, not only answers to practical questions about cognitive function in individuals with this condition, but also a distinct perspective on some theoretical questions about the architecture of cognition.

BIBLIOGRAPHY

Black, P. McL. (1990). The normal pressure hydrocephalus syndrome. In R. M. Scott (Ed.). *Concepts in neurosurgery.* Vol. 3: *Hydrocephalus* (pp. 109–14). Baltimore, MD: Williams & Wilkins.

Del Bigio, M. R. (1993). Neuropathological changes caused by hydrocephalus. *Acta Neuropathologica, 85,* 573–85.

Dennis, M., Fitz, C. R., Netley, C. T., Harwood-Nash, D. C. F., Sugar, J., Hendrick, E. B., Hoffman, H. J., & Humphreys, R. P. (1981). The intelligence of hydrocephalic children. *Archives of Neurology, 3,* 607–15.

Dennis, M., Jacennik, B., & Barnes, M. A. (1994). The content of narrative discourse in children and adolescents after early-onset hydrocephalus and in normally-developing age peers. *Brain and Language*, *46*, 129–65.

Fletcher, J. M., Brookshire, B. L., Bohan, T. P., Brandt, M. E., & Davidson, K. C. (1995). Early hydrocephalus. In B. P. Rourke (Ed.), *Syndrome of nonverbal learning disabilities: Neurodevelopmental manifestations* (pp. 206–38). New York: Guilford.

MAUREEN DENNIS

hyloagnosia Hyloagnosia is one of the forms of tactile agnosia (*see* TACTILE PERCEPTION DISORDERS) and is the inability to identify qualities, as in the nature of a material, from tactile information alone. It is therefore considered a primary disorder of touch, distinct from STEREOAGNOSIA.

hyperactivity A child's inattentive, impulsive and restless behavior can arise from constitutional causes and is termed hyperactivity, and more recently, attention deficit disorder. It is thought to be due to abnormalities of brain neurochemistry and to be for the most part genetically transmitted (Deutsch & Kinsbourne, 1990).

EARLY STUDIES

Though hyperactivity in children had previously been remarked upon, it was following the 1919 encephalitis lethargica epidemic that hyperactive and disinhibited behavior as a consequence of neurological injury came to medical attention. This notion of brain-based disinhibition was perpetuated in the concept of the "brain-injured child" applied to children who might or might not have neurological deficits such as cerebral palsy in association with their "hyperkinetic" behavior. The idea that a behavioral abnormality such as hyperactivity can not only be a sign of brain damage, but can be its only sign is now generally accepted, although the term brain dysfunction is preferred, to obviate any implication that the structure of the brain itself must be abnormal. Instead, an abnormality of neurotransmission is hypothesized. Correspondingly, the earlier emphasis on hyperactivity as a component of a syndrome including learning disabilities, clumsiness, and other abnormalities (MINIMAL BRAIN DYSFUNCTION) (Bax & McKeith, 1963) has been abandoned for a focus on the behavioral abnormality itself, though conceding that the abnormalities are often present in the same individual. In parallel with this increasing emphasis on the specific abnormal behavior has been a change of emphasis from the motor component "hyperactivity" to the concomitant abnormalities of attention; hence the term attention deficit, which underlies the several terms proposed by the diagnostic and statistical manual of the American Psychiatric Association (1980), namely attention deficit disorder with or without hyperactivity (DSM-III) and attention deficit-hyperactivity disorder (DSM-III-R). The diagnostic checklists that are presented as a basis for these diagnoses give common instances of the behaviors in question and, in the case of DSM-III, are organized under the three main headings of inattention, impulsivity, and hyperactivity. The SNAP questionnaire transforms this checklist into a rating scale and adds a number of peer interaction items to cover the frequent and important component of social difficulties that attend the syndrome. These four domains can serve as points of departure for a brief clinical description.

CHARACTERISTICS

Although attention deficit disorder with or without hyperactivity (ADHD) is in many cases life-long, school behavior usually serves to illustrate them. The *inattentive* schoolchild will fail to persevere on a task, be easily distracted, or even seek alternative occupation. He or she will fail to put forth intense mental effort when it is called for, will be easily bored, not listening but daydreaming. However, *impulsively*, the ADHD child will also dart from topic to topic, not stay in his or her seat, call out in class, not wait his or her turn, and tolerate frustration poorly. These outward-directed behaviors may well be attended by a motor restlessness termed *hyperactivity*, in which the child fidgets or jumps out of his or her seat or even roams as if driven by a motor. In peer *interactions*, ADHD individuals are either overly retiring or too pushy, and may be given to temper outbursts when their wishes do not prevail.

Most ADHD children are sensation-seekers (Zentall, 1975). They are most comfortable when a lot is going on, and when it is not they tend to complicate the situation until the stimulation level is to their liking. They will tend to choose hazardous occupations and pursuits, and are notably accident-prone.

Emotionally, ADHD children keep interactions at a superficial level. They appear not to be cognizant of the ways in which their behavior frustrates their own goals, although in time a dropping self-concept indicates that this point has struck home after all. They are generally not introspective, and do not much reflect either on cognitive or emotional issues. But the very personality patterns that generate the maladaptive difficulties are also at times seen as strengths, in an individual who can be perceived as bold, outspoken, enterprising, and innovative.

The outline above must be qualified. First, the inattentiveness and restlessness are not invariable. When ADHD children are doing things in which they are keenly interested, they then display a degree of attention that matches that of their attentionally normal peers. It can be generalized that all attention-deficient individuals at times display appropriate attentional skills and resources. The attention deficit is not fixed but task-specific. The child deploys a normal amount of attention when he or she is intrinsically interested in the task, or it is made salient or rewarding by experimental manipulations. It is when "incentive motivation" is called for, when current performance awaits a significantly delayed reward, that the phenomenon of attention deficit disorder is manifest.

LIFE-SPAN EVOLUTION

As a prelude, the preschool ADHD child is rambunctious, pushy, apt to grab other children's possessions, and attention-seeking. He or she is also apt to have frequent and severe temper tantrums. Even in infancy such a child may be prone to colic, irritability, and irregular sleep patterns. Restless movements may be noticed very early on, allegedly even before birth.

As the ADHD person enters adolescence, the motor hyperactivity may become less obtrusive but the inattention and impulsivity typically remain. They increasingly impair the child's achievements in school, as the latter depend more and more on close attention to instruction and time spent doing homework. Social failures on account of impulsive behavior and lack of planning and organization are also increasingly severe and are experienced as more serious by the teenager. These adolescents often appear under-

motivated, as they lose heart in falling more and more behind.

The adult "residual" ADHD individual is characterized by an impulsive inability to maintain long-term employment and sustain long-term relationships. Minor setbacks and frustrations are not tolerated and the individual frequently changes jobs and even careers, as well as partners. Early onset alcoholism involving "spree" drinking is a common accompaniment.

SUBTYPES

The syndrome of hyperactivity itself is being partitioned. Two approaches to subtyping have been suggested. One subdivides attention-deficient children with respect to the presence or absence of particular components associated with the disorder, and the other subdivides them in terms of their comorbidity with other psychopathologies (Biederman et al., 1991).

Many children with deficient attention are not notably hyperactive or have grown out of a phase in which they were. Many now believe that there are two attention-deficient syndromes, with and without hyperactivity. Whereas the former conformed to classical descriptions, the latter has been described at times as being the reverse of very active, namely sluggish, lethargic, and "spacey" (Lahey et al., 1984). In our view the important differentiation is not with respect to whether the individual is hyperactive but whether he or she is impulsive. It is the nonimpulsive attention-deficient children who appear to constitute a separate subtype, particularly in terms of comorbidity. Impulsive hyperactives are often also conduct-disordered and prone to aggressive and antisocial behavior (Loney et al., 1978), whereas the nonimpulsive inattentives are more likely to suffer from overanxious disorder or major depression.

ETIOLOGY

It is generally agreed that between 50 and 75 percent of attention deficit disorder is genetically transmitted (Cantwell, 1975). This is dramatically illustrated by the great propensity for children of nonrelative adoption to be hyperactive (when adopted into families where attention deficit is not to be found). It is presumed that the parents of the child offered for adoption transmit the relevant genes. Numerous other suggested but unvalidated causations for attention deficit disorder exist, including subclinical lead and maternal alcohol ingestion. Irritable, inattentive, and disinhibited behavior is at times triggered by a variety of foodstuffs and additives to the diet (Swanson & Kinsbourne, 1980). It is not clear whether when this occurs the disorder is any different from attention deficit disorder in general or whether these are simply aggravating factors in children who have attention deficit disorder in any case. Socioeconomic factors by themselves cannot be incriminated, but adverse social contexts do seem to determine whether comorbid conduct disorder is likely to arise in an attention deficit individual. Some supportive evidence for the early origin of attention deficit disorder is supplied not only by retrospective histories of behavioral difficulties in infancy, but also by the increased incidence of minor physical anomalies (Firestone et al., 1978).

DIFFERENTIAL DIAGNOSIS

Deficient attention is almost ubiquitous in developmental psychopathology, and certainly inattentiveness is a hallmark of major affective disorder and is prominent in the evolution of Tourette disease (GILLES DE LA TOURETTE SYNDROME). Head injuries and a variety of encephalitic disorders can also cause disinhibited behavior. Lapses of attention will less frequently emerge in the course of progressive brain degenerations of various kinds in children, and once in a while a case of petit mal in which innumerable momentary interruptions of consciousness occur is mistaken for attention deficit.

ASSESSMENT

There are no specific tests for attention deficit disorder, although an abnormally high level of errors of omission and commission on continuous performance tests (CPTs) may come close. The "freedom from distractibility" factor on the Wechsler scales (performance on arithmetic, digit span, and coding) is a highly unreliable index and, with respect to both psychometric and neuropsychological measures, the best evidences of attention deficit disorder derive from the clinician's observation of the quality of the performance rather than from scores on specific tests. Certainly, some standard tests are more liable to elicit inattentive or impulsive disorder performance than others, but this seems to be a function of how boring, monotonous and protracted they are, rather than anything about their categorical nature. The effects on performance of such tasks as the Stroop, Porteus Mazes, or the Wisconsin Card Sorting Test are quite inconstant. Tests requiring inhibition of predominant response dispositions (such as Luria's Go–No Go task) and tests calling for the spontaneous emission of fluent responses (Word Fluency Task; FAS) significantly discriminate between ADHD and control groups, but at nowhere near the level of sensitivity of tasks specifically designed to be either boring and monotonous or to call for substantial mental effort over lengthy periods of time.

In their test performance, as indeed in their classroom and everyday behavior, attention deficient individuals exhibit heightened variability, and this is very apparent on those tasks on which a continuity of attention and mental effort is called for. The computation of statistics reflecting variability of performance on CPT and mental effort tasks is a potent way of characterizing the attention deficient individual.

STIMULANT EFFECTS

Since Bradley's findings it has been known that stimulant drugs can be highly effective in correcting attention deficient behavior, and evidence has cumulatively supported the view that this is on account of their dopamine agonist potential. Dexedrine (dextroamphetamine), Ritalin (methylphenidate) and Cylert (pemoline) are all dopamine agonists, although the former two also have norepinephrinergic and perhaps some serotonergic activity. They are short-acting, with onset between half and one hour and offset of behavioral effect between four and six hours in most cases (Swanson et al., 1978). A voluminous literature attests to the striking improvement in attention, impulse control, and postural stability, as well as social interaction (Humphries et al., 1978) that the child can attain with the help of any of these medications (Barkley, 1977), and research has demonstrated that their effects are specifically to allow a child to approximate to a more normal attentional state. In contrast, normal people given stimulants within the same range of doses exhibit impairment of learning and memory (Wetzel et al., 1981). This normalizing effect is purely symptomatic in that, once the medication has worn off, the status quo ante is fully restored.

As used in usual clinical practice, none of these medications is cumulative in its effects, and the child on any of them is effectively off the medication for a large portion of each 24-hour period. This is a presumed safety factor which may in part account for the remarkably trouble-free nature of this particular form of pharmacotherapy.

The short-acting nature of the stimulant agents makes it possible to implement acute drug–placebo double-blind paradigms, in which one can both classify individual children in terms of their stimulant responsivity, favorable versus adverse, and demonstrate various characteristics of the attention-deficient state, using the child on medication as his own normalized control (Kinsbourne, 1983).

BRAIN BASIS

The efficacy of dopamine agonists in correcting attention deficit disorder spotlights dopamine-mediated projections in the brain. Of these the projections arising from the ventral-tegmental area seem the best candidates, particularly the mesolimbic-orbitofrontal projection which, based on animal experimentation, mediates incentive motivation. The putative involvement of frontal cortex in attention deficit disorder is suggested by metabolic studies, although their interpretation is not fully assured. In contrast, conclusions about any anatomical, morphological, or neurohistological abnormalities have not been drawn at this time.

MANAGEMENT

Given the susceptibility of attention deficit behavior to certain immediate rewards, behavior management systems of various kinds have been attempted (Patterson et al., 1965). These are not necessarily ineffective but their generality has yet to be determined. They are more likely to be effective when used in conjunction with stimulant therapy (Pelham et al., 1980). Stimulant therapy is the most widely used and clearly the most effective modality for attention deficit disorder. Some 80 percent of attention-deficient children respond favorably to stimulant medications, although over time many abandon treatment, for reasons which are not always medical. No alternative agent is as effective, but in some cases it is necessary to use other drugs. Where there is an element of depression and where there are tics which could be exacerbated by a dopamine agonist, it is customary to substitute a tricyclic, such as desipramine, or to use clonidine (Hunt et al., 1985). Comorbid anxiety can be treated with buspirone. The extent to which comorbid conduct disorder is amenable to pharmacotherapy is controversial. Caffeine does not appear to be effective (Garfinkel et al., 1981).

Many other treatments for attention deficit disorders have had their vogues (Silver, 1986) and their very number attests to their lack of demonstrated efficacy. Among these, diets that exclude certain foodstuffs or chemical additives do have some empirical support (Egger et al., 1985) but have never been shown to be a practical modality for the bulk of attention-deficient individuals.

OUTCOME

The outcome for a proportion of attention-deficient individuals is bleak, featuring not only continued attention deficit in the adult years, with its negative impact on employment and family dynamics, but also alcoholism (Blouin et al., 1978), psychopathy, and other serious psychopathologies (Menkes et al., 1967). A proportion of attention-deficient individuals function independently in adult years, but the follow-ups have not been clear on this point. Similarly, the educational prognosis of attention-deficient individuals is not good, but no satisfactory inquiry into how this might be improved by consistent long-term stimulant therapy has been published. Long-term use of stimulants has in itself not been shown to have important disadvantages.

BIBLIOGRAPHY

American Psychiatric Association (1980). *Diagnostic and statistical manual of mental disorders*, 3rd edn (DSM III). Washington, DC: APA.

Barkley, R. A. (1977). A review of stimulant drug research with hyperactive children. *Journal of Child Psychology and Psychiatry*, 18, 137–65.

Bax, U., & MacKeith, R. C. (1963). "Minimal Brain Damage" – a concept discarded. In R. C. MacKeith & M. Bax (Eds), *Minimal cerebral dysfunction* (foreword). London: SIMP with Heinemann.

Biederman, J. B., Newcorn, J., & Sprich, S. (1991). Comorbidity of Attention Deficit Hyperactivity Disorder with conduct, depressive anxiety, and other disorders. *American Journal of Psychiatry, 148*, 564–77.

Blouin, A., Bornstein, R., & Trites, R. (1978). Teenage alcohol use among hyperactive children: a 5 year follow-up study. *Journal of Pediatric Psychiatry, 3*, 188–94.

Cantwell, D. P. (1975). Genetics of hyperactivity. *Journal of Child Psychology, 16*, 261–4.

Deutsch, C. K., & Kinsbourne, M. (1990). Genetics and biochemistry in attention deficit disorder. In M. Lewis & S. M. Miller (Eds), *Handbook of developmental psychopathology* (pp. 93–110). New York: Plenum.

Egger, J., Graham, P. J., Carter, C. M., Gumley, D., Soothill, J. F. (1985). Controlled trial of oligoantigenic treatment in the hyperkinetic syndrome. *Lancet, 2*, 540–5.

Firestone, P., Peters, S., Rivier, M., & Knights, R. M. (1978). Minor physical anomalies in hyperactive, retarded and normal children and their families. *Journal of Child Psychology, 19*, 155–60.

Garfinkel, B. D., Webster, C. D., & Sloman, L. (1981). Responses to methylphenidate and varied doses of caffeine in children with attention deficit disorder. *Canadian Journal of Psychiatry, 26*, 395–401.

Humphries, T., Kinsbourne, M., & Swanson, J. M. (1978). Stimulant effects on cooperation and social interaction between hyperactive children and their mothers. *Journal of Child Psychology and Psychiatry, 19*, 13–22.

Hunt, R. D., Minderaa, R. B., & Cohen, D. J. (1985). Clonidine benefits children with attention deficit disorder and hyperactivity: report of a double-blind placebo-crossover therapeutic trial. *Journal of the American Academy of Child Psychiatry, 24*, 617–29.

Kinsbourne, M. (1983). Toward a model for the attention deficit disorder. In M. Perlmutter (Ed.), *Development of policy concerning children in special needs: The Minnesota symposium on child psychology*, Vol. 16 (pp. 137–66). Hillsdale, NJ: Erlbaum.

Lahey, B. B., Schaughency, E. A., Strauss, C. C., & Frame, C. L. (1984). Are attention deficit disorders with and without hyperactivity similar or dissimilar disorders? *Journal of the American Academy of Child Psychiatry, 23*, 302–9.

Loney, J., Prinz, R. J., Mishalow, J., & Joad, J. (1978). Hyperkinetic/aggressive boys in treatment: predictors of clinical response to methylphenidate. *American Journal of Psychiatry, 135*, 1487–91.

Menkes, M., Rowe, J., & Menkes, J. (1967). A 25-year followup study on the hyperkinetic child with MBD. *Pediatrics, 2*, 393–9.

Patterson, G. R., Jones, R., Whittier, J., & Wright, M. A. (1965). A behavioral modification technique for the hyperactive child. *Behaviour Research and Therapy, 2*, 217–26.

Pelham, W. E., Schnedler, R. W., Bologna, N. C., & Contreras, A. (1980). Behavioral and stimulant treatment of hyperactive children: a therapy study with methylphenidate probes in a within-subject design. *Journal of Applied Behavior Analysis, 13*, 221–36.

Silver, L. B. (1986). Controversial approaches to treating learning disabilities and attention deficit disorder. *Learning Disabilities, 140*, 1045–52.

Swanson, J. M., & Kinsbourne, M. (1980). Food dyes impair performance of hyperactive children on a laboratory learning test. *Science, 207*, 1485–7.

Swanson, J., Kinsbourne, M., Roberts, W., & Zucker, M. A. (1978). Time-response analysis of the effect of stimulant medication on the learning disability of children referred for hyperactivity. *Pediatrics, 61*, 21–9.

Wetzel, C. D., Squire, L. R., & Janowsky, D. S. (1981). Methylphenidate impairs learning and memory in normal adults. *Behavioral and Neural Biology, 31*, 413–24.

Zentall, S. (1975). Optimal stimulation as a theoretical basis of hyperactivity. *American Journal of Orthopsychiatry, 45*, 550–63.

MARCEL KINSBOURNE

hyperlexic state Hyperlexia, or a hyperlexic state, may be seen in children suffering from a developmental language disorder which is primarily receptive in nature. In this state, the child may call out words which have apparently been read, and may spell to dictation, but neither understands the words which have been called out, nor is able to converse in normal speech. The behavior may appear as young as 3 years of age, and may be present irrespective of the severity of the underlying learning disability, from children who are nearly autistic to some who express almost normal social behavior. The appearance of hyperlexic behavior may naturally raise false hopes of the acquisition of normal language, but these children comprehend what they read aloud no better than their very poor comprehension for what they hear.

hypertension Hypertension is an abnormal increase in blood pressure, and is most commonly caused by constriction of the smaller blood vessels. Insufficient blood flow to the brain may result in faulty control of the normal constriction and dilation of small blood vessels; an overactive thyroid gland may increase output from the heart, leading to hypertension; disorders of the kidney may similarly result in peripheral constriction of the blood vessels. In all forms of hypertension there is an increased risk of cerebral hemorrhage in addition to the likelihood of serious heart malfunction.

The constriction and dilation of the smaller blood vessels is controlled by a system of vasomotor nerves which arise in the spinal cord but are under the supervision of the HYPOTHALAMUS and regions of the frontal cortex. The ability to respond to very small changes in sensation, temperature, inhalation, drugs, and hormones is reflexive, but is also under the overall control of these higher brain centers.

Hypertensive changes in blood vessels in the brain may result in hemorrhage (*see* CERE-BROVASCULAR ACCIDENT), but acute hypertensive ENCEPHALOPATHY may also occur, resulting in massive edema and consequent pressure effects which are evident in generalized behavioral deficits, convulsions, and coma. It is considered by some that in milder cases of hypertensive disorder, which may lead to less dramatic cognitive changes, personality changes such as anxiety, irritability, depression, or paranoia may also be prominent and may precede awareness of the cognitive deficits.

Hypotension, an abnormally low blood pressure, has less dramatic consequences for cerebral function, but may be associated with fatigue, amnesia, fainting, convulsions, or impairments of specific cognitive functions.

hypnagogic phenomena Hypnagogic phenomena are hallucinations, mainly visual, which may occur in normal individuals during the period of falling into sleep. They have the subjective quality

of dreams, but there is at least a partial preservation of contact with reality. These phenomena may also occur in association with cerebral lesions and, because of the involvement of the PEDUNC-LES, are then sometimes termed *peduncular hallucinosis*. They are frequent in the Gelinau syndrome in association with CATAPLEXY and NARCOLEPSY. These hallucinations often have a rich scenic quality, but which is integrated in and continuous with the real external world. The patient may act as a spectator observing a spatially projected image, but is normally aware of the unreality of the vision.

hypokinesia *See* BRADYKINESIA.

hypomania Mania implies an unaccountably elevated mood of euphoria, increased activity, and the presence of self-important ideas or grandiose delusions. There is commonly a reduction in sleep, an increase in appetite and sexual desire, and pressure of speech and hallucinations occur. Less severe forms of mania are termed hypomania. As a psychotic illness, insight is lost. As any form of psychotic illness may accompany cerebral tumor, hypomania may be seen in cases of cerebral neoplasm, although other organic signs are normally present. However, hypomania may be mistaken for dementia when confusion and incoherence are the prominent features.

hypophonia Hypophonia is a reduction in the volume of spoken output so that the patient speaks in a barely audible whisper. It is most commonly seen as a stage in recovery following the period of acute muteness in APHEMIA, ANARTHRIA, or sub-cortical motor APHASIA. From being acutely mute, the patient passes through a stage of hypophonia until speech becomes soft, slow, but grammatically intact.

hypothalamus The hypothalamus is contained within that area of the brain known as the diencephalon, the literal translation being "between brain". The diencephalon contains all three thalamic structures: the THALAMUS, epithalamus, and hypothalamus; functionally it falls within the BRAIN STEM. The hypothalamus itself is situated immediately above the pituitary gland and below the thalamus. The optic chiasma marks its rostral boundary and the mammillary bodies its caudal. Relative to the brain as a whole the hypothalamus is extremely small; it is said to weigh only one-three-hundredth of the total weight of the brain. However, its small size does not reflect the number of functions that it serves.

The hypothalamus does not have well-defined boundaries; rather it is a collection of ganglion cells that have been differentiated into a number of nuclei, all with widespread connections to other parts of the brain. It has under its control the autonomic nervous system, as well as certain metabolic functions. It exerts its control by regulating hormone release, as well as through neural connections. The different nuclei making up the hypothalamus are frequently grouped and referred to according to their location within the structure. The main nuclei located within the anterior or rostral region include the preoptic, supraoptic, and paraventricular nuclei. The nuclei within the central part of the structure include the ventromedial, dorsomedial, and the arcuate nuclei. Within the posterior or caudal region lie the dorsal, posterior hypothalamic, and mammillary nuclei.

The hypothalamus receives information from the external environment via a number of afferent pathways that provide processed information from the peripheral sense organs of sound, taste, and smell, as well as somatic sensation. It also receives neural input from the viscera, allowing it to monitor certain aspects of the internal environment. In addition to receiving neural input it also contains cells that allow it to directly monitor variables such as blood temperature and salinity and hormone concentrations. The hypothalamus, as well as monitoring hormone levels, also produces two hormones of its own which are released directly into the bloodstream; these are antidiuretic hormone and oxytocin. In addition it produces chemicals known as regulating factors that are transported to the pituitary gland and serve to stimulate or inhibit the release of a corresponding hormone.

On the whole, localization of function within the hypothalamus is not specific to particular nuclei; there is considerable overlap of function between adjacent areas. This explains why hypothalamic functions tend to be attributed to regions. The following discussion will describe the more well-recognized activities of the hypothalamus, beginning with its basic life-sustaining functions. Nuclei in the anterior region (particularly the supraoptic nuclei) exert control over fluid balance in the body and the mechanisms of thirst. The area contains osmoreceptors that monitor the salinity of the blood. Control over these functions is achieved via the hypothalamo-hypophyseal tract that originates in the supraoptic and paraventricular nuclei and projects to the posterior lobe of the pituitary gland. Through this route the hypothalamus regulates the release of antidiuretic hormone (ADH), which controls water reabsorption in the kidneys. The hormones ADH and oxytocin are actually produced by the hypothalamus and stored in the posterior pituitary gland. A lesion within the anterior area of the hypothalamus can result in diabetes insipidus characterized by excessive thirst, polydipsia, and polyuria. The condition may improve or remain permanent. Lesions in this area can be induced by head injury or will occasionally occur spontaneously.

The ventromedial and lateral nuclei of the hypothalamus are involved in the control of eating. This control is exercised via regulation of pituitary growth hormone release. It would appear that these two nuclei monitor the concentration of blood glucose and regulate feeding behavior accordingly. In addition, feedback from the viscera and the senses of taste and smell are also relayed back to the hypothalamus and form part of the complex network regulating feeding behavior. Lesions in the ventromedial area will result in a voracious and unsatisfiable appetite (hyperphagia) leading to obesity. Lesions in the lateral nuclei have the opposite effect, with a loss of appetite resulting in a drop in food intake and eventual starvation. The ventromedial nuclei have been termed the "satiety center" and the lateral nuclei the "feeding center." The hypothalamus, therefore, can be seen to have a role in both the monitoring and regulation of internal functions such as glucose levels and visceral states, as well as the monitoring of external variables such as smell and taste. In addition, it plays a part in the control of autonomic responses, such as the release of saliva and digestive secretions, and indirectly on external behaviors, such as the act of eating. The role played by the hypothalamus in feeding provides a typical example of the multifunctional and complex contribution that the structure makes to life-sustaining behaviors.

The control of body temperature is another contribution the hypothalamus makes to maintaining homeostasis in the body. Certain cells in the structure serve as thermostats monitoring the temperature of the blood and will trigger changes that maintain body temperature at an optimal level. The anterior hypothalamus is largely concerned with the mechanism of losing heat. If this area is lesioned the body can no longer regulate its temperature in a warm environment, although it still retains its ability to regulate temperature in a cold environment. Heat loss is achieved through vasodilation of cutaneous blood vessels and by sweating. If the temperature of the blood is below normal it is the posterior hypothalamus that triggers changes that conserve heat, such as constriction of cutaneous blood vessels, shivering, and cessation of sweating.

Another important activity directly regulated by the hypothalamus and dependent upon its integrity is sexual behavior. It is the hypothalamus, by its control over the pituitary gland, which stimulates the gonads in both males and females to release the sex hormones testosterone and estrogen. It achieves this by stimulating the anterior pituitary to release FSH and LH into the bloodstream, which then travel to the gonads inducing production and release of the sex hormones. The hypothalamus, having triggered the release of the sex hormones, remains sensitive to their levels in the blood. Hormone-sensitive cells in the hypothalamus are activated by the gonadal hormones and initiate sexual behavior. It has been noted that lesions in the caudal nuclei will often result in increased sexual behavior whereas lesions in the ventromedial nuclei will often reduce sexual behavior or desire.

The hypothalamus also has a role in the expression of overt behaviors such as aggression. Experimental work on animals shows the posterior hypothalamus to be active in controlling certain aspects of sympathetic responses such as aggression, whereas stimulation of the anterior hypothalamus induces a dampening effect on both internal and external responses. The cortex, reacting to strong emotion, signals the hypothalamus which, through its connections with the autonomic nervous system and the pituitary gland, induces a series of changes that prepare an organism to react to changing situations such as threat. In this way the hypothalamus can be seen to mediate between higher cognitive states, such as the perception and recognition of threat, and the physiological responses that are necessary to cope with the situation. Much of the work on the role of the hypothalamus and the triggering of both physiological and behavioral changes has been carried out on animals. In humans it would appear that bilateral damage is necessary to induce significant changes in either behavior or physiological responses. This type of damage can result from head injury, subarachnoid hemorrhage, or hydrocephalus. It may also be a consequence of tumors such as craniopharyngioma or various forms of encephalitis.

The hypothalamus plays a part in maintaining appropriate levels of arousal as well as the sleep/wake cycle. Lesions of the anterior hypothalamus have been seen to induce states of extremely high arousal, whereas lesions of the posterior areas can induce states of unresponsiveness and hypersomnia. It is the suprachiasmatic nuclei in particular that have been observed to be involved in maintaining an appropriate balance between the states of sleep and arousal. This nucleus is thought to serve as the body's circadian clock. As an appropriate level of arousal is essential for efficient cognitive activity, disruption of this system can have significant implications for the everyday functioning of an individual. Cohen and Albers (1991) describe a patient who displayed inconsistent performance across time on tests of cognitive function, with the suggestion that these abilities were impaired by her body's inability to maintain consistent levels of arousal. This pattern contrasts with the consequences of cortical damage, where this inconsistency in performance across time would not be so apparent. These symptoms can serve a useful localizing function, suggesting that accompanying intellectual deficits may have diencephalic origins as opposed to cortical origins. Other disorders, such as raised intracranial pressure, may mimic these symptoms to some extent, so differential diagnosis is important.

Cohen (1993) reviews a number of studies looking at the attentional effects of hypothalamic lesions. It is observed that unilateral lesions of the lateral hypothalamus are associated with inattention to one side of space. These lesions can also result in disruption of an orienting and avoidance response to aversive stimuli. Cohen suggests that the hypothalamus has influence over attention because of the many basic behaviors, such as eating, drinking, and aggression, that it is able to activate. Satisfaction of these drives requires that an organism directs its attention and becomes sensitive to cues that may lead to a satisfaction of these needs. He suggests that the interaction between many of these rather basic and instinctive behaviors can form the basis of more complex cognitive processes.

Lesions within the diencephalon, particularly the posterior hypothalamus and neighboring midline structures, have for some time been associated with amnesic states. Damage to these areas by the growth of tumors or subarachnoid hemorrhage has been observed to produce amnesic states resembling in many respects the memory problems associated with KORSAKOFF SYNDROME. These problems have been particularly associated with damage to the posterior areas of the structure. On the whole the literature does suggest that memory problems are a relatively common consequence of hypothalamic damage, although it is not totally clear how much poor attention, which is also a possible consequence, contributes to this problem or indeed the metabolic problems that frequently accompany damage to the hypothalamus.

Discussions concerning the hypothalamus frequently give the impression that the various disorders associated with damage to this structure occur in relative isolation from each other. In fact, if damage does occur to this structure it is unlikely to be isolated to one area or specific nuclei. It is therefore more usual that hypothalamic damage results in a constellation of deficits and thus makes the identification of specific problems quite difficult, particularly with the higher-level functions such as memory and attention.

BIBLIOGRAPHY

Bannister, R. (1992). *Brain and Bannister's clinical neurology*, 7th edn. Oxford: Oxford University Press.

Carpenter, R. H. S. (1990). *Neurophysiology*. London: Edward Arnold.

Cohen, R. A. (1993). *The neuropsychology of attention*. New York: Plenum.

Cohen, R. A., & Elliot Albers, H. (1991). Disruption of human circadian and cognitive regulation following a discrete hypothalamic lesion: a case study. *Neurology*, *41*, 726–9.

Lishman, W. A. (1987). *Organic psychiatry: The*

psychological consequences of cerebral trauma. Oxford: Blackwell Scientific.

MARCUS J. C. ROGERS

hypotonia Hypotonia is a reduction in muscle tone, observed by testing the resistance of muscles to passive movement. Muscle tone is reflex in origin, and the relevant spinal reflex mechanisms are depressed by neural shock, so that following a lesion of either one of the cerebral hemispheres or the spinal cord, the paralyzed limbs remain for a considerable time hypotonic. Because the cerebellum also facilitates stretch reflexes, cerebellar dysfunction may also result in hypotonia.

hypoxia *See* ANOXIA.

hysteria The key phenomenon that the term "hysteria" can be used to identify is the presentation of symptoms, such as sensory loss, paralysis, and amnesia, that would normally be regarded as the result of some underlying physical pathology (or possibly mental pathology in the case of multiple personality) but where the appropriate pathological basis cannot be demonstrated. Indeed, such a pathological basis may be independently shown to be highly improbable. An example of the latter is where the claimed pattern of sensory loss runs entirely contrary to established anatomical distributions of sensory nerves, or where it can be clearly demonstrated that the subject's performance on a task is heavily dependent on the sensory system that is allegedly impaired (e.g. Grosz & Zimmerman, 1965).

This is a difficult, highly controversial topic, and there is not even agreement on terminology. Some have even questioned whether there is an underlying phenomenon to which the label can be applied (Slater, 1976). The term "hysteria" is used here because it carries the force of tradition. It is also as theoretically neutral as any of the usual alternatives, given that no one in present times would subscribe to the theory implied by its etymology (i.e. that hysteria is linked to the womb). Hysteria is of significance for neuropsychology in that a high proportion of those with hysterical symptoms present in neurological rather than psychiatric settings.

It is conventional to distinguish hysteria from

hypochondriasis on the one hand and malingering on the other. Hypochondriasis involves an excessive concern or anxiety about possible illness whereas the hysteric, or so it has been alleged, exhibits *la belle indifférence* for a symptom that is claimed to exist. Malingerers (otherwise known as having a factitious disorder) are those who deliberately simulate illness while it has normally been held that hysterics do experience a real symptom in that they are truly unable to move their paralyzed limbs or remember their names.

Another fundamental distinction is between hysterical symptoms and the hysterical (or histrionic) personality. The hysterical personality, characterized by over-dramatic and histrionic behavior, being egotistic, suggestible, and demanding, having a shallow affect, was once regarded as being closely linked to hysterical symptoms. More recent evidence indicates that hysterical symptoms are certainly not confined to those exhibiting these personality features and the usefulness of the whole concept of the hysterical personality can be disputed (Kendell, 1983a; Miller, 1988a). The hysterical personality will not be further considered here and those interested are referred to Kendell (1983a).

It has commonly been alleged that there is a strong link between hysterical symptoms and being female. It is true that most attempts to examine this issue do result in a preponderance of female cases (see Miller, 1988a). However, it also has to be noted that the sex ratio is linked to the type of hysterical symptom being manifested. In Whitlock's (1967) series there was an overall excess of females although, when individual symptoms were examined, hysterical fugues and amnesias emerged as being more common in men.

A feature of hysterical symptoms is that those exhibiting them show a definite tendency to mimic symptoms with which they are familiar, either as a result of their own illnesses or because the symptoms have occurred in people with whom they are in close contact. Evidence supporting this comes from a number of sources, including Roy's (1977) study of hysterical seizures, where an appreciable proportion of those exhibiting this phenomenon appear to have had real fits as well.

A number of different types of hysteria have been claimed (Kendell, 1983b; Miller, 1988a). These include mass or epidemic hysteria as well as Briquet's syndrome (also referred to in DSM

IV as the somatization disorder). The latter occurs almost exclusively in women and the individual presents with a large number of symptoms related to different bodily systems at different times, and usually to different physicians. Symptoms are dramatized so that the headache is always "excruciating," "agonizing," or something similar. One of the symptoms is almost always gynecological in nature.

A common distinction has been between so-called "conversion hysteria" and "hysterical dissociation." These are theoretically loaded terms which assume different underlying processes (Miller, 1987). Conversion is supposed to occur when an anxiety or conflict leads to repression, with the "conversion" of the released energy into symptoms (e.g. sensory loss or paralysis). Dissociation implies that some aspects of what would otherwise be part of consciousness become "dissociated" from the rest and therefore inaccessible to normal awareness. Hysterical symptoms normally associated with dissociation are such things as AMNESIA, FUGUE states or other disturbances of consciousness, and multiple personality.

The notions of conversion and dissociation have arisen from psychodynamic and related theories. What is generally lacking is any empirical evidence to support the existence of such processes. Such evidence as does exist has been discussed by Miller (1987).

AN ALTERNATIVE ANALYSIS

The use of the concept "hysteria" (or synonyms) has been taken to imply four things (Miller, 1988b):

(a) That patients present with symptoms where no pathological basis in the ordinary sense can be established or where the usual pathological mechanisms seem most unlikely to be involved. An example of the latter is when intact muscular functioning can be demonstrated in an allegedly paralyzed muscle group in the patient who, when lying on the back, cannot raise the legs from the bed but can use the same "paralyzed" abdominal muscles to sit up.

(b) The presence of *la belle indifférence* or a lack of anxiety about the symptom.

(c) The presence of "secondary gain," i.e. the patient achieves some gain from being "ill."

(d) The symptom is "real" in the sense that the patient genuinely cannot see with the blind eye or move the paralyzed limb.

All of the above assertions are open to dispute. As far as the first is concerned, Slater and Glithero (1965) carried out a follow-up study of patients diagnosed as having hysteria at the National Hospital for Nervous Diseases in London. At the time of follow-up an unexpectedly large number had died and others had been shown to have real illnesses with similar symptoms or had developed serious psychiatric disorder. This study raised the question of whether hysterical symptoms do exist as opposed to being nothing more than the manifestation of a true pathological process that cannot be identified at the time the label of hysteria is applied.

There are good reasons for being cautious in accepting such a conclusion. Other follow-up studies of diagnosed hysterics have not supported such an extreme picture. A proportion, albeit a minority, of Reed's (1975) cases appeared to have suffered from symptoms that could only be regarded as hysterical in nature. Watson and Buranen (1970) followed up 40 cases alleged to have hysterical symptoms and a similar number of matched neurotic patients. There was no excess of either morbidity or mortality in the hysterical group. Only a quarter of the original hysterics were considered to have produced any further indication that the primary problem was not hysterical in nature. In addition, detailed investigations of particular cases with alleged hysterical symptoms have demonstrated quite conclusively that the bodily system associated with the symptoms does function normally, or at least adequately enough to make the presence of the symptom impossible on the basis of normal pathological processes (e.g. Grosz & Zimmerman, 1965; Miller, 1986).

Errors in attribution or diagnosis do occur and it may be that a substantial proportion of those to whom the label "hysteria" is typically applied do turn out to have underlying pathological processes that would explain their allegedly hysterical symptoms. This does not in itself invalidate the concept of hysteria, although it does show that a hysterical attribution for symptoms is something that should only be made with caution. The point of relevance for the present discussion is that the balance of evidence indicates that some people do present with symptoms for which no underlying cause of a conventional kind appears to exist. Furthermore, situations arise where it is actually possible to demonstrate that the allegedly affected bodily system can function reasonably well and at least to a level incompatible with the claimed symptom. The first of the four features described above is therefore encountered.

La belle indifférence is one of the classical features of hysteria. Despite this, it is inevitably an unreliable sign. Judgment of its presence is highly subjective. Some people conceal anxiety more than others and it is difficult to know just how worried the patient ought to be about a symptom if it were real, given the patient's level of background knowledge. Furthermore, empirical investigations have indicated that anxiety levels are high in hysterical patients (Lader & Sartorius, 1968). Secondary gain may occur in hysteria but is not satisfactory as one of the defining criteria, since those with true physical illnesses can also experience secondary gain (e.g. because others in the environment may be more solicitous and helpful when someone is ill).

The final criterion, that those with hysterical symptoms experience these symptoms as real, is a basic feature in most conceptualizations of hysteria. In other words, the patient with hysterical paralysis is really unable to move the allegedly paralyzed limbs. In order to judge this point adequately, any examiner would have to have access to the patient's internal consciousness and this is something that is readily agreed to be impossible. This feature therefore has inherent problems.

The case for maintaining this criterion would be strengthened if it could be shown that patients with hysteria behave differently from those considered to be malingering or faking but with similar symptoms. As Miller (1988b) has pointed out, much of the available evidence runs contrary to this view.

For example, there have been many demonstrations using the "forced choice" methodology that those with hysterical sensory symptoms behave as if they were simulating. This technique essentially requires the person with an alleged sensory loss to make discriminations using the affected sensory system. In the original report of this technique, Grosz and Zimmerman (1965) required a man with hysterical blindness to repeatedly choose the odd one out of three visual stimuli, with the position of the key stimulus being varied within the array at random. If the patient had been blind and forced to guess he should have been correct on one-third of the trials just by chance. In repeated sessions he was correct at levels very considerably below that expected by chance. In effect this demonstrates that the subject was using visual information on which to base judgments. Similar results have been reported by others, sometimes using different bodily systems (e.g. Miller, 1968 & 1986; Pankratz et al., 1975). Aplin and Kane (1985) found that audiometric results of patients with alleged hysterical hearing loss were very similar in pattern to those obtained from normal subjects asked to deliberately simulate hearing loss.

Findings like the ones above cannot be taken as proving that hysteria is nothing other than deliberate dissimulation. It could be that processes of which the patient is unaware are still resulting in a lack of conscious awareness of functional systems linked to the symptom, but are also resulting in patterns of behavior similar to those exhibited in deliberate dissimulation. Such a hypothesis is very difficult, if not impossible, to test. At the very least, evidence of the type just described makes it unwise to rely strongly on the notion that those with hysterical symptoms experience their symptoms as "real" and it is probably safest to remain agnostic on this point. It also gives further cause to question explanatory models of hysteria, such as dissociation and conversion, which rely heavily on this assumption, as well as raising considerable doubts about the logical basis for distinguishing between hysteria and malingering.

EXPLAINING HYSTERIA

If explanations based on more psychodynamic models like conversion and dissociation are rejected, as argued above and in greater detail by Miller (1988a, b), what alternative approaches exist? One has been to see hysterical symptoms as behavior learned and maintained according to the principles of operant conditioning (Munford, 1978). Another is to view hysteria as an inappropriate assumption of the "sick role" (Parsons, 1951). Those who are regarded as ill can be relieved of responsibilities and others feel obliged to be especially considerate towards them. These processes may become distorted in hysteria. The hysterical person may perceive and evaluate symptoms inappropriately, as when a minor

twinge or sense of discomfort that most would ignore is elevated to the status of a major symptom (e.g. Mayou, 1976; Pilowsky, 1969). Alternatively, people may learn the rewards of the sick role, especially if these are particularly reinforcing for that individual (Kendell, 1983b). Contributing to the appeal of some sort of learning process underlying hysterical symptoms is the fact that such patients tend to mimic symptoms with which they are familiar (e.g. Roy, 1977).

The Mayou (1976) and Pilowsky (1969) versions of the sick role model emphasize a distorted way of evaluating or conceiving of minor symptoms of the kind which are frequently experienced by most people. This suggests the possibility of developing a cognitive model of hysteria similar to that used to explain depression, anxiety, and other psychiatric symptoms (e.g. Hawton et al., 1989) and Salkovskis (1989) has already started to explore the development of somatic symptoms in this way. It is interesting that Wilson-Barnett and Trimble (1985) present some indications that those with hysterical symptoms have a tendency to misperceive the significance of trivial symptoms.

Whether or not these alternative formulations do eventually turn out to be substantially correct, they do have one further advantage. This is that they suggest certain kinds of interventions, especially of the nature of those employed in cognitive therapy (Salkovskis, 1989), which might prove to be of value in resolving the problems produced by hysterical symptoms.

BIBLIOGRAPHY

Aplin, D. Y., & Kane, J. M. (1985). Variables affecting pure tone and speech audiometry in experimentally simulated hearing loss. *British Journal of Audiology*, *19*, 219–28.

Grosz, H. J., & Zimmerman, J. (1965). Experimental analysis of hysterical blindness. *Archives of General Psychiatry*, *13*, 256 –60.

Hawton, K., Salkovskis, P. M., Kirk, J., & Clark, D. M. (1989). *Cognitive behaviour therapy for psychiatric problems: A practical guide*. Oxford: Oxford University Press.

Kendell, R. E. (1983a). The hysterical (histrionic) personality. In G. F. M. Russell & L. A. Hersov (Eds), *Handbook of psychiatry*. Vol. 4: *The neuroses and personality disorders* (pp.

246–51). Cambridge: Cambridge University Press.

Kendell, R. E. (1983b). Hysteria. In G. F. M. Russell & L. A. Hersov (Eds), *Handbook of psychiatry*. Vol. 4: *The neuroses and personality disorders* (pp. 232–46). Cambridge: Cambridge University Press.

Lader, M., & Sartorius, N. (1968). Anxiety in patients with hysterical conversion symptoms. *Journal of Neurology, Neurosurgery and Psychiatry*, *31*, 490–5.

Mayou, R. (1976). The nature of bodily symptoms. *British Journal of Psychiatry*, *129*, 55–60.

Miller, E. (1968). A note on the visual performance of a patient with unilateral functional blindness. *Behaviour Research and Therapy*, *6*, 115–16.

Miller, E. (1986). Detecting hysterical sensory symptoms: an elaboration of the forced choice method. *British Journal of Clinical Psychology*, *25*, 231–2.

Miller, E. (1987). Hysteria: its nature and explanation. *British Journal of Clinical Psychology*, *26*, 163–73.

Miller, E. (1988a). Hysteria. In E. Miller & P. J. Cooper (Eds), *Adult abnormal psychology* (pp. 245–67). Edinburgh: Churchill Livingstone.

Miller, E. (1988b). Defining hysterical symptoms. *Psychological Medicine*, *18*, 275–7.

Munford, P. R. (1978). Conversion disorders. *Psychiatric Clinics of North America*, *1*, 377–90.

Pankratz, L., Fausti, S. A., & Peed, S. (1975). A forced choice technique to evaluate deafness in the hysterical or malingering patient. *Journal of Consulting and Clinical Psychology*, *43*, 421–2.

Pilowsky, I. (1969). Abnormal illness behaviour. *British Journal of Medical Psychology*, *42*, 347–51.

Reed, J. L. (1975). The diagnosis of "hysteria." *Psychological Medicine*, *5*, 13–17.

Roy, A. (1977). Hysterical fits previously diagnosed as epilepsy. *Psychological Medicine*, *7*, 271–3.

Salkovskis, P. M. (1989). Somatic disorder. In K. Hawton, P. M. Salkovskis, J. Kirk, & D. M. Clark (Eds), *Cognitive behaviour therapy for psychiatric problems: A practical guide* (pp. 235–76). Oxford: Oxford University Press.

Slater, E. T. O. (1976). What is hysteria? *New Psychiatry*, *2*, 14–15.

Slater, E. T. O., & Glithero, E. (1965). A follow-up of patients diagnosed as suffering from "hysteria." *Journal of Psychosomatic Research*, *9*, 9–13.

Watson, G. C., & Buranen, C. (1979). The frequency and identification of false positive conversion reactions. *Journal of Nervous and Mental Diseases*, *167*, 243–7.

Whitlock, F. A. (1967). The aetiology of hysteria. *Acta Psychiatrica Scandinavica*, *43*, 144–62.

Wilson-Barnett, J., & Trimble, M. R. (1985). An investigation of hysteria using the Illness Behaviour Questionnaire. *British Journal of Psychiatry*, *146*, 601–7.

EDGAR MILLER

I

ictal phenomenon, state   The ictal phenom-enon, seen in an ictal state, is one of the stages of an epileptic seizure, although the term is some-times used more loosely to refer to the complete epileptic event. The ictal phase is the period of the fit itself (the term is derived from rhythmical shaking movements), whatever the nature of the fit, to distinguish it from the *pre-ictal* phase when it occurs, otherwise known as the *aura*, and the *post-ictal* symptoms which follow the fit (*see* EPILEPSY).

ideational apraxia   *See* APRAXIA.

ideomotor apraxia   *See* APRAXIA.

idiopathic epilepsy   *See* EPILEPSY.

immune system   The immune system, more properly termed the *lymphatic system*, is composed of the spleen, lymph vessels and nodes, and lymph fluid, and it has the purpose of defending the body against invasion by injurious agents and removing worn-out cells.

Immune responses are affected by hormones secreted by the adrenal glands which are in turn regulated by hormones secreted by the pituitary gland and the HYPOTHALAMUS. There is also some degree of cortical control in that cognitively perceived stress may also have an effect on this system, with resulting reactive effects. Disorder of the immune system may also produce *autoim-munity* in which the system attacks the individual's own normal healthy cells. This mechanism is thought to be related to certain diseases of con-nective tissue such as rheumatoid arthritis, and also to migraine, allergies, thyroid, and gas-

trointestinal disorders. It has been suggested by Geschwind and Galaburda that these latter dis-orders are more commonly to be observed in individuals with abnormal LATERALIZATION (who are also more likely to be left-handers; *see* HANDEDNESS), the association being mediated by the fetal efects of testosterone. However, this hypothesis has not been clearly supported by the available data.

Direct and indirect associations between the brain and the immune system are also demon-strated by the neuropsychological consequences of AIDS.

imperviousness   Imperviousness characterizes a patient who responds only after repeated re-quests and often a considerable delay, and then often inappropriately and perhaps incompletely. This apparent apathy is classically associated with anterior callosal lesions, particularly the BUTTER-FLY GLIOMA. The symptom is probably not at-tributable to the involvement of the CORPUS CALLOSUM per se, but of the medial aspects of the frontal lobes and the anterior CINGULATE GYRI. Imperviousness is likely to render a subject uncooperative or relatively inaccessible to exami-nation.

impulsivity   Impulsivity, the tendency to act without careful forethought, may be an early sign of herpes simplex ENCEPHALITIS, particularly if accompanied by memory loss and an abnormality of emotional expression such as depression. This may be understood by the tendency for this inflammatory infection to affect the orbitofrontal and anterior temporal regions and hence have a widespread but selective effect upon the LIMBIC SYSTEM.

indifference The importance of indifference, an inappropriate lack of concern for the patient's own current state, accompanied by general emotional flattening, lies in the classical distinction between CATASTROPHIC and indifference reactions. Following a distinction first made by Goldstein, and elaborated by Gainotti and others, indifference reactions have been associated with lesions of the right hemisphere, while catastrophic reactions are associated with lesions of the left. While certainly an oversimplified classification of the emotional reactions, the distinction has received some empirical support. Explanations of indifference in being related to a denial of illness, or in being determined by associated right hemisphere cognitive deficits, have been shown to be incomplete, and disturbances of arousal also contribute to the indifference behavior.

infarct An infarct is an area of dead (necrotic) tissue usually resulting from the loss of the blood supply to the area as a result of STROKE or some other CEREBROVASCULAR ACCIDENT.

insula The insula is an area of phylogenetically old cortex hidden at the base of the SYLVIAN FISSURE and medial to it; it is only revealed when the anterior part of the temporal lobe is retracted. Structurally, it is the posterior continuation of orbitofrontal cortex behind the anterior temporal lobe. Being less vulnerable than more exposed areas of cerebral cortex, its functions are less well understood, although primary olfactory cortex is located in one region of the insula. Certain bilateral lesions resulting in facial AGNOSIA have been reported to involve the insula. Insulotemporal lesions in animals have been shown to affect discrimination of pure tonest and the discrimination of changes in temporal sequence in the visual and vibrotactile modalities, as well as the auditory modality.

intelligence quotient The intelligence quotient (IQ) is a standard index of general cognitive ability. As originally formulated by Binet and named by Terman in 1916, the mental age as determined by standardized test procedures was stated as a proportion of chronological age and

multiplied by 100 to give an index with a mean of 100 and a standard deviation of 16. Contemporary instruments have replaced this procedure with the "deviation IQ," which artificially establishes that the distribution of IQs in any age group has a mean of 100 and a standard deviation of 15 (in the case of the most commonly used Wechsler tests). As this index is constructed so as to be normally distributed, IQs can be accurately converted into percentile ranks. Intelligence quotients should never be regarded as an exact score, and should be interpreted with regard to the associated confidence interval which reflects the limited reliability of the test. IQs in the normal population range from about 70 to 130.

interhemispheric transfer *See* COMMISSUROTOMY; LATERALIZATION.

intermetamorphosis In the condition of intermetamorphosis, the patient believes that familiar individuals undergo a physical and mental metamorphosis, with the result that they become a different person. It is a very rare disorder, a combination of features of the CAPGRAS SYNDROME and the FREGOLI SYNDROME.

interthalamic connexus *See* MASSA INTERMEDIA.

intracarotid sodium amytal In the majority of people it can be assumed that language centers are located in the left hemisphere. In some people though, particularly left-handers, these centers may be found in the right hemisphere. In cases where elective surgery is required for the control of seizure activity it is essential that the surgeon be aware of the location of these centers to avoid disruption of language functions. It was to confirm which hemisphere subserved language that Wada and Rasmussen in 1949 pioneered the technique of selectively anesthetizing one side of the brain (the procedure became known as the Wada test). This was done by injecting sodium amytal, a fast-acting anesthetic agent, into the internal carotid artery feeding one hemisphere. This procedure results in temporary hemiplegia, hemianopia, and hemianesthesia on the side ipsilateral to the site of the injection. If the hemisphere dominant for speech has been anesthetized there will also be a temporary cessation of all language functions. After approximately five minutes a slow return of functions will be observed.

As well as being used to locate language centers prior to surgery, the technique has also been used to determine the effect of temporary ablation on different forms of memory and to investigate the lateralization of functions such as musical ability. Although a very useful procedure for the reasons outlined, it does present investigators with a number of problems. The effect of the anesthetic is relatively short-lived, thus limiting the time in which testing is possible. In addition, the presence of hemianopia, hemiplegia, and in some cases aphasia further restricts the type of investigation that can be carried out. It should also be remembered that the bulk of individuals used as subjects in experiments involving this technique do not have normal brains.

ischemia Cerebral ischemia follows insufficiency of the blood supply to the brain, resulting from narrowing or complete occlusion of an artery. Complete blockage will produce an INFARCT, but narrowing may produce temporary and reversible symptoms which can vary with blood pressure or local vascular spasm and include confusion, emotional instability, and decline in intellectual functions and memory.

Repeated episodes during which these symptoms appear and then subsequently resolve are known as *transient ischemic attacks* or *TIAs*. These periods are normally short, but are associated with a high risk of subsequent STROKE, which occurs in about one third of those suffering TIAs who go untreated. Generalized cognitive impairment may be observed in patients who suffer TIAs.

Where the ischemic attack is associated with insufficiency in the main arteries in the neck, commonly the carotid artery or the principal cerebral arteries, surgery may be performed to correct the blood flow by *carotid endarterectomy* or by arterial bypass surgery, although medical treatments are generally the first treatment of choice. Studies have shown that these forms of surgery may be effective in relieving the frequency and effects of the attacks, but neuropsychological assessment has generally failed to confirm improvements in cognitive status consequent upon these procedures.

J

Jacksonian fit   *See* EPILEPSY.

jamais vu   Jamais vu (literally "never seen") is the converse of DÉJÀ VU, a sense of strangeness with respect to familiar objects or places.

The more common use of the term relates to an altered perceptual experience during the aura preceding a temporal lobe seizure, often accompanied by other distortions of perception or feelings of derealization or depersonalization. The phenomenon is simply a change in the quality of recognition, with strong feelings of unfamiliarity for whatever is the current focus of attention. It is presumed that some dysfunction of the memory systems contained within the anterior temporal lobe results in the faulty attribution of novelty to familiar stimuli.

An alternative use of the term refers to the sensation in relation to visual HALLUCINATIONS, where the scene is clear and detailed in the sense of a vivid visual memory, yet the patient has the sense of never having previously had the experience, and may have feelings of anguish or disgust.

The term "jamais vu" is also used more loosely to refer to any sense of inappropriate unfamiliarity which may be reported by neurotic patients or even by normal subjects. Many normal subjects will report occasional sensations of jamais vu with respect to either objects or places, and the phenomenon alone in the absence of other neurological signs is not indicative of pathology. The conditions which produce jamais vu are similar to those which result in its converse, déjà vu.

jargon aphasia   *See* APHASIA.

K

Kennard principle The Kennard principle states that the younger the individual, the lesser will be the effects of a given cerebral lesion. The principle was originally developed by studying comparative lesions in infant and adult monkeys, but was seen to generalize to the human context in that children, particularly below the age of about 6 years, often suffer less dramatic sequelae from cerebral trauma or surgery. However, there are clear limits to the general validity of the principle, which depends upon the nature and site of the lesion, as well as upon the age of the individual.

Kleine–Levin syndrome The Kleine–Levin syndrome is a form of hypersomnia in which there is an increased tendency to sleep, although this tendency is resistible, unlike NARCOLEPSY. The syndrome occurs most commonly in adolescent males, when it is associated with episodes, lasting days or weeks, of excessive appetite and both behavioral and memory changes. The behavioral changes may include irritability and even frank aggression, uninhibited insolent behavior, confusion, muddled speech, vivid dreams and hallucinations. Attacks, occurring with an average frequency of about two per year, gradually diminish and become less frequent with time until they ultimately cease. The basis for this syndrome has not been determined.

Klüver–Bucy syndrome The Klüver–Bucy syndrome is a behavioral syndrome first documented in 1888 by Brown and Schaefer but "rediscovered" by Klüver and Bucy in 1939. They observed a number of dramatic behavioral changes in monkeys who had undergone bilateral anterior temporal lobectomies. The changes observed included the following: (1) tameness and placidity; (2) hyperorality involving the mouthing of inappropriate objects; (3) hypersexuality involving inappropriate partners and object choice; (4) visual AGNOSIA; and (5) a tendency to be overly reactive to every visual stimulus.

These observations led to increased interest in the role that the temporal lobes play in behavior, although the relative part played by the temporal neocortex as opposed to the limbic structures has not been well established. It would appear that bilateral removal of inferior temporal cortex as well as the amygdala is necessary for the full expression of the syndrome.

The syndrome has been seen to appear in humans with a variety of neurological conditions including head trauma, ENCEPHALITIS, and bilateral temporal LOBECTOMY. However, it is rare that the full and pure syndrome is seen in humans, possibly because damage, when it occurs, is frequently relatively diffuse.

MARCUS J. C. ROGERS

Korsakoff's psychosis *See* KORSAKOFF'S SYNDROME.

Korsakoff's syndrome In 1887–9 Korsakoff described a syndrome of characteristic memory disturbance, which he witnessed in over 30 alcoholic patients and 16 nonalcoholic cases. This occurred in a setting of clear consciousness: "At first, during conversation with such a patient . . . [he or she] gives the impression of a person in complete possession of his [or her] faculties; he [she] reasons about everything perfectly well, draws correct deductions from given premises, makes witty remarks, plays chess or a game of cards, in a word comports himself [or herself] as a mentally sound person." However, "the patient constantly asks the same questions and repeats the same stories . . . may read the same page over

428

and over again sometimes for hours . . . is unable to remember those persons whom he [or she] met only during the illness, for example, the attending physician or nurse." Characteristically, "the memory of recent events . . . is chiefly disturbed . . . everything that happened during the illness and a short time before." However, in some cases "not only memory of recent events is lost, but also that of the long past," in which case the impairment may involve memories of up to 30 years earlier. Moreover, he noted that, in some instances, events may be remembered "but not the time when they occurred" (temporal context memory impairment). He suggested that, in mild cases, personal memories are forgotten but "facts are remembered," whereas in more severe cases, "the memory of facts is completely lost."

Korsakoff drew attention to confabulation: "such patients invent some fiction and constantly repeat it . . . [for example] of conversations which have never occurred." However, he placed greater emphasis on the confusion of "old recollections with present impressions," another example of temporal context memory impairment. He gave several examples of this, including a woman who had confused a trip she had made to Finland before her illness with recollections of a journey to the Crimea.

The fact that Korsakoff obtained such findings in 16 nonalcoholic cases is important, and has often been forgotten. His sample included patients in whom the syndrome had developed following persistent vomiting (8 patients), postpartum (sepsis, macerated fetus), in acute or chronic infection (typhus, tuberculosis), after toxic poisoning (carbon monoxide, lead, arsenic), or after other chronic disease (neoplasm, lymphadenoma, diabetes). Moreover, Korsakoff noticed that the appearance of memory disorder often followed a period of prodromal confusion, ophthalmoplegia, nystagmus, and ataxia, and that peripheral neuropathy was commonly present (although not necessarily so) – these are all features of Wernicke's encephalopathy, described in 1881, although Korsakoff did not refer to Wernicke's writings.

SUBSEQUENT CLINICAL STUDIES

Subsequent clinical studies have confirmed the broad outline of Korsakoff's clinical description, and that a characteristic confusional state and/or neuropathological changes can result from a number of factors beside chronic alcohol abuse. For example, the variability and the general extensiveness of the retrograde memory loss has been emphasized by Victor among others. Victor and colleagues (1971) wrote that: "[While] it is true that remote memories were better preserved than recent ones . . . it was our impression that memories of the distant past were impaired to some extent in practically all patients with Korsakoff's psychosis and seriously impaired in most of them." Moreover, they followed Korsakoff in arguing that confabulation often results from the inappropriate recall of genuine memories, jumbled in temporal sequence. Spurning an emphasis on either a specific deficit of recent memory or the presence of confabulation, Victor and others (1971) defined the disorder as "an abnormal mental state in which memory and learning are affected out of all proportion to other cognitive functions in an otherwise alert and responsive patient." Contemporary diagnosis of the syndrome requires neuropsychological evidence of this disproportionate memory impairment and clinical evidence of an underlying alcoholic or nutritional etiology.

Two matters over which there has been some controversy are the mode of onset of the disorder and the prevalence of Wernicke features. Various authors have suggested that the disorder can have either an acute onset, frequently in association with Wernicke features, or an insidious onset, in which Wernicke signs occur more rarely. By contrast, Victor's group (1971) reported that 96 percent of their Korsakoff patients had previously manifested Wernicke signs, and only 10 per cent had exhibited an insidious onset. However, this may well have reflected the nature of their referrals within an acute neurological service; and more recent work indicates that some patients, in whom an autopsy diagnosis of the characteristic pathology is made, may have arrived in hospital in coma, whereas other cases may never have been diagnosed in life, although known to be heavy drinkers, surviving in the community with (presumably) a milder degree of memory impairment (see Kopelman, 1995). In short, it appears that the initial clinical manifestation of the disorder may vary from acute coma, through the classical Wernicke syndrome, to an insidious onset of memory impairment, and that, in some cases, the disorder may not be identified until the subject comes to autopsy.

Furthermore, various modern writers have confirmed that the Wernicke–Korsakoff pathology can result from a number of debilitating disorders, all of which produce malnutrition or malabsorption. De Wardener and Lennox (1947) provided a classical description of 52 prisoners of war in South-East Asia who developed a Wernicke encephalopathy as a result of malnutrition, of whom 32 patients (61.5 percent) developed loss of recent memory. The onset was 6 to 14 weeks after the start of captivity, and was usually preceded by episodes of diarrhea and vomiting, self-starvation, or concurrent infection. Interestingly, in the early stages, the subjects *complained* of wavering vision on looking sideways (a consequence of nystagmus), double vision (resulting from ophthalmoplegia), memory loss, and impaired time appreciation, indicating that "insight" was initially preserved. Other writers have described Wernicke symptoms and/or pathology occurring after self-starvation; intravenous feeding especially in the presence of a glucose load; the persistent vomiting of hyperemesis gravidarum; and carcinoma of the esophagus, stomach, or intestine.

Three recent papers have attempted to provide evidence of persistent memory impairment following onset of nonalcoholic nutritional depletion. Beatty and colleagues (1989) described a patient with a "Korsakoff-like amnesic syndrome" following severe anorexia and vomiting, but this patient had extremely abnormal liver function tests, including a very high gamma GT (not commented upon), which raises the suspicion of past alcohol abuse. Becker and others (1989) described a woman with malabsorption from an inflammatory cause in the small intestine, who had a past history of heavy drinking, although that seems to have resolved by the time of her amnesic disorder. Parkin and others (1991) described a patient who had had prolonged intravenous feeding, but this patient's amnesia arose after a surgical operation, in which she had to have a blood transfusion, and there were multiple small lesions in the deep white matter on MRI scan, thought to be vascular in origin, making the possible contribution of hypotension and/or hypoxia during the operation unclear. In short, it seems that it is surprisingly hard to find unequivocal cases of the amnesic syndrome from nonalcoholic nutritional depletion nowadays, presumably because of generally higher standards of nourishment than in Korsakoff's day. However, there is little doubt that nonalcohol causes

may complicate and compound alcoholic causation. The present author has seen cases of Korsakoff's syndrome in which the intake of alcohol has been compounded by either carcinoma of the stomach or a previous gastrectomy.

THE NEUROPATHOLOGY OF THE KORSAKOFF SYNDROME

Various authors have established that there is substantial overlap in the nature and distribution of the pathological lesions in Wernicke's syndrome and in Korsakoff's syndrome. There are abnormalities in the so-called "diencephalon," involving the paraventricular and peri-aqueductal gray matter of the brain, the walls of the third ventricle, the floor of the fourth ventricle, and the cerebellum, with the mammillary bodies and the thalamus among the sites most commonly affected. In these regions, there are micro-hemorrhages and endothelial proliferation (i.e. rupture and abnormal changes in the lining of blood vessels), together with focal areas of parenchymal necrosis, demyelination, gliosis, and variable degrees of neuronal loss (i.e. degeneration of brain cells and tissue and nerve fiber linings with associated scarring). In addition, cortical atrophy is commonly present, and attention has been drawn to the gross atrophy, reduced neuron count, and increased hydration in the frontal lobes at autopsy (for references see Kopelman, 1995).

Debate has ensued, however, regarding the critical lesion(s) for the development of an amnesic syndrome, the mammillary bodies and the thalamus being the sites most commonly implicated. Victor and colleagues (1971) pointed out that all 24 of their cases, in whom the medial-dorsal nucleus of the thalamus was affected, had a history of persistent memory impairment (Korsakoff's syndrome), whereas 5 cases, in whom it was unaffected, had a history of Wernicke features without a subsequent memory disorder. By contrast, the mammillary bodies were implicated in all the Wernicke cases examined, whether or not there was subsequent memory impairment. On the other hand, Mair and colleagues (1979) provided a careful pathological and neuropsychological description of two Korsakoff patients, whose autopsies showed lesions in the mammillary bodies and the midline and anterior portion of the thalamus, but *not* in the medial dorsal nuclei. Mair's group suggested that the lesions they described might "disconnect" a critical circuit running between the temporal lobes and the frontal cortex. Other studies have closely replicated the findings in the work of Mair and colleagues (1979). Severe anterograde amnesia has also been described, resulting from a traumatic lesion to the mammillary bodies.

Von Cramon and others (1985) examined the variability in the effects of thalamic lesions upon memory function. On the basis of a CT study, Von Cramon and his colleagues argued that the anterior thalamus, which receives input from the mammillo-thalamic tract, is always implicated in amnesic patients, whereas lesions confined to the dorsal medial nucleus do not usually produce amnesia. In short, it appears that the mammillary bodies, the mammillo-thalamic tract, and the anterior thalamus, rather than the medial dorsal nucleus, are critically involved in memory formation.

NEUROCHEMISTRY OF THE KORSAKOFF SYNDROME

Thiamine

The probable role of thiamine depletion in the etiology of the alcoholic Korsakoff syndrome was originally suggested both by experimental studies and by clinical observations. These suspicions appeared to be confirmed by the excellent De Wardener and Lennox (1947) study in malnourished prisoners of war. These patients exhibited mental changes in 78 percent of cases and loss of recent memory in 61 percent, generally occurring at the same time as other symptoms of thiamine depletion (approximately 6 to 14 weeks after captivity), but before the onset of illnesses resulting from the depletion of other vitamins. Moreover, the symptoms showed a very favorable response to thiamine treatment by injection, when this was available, but resulted in a very high mortality when thiamine was unavailable.

However, it is sometimes claimed that a *combination* of thiamine deficiency and a direct neurotoxic effect of alcohol is required to produce a *persistent* memory loss in the Korsakoff syndrome (Butters & Cermak, 1980). Against this, it should be noted that Korsakoff's own series included 16 nonalcoholic cases; and one of De Wardener and Lennox's (1947) and 3 out of 8 of Cruikshank's (1950) prisoners of war showed persistent mental

symptoms despite treatment. Moreover, in many other series, the follow-up details provided are insufficient to decide whether or not persistent memory impairment was present. It seems plausible that the nonalcoholic cases may show a better response to treatment than the alcoholic cases; and that the response to treatment is determined both by the abruptness of the onset of disorder and the rapidity with which treatment is instituted, and these may generally occur more rapidly in the nonalcoholic cases.

A genetic factor has been postulated to explain why only a minority of heavy drinkers develop the syndrome, which is far less common than the liver or gastro-intestinal complications of alcohol abuse. Blass and Gibson (1977) postulated a hereditary abnormality of transketolase metabolism, but other authors have reported wide variability in transketolase activity among Korsakoff and other alcoholics. There are now known to be up to six isoenzymes of human erythrocytic transketolase, with one study reporting that there is a particular pattern of isoenzymes associated with the presence of Wernicke–Korsakoff syndrome, although this in itself would not explain why these patients are particularly vulnerable to the effect of thiamine depletion (see Witt, 1985).

Witt (1985) has provided an excellent review of the possible ways by which thiamine depletion might predispose to the characteristic pathological lesions of the Wernicke–Korsakoff syndrome, although the precise mechanism involved is not known. Thiamine pyrophosphate (TPP), the active form of thiamine, appears to be involved in DNA synthesis as well as three enzymatic reactions which are essential for glucose metabolism and neurotransmitter production; and the metabolic heterogeneity of different brain regions might explain why some areas are more vulnerable to thiamine depletion than others. Six neurotransmitter systems are affected by thiamine depletion, either by reduction of TPP-dependent enzyme activity or by direct structural damage, and these neurotransmitters include acetylcholine and glutamate.

Acetylcholine

Particular interest lies in the possible contribution of cholinergic depletion to the memory disorder of the Korsakoff syndrome, in view of the evidence that cholinergic "blockade" in healthy subjects may induce memory impairment (Kopelman

431

& Corn, 1988), and that acetylcholine is depleted in Alzheimer's disease (Rosser et al., 1984). TPP depletion might be expected to produce diminished levels of acetyl-CoA, a precursor of acetylcholine, thereby resulting in diminished synthesis (Witt, 1985). There is some evidence that the inhibition of (TPP-dependent) pyruvate decarboxylase does indeed cause depleted acetylcholine *synthesis* and more substantial evidence of reduced acetylcholine *turnover* during thiamine deficiency.

Another possible link between Korsakoff's syndrome and the cholinergic system was suggested by Arendt and others (1983), who found a 47 percent reduction in neuron count in the basal forebrain of three Korsakoff patients at autopsy, which, it has been suggested, might be very important in producing the memory impairment. Subsequent studies reported basal forebrain lesions in other groups of amnesic patients. However, psychopharmacological studies of cholinergic blockade in healthy subjects suggest that cholinergic depletion would produce an anterograde amnesia without any retrograde loss, unlike the Korsakoff syndrome; and, more particularly, an autopsy of two Korsakoff patients failed to find any important changes within the basal forebrain (Mayes at al., 1988).

Noradrenaline and serotonin

McEntee and Mair have suggested an important role for the noradrenergic system in the memory disorder of the Korsakoff syndrome (McEntee et al., 1984). They found reduced MHPG (3 methoxy 4-hydroxy phenylglycol) levels in the CSF of Korsakoff patients, which were correlated with a measure of memory impairment. Clonidine administration produced a small but statistically significant improvement in memory test performance. However, later studies failed to replicate the finding of reduced MHPG or the clonidine finding. Animal studies implicate the adrenergic system in mechanisms mediating attention and arousal, rather than memory, and it seems very plausible that an attentional deficit might explain some of the personality and behavioral disorders seen in the Korsakoff syndrome (e.g. the characteristic apathy), but not the "core" memory disorder.

More recent studies have reported an improvement in free recall performance in five patients following administration of fluvoxamine, a sero-tonin-reuptake inhibitor. This finding requires replication in larger studies, especially in view of the observed failure of serotonin reuptake inhibitors to produce benefits in Alzheimer patients.

NEUROIMAGING STUDIES OF THE KORSAKOFF SYNDROME

Structural imaging

Three CT scan studies have employed planimetric or computerized measures of cortical atrophy. The first of these was by Carlen and others (1981), who found that alcoholic subjects (N = 93) showed significantly greater ventricular enlargement and sulcal widening than a non-alcoholic control group, but that differences between a Wernicke–Korsakoff group (N = 25) and other alcoholics were minimal and non-significant. Subsequently, Shimamura and colleagues (1988) reported significant enlargement of the third ventricle, and widening of the Sylvian fissures and the left frontal sulci, in 7 Korsakoff patients relative to 7 other alcoholics and 7 healthy controls. Within the Korsakoff group, a computerized measure of frontal sulcal enlargement showed a statistically significant median rank correlation (r = 0.43) with 12 memory measures.

In a much larger study, involving 38 Korsakoff patients, 100 alcoholic subjects, and 50 healthy subjects, Jacobson and Lishman (1987) found that a computerized measure of enlargement of the anterior interhemispheric fissure correlated with general intellectual decline (NART-IQ – current IQ). On the other hand, the degree of third ventricular enlargement was related to the severity of memory impairment (IQ-MQ).

There have also been reports of hypodensity in the thalamus of Wernicke–Korsakoff patients. However, density measurements are very prone to a number of important sources of artifact and, after controlling for these, Jacobson and Lishman (1990) found that thalamic density measurements were reduced in male Korsakoff patients only, and that there were no significant correlations with measures of memory performance.

Somewhat similarly, Christie and others (1988) found evidence of cortical atrophy in an MRI (magnetic resonance imaging) study, but they obtained only one significant correlation between measurements of cortical atrophy and a number of memory test scores. Squire and colleagues (1990) conducted an MRI study in four alcoholic Korsakoff patients, finding abnormally small mammillary nuclei, barely detectable by MRI, whereas the temporal lobes, hippocampi, and parahippocampal gyri were of normal size, contrasting with the findings in another group of amnesic patients of probable temporal lobe pathology.

Functional imaging

Hunter and others (1989) used single photon emission computerized tomography (SPECT) in Korsakoff and Alzheimer patients, finding that the Korsakoff group showed a general trend towards reduced tracer uptake throughout the neocortex, and there were significant rank correlations with clinical measures of orientation and recent memory on the CAMCOG assessment schedule. Fazio and others (1992) studied 11 patients with "pure amnesia," including 2 Korsakoff patients, using positron emission tomography (PET). They found significant bilateral reduction in glucose metabolism in the limbic-hippocampal regions, including the thalamic nuclei, as well as the frontal basal cortex. This metabolic impairment did not correspond to alterations in structural anatomy on MRI, and appears to have arisen irrespective of underlying etiology. More specific PET and MRI studies in Korsakoff patients are now under way in California and London.

THE NEUROPSYCHOLOGY OF THE ALCOHOLIC KORSAKOFF SYNDROME

The neuropsychology of the amnesic syndrome and of amnesic states is reviewed elsewhere in this volume. There are, of course, many studies of the pattern of impaired and preserved memory function in the alcoholic Korsakoff syndrome, and they will be reviewed here in brief.

Within primary or working memory, there are many investigations showing that performance on span tests (verbal and nonverbal) is preserved in the Korsakoff syndrome. Performance on short-term forgetting tasks is much more variable, with some studies showing preserved ability and some showing severe impairment. The consensus now appears to be that there is a variable pattern of performance on both verbal and nonverbal

tasks. It has been suggested that this variability in performance was correlated with the degree of frontal lobe dysfunction; whereas Kopelman (1992) argued that the impairments on verbal and nonverbal short-term forgetting tasks were correlated with left-hemisphere and right-hemisphere cortical atrophy respectively, as measured on CT scan.

By definition, there is a severe deficit in the explicit component of secondary memory. It is plausible that this results from an underlying dysfunction in some physiological process, such as "consolidation." However, various psychological deficits have been postulated, such as an impairment in the encoding of semantic information or in the encoding of contextual information. While there does indeed appear to be some degree of deficit in the processing or encoding of some types of semantic information, it seems unlikely that this accounts for the severity of the memory disorder in the Korsakoff syndrome. Similarly, although Korsakoff patients show a disproportionate deficit in the encoding of such aspects of context as temporal order, spatial location, modality of presentation, and source of information, such deficits sometimes appear incidental to the memory impairment for target information, being evident in some patients but not others. Moreover, the degree of contextual memory impairment shows a relatively low correlation (shared variance) with target memory performance. It may be that contextual information is particularly difficult to learn, but that it does not represent the "core" component of the amnesic disorder (for references see Kopelman, 1995).

Several studies have shown that rates of long-term forgetting are normal, once target information has been learned to an adequate level for as long as 10 minutes. Two possible qualifications to this finding are: (i) that all these studies have involved recognition memory, as "matching" is extremely difficult to achieve on recall tasks; and (ii) that it is plausible that there are differences in forgetting rates over shorter intervals than 10 minutes (Kopelman, 1992). In addition, there are many studies which reveal that Korsakoff patients show preserved capacity on tests of implicit memory, such as word-completion priming and procedural memory for perceptuo-motor skills (e.g. Tulving & Schacter, 1990). Such studies are generally interpreted as implying a distinct "implicit" memory system, preserved in amnesia and mediated by cortical structures (priming) and/or subcortical structures (procedural memory), from the (impaired) "explicit" memory system, mediated by limbic-diencephalic structures.

There is also, of course, an extensive retrograde memory loss in the Korsakoff syndrome, extending back several decades, as Korsakoff (1889) himself noted and modern neuropsychological studies have confirmed. This extensive retrograde loss involves memory for remote public or "semantic" information, facts about a patient's own life ("personal semantic memory"), and "autobiographical" memory for incidents or events from the patient's past (Kopelman, 1992). All these aspects of retrograde memory show a "temporal gradient" with relative sparing of the most distant memories, and the gradient is significantly steeper than that seen in dementing disorders such as Alzheimer's disease (Kopelman, 1992). The relative sparing of early memories may result from their greater salience and rehearsal, such that they become assimilated within semantic memory (Cermak, 1984). Consequently, there are two possible reasons why Korsakoff patients have a steeper temporal gradient than dementing patients: (i) semantic memory is relatively preserved in Korsakoff patients, allowing better retrieval of early memories than in dementing patients; and (ii) a progressive anterograde impairment during the Korsakoff patients' period of heavy drinking may have made the loss of recent memories particularly severe.

Although confabulation may occur in retrieving remote or autobiographical memories, it is relatively rare aside from fleeting intrusion errors, and it may result from certain types of concomitant frontal lobe damage. However, there appears to be a retrieval component to the retrograde deficit in the Korsakoff syndrome and several studies have shown that the severity of retrograde and anterograde memory impairments are poorly correlated in this group of patients (Shinamura & Squire, 1986; Kopelman, 1989, 1991b; Parkin, 1991). While performance on retrograde and anterograde tests showed 21 percent shared variance in one study, a regression equation based on three "frontal" tests predicted 68.5 percent of the variance on retrograde memory tasks (Kopelman, 1992). This suggested that frontal lobe dysfunction, resulting from the known

abnormalities in this region revealed in neuroimaging and autopsy studies, may contribute to a failure in the organization of retrieval processes for remote and autobiographical memories (Kopelman, 1992).

CONCLUSIONS

Korsakoff (1889) described a syndrome in which memory was profoundly impaired relative to other cognitive functions, but which was not always associated with alcohol abuse. Although Korsakoff himself recognized the association with some of the clinical features of Wernicke's encephalopathy, it now appears that a history of Wernicke's syndrome is not invariably present, and that coma or an insidious onset are alternative initial manifestations of the disorder. Moreover, alcoholic subjects, who have never been diagnosed during life, sometimes show the characteristic neuropathology at autopsy. While pathological features are found throughout the paraventricular and peri-aqueductal gray matter, there is agreement that lesions in either the thalamus or the mammillary bodies or both are critical in producing amnesia. The relative importance of the thalamus and the mammillary bodies is still debated, although the consensus seems to be that lesions in the anterior thalamus, mammillo-tract, and/or mammillary bodies are critical for memory disruption. The disorder is usually associated with cortical atrophy, particularly involving the frontal lobes, and this is evident in both neuroimaging and autopsy studies.

The belief that an alcoholic etiology is essential to produce a permanent memory impairment is not well established, even though "pure" non-alcoholic cases have been hard to find in recent times. A wide variety of causes of malnutrition or malabsorption have been described as giving rise to the characteristic neuropathology. The common factor underlying all these is almost certainly thiamine depletion, but why some subjects should be especially vulnerable to thiamine depletion, and its precise effect upon acetylcholine and other neurotransmitters, remains to be elucidated.

There is now general agreement concerning the pattern of the memory deficit in the Korsakoff syndrome, involving a severe impairment of new learning and an extensive retrograde loss with intact or well-preserved working memory, priming, procedural memory, and the rate of "long-term" forgetting. While structural lesions and/or neurochemical depletions within the diencephalon can account for anterograde amnesia, here it has been suggested that some other factor, such as frontal lobe dysfunction, must underlie the extensive retrograde memory loss characteristically found in this syndrome.

BIBLIOGRAPHY

Arendt, T., Bigl, V., Arendt, A., & Tennstedt, A. (1983). Loss of neurons in the nucleus basalis of Meynert in Alzheimer's disease, paralysis agitans and Korsakoff's disease. *Acta Neuropathologica, Berlin, 61*, 101–8.

Beatty, W. W., Baily, R. C., & Fisher, L. (1989). Korsakoff-like amnesic syndrome in a patient with anorexia and vomiting. *International Journal of Clinical Neuropsychology, 11*, 55–65.

Becker, J. T., Furman, J. M. R., Panisset, M., & Smith, C. (1990). Characteristics of the memory loss of a patient with Wernicke-Korsakoff's syndrome without alcoholism. *Neuropsychologia, 28*, 171–9.

Blass, J. P., & Gibson, G. E. (1977). Abnormality of a thiamine-requiring enzyme in patients with Wernicke-Korsakoff syndrome. *New England Journal of Medicine, 297*, 136–7.

Butters, N., & Cermak, L. S. (1980). *Alcoholic Korsakoff's syndrome: An information processing approach to amnesia.* New York: Academic Press.

Carlen, P. L., Wilkinson, D. A., Wortzman, G., Holgate, R., Cordingley, J., Lee, M. A., Huzzar, L., Moddell, G., Singh, R., Kiraly, L., & Rankin, J. G. (1981). Cerebral atrophy and functional deficits in alcoholics without apparent liver disease. *Neurology, 31*, 377–85.

Cermak, L. S. (1984). The episodic-semantic distinction in amnesia. In L. R. Squire & N. Butters (Eds), *The neuropsychology of memory* (pp. 55–62). New York: Guilford.

Christie, J. E., Kean, D. M., Douglas, R. H. B., Engleman, H. M., St Clair, D., & Blackburn, I. M. (1988). Magnetic resonance imaging in presenile dementia of the Alzheimer-type, multi-infarct dementia, and Korsakoff's syndrome. *Psychological Medicine, 16*, 319–29.

Cruikshank, E. K. (1950). Wernicke's encephalopathy. *Quarterly Journal of Medicine, 19*, 327–38.

De Wardener, H. E., & Lennox, B. (1947). Cerebral beriberi (Wernicke's encephalopathy): review of 52 cases in a Singapore PoW hospital. *Lancet, 1*, 11–17.

Fazio, F., Perani, D., Gilardi, M. C., Colombo, F., Cappa, S. F., Vallar, G., Bettinardi, V., Paulesu, E., Alberoni, M., Bressi, S., Franceschi, M., & Lenzi, G. L. (1992). Metabolic impairment in human amnesia: a PET study of memory networks. *Journal of Cerebral Blood Flow and Metabolism, 12*, 353–8.

Hunter, R., McLuskie, R., Wyper, D., Patterson, J., Christie, J. E., Brooks, D. N., McCulloch, J., Fink, G., & Goodwin, G. M. (1989). The pattern of function-related regional cerebral blood flow investigated by single photon emission tomography with ^{99m}Tc-HMPAO in patients with presenile Alzheimer's disease and Korsakoff's psychosis. *Psychological Medicine, 19*, 847–56.

Jacobson, R. R., & Lishman, W. (1987). Selective memory loss and global intellectual deficits in alcoholic Korsakoff's syndrome. *Psychological Medicine, 17*, 649–55.

Jacobson, R. R., & Lishman, W. A. (1990). Cortical and diencephalic lesions in Korsakoff's syndrome: a clinical and CT scan study. *Psychological Medicine, 20*, 63–75.

Kopelman, M. D. (1992). The "new" and the "old": components of the anterograde and retrograde memory loss in Korsakoff and Alzheimer patients. In L. R. Squire & N. Butters (Eds), *The neuropsychology of memory*, 2nd edn (pp. 130–46) New York: Guilford.

Kopelman, M. D. (1995). The Korsakoff syndrome. *British Journal of Psychiatry, 166*, 154–73.

Kopelman, M. D., & Corn, T. H. (1988). Cholinergic "blockade" as a model for cholinergic depletion: a comparison of the memory deficits with those of Alzheimer-type dementia and the alcoholic Korsakoff syndrome. *Brain, 111*, 1079–110.

Korsakoff, S. S. (1889 [1955]). Psychic disorder in conjunction with peripheral neuritis. Translated by M. Victor & P. I. Yakovlev. *Neurology, 5*, 394–406.

McEntee, W. J., Mair, R. G., & Langlais, P. J. (1984). Neurochemical pathology in Korsakoff's psychosis: implications for other cognitive disorders. *Neurology, 34*, 648–52.

Mair, W. G. P., Warrington, E. K., & Weiskrantz, L. (1979). Memory disorder in Korsakoff's psychosis: a neuropathological and neuropsychological investigation of two cases. *Brain, 102*, 783.

Mayes, A. R., Mendell, P. R., Mann, D., & Pickering, A. (1988). Location of lesions in Korsakoff's syndrome: neuropsychological and neuropathological data on two patients. *Cortex*, *24*, 367–88.

Parkin, A. J. (1991). Recent advances in the neuropsychology of memory. In J. Weinmann & J. Hunter (Eds), *Memory: Neurochemical and abnormal perspectives*. London: Harwood.

Rosser, M. N., Iversen, L. L., Reynolds, G. P., Mountjoy, C. O., & Roth, M. (1984). Neurochemical characteristics of early and late onset types of Alzheimer's disease. *British Medical Journal*, *288*, 961–4.

Shimamura, A. P., & Squire, L. R. (1986). Korsakoff's syndrome: a study of the relation between anterograde amnesia and remote memory impairment. *Behavioral Neuroscience*, *100*, 165–70.

Shimamura, A. P., Jernigan, T. L., & Squire, L. R. (1988). Korsakoff's syndrome: radiological (CT) findings and neuropsychological correlates. *Journal of Neuroscience*, *8*, 4400–10.

Squire, L. R., Amaral, D. G., & Press, G. A. (1990). Magnetic resonance imaging of the hippocampal formation and mammillary nuclei distinguish medial temporal lobe and diencephalic amnesia. *Journal of Neuroscience*, *10*, 3106–17.

Tulving, E. & Schacter, D. L. (1990). Priming and human memory systems. *Science*, *247*, 301–6.

Victor, M., Adams, R. D., & Collins, G. H. (1971). *The Wernicke-Korsakoff syndrome*. Philadelphia: Davis.

Von Cramon, D. Y., Hebel, N. & Schuri, U. (1985). A contribution to the anatomical basis of thalamic amnesia. *Brain*, *108*, 997–1008.

Witt, E. D. (1985). Neuroanatomical consequences of thiamine deficiency: a comparative analysis. *Alcohol and Alcoholism*, *20*, 201–21.

MICHAEL D. KOPELMAN

L

lacunar state The lacunar state results from repeated lacunar INFARCTS, minor strokes which are mild in their effects and from which, singly, there may be rapid recovery. However, the effect of an increasing number of these strokes is cumulative and results in a form of dementia with a gradual onset. The mental deterioration is said to lag behind the physical signs of weakness, slowness, and disturbances of gait, speech, and swallowing. Emotional lability with spasmodic laughing and crying is also associated with the lacunar state. Lacunar strokes are more common in hypertensive individuals, and where the lesions are predominantly in subcortical white matter, the condition is known as progressive subcortical encephalopathy (Binswanger's disease).

language disorders *See* AGRAPHIA; APHASIA; DYSLEXIA; SPELLING DISORDERS.

lateral cerebral asymmetry *See* LATERALIZATION.

lateral eye movements *See* LEMs.

lateralization The term lateralization derives from the Latin word *latus, lateris* (= side) and is currently used to define the process by which a neural function is "pushed to one side" of the brain. Lateralization is a concept which has a wide biological implication and can be applied to any side asymmetry in living organisms. Undoubtedly, the interest in this phenomenon is historically related to the discovery of lateralization of function in the human brain; however, there is growing evidence that many vertebrates share with humans the presence of lateralized structures and/or functions. Therefore, one cannot be wrong in stating that understanding brain lateralization is a prerequisite for grasping important general principles underlying the organization of the central nervous system.

EARLY HUMAN STUDIES

The French neurologist Paul Broca, in the second half of the last century, was the first who gave scientific credibility to the idea that cerebral functions were anatomically separated. Moreover, it was not long after having discovered that language production depended upon cortical areas corresponding to the third frontal convolution that Broca also realized that this was true only for the left hemisphere. In fact, post-mortem investigations had shown that the lesions of his first two aphasic patients encompassed areas beyond the third frontal convolution and extended to the inferior part of the parietal lobe and to the first temporal convolution. However, the crucial fact that the lesions were restricted to the left side of the brain did not escape him. In general, Broca's merit was in understanding that the lesion which impaired his patients' speech was related to a "center" for speech production that was distinct on the one hand from motor centers for the contraction of the phonation muscles and on the other from "higher-order" centers subserving ideas or linguistic memories. Broca's famous discovery was stimulated by the intense discussions taking place during those years between anthropologists, neuroanatomists, and clinical neurologists on the evolutionary emergence of the human mind and by the phrenological concepts of Gall. This author, at the beginning of the nineteenth century, was in some sense an originator of the modern neuropsychological concept of functional modules, believing, as he did, that the mind could be subdivided into different functions with different cerebral locations. As to the concept of cerebral lateralization, even before Broca, another French physician, Marc Dax, had extensively documented the association between left hemispheric lesions and language disturbances. However, it was Broca who pursued the topic and brought it to the attention of the scientific world.

Subsequently, at the beginning of this century, it became clear, following the pioneering studies of Liepmann on the syndrome of APRAXIA (i.e. an inability to execute purposeful skilled movements out of their natural context), that the left hemisphere was not only the site of language processes but also of the organization of complex volitional movements. The two functions, although partly related, are independent given that, among other things, they may show independent recovery following brain damage. Another major step in our understanding of brain lateralization occurred when, during the first half of this century, evidence began to be gathered about the important role of the right hemisphere in a range of cognitive functions characterized by their being mainly concerned with spatial perception, with little reliance on verbal mediation.

It was then that the earlier concept of *cerebral dominance* of the left hemisphere was replaced by the concept of *hemispheric specialization*, the term that is now more often used.

MAIN EXPERIMENTAL APPROACHES TO LATERALIZATION

Currently, lateralization studies are carried out following several lines of enquiry. The traditional approach of studying *patients with unilateral hemispheric lesions* is still of great importance and is being actively pursued. Another field of endeavor concerns patients who have undergone *transection of the corpus callosum and the other cerebral commissures* (see COMMISSUROTOMY). This approach, originated by Sperry and his co-workers (see Trevarthen, 1984; Nass & Gazzaniga, 1987), is extremely important because it permits a direct test of each hemisphere working in isolation from its fellow; unfortunately, it has an obvious limitation in the restricted number of subjects available and in the presence of severe pre-operative brain pathology in some of the patients. A further approach, the popularity of which is witnessed by the huge number of studies carried out in the last 25 years, is represented by studies in *normal subjects*, using the simple technique of restricting

sensory input initially to one or the other hemisphere. This is a relatively straightforward procedure for visual, auditory, somatosensory, and olfactory stimuli while, to my knowledge, few or no attempts have been carried out to lateralize gustatory stimuli. Such an approach allows testing of a great number of subjects, but suffers from the impossibility of directly relating the observed behavior to neural structures.

The above three methods have a common rationale, namely finding functions which are subserved differentially by the two hemispheres, but they differ in the way such asymmetries are tapped. In the unilateral lesion method, there are no laterality effects but hemispheric differences are inferred from the selective impairment following either a left- or a right-side lesion. The fundamental neuropsychological principles of *double dissociation of symptoms* can thus be usefully applied to this approach. Patients with a lesion in the left hemisphere will be impaired on a host of language-related functions while patients with a right-hemisphere lesion will be impaired on nonverbal, spatial tasks. The essential prerequisite for the principle of double dissociation is that the two groups must perform normally in the tasks which are supposed to tap the functions of their intact hemispheres. A broadly similar situation is present in patients with a section of the corpus callosum, where the performance in verbal tasks is dramatically decreased when sensory information is channelled to the isolated right hemisphere and the performance in visuospatial tasks is impaired when the sensory input is restricted to the left hemisphere. Studies with normal subjects, on the contrary, tap laterality effects by comparing the abilities of the sensory surfaces directly connected to the hemisphere which is competent for the task being investigated. Thus, the right visual hemifield, which is directly connected to the left visual cortex, is more accurate and rapid in handling visually presented linguistic material than the left visual hemifield. Conversely, the left visual hemifield, which is directly connected to the right visual cortex, is superior in handling visuospatial information.

Interesting contributions are also being provided by *morphological and functional studies of brain lateralization*; the former can be performed both at the macroscopic and at the cytoarchitectonic level while the latter can investigate electric, magnetic or metabolic brain activity during performance of specific cognitive tasks. Finally, an important field of endeavor encompassing all the above approaches concerns the *development of lateralization*, an issue which is crucial not only for an understanding of lateralization itself but also for a fuller comprehension of human psychological development in general.

The general picture emerging from such a variety of experimental approaches is difficult to synthesize in a few words and the neuropsychological community is still dwelling upon the best possible dichotomies to describe hemispheric differences. However, at least one undisputed finding has been obtained so far. The classic concept of *cerebral dominance*, with the left hemisphere dominating all cognitive functions, has been replaced by the concept of *opposite hemispheric specialization*, with the two hemispheres subserving different general cognitive operational modes. According to the latter concept, the two hemispheres share more or less equally the overall burden of cognitive life, with the left handling linguistic functions and the right nonverbal spatial operations. A widely (but not universally) accepted view is that the two hemispheres do not show differences in basic perceptual or motor operations, and only different cognitive modes characterize them. An interesting concept which has emerged from various studies with visual and auditory stimuli is that laterality effects in normal people are not rigidly contingent upon the stimulus itself but rather upon the way the stimulus is processed. Thus, perception of faces is subserved by the right hemisphere when unknown faces have to be discriminated, and the same holds true if subjects are to decide whether a face is unknown to them or not. However, facial recognition of well-known people yields an opposite left hemisphere superiority (see Marzi, 1989, for a brief review).

For a more detailed account of these approaches and the dichotomies invoked by the various authors to explain human lateralization see DIVIDED VISUAL FIELD TECHNIQUE, DICHOTIC LISTENING, DICHHAPTIC TASKS.

A few more words are in order to comment on the results of the two approaches which have yielded the most compelling evidence of lateralization in the human brain, namely HEMISPHERECTOMY (and focal unilateral lesions) and COMMISSUROTOMY.

HEMISPHERECTOMY

Obviously, the most dramatic, crude but straightforward clinical test of cerebral lateralization is to study patients who have undergone HEMISPHERECTOMY, i.e. removal of the cerebral cortex of one hemisphere. A number of such patients have been systematically studied. Some studies have dealt with right, others with left hemispherectomy patients, observing dramatically different neuropsychological impairments. Apart from the inevitable severe sensory and motor losses, after a *right hemispherectomy* patients have intact verbal capacities but visuospatial abilities are profoundly impaired. On the contrary, following a *left hemispherectomy* speech is reduced to a few isolated words, although usually a certain degree of language comprehension is left. This picture of the differential effect of right vs left hemispherectomy is typical of right-handers who have not suffered from disease in the remaining hemisphere before surgery. As demonstrated by studies on the plasticity of lateralization, there can be shifts of functions from one hemisphere to the other following early brain injury.

An interesting question concerns *the verbal capability of the right hemisphere* of dextrals. In principle, hemispherectomy cases represent a powerful source of evidence to decide between an *absolute* vs a *relative* lateralization of language. However, caution is in order in drawing inferences from hemispherectomy patients, as the number of cases is small and the duration of recovery is often short, because of the low survival due to the severity of the underlying pathology. Notwithstanding this, the picture seems to be reasonably clear: in the absence of the left dominant hemisphere some language comprehension is present, but language production is almost completely impaired (for a more complete account *see* HEMISPHERECTOMY).

There are two techniques that allow one to inactivate reversibly and for a brief period one or the other hemisphere, namely unilateral electroconvulsive therapy (ECT) and the unilateral carotid injection of the anesthetic sodium amytal (the so-called Wada technique; INTRACAROTID SODIUM AMYTAL). Both approaches have clearly shown that language functions are impaired by left rather than by right hemisphere inactivation. The latter is often used as a powerful diagnostic tool before cortical excisions and has yielded numerous indications on the lateralization of language as a function of handedness. Obviously, both methods have the intrinsic limitation of being affected by individual differences in the spread of the anesthetic (Wada) or current (ECT) to the other side of the brain, and by the short time available (this is especially true for the Wada technique) for testing during the inactivation period.

UNILATERAL LESIONS

The study of patients with focal lesions lateralized to one or the other hemisphere represents the oldest and perhaps richest source of evidence on functional lateralization, and a description of the huge number of studies gathered since the pioneering neurological observations of Broca and Wernicke is beyond the scope of this article. Information on the selective effects of left hemisphere lesions can be gathered from the following entries: ACALCULIA, AGRAMMATISM, AGRAPHIA, ALEXIA, APHASIA, APRAXIA, DYSLEXIA. In addition, it has been shown that memory deficits specific for verbal or visuospatial material are present in patients with either a left or a right temporal lobe and hippocampal damage respectively (see AMNESIA; AMNESIC SYNDROME).

THE EFFECTS OF COMMISSURAL SECTION

The contribution of the study of the so-called "split-brain" patients is twofold: (i) assessing laterality of function in the two isolated hemispheres; (ii) establishing the importance of the commissures for interhemispheric transfer of information.

The picture that has emerged following almost 30 years of research is that the two cerebral hemispheres differ not only in language processing but also in several other mental functions. The study of split-brain patients has been especially important for revealing the unique spatial abilities of the right hemisphere, as well as for giving clues to the degree of interhemispheric cross-talk necessary for normal mental functioning. Moreover, it allows an experimental investigation of philosophical issues, such as mechanisms of consciousness and volitional control, as well as the important question of right hemisphere language (for a more complete account of this fundamental approach to lateralization *see* COMMISSUROTOMY, DISCONNECTION SYNDROME).

THE GENERAL BIOLOGICAL FRAMEWORK OF LATERALIZATION

That lateralization of brain functions is not a unique human trait became definitively clear in the seventies when Nottebohm found that the left (but not the right) hemisphere of the canary subserves vocalization (see Nottebohm, 1979). By the early eighties the number of species showing various kinds and degrees of lateralized functions had multiplied and included not only birds but several mammals (see Denemberg, 1981). Finally, the early nineties are not only witnessing a continuous growth of interest in biological studies of lateralization but are also providing evidence of cognitive hemispheric asymmetries homologous to those found in humans.

ARE ASYMMETRIES IN NONHUMAN SPECIES HOMOLOGOUS OR ANALOGOUS TO LATERALIZATION OF HUMAN BRAIN FUNCTION?

Left–right asymmetries are present throughout the animal kingdom and left–right body axis formation in the vertebrates has been studied for many years. Recent observations (Yost, 1992) suggest that left–right axial information is contained in the extracellular matrix early in embryogenesis (gastrula stage); thus it is not surprising that there exist numerous examples of left –right asymmetries in visceral organs as well as in the nervous system. Heart, liver, gall bladder, and spleen are all "lateralized" organs; by the same token, harelip is more frequent on the left side and fingerprints are typically systematically different in right- and left-handers. As a consequence of these peripheral asymmetries, the nervous control of such organs also has to be lateralized; this fact may have some bearing on the emergence of asymmetries in the central nervous system. There is no doubt, however, that the onset of brain lateralization in humans is a major, further evolutionary step which has some resemblance but little homology with asymmetries of visceral organs.

An important question is whether nonhuman species show examples of lateralization of cognitive functions. Until a few years ago the answer to this question was typically negative; however, more recently, studies using new techniques have provided evidence of functional hemispheric asymmetries in monkeys and apes.

In monkeys with a section of the cerebral

commissures Hamilton and Vermeire (1988) found a differential lateralization of cognitive processing. The left hemisphere was better in the discrimination of slant while the right hemisphere was better at discriminating (monkey) faces. In language-trained chimpanzees Hopkins and colleagues (1991) demonstrated asymmetrical hemispheric activation using known and unknown warning stimuli (geometrical forms), some of which, through association, had been given some semantic value. Taken together, these findings show that hemispheric lateralization in nonhuman primates is not entirely dependent upon the emergence of human-like language, as was thought for a long time. They suggest instead that lateralization may be related to basic, phylogenetically old, neuropsychological systems.

WHY DOES LATERALIZATION OCCUR?

A fundamental question concerns the cause of lateralization, why certain functions are grouped in one hemisphere and others are common to both. A possible interpretation is that lateralization reflects the evolution of systems which have diversified because of their functional incompatibility. One major example could be provided by verbal and spatial skills which are kept segregated in the human hemispheres, perhaps because optimal performance in one of them is detrimental to optimal performance in the other. The advantage of keeping the two functions segregated might lie in the different requirements of verbal and spatial processing of information. Cues that are important for the former must be filtered out by the latter and vice versa. Environmental spatial cues are certainly irrelevant and potentially detrimental for discriminating a vowel from a consonant (both in the visual and the auditory modality) while, on the other hand, verbal cues are irrelevant for localizing the spatial source of either visual or auditory information.

Another important related question is *whether hemispheric asymmetries are casual or causal* (see Bryden, 1986). According to a commonly held interpretation of lateralization, the specialization of the left hemisphere for language is the *cause* of the specialization of the right hemisphere for spatial processing. This is either because of the necessity of keeping incompatible functions as separate as possible, as outlined above, or alternatively, because the "neural space" of the left hemisphere is mostly occupied by language and

other fundamental cognitive functions have to be housed elsewhere. This position is what Bryden (1986) defines as *causal complementarity*. However, in principle, another position is logically possible, namely that of *statistical (or casual) complementarity*. According to this view, the factors which bias the left hemisphere for mastering language and the right hemisphere for mastering spatial nonverbal skills might be independent of each other. Thus lateralization would arise for statistical not for causal reasons, i.e. for the simple fact that most people have language in the left hemisphere and visuospatial function in the right. It is important that the set of factors which lead to lateralization of language processes are totally independent from those leading to lateralization of spatial processes. Empirical support for this view comes from both studies on patients with unilateral brain lesions and from normal subjects. The hypothesis of causal hemispheric complementarity predicts a negative association between the incidence of aphasia and of visuospatial disorders. However, in a vast number of patients with unilateral left or right hemisphere lesions simply no association was found. By the same token, in normals no association could be found between the opposite laterality effects found for two dichotic listening tasks yielding a left ear (right hemisphere) or right ear (left hemisphere) superiority respectively. This is at odds with a causal complementarity explanation of lateralization, which would again have predicted a negative association between the two opposite laterality effects (see Bryden, 1986).

As is often the case when dichotomies are proposed, a compromise between the two possibilities is not unlikely. Thus it might be argued that certain lateralized functions possibly subserved by homologous cortical areas in the two hemispheres (see Geschwind & Galaburda, 1987) are indeed associated whereas others, subserved by non-homologous areas, are not.

Independent of these theories, establishing whether a given function is lateralized represents key information contributing to an understanding of the neuropsychological mechanisms underlying such a function. This, rather than merely adding new items to the list of known lateralized functions, is the main thrust of laterality research.

THE ONTOGENESIS OF LATERALITY

A crucial question for an understanding of lateralization is establishing the mechanisms of its onset. Early theories favored the idea that the two hemispheres are equipotential at birth and for the first two years of life and that a left hemisphere superiority for linguistic functions develops with age (Lenneberg, 1967). This viewpoint was based on the recovery of linguistic functions following early brain injury. More recently, studies of normal subjects employing different experimental paradigms, such as DICHOTIC LISTENING, DIVIDED VISUAL FIELD TECHNIQUES, as well as electrophysiological methods, mainly EVOKED POTENTIALS, have provided much information (see Hahn, 1987, for a review). Such findings have confirmed that some lateralization of function is present in newborns and add weight to the idea that lateralization is inborn rather than experience dependent. Moreover, the presence of a left hemisphere superiority at the time of birth is in keeping with a left–right asymmetry of the planum temporale at 31 weeks of fetal age (see Galaburda et al., 1990 for a recent review). It has also been established that the superiority of the left hemisphere for linguistic functions remains constant throughout childhood and that this is the case for both genders. As is often the case in laterality studies, the picture is somewhat less clear for the functional specialization of the right hemisphere. However, there is little doubt that some typically right-hemisphere features such as specific activation during musical sounds (Molfese et al., 1975) is present in infants.

The neurobiological mechanisms underlying onset of lateralization are still unresolved. Several intriguing theories have been proposed: Geschwind and colleagues (notably Behan and Galaburda) have proposed a complex theory in which they claim that fetal testosterone slows normal development of the left hemisphere and therefore modifies cerebral lateralization as well as development of other body processes, such as the immune system (see Geschwind & Galaburda, 1987). More recently, Galaburda and colleagues (1990) have specifically proposed that lateralization depends on a decrease in the number of neurons on one side of the brain while hemispheric functional symmetry entails equally large areas in both sides. In keeping with this idea, Witelson and Nowakoski (1991) stress the possibility that, in addition to a selective cell loss, an asymmetric pruning of callosal axons might be related (in males only) to onset of lateralization.

BIBLIOGRAPHY

Bryden, M. P. (1986). The nature of complementary specialization. In F. Lepore, M. Ptito, & H. H. Jasper (Eds), *Two hemispheres – one brain: Functions of the corpus callosum* (pp. 463–9). New York: Liss.

Denemberg, V. H. (1981). Hemispheric laterality in animals and the effects of early experience. *Behavioural and Brain Sciences, 4*, 1–49.

Galaburda, A. M., Rosen, G. D., & Sherman, G. F. (1990). Individual variability in cortical organization: its relationship to brain laterality and implications to function. *Neuropsychologia, 28*, 529–46.

Geschwind, N., & Galaburda, A. M. (1987). *Cerebral lateralization.* Cambridge, MA: MIT Press.

Hahn, W. K. (1987). Cerebral lateralization of function: from infancy through childhood. *Psychological Bulletin, 101*, 376–92.

Hamilton, C. R., & Vermeire, B. A. (1988). Complementary hemispheric specialization in monkeys. *Science, 242*, 1691–4.

Hopkins, W. D., Morris, R. D., & Savage-Rumbaugh, E. S. (1991). Evidence for asymmetrical priming using known and unknown warning stimuli in two language-trained chimpanzees (*Pan troglodytes*). *Journal of Experimental Psychology: General, 120*, 46–56.

Lenneberg, E. H. (1967). *Biological foundations of language.* New York: Wiley.

Marzi, C. A. (1989). Lateralisation of face processing. In A. W. Young & H. D. Ellis (Eds), *Handbook of research on face processing* (pp. 431–6). Amsterdam: North Holland.

Molfese, D. L., Freeman, R. B., & Palermo, D. S. (1975). The ontogeny of brain lateralization for speech and nonspeech stimuli. *Brain and Language, 2*, 356–68.

Nass, R. D., & Gazzaniga, M. S. (1987). Cerebral lateralization and specialization in human central nervous system. In F. Plum (Ed.), *Handbook of physiology. Section 1: The nervous system.* Vol. 5. *Higher functions of the brain, Part 1* (pp. 701–61). Bethesda, MD: American Physiological Society.

Nottebohm, F. (1979). Asymmetries in neural control of vocalization in the canary. In S. Harzad, R. W. Dory, L. Goldstein, J. Jaynes, & G. Krauthamer (Eds), *Lateralization in the nervous system.* New York: Academic Press.

Trevarthen, C. (1984). Hemispheric specialization. In I. Darian-Smith (Ed.), *Handbook of physiology. Section 1: The nervous system.* Vol. 3. *Sensory processes, Part 2* (pp. 1129–90). Bethesda, MD: American Physiological Society.

Witelson, S. F., & Nowakoski, J. J. (1991). Left out axons make men right: a hypothesis for the origin of handedness and functional asymmetry. *Neuropsychologia, 29,* 327–33.

Yost, H. J. (1992). Regulation of vertebrate left-right asymmetries by extracellular matrix. *Nature, 357,* 158–61.

C. A. MARZI

laughing, involuntary Involuntary laughter may result from lesions which interrupt the corticobulbar motor pathways bilaterally, thus releasing reflex mechanisms for facial expression, in the pontobulbar area, from cortical control. The emotional behavior, which may involve laughing, crying, or both, is stereotyped and the patient may report feeling normal emotions rather than the emotion expressed. The emotional behavior may be triggered by a variety of stimuli and can be neither initiated nor stopped under voluntary control.

Uncontrollable laughter may also occur in gelastic EPILEPSY, in which the seizure is preceded or accompanied by giggling or laughter. It may be that the laughter in this case is evoked by the emotional content of a brief temporal lobe aura.

lead poisoning Traditionally, the term lead poisoning has referred to any of a constellation of effects on various organ systems resulting from environmental or occupational exposures to high levels of lead (Pb). The central (CNS) and peripheral (PNS) nervous systems feature prominently in lead poisoning; other affected systems include the GI tract, the kidney, and the hematopoietic system. Today, different levels of lead poisoning are widely recognized with respect to neuropsychological outcome and can be construed as frank lead poisoning resulting in acute ENCEPHALOPATHY, frank lead poisoning in the absence of encephalopathy, and subclinical lead toxicity. In essence, this division might be thought of as a continuum along which the neuropsychological outcomes produced by lead exposure

decrease in magnitude and severity, i.e. a type of dose-effect function. Today, lead poisoning per se and accompanying acute encephalopathy occur infrequently as a result of regulation of exposure. The major concern instead is the neuropsychological impact of chronic low-level exposure resulting from environmental contamination.

LEAD USE AND EXPOSURE

The utilization of lead by man extends far back into history, as does the knowledge of its toxic properties. The Romans were major users of lead, not only for their aqueducts and water-pipe systems (many of which remain even today), but also their cooking practices and cookware. Together, these uses resulted in rather extensive contamination of the population and widespread geographical dispersion of lead into the environment.

An even more marked increase in the production and geographical dispersion of lead occurred during the Industrial Revolution, and was followed, in turn, in the early nineteenth century by a rising incidence of occupational lead poisoning, a problem which eventually provoked the implementation of industrial hygiene practices and standards for exposure. Occupational exposure levels have since been continually refined downwards as the definition of a safe level of occupational lead exposure has declined.

Current environmental lead exposure is derived primarily from the residual impact of two prior uses of lead, namely lead-based paints and leaded gasoline. Repeated episodes of acute and chronic lead poisoning in children during the first half of the twentieth century resulted from the ingestion of lead-based paint chips (a behavior known as pica). Although lead-based paints have since been banned in many countries, old layers of lead-based paint are continuously chipped off or are scraped off during repainting. Lead particles are then released into the atmosphere and eventually become incorporated into the surrounding dusts and soils, sometimes reaching extremely high concentrations. This remains a major source of exposure even today, particularly for children, who are prone to engage in hand-to-mouth behavior from which leaded dust and soil are subsequently ingested.

Lead released in automobile exhaust from leaded gasoline has been geographically dispersed and from there incorporated into the ecosys-

443

tem, and hence into our food and water supplies. This constitutes the major source of lead exposure for adults not occupationally exposed to it, with inhaled atmospheric lead making only a minor contribution. Although ingestion of lead-contaminated food and water is also a primary source of exposure for children, it is still secondary to that resulting from the ingestion of lead from dust and soil.

The most readily accessible and relatively noninvasive index of lead exposure in humans is the concentration of lead in blood, and many thresholds for effects or ranges of exposure for effects are reported on the basis of blood lead level (PbB). This measure, however, predominantly reflects recent exposure to lead. Because most of the lead burden resides in the skeleton, some studies have examined tooth lead levels to achieve a better estimate of total lead exposure.

DEVELOPMENTAL DIFFERENCES IN SUSCEPTIBILITY

Children demonstrate a greater vulnerability to lead than do adults. With respect to the CNS, for example, the threshold for lead-induced encephalopathy is lower and the residual neurological sequelae are more severe in children. This enhanced susceptibility arises from toxicokinetic, nutritional, behavioral, and developmental factors.

With respect to kinetics, uptake of lead, both from the GI tract and from the respiratory tract, and retention of lead in the body, is greater in children than in adults. In addition, less of the lead burden of children is stored in the skeleton, making greater amounts available to soft-tissue target organs such as the brain.

Deficiencies of many essential metals such as calcium, iron, and zinc can increase absorption of lead from the GI tract and may also alter distribution preferentially to soft tissues such as the brain. Nutritional deficiencies of calcium, iron and zinc are certainly not uncommon in childhood populations, and may be more prevalent among economically disadvantaged children who are already at increased risk if they reside in urban areas where old housing with lead-based paint is common.

Typical patterns of behavior early in development likewise serve to increase exposure to lead, especially hand-to-mouth activity. When children

become mobile, the contamination of hands and toys with lead-containing dust becomes an added bolus of lead which is ingested as a result of hand-to-mouth activity. As mentioned, pica for lead-based paint chips was a prominent factor in the episodes of childhood lead poisoning in the first half of the twentieth century.

A final factor proposed to enhance susceptibility to lead during the earlier stages of development is the immaturity of the blood–brain barrier in children. An undeveloped blood–brain barrier may be more permeable to toxicants such as lead, again with the net result being a functional increase in the dose of lead to the brain.

NERVOUS SYSTEM EFFECTS ASSOCIATED WITH OVERT LEAD POISONING

Overt lead poisoning results in a variety of adverse effects both on the nervous system and on other organs and systems of the body. It is the neurotoxic consequences of lead exposure, however, that tend to be the most severe. The most dramatic example of this is acute lead encephalopathy, a syndrome which can prove fatal. Early features of this syndrome include nonspecific signs and symptoms such as dullness, restlessness, irritability, attention lapses, headaches, and tremor. The syndrome may progress to more severe manifestations such as delirium and mania, convulsions, ATAXIA, and intractable seizures, and may then be followed by coma or even death. However, the more severe form of the syndrome is not always preceded by the less severe signs, and may start in the absence of any prior symptoms of lead toxicity and progress to fatality within 48 hours. This scenario seems to be particularly prevalent in young children, a fact which may reflect not only their enhanced vulnerability, but also the greater difficulty in detection and reporting of early symptoms in young children, such that the syndrome has progressed beyond the point of treatment prior to recognition.

The levels of lead exposure associated with acute encephalopathy actually vary quite widely, rendering it difficult to predict individuals at risk. In general, it is thought that acute encephalopathy is associated with PbBs (lead burdens) well in excess of 120 ug/dl in adults, but is manifest at 90–120 ug/dl in children, the same PbBs associated with death in children. Since the range for these effects is so broad, however, some individuals may exhibit levels as high as 700–800 ug/dl before encephalopathy ensues.

The neuropathological features of acute encephalopathy are not distinctive, in that no specific pathological lesion is characteristic of this syndrome, nor does any particular brain region appear to be involved. In fact, in some cases pathological changes are minimal. When neuropathology is noted, it frequently includes cerebral edema and damage to the cerebral vasculature, as well as glial proliferation. It has been stated that the damage to the cerebral vasculature is the basis for the edematous response. Studies of exposure to high levels of lead in experimental animals generally confirm this picture and also suggest reduced cortical thickness and a decline in the number of synapses per neuron and in axonal size.

Survivors of acute lead encephalopathy are highly likely to show residual neurological and behavioral impairment. The types of neurological sequelae observed have been stated not to differ from those produced by other diffuse brain injuries in children (e.g. severe head trauma, viral or bacterial ENCEPHALITIS, and MENINGITIS) and can include cortical ATROPHY, HYDROCEPHALUS, convulsive disorders, CEREBRAL PALSY, mental retardation, and blindness. Along with the lower thresholds for acute lead encephalopathy exhibited by children, residual permanent neurological sequelae occur more frequently. It has been estimated that at least one-quarter of the children who survive acute encephalopathy are left with multiple permanent neurological sequelae, a figure which can increase to nearly 100 percent if children return to the same lead-contaminated environment following the episode of acute encephalopathy. Proportions as high as 80 percent may be left with at least one residual neurological effect.

Even when lead poisoning occurs without acute encephalopathy, permanent neurological or behavioral sequelae as described can result, with as many as 37 percent of poisoned children being affected and 9 percent experiencing mental retardation. Also included among such residual effects may be unsatisfactory progress in school, short ATTENTION span, and behavioral disorders.

Another nervous system effect associated with lead poisoning is peripheral neuropathy, an effect more prevalent in adults than children, which manifests clinically as wrist drop. This may be more severe in the dominant hand and may be accompanied by ankle weakness as well. When severe enough in nature, the result may be permanent neurological damage. Peripheral neuropathy has been attributed to segmental demyelination and axonal degeneration secondary to an effect on the Schwann cell. As is the case with acute encephalopathy produced by lead exposure, there are wide individual differences in the PbBs at which peripheral neuropathy is observed.

NERVOUS SYSTEM EFFECTS AT LOWER LEVELS OF EXPOSURE

The controversial effects of lead are those attributed to lower levels of exposure. Studies carried out in the 1970s and 1980s in adults documented increased reports of various symptoms, both of the CNS (e.g. tiredness, irritability, and headaches) and PNS (muscle and joint pain, PARESTHESIA, weakness, and dropping of objects) at PbBs of 40–60 ug/dl, i.e. well below the 80 ug/dl figure that had previously been deemed safe for occupational lead exposures. As with many of the other reported effects of lead, individual differences in vulnerability to such symptoms were marked.

In addition, a variety of studies report neuropsychological impairments in occupationally exposed adults at 40–60 ug/dl PbBs in the absence of any indication of overt intoxication. These impairments include disturbances of occulomotor function, reaction time, eye–hand coordination, hand dexterity and visual–motor performance. Other studies found impairments in aspects of cognitive function as well, including changes in intelligence, memory, vigilance, acquisition, coding, spatial relations, distractibility, and vocabulary.

Neurophysiological effects of lead in occupationally exposed adults are described at PbBs below 70 ug/dl and possibly as low as 30 ug/dl. These effects were noted most consistently in the median motor nerve as a decrement in nerve conduction velocity. Comparisons of distribution of nerve conduction velocities indicated a shift of the values of workers exposed to lead toward the extreme (slowest) range of normal values.

Low-level effects of lead on neuropsychological outcome in children has without doubt been the subject of the most intensive examination, debate, and controversy. Many investigators are of the opinion that the available evidence favors the contention that PbBs as low as 10–15 ug/dl can adversely impact intelligence in children. Others contend that studies reporting such effects have overinterpreted data, used inappropriate statistical approaches, or not properly controlled for potential confounders or covariates of IQ. The earlier experimental approaches to this topic took the form of cross-sectional studies, including clinical studies of children with identified high lead levels, general population studies, and studies of children residing near lead smelters. Outcome measures generally include standardized IQ tests and subscales, as well as other psychometric tests of various functions. While many of the clinical studies suffer deficiencies in adequately controlling for some of the potential confounders and covariates of IQ, when taken together, their results were deemed by the US Environmental Protection Agency to be consistent with lead-induced decrements in IQ, as well as other neuropsychological functions at blood levels of 40 ug/dl and above in children who were otherwise asymptomatic. It has been estimated from these studies that the magnitude of the decrement in full-scale IQ score at PbBs of 50–70 ug/dl is 5 points.

Population studies have compared groups of children from the general population with lower lead exposures to those with higher lead exposures. When a simple comparison of the number of such studies reporting statistically significant effects to those not reporting statistically significant effects is undertaken, the outcome of these studies is mixed. Those reporting positive outcomes indicate that PbBs of 30 ug/dl and possibly less are associated with decrements in IQ scores and other neuropsychological functions, as well as differences in teacher rating scales of classroom behavior and HYPERACTIVITY. In one such study a particularly striking linear relationship between PbBs from 5 to 50 ug/dl and IQ was plotted, with 78 percent of the subjects exhibiting PbBs less than 30 ug/dl. Another such study reported deficits in IQ in school-age children at levels of 10–15 ug/dl and possibly lower without any apparent threshold.

In contrast, other population studies failed to find statistically significant effects of lead exposure, using the same or related measures. A summary of the results of studies undertaken in children residing near smelters has provided the same type of mixed outcome. This general balance between the number of studies reporting positive and negative results constitutes the basis for some investigators' claims for the lack of a convincing case relating lead exposure to IQ.

Others contend, however, that this mixed outcome between studies must be reevaluated when considered in relation to the fact that, even in most of the studies reporting no statistically significant effect, the mean IQ scores for the lead groups were lower than those of controls, and for many of the statistical outcomes, the resulting p values were actually less than 0.10. This consistency in the direction of effect across both "significant" and "non-significant" studies, i.e. the replication of an effect across different conditions in different studies, is a more powerful argument for the relationship between low-level lead exposure and cognitive impairment than is the net change in p values across studies. One must consider how likely it is that such a high proportion of such studies should evidence a similar magnitude and direction of effect across these different conditions. This conclusion was supported by the results of a meta-analysis undertaken using 12 of 24 of these investigations (some studies were excluded for methodological reasons). This meta-analysis provided strong statistical support for the hypothesized relationship between low-level lead exposure and IQ; its outcome was not influenced by the results of any single study included, nor by those which were excluded.

One of the major difficulties inherent in cross-sectional studies is the difficulty in evaluating total lead exposure. Most such studies have had to rely on assumptions about total exposure based on a single PbB. This increases the likelihood of inappropriate dose grouping of individuals and of group overlap in terms of total lead body burden. Prospective studies, going on in Boston, Cincinnati, Cleveland, New Zealand, Australia, and many countries in Europe, were initiated as a response to such problems. These prospective studies have followed longitudinally the neuropsychological progress of children, as well as their lead exposure levels.

Results reported to date from the longitudinal prospective studies provide compelling support for low-level lead-induced impairment in neuropsychological function. These studies indicate changes at PbBs of 10–15 ug/dl in indices of development and intelligence and in parent and teacher ratings of behavior which parallel those noted in the cross-sectional studies. They also suggest that some of the cognitive effects may represent developmental delays, such that by 4–5 years of age, lead-exposed children have achieved performance levels of controls. However, the degree of such compensation may be largely influenced by socioeconomic considerations, since children of lower socioeconomic status show a greater impact of postnatal lead exposure on neuropsychological outcome to begin with and less improvement over time than children from the higher socioeconomic classes.

These positive findings from human prospective studies are supported by the results of numerous studies in experimental animals reporting lead-induced changes in different aspects of cognitive function. Moreover, the PbBs associated with such behavioral effects are strikingly comparable, being less than 15 ug/dl in nonhuman primates and 15–20 ug/dl in rodents. The combined evidence from human prospective studies and the experimental animal literature led the Centers for Disease Control in the US to decrease the designated "safe" PbB to 10 ug/dl for children in 1991.

To date, the underlying neurobiological mechanisms of lead-induced changes in neuropsychological function have not been identified. It is clear that no specific neuropathology occurs to which such effects can be attributed, particularly at the very low levels of lead exposure that are currently associated with cognitive effects. Alterations in several different NEUROTRANSMITTER systems have been suggested as a basis for cognitive impairment, but confirming data have not yet been presented.

ANTIDOTES TO THE NEUROPSYCHOLOGICAL IMPACT OF LEAD EXPOSURE

While it is well known that administration of calcium disodium edatate (CaEDTA) can sometimes prevent the fatality associated with lead poisoning, its efficacy for reversing the neuropsychological effects associated with lower levels of exposure is unclear. Several past studies have reported that treatment with CaEDTA can ameliorate the residual neurological effects ensuing from previous lead poisoning in children. However, these studies have not included adequate control groups for the intervention procedures themselves (i.e. increased attention, hospitaliza-

tion, etc.) to rule out the possibility that the events associated with intervention were responsible for the improvement. This is particularly important, since placebo response rates can be quite high in clinical trials. Further research efforts are clearly warranted in this area.

BIBLIOGRAPHY

Anger, W. K. (1990). Worksite behavioral research: results, sensitive methods, test batteries and the transition from laboratory data to human health. *Neurotoxicology*, *11*, 629–720.

Bellinger, D. (1989). Prenatal/early postnatal exposure to lead and risk of developmental impairment. *Birth Defects*, *25*, 73–97.

Davis, J. M., Otto, D. A., Weil, D. E., & Grant, L. D. (1990). The comparative developmental neurotoxicity of lead in humans and animals. *Neurotoxicology and Teratology*, *12*, 215–29.

Smith, M. A., Grant, L. D., & Sors, A. I. (Eds). (1989). *Lead exposure and child development: An international assessment*. London: Kluwer.

US Environmental Protection Agency. (1986). *Air quality criteria for lead* (4 vols). Research Triangle Park, NC: Office of Health and Environmental Assessment, Environmental Criteria and Assessment Office.

US Environmental Protection Agency. (1989). *Supplement to the 1986 EPA air quality criteria for lead*. Volume I addendum. Washington: Office of Research and Development, Office of Health and Environmental Assessment.

DEBORAH A. CORY-SLECHTA

lemniscal system In somesthesis the distinction between EPICRITIC and PROTOPATHIC INNERVATION is retained in the concept of two distinct systems: the lemniscal and SPINOTHALAMIC systems. In the lemniscal system, cutaneous and subcutaneous receptors connect by relatively large myelinated fibers to the medial lemniscal tract, dorsal columns, and on to the posterior ventral nuclei of the THALAMUS and primary sensory cortex in the postcentral gyrus. This system is considered to be responsible for the discriminative aspects of somesthetic sensitivity. The information provided may be in terms of position, contour, or form, relates to a small defined receptive field, preserves somatotopic representation, and projects contralaterally from receptor to cortex.

LEMs   LEMs (*lateral eye movements*, also referred to as *conjugate lateral eye movements* or *cLEMs*) are consistent lateral deviations of gaze which, it has been proposed, may be related to activation of the cerebral hemisphere contralateral to the direction of deviation of conjugate gaze. LEMs have therefore been suggested as an index of lateralized cerebral activity, either in relation to transient activation or as a more enduring index of cognitive style. Both of these suggestions continue to be the subject of debate.

Lateral eye movements in response to specific questions were first reported by Day during clinical practice (although certain earlier reports were acknowledged). His observation was that the type of question asked influenced whether subjects deflected their gaze to the left or the right, a deviation away from eye contact with the questioner being a natural and well-established phenomenon in social interaction. This observation was subsequently investigated by Bakan, who established the hypothesis that this deviation of gaze during the period of preparing the response to a question is related to hemispheric asymmetry (*see* LATERALIZATION) and that "verbal" questions elicited a rightward deviation in gaze, while "spatial" questions elicited a leftward shift in gaze (Bakan, 1969). In this context, "verbal" questions are those which require the subject to perform mental arithmetic, solve logical puzzles, interpret proverbs, spell, or define the meaning of words. By contrast, "spatial" questions require the subject to visualize objects ("How many edges are there on a cube?" or "How many windows are there in your house?"), manipulate spatial relationships, or undertake musical tasks. Bakan's hypothesis (which related, as might be expected, only to right-handers) was that, as eye movements are controlled by regions of the FRONTAL LOBE, task engagement which leads to activation of one of the hemispheres will have the consequence of generating eye movements in the contralateral direction.

The hypothesis was further developed, and gained greater prominence, through the work of Kinsbourne (1972). Kinsbourne linked the phenomenon of lateral eye movements with his current proposals for an attentional explanation of laterality phenomena, suggesting that the eye movement reflected a shift in the gradient of attention towards the sensory hemispace contralateral to the activated hemisphere. LEMs were proposed as one index of the degree of the attentional shift which accompanied lateral cerebral activation.

A relatively intense period of investigation of LEMs followed these publications. Two things became clear: while the phenomenon could be observed, it was not found in all studies or reliably in all individuals, and various procedural variables influenced the appearance of the phenomenon. The most important procedural observation, which was thought partly to explain the inconsistencies appearing in the literature, was the effect of the location of the questioner (Gur et al., 1975). It was observed that, when subjects were confronted by the experimenter, they tended to move their eyes predominantly in one direction, which might be either left or right, regardless of the content of the question. However, when the experimenter sat behind and out of sight of the subject (centrally, to avoid any lateral bias) the content of the question elicited LEMs in the expected direction (rightward for verbal questions, leftward for spatial questions). Left-handers were also investigated in this study, but were found not to have consistent LEMs, in accord with the hypothesized lesser degree of cerebral lateralization in this group (*see* HANDEDNESS). Kinsbourne, in his earlier study, had incidentally sat behind the subject while presenting the questions, and this procedure became the standard practice in LEM research.

A more recent development has been the use of dark conditions and infra-red eye movement recording. The idea may have been stimulated by the observation of the standard pattern of LEMs in a blind subject, in whom, of course, all external visual influences on ocular-motor activity had been removed, although earlier reports employing relatively dark conditions had failed to obtain the expected effect. Raine, Christie, and Gale (1988) published the first report of LEM recording under dark conditions with infra-red recording, finding an unusually strong effect of verbal questions in generating rightward deviations of gaze, although they failed to find the expected leftward deviations contingent upon spatial questions. They suggest that this failure to observe LEMs following spatial questions might be the result of a reduced level of activation of the right hemisphere, which might be primed by the visual spatial stimulation which naturally occurs under lit conditions.

A very influential review of the literature on LEMs was published by Ehrlichman and Weinberger in 1978. On the basis of the evidence to date, they came to the clear conclusion that, while LEMs may be a reliable and consistent phenomenon (with some qualifications), they do not necessarily relate to hemisphere asymmetry. While they accepted that LEMs might occur under certain conditions and be related in some way to cerebral activity, they rejected the idea that LEMs may be used as some index of generalized lateral cerebral activation, and that the data derived from the study of LEMs may be cited as evidence for or against a hemisphere asymmetry model of lateral eye movements. Nevertheless, LEMs have continued to be employed in laterality research, albeit rather less enthusiastically since Ehrlichman and Weinberger's review, and the rather inconsistent pattern of findings has been upheld. There have, however, been sufficient reports emerging to maintain some association between LEMs and cerebral lateralization.

It is important to distinguish two different ways in which the association between LEMs and neuropsychological laterality has been discussed. The first is as an indicator of transient states of hemispheric activation; the second is as a more enduring index of an individual's neuropsychological style and is linked with cognitive style and with HEMISPHERICITY.

The evidence for an association between the transient state of lateral activation which is specifically contingent upon the momentary relative state of the hemispheres as evoked by the content of a question is substantial, if not strong. Having taken account of the appropriate procedural concerns, the phenomenon has been reliably demonstrated in sufficient studies for it to be taken seriously. Moreover, evidence which provides a degree of independent validation has more recently become available. Concurrent measurement of electrophysiological variables employing evoked potentials has linked lateralized components with LEMs, and the effect has also been seen in the ongoing EEG. BLOOD FLOW STUDIES have also been employed to validate the association between cerebral asymmetries and LEMs. Despite certain technical difficulties, these studies provide some independent support for the hypothesis that, under certain conditions, LEMs may reflect the relative activation of one of the lateral cerebral hemispheres.

A related hypothesis has been that LEMs may reflect current emotional state, reflecting lateral cerebral specialization for emotion. Interest in this aspect of neuropsychological organization originates with the report of Schwartz, Davidson, and Maer (1975) that not only the formal content of questions, but emotional states evoked by questions, which also might have a verbal or spatial dimension, could also generate LEMs. The verbal emotional questions were of the type, "Is anger or hate the stronger emotion?" but a typical spatial emotional question was, "When you visualize your father's face, what emotion first strikes you?" Schwartz and colleagues found that verbal emotional questions evoked more rightward LEMs as anticipated, although the converse was not found for spatial emotional questions. Over all questions, more leftward LEMs were produced by emotional questions than the control nonemotional questions, which was interpreted in the light of the hypothesis that there is a degree of right hemisphere cortical specialization for emotional processes. This finding has not been unequivocally supported by later work. A recent reappraisal of this area by MacDonald and Hiscock (1992) found that, while cognitive content affected the incidence of LEMs, emotional content did not do so, although it did affect subjective ratings of imagery. Neither variable, cognitive or emotional content, significantly affected the direction of LEM in any of their studies.

The second way in which LEMs have been used is as an index of more generalized neuropsychological organization as expressed in the concept of hemisphericity. This concept is that individuals tend to rely on modes of processing associated with one of the two hemispheres, that this relates to a predominant cognitive style, and can be observed in the general pattern of LEMs. The evidence for this concept is far less convincing than that for LEMs as a transient indicator of hemispheric activity (as it is for HEMISPHERICITY as a whole). Ehrlichman and Weinberger in their 1978 review were particularly clear in stating that there was no justification at that time for linking LEM patterns with hemisphericity. Beaumont, McManus, and Young (1984) extensively reviewed the concept of hemisphericity, including the use of LEMs as an index of the putative construct, but argued that there was no satisfactory validation for the use of LEMs as an index in the way in which they had been employed and that, in any case, the concept of hemisphericity lacked an adequate foundation. Nothing has appeared since their review fundamentally to change that conclusion. This conclusion is supported by the work of Raine (1991), who recorded LEMs in the standard way, but using infra-red recording in the dark, and also conducted measures of left and right hemisphere functioning. These measures included verbal and nonverbal DICHOTIC LISTENING, and indices derived from subtests of the Wechsler Adult Intelligence Scale. While these may not be the most sensitive tests of general hemispheric laterality, a weak association with the LEM indices might reasonably be expected. No such association was found; the validation measures were unrelated to the LEM laterality indices, although effects of question type on direction of LEM deviation were found. Raine's conclusion, that LEMs cannot provide a valid index of stable individual differences in hemisphere utilization, supports the conclusion reached by earlier work.

LEMs, lateral deviations of gaze contingent upon questions which may be inferred to evoke transient activation of one of the cerebral hemispheres, may under certain conditions provide a behavioral manifestation of that activation, although the phenomenon is not particularly robust or reliable within individuals. The hypothesis that LEMs may provide an index of hemisphericity, associated with stable trait asymmetries in hemisphere functioning, is not supported by the available evidence, and this may be attributable to the possibility that such stable trait asymmetries do not exist.

BIBLIOGRAPHY

Bakan, P. (1969). Hypnotizability, laterality of eye movement and functional brain asymmetry. *Perceptual and Motor Skills*, 28, 927–32.

Beaumont, J. G., Young, A. W., & McManus, I. C. (1984). Hemisphericity: a critical review. *Cognitive Neuropsychology*, 1, 191–212.

Ehrlichman, H., & Weinberger, A. (1978). Lateral eye movements and hemispheric asymmetry: a critical review. *Psychological Bulletin*, 85, 1080–101.

Gur, R. E., Gur, R. C., & Harris, L. J. (1975). Cerebral activation, as measured by subjects' lateral eye movements, is influenced by experimenter location. *Neuropsychologia*, 13, 35–44.

Kinsbourne, M. (1972). Eye and head turning indicates cerebral lateralization. *Science*, 176, 539–41.

MacDonald, B. H., & Hiscock, M. (1992). Direction of lateral eye movements as an index of cognitive mode and emotion: a reappraisal. *Neuropsychologia*, 30, 753–5.

Raine, A. (1991). Are lateral eye-movements a valid index of functional hemispheric asymmetries? *British Journal of Psychology*, 82, 129–35.

Raine, A., Christie, M., & Gale, A. (1988). Relationship of lateral eye movements recorded in the dark to verbal and spatial question types. *Neuropsychologia*, 26, 937–41.

Schwartz, G. E., Davidson, R. J., & Maer, F. (1975). Right hemisphere lateralization for emotion in the human brain: interactions with cognition. *Science*, 190, 286–8.

J. GRAHAM BEAUMONT

Lesch–Nyhan syndrome The Lesch–Nyhan syndrome is a disorder of uric acid metabolism which results in flexor spasms of the trunk, clonic movements, ATHETOSIS, HYPOTONIA, and fits. Self-destructive biting of the lips, fingers, and feet, head-banging, and face-scratching follow and mental retardation may result. The syndrome occurs early in life and in males, being an X-linked recessive trait.

lesion A lesion is any morbid change in the functioning or texture of a bodily organ; in practice, any injury or damage to the nervous system.

leukoencephalopathy Also called leucoencephalopathy or progressive multifocal leucoencephalopathy (PML), leukoencephalopathy is a form of ENCEPHALITIS caused by a papovavirus. It is an occasional complication of defective immune responses in certain chronic diseases, and is a neurological complication of HIV infection. The disease progresses rapidly to dementia and death within weeks or months.

limbic system   Anatomically, the central unifying concept of the limbic system is that, in a modular sense, the limbic cortex and its primary brain-stem connections constitute a functionally integrated system.

It should be noted at the start that there are those who claim that because of the brain's extensive interconnections there is no way to establish the limits of a system and therefore it makes no sense to speak of a "limbic system." The first part of this article will show, however, that such arguments can be disposed of, not only by the use of parsimonious, Occam-type, anatomical definitions, but also by citing comparative electrophysiological, biochemical, and other findings. The rest of the article will then give an overview of the development of different concepts of limbic function, concluding with an emphasis on latest findings pertaining to the role of the limbic system in the experience of affect and emotionally guided behavior. It helps to gain perspective of the diverse clinical and experimental findings if it is kept in mind that the history of the evolution of the limbic system is the history of the evolution of mammals and their family way of life.

DEFINITION

As background for defining the limbic system concept it will be helpful to begin with a short statement about the evolution of the mammalian forebrain. Based on the fossil record and comparative findings, it is inferred that the forebrain of human beings and other advanced mammals has evolved as a triune structure consisting of three neural assemblies that anatomically and chemically reflect ancestral commonalities with reptiles, early mammals, and late mammals (see MacLean, 1990). The neural assembly identified with early mammals is found as an intermediate development interconnected with the reptilian and neomammalian formations.

The term "limbic" derives from a paper published in 1878 by Paul Broca, who used it descriptively to refer to a large convolution surrounding the brain stem of mammals. It was Broca's special contribution to have examined the brains of many different mammals and provided evidence that the system exists as a common denominator of the mammalian brain.

Defining anatomical features   Broca explained his choice of the descriptive word limbic, commenting that, among other reasons, it did not "imply any theory" in regard to function. In proceeding now to define the *limbic system*, I should note that, in introducing this expression in a paper of 1952, I reverted to Broca's use of the word "limbic" for similar descriptive reasons.

Broca pointed out that in gyrencephalic animals the rhinal and limbic fissures ("scissure") mark the boundary between the limbic lobe and the rest of the hemisphere. Elliot Smith's paper of 1902 is a good source for details regarding terms for variations in Broca's *limbique scissure*. In addition to its location in the limbic lobe, the limbic cortex can be distinguished by its cytoarchitecture. A next step in reaching a definition of the limbic system is to characterize the distinctive features of the limbic cortex. By 1900 enough had been learned about the embryology and cytoarchitecture of the cortex to say that the limbic cortex "is phylogenetically and ontogenetically the oldest" (Schäfer, 1900, p. 765). But several years were to elapse before there was a clarification of and terminology for the distinctive features of the limbic cortex other than that of the hippocampus and adjacent structures.

The naming of different types of cortex developed somewhat accidentally. Using Reichert's term "pallium" for referring to the cerebral mantle, Elliot Smith (*1901*) referred to the temporal portion of the limbic lobe as "old pallium" and designated the cortex of the rest of the hemisphere as "neopallium." Much to his disgust (*1910*), the German neurologist Edinger translated the expression *old pallium* as "archipallium," for which archicortex later became a synonym. The neopallium became known as neocortex.

By including the cingulate cortex of the limbic lobe as neopallium, Smith (*1901*) seems to have predisposed others to overlook features indicative of a transitional development between archicortex and neocortex. Even Abbie (*1942*) adhered to the same characterization in elaborating his proposition that the cerebral cortex evolved by "successive waves of circumferential differentiation." It remained, however, for Maximilian Rose of the Vogt School to provide the first convincing clarification of the transitional nature of the cingulate cortex. Based on comparative embryological studies, he concluded that there were three main types of cortex that originated, respectively, from a basic two-, five-, and seven-layer stage (1926). He identified most of the cingulate cortex as originating from the five-layered type to which he gave the Latin name *quinquestratificatus* (*1927*). Regarding such cortex as being transitional between the archicortex and the neocortex, he referred to it as "mesocortex" (1926, p. 129). In the meantime Ariëns Kappers (*1909*) had introduced the term *paleo-cortex*, implying a "younger than" status of the olfactory piriform part of the hippocampal gyrus.

The next observation is so important and so germane to what has been described that it deserves to be set in a paragraph by itself. In his comparative study of 1926 Rose states that the five-layered cortex (*fünfschichtige Rinde*, p. 155) – i.e. his mesocortex – found in the cingulate gyrus *appears for the first time in mammals*.

Without going into detail about the subdivision of the limbic cortex into different cytoarchitectural areas, it may be said as a generalization that it consists of two concentric rings of cortex – an inner ring of archicortex and an outer ring of mesocortex.

Given the evidence that the limbic convolution is a common denominator of the mammalian brain, and given also the features that distinguish its enveloping cortex from that of the neocortex, one can then judge the validity of other anatomical criteria that were used in defining the limbic system. A first requisite for designating it, in a modular sense, as an integrated system was the

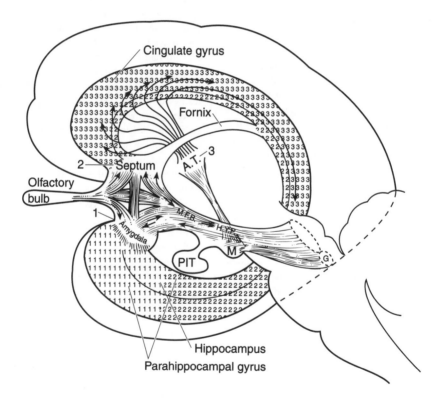

Figure 49 Three main subdivisions of the limbic system. The nuclear groups associated with the amygdalar, septal, and thalamocingulate divisions are respectively labelled with the large numerals, 1, 2, and 3, while the cortical sectors primarily associated with them are overlain with the smaller corresponding numerals. The numerals overlaying archicortical areas are somewhat smaller than those identifying the rest of the limbic cortex. AT, anterior thalamic nuclei; G, dorsal and ventral segmental nuclei of Gudden; HYP, hypothalamus; M, mammillary bodies; MFB, medial forebrain bundle; PIT, pituitary; OLF, olfactory. (After MacLean, 1990.)

inclusion *only* of the limbic-type cortex and its primary connections with the brain stem, including the amygdala and septum as telencephalic structures of the brain stem (MacLean, 1952). A second requisite pertained to the interconnectivity within the limbic lobe itself. The strength of such rules is illustrated by an anatomical study of the cingulate cortex of the macaque monkey by B. A. Vogt et al. (*1987*).

Electrophysiological evidence At this point it should be emphasized that nothing serves so well to illustrate that the limbic cortex and its primary brain stem connections constitute an anatomically and functionally integrated system than to map the propagation of neuronal after-discharges induced in limbic structures by electrical stimulation (Kaada, *1951*; Creutzfeldt, *1955*; MacLean, *1957*). In experiment after experiment, one finds that the propagating nerve impulses stay within the confines of limbic circuitry. Parallel observations have been made during therapeutic neurosurgical procedures (e.g. Feindel & Penfield, *1954*; Pagni, *1963*; Jasper, *1964*).

Biochemical evidence There also exist a number of chemical reasons for regarding the limbic cortex and its immediate connections as part of a system. Perhaps the earliest piece of evidence in regard to the entire lobe was the autoradiographic finding in rats that, following the parenteral injection of ^{35}S-labelled L-methionine, there was a high uptake of the agent in both the archicortex and cingulate mesocortex, which differentiated the limbic cortex from that of the rest of the hemisphere (Flanigan et al., *1957*). With respect to this observation, the recent findings of Levitt and colleagues are of particular interest (Levitt, 1984; Zacco et al. in Vogt & Gabriel, 1993, p. 4). They have identified what they refer to as a "limbic system-associated membrane protein (LAMP)" that is expressed throughout the limbic system. Such a localization of this protein raises the question of what relevance it might have to the long recognized predilection of certain viruses to invade the limbic cortex.

CONCEPTS OF LIMBIC FUNCTION

Because of its characteristic presence in the mammalian brain, Broca (1878, *1879*) was inclined to believe that the limbic lobe subserved animalistic functions, referring to it as a *cerveau brutal*. Moreover, because of the robust connections of the rostral parts of the limbic lobe with the

olfactory apparatus, he suggested that the *entire* convolution was perhaps implicated in olfactory functions. This latter interpretation gained rapid and wide appeal and, by the next decade, several textbooks were referring to the entire lobe as the "rhinencephalon."

Since the sense of smell was regarded as unimportant in human beings, the rhinencephalon received little attention in medical instruction. As one anatomist said as recently as 1957, the rhinencephalon has "probably not contributed greatly to the evolution of the human brain and will . . . not be considered further."

In a review, "Functions of the 'Olfactory Brain,'" which appeared in *1954*, Pribram and Kruger made the point that there was little experimental support for growing interest in the view that the greater part of the limbic lobe was involved in emotion. Their review did not take into account clinical developments providing the best evidence, and indeed the only subjective evidence, that the limbic system is basically involved in the experience and expression of emotional feelings. But they could not have foreseen developments that were to show that the cingulate cortex is involved in forms of behavior that, in an emotional sense, have been hewn in mammalian evolution.

Emotional functions Behavioral manifestations provide our only means of evaluating the subjective state of another individual. Descartes's word emotion serves as a suitable term for the outward expression for what we identify in ourselves and others as emotional feelings. In the realm of subjective experience a person's emotional feelings are referred to as affects. Affects may be qualified as agreeable or disagreeable feelings that "impart subjective information that is instrumental in guiding behavior required for self-preservation and preservation of the species" (MacLean, 1990, p. 425). Given such a definition, then the phenomenology of psychomotor epilepsy that will be considered later indicates that limbic structures are implicated in generating three main forms of affects that may be designated as *basic, specific,* and *general* affects (MacLean, 1990, p. 422 ff.). The *basic affects* apply to gradations of feelings associated with basic bodily needs, such as feelings of hunger and thirst. The *specific affects* are agreeable or disagreeable feelings identified with specific sensory systems. The *general affects* include what we commonly regard as emotional feelings. They are called "general" because they may pertain to individuals, situations, or things. Unlike the basic and specific affects, they do not depend on specific pathways to the sensorium and may occur and persist as the result of mentation. In case histories of psychomotor epilepsy, the words used in descriptions of feelings during the aura represent a virtual thesaurus of basic, specific, and general affects.

Despite the rhinencephalic stamp given to the limbic lobe, a few authors singled out certain limbic structures as possibly having other than olfactory functions. For example, in his Croonian Lectures, Elliot Smith (*1919*) suggested that olfactory structures of the temporal lobe, unlike those of other sensory systems, might provide "an affective tone" combining anticipation and consummation into one experience and thereby seed the germ of memory.

Prior to 1937, however, no author appears to have considered the entire limbic lobe with respect to functions other than olfaction. In that year Papez, at Cornell University, published a paper titled "A Proposed Mechanism of Emotion" (1937). Based on what had recently been learned about the role of the hypothalamus in the expression of emotion, Papez emphasized that structures of the limbic lobe on the medial wall of the hemisphere were the only ones known to have strong hypothalamic connections. He cited case material to support his proposal that "the central emotive process of cortical origin may be . . . conceived as being built up in the hippocampal formation and as being transferred to the mammillary body and thence through the anterior thalamic nuclei to the cortex of the gyrus cinguli. The cortex of the cingulate gyrus," he continued, "may be looked on as the receptive region for the experiencing of emotion as the result of impulses coming from the hypothalamic region, in the same way as the area striata is considered the receptive cortex for photic excitations coming from the retina" (p. 728). The loop formed by these serially connected structures became known as the Papez circuit.

Ten years after the appearance of the Papez paper, Gibbs and others (*1948*) published an article that in retrospect must be considered a landmark in the history of neurology and the knowledge of the cerebral substrate of emotion. They drew attention to an ictal condition called psychomotor epilepsy in which there may be no

convulsion, but during which the patient experiences a variety of emotional feelings, followed by amnesia and automatisms. With scalp electrodes they found that in most cases the epileptogenic disturbance appeared to involve the anterior temporal region. That same year the present author's own research required the recording of electrical activity at the base of the brain. Using an improved type of nasopharyngeal electrode and newly devised tympanic electrodes, Arellano and I recorded both the standard and basal electroencephalogram (EEG) in a group of patients with psychomotor symptoms, but no localizing signs in previous EEGs (MacLean & Arellano, *1950*). In recordings during light sleep (as recommended by Gibbs et al.) the majority of these cases showed spiking activity with maximum amplitude of the spike in recordings from one or the other nasopharyngeal leads. Because the nasopharyngeal electrode was the one nearest the medial aspect of the temporal lobe, it was suggested that the focus of the disturbance might be in the hippocampal formation.

Since the hippocampal formation was considered part of the olfactory system, how was one to explain the fact that the symptoms of psychomotor epilepsy included not only a wide range of emotional feelings with viscerosomatic manifestations, but also that these symptoms involved the visual, auditory, and somesthetic systems? It was then that I discovered the Papez paper and had the good fortune to visit him with the purpose of asking if he could provide an anatomic answer to these questions. In the human brain he pointed out cortical association pathways that could potentially connect visual, auditory, and somatic neocortical areas with the parahippocampal gyrus, which in turn connects with the hippocampus. Later our neuronographic studies in the monkey (Pribram & MacLean, *1953*) offered experimental support for such inputs to the hippocampal gyrus, and subsequent neuroanatomical studies gave confirmation to such stepwise connections (e.g. Jones & Powell, *1970*; Van Hoesen & Pandya, *1975*). Of greater interest, our recordings from single nerve units in squirrel monkeys and our anatomical studies provided evidence of more direct connections via the brain stem, not only for these modalities but also for interoceptive systems (see MacLean, 1990, for a detailed summary).

After visiting Papez, I wrote a paper citing new

experimental and clinical evidence in support of his theory of emotion (1949). Pointing out the possible connections of the visual, auditory, and somatic systems with the hippocampal formation, together with inputs from other extero- and interoceptive systems, I noted that there would be the possibility "for bringing into association not only oral ... sensations, but also impressions from the sex organs, body wall, eye, and ear." The thrust of the article was that this part of the limbic lobe derives information in terms of emotional feelings and "eludes the grasp of the intellect because its animalistic and primitive structure makes it impossible to communicate in verbal terms" (p. 348). "This situation," I suggested, "provides a clue to understanding the difference between what we 'feel' and what we 'know'" (p. 351). In the title of the paper I referred to the limbic lobe as the "visceral brain," as a means of reducing the accent on olfactory functions conveyed by the familiar term rhinencephalon. In its sixteenth-century meaning, visceral applies to strong inward feelings and their associated visceral manifestations. The word, however, proved to be subject to misinterpretation because of its more familiar use in reference solely to the viscera. As a way around this I took advantage of Broca's descriptive word limbic and referred to the limbic cortex and its primary brain-stem connections as *the limbic system*. This explains how the term was introduced into the literature (Mac-Lean, 1952).

COMPARATIVE NEUROBEHAVIORAL FINDINGS

As a preface to neurobehavioral studies, it is necessary to say a word about mammalian evolution. More appropriately one might say "directional evolution" because, in the evolution of some 20 orders of extant mammals, the same basic cerebral structures keep cropping up in all of them. In terms of bodily structures, however, there could be no better illustration of directional evolution than the mammal-like reptiles (therapsids) which are believed to be the antecedents of mammals. The fossil record shows that several lines of these animals were approaching the mammalian condition, so that finally the most reliable distinction is the presence in the therapsid jaw joint of two small bones that in mammals become the malleus and incus of the middle ear.

There are no extant reptiles directly in line with the therapsids. Consequently, for our neurobehavior studies we chose lizards because of the therapsid similarities of both their cranial and postcranial skeleton. In comparing lists of basic behavior in lizards and mammals, one finds that there are three kinds conspicuously missing in lizards, and this would apply to reptiles in general. There are three cardinal forms of behavior identified with the evolutionary transition from reptiles to mammals, namely (1) nursing, conjoined with maternal care, (2) audiovocal communication for maintaining maternal–offspring contact, and (3) play. The "separation cry" perhaps ranks as the most primitive and basic mammalian vocalization, serving originally to help assure maternal–offspring contact and then, as a later development, contact with members of an affiliated group.

Contrast this situation with that of lizards. Most lizards lay their eggs and then leave them to hatch on their own. And most lizards do not vocalize, which for the young hatchlings appears life-saving, because if they were to make a separation cry typical of mammals, the chances are that their parents or other adult lizards might seek them out and eat them. The young of the giant Komodo lizards must take to the trees for the first year of life to avoid being cannibalized.

The three cardinal forms of behavior typical of mammals appear to have depended on the progressive evolution of the limbic system.

FUNCTIONS OF THREE SUBDIVISIONS OF THE LIMBIC SYSTEM

On the basis of anatomy and functions, the limbic system can be divided into three main cortico-subcortical subdivisions, with each division consisting of a sector of limbic cortex having connections predominantly with a particular group of nuclei (see Figure 49 and MacLean, 1990, for a review). The cortical sectors predominantly associated with the nuclei of the amygdala and septum respectively comprise the so-called amygdalar and septal divisions.

Amygdalar division With respect to emotional behavior, it is first of all noteworthy that electrical stimulation in commonly used laboratory animals elicits angry or defensive forms of behavior. In addition, stimulation induces searching and sniffing and a wide range of oral responses, including those involved in feeding and alimentation.

As first shown in monkeys by Brown and

Schäfer in *1888* and rediscovered by Klüver and Bucy 50 years later (*1939*), bilateral temporal ablations including the amygdala and hippocampus induce a reverse effect of the above emotional changes seen with stimulation, resulting in a profound apathy marked by a loss of response to fear-inducing situations. Comparable changes have been observed in human beings.

In summary, the amygdalar division is primarily involved in oral-related behavior used in feeding and associated forms of self-preservation.

Septal division In contrast to the amygdalar division, the septal division appears to promote primarily procreative functions. At the most basic level, for example, electrical stimulation of the septum near the midline elicits genital tumescence at regular, short latencies in both male and female squirrel monkeys. Genital erection can also be elicited by stimulation in certain parts of the proximoseptal part of the hippocampus in squirrel monkeys and other laboratory animals. In male cats grooming, pleasure reactions, and other behavior seen in courtship has also been elicited by electrical or cholinergic stimulation of the proximoseptal part of the hippocampus. In summary, the septal division appears to be primarily concerned with primal sexual functions and behavior conducive to procreation. Apropos of the functions of the third subdivision, it should also be noted that there is evidence in rodents of an incipient involvement of the septum in maternal and nesting behavior.

Thalamocingulate division It is the thalamocingulate division that is of primary interest with respect to the evolution of the limbic system and the three forms of family-related behavior. This third limbic subdivision consists of the mesocortex of the cingulate gyrus and its associated thalamic nuclei. Significantly, there is no definite representation of any part of this division in the reptilian brain.

Stamm (*1955*) is the first to have made the important observation that ablations of the cingulate cortex interfere with the various acts of maternal behavior. His experiments were performed on rats and have since been confirmed by Slotnick (*1967*) and others.

We ourselves observed confirmation of their findings on maternal behavior in another kind of experiment which involved making cortical lesions in neonatal hamsters. While waiting for these animals to mature, we observed that the

cingulate cortex is implicated in another constituent of the behavioral triad. Those pups in which the entire neocortex proved to be absent grew and developed normally, manifesting every form of species-typical behavior. But unexpectedly and most notably, those with additional absence of the cingulate cortex failed to develop play behavior at the expected time or thereafter.

The third element of the family-related triad is audiovocal communication for maintaining maternal–offspring contact. The only studies known thus far to have focused on the cerebral representation of the cry have been performed on squirrel monkeys. The results of ablating areas of the medial frontal cortex indicated that a strip of rostral limbic cingulate cortex is necessary for the spontaneous production of the cry in adult monkeys isolated while being tested in a sound-reducing chamber (MacLean & Newman, *1988*).

A psychological condition that is especially painful for mammals is separation. In an evolutionary sense, the possibility suggests itself that the painful aspects of separation are traceable to the fatal consequences of separation of mother and offspring when nursing became a family way of life. In this respect it is notable that the rostral cingulate cortex implicated in the call is innervated by nuclei involved in the perception of pain. It is also relevant that the cingulate cortex has a high concentration of opioid receptors and that morphine eliminates the separation cry in monkeys, dogs, and other animals. It is of reciprocal interest that morphine also interferes with maternal behavior.

CLINICAL CONTRIBUTIONS

Crying and laughter Our findings, which implicated the cingulate cortex in the separation cry and in play, made it desirable to review clinical case material in regard to the localization of epileptogenic foci and lesions associated with epileptic crying and laughter, as well as locations where electrical stimulation resulted in these manifestations during neurosurgical intervention. The outcome of the review is too detailed to be described here, but it may be summarized by saying that, both with respect to the somatic manifestations and lacrimation, the structures involved were located along the "Papez circuit," involving the *rostral* hippocampal formation and adjacent amygdala; the mammillary bodies; the anterior thalamus; and the midline frontocingulate cortex (MacLean, 1990, pp. 534–8). Under ictal conditions, just as in everyday life, there may be an alternation of crying and laughter, suggesting that these manifestations have an underlying reciprocal innervation.

Experience of affects The affects provide subjective information instrumental in guiding behavior required for self-preservation and procreation. The study of psychomotor epilepsy provides the best evidence, inclusive of the only subjective evidence that the limbic system plays a basic role in the generation of affects. This evidence was derived from observations made during stimulation and recording of the exposed brain in the course of therapeutic neurosurgical procedures. The pre-eminent contributions in this respect were those of Penfield and Jasper (*1954*) and their colleagues at the Montreal Neurological Institute. With stimulation at the site of an epileptogenic focus in or near limbic structures, it has been possible to reproduce not only the patient's ictal symptoms, but also the subsequent automatism with its associated amnesia (e.g. Feindel & Penfield, *1954*).

Symptoms experienced during the aura include one or more of the *basic*, *specific*, and *general* affects defined above. Since feelings of separation may have been influential in the evolution of affects, it is of interest to cite the symptoms of a patient who experienced the basic affect of hunger that may accompany grief reactions. A factory worker described his aura to me as beginning with a feeling of sadness and wanting to cry. This was followed by a feeling of hunger and welling up of tears.

The experienced specific affects illustrate the capacity of limbic mechanisms to affect and modulate the intensity and amplitude of feelings and perceptions: sounds may seem to grow unusually loud or faint; as in delirium, an extremity may seem swollen to large proportions; things seen may seem near or far.

The general affects represent what are usually regarded as emotional feelings. At the beginning of an epileptic storm, the patient's mind may light up with feelings that in one case or another range all the way from intense fear or terror to ecstasy. The general affects fall into six main categories including (1) feelings of desire; (2) fearful feelings; (3) angry feelings; (4) dejected feelings; (5) gratulant feelings, and (6) feelings of affection. As noted later, gratulant affects include feelings that

have profound implications for epistemology. A patient may have eureka-type feelings of discovery; feelings of revelation; feelings of enhanced reality; feelings of conviction that what is being experienced is of the utmost importance, that it's the absolute truth, that it's what the world is all about. *Significantly, these feelings are free-floating, being unattached to any particular thing, situation, or idea*, and hence without regard for truth or falsity.

Finally, two indeterminate types of affects should be noted: (1) feelings of familiarity or strangeness (sometimes alternating as though by reciprocal innervation) and either one potentially pleasant or unpleasant and (2) affects associated with time and space.

Emotional expression During the automatism subsequent to the aura, the unconscious behavior may be in keeping with the remembered feelings of the aura. Following a horrifying feeling of fear or terror, for example, a patient may run screaming to someone for protection, or, after a feeling of anger, there may be angry vocalization and pugilistic behavior, with the arms flailing somewhat like those of a fighting chimpanzee. An opposite sort of behavior is that of a woman who would walk around her room showing marked affection to anyone present.

Insights into ontology and memory After the aura the patient develops automatic behavior that ranges from simple to very complex automatisms. Throughout that entire period there is absolutely no memory for anything that happened. Nevertheless, as illustrated by Jackson's famous case Z, the patient may be capable of skilled performance and cognition dependent on a functioning neocortex. Case Z was that of a physician who, during a limbic seizure found to result from a small cavity at the junction of the amygdala and hippocampus, examined a patient, and wrote a correct diagnosis and prescription – all with no memory of it afterwards (Jackson & Colman, *1898*).

Clinically, it has been recognized since 1900 (Bechterew) that bilateral damage or destruction of the hippocampus results in a loss of memory of ongoing experience (anterograde amnesia). Why the loss of memory for what happens during the automatism? I have suggested that a bilateral propagation of a limbic seizure amounts to a temporary "functional ablation" of the hippocampus and related structures involved in the registration and retention of ongoing experience. But still, why the loss of memory? This question calls for a further answer as to what accounts for a sense of individuality. Without a sense of personal identity there is, so to speak, no place to deposit a memory. Through introspection there results the realization that a sense of personal identity depends upon an integration of externally and internally derived experience. Whereas the neocortex receives its information primarily from the exteroceptive systems (somatic, auditory, visual), microelectrode studies have shown that the limbic cortex receives information not only from these systems but also from the olfactory, gustatory, and visceroceptive systems. It should be emphasized that all these systems converge on the hippocampus. Because of the regularity with which they found that automatisms and amnesia occurred with after-discharges triggered by medial temporal stimulation, Feindel and Penfield (*1954*) were of the opinion that the hippocampal formation and amygdala are requisite for the registration of memories.

CONCLUSION

Mention was made of the profound epistemic implications of the role of the limbic system in generating the affective feelings of conviction that we attach to our beliefs, regardless of whether they are true or false. It is one thing to have this primitive, untutored mind to assure us of the authenticity of food or mate, but how can we rely on its judgments for conviction in the truth of our ideas, concepts, and theories? The resulting unresolvable uncertainty is compounded by the artifactual consequences of the logical functions of the neocortex. These are the artifacts owing to the unavoidable self-reference that cannot be purged from logical systems of any complexity. As one writer has commented, the situation amounts to an endless hall of mirrors of self-reflection.

There is at least one compensation for the apparent inability of ever achieving certainty of knowledge, and this is the satisfaction that can be derived from human values for which there are no measures. For one such value, our eyes may look up to the evolving frontal neocortex that is strongly interconnected with the thalamocingulate division inferred to be involved in family-related behavior. It might be presumed that its tie-in with parental concerns may have favored the development of the capacity for altruistic and empathic feelings, and more than that, to imagine such concerns as working in future situations.

Remarkably, the reaches of the human brain have made it possible for the projection of concerns to generalize not only to one's own progeny, but also to the worldwide human family. More remarkably still, for the first time in the known history of biology, we are witnessing the evolution of beings with a concern for the future suffering and dying of all living things.

BIBLIOGRAPHY

Note All citations with italicized dates can be found in the author's book: *The Triune Brain in Evolution* (New York: Plenum Press, 1990).

Broca, P. (1878). Anatomie comparée des circonvolutions cérébrales. Le grand lobe limbique et la scissure limbique dans la série des mammifères. *Revue d'Anthropologie*, 1 Sér. *2*, 385–498.

Levitt, P. (1984). A monoclonal antibody to limbic system neurons. *Science*, *223*, 299–301.

MacLean, P. D. (1949). Psychosomatic disease and the "visceral brain." Recent developments bearing on the Papez theory of emotion. *Psychosomatic Medicine*, *11*, 338–53.

MacLean, P. D. (1952). Some psychiatric implications of physiological studies on frontotemporal portion of limbic system (visceral brain). *Electroencephalography and Clinical Neurophysiology*, *4*, 407–18.

MacLean, P. D. (1990). *The triune brain in evolution: Role in paleocerebral functions*. New York: Plenum Press.

Papez, J. W. (1937). A proposed mechanism of emotion. *Archives of Neurology and Psychiatry*, *38*, 725–43.

Rose, M. (1926). Über das histogenetische Prinzip der Einteilung der Grosshirnrinde. *Journal für Psychologie und Neurologie*, *132*, 97–160.

Schäfer, E. A. (1900). The cerebral cortex. In E. A. Schäfer (Ed.), *Text-book of physiology*, Vol. 2, (pp. 1–1365). Edinburgh and London: Young J. Pentland.

Vogt, B. A., & Gabriel, M. (Eds). (1993). *Neurobiology of the cingulate cortex and limbic thalamus*. Boston: Birkäuser.

PAUL D. MACLEAN

lingual gyrus The lingual gyrus is situated in the medial cortex of the occipital lobe, close to the calcarine fissure. Functionally it contains primary visual cortex, but it has also been associated with facial AGNOSIA in the case of bilateral lesions.

lissencephaly An abnormality of brain development in which the brain fails to form sulci and gyri is termed lissencephaly. The brain therefore lacks its normal corrugated appearance and remains like that of a 12-week embryo (*see* AGYRIA).

lobectomy (lobotomy) Lobotomy is the name given to the surgical procedure carried out on the brain with the intention of relieving severe psychiatric conditions. Although there is evidence that relatively primitive people carried out procedures involving the opening of the skull in the presumed hope of affecting some behavior change it was only in the 1930s, with the work of the neurosurgeons Egas Moniz and Pedro Almeida Lima, that interest in the procedure became widespread. After observing the behavior changes in monkeys following lesioning of the frontal lobes, Moniz came to believe that a similar operation might produce beneficial changes in humans displaying aberrant behaviors resulting from psychiatric disorders.

The operation they devised involved burring two holes in the front of the skull, inserting a steel blade (leucotome), and cutting the fibers connecting the frontal lobe to the subcortical areas. The procedure was taken up and modifications made by Freeman and Watts in the United States. Their procedure was adopted as the "standard leucotomy" operation. American writers prefer the term lobotomy to describe the procedure, English writers on the other hand prefer the term leucotomy. The two terms can largely be used synonymously.

The standard leucotomy operation was used to treat a range of psychiatric disorders ranging from depression and anxiety to schizophrenia. Later modifications of the procedure were devised, such as that developed by Scoville in 1948. His procedure involved the isolated cutting of the medial fibers connecting the frontal lobes to the thalamus. All the methods, though, were attempts at disconnecting the frontal lobes from subcortical areas. Some estimates put the number of such operations carried out worldwide as high as 100,000. The standard or modified versions of the procedure were carried out up until the late 1970s.

It soon became apparent that some of the patients experienced undesirable aftereffects, such as emotional flattening, as well as receiving little relief from the psychiatric problems for which the operation was carried out. Studies highlighting these problems, plus the introduction of antipsychotic medications in the 1950s, led to a gradual reduction in the number of such operations performed.

The term lobectomy as opposed to lobotomy (leucotomy) refers to a surgical procedure that involves the actual removal of brain tissue as opposed to the severing of connections. This procedure is most commonly carried out to tackle intractable seizures arising in the temporal lobe. Removal of the temporal lobe, particularly if the lesion is well circumscribed, can frequently result in a significant reduction in seizure activity.

MARCUS J. C. ROGERS

localization The relationship of function to structure is the subject of localization in physiology and neuropsychology. The fundamental issues of localization may be formulated as follows: (1) What is a neurophysiological or a neuropsychological function? (2) What are the anatomical structures necessary to carry out such a function in the normal brain? (3) What does a certain area of the brain do? (4) What other structures can compensate if certain parts of the brain are damaged? The major confounding issue in localization is that, even though the lesion can be accurately located, the function that is examined after injury does not reflect the simple equation of the normal function missing, but it represents a new state of reorganization of the brain. Jackson's warning, therefore, that only lesions and not functions can be localized must remain in the foreground of all localization studies. This, of course, does not mean that localizing lesions does not provide information about function. It has to be studied, however, with a great deal of sophistication in function analysis, biology, and localization technology, some of which will be discussed below.

The principle of "sensorium commune," developed in the nineteenth century, was based on the hypothesis that all functions in the brain are

459

connected in some fashion. This gave rise to a unitary theory of brain function, with subsequent modifications such as the equipotentiality theory of Lashley and even the denial of the need to study localization mainly by behaviorists or the mentalists who were satisfied to examine mental processes independently from brain activity. Some modern information processing and connectionistic models also consider the localization of lesions largely irrelevant. Nevertheless, the structuralists and localizationists continued to explore brain–behavior relationships within their technological limitations.

Nineteenth-century anatomists who described the regular patterns of gyri and their interconnections began to assign function to certain structures. At times this was related to empirical evidence, at other times to speculation, which led to PHRENOLOGY. New techniques of preserving the brain, discovering the cellular constituents (Cajal and Golgi), and developing the axonal and myelin stains (Weigert) provided a scientific base for exploring brain structure. The most important support for localization of function came from physiologists who observed the close relationship of stimulated cortical points and movements in animals (Fritsch and Hitzig, Goltz), the occipital cortex and vision (Munk), language and the perisylvian brain region (Broca, Wernicke), and clinicians studying the long tracts, sensorimotor function, and spinal disorders (Romberg, Charcot). These investigators opened a vast discipline of clinicoanatomical correlations which from the beginning and for the first 50 years relied almost entirely on autopsy. The discovery of X-ray VENTRICULOGRAPHY (Dandy) and ANGIO-GRAPHY (Moniz) supported in vivo localization, particularly of tumors and malformations in the nervous system. Animal studies that included lesions, as well as electrical stimulation, the development of the tracing methods of neuronal degeneration to study connectivity, and the recent development of radioactive tracers that allow functional analyses, all contributed to the study of human localization in parallel. The recent development of non-invasive neuroimaging methods enhanced in vivo localization of lesions exponentially. New sophistication in experimental techniques and new functional methods of localization represent the third major wave in technology that is expanding our knowledge of brain function.

ARE FUNCTIONS LOCALIZABLE?

The extent to which function is localizable is quite variable. The primary somatosensory and motor areas and the cortical areas for special senses, such as auditory and visual processing, have the greatest anatomical and structural correlations. A great number of psychological functions, such as planning, judgment, social adaptability, and general intelligence, have relatively widespread cortical localization, although frontal lobes are considered important in mediating some of these "executive" functions. Language and memory represent more intermediately localizable functions, as language networks are clearly related to perisylvian cortex on the left side and memory acquisition and retrieval are related to the limbic structures. Long-term memory storage, on the other hand, remains a most complex and widespread function that is dependent on context-related activation through multiple modalities and convergent, overlapping, networks throughout the neocortex.

Some of the physiological and anatomical correlations, such as the association of visual feature analysis with specific columnar organization in the visual cortex, carry functional localization to a cellular level (Hubel & Wiesel, 1968). However, much of the actual matching of cortical physiology with function remains controversial, albeit still an actively investigated area. Even the localization of primary motor functions in the precentral gyrus area has uncertainties regarding the functional units that are localizable. Instead of single muscle, movements as a whole seem to be represented. Even though some of the physiological experiments suggest a columnar organization for certain sensory functions in the brain, lesions were less successful in reproducing a specific functional loss that could be related to such an organization. Physiological maps in the cortex are not fixed representations; some recent work indicates a great deal of plasticity. Representation in the cortex is dynamic, changes with time, concurrent activity, context, and general alerting, attentional mechanisms. The diffuse nature of thalamocortical activation systems, the extraordinary degree of interconnectivity of some of the cortical areas, and the multiple areas that are functionally activated during the performance of a circumscribed psychological task suggest widely distributed processing even for relatively "simple" psychological function. Despite the changeability and plasticity of cortical organization, certain cortical modules subserving function appear to be well established, even though they are as yet only physiological realities. There is still a significant gap between connecting physiological phenomena to psychological function, let alone to lesion localization. The gap between lesions and normal function needs to be bridged in many areas, using divergent technology and accounting for the dynamic aspects of compensation and PLASTICITY after lesions.

WHAT IS FUNCTION? THE INTEGRATION OF BEHAVIOR

Physiologists, psychologists, and clinicians have different concepts about the same behavior and the definition of what constitutes a function is often arbitrary. In many instances, complex alternative theories are offered as to how function should be interpreted. Fractionation or reduction of complex behavior to its components on a theoretical basis is fraught with the hazard of losing the meaning and biological significance of the organism. Some psychological concepts, based on information processing theory, may not be appropriate to describe actual brain function or physiological connectivity. Anatomy and physiology, however, do not alone even provide the questions, let alone the answers about behavior.

The analysis of behavior after a lesion should be supplemented by studies in normals to corroborate conclusions about function. A detailed analysis of functions is necessary to understand the complex way a lesion may affect function, but even then there is no guarantee that lesion localization will provide the correct conclusions. The behavior observed after a lesion may not be analyzable in terms of normal function but, on the other hand, the functional analysis of normal cognitive systems may not provide enough background to test damaged or reorganized functions in patients. These discrepancies often prevent any direct conclusion being made about normal mechanisms based on pathological observations, therefore a great deal of caution is needed in the interpretation of pathological behavior as a model of brain function. At the same time, theoretical constructs based on normative data are insufficient by themselves to explain behavior after lesions. Nevertheless, the integration of the two types of modelling will probably be more successful in providing answers than either of them alone.

THE MEASUREMENT OF BEHAVIOR: TAXONOMIC ISSUES

The accurate, detailed measurement of a deficit is essential for meaningful localization. Unfortunately, much of the older clinicopathological literature is handicapped by rudimentary descriptions of the psychological or clinical deficits. Large collections of autopsied cases are difficult to analyze because of the lack of standardized examination or the uneven or scanty description. Some of the terminology covers different and even conflicting clinical pictures. When these are lumped together, localization will fail to produce consistent results. On the other hand, when extensive, individually designed testing is used in single case reports it becomes difficult to replicate it. The lack of standardized examination prevents meaningful comparison of individual cases. Standardized, practical, and consistently used tests are important in localization studies. Without reliable, relevant, and standardized measures of deficit, it is impossible to establish a reliable taxonomy, and without such a taxonomy, localization can be misleading. The analytical examination of single cases may represent isolated behavior and it is difficult to generalize from them. Often the conclusions are idiosyncratic and cannot be statistically evaluated, although single-case statistics have been developed. The syndrome approach represents reproducible, albeit complex, behavior, and some syndromes are difficult to define. More successful clinicopathological correlations have been done on complex syndromes, because they involve a network of functions that is related to a definable anatomical structure. More fractionated or isolated phenomena are difficult to localize. For example, word retrieval, a basic and common language function, is part of many other language behaviors and probably depends on a widespread network, proceeding from the prelinguistic notion on to semantic associations, assembly of phonology, and syntax, and elicitation of motor response. Such a function is less likely to be localizable than a syndrome that is defined by the impairment of several complex functions.

Definitions and taxonomy of behavior are crucial steps in localization. Many of the controversies are related to loosely applied terminology describing different behaviors. Sometimes the opposite error occurs and similar behaviors are grouped or classified differently. When the phenomenon is poorly defined and only described qualitatively it becomes difficult to replicate it. Nevertheless, there is a great reluctance to use standardized examination because of the restrictions and rigidity that it imposes on data collection. Complex syndromes are difficult to define and when attempts are made to apply a numerical taxonomy to behavior there is often a great deal of controversy about just where the line should be drawn. On the other hand, if only typical patients are examined for localization, a high proportion of unclassifiable patients detracts from the validity of the generalization. The choice of what is considered typical behavior may be selective or biased. Nevertheless, as long as behavioral criteria are clearly defined and standardized measurements are used, groups can be compared with reasonable efficiency. Single cases that are examined in great detail functionally complement this effort and the two methods used together in localization can be more productive.

BIOLOGICAL ISSUES

Biological differences between lesions and individuals who sustained these lesions will produce a significant variation in the extent of the deficit. Sudden removal of large areas of the brain due to ischemic lesions is quite different from a slowly growing tumor. The shock effect of a sudden deprivation of connected structures is called "diaschisis" (von Monakow, 1914) and the disappearance of this inhibitory effect on previously normal functioning tissue may account for some of the recovery of deficit. Rapidly expanding tumors produce different distant effects by virtue of interference with vascular supply, edema, and general increased intracranial pressure. In studies including different etiologies, lesions of the same size and even location will produce different deficits. Variation may also occur in the opposite direction. Different etiologies will produce the same deficit but with different localization, for example, the amnestic syndrome could be produced by dorsolateral thalamic or hippocampal lesions, or transcortical sensory aphasia may appear with a stroke in the posterior cerebral artery distribution or with diffuse cortical degeneration due to Alzheimer's disease. Therefore the quality of studies depends on how strictly the etiology of the lesions is controlled for.

TIME FROM ONSET

Functional alteration after lesions is often dynamic, changing with time. The evolution of deficits after a lesion also depends on the etiology. If localization is done on the basis of an early deficit following a stroke or trauma, then some of the findings may be related to edema, cellular reaction, or transient recoverable ischemia. If such cases are compared to a chronically established deficit then conflicting conclusions will be reached (Kertesz, 1979). The chronic deficit is influenced by the compensatory changes of the brain during recovery, usually including neighboring areas or homologous areas in the contralateral hemispheres. All efforts of localization have to pay careful attention to the time from the onset, because the recovery that occurs after stroke and trauma is substantial. Deterioration, on the other hand, may be observed with tumors or in neurodegenerative disease.

THE AGE OF THE ORGANISM

A major difference in the effect of a lesion is related to the age of the organism. In ablation experiments younger animals recover from cerebral damage to a greater extent. This is called the Kennard effect after a series of lesion experiments on infant animals by Margaret Kennard (1941). Children show a great deal more plasticity after lesions, even after hemispherectomy. For instance, prepubertal lesions produce only transient loss of language as a rule. This suggests a possibility of hormonal influence on plasticity. The so-called critical period of language acquisition coincides with the period of more rapid recovery. Others assume that the evolution of brain specification continues throughout the life span and even aging has an important effect on biological reorganization of cerebral function.

SEX HANDEDNESS AND INDIVIDUALITY

Sex differences have also been studied, although the supposedly more bilateral organization of language in women has not been substantiated reliably. Similarly, left-handers were assumed to have more bilateral representation. Although left-handers show some biological and psychological differences, this is still the subject of debate. Language lateralization has been examined through INTRACAROTID SODIUM AMYTAL infusion (the Wada test) and shown to be relatively independent of handedness. Approximately 5 percent of the subjects have bilateral language areas, 4 percent have language lateralization on the right, and the remainder are on the left. Lesion localization and sodium amytal injection evidence also indicates that even sign language and pictographic languages are lateralized in the left hemisphere in the majority of individuals. Anatomical differences may underlie some of the functional differences of the effects of lesions. The complexity of human cortex allows for a great deal of individual variation. Certain anatomical asymmetries between the left and right hemispheres have been explored in some detail, and some sex and handedness differences have been observed which could be the basis of variability in localization.

DISTRIBUTED NETWORKS

It has been recognized throughout the years that the same function can be represented by several areas in the brain and this is variously conceptualized as a redundancy of functional organization or hierarchical representation in functionally interconnected networks. The idea that completely unrelated structures in the nervous system can take over function is called "vicarious functioning." Although this cannot be disproved, there is little, if any, evidence for it. Most neuroscientists have favored certain principles of the network functioning of interconnected areas as a model of function for the brain: (a) a single function may be represented at several sites which are interconnected to form a network; (b) this representation is dynamic and to a certain limit changeable, according to the conditions of elicitation or alterations in the physiology of the network; (c) each cortical area contains the neural substrate for several distinct functions and may belong to several networks, therefore a lesion is likely to produce multiple deficits; (d) persisting impairment usually requires that a large portion of the network is damaged; (e) the same function may be impaired as a result of damage in different areas, each of which has some relationship to the network.

These principles are usually sufficient to explain the variability of findings in lesion localization studies and they also pertain to physiological stimulation or functional activation. Experiments on animals have the advantage of controlling the lesion size and location, in addition to other factors. This is not available to the same extent to neuropsychologists and clinicians, but complex behaviors after lesions that are unique to humans can be explored by in vivo localization techniques. The biological implications of human pathology need to be considered in their own right. The complexity of human behavior is matched only by the complexity of the human brain. When attempting to correlate functional changes with anatomy, alternative ways of explaining phenomena should be explored carefully. For instance, such anatomical issues as whether the target organ is damaged or whether only passing fibers are disconnected by lesions provide alternative interpretation in localization. In the remaining sections we shall examine the various methods of localization available at this time.

METHODS

Neuropathology and neuroanatomy

The clinicoanatomical correlation remains the basic method of localization, but often it can only be carried out after a significant amount of time has passed between the detailed functional examination and the availability of the brain at autopsy. By then, age and intercurrent illness may have altered the correlation beyond usefulness. This time interval and the lack of availability of the brain, in many instances where detailed examination has been accomplished, is a serious drawback. In addition, some well localized and described lesions at autopsy lack the desirable functional description in vivo. However, technical advances in preserving the brain and staining it post-mortem, and developments in cytoarchitectonics and myeloarchitectonics at the turn of the century, allowed pathologists to determine lesion location and extent with considerable accuracy. Axonal tracers of degenerating tracks, such as silver stains and horseradish peroxidase, autoradiography, and more recently transmitter and enzyme tracers, allow the detection of extraordinary detail in post-mortem localization and in animal experiments. The topographical localization of gyral and sulcal structures and fiber tracts, and the accurate determination of the extent of the lesion on post-mortem examination, remain the bench mark for all other localization studies.

Neurosurgery

Neurosurgical removal of tumors and the resection of epileptogenic scars have been used in localization extensively. Benign tumors tend to compress the brain in an insidious fashion and there is often a great deal of compensation for a slowly increasing lesion. This may, in fact, result in false negative conclusions concerning the role of certain areas of the brain. On the other hand, malignant tumors often infiltrate the brain tissue outside the area described at surgery, and their distant effect, related to edema and vascular interference, reaches far beyond the actual tissue removed. Epilepsy surgery may also have false negative effects because it is often performed on damaged brain which may not be fully functional and other parts of the brain may already have taken over the function of the removed area. Therefore the post-operative deficit could be less than that in a normal brain caused by a lesion in the same location.

Cortical stimulation

Cortical stimulation during neurosurgery has contributed interesting localizing information that is somewhat different from lesion removal. Some recent studies found that function is organized in a mosaic pattern. A few millimeters in the electrode placement made a great deal of difference in what functional alterations could be elicited. For instance, anomia in one language in a bilingual individual could only be produced by stimulating one site, and not in the immediate vicinity of where it was elicited in the other language. Some of this variability was attributed to individual differences in cerebral organization. The essential areas that would interrupt, for instance, naming would only be 2.5 cm^2 or less in most of the subjects. It was also suggested that language was organized concentrically around the Sylvian fissure rather than in a traditional anterior posterior fashion. One has to consider, however, the differences between stimulation of cortical points and the effect of large lesions. Cortical stimulation is usually done over limited exposures during epilepsy surgery, but recently subdural electrodes placed in ambulant patients have been used with success to obtain functional localization. The technique is complex and restricted to a few centers. It should also be remembered that although only small areas are stimulated at any particular point, they represent a group of cells (possibly a column) that are connected to other areas, therefore function may not be "located" at the site of stimulation only. This is the same caveat that was mentioned for lesions.

Neurophysiology

In vivo neurophysiological investigations include ELECTROENCEPHALOGRAPHY and event-related potentials. These are non-invasive methods that investigate "on-line" cerebral processing as it is actually taking place. There is a time restriction on the stimulus, which is usually very short and has to have a definite onset, duration, and off-set to connect with an evoked cerebral event. The actual localization is relatively poor, compared to other methods. EVOKED POTENTIALS are usually recorded over a large area of the scalp and the brain. Nevertheless, various cerebral maps have been constructed which are related to functional localization.

X-ray computerized tomography (CT)

Plain X-rays of the head only show bony structures, although even these may have indirect localizing value. Ventriculography is of only historical interest, and angiography is used mainly to identify vascular disease. The invasive nature of these tests precluded their widespread use for other than clinical indications. It was not until the introduction of radioisotope scans and computerized tomography (CT) that a significant break-through in the in vivo imaging of the nervous system was achieved. Strokes and tumors can be localized by these methods with a degree of reliability and practical availability that has truly revolutionized localization studies. The CT scan has become a widespread clinical tool; it takes relatively little time and there is no discomfort to the patient. The extent of strokes, hemorrhages, and tumors is reliably determined, although the exact anatomical localization is not as accurate as MAGNETIC RESONANCE IMAGING (MRI). Early strokes may be missed and a negative CT in the acute stages of stroke may be a source of error in CT localization studies. Most CT localization studies have transferred the lesions on the scans to a template of an idealized brain slice from an anatomical atlas. Much of the source of the variance is related to the angle of the CT scan slices, which have to be matched to the template. The better CT atlases provide anatomical examples at several CT angles. The image can be transferred free-hand, which requires that the operator uses experience, and the landmarks that are available in each given case to adapt the actual lesion seen to the idealized template. Various other methodologies, such as x/y plotting, measuring lesion contour against the contour of the surrounding brain, using a grid, or using a photographic enlarger with a predetermined ratio of enlargement that produces life-size images for tracing, have been used. Whatever the method, as long as it is consistently applied, it provides a fairly accurate estimation of the lesion size and lesion location. Further improvement can be achieved by three-dimensional reconstruction techniques of the actual image itself, which can be digitized. Three-dimensional reconstruction and rotation is particularly useful in MRI because more anatomical landmarks on the image can be identified. The identification of the various sulci and gyri still requires experience and operator involvement. The direct reconstruction method allows the direct visualization of each individual brain without interposing an idealized template. This method of lesion localization has practical applications in neurosurgery, where accurate preoperative identification of the lesion location is crucial.

Magnetic resonance imaging (MRI)

The amount of anatomical detail that is seen in MRI is truly astonishing and approximates what can be seen on autopsy. Furthermore, there is an ease of obtaining images in the coronal and sagittal sections, in addition to the usual axial ones that are available on CT. There is also less biohazard associated with it than with X-ray techniques, such as CT. The radiofrequency pulse sequences provide a variety of tissue-specific images that are still in evolution. Functional imaging with MRI is becoming a promising investigative tool. First a contrast material injection provided some measure of cerebral blood flow, but recent diffusion and perfusion imaging is capable of detecting changes in cerebral blood flow that are associated with normal function. MRI is better in detecting early stroke and demyelinating disease and, when contrast (gadolinium) is used, tumors.

MRI also has the potential to provide functional information because several parameters are influenced by function, such as changes in proton density, longitudinal and horizontal relaxation times, chemical shifts, magnetic susceptibility, and effects of flow on signal. Positive enhancement with gadolinium reflects a change in the function of the blood–brain barrier similar to contrast enhancement on CT. The signal loss that accompanies the transit of the contrast agent through a region of interest is proportional to the tissue blood volume. Maps of circulation obtained that way are similar to PET studies of blood volume obtained with F18 Fluoro-deoxyglucose and have been used to detect changes in cerebral blood volume induced during task activation paradigms, such as visual stimulation. Even more recently, an approach without contrast agents demonstrated real-time changes in MRI signal in response to functional activation. This method uses the decrease in AV oxygenation difference that accompanies the regional increase in blood flow. A reduction of deoxyhemoglobin concentration produces regional signal intensity enhancement in the area of activation. This way the oxyhemoglobin acts as the body's own contrast agent and allows regional tissue oxygen consumption to be measured. An example of the new types of pulse sequences used for detecting cerebral blood flow is the dynamic FLASH (fast low angle shot). This approach exploits the sensitivity of the gradient echo sequence to the varying concentrations of paramagnetic deoxyhemoglobin in the region of activation. The activation occurs 6 to 9 seconds after the psychophysical stimulus applied. After the stimulation is switched off, the MRI signal returns to basal value in a similar period of time. Furthermore, a decrease in the basal MRI signal was noted in the activated area after 60 to 90 seconds of persistent activation which was considered to be related to an autoregulatory adaptation of increased overall brain activity associated with information processing.

Echo planar imaging is another methodology that can detect task-specific changes in oxygenation. Preliminary MRI studies of brain activation included the visual systems, sensory motor areas, and language processing. Some of the functional activation maps of the visual cortex, for example, have been obtained at spatial resolutions almost two orders of magnitude better than positron emission tomography (PET). These new MRI approaches allow a noninvasive correlation of brain anatomy to function at a high level of spatial resolution and within a brief temporal interval. From the small amount of data available, a remarkable amount of intersubject reproducibility can be seen. Interindividual differences, however, are also detected, reflecting the differences in the anatomy of the cortex investigated. These techniques eliminate the averaging of results and using a geometrically standardized brain as employed with PET data.

Magnetic resonance spectroscopy (MRS) is sensitive to water moleculars (protons), lactate and phosphate compounds, and some amino acids, so could be used for localization of function. Although the chemical specificity is high, the sensitivity and resolution is low, and the relationship to function is at a biochemic level.

PET is a highly complex and expensive technique available at only a few centers, but it provides functional localization in vivo that has contributed a great deal to our knowledge of functional and structural correlations in the brain. Positron labelled metabolites, such as 18F-Deoxy-glucose, required sustained physiological or psychological activity for 20–40 minutes. Recently, the oxygen-15 technique allows briefer observations and repeated measurements in the same subjects and is capable of a temporal resolution of less than a minute. Brain areas selectively activated by a behavior task can be isolated by subtracting a paired control image from the task state, thereby removing areas not recruited by the task (Raichle, 1990). Another methodology applies statistical comparison of areas activated and correlates the degree of activation or decrease in flow. Mapping precision varies with intensity and focality of the task-induced cerebral blood flow change, which in turn is affected by task design.

PET studies have included measurements of cerebral blood flow, oxygen utilization, glucose metabolism, dopamine, opiate, serotonin, acetylcholine, glutamate, and gamma aminobutyric acid, neurotransmitter imaging, and various other pharmacological processes. Even though the resolution power of the PET scanners has been around 1 to 2 cm, recent devices have been built which brought it down to 2.5 mm. Some of these studies suggest that even subtle task differences can result in the recruitment of different cortical areas and that the connection between the areas is a dynamic balance of stimulation and inhibition, the interpretation of which may be quite difficult. Some of the activation studies have shown somewhat unexpected localization, such as semantic processing in the medial frontal regions on a word

association task. Anatomical information from MRI can be combined with functional information on the PET scan. The integration of standard regions of interest on the PET with MRI anatomical templates provides a visual image of the statistically significant changes on activation.

A less expensive measure of functional activation is single photon emission computerized tomography (SPECT), but the resolution is much less than that produced by PET. The correlation with function is less direct using SPECT, but as a technique it is more available and more widely used. SPECT tracers, such as radioactive isotopes of iodine and technetium are combined with lipophilic amines and cross the blood–brain barrier early. Some of them leave the brain slowly and their distribution represents a record of regional cerebral blood flow at the time of injection. Activation has to proceed and coincide with the injection. Imaging can be carried out several hours later without loss of information, and this flexibility is a useful feature in a clinical setting. SPECT is most often used to detect chronic alteration of cerebral blood flow associated with lesions or degenerative disease, rather than in activation studies.

The recent exponential development of imaging modalities heralds an exciting era of an expanding knowledge base in anatomical and structural correlations. Functional imaging may allow us a window on functional reorganization, further closing the gap between function and structure. Localization remains a most powerful tool and a large subject area in the study of neuropsychology.

BIBLIOGRAPHY

Alavi, A., & Hirsch, L. J. (1991). Studies of central nervous system disorders with single photon emission computed tomography and positron emission tomography: evolution of the past two decades. *Seminars in Nuclear Medicine, 21*, 58–81.

Belliveau, J. W., Kennedy, D. N., & McKinstry, (1991). Functional mapping of the human visual cortex by magnetic resonance imaging. *Science, 254*, 716–19.

Hubel, D., & Wiesel, T. (1968). Receptive fields and functional architecture of monkey striate cortex. *Journal of Physiology, 195*, 215–43.

Kennard, M. A. (1936). Age and other factors in motor recovery from precentral lesions in monkeys. *American Journal of Physiology, 115,* 138–46.

Kertesz, A. (1979). *Aphasia and associated disorders: Taxonomy, localization and recovery.* New York: Grune and Stratton.

Kertesz, A. (1983). *Localization in neuropsychology.* New York: Academic Press.

Monakow, C. von (1914). *Die Lokalisation im Grosshirn und der Abbau der Funktionen durch corticale Herde.* Wiesbaden: Gergmann.

Raichle, M. (1990). Exploring the mind with dynamic imaging. *Seminars in Neuroscience, 2,* 307–15.

ANDREW KERTESZ

locked-in syndrome   The locked-in patient is fully aware and conscious yet is unable to make any response. It results from a lesion, such as a vascular or hypoxic lesion of the midbrain or brain stem, which leaves the cortex intact yet interrupts the corticobulbar and spinal pathways so that the patient is unable to move or to speak. Occasionally movement of the eyes or the eyebrows may be preserved and permit the patient to operate a communication device. When this is feasible, it may be possible to demonstrate that normal or even superior intelligence is preserved. Such patients may be very highly dependent, but they may retain the capacity to operate technological aids to assist in overcoming their disabilities. The condition should be clearly distinguished from persistent VEGETATIVE STATE in which cortical function is not preserved.

lumbar puncture   Lumbar puncture permits measurement of the pressure of the CEREBROSPINAL FLUID (CSF) and removal of a sample of CSF. A needle is inserted either above or below the fourth lumbar vertebra while the spine is held flexed, until it enters the subarachnoid space containing the CSF around the spine. Once the needle is inserted, pressure in the CSF may be measured with a manometer, or a sample of CSF withdrawn for examination. A period of headache associated with reduction in CSF pressure following lumbar puncture is common.

M

macrogyria *See* MICROPOLYGYRIA.

macropsia Macropsia is a form of visual illusion or METAMORPHOPSIA in which objects appear to be increased in size. An alternative term occasionally employed is *megalopsia*, implying a more dramatic size increase. The illusion is frequent among the metamorphopsias and may be, but is not invariably, associated with a sense of being nearer to the object. It may involve selected objects in the visual array, and occasionally selected parts within the object. As with other metamorphopsias, it may be an epileptic phenomenon, associated with migraine attacks or, when persistent, present in the acute phase following cerebral trauma. An alternative cause is a peripheral ophthalmic disorder, and the problem is generally understood as a disorder of sensorimotor coordination affecting accommodation at either a peripheral or a central level.

macrosomatognosia Macrosomatognosia is parallel to MACROPSIA but in the somesthetic modality. This illusion of bodily transformation consists of a sense of increase of some aspect of the dimensions of the body, which seems heavier, taller, or of greater volume. While the illusion may affect the whole body, it is more commonly limited to a single body part, generally the distal portion of a limb. Macrosomatognosia occurs in association with epileptic events, during migraine attacks, and during the early recovery from cerebral trauma, but it has also been reported as an effect of hallucinogenic drugs, particularly LSD and marijuana. The posterior parietal lobe is implicated in this illusion, with evidence for contralateral representation.

macular sparing *See* STRIATE CORTEX; VISUAL FIELD DEFECTS.

magnetic resonance imaging Magnetic resonance imaging (MRI), also known as nuclear magnetic resonance (NMR), is one of the most recent techniques developed for noninvasive imaging of the brain. It does not require the use of X-rays or the injection of contrast media. It makes use of the magnetic properties of the nuclei of certain atoms and their tendency to resonate in response to rapidly changing magnetic fields.

When nuclei, usually hydrogen nuclei, are placed in a magnetic field they line up in parallel to the direction of that field. When radio frequency pulses are directed at right angles to the magnetic field they change the direction in which the nuclei spin. When the pulse ends the nuclei return to their low-energy state and in the process of this change they emit electrical signals which are picked up and analyzed by computer to reveal the location of the hydrogen atoms. The location of these atoms allows the computer to reconstruct images of the brain that resemble those obtained through computerized axial tomography (CAT).

MRI achieves a better quality image than CAT because of the contrast obtained between different soft-tissue types. This degree of contrast, for instance, reveals a strong differentiation between gray and white matter and can demarcate even quite small structures within the basal ganglia. Pathological changes such as infarctions, tumors, and the plaques of multiple sclerosis can be seen more clearly than with CAT scans. The most significant drawback with this technique is its cost, which still places considerable limits on its use. (*See also* SCAN; LOCALIZATION.)

MARCUS J. C. ROGERS

mammillary bodies The mammillary bodies (occasionally *mamillary*) are an element of the LIMBIC SYSTEM. These are easily seen on the base of the forebrain adjacent to the midline as a pair of spherical protrusions. The mammillary bodies are essentially a part of the HYPOTHALAMUS but they receive input from the HIPPOCAMPUS via the FORNIX and have important projections to the THALAMUS and to the AMYGDALA, which is just lateral and inferior to the mammillary bodies. These bodies play a role in general limbic functions, but are also particularly sensitive to certain toxins and to the effects of malnutrition, with the consequence that they have been linked to the amnesic states associated with chronic alcoholism.

marche à petit pas *Marche à petit pas* is a small-stepped slow and shuffling gait which is most characteristically seen in PARKINSON'S DISEASE but which may also result from bilateral lesions of the frontal white matter such as may occur in PSEUDOBULBAR PALSY or from normal pressure HYDROCEPHALUS.

Marchiafava–Bignami disease Marchiafava–Bignami disease is a rare condition which leads to severe dementia together with motor disorders, dysarthria, epilepsy, and changes in consciousness, in association with the degeneration of central white matter and in particular the CORPUS CALLOSUM. It is considered to result from a deficiency in thiamine and associated nicotinic acid depletion. The disease is more common among drinkers of cheap Italian red wines, although this evidence has probably been overstated. The presence of some dietary, possibly toxic, factor in the causation of the disease is, however, likely.

mass action The principle of mass action is that it is the quantity of cortical tissue destroyed which determines the effects of a lesion rather than its location; mass action is therefore directly related to the theory of *equipotentiality*, which holds that functions are not localized within the cortex.

The principle of mass action is normally associated with Lashley's influential investigations in animals, which showed that the behavioral deficit was determined by the mass of the experimental lesion and not its site. In human neuropsychology, these ideas were most notably taken up by Halstead and co-workers in the late 1940s to explain the effects of lesions in the frontal lobes in relation to his concept of "biological intelligence," where the extent of the lesion appeared more important than its location. The principle of mass action, as opposed to functional localization, is no longer accepted as valid, but is recognized to be a factor which contributes to the effects of lesions within the compromise of regional equipotentiality. The recent development of connectionist approaches to NEUROPSYCHOLOGY has renewed interest in mass action, at least within restricted regions of the brain.

massa intermedia The massa intermedia is a commissure which connects the THALAMUS in one hemisphere to that in the other. It is not present in all individuals, and there is some evidence that the absence of the massa intermedia may be associated with higher intelligence, although the evidence for this is not strong. The massa intermedia may or may not be divided in the COMMISSUROTOMY operation, depending upon the particular procedure employed.

maturation The maturation of cerebral neocortex consists of a series of morphogenetic processes whose characteristics raise two general questions. The first concerns the degree of heterogeneity and specificity of this structure at the cellular and supracellular level, the second is the old and more general problem of the role of innate and environmental factors in the development of neural structures. The following account mainly reflects studies on the primary visual, and, to a lesser extent, somatosensory areas in rodents, cats, and monkeys. Several essential aspects of the neocortex, in particular its cellular composition, and the distribution of the different cell types in layers, appear to be specified early, probably by intrinsic genetic determinants. Other aspects, including the detailed organization of dendritic and axonal arbors, the formation of synaptic patterns, and the cytoarchitectonic and columnar specialization of neocortical areas, are based on interactions between different cell populations and are open to environmental influences.

The maturation, phylogenesis, and pathology of neocortex are interrelated. While certain aspects of neocortical development may directly reflect evolutionary changes, more often development brings to light mechanisms whose regulation in the course of phylogenesis (here referred to as "phylogenetic regulation") may have been crucial for cortical evolution. On the other hand, maladaptive changes in the developmental mechanisms result in specific pathologies of the neocortex.

NEURONAL GENERATION AND MIGRATION: FORMATION OF LAYERS

Neocortical neurons are generated in the proliferative zone on the roof of the cerebral ventricles during a defined period whose duration and relationship with birth change across species. The initial divisions of neuroblasts (till E40 in the monkey) are symmetrical (each progenitor producing two dividing offsprings) and determine the extent of the proliferative layer and indirectly that of the future neocortex (Rakic, 1988). Later divisions are asymmetrical (each progenitor producing one dividing and one migrating offspring) and related to the radial neocortical dimension; in particular, they determine the thickness of the neocortical gray matter (Rakic, 1988) but also the cellular composition of neocortical laminae (see below). The molecular mechanisms controlling the onset and offset of neuronal generation are unknown. They must, however, have been under strong phylogenetic regulation since neocortical volume varies across the mammalian radiation, mainly owing to the tangential increase of neocortex, but also, in particular, at the transition between reptiles and mammals to its radial increase.

From the proliferative zone neurons migrate (Rakic, 1988) along spatially complex palisades of radial glial processes towards the surface of the brain, where they form three juvenile structures: the marginal zone, the cortical plate, and the subplate. The earliest generated neurons occupy the prospective marginal zone, located at the surface of the neocortex and the subplate, near and within the subcortical white matter. The cortical plate grows between the former two (Marin Padilla, 1978) by the progressive arrival of

newly generated neuronal cohorts; neurons generated later occupy more superficial positions (inside-out layering). Layers are conventionally numbered from I to VI along a direction perpendicular to the cortical surface. Layers II to VI originate from the differentiation of the cortical plate, layer I from the marginal zone. Neurons deriving from a common ancestor in the proliferative zone (a clone) come to occupy different neocortical layers and are often, but not always, relatively unscattered in the tangential cortical dimension (Rakic, 1988; Walsh & Cepko, 1992).

The role of neuronal death in the morphogenesis of cerebral neocortex is unclear. Neurons in the marginal zone and in the subplate, however, are to a large extent deleted by neuronal death.

The molecular mechanisms of neuronal migration are incompletely known. In a mutant mouse strain (the reeler) defective neuronal migration results in a scrambled and reversed order (outside-in layering) of neuronal birth dates in the neocortex (Caviness, 1980). The study of this mutant will probably clarify at least some of the mechanisms. Neuronal migration may have been phylogenetically regulated at the transition between reptiles and mammals. In the former, outside-in gradients of neuronal birth dates were found in the pallium, a cortical analogue (Goffinet et al., 1986). Defective migration is found in developmental pathologies of the human brain, characterized by clusters of neurons settling at ectopic positions along the migratory pathways. Neocortical neuronal ectopias may be related to learning disabilities, notably developmental dyslexia.

DIFFERENTIATION OF NEURONAL TYPES

The gray matter of the neocortex consists of a variety of neuronal types that differ in somatic size, dendritic morphology, position, connectivity, neurotransmitter and firing properties. A fundamental taxonomic dichotomy exists between pyramidal and nonpyramidal neurons. The former give rise to long cortico-cortical or cortico-subcortical excitatory projections, although their initial axon collaterals also distribute massively and locally in the neocortex; they are characterized by the presence of an apical dendrite, dendritic spines, and glutamate or aspartate as a neurotransmitter. Nonpyramidal neurons, with a few exceptions, possess nonspinous dendrites and give rise to local intracortical connections; they use gamma-aminobutyric acid as a neurotransmitter and are inhibitory. Several types of pyramidal and nonpyramidal neurons can be distinguished on the basis of their axonal and dendritic patterns and transmitter-related features. One type of nonpyramidal excitatory neuron, the spinous stellate neuron (spinous dendrites, no apical dendrite), is characteristic of layer IV of the sensory areas.

Pyramidal neurons and nonspinous nonpyramidal neurons originate from different clones (Parnavelas et al., 1991). Pyramidal neurons in different layers send their axons to different cortical or subcortical targets. Serial position in a clone (or birth date) determines, in a partially reversible way, the "laminar fate" (McConnell and Karnowski, 1991) of a neuron, that is, in which layer that neuron will settle and to which cortical or subcortical projection its axon will contribute.

The final pattern of dendritic morphology in the neocortex results from both progressive and regressive events. In pyramidal neurons, the apical dendrite grows and ramifies earlier than the basal dendrites. Pyramidal and nonpyramidal neurons, in general, undergo profound re-

organization of their dendritic arbors, including deletion and selective growth of dendritic branches. Deletion of the apical dendrite of early pyramidal-like neurons results in the acquisition of spinous stellate morphology by callosally projecting neurons in area 17 of the cat (Figure 50).

In sensory areas, thalamic afferents are important in determining the orientation of dendritic arbors and experiential factors can regulate the number and distribution of dendritic spines (Greenough & Chang, 1988). In contrast, unlike other neural systems, the role of retrograde "trophic" signals from the targets in the development and maintenance of dendrites of neocortical neurons is unclear. Callosally projecting neurons, for example, attain and maintain normal dendritic arbors in spite of ablation of their normal contralateral target. This target, therefore, may have no role in shaping dendritic arbors of callosally projecting neurons. Alternatively it may have no *specific* role, since callosal neurons send axon collaterals to ipsilateral cortical targets from which they may also receive trophic signals.

TRANSIENT NEURONAL STRUCTURES AND CONNECTIONS

Transient structures are produced during neo-

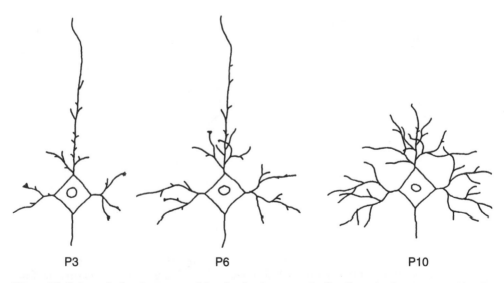

P3 P6 P10

Figure 50 Schematic drawing summarizing the development of callosally projecting neurons with spiny stellate morphology in areas 17 and 18 of the cat. Some neurons in upper layer IV bear a poorly ramified apical dendrite at early stages of development (postnatal days 3 and 6). They give rise to spiny stellate cells before P10, probably through deletion of an apical dendrite. (Vercelli et al., 1992.)

cortical maturation, a phenomenon usually known as developmental exuberance.

Transient circuits are established by a population of neurons in the marginal zone, the Cajal-Retzius cells and their cogenerated neurons in the subplate to which they are presumably synaptically connected (Marin-Padilla, 1978; Shatz et al., 1988). Both neuronal populations largely degenerate during neocortical maturation. Both layer I and the subplate are early sites of high synaptic density. They might provide transient targets for axons from the thalamus, from other parts of the cortex, and from still other brain regions.

In rodents, carnivores, and primates, developing neocortical neurons establish impressive arrays of transient projections to cortical or subcortical sites (references in Innocenti, 1991). These include projections from area 17 and/or 18 to the contralateral hemisphere, from auditory to visual areas, from visual areas and other areas to

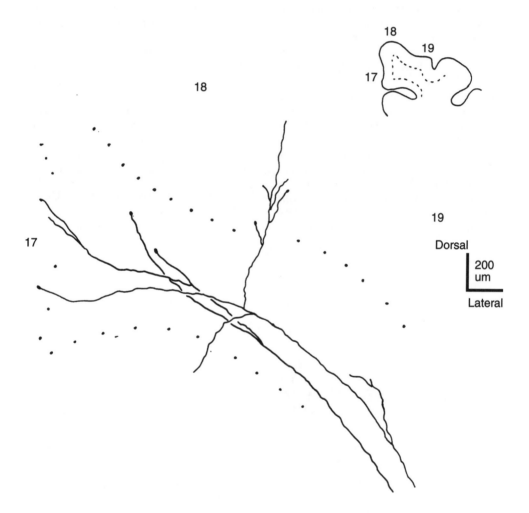

Figure 51 Transient callosal axons labelled by a localized injection of biocytin in the medial part of area 17 in a kitten injected at postnatal day 6.5, killed at postnatal day 8.5. Computer reconstruction from serial section of the region near the border between gray and white matter in areas 17, 18, and 19 (inset). Axons of this kind are usually deleted by the end of the first postnatal month. Notice the widely divergent pattern of axonal branches. The terminating arbor in area 19 is a very rare finding because the transient axons commonly end in layer VI and in the white matter. (Aggoun-Zouaoui & Innocenti, 1994.)

the spinal cord, and intrinsic projections within areas. Much of what is known of the development of neocortical connections comes from studies of interhemispheric (callosal) connections. In cats and rhesus monkeys, the total loss of callosal axons in development amounts to over 70 percent of the axons initially generated. In cats the axonal loss coincides with: (i) a pause in the growth of the corpus callosum; (ii) the fast phase of synaptogenesis in the neocortex (see below); and (iii) the elimination of projections. Most of the axons are eliminated before the onset of myelination. The elimination of transient projections is due to selective deletion of axonal branches and probably to the phagocytic action of cells of the microglial line, but it does not seem to involve neuronal death. In Man, a pause in the growth of the corpus callosum occurs roughly during the last two months of gestation, and extends over the first, and part of the second postnatal month. This pause has similar temporal relations with myelination and synaptogenesis to those found in the cat, therefore it may also correspond to the period of massive elimination of transient callosal projections. The elimination may continue at a slower pace afterwards.

It is unknown whether, morphologically or functionally, the transient axons are all of one kind. Species differences appear to exist in the relative distance spanned by individual transient axons. Axons involved in transient intra-areal or interhemispheric projections from area 17 of the cat form complex arborizations in the white matter and near the subplate, and occasional branches can be found in layer VI, and exceptionally above (Figure 51). Therefore the most likely synaptic target of these transient axons, if any, appears to be neurons in the cortical subplate or dendrites of layer VI neurons. Transient projections were found from the temporal neocortex to limbic structures in maturing rhesus monkeys; they may allow access to memory from levels of visual processing that do not have such access in the adult (Webster et al., 1991).

Several factors decide whether an axon will be maintained or eliminated. They include visual experience (for projections in visual areas), integrity of the sensory periphery and of the target areas, competitive and possibly cooperative interactions with other corticopetal axons, and thyroid hormones. A role for specific, possibly chemical, axon-target recognition mechanisms is suspected.

Developmental exuberance probably played a permissive role in the evolution of cerebral neocortex. Phylogenetic regulation of the selection of juvenile projections may have been instrumental in connecting newly emerged neocortical areas into pre-existing networks and in the establishment of hemispheric specialization. On the other hand, regulation of selection in ontogenesis does not necessarily have adaptive consequences. Developmental pathologies of the human brain, including strabismus, congenital cataract, anophthalmia, early brain injury, microgyria, fetal alcohol syndrome, hypothyroidism, and developmental epilepsy, have been reported to involve deviations from the normal pattern of selection of juvenile projections.

The axons which escape elimination undergo significant structural transformations, including the radial growth of some of them and their myelination, as well as changes in cytoskeletal compartments, notably the microtubules and the neurofilaments. The latter are paralleled by the progressive appearance of adult variants of cytoskeletal proteins, such as the heavy subunit of neurofilaments, and the proteins associated with the microtubule. These changes may correspond to the transition from the juvenile-labile to the adult-stable state of neocortical axons. In the human brain, perinatal massive degeneration of axons of neocortical origin has been described as part of a lethal developmental syndrome including cardiomyopathy, necrotizing myopathy, and cataracts (Lyon et al., 1990). This degeneration may be due to exaggeration of the normal developmental elimination resulting from failure of cortical axons to achieve their adult-stable state.

Synaptogenesis in the neocortex consists in general of a phase during which synapses increase at a fast pace and of a later period of partial elimination (references in Innocenti, 1991). The fast phase of synaptogenesis is cotemporaneous with the elimination of the transient projections which, however, continues into the later phase of synaptic loss. In the rhesus monkey, synaptogenesis appears to be synchronous across areas. This, however, does not exclude the possibility of important, profound, developmental reorganizations with age of the synaptic composition of each neocortical area.

Finally, the whole landscape of neurotransmitter receptors and neuromodulators undergoes profound developmental changes; these changes

473

may be controlled by afferents to the neocortex and may be related to its developmental plasticity (Cynader et al., 1990).

DIFFERENTIATION OF AREAS AND COLUMNS

Neocortical areas differ in architectonic features, notably in the size and type of constituent neurons, and in their distribution in different layers. These features are correlated with patterns of afferent and efferent connectivity with other cortical and subcortical sites. Each pattern is unique for a given area and determines its functional properties. Afferents of thalamic origin appear to play a crucial role in the differentiation of area-specific features, but it is unclear whether the neocortex can be freely "imprinted" by thalamic afferents or is intrinsically determined to acquire a given, restricted set of architectonic characteristics (Rakic, 1988).

Most areas, possibly all, are organized into "columnar" modules oriented perpendicular to the neocortical surface. Neurons in a "column" share functional properties, e.g. tactile submodalities, ocular dominance, orientation specificity, and color sensitivity. Columns share a common input from the thalamus and/or common patterns of afferent or efferent connectivity, in particular, with other neocortical areas.

Ocular dominance columns in the primary visual cortex emerge through the segregation of geniculo-cortical afferents. This process involves activity-controlled synaptic selection and stabilization. Activity caused by visual experience regulates the competition of axons receiving information from the two eyes (Wiesel, 1982) near their target in layer IV. Synaptic selection probably results in the elimination of certain branches of thalamo-cortical axons and in the additional growth of the branches that are maintained. Synchronous activation of pre- and postsynaptic neurons is responsible for synaptic selection and stabilization. This "Hebbian" mechanism appears to involve the activation of NMDA-receptors-coupled Ca^{2+} channels and unknown cascades of biochemical events (Singer, 1990).

"Barrels" are columnar cytoarchitectonic specializations of layer IV in the representation of mystacial vibrissae of the somatosensory cortex in several rodents, most clearly in mice. They consist of a cell-poor "hollow," which receives thalamic afferents, surrounded by a cell-rich "wall." Each "barrel" is anatomically and functionally related to one mystacial vibrissa. Barrel formation involves the shaping of terminal arbors of thalamo-cortical axons, controlled by information originating at the receptor surface (Van der Loos & Welker, 1985). The mechanisms are poorly understood. However, a critical minimal number of axons related to one whisker appears to be required for one barrel to appear.

Efferent columns are aggregates of neurons projecting to the same target, separated by neurons whose axons reach a different target. Detailed developmental analysis of efferent columns exists for the intrinsic and inter-areal projections of area 17 of the cat, and for callosal projections in the somatosensory cortex of the rat. In both systems, they appear to be sculpted out by selective loss of transient projections. Columns of cortico-cortical afferents are aggregates of axon terminals with the same origin, separated by spaces where axons of a different origin arrive. Selective growth of axons into the gray matter may be responsible for the formation of this type of column (references in Innocenti, 1991).

CONCLUSIONS AND PERSPECTIVES

Recent work on the development of the cerebral neocortex clearly demonstrates that certain characteristics of this structure may be due to somewhat rigid, intrinsic developmental programs, while others are more flexible and are decided by interactions with different brain structures and/or the environment. This does not imply that neocortical maturation escapes genetic control. Rather, the genes and their products must themselves be regulated according to rules which have presumably been selected in the course of evolution, on the basis of their adaptive value. In the evolutionary selection of rules and in their ontogenetic implementation there may be room for "downward causation" across the various levels (functional, structural, molecular, etc.) of nervous system organization.

Work over the last 15 years has given attention to the formation of transient structures in the maturation of cerebral neocortex. These include early generated and phylogenetically older layers such as the subplate, massive transient projections, some of which are now known to serve transient functions, and transient neuronal phenotypes. These findings emphasize the potential for developmental plasticity in cortical development. Nevertheless, maintenance or elimination of juvenile structures is decided according to precise, albeit not necessarily simple rules.

On the whole, cerebral neocortex appears to mature through successive stages, each with a different degree of organization. The full characterization of these stages in molecular, structural, and functional terms, and the rules controlling the transition across these stages, offer many promising areas for future investigations.

BIBLIOGRAPHY

Aggoun-Zouaoui, D., & Innocenti, G. M. (1994). Juvenile visual callosal axons in kittens display origin- and fate-related morphology and distribution of arbors. *European Journal of Neuroscience*, *6*, 1846–63.

Caviness, V. S., Jr. (1980). The developmental consequences of abnormal cell position in the reeler mouse. *Trends in NeuroSciences*, *2*, 31–3.

Cynader, M., Shaw, C., van Huizen, F., & Prusky, G. (1990). Transient receptor expression in visual cortex development and the mechanisms of cortical plasticity. In B. L. Finlay, G. Innocenti, & H. Scheich (Eds), *The neocortex: Ontogeny and phylogeny* (pp. 245–53). New York: Plenum.

Goffinet, A. M., Daumerie, Ch., Langerwerf, B., & Pieau, C. (1986). Neurogenesis in reptilian cortical structures: ^{3}H-thymidine autoradiographic analysis. *Journal of Comparative Neurology*, *243*, 106–16.

Greenough, W. T., & Chang, F. L. F. (1988). Plasticity of synapse structure and pattern in the cerebral cortex. In A. Peters & E. G. Jones (Eds), *Cerebral cortex* (Vol. 7): *Development and maturation of cerebral cortex* (pp. 391–440). New York: Plenum.

Innocenti, G. M. (1991). The development of projections from cerebral cortex. In *Progress in sensory physiology*, Vol. 12 (pp. 65–114). Berlin and Heidelberg: Springer-Verlag.

Lyon, G., Arita, F., Le Galloudec, E., Vallée, L., Misson, J.-P., & Ferrière, G. (1990). A disorder of axonal development, necrotizing myopathy, cardiomyopathy, and cataracts: a new familial disease. *Annals of Neurology*, *27*, 193–9.

McConnell, S. K., & Kaznowski, C. E. (1991). Cell cycle dependence of laminar determination in developing neocortex. *Science*, *254*, 282–5.

Marin Padilla, M. (1978). Dual origin of the mammalian neocortex and evolution of the cortical plate. *Anatomical Embryology*, *152*, 109–26.

Parnavelas, J. G., Barfield, J. A., Franke, E., & Luskin, M. B. (1991). Separate progenitor cells give rise to pyramidal and nonpyramidal neurons in the rat telencephalon. *Cerebral Cortex*, *1*, 463–8.

Rakic, P. (1988). Specification of cerebral cortical areas. *Science*, *241*, 170–6.

Shatz, C. J., Chun, J. J. M., & Luskin, M. B. (1988). The role of the subplate in the development of the mammalian telencephalon. In A. Peters & E. G. Jones (Eds), *Cerebral cortex*. Vol. 7: *Development and maturation of cerebral cortex* (pp. 35–58). New York: Plenum.

Singer, W. (1990). Search for coherence: a basic principle of cortical self-organization. *Concepts in Neuroscience*, *1*, 1–26.

Van der Loos, H., & Welker, E. (1985). Development and plasticity of somatosensory brain maps. In *Development, organization, and processing in somatosensory pathways* (pp. 53–67). New York: Alan R. Liss.

Vercelli, A., Assal, F., & Innocenti, G. M. (1992). Emergence of callosally projecting neurons with stellate morphology in the visual cortex of the kitten. *Experimental Brain Research*, *90*, 346–58.

Walsh, C., & Cepko, C. L. (1992). Widespread dispersion of neuronal clones across functional regions of the cerebral cortex. *Science*, *255*, 434–40.

Webster, M. J., Ungerleider, L. G., & Bachevalier, J. (1991). Connections of inferior temporal areas TE and TEO with medial temporal-lobe structures in infant and adult monkeys. *Journal of Neuroscience*, *11*, 1095–116.

Wiesel, T. N. (1982). Postnatal development of the visual cortex and the influence of environment. *Nature*, *299*, 583–91.

G. M. INNOCENTI

Mayer–Reisch phenomenon An alternative term for GEGENHALTEN.

maze learning Assessment of the ability to learn mazes, with or without visual guidance, has been widely used in experimental psychology and in clinical neuropsychology. A failure of this ability may be attributed to a disorder of visual perception, but as posterior right hemisphere lesions produce deficits in performing both visually and tactually guided mazes, an element of the performance is clearly supramodal. The deficit may also be associated with a disorder of spatial orientation, or result from an inability to follow rules, or from perseveration, both classically attributable to frontal lobe lesions. There is also a memory component so that learning a maze may be disrupted by bilateral hippocampal lesions; right temporal lobectomy may interfere with maze learning, but only when the resection involves the hippocampus.

medulla   The medulla (more properly *medulla oblongata*) is the portion of the BRAIN STEM immediately above the spinal cord. The functions of the medulla include maintenance of heart rate and respiration, together with other visceral functions. Tumors of this structure may cause hiccups and alterations of both the cardiac and respiratory rate and rhythm. Bilateral paralysis may occur in an advanced condition, but both ipsilateral and crossed HEMIPLEGIAS may result from lesions in this region depending on the exact site of the damage.

megalopsia   *See* MACROPSIA.

melodic intonation therapy   Melodic intonation therapy is a form of intervention for APHASIA. It relies upon intact rhythmical and intonation abilities for the new development of oral expression.

The approach of melodic intonation therapy relies upon the observation that many aphasics retain the ability to sing, as well as to recite previously well-rehearsed material such as nursery rhymes and popular poems. The therapy provides a systematic hierarchy for the development of phrases which are sung in unison with the therapist through to normal conversational speech production by gradual shaping and fading of the more exaggerated intonation associated with singing. There is some evidence for the effectiveness of melodic intonation therapy, especially in individuals who retain good compre-

hension, self-criticism, and motivation, but who may have poor repetition and restricted and stereotypic speech output.

Melodic intonation therapy has also been linked with theories of the relative LATERALIZATION of speech and musical abilities. The hypothesis is that, although the left hemisphere-based language systems may be dysfunctional, systems associated with music and song are supported by the right hemisphere and, being unaffected, may be employed to establish a new strategy for speech production. The effectiveness of the therapy does not depend on the validity of this hypothesis.

memory disorders   *See* AMNESIA; AMNESIC SYNDROME; KORSAKOFF'S SYNDROME.

meninges   The three layers of protective tissue which encapsulate the brain and spinal cord are collectively the meninges. The three layers, from outer to inner, are the *dura mater*, the *arachnoid layer* (occasionally *arachnoid mater*), and the *pia mater*. Rather poetically these terms indicate the "hard mother," the "spider-like" layer, and the "soft mother," cradling the brain. The meninges extend longitudinally down into the sagittal fissure between the hemispheres forming the *falx*, and between the cerebellum and the cerebrum forming the *tentorium*. These membranes, besides providing some mechanical protection, serve to contain the CEREBROSPINAL FLUID and provide support to the vascular system.

meningioma   Meningioma is a tumor not of the brain substance but of the MENINGES, normally originating in the arachnoid layer. Meningiomas form irregular single masses and may occur at any site over the convexity of the hemispheres. Their effects upon the brain are made by occupying space, so causing displacement of neural structures. Because they are slow-growing, and consequently allow for a degree of neural compensation, they may grow to a very considerable size (up to the size of an orange) before causing significant interference with functions, particularly if located over the right hemisphere, where the very gradual functional degradation of nonverbal abilities is less apparent in everyday life. Being external to brain tissue, their surgical removal is commonly easier and more likely to be successful.

meningitis Meningitis is an intracranial bacterial or viral infection that results in inflammation of the MENINGES of the brain or spinal cord, most specifically the leptomeninges (the arachnoid and pia mater). Viral meningitis is more common and is generally less serious than the bacterial variety, which includes the pyogenic and tuberculous forms. In most varieties pyrexia, headaches, stiffness of the neck, and vomiting quickly become apparent, with lumbar puncture being used to confirm the diagnosis.

Pyogenic meningitis is a life-threatening condition most frequently caused by the meningococcus bacteria. Within a period of 12 to 24 hours a patient's condition may progress from a severe headache to drowsiness, confusion, and finally into semicoma. Signs of delirium may be present and DIPLOPIA may be reported. In some cases there may be degenerative changes in the cerebral cortex resulting in blindness or deafness, with hydrocephalus sometimes leading to residual dementia and spastic paralysis. With prompt diagnosis and treatment complete recovery generally takes place, but particularly with children, delay can lead to severe learning difficulties and personality changes. In adults, depression can occur during the convalescent stage, with residual changes in intellectual functioning and personality being reported in some of the more severe cases.

Tuberculous meningitis is a subacute form of the disorder with symptoms similar to those of the pyogenic variety, but with onset being slow and insidious. In the early stages there may be fluctuating signs of general ill health including headache, vomiting, and anorexia, with later onset of fever. Mental changes often occur and may include irritability, apathy, and personality changes. As the condition progresses the patient may become disorientated and confused, with periods of delirium. Delay in treatment may result in complications such as diplopia, communicating HYDROCEPHALUS, or focal neurological signs with progression towards coma and death. With treatment, the period of confusion evolves into an amnesic stage with significant impairment in new learning capacity being prominent. Typically, the patient shows little concern and confabulation may be common. AMNESIA frequently exists for events before and during the illness. With recovery, memory and learning ability slowly return, but often less quickly than other cognitive functions.

Aseptic meningitis is the viral form of the disorder. Viral infection is the commonest cause of meningitis and is less serious than the bacterial variety. The onset is acute, with symptoms resembling those of the pyogenic form, but being less severe. The course of the disorder is rarely longer than ten days. No long-term residual cognitive impairments have been observed.

MARCUS J. C. ROGERS

metamorphopsia Metamorphopsia indicates a visual illusion in which there is some distortion of visual perception involving form, contour, size (MACROPSIA, MEGALOPSIA, MICROPSIA), distance (PELOPSIA, TELEOPSIA), number (DIPLOPIA, POLYOPIA), or movements of objects. Objects may also persist (PALIOPSIA) or lose their colour (ACHROMATOPSIA). Metamorphopsias are commonly PAROXYSMAL DISORDERS, or may occur in association with migraine attacks, although there may be peripheral as well as central causes. Critchley (1966) is the definitive source on the classification of these disorders.

BIBLIOGRAPHY

Critchley, M. (1966). *The parietal lobes*. New York: Hafner (facsimile of 1953 edition).

metamorphotaxis Metamorphotaxis is related to METAMORPHOPSIA, but in the tactile rather than the visual modality. The tactile illusion is of the deformation of a grasped object so that it is perceived as being larger or smaller than would normally be the case. This tactile illusion normally occurs in association with one or more of the metamorphopsias.

metastases Tumors which are secondary to a primary tumor elsewhere in the body are known as metastases (or metastatic tumors) and account for over half the cerebral neoplasms arising in the population. The most common primary sites

477

giving rise to these metastases are the lung, breast, stomach, prostate, thyroid, and kidney. Metastases are usually multiple, growing rapidly and carrying a very poor prognosis.

methodological issues Most theoretical and, slowly but increasingly, clinical questions currently investigated in neuropsychology are nowadays viewed, under the influence of the cognitive approach, as information processing problems. Accordingly, neuropsychological findings are regarded as potentially helpful in specifying independent processing components and their mutual arrangement in the cognitive system (the "functional architecture"). At a further level of detail (not aimed at or achieved often enough in the field, according to some critics; see Seidenberg, 1988; Grodzinsky, 1990) the description concerns the content and the format of the information encoded by a component (the representation) and the processes that transform one class of representation into another (note that representation and processes determine in turn the shape of functional architecture). The kind of theoretical model encompassing these descriptions is called "computational," after Marr (1982). Within this model, the correct level of clinical diagnosis is identified as the one referring to the damage of such components, at least ideally; however, most cases involve damage of varying degrees of severity to several components and do not lend themselves easily to such description.

It is thought that, with respect to other theoretical frameworks, information processing models are more suitable to the needs of neuropsychology and, vice versa, neuropsychological research can be more easily and directly viewed as a source of relevant data for building such models and constraining theories about them. In fact, information processing models can easily be lesioned conceptually; neuropsychological effects can then be matched against the predictions of the model, with benefits in both directions. It is less obvious how this mutual exchange could have worked with other theories, for example, with Gestalt (no wonder, therefore, that the highest fortune of Gestalt theory corresponded, in the history of psychology, to a relatively obscure period for neuropsychology). The result of this interaction is that neuropsychology has become a respectable

partner of the other disciplines that make up cognitive science and the convergence of normal and neuropsychological findings is actively pursued. The common goal is the development of a cognitive theory, a theory that has to specify the inherent contents of a given cognitive task. On the other hand, localization of cognitive functions, one of the historical aims of neuropsychology, will, it is believed (Shallice, 1988; Semenza et al., 1988; Olson & Caramazza, 1991), progress only when the level of detail achieved by the functional theory will allow it. At present the proper scale for matching functional and anatomical description is not even known. As a consequence, cognitive neuropsychologists, while not indifferent to neuroanatomical problems in general and to the progress brought about by new instrumental techniques, tend to avoid the issue of localization.

OBJECTIONS TO NEUROPSYCHOLOGY

Repeated objections are raised against the use of neuropsychological data in constraining theories of normal cognitive processing. Basically there have been three such objections. First, it has been contended that brain injury might cause a global decrease in cognitive resources, so observed focal effects could be due to spurious variations that say nothing about normal functions. However, observations impermeable to this criticism are reported in the neuropsychological literature, consisting of very selective disturbances, where patients perform normally on some tasks although they fail in others. More to the point, it is often the case that other patients exhibit the opposite pattern with respect to the same tasks, being normal where the others fail. Indeed, it is through seeking findings of this sort (so-called double DISSOCIATIONS) that in most cases neuropsychology makes significant progress (Shallice, 1988).

Another objection, coming in various forms, is that there is no way to demonstrate that brain insult does not fractionate a particular cognitive subsystem arbitrarily. Marin and others (1976) have countered this criticism by arguing that nobody can tell a priori that brain damage fractionates cognitive processes more arbitrarily than the artifices of laboratory experiments. Indeed, as has been argued by Caramazza (1991), it might very well turn out that the functional organization of the brain is such that the analysis of impaired performance following brain damage will not be helpful for the task of constraining cognitive theory. But again, this is a matter that cannot be decided a priori and the justification for undertaking the enterprise must ultimately be based on pragmatic considerations. Vis-à-vis more than a hundred years of neuropsychology, pessimism does not seem to be justified. Observations on brain organization exist that independently support theories based on findings in normal subjects. Conversely, the significance of neuropsychological findings has often been, as indeed it should always be, independently corroborated through investigation of normal subjects. The heuristic value of neuropsychological research has been thus underlined by Semenza and colleagues (1988, p.15; but see Shallice, 1988, 1991, for a similar view): "the investigation of neuropsychological disturbances forces one to ask questions that are often very different from those arising with respect to normal subjects or artificial systems. Neuropsychological diseases are accidents of nature that are blind with respect to our epistemic perspectives. Investigating such impairments of cognition can, therefore, direct our attention to the relevance of phenomena that we otherwise might overlook." Furthermore, as Shallice (1988) pointed out, neuropsychological findings often compare favorably (because of their robustness and the size of their effects) with findings in the study of normals, where observed effects are slippery and a myriad of inessential aspects of the experimental situation may be wrongly taken as critical.

A third, more insidious objection concerns the possibility that a critical reorganization of functions may take place after the lesion, such that new cognitive operations would appear as a consequence of brain damage. This would set the interest of neuropsychology back within the limits of the clinical field (Shallice, 1991, p. 434). However, although no positive evidence exists that perverse new mechanisms do not develop, the possibility that the destruction of brain tissue would result in completely new and efficient processing mechanisms is rather unlikely. In the particular case of a double dissociation, Shallice (1991) argues that it is impossible that reorganized systems with opposing characteristics should substitute for the original one in different patients. Note that the eventuality of functional reorganization is not denied; in fact, it seems unlikely that the performance of neurological patients merely represents a combination of intact

and lacunae patterns of behavior. Their performance may reflect a reorganization that highlights the peculiarities of the residual system in its regular functions as well as its hidden potentialities (Marin et al., 1976). If this makes neuropsychological investigation more difficult (but it can also facilitate it!) it does not limit at all its relevance for universally valid cognitive theory. To address these and other criticisms, cognitive neuropsychologists have specified a set of theoretical assumptions and developed a vast methodological apparatus.

BASIC ASSUMPTIONS: THE ISSUE OF MODULARITY

The single concept that has come out most prominently in discussions concerning the rationale behind (neuro)psychological studies is that of modularity. It refers to the assumption that any complex computation (and, by extension, any complex organic system) is constituted of a collection of smaller subparts that are as independent of one another as the task and the medium allow (Simon, 1962; Shallice, 1981; Marr, 1982; Fodor, 1983). Arguments and empirical support for this position come from a number of different sources (e.g. computational, linguistic, physiological, and psychological) that are indicated in detail in Fodor (1983) and Shallice (1988). However, despite widespread agreement on the meaning of this assumption at an intuitive level, there exist divergent views about the precise meaning of the word "module," and about the extent to which the concept may be useful to the neuropsychological enterprise.

The most detailed theory about modules and the one that has received the most attention is that of Fodor (1983). A module, for Fodor, is a device characterized by a precise set of properties: it is domain-specific, mandatory, fast, computationally autonomous, informationally encapsulated, hardwired, innate, and has a characteristic pattern of development. By computationally autonomous, Fodor means that a module does not share attention, memory, and other general-purpose processes with other modules. By informationally encapsulated, the most essential quality, he means that modules are resistant to top-down cognitive influences – knowledge of the world cannot affect the operations. The output of modules is thus indicated as shallow, since it does not convey any information about how it has been

479

derived or about its relation with world knowledge. Another important feature of Fodor's theory is the distinction he sets between modular systems, which he thinks include just input and presumably (see Marshall, 1984) output devices and central systems that are not organized in a modular fashion. Fodor's contention is that central systems are not suitable to psychological research simply because they are not modular.

Ample reviews and criticisms of Fodor's theory from neuropsychologists can be found in Marshall (1984) and Rosenthal (1988). To some authors (see Shallice, 1988), Fodor's defining criteria appear too specific, and the systems to which they are supposed to apply too limited for neuropsychological purposes. Shallice favors instead, perhaps more along the lines indicated by Marr (1982), a less explicit and indeed a looser view of modules seen as isolable (dissociable) subsystems, where the amount of interaction among systems may be considered relatively negligible. Shallice's view of modules therefore seems to allow a broader use of the concept of modularity. However, as dissociations appear also to concern what Fodor considers non-modular (central) processes, Shallice seems to retreat from extending the domain of modular systems beyond a certain point. He admits that in some cases what forms isolability remains unclear, and certain dissociations may turn out to be explicable in terms other than the existence of separate modules.

Other neuropsychologists pursue Fodor's pathway more closely. Thus Moscovitch and Umiltà (1989), although critical of Fodor's theory in some respects, expand the modularity theory by distinguishing three possible kinds of modules. The basic ones, type I modules, are those more similar to the ones proposed by Fodor: they alone carry out a single function. Among these would-be modules are those for the perception of basic sensory features in each modality and perhaps others that pick up complex sensory information, such as faces. Type II modules consist of a collection of simpler modules whose organization is innately given and whose output is integrated or synthesized by a non-modular processor dealing only with information coming from that particular group of modules. They are capable of modification or learning. Examples of functions mediated by such modules would be object recognition or linguistic abilities, like syntactic ones. Type III modules are experientially assembled modules in which a central processor assembles the component basic and type II modules; they assume full integration and automatization with repeated use. Examples of these modules are those concerned with reading and learned, skilled, motor sequences. By these distinctions Moscovitch and Umiltà seem to rescue for neuropsychological inquiry most processes that Fodor would consider central and therefore relatively unsuitable for (neuro)psychological scrutiny.

Positions as different as those just outlined seem to determine more or less directly not only the extent of application of the modularity concept but also the strategy of the researcher. The dissociation approach is certainly the most widely used and the underlying assumptions, seldom made explicit, seem to be of the type endorsed by Shallice (1988). Perhaps surprisingly few, compared to Fodor's success (but remember Shallice's warning about the complexity of Fodor's approach), are the studies more directly concerned with the functioning of Fodor's encapsulated modules (e.g. Swinney et al., 1989). One of the difficulties is that a line of research fully adherent to Fodor's criteria may require unusual techniques. In fact, supporting evidence (paradoxically, the example advocated by Fodor) for encapsulated modules' reliance on fixed localizable neuropsychological architecture is based on the gross anatomical correlate of clinically observed deficits. However, these data are far removed from the millisecond speeds of modular system operations (one of the reasons for the existence of modules is fast processing). It may be that, as Swinney and others (1989) suggest, the lesion localizing value of disruptions to modular information processing systems would emerge more clearly from on-line analyses of processing, an unfamiliar method to most neuropsychologists (which may also be difficult to handle in a clinical setting).

A less impervious pathway is indicated by Moscovitch and Umiltà. They argue that, at a neuropsychological level, a function may be considered to be modular if it can be selectively impaired after focal brain damage (domain specificity) and selectively spared in cases of dementia caused by degenerative brain damage (informationally encapsulated). In fact, if a particular function remains intact despite evidence of gross intellectual loss, one can assume that it is informationally encapsulated because the malfunctioning of a central cognitive system, which is a repository of general knowledge, has no effect on that function. The only problem with this approach, as Moscovitch and Umiltà clearly state, is that the conditions that give rise to the general intellectual deficit in dementia are also likely to affect each particular module. Even if some modules are not affected, it may not be possible to evaluate their state because of the patient's inability to follow instructions. Therefore failure to find that a particular modular function is spared, in the face of a general intellectual loss, does not constitute evidence against informational encapsulation. Only positive evidence counts. This approach is new and it is too early to harvest any fruit, as may well be expected, from its applications.

The question of modularity remains at present an open one. Whichever view one wishes to entertain about it, a word of caution is proper. Without a theory of a given task, the principle of modularity applied to that task is conceptually empty and has no empirical ramification because anything may be viewed as a module. Finally, the value of the modularity principle probably transcends the likelihood of the nervous system implementing cognitive functions in a modular way. It seems, in fact, to honor a longstanding scientific tradition of decomposing complex entities into their basic functional components, a method that has often been shown to be successful in the physical sciences.

THE FRACTIONATION AND SUBTRACTION ASSUMPTION

Modularity has no consequences in neuropsychology if further assumptions are not made. One assumption (the "fractionation" assumption; see Caramazza, 1984) is that brain damage may result in the selective deficit of one or more processing units, leaving the others intact. The other is the "subtraction" or "transparency" assumption. According to earlier formulations (e.g. Caramazza, 1984), the primary concept underlying this assumption is that there is a transparent relationship between an observed deficit D and processing components P that are supposedly "removed" as a consequence of brain injury, so a selective deficit D can be held as a demonstration that P normally exists. Further considerations, however,

may lead to the conclusion that this first formulation is too bold. It seems to entail a paradox: what becomes transparent (thus more understandable) after a brain lesion is that which is lost! As Semenza and others (1988) later observed, the identification of a deficit does not necessarily imply that what is seen is the lack of a definable, separate, processing component. A more satisfactory, though perhaps less strong formulation of the transparency assumption may stress the fact that brain damage allows one to spot more easily the working of processes that are opaque in normals' flawless performance. The paradox would disappear: what is transparent is what is left. To take this view does not just mean to avoid logical fallacies; consequences are there, inherent in this position for neuropsychological work. First, symptoms may be understood better in terms of factors concerning the use of information rather than in terms of the loss of one or another type of information (Semenza et al., 1987; Margolin et al., 1985). This would help to avoid the recurrent danger of taking seriously associations of deficits that are only casually related to each other (see below). Second, since the stress would be more on what the patient does rather than on what he or she does not do, the analysis of errors becomes more important. Third, whatever the patient does (instead of doing nothing) may be viewed as a way to overcome the deficit based on residual abilities. In any case, it is important to stress (Caramazza, 1991) that the relation between impaired performance and normal cognition becomes a transparent one as long as the hypothesized modifications of the normal processing system are tractable within a proposed theoretical framework.

THE PROBLEMS OF INDIVIDUAL VARIABILITY, PATIENT'S STRATEGY, AND TASK DIFFICULTY

Caveats to go with the transparency assumption were provided by the earlier formulators. If one wants to draw conclusions from patients' behavior, normal individual variability should be taken into account. Group data may deal better with this problem than data from a single case, but there are overwhelming reasons to consider single cases as the most revealing under the cognitive neuropsychology approach. A single patient, however, may have been weak at certain tasks before illness. Shallice (1988) argues that if the dissociation is *classical* (all other tasks in this case are performed normally), then an account using individual differences is less plausible. More problematic would be the case, not infrequent, where patients' performance on the tasks they carry out better is still below the normal range. All in all, the consideration prevails that individual differences among normal subjects in the extent of the resources available are small, compared to the destructive effects of neurological disease on resources.

A second problem regards the patient's strategy. Quite frequently, unimpaired processes are used to compensate for a deficit in other processes (e.g. pragmatic abilities in certain forms of agrammatism). This compensation may occur more or less actively and more often than not unconsciously. It may be more or less effective and occasionally misleading. Sometimes functional shifts occur to other much less efficient systems unlikely to be used in normals (e.g. letter by letter reading in certain forms of dyslexia). This matter is treated at some length in Semenza, Bisiacchi, and Rosenthal (1988) and Semenza, Panzeri, and Butterworth (1987). The fact is stressed that compensation may not always become a complicating factor. On the contrary, it may highlight residual systems, for instance. When this is not the case, a number of methodological heuristics such as using strategy control tests, training the patient in the appropriate procedure, and using converging operations have been proposed to make the processes used by the patient more transparent (see Shallice, 1991).

Another complication may result from the fact that tasks are often of different levels of difficulty. A single dissociation in performance in two tasks, one being spared, the other impaired, may simply reflect the fact that the second task, while relying on the same cognitive ability, is intrinsically more difficult than the first. The classic solution is to seek a complementary dissociation and thereby demonstrate a double dissociation (some difficulties with this method, indicated in the next section, do not essentially hamper its validity).

DISSOCIATIONS AND ASSOCIATIONS

DISSOCIATION is a type of neuropsychological finding that is considered universally important. Methodological accounts of this topic date back to Teuber (1955) and full exploitation of the virtues of the dissociation approach constitutes the core

of Shallice's book *From neuropsychology to mental structure* (1988) to which the reader is referred for a detailed description. As already mentioned, a *dissociation* occurs when a patient performs extremely poorly on one task – preferably way outside the normal range – and at a normal level, or at least at a very much better level, on another task; a *double dissociation* occurs if another patient is observed who shows the opposite pattern, i.e. is impaired where the first patient is unimpaired and does well where the first patient has difficulties. Given the fractionation assumption, dissociations (the more selective the better) are seen as informative about the organization of the cognitive system. In particular, double dissociations observed on two tasks may indicate that the two tasks require a different set of processing systems or at least some degree of functional specialization within a system. Note that a single dissociation may simply mean that one task is easier than the other, and therefore, observing a double dissociation allows in general much safer conclusions. It should be clear, however, that in order to draw safe conclusions it is not enough that a double dissociation has just the form of two complementary dissociations (a patient does significantly better in task A than in task B and the other patient does the reverse). Differences in the performance/resource functions for different tasks (e.g. one steeper than the other) may determine a double dissociation perfectly explicable by damage to a single unspecialized subsystem. To avoid this problem the necessary condition is that one patient is *significantly superior to the other patient in one task* while the other patient is *significantly superior to the first in the second task* (Shallice, 1988).

Another source of information that is similar to the dissociation approach is the so-called "critical variable method" (Shallice 1988, 1991), where the performance of a certain type of task is affected in one patient by a change in variable x but not in variable y, and the complementary effect is observed in another patient. Difficulties with this approach parallel those described for double dissociations.

Associations are as important as dissociations, provided they are considered in a theoretically sound framework. Theoretically valid associations are those whose interpretations cannot be undermined by the observation of a dissociation of their components. Of course, it is easy to show that certain association symptom complexes, like the Gerstmann syndrome, have no inferential value for the understanding of normal processes simply because their components are also observed in isolation and no common factor (except anatomical contiguity) can be advocated. However, this is not always the case. For instance, patients have been described who make semantic errors of the same kind on various types of lexical processing tasks (reading, writing, naming, and comprehension) at virtually identical rates, regardless of the modality of stimulus or response (Caramazza & McCloskey, 1991). The finding, interpreted as evidence of selective damage to a semantic system common to all lexical processing, is not hampered by the observation of patients who show the same effect only in one modality. According to current models, this latter patient may be disturbed at the level of one of the peripheral lexicons. Associations cannot be treated, in principle, as determined by mere coincidence; it is clear that in many cases a coincidence is the least likely reason for the association. Consider, for instance, the fact that published cases of anomia for proper names affect both oral and written naming in the same way. Note also that these patients have clearly retained all information on a given item except for the name itself (therefore a putative "central" semantic system is intact). This fact forces one to specify further either that (a) the phonological and the orthographical output lexicons interact to a certain extent, or (b) intermediate processes between the semantic system and the peripheral lexicons are sensitive to categorical information. What one cannot do is dismiss the association of such peculiar deficits (a selective deficit to the same semantic category) in the oral and written modalities as casual, even if in future a patient is described who shows this particular anomia only in one modality. These are what one could indicate as strong, theoretically valid, associations. However, other recurrently observed but loosely defined symptom complexes (e.g. Broca's aphasia) should not, according to some authors, be disregarded on the grounds that they do not seem to fit a proper theory. As Zurif and others (1991) put it, the neuropsychologist is in the position of the astronomer. In observational sciences like astronomy and, as they claim, cognitive neuropsychology, practitioners may often get by without having control over experimental

manipulation. All they may have is given phenomena that may lead to a theory and therefore to predictions for further investigation. Observed recurrent symptom associations may at the very least start a theoretical process. Finally, indications exist (Shallice, 1991) that the rejection of certain symptom complexes based primarily on the association of some error types (e.g. deep dyslexia) may be or may have been premature. In fact, it can now be demonstrated that some of them are predictable on the basis of new (connectionist) models. Again, the appropriate methodology will depend on the general type of model of the cognitive system being considered.

An important addendum has to be included in the discussion about dissociations and associations. In most cases these phenomena are observed in order at a specific testing date and are not considered in their evolution. It is becoming a widespread opinion, however, that longitudinal studies of dissociations and associations may add value to the method. On one hand, hidden dissociations of functions may thus be revealed. On the other, if a functional dependency is hypothesized between two tasks, this may be better shown by studying the evolution of the performance in the two tasks. Both recovery and deterioration are suitable for longitudinal investigation. Of particular interest may also be the comparison between the evolution of a neuropsychological patient and that of a computer-simulated neural network which is "lesioned" in a way that is thought to parallel the patient's problem. Studies of this sort are just starting at present.

Finally, an experimental paradigm that could provide an analogue of the dissociations in clinical neuropsychology is the DUAL TASK technique. In this situation subjects are asked to perform a primary task while at the same time performing a second task. The prerequisite for being able to combine two tasks is that they use separate functional subsystems, hence the analogy with the dissociation method. A significant decrement in performance is expected when both tasks occupy the same part of the system.

SINGLE CASE AND GROUP STUDIES

Perhaps the argument that has been most furiously debated since the rise of cognitive neuropsychology is the relative benefit of single and group studies in providing information, as far as inference to normal functions is concerned. The problem is extensively treated in books and journals (e.g. Shallice, 1988; see also a special issue of *Cognitive Neuropsychology* in 1988) to which the reader is referred for details.

The prevalent bias is in favor of single-case studies because group studies, emphasizing the average performance, are unlikely to enhance the discrimination of subtle but interesting effects; patients showing the clearest effects would go easily unnoticed. Problems exist for the inclusion of patients in a group; several selection artifacts are likely to influence the results due to poor control of factors like age, time of the onset and time of the disease, patients' understanding of the instructions (which biases, for instance, any study concerned with right/left hemisphere differences because of the presence of severe aphasia in the left hemisphere group), and so on. Grouping according to different syndromes also seems arbitrary, both because in many instances there might be classification problems and because, as has already been argued when speaking of symptom association, syndromes may turn out to be theoretically unmotivated. Other reasons why people prefer single-case studies are pragmatic: group studies take a long time and are difficult to conduct for people who are not directly working in a clinical setting, which is increasingly the case for investigators in the field. The advantages of the single-case approach are so unanimously recognized that, indeed, the debate may be more accurately described as going on between those authors who just prefer single-case studies and those who do not admit any other method in cognitive neuropsychology.

Some authors (e.g. Caramazza, 1986), in fact, claim that group studies do not provide a valid database for generalizing to normal functions. The main argument underlying this claim lies in the difficulty or impossibility of having a group of patients which is sufficiently homogeneous. In normals, one can assume that subjects are homogeneous with respect to the cognitive apparatus. In cognitive neuropsychology, a homogeneous group would consist of patients who share the same disruption to the cognitive system. However, as Caramazza puts it, it is in principle impossible to specify the locus of damage to the functional architecture before testing each patient in the group on all the relevant tasks. This reduces the group study to case studies and makes

grouping irrelevant. Critics of this position (Shallice, 1988; Zurif et al., 1989) argue that, on one hand, based on the same rigidly taken grounds (lack of homogeneity) one should not even use average results from normals. On the other hand, they claim that a priori grouping on the basis of some observed interesting feature would help focus a problem and that further divisions among patients are expected as a result of the experimental treatment. Other criticisms of the "single-case-only" approach point out that group results are less prone to get misleading results due to patients' idiosyncratic strategies. Also group studies require fewer items, which has the double advantage of (a) allowing investigations of domains that do not have numerous stimuli and (b) minimizing the possible confusion induced by strategies developed by the patient over several trials.

The problem of cross-patient replication is also viewed differently according to various authors. By the same logic leading to the claim that single-case studies are the only valid ones, the direct replication of the finding is declared impossible in neuropsychology and therefore the problem nonexistent. This is probably the single point which even people sympathetic with the single-case-only approach find most difficult to concede.

It should finally be pointed out (it may be obvious but, given the present climate, it is better to remember it) that drawing inferences on normal performance is just one, albeit the more important, aim in neuropsychology. Some problems of clinical order can only be solved via group studies, for example, the study that clarified and first empirically demonstrated the role of unilateral spatial neglect in hampering recovery from left hemiparesis (Denes et al., 1982) had to be a group study. Its value, based on a regression analysis isolating the significant contribution of neglect among other factors in delaying recovery, would clearly not be undermined by sporadic cases of patients suffering from neglect and yet rapidly recovering from hemiparesis.

NONMODULAR SYSTEMS: FROM CONNECTIONISM TO NEUROPSYCHOLOGY

Although the strategy explicitly based on the modularity and fractionation assumptions has allowed neuropsychology to flourish in the recent past, compelling reasons also exist to consider nonmodular views of the cognitive system. First of all one should not forget that, despite collected empirical evidence, modularity is essentially a working hypothesis. Second, even in strong modularist views like Fodor's (1983) there is space left for nonmodular organization (in Fodor's case it would concern "central" processes). Third (and quite distinct from Fodor's particular view) modular and nonmodular organization may turn out to coexist in the cognitive system (and in the brain). As is more and more frequently spelled out, while modular organization would be better able to describe functional architecture at a "coarse-grain" level (Shallice, 1988), nonmodular organization may apply to describe the "inside" of modular isolable parts of the cognitive system at a finer-grain level (what goes on within the box, as Farah and McClelland (1991) put it). In fact most of the work in connectionist (the prototypical "nonmodularist") modelling is concerned with "connectionist modules," that is, with small specialized and relatively encapsulated parts of some hypothetical larger processing structure. Fourth, a widespread feeling exists that a connectionist model would be closer to the actual working of the brain (parallel distributed processing computers, which allow connectionist models to be simulated, are indeed more directly inspired by the brain than their predecessors). Along with the feeling of biological plausibility, the idea exists that connectionist models may be better able to capture the level of description concerned with the implementation theory of a task (or the algorithm, in Marr's (1982) terms: how something is computed) beyond the task theory itself (the computational theory: what is computed and why). A final reason to take nonmodular views seriously is that some connectionist models, artfully "lesioned," recently allowed (as reported in Shallice, 1991; see also Farah & McClelland, 1991) successful computer simulation of some neuropsychological impairments.

The range of possible nonmodular architectures has been described in various ways. Kosslyn and Van Kleek (1990) summarized eight possible patterns of neural organization, resulting from the combination of the following three binary distinctions:

(a) clustered versus distributed neurons: functionally homogeneous neurons are either spatially clustered or spatially distributed;

(b) shared versus dedicated neurons: neurons are either shared across functions or dedicated to a specific function;

(c) large versus small numbers of neurons subserving a given function.

It is obvious that the modularist/fractionation assumption would work better when the maximum likelihood exists that a focal brain lesion would result in a selected cognitive disorder, which is the case where a function is realized by a large number of dedicated, clustered neurons. The worst possible case would occur where a function is realized by a small number of shared, distributed neurons. In this latter case, focal brain damage would hardly allow a revealing analysis about the organization of the cognitive system. From this scenario, Kosslyn and Van Kleek (1990) draw pessimistic conclusions about the enterprise of using impaired performance to constrain theories of normal cognition. However, they have recently been countered by Caramazza (1991). As mentioned above, the ultimate answer about the utility of neuropsychological research cannot be given a priori but must be based on considerations about the productivity of the enterprise; furthermore, independently of logical possibilities, the empirical evidence is that focal brain damage frequently results in highly selective disorders that allow what appear to be sound enough analyses.

A more constructive attitude is taken by Shallice (1988) who considers examples of nonmodular systems with the concern of establishing whether double dissociations could reflect damage to such organizations. He identifies five types of nonmodular systems. The first would be based on a continuum of processing space; a concrete example would be the visual cortex. Damage in two different parts of this system would provide a sort of double dissociation between processes that do not interact but are not themselves units, being merely different sections of a continuum of processes. The second type of nonmodular system, for which no concrete example can be provided, would consist of at least two partially overlapping processing regions. Distinct lesions to nonshared spaces would give rise to a double dissociation that would not reflect damage to functionally isolable subsystems. The third type would consist of two subsystems that, while receiving different inputs, are highly interactive and not computationally autonomous. Appropriate damage to such a system can give rise to a double dissociation. Such findings would not indicate the operation of two different systems, but rather a certain degree of functional specialization. The fourth type is called "semimodules"; this term would indicate a processing region that has several inputs and outputs, some of which are privileged over the others. If damaged, this system would produce dissociations. The last category of nonmodular systems encompasses multilevel "interactive" systems. Models of these systems are currently widely used for the simulation of cognition (e.g. Hinton & Anderson, 1981; McClelland & Rumelhart, 1985). Two types of these models have been employed to account for observations in neuropsychology. The first are "cascade" models (McClelland & Rumelhart, 1981) that can be viewed as an intermediate conceptual step between the discrete stage, serially working models, and the second type of interactive models, the so-called "distributed memory" models. In cascade models subprocesses at different levels, although working in a feed-forward manner, overlap in time. The pattern of activation that each level feeds into the next is also not all or none. Nontarget competitors within these levels may also become activated to the extent that their underlying representations are similar to the target. Correct performance is possible when target representations reach a high enough level of activation to inhibit all competitors. Cascade models have been used to account for various neuropsychological phenomena like anomia, agnosia, agrammatism, and deep dyslexia.

According to distributed memory ("connectionist") models, an entity to be represented is not represented in discrete elements but rather by a pattern of activity distributed over many elements, and each element is involved in representing many different entities. This abstract description may be envisaged more concretely by substituting "computing elements" for neurons. So one may say that a given function is performed over many neurons (a "neural network") and each neuron is involved in many functions.

Damage to such systems is thought (Shallice, 1988) to be able to reliably produce dissociations only if the network is imperfectly distributed or if it operates on more than one type of input or output and the damage is close to the input or output. Dissociations would then indicate some sort of functional specialization within the system. Different effects would also result from different kinds of damage, for instance, a loss of the elements of the network, a loss or noise in their connections.

As has already been mentioned, connectionist models have recently allowed successful computer simulation of a number of neuropsychological disorders. This adds momentum to the general feeling pervading cognitive science that, only with connectionist models, a fruitful loop between simulation, theory, and standard data has begun. However, problems that have to be solved exist with the explanatory transparency of distributed memory networks. As Olson and Caramazza (1991) have observed, the working of most networks is opaque. When a model fails there is nothing that ties the level at which success or failure is judged to the level that changes the network's performance. Without such a connection it cannot be predicted how changes in the network will affect performance. The understanding of these connections will help in putting this kind of model to good use for the neuropsychologist.

BIBLIOGRAPHY

Caramazza, A. (1984). The logic of neuropsychological research and the problem of patient classification in aphasia. *Brain and Language, 11*, 9–20.

Caramazza, A. (1986). On drawing inferences about the structure of normal cognitive processes from patterns of impaired performance: the case for single-patient studies. *Brain and Cognition, 5*, 41–66.

Caramazza, A. (1992). Is cognitive neuropsychology possible? *Journal of Cognitive Neuroscience, 4*, 80–95.

Caramazza, A., & McCloskey M. (1991). The poverty of methodology. *Behavioral and Brain Sciences, 14*, 444–5.

Denes, G., Semenza, C., Stoppa E., & Lis, A. (1982). Unilateral spatial neglect and recovery from hemiplegia: a follow up study. *Brain, 105*, 543–52.

Farah, M., & McClelland, J. L. (1991). A computational model of semantic memory impairment: modality specificity and emergent category specificity. *Journal of Experimental Psychology: General, 120*, 339–57.

Fodor, J. A. (1983). *The modularity of mind*. Cambridge, MA: MIT Press.

Grodzinsky, Y. (1990). *Theoretical perspectives on language deficits*. Cambridge, MA: MIT Press.

Hinton, G. E., & Anderson, J. A. (Eds). (1981). *Parallel models of associative memory*. Hillsdale, NJ: Erlbaum.

Kosslyn, S. M., & Van Kleek, M. (1990). Broken brains and normal minds: why humpty dumpty needs a skeleton. In E. Schwartz (Ed.), *Computational neuroscience* (pp. 48–50). Cambridge, MA: MIT Press.

McClelland, J. L., & Rumelhart, C. A. (1981). An interaction model of context effects in letter perception. Part 1. An account of basic findings. *Psychological Review*, *88*, 375–407.

McClelland, J. L., & Rumelhart, C. A. (1985). Distributed memory and the representation of general and specific information. *Journal of Experimental Psychology: General*, *114*, 159–88.

Margolin, D. J., Marcel, A. J., & Carlson, N. R. (1985). Common mechanisms in dysnomia and postsemantic surface dyslexia: processing deficits and selective attention. In K. E. Patterson, J. K. Marshall, & M. Coltheart (Eds), *Surface dyslexia* (pp. 139–74). Hillsdale, NJ: Erlbaum.

Marin, O. S., Saffran, E. M., & Schwartz, M. (1976). Dissociation of language in aphasia: implications for normal functions. *Annals of the New York Academy of Sciences*, *280*, 868–84.

Marr, D. (1982). *Vision*. San Francisco: Freeman.

Marshall, J. C. (1984). Multiple perspectives on modularity. *Cognition*, *18*, 209–42.

Moscovitch, M., & Umiltà, C. (1989). Modularity and neuropsychology. In M. Schwartz (Ed.), *Modular processes in Alzheimer's disease* (pp.1–59). Cambridge, MA: MIT Press.

Olson, A., & Caramazza, A. (1991). The role of cognitive theory in neuropsychological research. In, F. Boller & J. Grafman (Eds), *The handbook of neuropsychology* (pp. 287–309). Amsterdam: Elsevier.

Rosenthal, V. (1988). Does it rattle when you shake it? Modularity of mind and the epistemology of cognitive research. In G. Denes, C. Semenza, & P. S. Bisiacchi (Eds), *Perspectives on cognitive neuropsychology* (pp. 31–58). Hillsdale, NJ: Erlbaum.

Seidenberg, M. S. (1988). Cognitive neuropsychology of language: the state of the art. *Cognitive Neuropsychology*, *5*, 403–26.

Semenza, C., Bisiacchi, P. S., & Rosenthal, V. (1988). A function for cognitive neuropsychology. In G. Denes, C. Semenza, & P. S. Bisiacchi (Eds), *Perspectives on cognitive neuropsychology* (pp. 3–30). Hillsdale, NJ: Erlbaum.

Semenza, C., Panzeri, M., & Butterworth, B. (1987). Sull'interpretazione delle conseguenze del danno cerebrale, revisione critica del cosidetto "principio di trasparenza." (On the interpretation of the consequences of brain damage: a critical revision of the so-called principle of transparency.) In *Atti XXI Congresso Società Italiana di Psicologia* (pp. 65–9). Milan: Guerrini.

Shallice, T. (1981). Neurological impairment of cognitive processes. *British Medical Bulletin*, *37*, 187–92.

Shallice, T. (1988). *From neuropsychology to mental structure*. Cambridge: Cambridge University Press.

Shallice, T. (1991). Precis of "From neuropsychology to mental structure." *Behavioral and Brain Sciences*, *14*, 429–69.

Simon, H. A. (1962). The architecture of cognition. *Proceedings of the American Philosophical Society*, *106*, 467–82.

Swinney, D., Zurif, E. B., & Nichol, J. (1989). The effects of focal brain damage on sentence processing: an examination of the neurological organization of a mental module. *Journal of Cognitive Neurosciences*, *1*, 25–37.

Teuber, H. L. (1955). Physiological psychology. *Annual Review of Psychology*, *9*, 267–96.

Zurif, E. B., Gardner, H., & Brownell H. H. (1989). The case against the case against group studies. *Brain and Cognition*, *10*, 237–55.

Zurif, E. B., Swinney, D., & Fodor, J. A. (1991). An evaluation of assumptions underlying the single patient only position in neuropsychological research: a reply. *Brain and Cognition*, *16*, 198–210.

C. SEMENZA

microcephaly, microencephaly Microcephaly results from an abnormality of the development of the brain in which the resulting cerebrum is abnormally small and rudimentary in formation. The condition is invariably associated with intellectual deficit.

microgenesis The term microgenesis has been proposed for the continuous formative activity which underlies cognition. Implicit in the concept is the idea that microgenesis reflects the sequences of phylogenetic and ontogenetic development. Use of the term encapsulates the idea that, as a reflection of cognitive elaboration, neural development occurs in a dynamic and adaptive way, distributed across most areas of the brain, and governed by general principles of phylogenetic and ontogenetic evolution.

micropolygyria Micropolygyria describes a result of abnormal development of the brain in which the cortical gyri are smaller and more numerous than in the normal brain. It is contrasted with *macrogyria* in which the gyri are larger but less numerous than normal.

micropsia A visual illusion, the converse condition to MACROPSIA, micropsia is a form of METAMORPHOPSIA in which objects are perceived as smaller in size than normal. The associated phenomena and causes are as for macropsia.

microsomatognosia Microsomatognosia is parallel to MICROPSIA, but in the somesthetic modality. The illusion is the converse of MACROSO-MATOGNOSIA, so that an illusion of a decrease in some dimension of the whole body or selected body parts results. The associated phenomena and causes are as for macrosomatognosia.

mind–body problem The so-called mind–body problem boils down to the twin question, "What is mind and how is it related to the body?" This is an ancient problem in theology, philosophy, science, and medicine. It has fascinated philosophers such as Aristotle, Spinoza, and Russell; psychologists such as Fechner, Wundt, and Hebb; neuroscientists like Cajal, Sherrington, Penfield, Eccles, and Mountcastle; physicians such as Hippocrates, Galen, and Hughlings Jackson; and theologians like St Augustine and St Thomas Aquinas – to name but a few eminent men. And the problem is of course at the very heart of the work of all neuropsychologists, psychiatrists, and philosophers of mind.

A large number of distinguished scientists and philosophers have claimed that we shall never solve the problem – it is insoluble. For example, in 1872 Emil Du Bois-Reymond, the founder of modern electrophysiology, stated his famous formula: *ignoramus et ignorabimus* – we ignore and shall forever ignore the root of mental phenomena. A few years later the neo-Hegelian Francis Bradley denied that "the connection of soul and body is really either intelligible or explicable." Ludwig Wittgenstein went to the extreme of claiming that the hypothesis that we think with the brain is "one of the most dangerous of ideas for a philosopher." Characteristically, he did not explain why. All three men adopted tacitly psychoneural dualism, i.e. the view that mind and body are separate entities.

The great neuroscientist Sir Charles Scott Sherrington (1941) leaned toward psychoneural dualism. He wrote about the "collaboration of brain with psyche" and he asserted confidently that the visual images which come from the left and right angles are conjoined by the mind, not by the brain. However, he did not write off monism in a conclusive way. Thus he admitted that it is practical "to subsume mind under life" (1941, p. 191). And on the next page he wondered how much longer men would go on using the metaphor that mind is the master and body the servant – the animistic metaphor adopted by Plato and revived in our days by Sir John Eccles and Sir Karl Popper (1977). Sherrington was aware that this is just a metaphor, hence no part of a scientific theory, yet he despaired of getting rid of it.

If hard-nosed neuroscientists can adopt uncritically the ancient myth of the immaterial soul or mind, it should come as no surprise to learn that a well-known contemporary psychologist is said to have declared that "All you need to know about brains is how to cook them." An equally well-known philosopher has written that neuroscience is irrelevant to psychology, to the point that "We could be made of Swiss cheese and it wouldn't matter." Many others find comfort in the idea that the mind is a collection of computer programs, and that to undergo a cognitive process is to compute something. This allows them to ignore neuroscience and all the non-cognitive mental functions.

It might be thought that the successes of neuropsychology and biological psychiatry over the past three decades would have discredited psychoneural dualism. But such an impression rests on the tacit hypothesis that everyone interested in the mind–body problem is curious over recent findings about the two aspects of the problem, i.e. the psychological and the physiological. (Notice that the problem is said to have two aspects, not that mind and body are two aspects or manifestations of the same thing – the thesis of neural monism.) But obviously that hypothesis is false. People do tend to focus on a single side of every problem, however many-sided it may be. The consequence is that here, as elsewhere, the sectoral approach leads to monocular vision, which in turn prevents depth perception.

We have mentioned only a few views on the mind–body question. It is time to exhibit the whole family.

TEN PHILOSOPHIES OF MIND

There are at least ten different views, or rather species of doctrine, on the nature of mind and its relation to body. These species can be grouped into two broad genera: monism and dualism. Monists assert the unity and dualists the separateness of mind and body. However, there are important differences between the various species in each genus. The list below summarizes the main theses.

1 *Psychoneural monism*

1.1 *Idealism (spiritualism): Everything is mental* (Berkeley, Fichte, Hegel, Fechner, Mach, the later W. James, Whitehead, Teilhard de Chardin, and B. Rensch).

1.2 *Neural monism or double aspect doctrine: The mental and the physical are so many manifestations of an unknowable neutral substance* (Spinoza, at one time W. James, B. Russell, R. Carnap, M. Schlick, H. Feigl, and radical informationism, or the thesis that everything in the world is information).

1.3 *Eliminative materialism: Nothing is mental* (J. B. Watson, B. F. Skinner, and A. Turing).

1.4 *Physicalism or reductionist materialism: Mental events are physical or physico-chemical* (Epicurus, Lucretius, Hobbes, La Mettrie, d'Holbach, I. P. Pavlov, K. S. Lashley, J. J. C. Smart, D. Armstrong, W. V. Quine, and possibly the connectionist models currently in vogue, since they are said to apply equally to brains and computers).

1.5 *Emergentist materialism: Mental processes constitute a subset of processes in brains of higher vertebrates* (Diderot, Darwin, Ramón y Cajal, T. C. Schneirla, C. Judson Herrick, D. Hebb, D. Bindra, T. H. Bullock, R. W. Doty, G. M. Edelman, V. Mountcastle, J. Olds, W. R. Uttal, H. Jerison, S. Dimond, R. F. Thompson, and J. Wolpe).

2 *Psychoneural dualism*

2.1 *Autonomism: The mental and the neural are unrelated* (F. H. Bradley and L. Wittgenstein).

2.2 *Psychophysical parallelism: Every mental event is accompanied by a synchronous neural event* (Leibniz, R. H. Lotze, W. Wundt, H. Jackson, the young Freud, and some Gestaltists).

2.3 *Epiphenomenalism: Mental events are caused by neural ones* (T. H. Huxley, C. Vogt, C. D. Broad, A. J. Ayer, and R. Puccetti).

2.4 *Animism: Mental events cause neural or physical ones* (Plato, St Augustine, and computationalist cognitive psychology, according to which people and computers are run by immaterial programs).

2.5 *Interactionism: Mental events cause or are caused by neural or physical ones, the brain being only the tool or "material basis" of the mind* (Descartes, W. McDougall, the mature Freud, W. Penfield, R. Sperry, J. C. Eccles, K. R. Popper, and N. Chomsky).

In short, at least ten solutions to the mind–body problem have been sketched, and every one of them is part of some philosophical school. But, of course, this does not entail that only philosophers are competent to handle the problem. On the contrary: when cacophony reigns in a philosophical field, it may be the chance for scientists to step in and introduce some order.

THE RELEVANCE OF SCIENCE TO PHILOSOPHY

We shall argue that science is relevant to philosophy and, in particular, to the problem of settling the disputes among the ten philosophies of mind outlined in the previous section.

Let us see what science has to say about these philosophies. To begin with 1.1 or idealism, it is untenable for it entails that all the sciences are reducible to mentalist psychology. This thesis, which was actually held by Ernst Mach, is manifestly false, if only because psychologists do not investigate atoms, electromagnetic fields, chemical reactions, cell division, and the like, except insofar as these things affect sentient beings.

As for 1.2 or neural monism, it is not a scientific doctrine because it postulates that the neural substance cannot be investigated, and because it does not explain how that unknowable substance can now appear as physical, now as mental.

Eliminative materialism (1.3) is at variance with our raw experience of mental processes, as well as with the fact that psychologists happen to investigate these and have even discovered some regularities concerning memory, learning, affect, and other kinds of mental phenomena.

Physicalist or reductionist materialism (1.4) is too simplistic to be true. Indeed, it makes no room for the emergent properties of nervous tissue or even for the peculiarities of organisms vis-à-vis physical or chemical systems.

The elimination of the first four monistic views leaves us with 1.5, or emergentist materialism. It holds that mental functions are brain functions that emerge in the course of individual development, and which have emerged in the course of evolution. (More precisely, every mental function is a process in some brain subsystem. Hence, if the latter alters in any way, so does the function it discharges.)

This view is attractive for being no less than the philosophy underlying physiological psychology. Indeed, the goals of this science are precisely (a) to identify the neural systems that perform the known psychological functions, (b) to discover the possible psychological functions of certain neural systems, in the hope of enriching the list of mental phenomena, (c) to explain the mental in terms of neurophysiological mechanisms such as long-term potentiation and dendritic sprouting and pruning, and (d) to supply to psychiatry the knowledge required to treat mental illness by acting upon the nervous system.

Even a quick perusal of the recent scientific literature should convince anyone that this enterprise has been highly successful, not only in terms of findings but also for having opened up a huge mine of intriguing scientific and medical problems likely to be tackled in the course of the next few decades. Suffice it to recall the following ones: At what point in evolution did ideation begin? At what stage in human development does reasoning start? Which are the smallest neuron assemblies capable of performing mental functions? Where and how do the outputs of the various visual systems (those perceiving shape, color, texture, and motion) become synthesized into percepts? Which subsystem of the human brain can perform computations proper? How do emotions drive or inhibit imagination and reasoning? How do mental processes affect the immune system? Which are the mechanisms of the actions of drugs on the various mental processes? Is there a cure for depression? What are the mechanisms of Alzheimer's disease and how can they be blocked? Can live prostheses replace damaged parts of the human brain?

Notwithstanding the achievements and heuristic power of emergentist materialism, we have yet to examine its dualist rivals, to which we now turn.

Autonomism, or 2.1, is too far-fetched to be believable. Even folk psychology knows of psychosomatic effects, such as blushing and the increase in morbidity caused by grief, as well as the mental deficits caused by brain injuries such as strokes.

Psychophysical parallelism, or 2.2, is too vague. It does not tell us what makes the mental peculiar or what the synchronization mechanism could be. In fact, it is so vague that it may be regarded as being confirmable by any data about the "correlation" of the mental and the physiological. Still, given its popularity, we shall have to take a closer look at it later.

The third dualistic view, epiphenomenalism or 2.3, leaves the mental unexplained and involves the obscure notion of one of the "substances" acting upon the other. Now, the notion of action is clear for concrete things such as photons, molecules, cells, and whole organisms, because in these cases we can often describe their states and changes of state, as well as the mechanisms of such changes. For example, we understand, at least in principle, what it is for a center of the will, located in a frontal lobe, to act upon the motor strip; or for an organ of emotion, belonging to the limbic system, to act upon the immune system. But the idea of something material acting upon, or even secreting, an immaterial entity, or the converse, is obscure. Moreover, such a hypothesis is experimentally untestable, because laboratory tools can only alter or measure properties of material objects.

What holds for epiphenomenalism holds for animism or 2.4, as well as for interactionism or 2.5. In fact these two views share the concept of mind that occurs in ordinary discourse and they do not bother to elucidate the even fuzzier idea that the mind acts on the brain or the other way round.

Let us go back for a moment to psychophysical parallelism or 2.2. This is the most attractive of all the varieties of psychoneural dualism for the following reasons. First, it jibes with the popular idea that, although mind and body are separate, they are somehow related to one another. Second, it allows physicists, chemists, and biologists to go about their business without bothering about the possibility that their mental processes directly influence their laboratory operations. Third, it forgives those psychologists who take no interest in the brain.

Still, parallelism and the other varieties of psychoneural dualism have several fatal flaws. First, because dualism takes the mental for granted, it writes off the problem of accounting for its emergence in the course of evolution and individual development. Second, it blocks research into the neural mechanisms of mental processes, as well as into the interactions between such processes, on the one hand, and muscular, visceral, endocrine, and immune processes on the other. Third and consequently, dualism hinders the advancement of psychiatry, psychosomatic medicine, and clinical psychology. In sum, psychoneural dualism is worse than barren. It is an obstacle to the advancement of science and medicine. Fortunately, this obstacle can easily be removed with a bit of philosophical analysis, as will be seen.

CRITERIA FOR CHOOSING AMONG RIVAL VIEWS

How does one choose among rival scientific hypotheses or theories, particularly when two or more of them seem to fit the known facts equally well? When evaluating any view concerning a domain of facts, one should check whether it complies with the following requirements: (1) *Intelligibility*: Is the view clear or obscure? If somewhat obscure, can it be elucidated and eventually formalized, or is it inherently fuzzy and therefore not susceptible to development? (2) *Logical consistency*: Is the view internally consistent or does it contain contradictions? If it does contain inconsistencies, can these be removed by altering or dropping some of the assumptions without giving up the most important ones? (3) *Systemicity*: Is the view a conceptual system (in particular a theory) or part of one, or is it a stray conjecture that cannot enjoy the support of any other bit of knowledge? If a stray, can it be developed into a hypothetico-deductive system or embedded in one? (4) *Literalness*: Does the view make any literal statements or is it just a metaphor? If an analogy, is it shallow or deep, barren or fertile? And is it indispensable or can it be replaced with a literal account? (5) *Testability*: Can the view be checked conceptually (against previously accepted items of knowledge) or empirically (by observation or experiment), or is it impregnable to criticism and experience? (6) *Empirical support*: If the view has been tested, have the test results been favorable, unfavorable, or inconclusive? (7) *External consistency*: Is the view compatible with the bulk of knowledge in all the fields of scientific research? (8) *Originality*: Is the view novel? And does it solve any outstanding problems? (9) *Heuristic power*: Is the view barren or does it raise new and interesting research or application problems? (10) *Philosophical soundness*: Is the view compatible with the philosophy underlying scientific research, i.e. is it epistemologically realistic or does it involve subjectivism or apriorism (e.g. conventionalism)? And is the view naturalistic or does it posit ghostly items such as immaterial entities or processes beyond experimental control?

Let us check which of the ten philosophies of mind mentioned above comes closest to satisfying these desiderata. Let us start with psychoneural dualism. All five varieties of it are unclear for failing to clarify the very notion of mind, which they take from ordinary knowledge. Epiphenomenalism, animism, and interactionism are afflicted with an additional obscurity, namely the notion of the action of matter on mind or the converse, which is undefined. Because of such a lack of clarity neither of these views can be said to be, or fail to be, internally consistent. Nor do they satisfy the systemicity condition. Indeed, no dualistic hypothetico-deductive system is known. Furthermore most dualists cannot dispense with metaphors. Thus parallelists use the metaphor of the two independent synchronized clocks; animists are fond of the Platonic proportion (mind is to matter what the pilot is to the ship), and psychoanalysts use plenty of physical and anthropomorphic metaphors. But the worst defect of dualism is that, strictly speaking, it is untestable by scientific means. Indeed, if the mind is immaterial, then, unlike the minding brain, it is inaccessible to electrodes, drugs, lancets, and other tools. Moreover, epiphenomenalism, animism, and interactionism are at odds with physics, for they violate the conservation laws. (Epiphenomenalism involves energy loss, whereas animism and interactionism involve energy gain out of nothing material.) Far from being novel, dualism is as old as religion and idealistic philosophy. It is not heuristically powerful either, for it suggests no new experiments and no new conjectures. Finally, dualism is not philosophically sound, for it posits ghostly entities. In sum, dualism fails to pass at least eight out of the ten scientificity tests listed above.

The monistic views, except for neural monism, are reasonably clear, consistent, systemic, literal, and testable. But only emergentist materialism seems to possess the five additional virtues. In fact, it enjoys empirical support – namely all of the findings of psychobiology; it is consistent with what is known in psychology and neuroscience; without being brand new, it is far newer than its rivals; it is heuristically powerful, since it underlies an entire research project, namely that of psychobiology; and it is philosophically sound for being realistic and naturalistic.

Although emergentist materialism postulates that the mind is a set of brain functions, it does not claim that neuroscience is enough to explain subjective experience. Rather it suggests that, because brains are sensitive to social stimuli, mental processes are strongly influenced by society. This implies that neuropsychology must be supplemented by sociopsychology. In technical jargon, emergentist materialism is ontologically halfway reductionist, and in matters epistemological it fosters the merger of psychology with neuroscience rather than the full reduction of the former to the latter. It thus promotes the vigorous interaction of all the branches of psychology.

BIBLIOGRAPHY

Borst, C. V. (Ed.). (1970). *The mind–brain identity theory*. London: Macmillan; New York: St Martin's Press.

Bunge, M. (1980). *The mind–body problem*. Oxford and New York: Pergamon.

Bunge, M., & Ardila, R. (1987). *Philosophy of psychology*. New York: Springer.

Hebb, D. O. (1980). *Essay on mind*. Hillsdale, NJ: Erlbaum.

Hook, S. (Ed.). (1960). *Dimensions of mind*. New York: New York University Press.

Popper, K. R., & Eccles, J. C. (1977), *The self and its brain*. New York: Springer.

Sherrington, C. S. (1941). *Man on his nature*. Cambridge: Cambridge University Press.

Smythies, J. R. (Ed.). (1965). *Brain and mind: Modern concepts of the nature of mind*. London: Routledge & Kegan Paul.

Vesey, G. N. A. (Ed.). (1964). *Body and mind*. London: George Allen & Unwin.

MARIO BUNGE

minimal brain dysfunction (MBD) This term is used to attribute any of a broad class of childhood learning and behavior problems to deviations in brain status.

The ten most frequent symptoms of MBD are HYPERACTIVITY, perceptual-motor impairments, emotional lability, general coordination deficits, disorders of attention, IMPULSIVITY, disorders of memory and thinking, specific learning disabilities, disorders of speech and hearing, and equivocal neurological signs and electroencephalographic irregularities (Clements, 1966). A variety of other relatively specific problems in personality and development, and even psychometric test scatter, are also subsumed within the MBD classification. Problems related to mental retardation, psychiatric disturbance, or frank neurologic injury or disease are explicitly excluded from this category. Although the lack of clear boundaries for the MBD classification makes it difficult to estimate incidence rates, as many as half of the children referred to mental health centers may qualify (Taylor, 1984).

Prior to the guidelines set forth by the MBD Task Force on Terminology and Identification (Clements, 1966), a wide range of terms were used to refer to this category of disorders. Examples included "organic drivenness," "organic behavior disorder," "minimal brain injury," and "minimal cerebral palsy." Terms referring to more specific handicaps were also used, such as "hyperkinetic behavior syndrome," "psychoneurological learning disorders," and "perceptual handicap."

Recognizing that these and other labels made a presumption of brain abnormality in cases where such abnormality could not be proved, the MBD Task Force recommended that the term "Minimal Brain Dysfunction Syndrome" refer to "children of near average, average, or above average general intelligence with certain learning and behavioral disabilities ranging from mild to severe, which are associated with deviations of function of the central nervous system" (Clements, 1966, p. 9). The Task Force report further stipulated that such deviations of function "may manifest themselves by various combinations of impairment in perception, conceptualization, language, memory, and control of attention, impulse, or motor functions" (pp. 9–10).

Analysis of the MBD concept suggests that its meaning is best understood by considering the rationale for this definition (Taylor, 1984). The requirement that children within the MBD category have "near average" or higher intelligence was based on an interest in contrasting major forms of disability, such as mental retardation, with the more minor deviations of function associated with MBD. Parallel contrasts were drawn between (a) the motor incoordination of children with MBD, compared to the outright movement disorders of children with cerebral palsy; (b) the more subtle perceptual and language disabilities of these children, as compared to the primary sensory and language disorders associated with deafness, blindness, or aphasia; (c) the more selective problems in attention, impulse control and affect of children with MBD, compared to the gross deficits in affect and attention observed in children with autism or mental retardation; and (d) the more equivocal deviations of function observed in sensory-motor, cognitive, or electrophysiological examinations of these children, compared to clear-cut abnormalities on the neurological exam or EEG. Examples of equivocal or "soft" neurological findings include gross motor incoordination, poor balance, motor impersistence, difficulties in performing alternating or repetitive motor movements, synkinesias, oculomotor abnormalities, and difficulties in sensory or somatosensory testing (e.g. difficulties in tactile recognition or in two-point discrimination). According to the Task Force report, these and other characteristics of MBD exist "in the absence of findings severe enough to warrant inclusion in an established category, e.g. cerebral palsies, mental subnormalities, sensory defects" (Clements, 1966, p. 9). In essence, the MBD

category was created to recognize the feasibility of a constitutional basis for a broad class of disorders that did not fit into already established diagnostic groupings.

Use of the expression "deviations of function of the central nervous system" served to acknowledge the possibility that biological factors could influence children's learning and behavior, even when outright neurologic impairment was absent. The MBD term, in other words, connoted the conviction that the central nervous system need not be frankly damaged in order for there to be a biological basis for children's learning or behavior disorders. It was appropriate to hypothesize undetected neurological abnormalities, or even nonpathological variations of brain status, as potential explanations for these disorders. According to the Task Force report (Clements, 1966), such neurological abnormalities may involve "genetic variations, biochemical irregularities, perinatal brain insults or other illnesses or injuries sustained during the years which are critical for the development and maturation of the central nervous system, or from unknown causes" (p. 10).

Reference to "various combinations of impairment" underscored the fact that this category of disorders was not well understood and there was considerable overlap of symptomatology. The Task Force report called for further study of specific disorders within the MBD category, in order that subtypes be identified and the full extent of children's problems be appreciated.

Choice of the word "dysfunction," in contrast to "damage," highlighted the fact that the MBD concept was not meant to apply to cases in which impairment was associated with outright disease or injury. By adding the adjective "minimal," the Task Force distinguished the severity of disabilities observed in cases of frank neurological disorder from what were believed to be the more subtle manifestations of MBD. The latter term was also a tacit acknowledgement of the insufficiency of evidence for actual brain abnormality (Benton, 1973).

HISTORICAL BACKGROUND

Reviews of the MBD concepts suggest this term originates most directly from recognition of the fact that demonstrable brain disease frequently has distinct effects on children's behavior and cognition (Taylor, 1984). These effects include learning problems, impulsivity, difficulties in abstract thinking, perseverative tendencies, and perceptual disturbances, all of which may occur in the context of grossly normal intelligence. Observations of similar patterns of disability in patients without demonstrable brain disease, made earlier in the twentieth century, lead investigators to presume underlying central nervous system abnormalities. Strauss and Lehtinen (1947) were among the first to purport that cognitive deficits similar to those seen in brain-injured children justified the diagnosis of "minimal brain injury." Later notions of a "biological gradient of disease" and a "continuum of reproductive casualty" were based on similar logic. According to this view, learning and behavior disorders that were less marked or pervasive than disabilities arising from obvious forms of brain disease were considered to be expressions of milder or subclinical brain pathology.

Other reasons for hypothesizing underlying brain pathology included documentation of specific effects of brain damage on language abilities, personality traits, and academic skills in children of normal intelligence, as well as specific learning and behavior disorders in children without histories of brain disease (Benton, 1973; Taylor, 1984). By the 1960s there was also a growing dissatisfaction with prevailing psychodynamic accounts for children's learning and behavior problems. Organic explanations, in contrast, were becoming increasingly credible. The concept of MBD was meant to complement rather than supplant psychosocial interpretations of these problems. Nevertheless, it had become clear that certain disabilities were difficult to explain solely in terms of family or psychogenic factors. Increasing acceptance of an organic etiology came with observations of similar disorders in other members of the child's family, with the discovery of elevated rates of disorder in children with perinatal complications and in males compared to females, and with demonstration of a positive response to stimulant medications in children with attention deficits.

LIMITATION OF THE MBD CONCEPT

An unfortunate consequence of the term MBD is that it has perpetuated several misconceptions about brain–behavior relationships (Rutter, 1982; Taylor, 1984). According to Denckla (1977), use of the term serves to draw a "loose organic line"

around certain childhood learning and behavior disorders, rather than to indicate a specific diagnosis. Many researchers and clinicians have failed to appreciate this distinction. Use of the term has also been misinterpreted to signify both proof of brain pathology and the existence of a single MBD syndrome. Subsequent analyses have made it clear that the presence of neurological, electrophysiological, or cognitive impairments do not constitute direct proof of underlying neuropathology. There also is no such thing as an MBD syndrome (Benton, 1973; Taylor, 1983). The term MBD itself has contributed to these misconceptions by suggesting that it is the brain, rather than behavior, that is dysfunctional.

Critical reviews of the term also reveal several conceptual flaws. First, MBD symptoms in persons without established brain disease, mental retardation, or emotional disturbance are effectively excluded from consideration. Although the MBD Task Force (Clements, 1966) recognized cases in which MBD symptoms were present in children with frank neurological insults, the concept is overly restrictive. By confining application of the term MBD to children without other diagnoses, the concept precludes study of the association of MBD symptoms to brain disease, mental retardation, and emotional disorder. In so doing, the concept also implies that these symptoms are unique to the MBD category. Both connotations are unfortunate. Study of MBD symptoms found in association with known brain disease or emotional disorder is relevant to an understanding of the sources of these symptoms. Furthermore, relatively isolated impairments in cognitive skills, such as memory and attention, are common sequelae of brain insults, and are frequently found in children without residual neurological abnormalities or general mental deficiency.

A second and related conceptual limitation is the restriction of the MBD label to children of at least near average intelligence. Brain disease in children commonly results in depressed IQ scores in combination with relatively selective cognitive impairments. Requiring at least near average intelligence tends to discourage consideration of biological factors in cases where these factors may be especially relevant.

Third, there is little justification for the concept's assumption of a brain–behavior isomorphism. Mild forms of behavioral deviation do not, in fact, imply milder or subclinical forms of brain pathology. The pathology associated with the types of behavioral deviations included in the MBD category may be just as extensive as that associated with classic neurologic signs. According to Benton (1973, p. 30), the

> mass of evidence points to the fact that cerebral lesions in children must either be quite extensive or have specific disorganizing functional properties in order to produce important behavioral abnormalities. It follows, I think, that if the behavioral deviations defining MBD are to be ascribed to brain damage or dysfunction, then that damage or dysfunction can hardly be minimal in character. Nor is there evidence that it is less extensive than the cerebral alterations underlying mental efficiency or cerebral palsy; the differences may well be qualitative in nature.

A fourth conceptual limitation relates to the fact that the symptoms of MBD are as likely to reflect social and emotional influences on the child as they are to be a manifestation of brain integrity. By failing to acknowledge this fact, the MBD concept stifles interest in potential psychosocial determinants on children's learning and behavior problems. Personality characteristics, such as self-esteem, motivation, and temperament, may also contribute to problems of this nature, even in children who do not qualify for formal behavioral or psychiatric diagnoses.

Fifth, the concept is vague and overly inclusive. Apart from the testimony it gives to biological influences on learning and behavior, it provides no guidance as to how meaningful diagnoses might be established. As Rutter states, "the diagnosis of minimal brain dysfunction, at best, is just an uncertain hypothesis, which usually is not open to testing in the individual child, and, at worse, creates a neuromythology, which provides a rather pretentious cloak to cover ignorance" (1982, pp. 25–6).

Finally, the definition of MBD is essentially exclusionary, raising the specter of biological influences in cases where other etiologies are regarded as untenable. The concept is so broad and ambiguous as to include almost any instance of behavioral deviation not easily explained in other ways. A major disadvantage of definitions of this sort is that they create "wastepaper basket" categories of disabilities, inclusion in which is based on uncertainty regarding antecedent conditions rather than on positive evidence. Additional disadvantages of the definition of MBD include

the fact that its use inspires a false sense of confidence with regard to the basis of the child's problems; and that it encourages pathological accounts of individual differences (Satz & Fletcher, 1980).

CONTEMPORARY SIGNIFICANCE

Despite these limitations and the eventual abandonment, by 1980, of the term MBD, the working hypothesis of a constitutional basis for childhood learning and behavior disorders remains viable. The search for pathological correlates of specific developmental disorders, such as attention deficit disorder and learning disabilities, has led to a number of new findings, including the discovery of anomalies in the cellular structure of the brain in individuals with histories of dyslexia (Galaburda, 1989). Indirect evidence for constitutional influences has also accumulated. There is now substantial support for the heritability of some forms of learning disability (Pennington & Smith, 1988). Birth complications – most notably, very low birth weight – have been linked to later difficulties in attention and to other MBD symptoms, even in children with normal neurological histories. MBD-type disorders have also been linked to EEG abnormalities, "soft" neurological findings, deficits in neuropsychological testing, and developmental delays (Taylor & Fletcher, 1983).

In many ways, the MBD concept has had a positive influence on the study of children's learning and behavior problems. This concept has focused attention on a variety of childhood disabilities that do not fall into other clinical classifications. It also has encouraged study of individual differences and of the psychological correlates of learning and behavior problems. In this sense, the term has been an essential stimulus to the creation of the field of child neuropsychology.

CONCLUSION

Although the term MBD has generated substantial confusion in the literature on children's learning and behavior problems, the concept behind the term is both meaningful and historically significant. Contrary to the manner in which the term MBD has been applied in much of the clinical and research literature, classifying a child with MBD does not mean that a biological basis for a given problem can be proved. The term is not intended to refer to a single diagnosis or behavioral syndrome. The concept is construed more fairly as a prediagnostic classification. Viewed from a historical perspective, the term signifies the conviction that organic factors contribute to a number of more or less specific developmental disabilities – that is, those not attributable to outright neurological or sensory defect, mental retardation, or psychiatric disturbance. Attention deficit hyperactivity disorder, and specific learning and language disabilities are contemporary examples of disorders that fall into the MBD category. Other behavioral manifestations of MBD include cognitive deficiencies, equivocal neurological findings, and electrophysiological abnormalities.

The presumption that disorders in the MBD category are constitutionally determined is based on a variety of circumstantial findings. Children to whom the label has been applied often have a family history of similar problems or complicated birth histories. They exhibit abnormalities in psychological, neurological, or electrophysiological testing that are similar to the sequelae of documented brain disease. Finally, one has difficulty accounting for the problems of these children by reference to psychosocial factors alone. Circumstantial evidence of this type continues to be credible and provides some measure of justification for the concept.

In other respects, however, the MBD concept is difficult to defend. Symptoms of MBD are not unique to children in this category, but are found in association with a variety of other developmental and psychiatric disorders. The MBD concept is also based, in part, on the fallacy that there is a direct relationship between the severity of behavioral or developmental impairment and the degree of physiological damage to the brain. Finally, the concept is vague and overly inclusive. The concept tends to be applied whenever reasons for a child's disability are unknown or uncertain, rather than on the basis of identifiable characteristics. By stressing the relevance of constitutional factors alone, the concept discourages multifactorial approaches to the understanding of clinical disorders.

Critical reviews of the MBD concept concur with a need to abandon this term in favor of more descriptive definitions of childhood learning and behavior problems (Benton, 1973; Rutter, 1982;

Taylor, 1983, 1984). These reviews also indicate that it is reasonable for the clinician or the researcher to consider constitutional determinants for disorders in the MBD classification, so long as one admits that the evidence for suspecting biological influences is circumstantial and that such an etiology cannot be proved (Rutter, 1982).

Reviews of the MBD concept have also stressed the importance of distinguishing operational definitions of children's disabilities (e.g. based on level of academic achievement or on clinical symptoms) from cognitive and behavioral correlates of purported etiological significance. This distinction often has been blurred by a tendency of the MBD label to be applied to children on the basis of associated or secondary symptoms alone, such as "soft" neurological signs or cognitive deficits, without reference to the child's learning or behavioral status. Researchers have also emphasized the need to pay more attention to developmental changes and to assess learning and behavioral problems in relation to normative standards (Satz & Fletcher, 1980; Taylor, 1984).

Positive outgrowths of the concept of MBD include: (a) a continued focus on specific disabilities in learning and behavior; (b) the use of neurobehavioral and electrophysiological techniques to investigate subtypes of these disorders; (c) further research on the consequences of documented brain disease in children; and (d) more intensive study of the influences of overall cognitive level, personality characteristics, and psychosocial and environmental variables on children's learning and behavior (Benton, 1973; Taylor, 1984). As Benton (1992, p. 19) states, "although the global concept has proved to be defective, it is serving us well as a starting point for the empirical verification of more meaningful limited forms of organically conditioned behavior disorders."

BIBLIOGRAPHY

Benton, A. L. (1973). Minimal brain dysfunction from the neuropsychological point of view. *Annals of the New York Academy of Sciences, 205*, 29–37.

Benton, A. L. (1992). Developmental neuropsychology: its present status. In A. Benton, H. Levin, G. Moretti, & D. Riva (Eds), *Neurophisologia dell'eta: evalutiva/Developmental*

Neuropsychology (pp. 11–25). Milan: Franco Angeli.

Clements, S. D. (1966). *Minimal brain dysfunction in children – terminology and identification*. NINDB Monograph No. 3. Washington: US Public Health Service.

Denckla, M. B. (1977). The neurological basis of reading disability. In F. G. Roswell & G. Natchez (Eds), *Reading disability: A human approach to learning* (pp. 25–47). New York: Basic Books.

Galaburda, A. M. (1989). Ordinary and extraordinary brain development: anatomical variation in developmental dyslexia. *Annals of Dyslexia, 39*, 67–80.

Pennington, B. F., & Smith. S. D. (1988). Genetic influences on learning disabilities: an update. *Journal of Consulting and Clinical Psychology, 56*, 817–23.

Rutter, M. (1982). Syndromes attributed to "minimal brain dysfunction" in childhood. *American Journal of Psychiatry, 139*, 21–33.

Satz, P., & Fletcher, J. M. (1980). Minimal brain dysfunctions: an appraisal of research concepts and methods. In H. E. Rie & E. D. Rie (Eds), *Handbook of minimal brain dysfunctions: A critical review* (pp. 667–715). New York: Wiley.

Strauss, A., & Lehtinen, L. (1947). *Psychopathology and education of the brain-injured child*. New York: Grune & Stratton.

Taylor, H. G. (1983). MBD: meanings and misconceptions. *Journal of Clinical Neuropsychology, 5*, 271–87.

Taylor, H. G. (1984). Minimal brain dysfunction in perspective. In R. E. Tarter & G. Goldstein (Eds), *Advances in clinical neuropsychology*, Vol. 2 (pp. 207–29). New York: Plenum.

Taylor, H. G., & Fletcher, J. M. (1983). Biological foundations of "specific developmental disorders": methods, findings, and future directions. *Journal of Clinical Child Psychology, 12*, 46–65.

H. GERRY TAYLOR

monism *See* MIND–BODY PROBLEM.

morphagnosia Morphagnosia is one of the forms of tactile agnosia (*see* TACTILE PERCEPTION DISORDERS) and is the inability to identify form from tactile information alone. It is therefore considered a primary disorder of touch, in distinction from STEREOAGNOSIA.

motor aphasia *See* APHASIA.

motor cortex *See* SENSORIMOTOR CORTEX.

motor skill disorders Disorders of the motor system involve a very wide variety of syndromes in which there is disturbance of the ability to plan, initiate, execute, coordinate, sequence, terminate, or inhibit movement. The movement involved may be reflexive, involuntary, or voluntary, it may be simple or complex, it may be observable or private to the individual concerned, and it may or may not be subordinated to a plan which is goal-directed.

All motor behavior and hence all motor disorder is multimodal, and is intimately dependent upon sensory feedback. Coordinated and skilled motor acts cannot be completed without sensory input and feedback. Motor dysfunction may occur primarily as a result of sensory input deficit, sensorimotor system integration disorder, or sensory feedback inefficiency or interruption, as well as motor output deficit per se. Some motor dysfunction syndromes involve various combinations of these dysfunctional modular units. Skilled motor movement requires input from a variety of sensory modalities (tactile, auditory, visual, spatial, proprioceptive, kinesthetic, and others) which provide direction and feedback, as well as cues for goal-directed behavior. Motor skill production does not exist in isolation from other neural systems. Analysis of motor system disorders therefore cannot be complete without a more general analysis of hierarchical functional neural systems that influence behavior at a variety of levels (Luria, 1973, 1980). In fact, motor function is influenced by all other forms of neural activity at all levels of neural organization (Aronson et al., 1971).

The nature of movement must be very broadly conceptualized, however, if one is to appreciate the host of disorders which have an integral motor component. The motor system is influenced by input from all other portions of the nervous system, since it constantly and synergistically interacts with them through voluntary and involuntary feedback loop pathways. The motor system serves as the effector pathway of all observable behavior. Dysfunction of various of its components is manifested as the range of syndromes of clinical neurologic and psychiatric disorders. The range of objective neurologic signs which are partially or totally dependent upon motor function is extensive. A thorough analysis of the many components of motor function constitutes an integral and complex portion of the standard neurological and neuropsychological examinations (for reviews see DeJong, 1967; Luria, 1980).

The very act of thought has been conceptualized as subvocal speech, a motor act, without phonation (Luria, 1973, 1980). Even auditory hallucinations have been shown to be a form of disinhibited subvocal speech. When hallucinating psychotic patients have their subvocal speech recorded with an ultrasensitive microphone placed over their vocal cords, and the speech is then amplified and played back to them, they recogize the recorded voice as that of their auditory hallucination (for review see Salzinger, 1986, p. 129).

The motor system is functionally and hierarchically organized (Luria, 1980). Its syndromes can be best understood when they are multiply analyzed through a variety of anatomic and cognitive-behavioral functional system schemas. This review will employ both approaches to the material. Neurologic motor disorder syndromes commonly present with signs that involve muscular atrophy, abnormal muscular tone as in spasticity or flaccidity of voluntary muscles, pathologic reflex activity, incoordination, motoric sequencing difficulty, sensorimotor integration disturbance, disinhibition with such complex behavioral motor syndromes as impulsiveness and hyperactivity, and executive planning difficulties that lead to such signs as motor perseveration.

A recently reclassified group of progressive, degenerative, subcortical neurologic disorders of the brain produce similar dementing syndromes, and all of them are associated with various forms of movement disorder due to dysfunction of various elements of the extrapyramidal motor system. Some of these signs and symptoms of motor system disorder will be noticed in routine clinical observation; others, particularly the complex behavioral motor disorders such as the APRAXIAS, may require specialized testing to be recognized.

NEUROLOGIC MOTOR SYNDROMES

Neurologic syndrome analysis of motor disorders traditionally divides them anatomically into those that involve dysfunction of the upper or lower motor neurons. The syndromes that are associated with each of these lesion categories are diagnostically distinct. They are important to recognize clinically since this level of analysis generally distinguishes syndromes that are characteristic of lesions of the brain and the brain stem from those that are associated with lesions of the spinal cord and the peripheral nerves.

Upper motor neuron syndrome The upper motor neuron (UMN) complex involves any motor neuron that originates in the central nervous system above the level of the spinal cord and which synapses either directly or through interneuronal relays on an anterior horn (motor) cell of the spinal cord. UMN circuits are located entirely within the central nervous system. Influences on the motor system by way of the UMN system include the input from the cerebral cortex, the basal ganglia, and the cerebellum. The corticospinal or pyramidal tract is involved in all voluntary movement of skeletal muscle of the torso, arms, and legs. The corticobulbar tract is the portion of the voluntary motor pathway that innervates the skeletal muscle groups of the soft palate, larynx, pharynx, tongue, portions of the neck, the mouth, cheeks and lips, and the eyelids from motor nuclei in the pontine and medullary brain stem. A lesion of any portion of the corticospinal or corticobulbar tracts of the UMN functional system thus can effect interaction and feedback among a wide variety of effector organs and body parts that are intimately involved in speech, emotional expression, and gross motor behavior. It should also be noted that disturbance in any key portion of the UMN system will also change the integrative unity and functional integrity or balance of the UMN system as a whole, but the system is hierarchically organized and can provide compensatory adjustments for the dysfunctional elements. The nature of these patterns of dysfunction and sparing of motoric functional systems forms the basis of motoric syndrome analysis in neurologic and psychiatric disorder.

Upper motor neuron: corticospinal/corticobulbar syn-

dromes Neurologic clinicians typically limit UMN syndrome analysis to discussion of the clinical effects of lesions of the corticospinal or corticobulbar tracts. A complex of symptoms classically characterizes lesions that involve the corticospinal tract, although variants from the full syndrome occur clinically. These symptoms include abnormally increased muscle tone at rest which may be associated with SPASTICITY, paralysis or weakness (paresis) of the face and/or extremities (arm held in flexion, leg in extension) contralateral to the side of the brain lesion, relative absence of atrophy (unless due to disuse), pathologic briskness or increase in magnitude of muscle stretch (deep tendon) reflexes, loss of cutaneous reflexes, and presence of pathologic reflexes, particularly the reflex sign of Babinski (lifting of the great toe and fanning of the small toes when the base of the foot is stroked).

With a lesion of the voluntary motor nuclei of the brain stem or of the corticobulbar tracts which innervate them one should examine and question the patient as well as consult the medical history to identify difficulties with swallowing (dysphagia), difficulties with phonation such as hoarseness, and impairment of speech production due to weakness or paralysis of the mouth, tongue, cheeks, or lips that can lead to speech slurring or garbling in the syndromes of DYSARTHRIA (partial motor speech impediment) or ANARTHRIA (speech incoherence due to severe oral-facial motor impairment).

Upper motor neuron: cerebellar syndrome Normally the cerebellum coordinates muscular activity of antagonistic muscle groups (flexors and extensors) through relaxation of one portion of the muscular functional system while the opposed portion of the system contracts. This synergistic muscular coordination allows for the smooth and precise action of voluntary movement once the basic motor skill learning period for the activity has been accomplished. In disease of cerebellar origin there is a complex of associated signs that show disruption of this normal voluntary muscular coordination activity. The affected patient shows a complex syndrome that includes "ATAXIA, rebound, dysmetria, inability to perform rapidly successive movements (adiadochokinesia) and a gross tremor on voluntary movement" (Aronson et al., 1971). ATAXIA is a general term that involves the incoordination of muscles or associated muscular groups so that coordinated

voluntary activity is disturbed. The concept of ATAXIA is frequently used in analysis of disorders of GAIT, which will be considered as a group of syndromes in a subsequent section of this review. The action or intention tremor noted as a sign of cerebellar disease is discussed with the syndromes of tremor.

Rebound refers to inability to return the limb accurately to its original position (usually the arm) after it has been suddenly displaced. To test for this sign the examiner has the patient sit with the eyes closed and the arms extended horizontally forward from the shoulders with the palms downward. The patient is instructed to hold the arms in this position and to return them to this position if they are moved. A light tap to the back of the wrist produces a small displacement and a rapid return to the original position in a normal individual. In the patient with diffuse cerebellar disease the same light tap stimulus produces a large downward movement of the arm and oscillating movement of the arm above and below the original position as the patient attempts to steady it. The excessive movement of the limb when lightly touched is a sign of impairment of *motor check*. The oscillatory movement about the original static position of the arm is the *rebound* sign of cerebellar disease.

Dysmetria is "a disturbance of the trajectory or placement of a body part during active movements. Hypometria refers to a trajectory in which the body part falls short of its goal, and hypermetria indicates a trajectory in which the body part extends beyond its goal" (Gilman et al., 1981, p. 206). To test for dysmetria affecting the arms, the patient is asked to alternately touch his or her own nose and the finger of the examiner held at arm's length from the patient's face. As the patient succeeds in reaching the target, the examiner quickly moves the target finger to a new static position and the patient dynamically continues the task of trying to touch the examiner's finger in the new target position. In the legs, dysmetria can be tested by asking the patient to bring the heel of one leg to the knee of the other and to move the heel of the flexed leg from the knee to the ankle of the other leg and back again to the knee. Alternatively, this sign can be tested in one leg at a time by having the patient recline on his or her back, bend the knee of one leg that is raised about two feet above the hip, and point with the great toe of the elevated foot to the finger of the examiner, which is held within reach of the patient's toe in this position (Aronson et al., 1971).

Adiadochokinesia is a general term that literally means impairment of the ability to perform a series of movements. It is important to avoid confusion of the localizing significance of signs of neurologic disease of cerebellar origin with syndromes of motor sequencing that involve complex motor planning associated with cerebral cortical dysfunction of the premotor areas. Cerebral cortical motor sequencing tasks involve planning and verbal mediation as a rule; cerebellar-mediated tasks do not. Cerebellar testing for this syndrome therefore involves simple, repetitive movement sequences. Testing for this syndrome can be carried out separately for the arms, legs, and oral-facial muscles, particularly the tongue.

Alternate, rapid pronation and supination of one or both open hands is a common test for this sign *in the arms*. An alternative method of testing for this sign in the arms is to ask the patient to extend the hands in front of the chest with the elbows bent and to wiggle the fingers vertically in the manner of typing or playing the piano. The examiner demonstrates the behavior and the patient imitates it. It is important to include this feature, since the various forms of APRAXIA involve inability to carry out the action voluntarily to command without impairment of the ability to imitate the action when it is seen. Imitation of the action of the examiner also eliminates the possibility of error due to an auditory comprehension deficit that could impair the patient's ability to understand the task if it were presented verbally without demonstration. Allowance should be made for greater speed and dexterity of the dominant hand in each case of manual motor coordination.

In the legs the syndrome can be assessed by asking the patient to sit in a chair so the heel and toe of the foot are flat on the ground and then to tap rapidly with the ball of the foot on the floor without raising the heel from the floor.

In the mouth the syndrome is examined by asking the patient to open the mouth, extend the tongue beyond the lips, and move it from side to side as rapidly as possible. In the case of oral-facial weakness without involvement of the tongue, the patient alternatively may be asked to protrude and retract the tongue rapidly and repeatedly.

It is important to emphasize that the cerebellar syndromes are not isolated motoric dysfunction phenomena. The cerebellum receives rich sensory input by way of the spinocerebellar tracts through the inferior cerebellar peduncles, which convey specific proprioceptive and kinesthetic information about muscle tone and joint movement and position sense. By way of the middle cerebellar peduncle (brachium pontis) the cerebellum also receives input from the cerebral cortex that subordinates cerebellar activity to goal-directed activity, which is accomplished with the aid of verbal mediation or thought, which is a subvocal form of motor speech. Syndrome analysis also requires appreciation of the numerous modular elements of the motoric functional system of which the cerebellum is an integral part. Lesions of skeletal "muscles, of peripheral nerves, of posterior (spinal) columns, and of the frontal and postcentral cerebral cortex" (Aronson et al., 1971) can all individually or jointly produce a behavioral syndrome that can be confused with central cerebellar dysfunction. The dysfunction of the muscular coordination functional system can clearly be seen to involve sensory pathways (posterior columns, postcentral cerebral cortex, sensory peripheral nerves) as well as primarily motor elements. The integrity of sensorimotor function and the dependence of coordinated movement on accurate sensation is important to appreciate in all forms of voluntary activity.

Lower motor neuron syndrome The lower motor neuron (LMN) involves the anterior loop of the spinal reflex arc, the anterior horn cells of the spinal cord, the anterior spinal roots, and the peripheral motor nerves. LMN signs common to all lesions of this functional system involve flaccid, focal paralysis of anatomically localized muscular groups that are innervated by the lesioned cord level segment or dermatome, the presence of muscular atrophy or wasting, diminution or abolition of deep tendon reflexes (due to loss of the motor portion of the spinal reflex arc at the affected level), and intact sensation.

Extrapyramidal motor disorders Motor tracts of UMN origin that do not pass through the medullary pyramids with the corticospinal tract are collectively grouped as the extrapyramidal motor system. The extrapyramidal motor system anatomic structures are subcortical and include the caudate nucleus, putamen, globus pallidus, subthalamic nucleus, red nucleus, and substantia nigra. Some authorities also include the thalamus and the cerebellum in the extrapyramidal system.

The extrapyramidal motor system subunits are complexly and systemically interactive with each other and with the corticospinal tract (for a review see Adams & Victor, 1989). When the corticospinal tract is lesioned in clinical syndromes the extrapyramidal tracts are often affected as well, either directly or collaterally, through their intermingled anatomic pathways in the corona radiata, which course together with each other and with the corticospinal tract in this region. Current neuroscientific evidence attributes the signs of spasticity associated with the typical UMN lesion to dysfunction of the extrapyramidal system, since experimental animal models of pure corticospinal tract lesions do not produce spasticity. Also of interest from the experimental animal and human clinical literature is the finding that extrapyramidal tract sparing in the presence of focal, unilateral corticospinal tract lesions produces an initial period of flaccid hemiplegia with subsequent recovery of a considerable variety of voluntary movements. Remaining movements that return after recovery are typically slow relative to the premorbid state, and fine finger movements that are dependent upon corticospinal tract input remain dysfunctional permanently as a result of the focal corticospinal lesion (Adams & Victor, 1989, p. 44). These syndrome analytic findings highlight the general principles that the central nervous system's hierarchical organization of motor functions allows for at least partial compensation of dysfunctional elements of the system as a whole in the presence of disease, and that many voluntary motoric behaviors are significantly dependent upon the pyramidal as well as the extrapyramidal motor systems for their execution.

Extrapyramidal motor disorders associated with dementia Many of the extrapyramidal syndromes involve involuntary movement abnormalities which are among the primary signs of these degenerative neurologic disorders. Some of these movement disorder syndromes also involve associated cognitive deficits, symptoms of pathologic mood and personality alteration, memorial impairment, abstract and conceptual reasoning difficulty, and inefficient, slowed mental processing. These are the key symptoms that have been associated with the newly recognized generic syndrome of subcortical DEMENTIA (Cummings, 1990).

Neurologic disorders with extrapyramidal motor dysfunction in which the syndrome of subcortical dementia has been identified include PARKINSON'S DISEASE, HUNTINGTON'S DISEASE, progressive supranuclear palsy, familial and idiopathic calcification of vessels in the basal ganglia, spinocerebellar degenerative syndromes, THALAMIC SYNDROME degeneration, LACUNAR STATE, Binswanger's disease (a multi-infarct dementia syndrome with subcortical vascular encephalopathy), WILSON'S DISEASE (hepatolenticular degeneration), multiple sclerosis, AIDS encephalopathy, subcortical sarcoidosis, normal-pressure hydrocephalus, dementia pugilistica, and Bechet disease with neurologic complications (Cummings, 1990; Adams & Victor, 1989).

Involuntary motor disorders of the extrapyramidal system commonly involve symptoms or symptom complexes of CHOREA, ATHETOSIS, DYSTONIA, ATAXIA, ballism (called hemiballism or HEMIBALLISMUS when one side of the body is affected; called monoballism when only one limb is affected), and a variety of disturbances of GAIT. Ataxia is discussed earlier in this article under the cerebellar syndrome portion of the UMN category presentation, since it is a cardinal sign of cerebellar disorder. The differential diagnosis of involuntary movement disorder of neurologic origin is complex but has been well summarized in the standard psychiatric diagnostic nomenclature (American Psychiatric Association, 1987, p. 79) as follows:

Choreiform movements are dancing, random, irregular, nonrepetitive movements. *Dystonic movements* are slower, twisting movements interspersed with prolonged states of muscular tension. *Athetoid movements* are slow, irregular, writhing movements, most frequently in the fingers and toes, but often involving the face and neck. *Myoclonic movements* are brief, shocklike contractions that may affect parts of muscles or muscle groups, but not synergistically. *Hemiballistic movements* are intermittent, coarse, large amplitude, unilateral movements of the limbs. *Spasms* are stereotypic, slower, more prolonged than tics, and involve groups of muscles. *Hemifacial spasm* consists of irregular, repetitive, unilateral jerks of facial muscles. *Synkinesis* consists of movements of the corner of the mouth when the person intends to close the eye, and its converse. *Dyskinesias*, such as tardive

501

dyskinesia, are oral-buccal-lingual masticatory movements of the face and choreoathetoid movements of the limbs.

Disorders of gait A number of specific clinical disturbances of gait that are typical of neurologic disease have been identified. Observation of these gait disorders *as motor behaviors* need not require specialized testing, but appreciation of this portion of motor syndrome analysis is rare in neuropsychological evaluation. It tends to be the province of the neurologist or neurosurgeon. Knowledge of gait disorders and their neurologic implications will increase the neuropsychologist's acumen and will aid in the initial assessment of the level and kind of neurologic dysfunction that affects the central or peripheral nervous system. For a thorough summary of gait disorders and their relevance to neurologic differential diagnosis see Adams and Victor (1989) or Aronson et al. (1971).

Normal gait is typified by its automatic, effortless quality, the alternate shifting of the weight from one leg to the other, the right-angle association of the pelvis to the weight-bearing leg, erectness of posture, and the presence of arm swing opposite to the stepping foot. In *hemiplegic gait*, in contrast, the affected spastic leg is stiff due to the contralateral UMN lesion, and there is no free movement of the joints of the affected leg. The arm on the paralyzed side of the body is typically spastic as well, which prevents normal arm swing and may affect balance. The toe of the spastic leg tends to face downward, and the spastic leg is moved in a toe-down, stiff circular motion (circumduction), as though the person were trying to trace an arc on the floor with the toe. A *spastic or scissors gait* is one in which both legs are spastically involved, and produces extreme incoordination of the body as a whole. The legs advance in a bilaterally stiffened, jerking fashion which generally affects balance. The affected patient usually tries to maintain a tenuous sense of balance through "compensatory" movements of the arms and trunk. An *ataxic gait* is typically wide-based, clumsy, uneven in stride, swaying, and worsened by eye closure so that visual cues cannot be used to compensate for the motor coordination difficulty. In *steppage gait* the patient has weak ankle flexors so that the foot drops limply and must be raised from the knee to avoid stumbling over the toe. The tendency to appear to be stepping over an invisible obstacle in the manner of a horse accounts for the name of the syndrome. A *waddling gait* results from "weakness of the trunk and pelvic muscles (that) results in a sway-backed and potbellied posture" (Aronson et al., 1971, p. 117) so that the pelvis inclines toward the stepping foot and the torso moves toward the weight-bearing side. The result is a short-step, swaying gait in the manner of a duck. The *propulsive gait* of PARKINSON'S DISEASE is typically accompanied by a stooped posture and a gradually increasing speed of small, shuffling steps so that in the full syndrome the patient appears to be jogging or running in an effort to keep from falling forward. Loss of arm swing and imbalance due to rigidity and stooped posture associated with the disorder may compromise balance and produce lateral or retrograde motion as well in the advanced stages of the disorder, when balance is disturbed due to leaning too far in one direction or the other.

Tremor Disorders which present with tremor as a sign may be seen in some syndromes of extrapyramidal disorder, particularly those of basal ganglionic and cerebellar origin. Tremor involves involuntary, nonpurposive movements of the hands, legs, or occasionally the head or trunk. A number of characteristic motor syndromes of tremor that may be encountered in clinical practice are outlined by Aronson et al. (1971, pp. 109–10). The summary which follows is based on their traditional symptomatic classification schema.

Tremor at rest of a "pill-rolling" variety is typical of patients with Parkinson's disease.

Tremor of cerebellar origin is associated with a lesion of the dentate nucleus and is characterized by increased tremulousness when voluntary movement is attempted. As the patient reaches more and more closely toward the object to be grasped, the severity of the cerebellar tremor increases. Because of the association of the tremor with the attempt to carry out a voluntary act, this sign has been called an action, kinetic, or intention tremor.

In Wilson's disease a "wing-beating" tremor may be observed. A mild, resting tremor may be present, but it is greatly worsened by the attempt to raise the arms horizontally with the elbows bent at the level of the shoulders. In this position a dramatic vertical tremor is produced in these patients which resembles a "wing-beating" movement of a flying bird.

An unusual "wrist-flapping" tremor syndrome has been reported in patients suffering from advanced liver disease. With the arms outstretched the affected patient alternately flexes and extends the wrists. The fingers also may be alternately spread apart and joined as part of this tremulous syndrome.

Senile tremor is similar to the Parkinsonian syndrome in the features of "degree, amplitude, rate, and occurrence at rest. However, it most commonly affects the head, jaws and lips. The head may nod to and fro or from side to side. Increased muscular tone and other evidences of Parkinson's disease are not observed" (Aronson et al., 1971, p. 110).

A final group of tremulous syndromes is not associated with neurologic deficit. These conditions are collectively grouped as "'essential,' 'tension,' or 'familial,' [and] are absent at rest, appear when the muscles are brought into action to support or move an extremity, and are not intensified toward the termination of movement. Furthermore, they are not associated with rigidity or other evidences of neurologic disease" (Aronson et al., 1971, p. 110).

NEUROPSYCHIATRIC MOTOR SYNDROMES

Tic disorder is a group of related, complex, involuntary neuropsychiatric disorders of probable genetic origin. The stereotyped behavior pattern associated with TIC disorder may involve nonpurposive movement or vocalization and may be simple or complex. Examples of various tic behaviors are given with this general definition of this class of disorders in the standard psychiatric nomenclature (American Psychiatric Association, 1987, p. 78):

A tic is an involuntary, sudden, rapid, recurrent nonrhythmic, stereotyped, motor movement or vocalization. It is experienced as irresistible, but can be suppressed for varying lengths of time. All forms of tics are often exacerbated by stress and usually are markedly diminished during sleep. They may become attenuated during some absorbing activities, such as reading or sewing.

Perhaps the best known of the developmental period onset tic disorders is Tourette's disorder or GILLES DE LA TOURETTE syndrome. This variant of the tic syndrome presents with one or more vocal tic behaviors and multiple motor tic behaviors on a regular, usually more than daily basis. The frequency, specific nature, and combination of vocal and motor tics is changeable and unpredictable in individual cases.

Akathisia is a syndrome of motor restlessness which is commonly encountered as a side effect of neuroleptic medication for psychiatric disorders. The affected patient subjectively feels impelled to remain in constant motion. Common symptoms of the disorder involve pacing and restless, nonpurposive movements of the hands and feet.

CEREBRAL CORTICAL MOTOR SYNDROMES

Syndromes of cerebral cortical dysfunction are typically expressions of disinhibition and stimulus-bound response which is not subordinated to a goal-directed plan. Such plans normally are formulated with the aid of explicit or implicit language (thought). The cerebral cortex can normally control its sensory input from brain stem and even spinal levels through reciprocal feedback loops that allow only information that is relevant to the current task to reach consciousness. In cerebral dysfunction syndromes, particularly those of the frontal lobes, these inhibitory mechanisms are disturbed and the patient may respond to task-irrelevant stimuli simply because they are perceptually salient.

Simple motor cortical dysfunction appears as slowing of *fine motor speed*, as in slowed finger tapping. Multistep, novel motor sequences that require sequential organization become desynchronized or disorganized in the patient with a lesion of the premotor frontal zone, even though related single-step-component motor tasks and goal-directed, evaluative skills remain unimpaired. A lesion of the oral portion of the premotor area may result in speech dysfluency since individual words cannot be motorically sequenced. Visual-spatial-motor cortical dysfunction is often manifested as *echopraxia*, a sign in which patients passively mirror-image the hand or arm positions of a confronting examiner when they are asked to perform them with the same hand, which requires a response opposite to the perceptual stimulus. *Perseveration* occurs when the cortically disinhibited patient fails to suppress stimulus-bound, impulsive guesses at initial solutions and subsequently fails to make use of feedback to compare response outcome with the original response goal.

503

Failure to self-correct errors using feedback based on prior performance evaluation leads to repetition of the initial impulsive guess at the task solution, which is usually based on incomplete, inaccurate information. Replacement of accurate, goal-directed motor behaviors with stereotyped responses is particularly common in perseverative patients with lesions of the frontal lobes. For extensive discussions of motor syndrome variants associated with cerebral cortical lesions and their underlying mechanisms, see the reviews by Luria (1973, 1980).

BIBLIOGRAPHY

Adams, R. D., & Victor, M. (1989). *Principles of neurology*, 4th edn. New York: McGraw-Hill Information Services (Health Professions Division).
American Psychiatric Association. (1987). *Diagnostic and statistical manual of mental disorders*, 3rd edn, rev. Washington: American Psychiatric Association.
Aronson, A. E., Bastron, J. A., Brown, J. R., Burton, R. C., Corbin, K. B., Darley, F. L., Engel, A. G., Goldstein, N. P., Gomez, M. R., Groover, R. V., Howard, F. M. Jr., Klass, D. W., Lambert, E. H., Millikan, C. H., Mulder, D. W., Rooke, E. D., Rushton, J. G., Sandok, B. A., Siekert, R. G., Thomas, J. E., Waltz, A. G., & Whisnant, J. P. (1971). *Clinical examinations in neurology*, 3rd edn. Philadelphia: W. B. Saunders.
Cummings, J. L. (Ed.). (1990). *Subcortical dementia*. New York: Oxford University Press.
DeJong, R. N. (1967). *The neurologic examination: incorporating the fundamentals of neuroanatomy and neurophysiology*, 3rd edn. New York: Harper & Row (Hoeber Medical Division).
Gilman, S., Bloedel, J. R., & Lechtenberg, R. (1981). *Disorders of the cerebellum*. Philadelphia: F. A. Davis.
Luria, A. R. (1973). *The working brain: An introduction to neuropsychology*. (Basil Haigh, Trans.). New York: Basic Books.
Luria, A. R. (1980). *Higher cortical functions in man*, 2nd edn. New York: Basic Books.
Salzinger, K. (1986). Diagnosis: distinguishing among behaviors. In T. Millon & G. L. Klerman (Eds), *Contemporary directions in psychopathology: Toward the DSM-IV* (pp. 115–34). New York: Guilford.

JAMES A. MOSES JR.

mouthing movements Mouthing movements are abnormal involuntary movements of the mouth and tongue similar to the movements normally employed in chewing, although other movements similar to licking, kissing, and pouting may also occur. The phenomenon occurs most commonly in *tardive dyskinesia*, which is a chronic neurological disorder secondary to the administration of neuroleptics (major tranquillizers), but mouthing movements also occur in CHOREA and DYSTONIA, in conditions which include post-encephalitic states (*see* ENCEPHALITIS), GILLES DE LA TOURETTE SYNDROME, HUNTINGTON'S DISEASE, and WILSON'S DISEASE. In common with the pathology of all these disorders, mouthing movements are associated with lesions of the basal ganglia.

movement disorders *See* APRAXIA; ATAXIA; GAIT; HEMIPLEGIA; SPASTICITY.

MRI *See* MAGNETIC RESONANCE IMAGING.

multi-infarct dementia *See* DEMENTIA.

multiple sclerosis Multiple sclerosis (MS) is the most common neurodegenerative disease affecting young adults. A prevalence rate of 1 in 2,000 has been recorded. MS ranks as the greatest cause of neurological disability in adults under 50 years old.

One of the most striking features of the disease is its variability; this applies both to the clinical symptomatology and to the disease course. Some of the initial signs include weakness in one or more limbs (40 percent), optic neuritis (22 percent), paresthesia (21 percent), diplopia (12 percent), vertigo (5 percent), and disturbance of micturition (5 percent), (Swash & Schwartz, 1989). Although the disease course cannot be predicted with certainty, a classification of two types has evolved to assist clinical and research work. In the first type, the disease pursues a malignant course, devoid of any significant remission of symptoms, with death usually occurring within five years. This specific form of the disease, known as the chronic progressive type, pertains to approximately 10 percent of the entire MS population. In the remaining 90 percent, the disease course is characterized by periods of successive attacks and improvements and is known as the relapsing remitting type. In 5 to 15 percent of the latter group, relapses may be 20–25 years apart, with such patients not enduring any significant disability from initial onset. In the advanced stages of the disease, patients are often wheel-chair-bound. Spasticity, fatigue, ataxia, sensory loss, and urinary incontinence are common symptoms and patients almost invariably present with visual deficits.

NEUROPATHOLOGICAL CORRELATES OF MULTIPLE SCLEROSIS

MS is a multifocal demyelinating disease characterized by damage to or loss of myelin throughout the central nervous system. Early lesions tend to occur as an area of edema centered on a small vein a few millimeters in diameter, with inflammation and an infiltrate of plasma cells, lymphocytes, and macrophages. Myelin is destroyed, so nerve conduction is slowed or blocked, although axons remain relatively preserved. This early inflammatory lesion is later replaced by a gliotic scar or plaque (Warlow, 1991). The pathological presence of multiple sclerotic plaques or lesions is the source of the name for the disease. The identification of the exact size, nature, and location of lesions has become more accurate with the development of techniques such as computerized tomography (CT) and MAGNETIC RESONANCE IMAGING (MRI). Common sites for these lesions include the periventricular white matter, the optic nerve, the pons, the medulla, and the spinal cord. MS lesions are generally confined to the white matter although lesions of the white–gray matter junction and the gray matter have been reported (Rao, 1986). The severity of the clinical symptoms depends at least in part on the size and location of each lesion. There is also evidence that not all lesions produce symptoms of neurological dysfunction. In some patients on whom MRI was performed, a number of lesions were in place for which no clinical signs were recorded during the course of the disease. Similar evidence has also been reported following the autopsy of undiagnosed patients. Another peculiarity is that some patients report an almost complete recovery of function following an acute relapse. While the mechanisms underlying this remission of symptoms are poorly understood, it is generally believed to result from the resolution of edema, thereby leading to improved conduction down the axon.

DIAGNOSING MULTIPLE SCLEROSIS

There are no specific clinical tests for diagnosing MS. One of the greatest difficulties is that the initial symptoms can individually or collectively mimic other conditions. The diagnosis can therefore be seen as one of exclusion, making a neurological examination of current signs and symptoms, as well as an extensive clinical history, quite crucial. The dissemination of lesions in time and place forms the basis for the clinical diagnosis. It is now widely recognized that MRI provides the most sensitive technique for diagnosing MS.

GEOGRAPHIC AND DEMOGRAPHIC FEATURES OF MULTIPLE SCLEROSIS

The geographical distribution of the disease remains a puzzling feature of MS, with the highest rates occurring in temperate zones. Kurtzke (1980) has reported that the highest prevalence occurs in latitudes 43 to 65 degrees north in Europe, 37 to 52 degrees north in the Americas, and 34 to 44 degrees south in Australasia. Moderate then low prevalence rates occur both north and south of these latitudes, as the poles and the Equator are approached. This north/south divide is also apparent within countries. While a prevalence rate of 100 per 100,000 has been reported in the UK, higher incidence rates are reported in the northeast of Scotland with 140 per 100,000, compared with London's 90 per 100,000. Migration studies have revealed that individuals migrating from a high-risk zone to a low-risk zone will take the risk factor of the new country if they migrate prior to reaching 15 years of age. Individuals migrating after this critical age will carry with them the risk factor of their place of birth.

A low prevalence rate among non-Caucasians is an important demographic feature of multiple sclerosis. Women also tend to be more susceptible than men, with a ratio of 1.5:1. Another important demographic feature is the age of onset of MS. Onset generally occurs between the ages of 20 and 50 years with mean age of onset from 29 to 33 years. This particular characteristic has important diagnostic value, as it helps to distinguish MS

505

from other neurodegenerative disorders (e.g. Parkinson's disease).

THE ETIOLOGY OF MULTIPLE SCLEROSIS

The cause of multiple sclerosis is unknown. Extending from the epidemiological factors discussed, much research has attempted to link the etiology of MS with environmental factors. This hypothesis has been supported by the migration studies mentioned above. Others believe a genetic component is responsible, since the frequency of the disease is 30 times greater among the siblings of MS sufferers. Both viral and immunological factors are also influential variables in the bid to find the cause of MS. However, a multifactorial etiology is now more generally accepted. A genetically induced deficiency in immune mechanisms permits the persistence of a "slow virus" infection contracted before the age of 15 years. In adult life the virus is activated (given exposure to specific environmental factors), leading to myelin destruction resulting from harmful auto-immune reactions to some product of myelin breakdown. For the interested reader an excellent review of causation in MS is found in Matthews (1978).

THE NEUROPSYCHOLOGY OF MULTIPLE SCLEROSIS

Cognitive impairments in MS have been recognized since the writings of Charcot in 1877. In his lecture on "The diseases of the nervous system" he said of his MS patients: "The look is vague and uncertain . . . There is marked enfeeblement of the memory; conceptions are formed slowly; the intellectual and emotional faculties are blunted in their totality" (p. 194). Since this time numerous studies have endeavored accurately to estimate the prevalence of cognitive dysfunction in the MS population. Many of these studies have administered a wide range of intelligence tests to preselected groups of MS patients. The results were inconclusive, being as much a reflection of the tests employed and the nature of the MS patients recruited as they were of the cognitive deficits being investigated. Recently the development of more neuropsychological assessment tools has permitted more precise assessments of cognitive dysfunction. A recent study by Grossman and others (1994) reported intellectual functioning to be compromised in 30 to 70 percent of patients

with MS. This wide range is characteristic of the marked variability which typifies all aspects of MS.

Intelligence tests   In a bid to understand the nature of impaired and intact cognitive functioning in MS, many studies have administered general tests of intellectual functioning such as the Wechsler Adult Intelligence Scale Revised (WAIS-R). While comparisons with normal matched controls, other neurologically impaired patients, and psychiatric patients have been reported, the most significant finding to have emerged from these studies has been a consistent significant discrepancy between verbal IQ (VIQ) and performance IQ (PIQ) in the majority of MS patients. In general PIQ has been reported to be between 7 to 14 points lower than VIQ. While lower PIQ scores are generally indicative of impaired visuospatial abilities, it has to be pointed out that success on these subtests depends on fine motor control, coordination, and rapid information processing, in addition to a heavy reliance on visual cues, all of which are likely to be disrupted, given the nature of the neuropathology in MS. Performance tests are also timed and patients with MS can fail the subtests due to pressure of time rather than a failure to conceptualize how the problem ought to be solved. It is therefore not surprising that poor performance is often observed on the digit symbol subtest, a test specifically designed to assess psychomotor speed, sustained attention, visuomotor coordination, and motor persistence. In contrast to performance subtests, verbal subtests are sensitive to the level of education attained and the fund of general knowledge, and are generally not timed. The verbal subtest on which MS patients have the most difficulty is the digit span subtest. Poor performance on this measure reflects deficits in attention/concentration and immediate memory. The common interpretation from these studies is that MS "disrupts dynamic, novel, and conceptual problem-solving abilities, leaving static, over-learned, routinized skills relatively well preserved" (Rao, 1986, p. 513). More recent neuropsychological literature pertaining to cognitive dysfunction in MS has focused on more specific aspects of cognition rather than patterns of general intellectual impairments.

Memory   Impairments of memory are among the most frequently reported deficits in MS patients. While many studies have systematically investigated the nature of memory impairment in MS, there has been considerable variability in findings both between studies and between patients. The source of this variability is twofold: investigators have used different methods for assessing the same and different types of memory and MS patients can present with a broad spectrum of memory impairments, ranging from severe amnesia to no apparent dysfunction. Given the heterogeneity of any group of MS patients, it has been difficult to extract a clear account of the nature of memory disturbances in this disorder. In some of the earlier studies memory was assessed on dimensions such as short-term vs long-term memory or visual vs verbal memory. They used single and multitrial learning paradigms assessing immediate, delayed, and recognition memory. The majority of studies reported that MS patients were more impaired in their ability to learn and recall information than matched normal controls, non-brain-damaged control patients with chronic disabling conditions, and psychiatric patients. The general pattern which emerged from these studies was that short-term and recognition memory capacity were intact, but retrieval strategies from long- and short-term memory were impaired. (A review of these studies can be found in Rao, 1986.)

More recent studies have attempted to elucidate the complex mechanisms underlying impairments of memory in MS. Rao and his colleagues (1989) assessed learning and memory using measures such as the Brown–Petersen distracter task, the story recall test, the free verbal recall test, and the selective reminding test. Their results showed that disturbances of memory in MS patients resulted from an impaired ability to access information from long-term memory while encoding and storage capacity was preserved. A more recent study by Deluca and others (1994) examined whether memory impairments in MS reflect an impairment in the initial acquisition of the information or whether retrieval strategies were at fault, as Rao (1989) had suggested. Verbal memory was assessed by using a selective reminding (SR) task. SR is a verbal list-learning task in which the subject is asked to freely recall a list of 10 words over a maximum of 15 presentations. Subjects continued with the task until all 10 words had been learned and recalled on two consecutive occasions. This ensured that all subjects had learned the complete list and were not beginning the second stage of the task (the recall stage) with an incomplete list of words. Using this procedure DeLuca and his colleagues reported that, while MS patients required a greater number of trials to commit the list to memory relative to normal controls, the two groups did not differ in terms of recall and recognition. They concluded from this study that memory disturbances in MS patients result from impaired acquisition of information in the initial learning phase and not from impaired retrieval, as Rao and others (1989) had suggested.

Other studies have equated the memory impairment observed in MS as comparable to the type of memory disturbances seen in patients with frontal lobe damage. The link is more than coincidental, as MS patients also perform poorly on tests of verbal fluency and measures of concept formation and switching, such as the Wisconsin Card Sorting Test (WCST), both of which are known to be sensitive to frontal impairment. Beatty and colleagues (1989) examined whether the memory impairments in MS patients resembled those in frontal lobe-damaged patients, where there is a failure to benefit from semantic cues which assist learning at the encoding stage. A modification of Wicken's paradigm assessing release from proactive interference (PI) was employed. The result showed that even the MS patients who performed poorly on measures of frontal dysfunction showed a normal release from PI. This meant that MS patients, unlike frontal lobe-damaged patients, do not show impairment in semantic encoding but rather show deficits in processing information rapidly.

It is clear therefore that, while memory impairments are well recognized in MS patients, the mechanisms underlying the disturbance are still poorly understood. Patients differ considerably in the severity of the memory problem with which they present and this variability results in much inconsistency in the literature.

Conceptual reasoning Deficits in conceptual reasoning are also frequently reported in patients with MS. Patients appear to have difficulty forming new concepts, shifting set, and benefiting from environmental feedback. This has regularly been reported on the test of verbal fluency (forming new concepts), and on assessments such as the WCST (Wisconsin Card Sorting Test). On tests of verbal fluency, patients are required to spontaneously produce as many words as possible in a given time (usually 1 minute) in either a specific category (e.g. animals) or beginning with

507

a specific letter (e.g. F, A, or S). A number of studies have reported that MS patients produce fewer words than normal controls. In the WCST, subjects are required to sort cards according to a rule which they discover by trial and error on the basis of feedback from the assessor. On this measure MS patients tend to make more perseverative errors and appear to be generally poorer at "abstracting" the correct concept than are normal controls. While some investigators have speculated that poor performance on this measure might be a function of poor motivation, or impaired attention and memory, the majority of relevant studies have not found a significant correlation between these variables and patients' poor performance.

Other cognitive deficits Other cognitive abilities which are reported to be impaired in MS patients include visuospatial and visuoconstructional functioning. Patients perform well below premorbid levels of ability on performance subtests of the WAIS-R in comparison to normal matched controls. It is unclear from the existing evidence whether poor performance results from an impairment in processing complex visuospatial information or whether poor performance results from primary motor or sensory deficits. Since one of the initial symptoms in MS is optic neuritis, it is not uncommon for MS patients to present with visual deficits. Impairment on measures such as the PASAT (Paced Auditory Serial Addition Test) indicate that some MS patients perform poorly on measures of sustained attention and executive functions. PASAT is an addition task in which subjects are aurally presented with a series of numbers at a speed of one number every two seconds. The task for the subject is to add each number to the number which directly preceded it (e.g. if the subject was presented with 3, 6, 2, 3, the subject would respond 9, 8, 5).

Language Language functions are generally believed to be preserved in patients with MS although a handful of studies have reported dysphasia in a selective number of cases (see Rao, 1986, for review). Since all MS studies are group studies, and averages are usually calculated per MS subgroup, isolated impairments of this kind might well go unnoticed.

In summary, MS patients present with impairments of memory, conceptual reasoning, visuoperceptual abilities, and on tasks requiring rapid processing of information, all within the context of generally preserved language ability. This pattern of impairments has led some investigators to classify MS as a subcortical dementia. It contrasts sharply with dementias of the cortical gray matter which are characterized by prominent amnesia and aphasia, and agnosia (e.g. dementia of the Alzheimer's type). It is unclear from the literature whether such a classification is of any clinical benefit since some studies propose that MS shows characteristics of both cortical and subcortical dementia (see Rao et al., 1991, for a more detailed discussion).

A substantial number of studies have investigated the relationship between cognitive impairment in MS and variables such as disease course, degree of disability, duration of illness, medication usage, and emotional status. The relationship is controversial, with many of the studies reporting conflicting results. However, the majority of investigators have found no association between degree of disability, duration of illness or medication usage, and cognitive dysfunction. Some studies have reported that cognitive performance in depressed MS patients is more impaired than in nondepressed MS patients, although this discrepancy is rarely significant. Others have attempted to link poor performance with patients' fatigue and consequent low motivation. It is well established that low motivation can adversely affect cognitive performance, but this is unlikely to account for all the cognitive difficulties found in MS, since in the majority of studies disease course was found to be unrelated to cognitive impairment. Grossman and others (1994) systematically investigated whether relapsing-remitting (RR) or chronic progressive (CP) MS patients showed significantly different patterns of cognitive impairment. In general, CP patients were more severely impaired than patients in the RR group, but the overall pattern of deficits was not grossly dissimilar in the two groups.

Many studies have investigated the relation between cognitive performance in MS patients with quantified lesion scores derived from MR imaging. As expected, the extent of cerebral demyelination correlates significantly with severity of cognitive impairment. Swirsky-Sacchetti and others (1992) employed "lesion severity variables" such as total lesion area (TLA), ventricular-brain ratio, and size of corpus callosum, as well as ratings of lesion site (e.g. frontal, temporal, and parieto-occipital regions) and correlated them with performance on a broad range of neuropsychological tests. They found neuropsychological test scores to be highly related to all measures of degree of cerebral involvement, with TLA being the best predictor of neuropsychological deficit. They reported mean lesion area for the cognitively impaired group to be 28.30 cm^2 and mean lesion area for the cognitively intact group to be 7.41 cm^2. Lesion sites also correlated significantly with impairment on specific cognitive tests.

BIBLIOGRAPHY

Beatty, W. W., Goodkin, D. E., Beatty, P. A., & Monsoon, N. (1989). Frontal lobe dysfunction and memory impairment in patients with chronic progressive multiple sclerosis. *Brain and Cognition, 11*, 73–86.

Charcot, J. M. (1877). Lectures on the diseases of the nervous system delivered at La Salpétrière. London: New Sydenham Society.

DeLuca, J., Barberi-Berger, S., & Johnson, S. K. (1994). The nature of memory impairment in multiple sclerosis: acquisition versus retrieval. *Journal of Experimental and Clinical Neuropsychology, 2*, 183–9.

Grossman, M., Armstrong, C., Onishi, K., Thompson, H., Schaefer, B., Robinson, K., D'Esposito, M., Cohen, J., Brennan, D., Rostami, A., Gonzalez-Scarano, F., Kolson, D., Constantinescu, C., & Silberberg, D. (1994). Patterns of cognitive impairment in relapsing-remitting and chronic progressive multiple sclerosis. *Neuropsychiatry, Neuropsychology, and Behavioral Neurology, 3*, 194–210.

Kurtzke, J. F. (1980). Multiple sclerosis: an overview. In F. Clifford Rose (Ed.), *Clinical neuroepidemiology* (pp. 63–7). Tunbridge Wells: Pitman Medical.

Matthews, W. B. (1978). Miscellaneous topics: multiple sclerosis. In W. B. Matthews & G. H. Glaser (Eds), *Recent advances in clinical neurology 2* (pp. 1–9). Edinburgh: Churchill Livingstone.

Rao, S. M. (1986). Neuropsychology of multiple sclerosis: a critical review. *Journal of Clinical and Experimental Neuropsychology, 5*, 503–42.

Rao, S. M., Leo, G. J., & St. Aubin-Faubert, P. (1989). On the nature of memory disturbance in multiple sclerosis. *Journal of Clinical and Experimental Neuropsychology, 5*, 699–712.

Rao, S. M., Leo, G. J., Bernardin, L., & Unverzagt, F. (1991). Cognitive dysfunction in multiple sclerosis: frequency, patterns, and predictions. *Neurology, 41*, 685–91.

Swash, M., & Schwartz, M. S. (1989). *Neurology: A concise clinical text*. London: Baillière Tindall.

Swirsky-Sacchetti, T., Mitchell, D. R., Seward, J., Gonzales, C., Lublin, F., Knobler, R., & Field, H. L. (1992). Neuropsychological and structural brain lesions in multiple sclerosis: a regional analysis. *Neurology, 42*, 1291–5.

Warlow, C. (1991). *Handbook of neurology*. Oxford: Blackwell Scientific.

MARIE MCCARTHY

mutism Mutism is the term for the complete absence of speech, often with the implication that no attempt to speak can be inferred, in a patient who is conscious and is neither aphasic nor anarthric.

Mutism may occur as one form of HYSTERIA, usually in the company of other hysterical symptoms, but it may also occur as a severe organic condition called *akinetic mutism*. Akinetic mutism occurs as a state of total unresponsivity in a patient who is awake, looks around, and is apparently aware and conscious, but simply does not speak and may not make any other voluntary response. It should therefore be distinguished from the VEGETATIVE STATE, in which the patient, although awake, makes no response beyond certain reflexive behaviors and is apparently unaware, and the LOCKED-IN SYNDROME, in which the patient is awake and conscious but is unable to speak or make any response because the effector systems have been interrupted. Akinetic mutism is associated with cysts of the third ventricle, and is also used for patients with bilateral frontal or cingulate lesions who show a lack of any drive or initiation of action. Affective indifference also accompanies this state, particularly if it results from bilateral frontal lesions. A period of mutism, often lasting several days, also typically follows COMMISSUROTOMY in the acute phase of recovery, probably resulting from surgical disturbance of the area around the third ventricle.

myoclonic epilepsy *See* EPILEPSY.

myoclonic jerks Myoclonic jerks (also *myoclonus*) are brief shock-like muscular contractions which involve a whole muscle or specific muscle fibers. One or many muscles may be affected, and the phenomenon is familiar to many normal individuals as an occasional sudden jerk while falling asleep, when it is of no clinical significance. In abnormal cases, the jerk may be so slight as to be insignificant, or it may involve large groups of muscles and be sufficiently severe to throw the patient to the ground. It is most commonly associated with EPILEPSY but in rarer cases may be a feature of encephalomyelitis, ENCEPHALOPATHY (especially following an anoxic incident), or CREUTZFELDT–JAKOB DISEASE. Nonepileptic myoclonic jerks have been attributed to disorders of the olivodentate system.

N

narcolepsy In narcolepsy the patient suffers an attack of falling asleep even though the circumstances may be inappropriate and there may be no sense of fatigue. An important feature of the attack is that it is felt to be irresistible. Once asleep, the patient may be aroused as if in normal sleep. The cause may be a lesion in the region of the third ventricle, but it may also result from an epileptic lesion of which the narcolepsy is the only sign. The attacks are often compared to CATA-LEPSY although consciousness is not affected in the latter condition.

neglect Unilateral neglect is a neurological condition, characterized by an unawareness and subsequent failure to orient or respond to events in the contralesional hemispace, which cannot be explained by primary sensory or motor deficits.

Reference to the syndrome of unilateral neglect was first cited in medical journals just over a century ago. While Jackson (1876) is reported to have been the first to present a well-documented account of the neglect syndrome, the disorder was later expanded by Holmes (1918), Poppelreuter (1923), and Riddoch (1935), and extensively described by Brain (1941).

Following a rather stagnant 30-year period in which few papers were recorded, the beginning of the 1970s witnessed a resurgence of interest in the neglect phenomenon. A proliferation of scientific papers investigating various aspects of neglect emerged. The complexity of the disorder was soon reflected in the numerous terms devised to describe what appeared to be the same behavioral impairment. Terms such as unilateral spatial agnosia; amorphosynthesis; left-sided fixed hemianopia; hemi-inattention; hemineglect; unilateral neglect; hemispatial agnosia; contralesional neglect; dyschiria and directional hypokinesia were all used interchangeably to describe

the neglect disorder (cited in Halligan & Marshall, 1993).

The overwhelming growth of interest in the neglect phenomenon was partly due to the unique opportunity it provided to increase understanding about the normal cognitive processes underlying spatial and selective ATTENTION. Additionally, clinical therapists were being challenged to find ways of helping patients compensate for the disabling consequences of the disorder.

Today unilateral neglect is seen more as an umbrella term for a broad range of component deficits which are not necessarily manifested in any consistent pattern of dysfunction. An attempt to provide a unitary explanation for the disorder has long been dismissed since perceptual, motor, intentional, motivational, and representational factors are all critical, both in the qualitative manifestation and the severity of the condition. (The most comprehensive review of current research can be found in Robertson and Marshall, 1993.)

THE CLINICAL PRESENTATION OF NEGLECT

The presence of florid unilateral neglect is both dramatic and unmistakable. Typically, neglect is a consequence of damage to the right hemisphere, and is characterized by a failure to respond to stimuli and events in the left half of space. For example, if addressed from the left side the patient may fail to respond, or begin hopelessly searching for the source of the speaker on the right side. Patients may groom and dress only the right side of the body and others may even fail to eat food from the left side of the plate. Mesulam (1985) comments that "when neglect is severe, the patient may behave almost as if one half of the universe had abruptly ceased to exist in any meaningful form" (p. 142). If mobility is not compromised by hemiparesis, neglect patients may often bump into objects on the left side and sometimes lose their sense of direction as a result of their failure to attend to left-sided cues.

Patients demonstrate errors of spatial bias or neglect on many conventional and everyday tasks. They may fail to copy the features on the left side of a multi-element picture; produce only one side of a figure on tasks of spontaneous drawing; tend to err to the ipsilesional hemispace on measures of line bisection; show a curious tendency to leave an extra wide left margin if requested to write or copy a script, and fail to detect left-sided stimuli in typical cancellation tasks. It appears as if their whole world "left of center" is missing.

The frequent co-occurrence of hemianopia and hemiparesis in patients with the neglect condition raised some concern as to whether neglect merely reflected an arbitrary grouping of sensory motor deficits. This proposition is contestable on a number of grounds. First, patients who show severe visual neglect on line bisection and cancellation tasks do not always show evidence of visual field deficits on confrontation. Second, there is evidence that hemiparesis and neglect may be doubly dissociated. Third, patients also show neglect for the contralesional hemispace even when they are instructed to use the ipsilesional intact limb for the execution of exploratory tasks. Mesulam (1985) comments that "neglect is not a deficit of seeing, hearing, feeling, or moving but one of looking, listening, touching, and searching" (p. 142). (Bisiach and Vallar (1988) and Barbieri and De Renzi (1989) provide good discussions of the pattern of neglect dissociations.)

SUBTYPES IN UNILATERAL NEGLECT

Motor neglect refers to the condition where patients demonstrate a complete poverty of spontaneous movement in the contralesional limb without evidence of pathology in the motor cortex. Patients may raise only one hand in response to a command to raise both. Barbieri and others (1989) report that such patients "show a dissociation between the normal strength exerted with these limbs when they are implicitly instructed to attend to them and their failure to use them spontaneously in bi-manual and even automatic tasks" (p. 14). Motor neglect therefore concerns the contralateral side of the body and not the

contralateral environment as in the typical case of unilateral spatial neglect.

Neglect dyslexia A number of papers have been published in which neglect dyslexia was present independent of any other spatial bias tendencies on regular tests of neglect. However, many patients with left visual neglect following right hemisphere damage may fail to read the left part of single words and sentences. They read "smile" as "mile" or "belief" as "grief." Errors tend to be either complete omissions of the initial letter (particularly when the remaining letters form a real word in their own right) or they may be substitutions of the initial letters to form a real word. Similar errors have also been reported on the right side following left brain damage. For example, patients may read "south" as "soup" or "modern" as "modest." When reading a prose passage patients may begin from the center of the text, and fail to orient their attention to the left side despite the meaninglessness of the text. (See Ellis et al., 1993, for review.)

Neglect dysgraphia Patients show a curious tendency to begin writing at a central point on the page, leaving an extraordinarily large left margin, and proceed to squeeze their text into the right side. In spelling words aloud Ellis and colleagues (1993) report a patient who spelled "sneeze" as "sneed" and "events" as "evenis." When the same patient was instructed to write, she wrote "floor" as "floore" and "jury" as "jurd." Other common writing errors include examples of patients failing to dot their "i's" and cross their "t's."

The patterns of errors in neglect dyslexia and neglect dysgraphia are not fixed. Some cases have been reported in which patients show various combinations of errors, and both conditions do not always co-occur. (See Ellis et al., 1993, for a more detailed discussion.)

Facial neglect Young and others (1990) describe a unique case of a domain-specific form of unilateral neglect. They describe a patient who showed a deficit in the recognition of normal faces, chimeric faces, and half-faces presented in isolation whether upright or inverted. The deficit extended to both internal and external facial features and was later demonstrated on judgments of facial expressions and of resemblance between faces. The disorder was thought to result from a failure to attend to the left side of faces only, since normal performance in the recognition of everyday objects was reported. The authors interpreted the finding as a domain-specific form of unilateral neglect.

Auditory neglect Although a small number of papers are in vogue, claiming to have identified auditory neglect, there remains some controversy regarding the criteria for diagnosis. Since the auditory system is not as neatly lateralized as the visual system, it is exceedingly difficult to demonstrate complete unresponsiveness for unilateral aural stimuli, since processing in the ipsilesional pathways cannot be controlled. Some research in this area has identified auditory neglect as a failure to respond to stimuli presented in the left hemispace under conditions of bilateral simultaneous presentation. This deficit, better known as extinction, also occurs in patients with other cerebral pathologies and remains insufficient evidence in isolation to warrant the diagnosis of unilateral auditory neglect. While some may argue that extinction merely represents a more attenuated form of neglect, the issue is challenged by the findings of Barbieri and De Renzi (1989), who reported extinction and neglect to be doubly dissociated. More recent evidence has identified separate anatomical areas responsible for unilateral neglect and extinction.

Tactile neglect This is considered to be a rarity, not closely associated with right cerebral lesions. It typically refers to a behavior in which patients show a reluctance to manually explore their environment in search of a target stimulus. The condition is not simply contingent upon a lack of visual input as it may also be seen if the patient is blindfold. It is worth emphasizing that, while neglect may be demonstrated in more than one modality, it is currently more typical to find it confined to the visual modality.

Like many other neuropsychological disorders the phenomenon of neglect continues to be fractionated and dissociations for different spatial dimensions are reported. These include dissociations between vertical and horizontal neglect and neglect for near and far space. Mennemeier and colleagues (1992) refine these dissociations and provide evidence for separable anatomical involvement.

RELATED DISORDERS

Unilateral neglect has also been closely associated with a number of related disorders concerning contralateral space. These include ANOSOGNOSIA (ranging from a total denial of any impairment to a reluctant admission of some minor impairment on the contralateral side); ANOSODIAPHORIA (referring to an awareness of the contralateral deficit despite an apparent lack of concern regarding the disability); ALLESTHESIA or ALLOCHIRIA (a failure to detect unilateral tactile stimuli; typically, tactile sensations delivered to the contralateral side of the body are referred to the same position on the ipsilesional side); EXTINCTION (a failure to identify both stimuli in the presentation of bilateral simultaneous stimulus presentation); Bisiach and Vallar (1988) provide a good review of related disorders.

ETIOLOGY AND NEURO-PATHOLOGICAL CORRELATES

In the vast majority of cases the cause of unilateral neglect tends to be vascular or neoplastic in origin. However, unique case reports of the presence of neglect following traumatic brain injury, right temporal lobe seizures, and right ventrolateral thalamotomy have been cited. Neglect following subcortical lesions has also been reported and this typically results from an intracerebral hemorrhage. It is rare to see neglect as a result of a neurodegenerative disease (e.g. MULTIPLE SCLEROSIS, PARKINSON'S DISEASE, HUNTINGTON'S DISEASE, or motor neuron disease) as these diseases are often bilateral and insidious.

Neglect is most common following lesions of the inferior parietal lobule. Other cerebral regions where lesions produce neglect include the dorsolateral frontal lobe; cingulate gyrus; neostriatum; basal ganglia, and thalamus. Vallar (1993) provides an excellent review of the anatomical basis of spatial unilateral neglect.

INCIDENCE OF NEGLECT FOLLOWING RIGHT AND LEFT CEREBRAL LESIONS

Numerous studies have endeavored to quantify the incidence of neglect following unilateral lesions of the right and left hemisphere. Such studies have encountered many methodological problems, such as the variability in the tests employed, the etiology, and the time since injury. Typically, neglect is more prevalent and more severe following lesions of the right hemisphere. Some studies have disputed this and claimed that the marked asymmetry in the incidence of neglect results from a sampling bias due to the exclusion of aphasic patients. However, in studies recruiting unselected samples of right and left hemisphere damaged patients, the incidence and severity is always greater in those with a right hemisphere lesion. Stone and colleagues (1991) estimate the frequency of visuospatial neglect to range from 33 to 85 percent in right hemisphere damage and from 0 to 25 percent in patients with left hemisphere damage.

DIAGNOSIS AND PROGNOSIS

Florid visuospatial neglect is unmistakable. As well as marked disruption in everyday behavior, due to a failure to be aware of the left hemispace, patients typically show neglect on classic tests such as line bisection and cancellation, copying, spontaneous drawing, and visual search tasks. Assessing more subtle forms of neglect (like those previously discussed) requires more creativity and skill. Patients may demonstrate neglect on some of the classic tests while performing at their age equivalent on other tasks. The Behavioural Inattention Test (BIT) provides a standardized assessment tool for assessing neglect. It comprises six conventional subtests, such as line bisection and letter cancellation, and nine behavioral subtests reflecting everyday tasks which might cause difficulty for patients. Examples of these include telephone dialling, menu reading, and map navigation.

A number of studies have correlated specific pathological variables with the severity and recovery of neglect. Levine and others (1986) reported lesion size and premorbid brain atrophy to be important factors in estimating the severity and recovery of neglect 2–4 weeks post-insult. They found no correlation between the severity of neglect and either the locus of the lesion or the age of the patient. Subsequent studies have failed to replicate these findings. The mechanisms underlying recovery in neglect are poorly understood. Some attribute recovery to the intactness of the left hemisphere while others speculate that the callosal fibers play an important role. Nevertheless, there is still some recovery even when these callosal fibers are damaged, indicating that recovery is not solely contingent on the integrity of the callosal pathways. Levine and colleagues (1986) speculate that "other commissural pathways, perhaps at the midbrain level, are capable of

mediating reequilibration from the undamaged hemisphere" (p. 366) or even that ipsilateral pathways from the undamaged hemisphere to appropriate motor units may be responsible. Vallar (1993) reviews both the human and animal studies relating to severity and recovery in neglect.

MECHANISMS UNDERLYING UNILATERAL NEGLECT

The precise mechanisms underlying hemispatial neglect are still unclear. The literature is divided loosely into those who support representational accounts (in which proponents believe that neglect results from a disturbance in the patient's central representation of space) and those who support attentional accounts (believing that neglect results from a disruption in the attentional or orienting systems). (See Robertson and Marshall (1993) for specific references cited in the following accounts and for extensive discussion.)

REPRESENTATIONAL ACCOUNTS

Zingerle (1913) was the first to propose that the spatial representation of neglect patients in relation to their body was confined to the right side. When research into neglect again became fashionable in the early 1970s this spatial representation account was resurrected and the dramatic studies of Bisiach and colleagues helped to popularize it. Bisiach and Luzzatti (1978) argued that the posterior parietal cortex contains an elaborate spatial representation of the external world. It followed that unilateral injury to this area of the cortex would cause a unilateral loss of this spatial representation and hence neglect of that area of space. In one of their studies Bisiach and Luzzatti asked two of their patients (both with injury to the right cerebral cortex and left unilateral neglect) to describe the Piazza del Duomo in Milan, a place familiar to both subjects. Subjects were instructed to verbally describe the landscape from two separate, imagined viewpoints. On both occasions subjects failed to include the landmarks which were on the imagined left side of the scene. Since the descriptions were not contingent upon direct sensory input Bisiach and colleagues interpreted the findings to imply that the patient's internal spatial representation was impaired.

Bisiach and others conducted further studies to corroborate this hypothesis. In one of these studies, subjects were asked to give descriptions of the Piazza del Duomo (free recall condition) and then to describe the right and left side of the scene independently. While neglect patients appeared to improve in the cued condition, they continued to omit far more detail on the left side relative to the right side in comparison to matched control groups. Bisiach and colleagues (1981) proposed that imagined space is topographically represented across the hemispheres in a manner analogous to that of external space. When one hemisphere is damaged, that side of the represented space would not be reported. An equally convincing argument is that the representation of imagined space is preserved in neglect patients, but their ability to scan it spontaneously or automatically is impaired. This would explain their improved performance in the cued condition. A final study by Bisiach and others (1979) required a cohort of neglect patients with right cerebral damage to detect differences within pairs of successively presented patterns. By comparison with a non-brain-damaged control group, the neglect patients were more impaired at detecting differences on the left side than the right side of the patterns. In a final experiment, subjects made a same or a different judgment about two stimuli presented sequentially. Stimuli consisted of random cloud-like shapes which were only visible while moving past a small vertical slit in a display. Subjects had to construct a mental image of the stimulus as a prerequisite to this judgment, since only partial information was available to central vision at any one time. Patients with neglect made significantly more errors by identifying stimuli as the same when they were different.

The evidence appears convincing, but some concern has been raised as to how the data should be interpreted. It remains unclear whether the findings of Bisiach and others are indicative of patients having an impaired representation of space, whether they are impaired at scanning a preserved representation, or whether the results point to patients' inability to attend to the contralesional hemispace. Clearly the fact that cueing patients to the left side reduces the severity of the neglect errors points to some attentional involvement, and this is not readily accommodated in the representational account.

ATTENTIONAL HYPOTHESES

Attention is a complex construct and several scientists have speculated about the specific aspect of attentional mechanisms thought to be disrupted in unilateral neglect. (See Rizzolatti & Camara, 1987; Rizzolatti & Barti, 1993, for review and specific references.)

Heilman's unilateral akinesia hypothesis

Heilman proposes that neglect results from a decreased activation of the arousal systems of the damaged hemisphere (in particular although not exclusively) to lesions of the cortico-limbic reticular activating loop (Heilman & Watson, 1977). The effect of such a unilateral decrease in arousal is thought to be the selective loss of the orienting response to the contralateral side of space. Since it is assumed that the orienting response to the opposite side of space is represented in the contralateral hemisphere, Heilman and others proposed that the damaged hypoaroused hemisphere is rendered akinetic. The preponderance of neglect following lesions of the right hemisphere is also accommodated by Heilman's hypothesis. Heilman and his colleagues proposed that attentional mechanisms are asymmetrically represented such that the right hemisphere surveys and attends to both halves of space while the left hemisphere remains exclusive to the right hemispace. It therefore follows with a left hemisphere lesion that the capacity to orient to the contralateral hemispace is compensated for by the bilateral attentional mechanisms of the right hemisphere, while a right hemisphere lesion would leave the patient unable to orient contralaterally. The result is unilateral neglect.

Heilman's hypothesis revolutionized the way in which the neglect phenomenon was conceptualized and deserves credit for the emphasis it placed on the importance of attention. However, some unresolved issues remain. While this theory predicted that the most severe forms of neglect should result from lesions of the reticular formation, more recent evidence suggests that neglect is most severe following lesions of the right inferior parietal lobule. In addition, some remained unconvinced that a lesion in one of the many areas projecting to the reticular formation is sufficient to completely inactivate the structure and render the entire hemisphere akinetic. Finally, the subsequent rise in the number of studies claiming to have reduced the severity of neglect by cueing patients to the left side is not readily explained by Heilman's hypothesis. Neglect remains a more complex disorder, which is not fully explained by the hypo-arousal of one hemisphere.

Kinsbourne's attentional hypothesis

In Kinsbourne's (1978) hypothesis, it is argued that activation of one hemisphere causes inhibition of homologous functions in the other. He argued that the consequence of within-hemisphere activation could lead to a perceptual bias toward the contralateral side of space and transhemispheric inhibition. Hence right hemisphere damage might produce a general bias toward right-sided stimuli and away from left-sided stimuli, even within the intact right hemispace. While Kinsbourne's hypothesis finds support in a number of clinical studies identifying neglect in the left side of a stimulus array presented in the right hemispace, as well as in the left hemispace, other studies have been reported in which this phenomenon has not been documented.

Posner's covert orienting hypothesis

According to Posner and others (1982, 1984), neglect results from an impairment in the mechanisms which allow attention to be shifted away from the intact hemispace, rather than an inability to move attention toward the impaired side of space. In Posner's cue validity paradigm, subjects detect a target stimulus which is validly cued on 80 percent of all trials and invalidly cued on the remaining 20 percent of trials. Generally, as one would expect, reaction times for invalid trials are slower, reflecting the time taken for attention to be directed to the other visual field. In a cohort of neglect patients Posner and colleagues found that the most striking result was that, once miscued, patients found it remarkably difficult to disengage attention from the ipsilesional hemispace and move attention to the contralesional hemispace.

Posner's hypothesis was the first to accommodate findings that left-sided cueing reduced the severity of neglect errors. However, a selective deficit in visual attention cannot explain all the

findings since we know that neglect is not specific to the visual modality. In addition, Posner's hypothesis cannot account for the multiplicity of lesions which give rise to neglect, or for the anatomical independence of the regions which, if lesioned, produce neglect.

Mesulam's cortical circuit hypothesis for directing attention

Unlike the previous hypotheses where a single component deficit in the attentional system was proposed to explain the presence of neglect Mesulam (1981, 1985) avoids specifying the impairment of a single unitary function and instead proposes that an attentional circuit responsible for directing attention in the contralateral hemispace is disrupted. The hypothesis discards the notion that spatial attention is a localized single function in the inferior parietal lobe and instead introduces the idea that attention is a functional circuit subserved by several brain regions.

The starting point for Mesulam's hypothesis is the observation that lesions of the inferior parietal lobe, the frontal eye field, and the cingulate gyrus consistently result in the neglect phenomenon. Mesulam's observation that these three areas are reciprocally linked to each other *en route* from the reticular structures, led him to propose that the distribution of attention to extrapersonal targets is mediated by a neural circuit founded on these cortical regions. According to this hypothetical model, the effective distribution of attention within the extrapersonal space requires a flexible interaction between these three representations: the posterior parietal cortex for a sensory representation of the extrapersonal world; the frontal eye field, which may contain a map for the distribution or orientation of exploratory movements in the extrapersonal space; and the cingulate cortex, which may contain a map for the distribution of expectancy and relevance. Mesulam proposes that each of these representations receives a set of reticular inputs, and the entire circuitry, motivated by the cingulate cortex, directs attention to the target stimulus. According to Mesulam, damage to any one of these regions, to their interconnections, or to the thalamic and striate regions with which they are connected may give rise to unilateral neglect. Mesulam comments that "the clinical flavor of the resulting neglect syndrome in each case could reflect the anatomical site of involvement; but of course it would be unreasonable to expect rigid distinctions, since components of the network are tightly interconnected" (Mesulam, 1985, p. 158). Mesulam's hypothesis was the first model of neglect to account for the multiplicity of lesions and the anatomical independence of the regions which give rise to neglect. It can also account for the growing number of studies documenting variations in the manifestation of the neglect phenomenon.

Despite the limitations of many of these hypotheses, their purpose was well served in highlighting the role of spatial and attentional factors in understanding the complex dynamics underlying neglect. While much of the current research continues to employ many of these hypotheses, it is now widely accepted that neglect is a heterogeneous disorder and cannot be explained at a unitary level. The central focus has moved towards attempting to understand the relative contribution of spatial, attentional, perceptual, motor, and intentional variables in the specific type of neglect being manifested. In many of the current studies, the emphasis appears to be concentrated on modulating the expression of neglect, either by manipulating the nature of the task or the strategy employed in executing it. For example, some authors have analyzed neglect performance on lines of variable length; others have looked at whether the hand employed, or the hemispace in which the task is executed, increases or reduces the severity of neglect errors. Some papers have also been reported in which the motor component or the perceptual component are independently manipulated. These include studies where manual versus nonmanual line bisection performances have been analyzed or studies in which performance on line bisection has been altered by changing the focal and global characteristics of the task. Others have concentrated on the role of right-sided stimuli in the expression of neglect. It may be said that much of the research is specific to analyzing separable component deficits in visuospatial neglect.

Perhaps one of the most intriguing questions facing neglect researchers is whether any of the neglected stimuli are processed. While many had suspected that neglected stimuli underwent far more processing than was initially believed, the work of Marshall and Halligan's (1988) classic paper highlights the fate of neglected stimuli. Their patient PS failed to report bright red flames emerging from the left-hand side of a drawing of a house, and asserted that this drawing was the same as another drawing that had no flames. However, she consistently chose the non-burning picture as the one she would prefer to live in. Covert awareness has been demonstrated in more recent studies of associative priming in the neglected space: response to a word in the right visual field was faster when the word was preceded by the brief presentation of an associated word in the neglected field. Ladavas and colleagues (1993) report that, when their patient was instructed to orient to the left side of a computer, he was unable to detect the presence of, read aloud, or judge the lexical status or semantic content of left-sided stimuli. These workers interpreted the result to mean that their patient was able to perform a covert post-perceptual processing of the neglected stimuli, but was unable to demonstrate this when explicitly instructed.

There is no doubt that the mechanisms underlying neglect are extremely complex. It is probable that different functional components are disrupted in different forms of neglect, so a true understanding remains contingent on the specific variant or subtype of neglect being analyzed. Given the quantity and quality of neglect papers in current journals, there seems little doubt that a purer understanding of the disorder will be forthcoming.

REHABILITATING UNILATERAL NEGLECT

Few neuropsychological disorders (with the exception of memory and language) have attracted as much theoretical comment in rehabilitation studies as unilateral neglect. The reason is probably because of the unique opportunity which such studies provide in strengthening our understanding of the mechanisms disrupted in neglect and also in refining our understanding of the normal processes of spatial attention. Numerous studies investigating various forms of cueing techniques (typically on line bisection tasks) have been reported. Examples of such studies include placing a red strip on the left side of the page; having patients report a letter on the left or right side prior to commencing the task; manipulating the stimulus configuration on the right and left side; altering the starting position or hand employed; having patients guide the examiner through the bisection task, or altering the length or thickness of the line. These studies have reported mixed success in reducing the severity of neglect on the affected side. For those in whom an improvement is demonstrated, there is little generalization to other tasks. Similar results have been reported in vestibular stimulation studies. While some initial improvement can be seen immediately following treatment, the reduction in neglect rarely generalizes to other tasks and generally reverts to baseline performance within 15–30 minutes following treatment.

So far the most effective strategy for reducing the disabling consequences of neglect on a patient's quality of life has been contralateral limb activation therapy. A small number of studies report beneficial effects of left limb activation on the performance of various tasks. A theoretical debate has evolved as to whether the noticeable improvement resulting from limb activation could be attributed to activation of the damaged hemisphere or by a spatiomotor cueing explanation. Robertson and others (1992) pursued the issue and investigated the therapeutic benefits of limb activation and spatiomotor cueing on the performance of a range of tasks with three single-case studies. In the first two cases, a combined training program using limb activation and perceptual anchoring was employed. The results were positive and generalized outside the training environment. In the third case, limb activation was used in isolation from any explicit instruction to use the left limb as a perceptual anchor. Again a positive result was reported. As a result of later studies Robertson and Marshall (1993) report "the potent effect of treatment was not the perceptual anchoring of the left arm, but rather the fact of mobilising a part of the hemiplegic side" (p. 287).

BIBLIOGRAPHY

Barbieri, C., & De Renzi, E. (1989). Patterns of neglect dissociations. *Behavioural Neurology, 2*, 13–24.

Bisiach, E., & Vallar, G. (1988). *Hemineglect in humans*. In F. Boller & J. Grafman (Eds), *Handbook of neuropsychology*, Vol. 1 (pp. 195–222). Amsterdam: Elsevier.

Ellis, A. W., Young, A. W., & Flude, B. M.

(1993). Neglect and visual language. In I. H. Robertson & J. C. Marshall (Eds), *Unilateral neglect: Clinical and experimental studies* (pp. 233–56). Hove: Erlbaum.

Halligan, P. W., & Marshall, J. C. (1993). The history and clinical presentation of neglect. In I. H. Robertson and J. C. Marshall (Eds), *Unilateral neglect: Clinical and experimental studies* (pp. 3–26). Hove: Erlbaum.

Ladavas, E., Paladini, R., & Cubelli, R. (1993). Implicit associative priming in a patient with left visual neglect. *Neuropsychologia, 31*, 1307–93.

Levine, D. N., Warachy, J. D., Benowitz, L., & Calvanio, R. (1986). Left spatial neglect: effects of lesion size and pre-morbid atrophy on severity and recovery following right cerebral infarction. *Neurology, 36*, 362–6.

Marshall, J. C., & Halligan, P. W. (1988). Blindsight and insight into visuospatial neglect. *Nature, 336*, 766–7.

Marshall, J. C., Halligan, P. W., & Robertson, I. H. (1993). Contemporary theories of unilateral neglect: a critical review. In I. H. Robertson & J. C. Marshall (Eds), *Unilateral neglect: Clinical and experimental studies* (pp. 311–29). Hove: Erlbaum.

Mennemeier, M., Wertman, E., & Heilman, K. M. (1992). Neglect of near peripersonal space: evidence for multidirectional attentional systems in humans. *Brain, 115*, 37–50.

Mesulam, M. M. (1985). Attention, confusional states, and neglect. In M. M. Mesulam (Ed.), *Principles of behavioral neurology*. Philadelpia: Davies.

Rizzolatti, G., & Berti, A. (1993). Neural mechanisms of spatial neglect. In I. Robertson & J. C. Marshall (Eds), *Unilateral neglect: Clinical and experimental studies* (pp. 87–106). Hove: Erlbaum.

Rizzolatti, G., & Camarda, R. (1987). Neural circuits for spatial attention and unilateral neglect. In M. Jeannerod (Ed.), *Neurophysiological and neuropsychological aspects of spatial neglect: Advances in Psychology*, 45 (pp. 289–313). Amsterdam: Elsevier.

Robertson, I. H., & Marshall, J. C. (1993). *Unilateral neglect: Clinical and experimental studies*. Hove: Erlbaum.

Robertson, I. H., North, N. T., & Greggie, C. (1992). Spatiomotor cuing in unilateral left neglect: three case studies of its therapeutic effects. *Journal of Neurology, Neurosurgery and Psychiatry*, *55*, 799–805.

Stone, S. P., Wilson, B., Wroot, A., Halligan, P. W., Lange, L. S., Marshall, J. C. & Greenwood, R. J. (1991). The assessment of visuo-spatial neglect after acute stroke. *Journal of Neurology, Neurosurgery and Psychiatry*, *54*, 345–50.

Vallar, G. (1993). The anatomical basis of spatial hemi-neglect in humans. In I. H. Robertson & J. C. Marshall (Eds), *Unilateral neglect: Clinical and experimental studies* (pp. 27–59). Hove: Erlbaum.

Young, A., DeHaan, E. H. F., Newcombe, F., & Hay, D. C. (1990). Facial neglect. *Neuropsychologia*, *28*, 5, 391–415.

MARIE MCCARTHY

neurology Neurology is the specialty of medicine that deals with the diagnosis, study, and treatment of the diseases of the nervous system. All pathogenetic mechanisms may affect the nervous system, such as infections, tumors, trauma, toxins, and metabolic disorders. Thus the diseases range widely. Diseases not arising in the nervous system may also have their major effect on the nervous system. Diabetes, for example, may initially affect the peripheral nervous system, and this peripheral neuritis may be the most disabling part of the disease. Disease of the heart and blood vessels may be first manifested by nervous system dysfunction because of blocking the blood supply to the brain. This blockage, stroke, continues to be one of the major causes of disability and death. Neurological disorders are becoming more prevalent as the population continues to age. Aging is a major risk factor for DEMENTIA, stroke, and other disabling disorders, such as PARKINSON'S DISEASE.

CLINICAL EVALUATION

The clinical evaluation, that is, the history of the disorder and the neurological examination, is essential for establishing the diagnosis so that proper treatment may follow. A careful elicitation of the patient's problem, even before the neurological examination, will often lead to the diagnosis or to establishing the general category of disease. Even if the disease process is still obscure, a careful history will act as a guide for the clinician to pursue a rational plan for further

study. The history-taking is also important as a means for assessing the patient's mental status, language capabilities, and behavior. During history-taking, it is necessary that the clinician and the patient establish common understanding about certain descriptors. For example, "numbness," "blackout," "weakness," and "dizziness" may have very different meanings for the patient and for the physician.

The neurological examination is divided into the assessment of different neural systems. The mental status examination is very important as disorders of the nervous system may show up as changes in behavior, memory disturbances, language disturbances, and alterations in cognition. The presence and extent of these changes may become obvious during the history-taking. When changes are detected, greater attention may be directed to that area. The information may lead to a need for formal neuropsychological testing for greater definition and quantitation of the deficit.

The rest of the neurological examination can be broken down into various systems, such as cranial nerve examination, reflex testing, motor and sensory system assessment, and examination of coordination and balance. Clinicians vary in their approach to the neurological examination, but thorough testing of all systems is important. Interpretation of the findings depends upon the clinician's knowledge of what is normal and abnormal, and this is often the product of experience.

A lesion of the nervous system in one area, irrespective of the cause, will often manifest itself in similar ways. For example, a tumor, a stroke, or an injury in the occipital lobe will cause a visual defect that can be detected by the physical examination. The history of the illness will have established the time course of progression. Combining the historical information and findings will identify the process: a slow and gradually worsening course often indicates an enlarging mass, such as a tumor or an abscess; a sudden onset is much more common with disease of the vascular system, such as thrombosis of a vessel or a hemorrhage; and the history of a blow to the head for an injury.

In this era of high technology, history-taking and physical examination are becoming less extensive and sometimes even neglected. This neglect leads to mistakes in diagnosis, delay of treatment, and escalation of costs. The history, for example, of the patient with migraine is much more important for evaluation and proper treatment than complicated and expensive tests like COMPUTERIZED TOMOGRAPHY or MAGNETIC RESONANCE IMAGING, both of which will be of little help.

DIAGNOSTIC TESTING

It is the experience of the clinician that the diagnosis can usually be established by the history and the examination. However, there are many laboratory procedures that can improve and refine the clinical impression.

One of the oldest and most useful tests is the examination of the spinal fluid. This test is almost a hundred years old. The fluid is obtained by insertion of a needle into the space around the nervous system, usually into the subarachnoid space at the lower end of the spine. It is particularly important for detection of infections of the nervous system. Many infections of the nervous system, such as polio, have decreased; however, more and more obscure infections are being described. It is particularly important with infections in the central nervous system that therapy should be prompt, and often the spinal fluid will give the quickest and easiest answer.

ELECTROENCEPHALOGRAPHY, introduced by Hans Berger, is the recording of the electrical impulses of the brain, usually by electrodes placed on the scalp. The original notion of Berger, a psychiatrist, was to differentiate various mental disorders by characteristic patterns of the brain waves. This approach to the study of mental illness was disappointing, though it did prove to be useful for assessing many conditions affecting the nervous system.

It is particularly valuable in the detection and study of seizure disorders. Electrodes placed in the brain substance itself can often detect epileptogenic lesions that may be removable. Removal of these abnormal areas within the brain may cure or greatly improve the seizure status of the patient.

Imaging of the nervous system is used for the detection of lesions within the nervous system or in its vascular supply. The first brain imaging techniques were VENTRICULOGRAPHY and PNEUMOENCEPHALOGRAPHY. The brain was outlined by X-ray when air was substituted for the spinal fluid. This could be done by introducing the air into either the ventricular system (ventriculography) or the subarachnoid space (pneumoencephalography). These imaging techniques were often uncomfortable and carried some risk of morbidity and mortality, but they did provide much information about the location and extent of brain lesions, contributing greatly to the safety of neurosurgical procedures.

The vascular system of the brain is studied by injecting radiopaque contrast material into the vascular supply of the brain (ANGIOGRAPHY). Angiography is very useful for detecting vascular abnormalities of the brain, such as ANEURYSMS or angiomatous malformations. Blockages of the blood vessels and displacement of blood vessels by mass lesions are also detectable.

Imaging of the brain has taken great strides forward in the past 20 years with the introduction of computerized axial tomography (CAT) and magnetic resonance imaging (MRI). Refinements of these techniques can now localize and establish the extent and nature of many different disease processes. The resolution of these techniques has now made it possible to detect abnormalities of only a few millimeters in extent. Variation of these techniques also makes it possible to study blood flow and the vasculature of the brain.

POSITRON EMISSION TOMOGRAPHY (PET) using radiolabelled drugs or metabolites can detect changes in the functional activity of different parts of the brain. For example, the speech areas in the left hemisphere show increased glucose metabolism during tests of verbal function. The ability to combine this visualization of functional activity with various neuropsychological techniques has been a very important tool in anatomical and clinical correlations.

There are many other tests, such as nerve conduction velocities, electromyography, ultrasonography, and others which extend diagnostic capabilities. However, the use and interpretation of all these tests must be the responsibility of the clinician who assigns their proper place in the overall evaluation.

TREATMENT

Treatment has lagged behind diagnosis and our fundamental understanding of neurological disorders, but this is rapidly changing. The advent of better anticonvulsants has greatly changed the prognosis in epilepsy. Antibiotics have prevented, cured, or modified the course of many infectious diseases of the nervous system, such as SYPHILIS and bacterial MENINGITIS. An accelerated interest in vascular disease, beginning in the 1950s, has led to much better surgical and medical management of these disorders. Treatment involving the replacement of certain neurotransmitters has greatly modified the course of PARKINSON'S DISEASE. Adrenal medullary tissue, a source of neurotransmitter, has been placed in the brains of some patients with Parkinsonism. There has been some limited success reported with this procedure. Cholinergic drugs and nerve growth factor have been infused into the cerebrospinal fluid of patients with Alzheimer's disease. The rationale for this procedure has some basis in animal experimentation, but the number of human trials has been too few to predict any benefit. Recently, newly developed drugs and vaccines hold prospects of treating the demyelinating disorders, such as multiple sclerosis. Gene therapy is useful in some of the rare metabolic disorders affecting the nervous system.

It is heartening to note the increased number of drug and procedure trials for treatment of various nervous system disorders. Experience is showing that more and more neurologic diseases have a genetic basis. It is also likely that many of these disorders may have interacting nongenetic causes that make the disease manifest. Fundamental work on the genetics of neurodegenerative disorders, such as Alzheimer's and HUNTINGTON'S DISEASE, has provided information that is useful in detection, and may provide clues to treatment. It is now possible to detect defects that will lead to some of these genetic disorders later in life. All of this newly acquired knowledge will be helpful in devising strategies to treat or eliminate various disorders. It also raises many ethical dilemmas, as we now have the ability to detect untreatable disorders in yet asymptomatic patients.

HISTORY OF NEUROLOGY

The clinical specialty of neurology started in the last half of the nineteenth century. Before then much knowledge about the anatomy and the physiology of the nervous system had been accumulated. However, there was very little systematic information about patients with diseases of the nervous system. It was about that time that these patients were sequestered into wards of large hospitals or into special hospitals. This enabled clinicians to observe the diseases, some over many decades. Many became master describers and classifiers of disease, such as Charcot in France and Gowers in England. Others, such as Hughlings Jackson, were more interested in the disturbed physiology of the nervous system. Most of our fundamental knowledge about neuropathology came from the great mental hospitals, as in Germany, where the clinicians were interested in finding brain disorders as a cause of mental disease.

The links between psychiatry and neurology became gradually stretched as Freudian principles and psychoanalytical techniques became more popular. However, the links were never completely sundered as there developed a hybrid of neuropsychiatry that was popular in the first half of this century. Indeed, in the United States, the certifying boards of psychiatry and neurology are still joined, although the examinations are separate. In the last few decades advances in neurochemistry, neuropharmacology, imaging, and genetics have brought the two disciplines closer together.

The clinical specialty continued to grow despite the paucity of treatments for the disorders that were observed. However, this gradually changed, particularly with the introduction of antibiotics so that syphilis of the nervous system and common bacterial infections were treatable. Recently, the prospects for a basic understanding of neurological disorders have been greatly expanded by the use of molecular biological techniques. Various genes for different neurological disorders have been detected, and this has already led to new modes of therapy.

THE CONTRIBUTION OF NEUROLOGY TO THE UNDERSTANDING OF BRAIN FUNCTION

Physicians interested in the nervous system, particularly the diseased nervous system, have supplied a good deal of our fundamental knowledge of how the brain works. The fundamental contribution was the correlation of anatomical disturbances with disordered function. These anatomical and clinical correlations stemmed from centuries of clinical observations.

521

Early views of brain function

Early Greek and Roman views on the localization of brain function centered around a tripartite model. Baser instincts were assigned to the abdominal viscera, emotions to the heart, and rational thought to the brain. The view of the heart as a supplier of emotional tone was even repeated by Harvey in the seventeenth century.

The mechanics of brain function are often explained on the technological models of the time. For example, early in the twentieth century the telephone switchboard was often the model for neural functioning, just as the brain is likened to a computer today. In Greek and Roman times, some of the most advanced technology centered around the waterway system with its canals, aqueducts, and sewers. Thus the fluid-filled ventricles with their various passages were evoked as the mechanism of brain functioning. The anterior or lateral ventricles were a repository for sensory information, the fourth ventricle for memory, and the third ventricle was the mixing place for current impressions and past experience, so that this was the seat of rational thought. The ventricular theory of brain function persisted until the Renaissance and the time of Thomas Willis. Willis dismissed the fluid-filled ventricles as not essential in this process, and constructed his own view of the localization of function, utilizing the basal ganglion as the gatherer of sensory impressions (sensus commune), and cerebral cortices as repositories for memory. Willis' seminal contribution of relating mental functioning to brain tissue earned him the accolade of Sherrington, who noted that Willis was "the inventor of the nervous system."

Most of the thinking about brain function prior to the nineteenth century was holistic. Functions such as language and movement were not localized in an area of the brain substance, but proper brain function was dependent upon the integrity of the brain as a whole. This view was fortified by the influence of Flourens, the French physiologist, based on his animal experiments.

Franz Josef Gall, an Austrian physician, was responsible for the pseudoscience of PHRENOL-OGY. While this was not based on sound anatomical or clinical relations, it did advance the view that various functions of the brain could be assigned to different anatomical parts of the brain. For example, memory for words was assigned to the frontal lobes. This assignment was made as Gall observed that his classmates with good memories for words had prominent eyes. This, he reasoned, was due to large frontal lobes subjacent to the orbits.

Gall's observation of the parcelling of function within the brain led others to further discoveries based on clinical observation. Bouillaud, a prominent French physician, noted language disturbances in patients with lesions of the frontal lobes. Another landmark in the correlation of psychological changes with brain damage was made by an American practitioner, Harlow. He described personality changes following a lesion of the frontal lobe in his famous case of Phineas Gage. These observations led to Broca's findings based on solid anatomical and clinical correlations.

Paul Pierre Broca, a French surgeon, demonstrated that loss of language did correlate with frontal lobe lesions. His report followed the autopsy of a patient with severe loss of speech, and several other cases of a similar nature came to his attention. Broca not only provided scientific correlation for the location of speech function, but also lateralized this to the left hemisphere. This lateralization of function was contrary to anatomical and physiological notions of biological organization. It was thought that anatomically duplicate organs should have similar functions, such as the two kidneys. Thus the idea that the two halves of the nervous system should have different functions was not readily accepted. However, the evidence was overwhelming for speech function being localized to the left hemisphere. This was followed by the observations of Hughlings Jackson that spatial function was probably preponderant in the right hemisphere. The study of patients with corpus callosum sections by Sperry and his co-investigators has clarified the view of asymmetrical functioning in the nervous system.

The amalgamation of neurology and psychology took place largely after World War II. Neurologists had contributed carefully studied single observations correlating the injured brain anatomy with some cognitive defect. However, these single isolated observations did not have the strength of larger series of patients. Psychologists were able to supply this, along with rigorous and innovative testing methods. The collaboration of these two disciplines has led to the great advances in our knowledge of how the brain works.

BIBLIOGRAPHY

Clarke, E., & O'Malley, C. D. (Eds). (1968). *The human brain and spinal cord*. Berkely: University of California Press.

Haerer, A. F. (Ed.). (1992). *DeJong's The neurologic examination*, 5th edn. Philadelphia: J. B. Lippincott.

Joynt, R. J. (Ed.). (1988). *Clinical neurology*. Philadephia: J. B. Lippincott.

ROBERT J. JOYNT

neuromagnetometry Neural activity generates not only electrical fields but also magnetic fields; the technique by which these fields may be recorded is known as neuromagnetometry. As in the electroencephalogram (EEG), although the activity associated with a single neuron is very small, the field generated by the concerted action of groups of neurons may be sufficiently great to be detected and recorded outside the skull.

A SQUID (superconducting quantum interference device) is employed to detect the magnetic fields at the scalp and either a single detector is moved around the head or else an array of detectors is employed. As the SQUID has to be maintained in liquid helium and the recording conducted in a magnetically shielded environment, the technique is not widely available, but it is capable of producing three-dimensional magnetic isocontour maps of the brain. Clinically the technique is capable of resolving epileptic foci with a greater resolution than EEG recording, and in research the technique has already proved a useful counterpart to the evidence obtained from EEG recordings. (*See also* LATERALIZATION; SCAN.)

neuropsychiatry Neuropsychiatry, also termed *organic psychiatry* and closely linked with *liaison psychiatry*, is the specialism within psychiatry which deals with abnormal behavior attributable to demonstrable organic causes in the brain. Its borders are ill-defined, and it shares much in common with *behavioral neurology*, adopting a slightly different perspective, from psychiatry rather than neurology.

Part of the problem of circumscribing this field arises in the inevitable dualist perspective which the terms imply (*see* MIND–BODY PROBLEM); yet a monist perspective is more commonly adopted. It is generally accepted that even the "functional" or mental causes of psychiatric disorder are at some level operating through processes in the brain and are therefore organic in nature. That an abnormal behavior has a gross cerebral lesion as its apparent cause does not mean that psychological mental processes are not involved in its expression. It is more contentious to suggest that all psychiatric disorders might be understandable purely in terms of brain processes, if only our knowledge were adequate to provide the required explanations; but it might be generally acceptable to propose that the distinction between "functional" and "organic" disorders in psychiatry is made in terms of the level of description which is convenient, given our current state of knowledge about abnormal behavior.

In practice, neuropsychiatrists deal with behavioral disorders of a type which in other contexts might be understood in terms of functional processes, but which can be attributed to disorders of the nervous system: psychoses, neurotic reactions, personality change, disinhibited and asocial behavior, failures of personal adjustment to illness and disability, and the behavioral consequences of epilepsy. Their expertise is particularly required in the differential diagnosis between neurological and psychiatric factors in these disorders, and in the physical and pharmacological treatments traditional in the practice of psychiatry, when these are applied as interventions in the management and rehabilitation of individuals with cerebral lesions.

J. GRAHAM BEAUMONT

neuropsychological rehabilitation *See* REHABILITATION.

neuropsychology *Si monumentum requiris, circumspice* ("if you seek a monument, look around") is the inscription in St Paul's Cathedral, London, attributed to the son of Sir Christopher Wren, its architect. By the same principle, a definition of neuropsychology may seem superfluous in a dictionary of neuropsychology; the field is defined by its knowledge base, which is essentially the contents of this volume. Nevertheless, in promoting a perception of the wood as distinct from the trees, some discussion of neuropsychology as an identifiable scientific and clinical field (to mix the metaphor) seems appropriate.

If psychology is the science of mental life, to use George Miller's ingenious description, then neuropsychology is the scientific study of the relationship between the brain and mental life. It is common to see neuropsychology described as the study of brain–behavior relationships, but this is too limited a definition, in the way that contemporary psychology aspires to more than an understanding of overt behavior.

Such a definition immediately raises fundamental philosophical issues. It may be that the object of relating mental processes and physiological events is fundamentally flawed and unobtainable. It may be that the human brain is inadequate, as a matter of principle, to understand itself; self-knowledge may be inherently limited. These issues are discussed elsewhere (see MIND–BODY PROBLEM) and are addressed in certain respects below. However, whatever the philosophical position adopted by neuropsychologists, and most neuropsychologists implicitly adopt some form of psychoneural monism (that there is some degree of identity between mental and neural processes), two factors support the continuing effort to develop neuropsychological understanding. The first is that this is a legitimate field of scientific enquiry, the empirical pursuit of answers to the philosophers' questions. The second is that neuropsychology is of practical clinical utility. It will be clear from the contributions in this volume that, challenged by the human problems of neurological disease, injury, and disability, neuropsychology can be applied to the benefit of those who suffer from these conditions.

HISTORICAL PERSPECTIVE

What we now recognize as neuropsychological issues have been addressed in all societies throughout history. In ancient civilizations records survive of the interest in the behavioral functions of the brain, of which the Edwin Smith surgical papyrus, thought to date from between 2500 and 3000 years B.C., is an eloquent example. Even in preliterate societies the practice of craniotomy and trephination, from ancient as well as modern times, suggests a recognition of links between the brain and behavior.

In classical Greece, to which much of modern Western thought can be traced, the writers of the Hippocratic school accurately described a number of the basic neuropsychological phenomena which would still be accepted today. Nevertheless, it was the work of Aristotle, and subsequently the physician Galen, which was taken up by the Church fathers Nemesius and Saint Augustine around the turn of the fourth century A.D. and was to influence Western ideas up until modern times. Their hypothesis, the cell doctrine of brain function, was that mental faculties were located in the VENTRICLES of the brain, within which the animal spirits controlled behavioral functions. Anatomical illustrations which represent this hypothesis continued to appear well into the eighteenth century, and the ideas were also incorporated in the influential writings of Descartes in the seventeenth century. (An excellent introduction to this history is to be found in Walsh (1978), and more detailed information in Clarke and Dewhurst (1972), and Clarke and O'Malley (1968).)

While earlier writers had begun to speculate on the possible functional significance of the cerebral cortex, it was not until the nineteenth century that the role of the cortex was universally recognized. This recognition was due to three main influences. The first was the work of Flourens, who, experimenting mainly with birds, demonstrated the effects of neural ablations, the process of recovery, and the relative equipotentiality of neural tissue. The second was the demonstration by Broca in 1861 of the link between expressive aphasia and the region now called Broca's area. (Although credit is now also given to Bouillaud and to Dax for similar observations made about 30 years earlier, it was Broca's contribution which was influential.) The third was the development of phrenology by Gall, which maintained that separate mental faculties were located in the cortex of the brain, that development of these led to prominence of the overlying skull, and that palpation of the resulting "bumps" could reveal mental development and propensities. Phrenology had two significant vogues, the first scientific and the second more popular, lasting over almost a century. While fundamentally flawed it was, in

Boring's memorable phrase in his classic *History of Experimental Psychology*, "an instance of a theory which, while essentially wrong, was just enough right to further scientific thought."

In the final quarter of the nineteenth century these developments were built upon by Wernicke, Hughlings Jackson, Lichtheim, and Déjerine, among others, to form the foundations of modern neuropsychology. At first the identification of functional relationships with discrete cortical areas led to increasingly specific and detailed cortical mapping of mental abilities. This localizationist approach was the dominant school until well after World War I, when it became apparent that the detailed cortical maps were unsupported by clinical observation. Head's classic work on aphasia is a clear example of the criticism being raised of the extreme localizationist approach of the "diagram makers." In the same period, the work of Lashley in demonstrating the principle of mass action resulted in a reversal of thinking about neuropsychological organization. In human neuropsychology, the result was the adoption of a rather vague principle of "relative localization" in which general mental abilities were assigned to regions of the cortex, but with some degree of EQUIPOTENTIALITY or flexible organization being accepted within that region. The idea that functions at the level of psychological description might be only relatively localized, allowing for the possibility that component sub-functions might not be observable but more discretely localized, had in fact been prefigured in the work of Hughlings Jackson. This position fitted reasonably comfortably with clinical observation, and could be argued to be consonant with contemporary theoretical views of brain function which, by about 1960, adopted the early forms of information processing models.

MODERN NEUROPSYCHOLOGY

While neuropsychology had been an identifiable clinical specialty, allied to neurology, throughout this century, stimulated notably by the cases of missile wounds in the two World Wars, the recognition of neuropsychology as an independent field and its very rapid development have been relatively recent phenomena.

Contemporary neuropsychology can be divided into two main areas: clinical and experimental. *Clinical neuropsychology*, which is the branch of neuropsychology concerned with the psychological assessment, management, and rehabilitation of neurological disease and injury, has the longer history, which has led to the development of three identifiable traditions, although these traditions are becoming less distinct with the growth of international communication and collaboration.

The first tradition may be characterized as the behavioral neurological approach, and is historically the earliest. In modern times it has been most prominently linked with Luria, and it is European in origin. Essentially it relates distinct functional abnormalities (signs) to neuropsychological entities (conditions or syndromes), which belies its neurological foundation. A sign is dichotomous in state, being either present or absent, and there is no concept of a continuum of performance between the normal and the pathological. The patient either passes or fails the test, which is most commonly a simple elementary task designed to elicit the sign. In the hands of a skilled clinician such an approach is efficient and elegant, but it depends heavily on the identification of valid and easily assessable signs as indicators of abnormal function.

The second tradition is essentially psychometric and was developed most energetically in North America, in association with names such as Halstead and Reitan. Given the preoccupation of American psychology with the psychometric measurement of human abilities, the extension of the methodology to neuropsychology is hardly surprising. The result has been the creation of a number of widely used batteries which seek to survey a broad range of psychological functions, and then to draw conclusions from the detailed pattern of results, employing psychometric methods. While systematic and thorough, this approach is not always the most efficient in the use of precious clinical time, and may be inflexible in its application to individual patients. The power of the approach is naturally only as great as the validity yielded by the psychometric techniques, and the approach has been difficult to adapt to the rapidly changing nature of neuropsychological findings and theory. The clearest exemplars of the approach are the Halstead–Reitan Neuropsychological Test Battery and the Luria–Nebraska Neuropsychological Battery. The widespread use of the Wechsler Adult Intelligence Scale (WAIS) as a neuropsychological instrument is in part attributable to this tradition.

The third tradition is the individual-centered normative approach, associated with neuropsychology in the United Kingdom and the traditions of the British empirical approach, which led to extensive work on human performance and experimental cognitive psychology. This tradition seeks to employ specific tests which make use, where possible, of psychometric standardization, but which are combined flexibly in the investigation of a hypothesis about the patient's difficulties. The ethos of the approach is scientific detective work rather than medical examination (behavioral neurology) or formal assessment (psychometric battery). The clinician may use a general initial screening procedure (not infrequently the WAIS) or may simply rely upon current clinical information to construct hypotheses about any deficits which may be present, which are then tested, using individual test procedures or single-case empirical investigations. The approach can be efficient by being focused on the areas of dysfunction, and can also be finely tuned to investigate the exact parameters of abnormal performance. It does, however, rely upon an unusually high degree of knowledge and expertise on the part of the clinician for its general validity.

The clinical practice of most neuropsychologists is, of course, informed by all three of these traditions, which may be employed in the appropriate circumstances, yet to some degree these geographical traditions nonetheless persist. Whatever the approach adopted, however, the object is the same: the generation of a psychological description of the patient's behavioral deficits. Until the 1970s the practice of most neuropsychologists was principally concerned with the diagnosis of lesions and the determination of neuropsychological conditions. This was radically affected by the introduction of modern medical imaging, first with CT scans and subsequently with more advanced technologies (see SCAN). The role of neuropsychologists in assisting the neurologist and neurosurgeon with diagnosis became obsolete almost overnight. Far from a tragedy for neuropsychology, the result was a liberation from an over-narrow view of its purposes and application. Clinicians are now free to concentrate on creating functional descriptions in neuropsychological (rather than neuroanatom-

ical) terms, which in turn are of greater utility in permitting the development of strategies for interventions in management and rehabilitation. The interest of neuropsychologists in rehabilitation dates almost completely from the introduction of CT, bringing to an end the disgraceful neglect of this area by neuropsychology (see REHABILITATION).

Experimental neuropsychology remains a relatively independent branch, although naturally clinical and experimental neuropsychology inform each other. Leaving aside experimental work with nonhuman species (which might be thought to constitute a third branch of the discipline, but is not the subject of this volume) interest in experimental neuropsychology can be considered to date from 1960 and the publication of the first "split-brain" studies (see COMMISSUROTOMY). Although conducted with clinical patients, the importance and influence of these studies is not in the clinical field, but as having been the germ of a methodology for studying the neuropsychological organization of normal subjects within the neuropsychology laboratory (see DICHOTIC LISTENING, DIVIDED VISUAL FIELD TECHNIQUE). As a result, a vast literature on hemisphere differences was generated over the following two decades, which in turn was responsible for the general growth and prominence of the field.

At about the same time as the first "split-brain" studies appeared, there was a shift in the paradigms employed by psychologists interested in general aspects of human performance. Previously regarded as "experimental psychologists," these scientists became "cognitive psychologists," and cognitive psychology became the dominant mode at the core of academic psychology. This shift involved not only a renewed interest in cognitive processes such as perception, memory, language, thinking and reasoning, but a realization that data concerning abnormal cognitive processes (neuropsychological in nature) could inform the development of theories about normal cognitive processes. In turn the development of such theories of normal function was a considerable stimulus in the elaboration of neuropsychological theories, and the result has been a highly fruitful interchange between the two fields of psychology, and the creation of an identifiable area of *cognitive neuropsychology*.

Cognitive neuropsychology has not supplanted

the more traditional approaches in clinical and experimental neuropsychology, but rather stands alongside these approaches. Within experimental neuropsychology, the models derived from cognitive psychology are widely employed as a framework to study the neuropsychological characteristics of relevant processes. Within clinical neuropsychology, both the methods and the models of cognitive neuropsychology are employed in the assessment and description of neuropsychological abnormalities, most notably in the areas of reading, spelling, comprehension, object and face recognition, and memory: the areas in which relatively detailed cognitive psychological models now exist. The emphasis has shifted from group studies of deficits to the intensive investigation of single cases as the most commonly published methodology in neuropsychological research. In clinical practice the cognitive neuropsychological approach has made a less obvious impact, but the two approaches, traditional and cognitive, may be regarded as complementary facets of contemporary neuropsychology, both of considerable importance.

One issue which has been prompted by the growing influence of cognitive neuropsychology is the degree to which neuropsychology need have any reference to the brain at all. That this question arises illustrates the shift which has occurred in neuropsychology over the past 20 years. In one sense, if a cognitive neuropsychological approach is adopted, so that all neuropsychological constructs and resulting neuropsychological descriptions are couched in terms of cognitive psychological processes, then any reference to the brain is indeed unnecessary. There are, however, still those who consider that reference to neuroanatomy and neuropathology can provide information which assists the development of neuropsychological theories, and permits their neurobiological validity to be assessed. There is also a sense that neuropsychology entirely divorced from the brain would also be deficient in the sense that the central purpose of the field, understanding the relationship between mental processes and physiological events, would have been abandoned (*see* METHODOLOGICAL ISSUES).

Finally, it must be recognized that neuropsychology has a place within the burgeoning general field of neuroscience, which is probably the most exciting scientific frontier of the current decade.

Significant developments within neurobiology, neurogenetics, and neurochemistry are all enriching the ways in which the brain is being understood. The greatest impact from among the cognate fields of neuroscience is, however, probably being made by cognitive science, where the development of connectionist (neural network) models of intelligent functions is having an influence in two respects. The first is in the availability of purely computational connectionist models of functional deficits, which seem set to greatly refine our ability to conceptualize neuropsychological deficits. The second is by providing a new conceptual model for the nature of brain processes. A strictly computational, yet distributed (that is, not localized) model for cerebral functions has provided an alternative to the previous serial algorithmic information processing models, and a stimulus to new ways of thinking about the brain and how psychological functions are supported by that structure.

CONCEPTUAL ISSUES

Neuropsychology is in a conceptual morass. Neuropsychologists seek to study the relationship between brain and mind, but without ever really addressing the status of these two constructs, or what potential forms the relationship between them might take. It is conventional to adopt the behaviorist sleight of hand and propose that what we are studying is the relationship between brain and behavior, but this has become decreasingly tenable with the advent of cognitive neuropsychology and, more recently, the impact of connectionist modelling from cognitive science. It is no longer possible to escape the fact that neuropsychologists are studying psychological and not neurophysiological constructs, and what they are interested in is not just behavior, but the mind.

Bertrand Russell said of mathematics that it was the subject in which nobody knows what they are talking about. He no doubt meant to imply not that mathematicians are fools, but simply that the subject matter of mathematics is philosophically problematic, just as it is in neuropsychology.

Neuropsychologists have always, throughout the history of the discipline, tended to adopt a functionalist approach; but the problems of this approach have been exposed by the descriptive terms of neuropsychological explanations shifting from behavioral descriptors to cognitive descriptors, under the influence of cognitive neuropsychology. The introduction of mentalistic constructs such as logogens, semantic networks (the apparent neural reference of this term is unfounded), schemas, and other forms of mental representation has highlighted the fact that neuropsychologists deal no longer (and may never have dealt) with the processes of the brain. As already noted, that the question of whether neuropsychology without reference to the brain is possible can be raised is sufficiently indicative. That the answer, for at least some neuropsychologists, is "yes" confirms my thesis.

The dominant empirical thrust of neuropsychology in the last decade has been directed to psychological competence rather than performance, concerned with task analysis rather than with the nature of the processes involved. This has been unfortunately restrictive, because psychologists in general are interested not only in what tasks the mind can accomplish, but also what goes on in the mind, how, and when. The problem has been to find a way of specifying what these processes might be, and that problem arises out of a failure to think clearly about both the levels of analysis at which any given construct arises and the nature of the description of the relevant processes.

Marr's distinction between Type 1 and Type 2 theories may be relevant here. Marr was concerned with what he called "computational" theories, but this term is unfortunate (and provocative to some psychologists) because he is really referring to what previous writers had called task-analysis or competence. For Marr, a Type 1 theory is computational by providing an abstract identification of the task concerned; a Type 2 theory applies when information is processed by "the simultaneous action of a considerable number of processes, whose interaction is its own simplest description." Marr considered that these two types accounted for all scientific explanations. Type 2 explanations are important for psychology, because we may suspect that certain psychological phenomena are only describable in these terms: by a complete description of all the processes responsible for a given phenomenon. What happens, happens; nothing more can be said in explanation of why it happens. This has been challenged, of course, either by those who believe that formalism will allow for the development of Type 1 theories to account for the relevant phenomena or by those who wish to argue that other types of theory may exist.

Fodor is certainly the most prominent of those who argue for a formalist approach, believing that a computational psychology is the only theoretical psychology we can hope to achieve. Such a psychology treats mental processes as operations defined in terms of formal manipulations of formally described representations. Mental processes can only be viewed as operations within an uninterpreted logical system. The conclusion must be that, although such computational theories can describe mental states and processes, they cannot have anything to say about how mental states map onto the world. For psychological research, there is no point in trying to discover the mapping between the mind and the world, because how the world is makes no difference to one's mental states. In Putnam's phrase, this leads to methodological solipsism. Causal processes within the nervous system may well mediate between thought and action; there may be an abstract mapping between the mental representation and actual or possible worlds; the psychological calculus may map onto the environment and our activities within it, but, if we follow Fodor, such matters lie outside the formal syntactic concerns of a computational theory.

The diametric viewpoint is most commonly illustrated by Searle and his Chinese Room "thought experiment." He imagines himself locked in a room, in which there are various slips of paper with doodles on them; an opening through which further doodle-papers can be passed to him, and through which he can pass papers out; and a book of rules telling him how to pair the doodles, which are identified by their shape or form. An example of one of these rules might be that when squiggle–squiggle is passed into the room to him, he should pass out squoggle–squoggle. There are more complex sequences of doodle pairing, some requiring comparison of doodle pairs already inside the room. So far as Searle, inside the room, is concerned the squiggles and squoggles are mere meaningless doodles. However, unbeknown to him, they are Chinese characters and the people outside the room, being Chinese, treat them as such. The doodles passed in are, in fact, questions, and the doodles which he passes out are, in fact, answers. Although the answers are sensible answers to the questions, Searle himself, inside the room, knows nothing of this.

The point of Searle's analogy is that in the room he is instantiating a computer program; he is performing formal manipulations of uninterpreted patterns; it is all syntax and no semantics. Searle argues that no formal system can understand anything solely by virtue of its instantiating an algorithmic procedure. If it could, Searle in the room would understand Chinese; hence theoretical psychology (because it implies understanding) cannot be grounded in computational concepts, and semantic abilities can never be captured by a formalist description. There are well-known defences of the Chinese Room analogy (see Boden, 1988): the "Robot reply" and the "English reply," although most neuroscientists are likely to find them unconvincing. The one aspect upon which we should focus is the critical role of intentionality.

Searle's argument proposes that no system can possess understanding unless it also possesses intentionality, which, he declares, is a biological phenomenon. It depends upon the underlying biochemistry, as do photosynthesis and lactation. He accepts that neuroprotein may not be the only substance in the universe capable of supporting mental life, but he believes it to be intuitively obvious that inorganic substances are essentially incapable of supporting mental functions.

The problem is that we do not know whether intentionality is comparable to photosynthesis. Just what intentionality is, is philosophically controversial. We cannot even be entirely confident that we can recognize it when we see it. It is generally agreed that the propositional attitudes are intentional, and that feelings and sensations are not, but there is no clear consensus about the intentionality of emotions. The critical point is that an understanding of intentionality is critical for a resolution of the issue of the nature of mind, and the kind of processes which might be considered to support mental understanding.

It is common to speak of connectionist models as neurally inspired, and their units as neuron-like, although in some ways the biological metaphor is now more distant than in the early days, when these models were commonly referred to as neural networks. However, certain similarities between nervous systems and connectionist devices remain intriguing. For example, both neurons and connectionist units are elementary processing units which combine inputs from some units and send outputs to yet other units. In both connectionist networks and nervous systems it is the connectivity which seems to be the principal determinant of behavior. The characteristic of graceful degradation under insult is another common feature. These lend plausibility to the assumption that connectionist architectures can provide a model for certain aspects of the performance of nervous systems.

A rather tangled set of claims has resulted as to how connectionist models of the abstract, cognitive variety relate to neuropsychological theories. Some view connectionism as an explicitly neural model, as a branch of neural research, which facilitates the reduction of cognitive investigations to neural theorizing. An alternative view is to conceive of connectionism, at least from its cognitive science perspective, as related to but not identified with neural research. The choice of view depends critically upon the proper relation between cognitive theories and neuroscience theories.

Philosophers such as Putnam have opposed reductionistic mind–brain identity because of the independence of the symbolic structures and their implementation. From this leads another argument to the functionalist theory of mind, here characterizing mental states as understandable in terms of their interactions with other mental states, rather than in terms of their physical embodiment. By this argument, symbolic theories are functional theories par excellence.

With regard to the issue of theory reduction, Fodor has argued that the theory reduction model is inappropriate for what he calls the "special sciences," of which psychology is one. The argument is a familiar one, and it is that law-like regularities in nature are not reducible to the laws of the more basic sciences, because the concepts used to state these regularities cannot be translated into the concepts of the more basic sciences. His example is drawn from economics; it is that one cannot specify, in terms of the more basic sciences, what conditions must be met for something to count as "money," and yet there are law-like regularities in economics that refer to money. In the same way, there are regularities in the behavior of organisms that might be able to be stated in psychological terms, but not in the vocabulary of the more basic sciences.

This so-called strong autonomy position seems to entail that there can be no fruitful interaction between the special sciences and more basic sciences. Since the categories employed in cognitive psychology and in neuroscience are incompatible with each other, we cannot learn about cognitive processes by studying how they are instantiated in the brain. However, the history of the discipline already provides fruitful interactions between cognitive psychology and neuroscience, certainly at the level of peripheral processes (such as vision), but also at the cognitive level (for example, neurolinguistics).

So, are we forced to return to a reductionist approach? There may be an alternative. The interaction between sciences may be facilitated by what Darden and Maull have termed "interfield theories," theories which relate phenomena which are primarily studied in different disciplines. Their example is the chromosomal theory of inheritance, which relates Mendelian factors (understood functionally in terms of traits) with chromosomes. If we do not need reduction to relate disciplines, fruitful interaction might nevertheless be possible between cognitive psychology and neuroscience, even if cognitive science entities cannot be defined in neuroscience terms.

The second view of the relation between cognitivist and neuroscience theories is to see cognitive science models as more abstract than neural models. One reason for adopting this position is that it is critical for cognitive theorizing that connectionist networks (or any other functionalist architectures) carry a semantic interpretation. Very little is known at present about how this can be achieved at a neural level. Another reason is that, despite propaganda to the contrary, there are still many features of the brain which are not replicated in connectionist systems. Smolensky is among those to have pointed out that connectionist architectures are increasingly being dictated by mathematical considerations and decreasingly by neural ones.

It is only fair to acknowledge that many connectionists place little priority on the neural realism of their theories. Models are frequently explored because they seem capable of performing interesting cognitive tasks; and it is not clear how, for example, one might find a neural implementation of certain techniques, such as back-propagation. But if connectionist models do not model activity in the nervous system, what are they models of? The most common assumption is that they are relatively abstract models of the processing that occurs in the nervous system, and that they model the sort of information processing which the nervous system is capable of performing.

My most influential mentor, the late Professor Stuart Dimond, used an appealing metaphor. He likened the study of the brain to walking into a vast Gothic cathedral: a complex, sophisticated, and multidimensional machine, which is open to analysis in many differing ways. One might perform a purely structural analysis of the forces transmitted by the vaults down through the walls, piers, and buttresses. One might perform an analysis of the constructional techniques of the masonry, of the acoustic properties, or the visual aesthetics. Others might be concerned with air movement and thermal dynamics; or the social functions the building supports; and there are affective and spiritual components which merit analysis. None of these analyses alone provides an account of this particular machine and its individual properties; even together they provide only a limited insight into our understanding of the building.

The discipline of neuropsychology has taken on a hardly less daunting task in attempting to understand the brain from within the discipline of psychology. What is clear is that progress with the task will be limited and confused unless certain central issues are recognized and tackled.

First, it must be acknowledged that the constructs under study relate to the mind, and that this implies facing the very considerable philosophical issues which this entails. At the least, neuropsychologists must adopt an explicit theory of mind, and ensure that neuropsychological explanations are congruent with the position which has been adopted.

Second, it must be recognized that the descriptive form of the nature of neuropsychological processes is central to any adequate understanding of the relation between brain and mind. Pure functionalism is inadequate, and we must determine whether formalism is adequate to the representation of these neuropsychological approaches.

Third, the core position of intentionality should be acknowledged, and it is perhaps time that psychology saw a revival of interest in motivation. Cognitive theories will remain psychologically sterile without a new formulation of the concepts of drive, intention, and will. Conation demands to be reinstated alongside cognition and affect in psychological endeavor.

Finally, we must be clearer about the contribution which cognitive science approaches, and particularly connectionism, may make to neuropsychology, and the relationship between models cast in these terms and those cast as more purely psychological models of mental processes. Neuropsychologists should not lose sight of the fact that they have the intention of studying the mind, rather than simply behavior or cognition, for then neuropsychology would eventually be much the richer.

Note I acknowledge material drawn from Boden (1988) and Bechtel and Abrahamsen (1991) used in the preparation of this entry. *See also* the list of general neuropsychological references given on p. xix.

BIBLIOGRAPHY

Bechtel, W., & Abranhamsen, A. (1991). *Connectionism and the mind*. Oxford: Blackwell.
Boden, M. A. (1988). *Computer models of mind*. Cambridge: Cambridge University Press.
Clarke, E., & Dewhurst, K. (1972). *An illustrated history of brain function*. Oxford: Sandford.
Clarke, E., & O'Malley, C. D. (1968). *The human brain and spinal cord*. Berkeley: University of California Press.
Walsh, K. W. (1978). *Neuropsychology: A clinical approach*. Edinburgh: Churchill Livingstone.

J. GRAHAM BEAUMONT

neurotransmitters Neurotransmitters are chemicals that act on receptor sites at postsynaptic membranes after their release from nerve terminals to produce either excitation or inhibition of the target cell. These changes are produced by alterations in the distribution of ions across the postsynaptic membranes of neurons, muscles, and glands. Chemically mediated neurotransmission is the primary way in which signals are transferred from one neuron to another, or from neurons to muscle or gland cells. Electrically mediated transmission of signals can also occur at certain electrical synapses, but it is a relatively rare form of neurotransmission that occurs mainly in situations where it is important for two neurons to synchronize their activities exactly, such as synapses controlling rapid escape movements in certain fish and invertebrates. Chemically mediated transmission involves the following steps, all of which must occur for the substance to meet all the criteria for definition as a neurotransmitter:

1 *Synthesis at the presynaptic neuron*
The putative transmitter must be synthesized in the presynaptic neuron. This usually occurs in the synaptic terminal, although peptides are synthesized in the soma and transported via the axon to the terminal.

2 *Storage in the presynaptic terminal*
The putative transmitter must be stored in the terminal, either in bound form within synaptic vesicles or in unbound form in the cytoplasm.

3 *Release into the synaptic extracellular space*
The terminal should release the transmitter in a pharmacologically identifiable form. Not every substance released, however, is necessarily a neurotransmitter.

4 *Recognition and binding by postsynaptic receptors*
At the postsynaptic neuron, the putative neurotransmitter should reproduce exactly the transmission events produced by stimulating the presynaptic neuron and the effects should be obtained at concentrations as low as those present after release by nerve stimulation. The effects of a putative transmitter should also be blocked by competitive antagonists in a dose-dependent manner, similar to that observed with neuronal stimulation.

5 *Inactivation and termination of activity*
There should be mechanisms to terminate the action of the substance. These include an active reuptake mechanism which transports the substance back into the presynaptic terminal and degradative enzymes. Monoamines are either degraded or transported back into nerve terminals; amino acids are taken up into the nerve terminal or into adjacent glial cells (or both); peptides are degraded by peptidases.

531

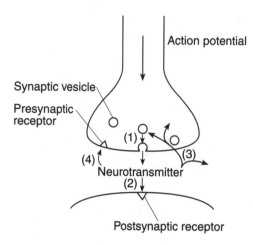

Figure 52 Chemical signalling at the synapse (synaptic transmission). The diagram shows the key stages in synaptic transmission: (1) release of neurotransmitter in response to depolarization of nerve terminal by the action potential; (2) interaction of neurotransmitter with postsynaptic receptor to cause a change in the postsynaptic cell; (3) the action of the neurotransmitter is terminated by either taking it back into the nerve terminal or be destroying it in the synaptic cleft; (4) synaptic receptors may exist to control release of the neurotransmitter.

TYPES OF NEUROTRANSMITTERS

More than 50 different chemicals are now known to function as transmitters in the brain, and research has been gradually adding to the list of known and putative transmitters. The three main categories of neurotransmitters are the biogenic amines or monoamines (which contain a single NH_2 group), the amino acids, and the peptides. One of the major differences between these types of neurotransmitters is in terms of molecular weight. The monoamine and amino acid neurotransmitters generally weigh less than 200 whereas peptides are relatively large and weigh considerably more. The functional significance of most of the monoamines and amino acids, and some of the peptides, is relatively well understood, and is summarized in Table 12.

There are at least 20 other identified peptide neurotransmitters including: adrenocorticotropic hormone, arginine vasopressin, arginine vasotocin, atrial natriuretic polypeptide, bradykinin, calcitonin, calcitonin gene-related peptide, L-carnosine, corticotropin-releasing hormone, gonadotropin-releasing hormone, growth hormone-releasing hormone, alpha-melanocyte-stimulating hormone, neuropeptide, neurotensin, oxytocin, thyrotropin-releasing hormone, and vasoactive intestinal peptide.

HISTORY

The first suggestion that chemical substances might be involved in neural transmission was probably made by Emil Du Bois-Reymond in 1877. Subsequent work by physiologists such as Langley (1901), Elliot (1904), Dixon (1907), and Dale (1914) led to the identification of adrenaline (epinephrine) and acetylcholine (ACh) as neurotransmitters in the peripheral nervous system. However, it was not until 1921 that Otto Loewi presented the first incontrovertible proof for the chemical mediation of nerve-impulse transmission. Loewi took the hearts out of two frogs and suspended them from a frame. Since the rate at which a heart beats is controlled by nerves that lead to the heart from the brain, Loewi electrically stimulated the nerve leading to one of the two hearts. He found that such stimulation slowed the rate at which the heart beat. He then took fluid that had been dripped over the heart that he had stimulated and dripped it over the second heart (which was not being stimulated) and found that its rate also became slower. This demonstrated that electrical stimulation of the nerve leading to one heart caused the release of a chemical that could slow the rate of the other heart, the nerves of which were not stimulated, proving that nerves exert their effects by releasing chemicals that act on the structure that the nerves innervate. Loewi subsequently identified this substance as ACh.

IONOTROPIC, METABOTROPIC AND NEUROMODULATORY EFFECTS

Neurotransmitters can affect other neurons in a number of ways. For the sake of clarity, three major types of effects will be distinguished: ionotropic, metabotropic, and neuromodulatory.

Ionotropic neurotransmitters

Some neurotransmitters such as ACh, glycine, glutamate, and gamma-aminobutyric acid (GABA), have "inherent" biological activity such that the neurotransmitter directly increases the conductance of certain ions across the postsynaptic membrane. Neurotransmitters of this

Table 12   Functional significance of neurotransmitters.

Category	Transmitter	Functional significance
	Acetylcholine (ACh)	Principal peripheral transmitter at neuromuscular junctions, and neural-neural synapses of the autonomic nervous system. Major central roles include modulation of arousal, attention, learning, and memory. Decreased in the neocortex and hippocampus in patients with Alzheimer's disease.
Monoamines	Serotonin (5-HT)	Major central roles include modulation of information processing, body temperature, blood pressure, sleep, pain, aggression, mood, movement, sexual behavior, and endocrine secretion. Peripheral actions include mediation of satiety.
	Histamine	Central effects include regulation of arousal, body temperature, and biological rhythms. Peripheral effects include hypotension, bronchoconstriction, and gastric release of hydrochloric acid.
(Catecholamines)	Dopamine (DA)	Central effects include modulation of reward, positive reinforcement, and locomotor activity. Implicated in the etiology of substance abuse, Parkinson's disease, and schizophrenia.
	Noradrenaline (Norepinephrine) (NA or NE)	Principal transmitter at neuroeffector junctions of the autonomic nervous system. Central roles include modulation of arousal, feeding, and mood.
	Adrenaline (Epinephrine) (A or E)	Produced in periphery by adrenal medulla. Stimulates sympathetic division of the autonomic nervous system to produce "fight or flight" responses.
Amino acids	Glutamate	The major excitatory transmitter in the mammalian CNS. Implicated in neural plasticity, learning, and memory. Excessive activity is associated with eleptogenesis and excitotoxicity.
	Aspartate	Another excitatory transmitter that plays a similar role to glutamate, although it is less abundant.
	Gamma-aminobutyric acid	The major inhibitory amino acid in the mammalian CNS. Enhanced activity produces sedative, anxiolytic, and anticonvulsant effects.
	Glycine	Another inhibitory amino acid that may play a modulatory role at interneurons in the spinal cord.
Peptides (endogenous opioids)	Leu-Enkephalin	The functional properties of the endogenous opioids can best be characterized as a group by stating that their effects are similar to plant-derived and synthetic opiate alkaloids. Their physiological roles include pain perception, stress mechanisms, respiratory regulation, temperature control, tolerance development, and physical dependence.
	Met-Enkephalin Beta-endorphin Dynorphin A	
Other peptides	Substance P	A mediator of inflammation, as well as a neurotransmitter in primary afferent fibers carrying pain signals.
	Cholecystokinin Octapeptide (CCK-8)	Central effects include modulation of opioid analgesia. Peripheral effects include modulation of satiety.
	Vasopressin	Also known as antidiuretic hormone (ADH) and acts peripherally to facilitate water reabsorption by the kidneys. May play a role in memory consolidation.
	Somatostatin	Central activities include modulation of heat, pain, sleep, and locomotor activity. Greatly reduced in cerebral cortex of patients with Alzheimer's disease.
	Angiotensin II	Has potent vasoconstrictor activity in the periphery. Central actions include stimulation of pressor responses and drinking.

that the neurotransmitter directly increases the conductance of certain ions across the post-synaptic membrane. Neurotransmitters of this type are classified as "ionotropic" transmitters. For example, glutamate opens sodium channels, thereby enabling sodium ions to enter the post-synaptic cell. The sodium ions, bringing with them a positive charge, partially depolarize the membrane, making it easier for an action potential to be generated. Consequently, glutamate is an excitatory neurotransmitter.

ACh exerts ionotropic effects at some synapses but not at others. The synapses at which it produces ionotropic effects are known as nicotinic synapses because they can be stimulated by nicotine. When ACh attaches to a nicotinic receptor it opens sodium channels to allow sodium ions to cross the membrane for about 1 to 3 msec. Ionic effects at synapses are rapid but short-lived. Typically the transmitter opens the ion channels within 10 msec after its release and keeps them open for about 10 to 20 msec. Ionotropic synapses are therefore useful for conveying information about rapidly changing events, such as those associated with visual and auditory stimulation, and certain muscle movements. GABA is another neurotransmitter that exerts ionotropic effects, but its effects are inhibitory. When GABA binds to its receptors, it opens chloride channels, enabling chloride ions, with a negative charge, to cross the membrane into the cell more rapidly than usual.

Metabotropic neurotransmitters

Other neurotransmitters, such as norepinephrine, dopamine, and serotonin, have no direct activity but act through a "second messenger" system to cause metabolic changes in the postsynaptic membrane, leading to changes in conductance of particular ions or other biological effects. Neurotransmitters of this class are known as "metabotropic" transmitters. Since these effects take place through a sequence of metabolic reactions they are slower, last longer, and are more complicated than ionic effects. The effects emerge about 30 msec after the release of the transmitter; they may last seconds or in some cases much longer.

For example, epinephrine is a neurotransmitter that exerts metabotropic effects. When an epinephrine molecule attaches to its receptor, it alters the configuration of the receptor protein. The altered protein allows part of the protein inside the

neuron to react with other molecules. A series of chemical steps then produces an increased concentration of the second messenger cyclic AMP (adenosine monophosphate) inside the neuron. The second messenger carries a message to several areas within the postsynaptic cell. Cyclic AMP provides the energy to alter (phosphorylate) certain proteins. Exactly which proteins are altered, and how they are altered, varies from one cell to another. In some cases the altered proteins open or close one type of ion channel in the membrane. In other cases the proteins alter the structure of the cell or change its metabolic activity. It is believed that these relatively slow and long-lasting changes are involved in processes such as learning and memory.

Neuromodulators

A neuromodulator is a substance that works at the synapse to modulate the normal effect of the neurotransmitter at that synapse. It may either increase or decrease the action of the neurotransmitter, or it may shorten or prolong its activity. In most cases, like the metabotropic neurotransmitters, neuromodulators exert their effects by second messengers. Most neuromodulators are peptides. Some peptides that play a neurotransmitter role at some synapses can also play a neuromodulatory role at others. These peptides often have additional physiological effects that are related to their origins in the stomach, intestines, or other visceral organs.

Most neurons release two or more chemicals from their terminals (colocalization). In many cases one of them is a neurotransmitter such as ACh and the other is a peptide neuromodulator. Such a combination can be highly adaptive. For example, ACh triggers salivation and a peptide neuromodulator (vasoactive intestinal peptide – VIP) released with it causes the salivation to continue. The effect of ACh by itself would be too brief, and the effect of the peptide by itself would be too weak and too slow. In other cases a peptide may reduce or halt the effect of ACh.

NEUROTRANSMITTERS AND DRUGS

Most psychoactive drugs affect behavior by altering neurotransmission. Some drugs known as "agonists" mimic or increase the activity of a given neurotransmitter at the postsynaptic membrane and activate the postsynaptic neuron. Other drugs known as "antagonists" bind to postsynaptic receptors to block the effects of a neurotransmitter. There are also drugs which can affect the production or release of a neurotransmitter, modify the availability of the neurotransmitter in the synaptic cleft, or modulate the activity of second messenger systems in the postsynaptic membrane.

The various synaptic sites at which drugs or dietary manipulations can act to modify neurotransmission include: the axonal membrane; axonal transport; precursor availability; presynaptic synthesis, storage, and release mechanisms; presynaptic autoreceptors; postsynaptic receptors; reuptake mechanisms; enzymatic inactivation mechanisms; and postsynaptic "second messenger" mechanisms.

The local anesthetics (or membrane stabilizers) are one class of drugs that prevent depolarization of the axonal membrane and prevent action potentials being propagated down axons. Other drugs, such as colchisine, nonselectively interfere with axonal transport of neurotransmitters from the soma to the synaptic terminal where it is released. Yet other drugs produce their effect by inhibiting the actions of enzymes found in presynaptic terminals which, together with cofactors and necessary ions, catalyze the synthesis of neurotransmitter from its precursor. Inhibition of the activity of these enzymes decreases the amount of neurotransmitter available for release. For example, the drug AMPT blocks the synthesis of the catecholamines: dopamine, norepinephrine, and epinephrine. Tyrosine from the diet is normally converted into dopa, which is a precursor to the catecholamines. AMPT is similar enough to tyrosine for it to attach to the same enzyme. When it does so, it blocks the enzyme from attaching to tyrosine; as a result, very little tyrosine is converted to dopa. Synthesis inhibitors such as AMPT are used mainly for research purposes.

It is also possible to modify the synthesis of neurotransmitters by changing the availability of certain precursors in the diet. Normally the brain maintains fairly constant levels of each neurotransmitter. However, in some cases precursor availability becomes the "rate limiting step" in transmitter synthesis. This is particularly true of the precursor for serotonin (5-HT) – tryptophan. The brain has an active transport system that carries tryptophan into neurons and is also used to transport other amino acids that are almost always more prevalent in the diet. Thus, after a meal rich in protein, the level of tryptophan reaching the brain is often reduced by competition from other amino acids. Since serotonin synthesis is dependent on the availability of tryptophan, the effect of such competition is to reduce the synthesis of serotonin. One way to increase the amount of tryptophan entering the brain is to eat carbohydrates. Carbohydrates increase release of the hormone insulin, which takes several competing amino acids out of the bloodstream and into cells throughout the body, thus decreasing the competition against tryptophan for entry into the brain and promoting serotonin synthesis. The relative sensitivity of serotonin synthesis to dietary manipulation suggests that some disorders associated with low levels of serotonin (e.g. affective disorder) may be amenable to this alternative to pharmacological intervention.

Within the presynaptic terminal, neurotransmitters are stored either within vesicles or in the cytoplasm. Reserpine, a drug that has been used as an antihypertensive and as an antipsychotic, is an example of a drug that disrupts vesicular storage. Reserpine causes prolonged release of brain amines, especially catecholamines, from vesicles, resulting in a significant depletion of brain catecholamines for several days after a single dose. A more transient increase in the release of catecholamines, especially dopamine, is produced by amphetamine, which also inhibits the reuptake of catecholamines. Drugs that alter the synaptic availability of a transmitter, rather than mimic the transmitter, are known as indirect agonists. Thus, amphetamine is an indirect dopamine agonist.

The terminal of an axon has voltage-dependent calcium channels. When the membrane is at rest, these channels are closed and calcium stays outside the cell. When an action potential reaches the end of an axon, however, the consequent depolarization opens the calcium channels. The increased calcium concentration inside the presynaptic cell causes the cell to release a certain amount of its neurotransmitter during the subsequent 1 or 2 milliseconds. This calcium-dependent release mechanism provides another opportunity for modulation by a class of drugs known as calcium channel antagonists.

All the sites of drug action described hitherto are presynaptic. There is one remaining significant target of presynaptic drug action – the autoreceptor. Autoreceptors are similar to post-synaptic receptors in that they both bind neuro-transmitters in a fashion analogous to a key (the transmitter) fitting into a lock (the receptor). However, unlike postsynaptic receptors, which bind transmitters released from other neurons, autoreceptors bind transmitters released from their own terminal. Consequently, autoreceptors are able to detect the presynaptic output of a given transmitter and are believed to play a role in feedback systems governing the release or synthesis of neurotransmitters. Autoreceptors tend to differ in their sensitivity to neurotrans-mitters in comparison with the corresponding postsynaptic receptor. This means that it is sometimes possible to modulate synaptic activity by employing a concentration of a drug that will preferentially bind to the autoreceptor rather than the corresponding postsynaptic receptor.

The most important synaptic site of drug action is the postsynaptic receptor. This is where the majority of drugs have their activity, either as agonists or as antagonists. In recent years a variety of receptor subtypes have been identified for each of the monoamines and amino acids. Examples of selective agonists and antagonists at specific monoamine and amino acid receptor subtypes are presented in Table 13.

After its release a neurotransmitter would continue to stimulate receptors if a mechanism for its inactivation did not exist. Two main types of inactivation occur. Enzymatic inactivation is med-iated by enzymes that occur within the synaptic cleft. For example, acetylcholinesterase is an enzyme that inactivates ACh. It can be reversibly

Table 13   Examples of selective agonists and antagonists at the receptor subtypes of monoamine and amino acid neurotransmitters.

Category	Transmitter	Receptor	Agonist	Antagonist
	Acetylcholine	Nicotinic	Nicotine	Mecamylamine
		Muscarinic	Muscarine	Scopolamine
		M_1	McN-A-343	Pirenzepine
		M_2	—	Methoctramine
		M_3	—	Hexahydrosiladifenidol
Biogenic amines	Serotonin	$5HT_{1A}$	8-hydroxy-DPAT	Propranolol
		$5HT_{1B}$	Isapirone	—
		$5HT_{1C}$	α-methyl-5HT	Propranolol
		$5HT_{1D}$	Sumatriptan	Cyanopindolol
		$5HT_2$	LSD	Ritanserin
		$5HT_3$	2-methyl-5HT	Ondansetron
		$5HT_4$	2-methyl-5HT	Tropisetron
	Histamine	H_1	Histamine	Diphenhydramine
		H_2	Histamine	Cimetidine
(Catecholamines)	Dopamine	D_1	SKF38393	SCH23390
		D_2	Quinpirole	Haloperidol
		D_3	Quinpirole	Spiperone
		D_4	—	Clozapine
		D_5	SKF38393	SCH23390
	Noradrenaline	$\alpha 1$	Phenylephrine	Prazosin
		$\alpha 2$	Clonidine	Yohimbine
		$\beta 1$	Dobutamine	Metoprolol
		$\beta 2$	Salbutamol	Butoxamine
Amino acids	Glutamate	Kainate	Kainic acid	DNQX
		AMPA	AMPA	—
		NMDA	AMAA	MK-801
	Gamma-amino-butyric-acid	$GABA_A$	Muscimol	Bicuculline
		$GABA_B$	Baclofen	Phaclofen

inhibited by acetylcholinesterase inhibitors, such as physostigmine, which have the effect of increasing ACh activity (and therefore act as indirect agonists). Monoamine oxidase (MAO) and catechol-O-methyltransferase (COMT) are two other enzymes that are primarily responsible for the inactivation of catecholamines. MAO inhibitors like deprenyl (selegiline), or COMT inhibitors such as pyrogallol, have the effect of prolonging the action of released catecholamines.

The other major mechanism of inactivating neurotransmitters in the synaptic cleft is reuptake back into the presynaptic terminal. This is an active process that has the advantage of recycling the transmitter so that it is available for release on a subsequent occasion. Cocaine, and certain antidepressants, are examples of drugs that inhibit reuptake, and thereby prolong the effects of released catecholamines and/or serotonin.

Finally, it is increasingly clear that there is also considerable scope for drug action "downstream" from the postsynaptic receptor at the level of second messenger systems. The three major second messenger systems are the cyclic AMP system, the cyclic GMP system, and the calcium system. All three systems are intermediates between neurotransmitter "first messengers" and protein phosphorylation, which is both a final common pathway and a prerequisite for diverse biological responses. Many drugs regulate protein phosphorylation, and thus behavior, by affecting the ability of neurotransmitters to alter second-messenger levels.

IMPLICATIONS FOR NEURO-PSYCHOLOGY

A knowledge of neurochemistry has become increasingly important to the discipline of neuropsychology as a result of advances in the identification and localization of specific neurotransmitter systems and receptor subtypes in the brain through the use of sensitive and specific biochemical, histochemical, and neuroimaging methods (e.g. positron emission tomography – PET). Indeed, since the discovery of the association between PARKINSON'S DISEASE and a deficiency in nigrostriatal dopamine (Hornykiewicz, 1960), a progressively more detailed picture of the neurochemical bases of other neurodegenerative disorders, including Alzheimer's disease and HUNTINGTON'S DISEASE, has emerged. There are also numerous hypotheses concerning the nature of the neurochemical dysfunction underlying many other neurological and psychiatric disorders such as EPILEPSY, SCHIZOPHRENIA, depression, anxiety, and obsessive-compulsive disorder. Knowledge of neurotransmitter systems is also increasingly relevant to the study of neurological lesions, since it is now possible to infer, or actually observe with PET or other functional neuroimaging techniques, the neurochemical consequences of such lesions. This additional information could then provide the basis for a significant improvement in clinical assessment and treatment.

BIBLIOGRAPHY

Bloom, F. E., & Kupfer, D. J. (Eds). (1995). *Psychopharmacology: The fourth generation of progress*. New York: Raven.

Carlsson, A. (1987). Perspectives on the discovery of monoaminergic neurotransmission. *Annual Reviews of Neuroscience, 10*, 19–40.

Cooper, J. R., Bloom, F. E., & Roth, R. H. (1991). *The biochemical basis of neuropharmacology*, 5th edn. Oxford: Oxford University Press.

Feldman, R. S., & Quenzer, L. F. (1984). *Fundamentals of neuropsychopharmacology*. Sunderland, MA: Sinauer.

Gilman, A. G. et al. (Eds). (1990). *The pharmacological basis of therapeutics*. London: Macmillan.

Green, A. R., & Costain, L. (1986). *Pharmacology and biochemistry of psychiatric disorders*. Chichester: Wiley.

Leonard, B. E. (1992). *Fundamentals of psychopharmacology*. Chichester: Wiley.

Stone, T. N. (1995). *Neuropharmacology*. New York: W. H. Freeman.

Strange, P. G. (1992). *Brain biochemistry and brain disorders*. Oxford: Oxford University Press.

Webster, R. A., & Jordan, C. C. (Eds). (1989). *Drugs, neurotransmitters and disease*. Oxford: Blackwell.

MICHAEL J. MORGAN

nonfluent aphasia *See* APHASIA.

nystagmus Nystagmus is an abnormal rhythmic oscillation of the eyes, which may occur in the vertical or the lateral plane, or may be rotational (*rotational nystagmus*). The speed of movement may be the same in both directions, or it may be quicker in one direction when the more rapid deviation is taken as the direction of the nystagmus. It may occur at rest, on convergence, when gaze is directed in a specific direction, or only when the head is placed in certain positions (*positional nystagmus*).

There are various causes of nystagmus, which may not necessarily be pathological, as nystagmus may occur in a familial and congenital form. It may also be secondary to prolonged working in dim light, as in miner's nystagmus, which is understood as a chronic adaptation which attempts to maintain a compromise between central high acuity vision and peripheral vision which is more effective at low levels of light. Miner's nystagmus is of retinal origin, and retinal defects may also produce nystagmus. However, nystagmus may also be associated with disorders of the labyrinth (this form is also related to the nystagmus produced by CALORIC STIMULATION), and with central lesions of the CEREBELLUM and BRAIN STEM. Nystagmus in the vertical plane is always associated with lesions of the brain stem. MULTIPLE SCLEROSIS is a common central cause of nystagmus.

O

object agnosia *See* AGNOSIA

occipital eye field   The occipital eye field is the region of the occipital lobe involved in the control of EYE MOVEMENT. It is less clearly defined than the FRONTAL EYE FIELD.

occipital lobe   The occipital lobe is situated in the most posterior portion of the cerebral cortex. Unlike the temporal, parietal, and frontal cortices, the occipital lobe is almost exclusively devoted to a single sensory system – namely vision. Although its special involvement in visual processing was clearly recognized by the middle of the 1800s, only during the past three decades have some of the most important details concerning the anatomical connections and physiological functions of the visual cortical areas been discovered.

BASIC ANATOMY

The occipital lobe encompasses the region extending anteriorly from the calcarine fissure, located at the posterior poles of the left and right cerebral hemispheres. Its anterior boundary is framed by the parieto-occipital sulcus dorsally and by the inferior preoccipital sulcus ventrally (Bailey & Von Bonin, 1951). It is primarily composed of three cytoarchitectonically distinct areas – striate cortex (area 17), parastriate cortex (area 18), and peristriate cortex (area 19).

The striate cortex, also known as V1, is so named for the distinctive lamination pattern (including the "stria of Gennari") in its greatly enlarged layer 4. Often referred to as the "core" of the occipital lobe, area 17 houses primary visual cortex in the area in and immediately surrounding the calcarine fissure. The calcarine region has attained special prominence only in primates, but its precise size and shape and the manner in which

the visual world is represented in it exhibit striking variability, even among individual humans (Miller, 1982). V1 contains an exquisitely precise topographical "map" of the visual world, derived from the lateral geniculate nucleus (LGN) inputs that project almost exclusively to it. The striate area is remarkably similar morphologically across the various primate species, but it constitutes a much higher overall percentage of the cerebral cortical surface in monkeys than in humans (more than 15 percent vs less than 5 percent), despite being physically twice as large in humans. This feature can be mainly attributed to the great expansion of the association regions of the human cortex.

The parastriate area forms a belt around the striate zone and is believed to contain several functionally distinct visual areas. One of these is known as V2, whose visual map forms a mirror image of that found in V1, except that the representation of the horizontal meridian is split into V2's dorsal and ventral segments. Area 18 receives very few direct geniculate projections in the primate, but has important topographically organized connections with the pulvinar and other subcortical structures. The peristriate cortex located anterior to area 18 forms yet another belt that contains still more visual areas (including V4) that provide topographical maps of the visual world, albeit coarser ones than those found in area 17. The number of primate cortical visual areas continues to proliferate, with at least two dozen visual areas and 300 interconnections having been documented thus far in the macaque monkey. Much of this neural circuitry lies outside the boundaries of the occipital lobe itself.

Several anatomical features are prominent in the striate and prestriate regions of the occipital cortex. One of these is the radial columnar structure ubiquitous throughout the cerebral cortex, which in V1 (and to a lesser extent in V2) is associated with ocular dominance and orientational selectivity (see discussion on V1 functional physiology). The complex lamination is associated with different patterns of anatomical connectivity in that: (a) projections to "higher" cortical centers emanate mostly from the three most superficial layers; (b) projections to "lower" cortical and subcortical areas originate to a greater extent in the deepest two layers; and (c) intermediate layer 4 receives projections from "lower" visual regions (Van Essen & Maunsell, 1983). In V1, the greatly enlarged granular layer 4 is subdivided into several smaller layers, one of which (layer 4C) contains parallel visual projections from the magnocellular and parvocellular LGN layers (located in layers 4Cα and 4Cβ respectively). A more recent discovery is that cytochrome oxidase (CO) blobs in V1 contain primarily monocular, color-selective cells with little orientation preference. These blobs connect with corresponding CO stripes in V2 in a functionally significant manner, discussed below. All of these features are present at birth and do not appear to depend greatly on visual experience, although visual disruption during development clearly affects the size and functional properties of occipital cortex, especially in the prestriate regions.

REPRESENTATION OF THE VISUAL FIELD IN V1

The representation of the visual field in V1 reflects both the "inverted" topography of the retinal image and the decussation of the visual pathways at the optic chiasm. Thus the lower-field and upper-field projections are located in the upper and lower lips of the calcarine fissure respectively, while the right half of the visual field in both eyes is represented in the left striate cortex, and vice versa. The V1 representational map is depicted in Figure 53. The central portion of the visual field is confined to the occipital pole region in humans, whereas the peripheral visual field lies buried deep within the anterior portion of the calcarine fissure. In monkeys the entire visual map is shifted laterally, such that the foveal representation lies just posterior to the lunate sulcus in the lateral face of the occipital lobe.

One important feature of the retinotopic map of V1 shown in Figure 53 is the disproportionately large amount of neural area devoted to the central visual field. Indeed, one visual degree lying along the horizontal meridian at the center of the visual field occupies over 6 mm of cortical surface, whereas 10 degrees or more of the peripheral visual field are compressed into less than 1 mm of visual cortex. This feature is known as the cortical magnification factor, and parallels the receptor density distribution on the retina and the reduction in visual acuity from the fovea to the periphery.

The topography of the cortical visual map explains the nature of the visual field defects characteristic of area 17 damage. Homonymous HEMIANOPIAS (loss of one half-field in both eyes) are more likely to be produced by damage to primary visual cortex than anywhere else, and *quadrantanopias* (loss of either the upper or lower visual quadrant on the left or right side) can also occur. Damage to the left and right calcarine regions leads to right- and left-sided hemianopias respectively, whereas unilateral damage confined to the lower and upper lips of the calcarine fissure produces superior and inferior quadrantanopias respectively. Altitudinal hemianopias in which either the lower or upper visual fields are affected bilaterally may also occur, but these are rarely observed except when trauma damages the calcarine region (usually the superior portion, since injury to the ventral portion more often proves fatal). Prestriate occipital damage extending into the temporal and parietal lobes is also likely to produce hemianopias and especially quadrantanopias, primarily due to selective damage to the optic radiations lying beneath the gray matter. But the field defects are generally more congruous (i.e. matching in the two eyes) when they are created by posterior occipital damage (Miller, 1982).

Central visual field losses arise from posterior striate damage, whereas anterior striate damage produces visual defects that may break out into the periphery. However, a phenomenon known as macular sparing occurs with many occipital lesions, due mostly to the fact that the occipital pole area representing the macula is served by two major blood supplies from the middle and posterior cerebral arteries and is therefore less likely to sustain an infarct. But since nonvascular damage to the posterior occipital lobe can also yield a limited degree of macular sparing, it is believed that an overlap of 1–3 degrees in the cortical representations of the left and right visual fields is also partly responsible for this phenomenon.

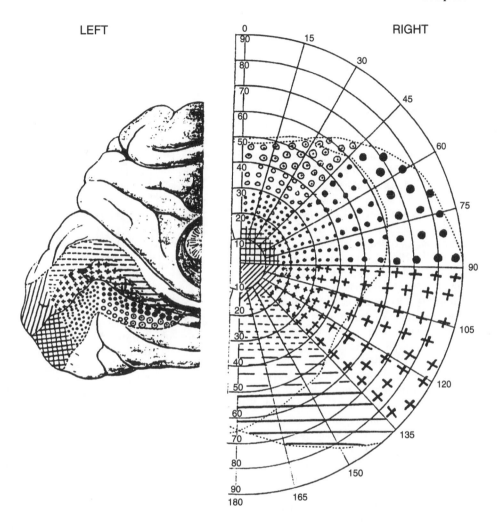

LEFT   0   RIGHT

Figure 53 The projection of the visual field (right) onto the surface of the contralateral striate cortex. The calcarine fissure has been opened up to expose a large portion of its medial surface. (From Figure 453 of S. Duke-Elder & G. I. Scott, *System of ophthalmology*. Vol. 12: *Neuro-ophthalmology*. St Louis: Mosby, 1971, with permission.)

In addition to the field defects described above, small visual field losses known as SCOTOMAS can be created by localized occipital lobe lesions, whereas bilateral visual field losses that can extend over large portions of the visual field accompany more substantial posterior occipital lesions. Small scotomas are rarely acknowledged by the patient, and even large-field visual losses often go unrecognized (in a condition known as ANTON'S SYNDROME), possibly due to attentional disturbances arising from collateral prestriate damage. Indeed, visual attentional neglect in one half of egocentric (i.e. body-centered) visual space can often masquerade as a hemianopia unless measures are taken to vary eye position independently of the head and body axes during visual performance assessment.

FUNCTIONAL PHYSIOLOGY OF THE OCCIPITAL LOBE

An explosion of knowledge concerning the functional architecture of visual cortex began with the

541

advent of single-neuronal recording in the late 1950s and has continued unabated to the present time, as new neurochemical and neurophysiological assays have been steadily introduced (see Peters & Jones, 1985; DeYoe & Van Essen, 1988). The general picture that has emerged is of steadily increasing processing complexity from V1 through the higher visual regions, intermixed with a significant amount of parallel processing.

Neuronal processing of visual information has been most widely studied in area 17, beginning with the work of Hubel and Wiesel in the 1960s. It has been shown that V1 neurons respond to relatively simple aspects of the visual environment in a highly organized fashion. Some of the stimulus attributes coded by V1 neurons include orientation, direction of motion, spatial frequency, color, luminance contrast, and binocular disparity. A major distinction has been drawn between simple and complex cells, both of which are found throughout V1. Simple cells respond to a properly oriented line located in a specific region of their receptive field in a highly precise (i.e. linear) manner, whereas complex cells respond well to a properly oriented stimulus placed anywhere within their receptive field (i.e. in a nonlinear manner). In most other respects, simple and complex cells overlap in their processing of visual information. In the primary geniculate recipient zones of layer 4, concentrically organized neuronal receptive fields with properties similar to those in the LGN are encountered.

Visual processing in V1 appears to be carried out in a modular fashion (see Figure 54). Neurons responsive primarily to one eye or the other are located in adjacent columns, whereas different stimulus orientations are coded in additional columns running perpendicular to the ocular dominance ones. A more recent finding is that neurons in CO "blobs" (rod-type subcolumns that do not traverse all cortical layers) are located in the center of ocular dominance columns and are much more selective for the color of the stimulus than its orientation. While much remains to be discovered about the way in which V1 codes the various features of the visual world, it is generally believed that all information contained within a particular region of the visual field is processed in a 1-mm^2 hypercolumn, although the number of hypercolumns per degree of visual field varies with eccentricity, according to the previously described cortical magnification factor.

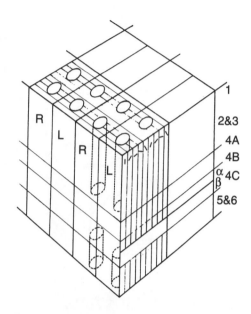

Figure 54 A model of monkey striate cortex, showing the columnar structure of ocular dominance (R-L) and orientational selectivity, and the existence of CO blobs (rod-like columns). (From Figure 34 of M. S. Livingstone & D. H. Hubel in *Journal of Neuroscience*, *4*, 1984, 309–56, with permission.)

The complexity of neuronal processing increases in areas beyond V1. Besides engaging in some of the same basic visual processing carried out in V1, V2 neurons are involved in higher-order disparity processing; illusory contour, end-stopping and other types of "texture" processing; and velocity (speed) detection. While segregated somewhat into different CO and [^{14}C] -2-deoxy-glucose (2-DG) stripes running parallel to the cortical surface, processing in V2 does not appear to be as tightly modularized into columns as in V1. Receptive fields of V2 neurons are also about twice as large as those of V1 neurons.

An even greater level of complexity is achieved by neuronal processing in visual areas anterior to V2. Nonretinal influences related to attention and eye movements become more prevalent, and complex interactions within extended portions of the cell's receptive field occur (see Maunsell & Newsome, 1987). For instance, some V4 neurons respond best when different spatial frequencies and/or colors are presented in the center and surround portions of their receptive field, with some surround influences extending over as many as 30 degrees of the visual field. Similarly, in the middle temporal area (referred to as either MT or V5) located at the border of the occipital and temporal lobes in the monkey, many neurons have been shown to prefer opposite motion in the center and surround portions of the receptive field. As one moves up the hierarchy of prestriate visual areas, substantial increases in receptive field size and complexity accompany a loss of topographical precision. The full visual map contained in V1 is typically replaced by ones that emphasize only a portion of the visual field, as exemplified by V4's confinement to the central 35–40 degrees. As will be discussed below, marked asymmetries and specialization in various visual areas – as well as in the dorsal and ventral subdivisions of the same visual area – also emerge.

The above single-neuronal findings are consistent with the type of hallucinations produced by stimulation or lesioning of the occipital lobes in humans (Gloning et al., 1968). Most elementary hallucinations (photisms) are generated in the occipital lobe; these include both colored and noncolored points, flashes, stars, wheels, flicker, and diffuse light, that may be either stationary or moving. Lesions of the calcarine region in particular appear to give rise to the occurrence of hallucinated lines, which corresponds to the known line-orientational specificity of V1 neuronal columns. More complex visual hallucinations such as objects and visual scenes are more likely to be generated by disturbances in the occipitotemporal regions.

PARALLEL PATHWAYS IN THE VISUAL CORTEX

Although functional specialization in the higher visual areas has been recognized for several decades, the existence of parallel neuronal pathways performing functionally distinct visual processing, clear from the retina to the highest visual cortical stages, has only recently been postulated.

The concept of parallel cortical visual processing grew out of two major sources. One was the "two visual systems" hypothesis that was first articulated by Schneider in 1968 on the basis of hamster data and transferred to primates by Trevarthen (see Ungerleider & Mishkin, 1982). This hypothesis argued for the existence of two anatomically distinct visual systems – one used for pattern recognition in central vision (i.e. which determines *what* the object is) and another, more peripheral system engaged in visual orientation and spatial perception (i.e. which tells us *where* the object is located). The geniculostriate pathways leading from the retina to the LGN and on into striate cortex allegedly constituted the "what" system, and their final termination was postulated to be the inferior temporal lobe, which was known to be important for pattern recognition functions. The secondary "where" system was termed the "tectopulvinar" one since it supposedly used the pathways leading from the retina to the superior colliculus (optic tectum) and on into the thalamic pulvinar nucleus, before finally terminating in the posterior parietal lobe. The organization of the second visual system was later modified by Ungerleider and Mishkin (1982) so as to involve predominantly the peripheral portions of striate cortex, a change that brought the model into a better fit with the greatly expanded role of striate cortex in the primate.

A second basis for the parallel pathways notion were the neurophysiological distinctions used to explain the properties of cat retinal ganglion cells. These schemes classified one type of ganglion cell (the Y-cell) as a spatially nonlinear and transient responder, and the other major cell type (the X-cell) as a linear, sustained responder. These distinctions were then shown to loosely correspond to the functional specializations of the magnocellular and parvocellular layers of the monkey LGN, since transient/nonlinear cells are found to a greater extent in the "magno" layers than in the "parvo" ones. The properties of such cells render them more ideal for motion and visuospatial operations, whereas the linear, color-sensitive neurons dominating the parvo layers appear better suited to pattern recognition (*see* Livingstone & Hubel, 1988; Previc, 1990).

In the late 1970s and early 1980s, several sets of investigators began to close the gap between the parallel visual processing evidenced in the monkey LGN and that found in the temporal and parietal visual areas. Using a variety of techniques, it was shown that the magno LGN layers project to layer $4C\alpha$ and then to layer 4B of V1, whereas the parvo layers project to layers 4A and $4C\beta$ and into the superficial layers of V1. In turn, magno-recipient layer 4B projects to V2's thick CO stripe regions and to dorsal V3 and MT, all of which seem to be preferentially involved in motion (transient) processing, low spatial frequency, and low-contrast analysis, and other magno-related functions. In contrast, the more superficial V1 layers (which also receive some magno input) appear to project to the thin and pale CO stripes of V2, which in turn transmit information primarily to V4, which is believed to be specialized for form and color processing. Parvo outputs are also known to be better represented in the upper-visual-field processing regions located in ventral prestriate cortex than in the lower-field representations found in dorsal prestriate cortex. Out of these collective research findings emerged the concept of partially segregated magno and parvo *streams of processing* leading clear from the retina to the highest levels of dorsal and ventral posterior association cortex (Van Essen & Maunsell, 1983).

Evidence of functional specialization in the occipital lobes of humans also exists, although it is less definitive. Localized anterior prestriate areas surrounding the lingual and fusiform gyri in the inferior and medial occipital lobes are believed to be important in selectively processing higher-order aspects of color, and in facial and other specific types of visual pattern discriminations (Damasio, 1985). Deficits in visual object recognition (object AGNOSIA) probably require more extensive ventral prestriate damage spreading more laterally and dorsally. Although anterior ventral occipital damage on the left side is also associated with reading loss (ALEXIA) – which is, in turn, often accompanied by color agnosias, as in Potzl's syndrome – pure alexia is believed to be mainly due to a disconnection of visual inputs from the left temporoparietal language areas.

Conversely, deficits in visually guided reaching and certain types of motion and temporal processing, SIMULTANAGNOSIA (the inability to see all parts of an object at once, possibly due to temporal fading of the image), and impaired visual orientation functions are confused, primarily by superior occipital damage. Indeed, it is rare for ventral-type deficits such as PROSOPAGNOSIA (impaired facial recognition) to accompany impaired visual reaching and other types of dorsal deficits, although both occipitoparietal and occipitotemporal damage may result in topographical visual loss (i.e. impairment in remembering and/or navigating through one's surrounding environment).

Unfortunately, the clinical evidence for parallel processing in the occipital lobe of humans is clouded by several factors. For one, the extent to which occipital damage by itself leads to many of the above deficits is still debated. Nor are the precise homologues of monkey areas MT and V4 known in humans, although they are probably located somewhat more inferiorly and caudally than in the monkey (Kaas, 1992), due to the tremendous expansion of the supramarginal gyrus in the higher primates. A further complicating factor in humans involves the issue of asymmetric cerebral function – i.e. whether the left or right occipital areas are damaged in a particular individual. It is generally accepted that right-sided occipitoparietal lesions produce more severe dorsal-type visual deficits, but the laterality of most occipitotemporal symptoms is less agreed on (although many researchers believe that prosopagnosia depends more on right-sided ventral occipital damage). Whether POSITRON EMISSION TOMOGRAPHY (PET) scanning – which provides a measure of brain metabolic activity in normal humans as they view various visual inputs or perform different visual tasks – can significantly clarify the clinical findings concerning parallel processing remains to be seen, but the preliminary evidence obtained thus far is encouraging.

It is probably fair to state that a consensus of opinion now holds not only that some degree of parallel visual processing exists in humans, but that it is probably manifested in the occipital lobes as well as in the higher visual areas lying anterior to it. But the best characterization of dorsal and ventral processing differences remains a topic of active debate. Many theorists agree with Ungerleider and Mishkin (1982) that the dorsal stream is primarily involved in peripheral spatial analysis, while the ventral system is more involved in central object perception. Others favor the emphasis of Van Essen and Maunsell (1983) and Livingstone and Hubel (1988) on the pre-eminent color and form analyses performed by the occipitotemporal pathways vs the specialization of the occipitoparietal system for motion and possibly depth processing. More recently, Previc (1990) proposed that the dorsal visual pathways are primarily concerned with processing in peripersonal (near-visual) space, which includes visually guided reaching and many related visuospatial processes, whereas the occipitotemporal system is more devoted to extrapersonal (far-visual) space, in which object, color, and face recognition primarily occur. This theory is based largely on the ecological relationship of the lower and upper visual fields to near and far vision, and on the disproportionate emphases of the occipitoparietal and occipitotemporal systems on the lower and upper visual fields respectively. In a somewhat related theory, Goodale and Milner (1992) distinguish between the ventral and dorsal pathways in terms of their *output* specializations (perception vs action) rather than their input ones. In their scheme, the ventral system is the "what" system concerned with perceptual recognition of the visual environment, whereas the dorsal stream is the "how" system that uses the same visual inputs to organize and direct skilled visuomotor activity.

In summary, the existence of parallel processing in the primate visual system is now widely accepted, but its essential nature and origins are still subject to considerable speculation. Several theories that share many tenets in common have been put forth, but further research will undoubtedly be required before a firm theoretical consensus can emerge.

STRIATE CORTICAL LESIONS AND THE ISSUE OF BLINDSIGHT

As noted earlier, the dependence of most visual functions on the integrity of V1 has dramatically increased in primates, especially humans. Not only does damage to the tectopulvinar visual pathways by itself produce almost no permanent visual impairment in primates, but much of the visual responsiveness in these structures is maintained by downstream projections from striate and prestriate visual cortex. Unlike the situation in the cat, in which the Y-cell system sends a large projection directly to V2, 99 percent of all primate LGN fibers terminate in V1. Thus one would expect a major disruption of visual function following striate damage in humans, as is indeed the case.

In most instances involving only partial V1 damage, visual function is slowly restored, beginning first with rather primitive luminance sensations and concluding with the return of form perception. But the amount of residual visual function following *complete* striate cortical removal in humans is more debatable. Striate patients are almost uniformly unaware of the return of their visual capabilities, and researchers initially concluded on the basis of self-report studies that no visual functions survive the removal of primary visual cortex. But many researchers who have

carefully tested striate patients, using forced-choice and other "objective" techniques, claim to have demonstrated significant visual capabilities, ranging from simple localization and movement detection to color and form perception and even limited word recognition. A general term for the spared visual capabilities that do not reach conscious awareness is BLINDSIGHT. Blindsight is typically more limited when the entire occipital lobe – rather than just V1 – is damaged, but even in this case some residual visual function has been alleged.

Various theories have been put forth to explain the existence of blindsight (see Cowey & Stoerig, 1991). One possibility is that the tectopulvinar pathways mediate the remaining visual function, as these fibers apparently reach area MT and reputedly account for the continued visual activity of neurons in that structure. While some evidence favors this notion, other findings suggest that some blindsight survives even combined striate-collicular removal. Moreover, it is not clear how wavelength and motion discriminations are carried out using only tectal inputs, given that primate collicular neurons are neither color-selective nor direction-selective in their responding. Because, however, all residual visual responsiveness in MT neurons after V1 ablations in monkeys is abolished with additional collicular lesions, it is possible that direction selectivity is created from tectal inputs at a later stage.

Several other more primitive pathways lying outside the geniculostriate system (such as the accessory optic system) have also been invoked to explain blindsight. But the most widely accepted alternative to the tectopulvinar hypothesis is that the tiny remnant of LGN cells that survive striate removal is sufficient to carry out most blindsight functions. How they reach the higher cortical centers is not certain, but it is now believed that at least some direct projections exist from the LGN to prestriate visual regions such as V4. This would account for why damage to both striate and prestriate occipital cortex is more likely to lead to permanent and total blindness than is striate damage by itself. Indeed, it has been shown that prestriate damage by itself can produce functional blindness, even when sparing of V1 occurs and the early components of the visual evoked potential that are believed to emanate from V1 are present. This is presumably because both the V1 transcortical projections and the LGN-prestriate connections are destroyed in this case.

While it remains an open question as to whether the tectopulvinar system in humans possesses the capability for most blindsight functions, it is clear that neither it nor any of the other extrastriate visual pathways exclusively mediates *conscious* visual perception. Nor, obviously, does visual awareness reside in the isolated primary visual cortex. It can only be concluded, therefore, that "visual consciousness" is mediated by the combined outputs of striate and prestriate cortex or, as seems even more likely, the additional involvement of higher visual association cortical areas lying outside the occipital lobe. It has even been suggested that the ventral system alone is the source of conscious visual awareness (Goodale & Milner, 1992).

CONCLUSIONS

The tremendous advances of the past several decades concerning our knowledge of the primate cortical visual areas have led to new perspectives on the functioning of the occipital lobe. Although V1 continues to be viewed primarily as a region that transforms a streamlined visual transmission from the LGN into a greatly expanded functional analysis at every location in visual space, the remaining portion of occipital cortex is now believed to be the site of numerous visual areas that hierarchically increase in their processing complexity as well as their affinities to either parietal or temporal cortex. The occipital lobe represents, therefore, a critical link in two great visual systems that flow clear from the retina to their partially segregated termination sites in the parietal and temporal lobes. Without the impressive functional analysis provided by V1, neither cortical system could attain its maximum capability and would be forced into very rudimentary interactions with the visual world. But V1 by itself does not provide the conscious effort required to transform elementary sensations into perceptual experience, although it is probably more involved in such processes than was once suspected. Whether the occipital lobe will be viewed by future researchers as a distinct functional (as opposed to anatomical) entity depends on the extent to which its unique visual information processing capabilities continue to overshadow the increasingly prominent anatomical

and functional links of specialized subareas within it to the parietal and temporal lobes.

BIBLIOGRAPHY

Bailey, P., & Von Bonin, G. (1951). *The isocortex of man.* Urbana, IL: University of Illinois Press.

Cowey, A., & Stoerig, P. (1991). The neurobiology of blindsight. *Trends in Neurosciences, 14,* 140–5.

Damasio, A. R. (1985). Disorders of complex visual processing: agnosias, achromatopsia, Bálint's syndrome, and related difficulties of orientation and construction. In M.-M. Mesulam (Ed.), *Principles of behavioral neurology* (pp. 259–88). Philadelphia: Davis.

DeYoe, E. A., & Van Essen, D. C. (1988). Concurrent processing streams in monkey visual cortex. *Trends in Neurosciences, 11,* 219–26.

Gloning, I., Gloning, K., & Hoff, H. (1968). *Neuropsychological symptoms and syndromes in lesions of the occipital lobe and the adjacent areas.* Paris: Gauthier-Villars.

Goodale, M. A., & Milner, A. D. (1992). Separate pathways for perception and action. *Trends in Neurosciences, 15,* 20–5.

Kaas, J. H. (1992). Do humans see what monkeys see? *Trends in Neurosciences, 15,* 1–3.

Livingstone, M., & Hubel, D. (1988). Segregation of form, color, movement, and depth: anatomy, physiology, and perception. *Science, 240,* 740–9.

Maunsell, J. H. R., & Newsome, W. T. (1987). Visual processing in monkey extrastriate cortex. *Annual Review of Neuroscience, 10,* 363–401.

Miller, N. R. (1982). *Walsh and Hoyt's clinical neuro-ophthalmology,* 4th edn. Baltimore: Williams & Wilkins.

Peters, A., & Jones, E. G. (Eds). (1985). *Cerebral cortex,* Vol. 3: *Visual cortex.* New York: Plenum.

Previc, F. H. (1990). Functional specialization in the lower and upper visual fields in humans: its ecological origins and neurophysiological implications. *Behavioral and Brain Sciences, 13,* 519–75.

Ungerleider, L. G., & Mishkin, M. (1982). Two cortical visual systems. In D. J. Ingle, M. A. Goodale, & R. J. W. Mansfield (Eds), *Analysis of visual behavior* (pp. 549–80). Cambridge, MA: MIT Press.

Van Essen, D. C., & Maunsell, J. H. R. (1983).

Hierarchical organization and functional streams in the visual cortex. *Trends in Neurosciences, 6,* 370–5.

FRED H. PREVIC

oculomotor apraxia   Oculomotor apraxia (also *ocular apraxia*) is one of a number of closely related phenomena which may be generally termed "psychic paralysis of gaze," in which there is paralysis of conjugate gaze. The patient is unable to shift gaze voluntarily from the point of fixation and stimuli appearing peripheral to the point of gaze fail to capture visual attention. The clearest example of the disorder is of a patient who, asked to name the color of the examiner's tie, named the color of another person's tie at which he was looking at the moment of the question. Other patients have been described who pour water from a bottle onto the table instead of into a glass upon which their gaze is fixated, or fail to accurately locate a lighted match while fixating on the tip of their cigarette. When not actively engaged, fixation appears to wander in an uncoordinated fashion, and to be readily captured by an object passing into view.

A closely related problem involving a failure of reaching is more commonly termed OPTIC ATAXIA and both are associated with BÁLINT'S SYNDROME.

oedema   *See* EDEMA.

olfaction   Olfaction, the sensation and perception of smell, is relatively poorly understood and under-researched. Olfaction is served by the first CRANIAL NERVE which passes information to the olfactory bulbs located below the base of the frontal lobes and then by the olfactory tract to the cortex in the region of the uncus in the PYRIFORM CORTEX. It is the only sensory system which does not pass through the THALAMUS on the route from receptors to cortex, presumably because it is part of a phylogenetically older system. Disorders of the sense of smell, which are also closely involved in disorders of taste, are associated with two causes. Bilateral *anosmia* sometimes follows head injury and, if it does not resolve within a few weeks, may be a permanent and unexpectedly distressing consequence. Unilateral anosmia may be the early sign of a tumor, particularly a MENINGIOMA of the olfactory groove, which presses upon the olfactory tract and may, if untreated, progress to bilateral anosmia.

oneirism   Oneirism is a form of complex visual hallucination associated with disturbances of consciousness which may range from drowsy, dream-like states to severe confusional states with emotional disturbances. Oneirism is more frequent following infection or toxic-metabolic disorders, but may also occur with certain subcortical lesions. Its association with CATAPLEXY and NARCOLEPSY supports the idea of a subcortical location. The hallucinations are generally highly organized and rich, and may be continuous with the external world and recruit hallucinations in other sensory modalities, provoking an emotional response which is commonly one of anxiety. Delirium tremens is an extreme form of oneirism. The parallels with dreams are obvious and, as with dreams, amnesia for the episode is often complete.

optic aphasia   *See* APHASIA; DYSLEXIA.

optic ataxia   One of the phenomena which may be grouped as "psychic paralysis of gaze," optic ataxia is a failure of reaching or grasping for an object within the visual field, although the term is sometimes used more broadly for any failure of action attributable to defective visual guidance. Such failures may even extend to faulty visuoconstructional performance. The failure is attributable to an inability to perform coordinated conjugate eye movements solely under visual control; eye movements may be executed normally when under proprioceptive control. The deficit is related to OCULOMOTOR APRAXIA and both are associated with BÁLINT'S SYNDROME. However, optic ataxia may appear as an isolated deficit and is more commonly unilateral in the hand affected, which may be either ipsilateral or contralateral to the side of the lesion, depending on its precise location within the visuomotor pathways.

optic chiasm   The optic chiasm (or, occasionally, *optic chiasma*) is where the optic nerves from the two eyes meet, partially decussate, and then form the left and right optic tracts projecting back within each hemisphere. It is located on the ventral surface (base) of the brain at the anterior extremity of the HYPOTHALAMUS and anterior to the pituitary, close to where the internal carotid artery reaches the brain.

The partial decussation of the optic pathway at the chiasm provides an arrangement whereby visual stimuli appearing to the left of fixation (in the left visual half-field) are projected to the right occipital cortex, while stimuli in the right visual half-field are projected to the left occipital cortex. In order to achieve this, the fibers in the optic nerve from the temporal hemiretinae (the outer half of each retina) do not cross but pass directly back on the same side. However, the fibers from the nasal (inner) hemiretinae decussate (cross) and pass back into the opposite hemisphere. Therefore the hemiretinae receiving stimuli from the left visual half-field, the nasal hemiretina of the left eye and the temporal hemiretina of the right eye send fibers back to the right side of the brain, those from the nasal hemiretina crossing over to join those from the temporal hemiretina which do not cross.

This arrangement is of significance in the diagnosis of lesions affecting the optic pathways (*see* HEMIANOPIA), and also in providing the opportunity for the application of the DIVIDED VISUAL FIELD TECHNIQUE.

optokinetic nystagmus A form of NYS-TAGMUS which may be elicited by prolonged exposure to a slowly but constantly moving display, usually presented as lateral movement. The nystagmus is not dissimilar from that produced by CALORIC STIMULATION, and is a nystagmus in the direction of movement of the display.

It has been demonstrated that NEGLECT may be reduced when a task such as line bisection is performed against the background of a leftward moving display which produces optokinetic nystagmus. It is presumed that the nystagmus is accompanied by an attentional shift to the left.

orienting reflex The orienting reflex, or *orienting response*, is a term generally used to refer to any turning of the body with reference to the position of a specific stimulus. However, the term is used in a rather stricter sense to apply to an attentional response contingent upon the onset of a stimulus (for example, head-turning or ear-raising); in this context "reflex" is more likely to be employed than "response." The implication is usually that the reflex or response serves to bring the individual into a position appropriate for optimal exposure to the stimulus. While not a true reflex, although in the stricter sense in which it is used it may involve reflexive components, the phenomenon is important in studies of attention, and as one of the signs of emergence from a VEGETATIVE STATE.

P

pachygyria Pachygyria is a less severe form of AGYRIA, in which there is a reduced number of abnormally broad convolutions across the cerebral CORTEX. However, the cortex is not uniformly affected, with the parietal, temporal, and occipital regions of the cortex being more severely affected than the frontal or medial cortical areas. This abnormality is a HETEROTOPIA, resulting from abnormal neuronal migration from the fourth month of gestation. It may result in behavioral and cognitive abnormalities, depending on the degree of the pachygyria.

pain Pain research and therapy have long been dominated by "specificity theory," which proposes that pain is a specific sensation and that its intensity is proportional to the extent of tissue damage. Recent evidence, however, shows that pain is not simply a function of the amount of bodily damage alone. Rather it is a subjective experience which is influenced by cultural learning, the meaning of the situation, attention, and other cognitive activities.

The "gate control theory" of pain, proposed by Melzack and Wall (1988), suggests that neural mechanisms in the dorsal horns of the spinal cord act like a gate which can increase or decrease the flow of nerve impulses from peripheral fibers to the spinal cord cells that project to the brain. Somatic input is therefore subjected to the modulating influence of the gate *before* it evokes pain perception and response. Recent physiological evidence supports the concept.

The dorsal horns, which receive fibers from the body and project impulses towards the brain, provide valuable clues about information processing at the spinal cord level. The dorsal horns comprise several layers or laminae, each of which is now known to have specialized functions. The substantia gelatinosa (laminae 1 and 2) is of particular interest because it represents a unique system on each side of the spinal cord. Many afferent fibers from the skin terminate in the substantia gelatinosa, and the dendrites of many cells in lower laminae, whose axons project to the brain, lie within the substantia gelatinosa. This region is situated between a major portion of the peripheral nerve fiber terminals and the spinal cord cells that project to the brain. Convincing physiological evidence shows that the substantia gelatinosa acts as a gate, so that small-fiber inputs evoked by intense somatic stimulation facilitate transmission to the brain while large-fiber inputs evoked by gentle stimulation, or descending influences from the brain, inhibit transmission.

Although cells in all laminae undoubtedly play a role in pain processes, lamina 5 cells are particularly responsive when noxious stimuli are applied within their receptive fields. They respond with characteristic firing patterns to stimulation over a wide range of intensities, and receive inputs from the skin, from deeper tissues such as blood vessels and muscles, and from the viscera. Dorsal horn cells project to the brain through multiple ascending systems.

THE DIMENSIONS OF PAIN EXPERIENCE

Pain is usually labelled as a sensory experience, yet it also has a distinctly unpleasant affective quality. It motivates or drives the organism into activity aimed at stopping the pain as quickly as possible. These considerations suggest that there are three major psychological dimensions of pain: sensory-discriminative, motivational-affective, and cognitive-evaluative. Melzack and Casey have proposed that they are subserved by physiologically specialized systems in the brain.

Physiological and behavioral studies suggest that several rapidly conducting systems – the neospinothalamic tract, the spinocervical tract, and the postsynaptic neurons in the dorsal column

549

system – contribute to the sensory-discriminative dimension of pain. Studies in human patients and in animals, taken together, suggest that the rapidly conducting projection systems (which ascend in the lateral brain stem) have the capacity to transmit precise information about the spatial, temporal, and magnitude properties of the input that characterizes the sensory-discriminative dimension.

There is strong evidence that the brain-stem RETICULAR FORMATION and the LIMBIC SYSTEM, which receive projections from the spinoreticular and paleo-spinothalamic components of the anterolateral somatosensory pathway, play a particularly important role in the motivational-affective dimension of pain. These medially coursing fibers tend to be short and connect diffusely with one another during their ascent from the spinal cord to the brain. Their target cells in the brain usually have wide receptive fields, sometimes covering half or more of the body surface. In addition to the convergence of somatosensory fibers, inputs from other sensory systems, such as vision and audition, also arrive at many of these cells.

It is now firmly established that the limbic system plays an important role in pain processes. Electrical stimulation of the hippocampus, amygdala, or other limbic structures may evoke escape or other attempts to stop stimulation. After ablation of the amygdala and overlying cortex, cats show marked changes in affective behavior, including decreased responsiveness to noxious stimuli. Surgical section of the cingulum bundle, which connects the frontal cortex to the hippocampus, also produces a loss of "negative affect" associated with intractable pain in human subjects. In animals, local anesthetic block of the anterior cingulum produces striking decreases in pain. This evidence indicates that limbic structures, although they play a role in many other functions, provide a neural basis for the aversive drive and affect that comprise the motivational dimension of pain.

Cognitive activities such as cultural values, anxiety, attention, and suggestion all have a profound effect on pain experience. These activities, which are subserved in part at least by cortical processes, may act selectively on sensory processing or motivational mechanisms. In addition, there is evidence that the sensory input is localized, identified in terms of its physical properties, evaluated in terms of past experience, and

modified *before* it activates the discriminative or motivational systems.

The physiological and behavioral evidence described above led Melzack and Casey to extend the gate control theory to include the motivational dimension of pain. They propose that: (1) the sensory-discriminative dimension of pain is influenced primarily by the rapidly conducting somatosensory systems; (2) the powerful motivational drive and unpleasant affect characteristic of pain are subserved by activities in reticular and limbic structures which are influenced primarily by the slowly conducting spinal systems; and (3) neocortical or higher central nervous system processes, such as evaluation of the input in terms of past experience, exert control over activity in both the discriminative and motivational systems. These three forms of activity are reflected in the three dimensions of the McGill Pain Questionnaire, which is the most commonly used measuring instrument in pain research with human subjects.

CHRONIC AND ACUTE PAIN

The time-course of pain is profoundly important in determining its psychological effects on an organism. Acute pain, which is usually associated with a well-defined cause (such as a burned finger or a ruptured appendix), normally has a characteristic time-course and vanishes after healing has occurred. The pain usually has a rapid onset – the *phasic* component – and a subsequent *tonic* component that persists for variable periods of time.

Chronic pain states – such as low back pain, the neuralgias, or phantom limb pain – may begin as acute pain and pass through both the phasic and tonic phases. The tonic pain, however, may persist long after the injury has healed. It is then labelled as "chronic pain" and appears to involve neural mechanisms that are far more complex than those of acute pain. The pain not only persists but may spread to adjacent or more distant body areas. It is resistant to surgical control and its prolonged time-course is characteristically associated with high levels of anxiety and depression.

The rapidly conducting pathways described above seem to be particularly well suited to conveying phasic information. The value of rapidly conducting, direct pain-signalling systems is obvious: unless an organism reacts quickly, a stimulus which only threatens tissue damage may become overtly damaging. The slowly conducting pathways are unlikely to signal the need for immediate action. Instead, they are more likely to play a role in chronic, deeply unpleasant, diffuse pain, as well as in a longer-lasting motivational-affective dimension of pain. These pathways continue to send messages as long as the wound is susceptible to re-injury. The continuing pain may prevent further damage, and foster rest, protection, and care of the injured areas, thereby promoting healing and recuperative processes.

MEMORY AND PAIN

A memory-like mechanism may account for pain in the absence of a detectable lesion or any other peripheral input that could cause the pain. A patient in whom a memory-like mechanism such as this is active may be diagnosed as a malingerer or a conversion hysteric when, in fact, a central neural mechanism, such as self-sustaining neural activity, may be the major underlying cause of the pain.

There is now a growing literature on the neural mechanisms of prolonged, memory-like activity related to referred pain. An injury of a hindpaw in the rat produces a prolonged, heightened sensitivity to pain (hyperalgesia) in the same paw *and* in the opposite paw. Surprisingly, the hyperalgesia in the contralateral paw persists even after all the nerves from the injured area are completely sectioned. These results show clearly that the persistent hyperalgesia is dependent on abnormal activity in the central nervous system. There is excellent evidence, moreover, that the changes in central neural activity continue for many weeks or longer after injury. Thus there is a growing body of data to show that surgical patients who receive an epidural block, in addition to a general anesthetic, have significantly less pain and fewer pain-related complications during and after recovery than patients who have surgery with only a general anesthetic.

HYPERSTIMULATION ANALGESIA

It is well known that short-acting, local anesthetic blocks of trigger points often produce prolonged, sometimes permanent relief of some forms of myofascial or visceral pain. Astonishingly, brief, intense stimulation of trigger points by electrical stimulation, acupuncture, intense cold, or injection of normal saline often produces prolonged relief of some forms of myofascial or visceral pain.

This type of pain relief, which is generally labelled as "hyperstimulation analgesia," is one of the oldest methods used for the control of pain. It is sometimes known as "counter-irritation" and includes such methods of folk-medicine as application of mustard plasters, ice packs, hot cups, or blistering agents to parts of the body.

The relief of pain by brief, intense stimulation of distant trigger points (or acupuncture points) can be explained physiologically in terms of the gate control theory. The most plausible explanation seems to be that the brain-stem areas which are known to exert a powerful inhibitory control over transmission in the pain signalling system may be involved. The descending controls, which have been labelled as a "central biasing mechanism" or as "diffuse noxious inhibitory controls," receive inputs from widespread parts of the body and, in turn, project to widespread parts of the spinal cord. The stimulation of particular nerves or tissues by transcutaneous electrical nerve stimulation or any other form of stimulation that activates small fibers could bring about an increased input to the central biasing mechanism, which would close the gates to pain signals from selected body areas.

There has been convincing support for this hypothesis. Direct electrical stimulation of the brain-stem areas which produce behavioral analgesia inhibits the transmission of nerve impulses in dorsal horn cells that have been implicated in gate-control mechanisms. Furthermore, the analgesia-producing brain-stem areas are known to be highly sensitive to morphine, and the effect of stimulation is partially reduced by administration of naloxone, an opiate antagonist. The demonstration that naloxone also reduces the analgesic effects of transcutaneous electrical stimulation and acupuncture is consistent with the hypothesis that intense stimulation activates a neural feedback loop through the brain-stem analgesia-producing areas.

CENTRAL PATTERN-GENERATING MECHANISMS

The complexity of the interacting sensory and psychological factors in pain and its management is highlighted by studies of chronic phantom body pain in paraplegics with total spinal cord lesions. Melzack and Loeser reviewed cases of patients who had sustained total spinal cord sections at thoracic or lumbar levels, yet continued to suffer severe pain in the abdomen, groin, or legs. The completeness of the lesion was verified visually during surgical removal of injured tissue or as a result of segmental cordectomy (the removal of an entire section of the spinal cord) to prevent nerve impulses produced by injured tissues from reaching the brain. Nevertheless, the pain was usually felt in definite parts of the phantom body and was often described as burning, crushing, or cramping. The sympathetic ganglia – the only other possible route for nerve impulses from the legs – were also blocked in several patients without effect on the pain.

Since there is no known anatomical substrate for sensory input from the lower abdomen or legs to enter the spinal cord above midthoracic levels, it is evident that peripheral input from levels below the total transection is not the cause of pain in these patients. Although many of the patients were severely depressed by their physical status as paraplegics, there was no evidence that the pain was caused by depression or neurosis. On the basis of the clinical data, Melzack and Loeser proposed that the loss of input to central structures after deafferentation may play an important role in producing pain.

The effects of deafferentation on the activity of central neurons have been investigated in several contexts. Loeser and Ward showed that cutting several dorsal roots in the cat produces abnormal bursts of firing in dorsal horn cells that persist for as long as 180 days after the root section. Furthermore, single shock pulses to adjacent intact roots produce prolonged firing that persists for hundreds of milliseconds. The abnormal firing patterns observed in the deafferented spinal cord in cats have also been observed in Man.

These observations led Melzack and Loeser to suggest a concept of pain to explain these clinical data. They proposed that neuron pools at many levels of the spinal cord and brain can act as "pattern generating mechanisms." In paraplegics, these mechanisms must lie above the level of spinal transection or cordectomy. Furthermore, those regions responsible for pattern generation are assumed to project to the regions of the brain involved in precise localization of sensory inputs – that is, those neural areas that subserve the body schema – as well as to the areas that subserve the affective dimensions of pain.

The concept of central pattern-generating mechanisms provides an explanation for those pain states which are characterized by degeneration of sensory nerve fibers, dorsal root pathology, or spinal injury. Many of the neuralgias, causalgia, and phantom limb pain are associated with nerve damage.

Katz has described "pain memories" in phantom limbs – that is, phantom limb sensations which resemble somatosensory events experienced in the limb before amputation. These somatosensory memories are predominantly replicas of distressing pre-amputation lesions and pains which were experienced at or near the time of amputation, and are described as having the same qualities of sensation as the pre-amputation pain. The patients who experience these pains emphasize that they are suffering real pain which they can describe in vivid detail, and insist that the experience is not merely a cognitive recollection of an earlier pain. Among the somatosensory memories reported are cutaneous lesions, deep tissue injuries, bone and joint pain, and painful pre-amputation postures. These findings suggest that somatosensory inputs of sufficient intensity and duration can produce long-term changes in central neural structures.

These data have recently received support from studies with animals. Peripheral neurectomy in rats is followed by self-mutilation (autotomy) in which the animal chews and scratches the distal portions of the insensitive paw to the point of amputation. It is well established that autotomy is a response to painful or dysesthetic sensations referred to the denervated limb. Several studies have found that the onset of autotomy is earlier if the paw is injured prior to nerve section. Furthermore, electrical stimulation of the sciatic nerve prior to neurectomy results in a significantly greater incidence of autotomy and even changes the pattern of autotomy. These results suggest that the central excitability produced by sciatic nerve stimulation prior to nerve section is retained in CNS structures as a somatosensory pain memory. They complement reports of amputees with phantom limb pain characterized by the persistence of a painful pre-amputation lesion.

BIBLIOGRAPHY

Coderre, T. J., Katz, J., Vaccarino, A. L., & Melzack, R. (1992). Contribution of central neuroplasticity to pathological pain: review of clinical and experimental evidence. *Pain, 52,* 259–85.

Katz, J., & Melzack, R. (1990). Pain "memories" in phantom limbs: review and clinical observations. *Pain*, *43*, 319–36.

Katz, J., Vaccarino, A. L., Coderre, T. J., & Melzack, R. (1991). Injury prior to neurectomy alters the pattern of autotomy in rats. *Anesthesiology*, *75*, 876–83.

Melzack, R., & Wall, P. D. (1988). *The Challenge of pain*, 2nd edn. London: Penguin.

Wall, P. D., & Melzack, R. (1994). *Textbook of pain*, 3rd edn. Edinburgh: Churchill Livingstone.

RONALD MELZACK

paliacousia   Paliacousia is a form of complex auditory verbal hallucination in which, during a real conversation, a particular spoken word or words is heard repeated several times. It may be similar to the hallucinatory phenomenon in which a thought is "heard" over and over again, but in the case of paliacousia there is an objective stimulus which forms the content of the hallucination. As with almost all auditory hallucinations associated with cortical pathology, paliacousia is a sign of epilepsy, most commonly of the temporal lobe and more frequently lateralized to the left.

palilalia   Palilalia (occasionally *pallilalia*) is a rare disorder of speech in which a phrase is repeated reiteratively and with increasing rapidity. It is then associated with Parkinsonism, the general set of symptoms seen in PARKINSON'S DISEASE. The term is also sometimes used for the perseverative repetition of a single word (with ECHOLALIA then being used for the repetition of phrases), *logoclonia* being the term for the repetition of a final syllable. When the term is used in this way it descriptively implies no more than a high-level motor output dysfunction of speech.

paliopsia   Paliopsia is a rare form of META-MORPHOPSIA in which visual perseveration in time occurs; there is an illusory re-occurrence of the visual perception after the stimulus object has been removed. Illustrative case studies give reports of a person being seen again to walk past

the patient, moments after they were first seen to do so; or objects familiar or recently seen being perceived to float past the patient. The lesion giving rise to this phenomenon is normally on the borders of the occipital lobe with the parietal or temporal lobe, but may be on the left, right, or bilateral. Other VISUAL FIELD DEFECTS may be present, as may visual AGNOSIA.

palmomental reflex   The palmomental reflex is elicited by scratching or stroking the palm of the patient, which evokes a twitch of the mentalis muscle near the angle of the chin. An abnormal cutaneous reflex, it is the result of an upper motor-neuron lesion on the side contralateral to the reflex. It may appear as an early sign of dementia in association with cognitive decline, and may be attributed to a loss of inhibition of such rudimentary reflexes and the consequent appearance of *frontal release signs*, of which the palmomental reflex is one.

palsy   Palsy is an outmoded term for paralysis, although its use has included other motor disorders; for example, Parkinson's original description of the disease which bears his name was "shaking palsy."

The term persists in current usage in *progressive supranuclear palsy* (or the *Steele–Richardson syndrome*), which is a progressive neurological disease with ocular, motor, and mental symptoms. The ocular symptoms include paralysis of the external eye movements resulting in gaze being centrally fixed, and the motor signs are widespread rigidity of the neck, trunk, and limbs. There is commonly also DYSARTHRIA, and the whole clinical picture results from pathological changes in the BASAL GANGLIA, BRAIN STEM, and CEREBELLUM, with the cerebral cortex being little affected. Onset is usually after the age of 50, with fairly rapid progression to death.

The cognitive changes, palsy being a subcortical DEMENTIA, are characterized by psychomotor retardation and general slowing of thought, affected individuals often being able to correctly complete intellectual tasks, given sufficient time and motivation. The apparent effects upon memory can be reduced by providing encouragement and an abnormally lengthy period for recall. Aphasic deficits, or specific apraxias or agnosias are rare, although some other high-level abstract processes may be affected. There may also be changes in personality or affect, which may include outbursts of rage, or inappropriate laughing or crying. The links with the intellectual impairments in other subcortical dementias such as PARKINSON'S DISEASE and HUNTINGTON'S DISEASE are clear, and it has been pointed out that all these disorders clearly demonstrate that the cerebral cortex does not have to be primarily affected for cognitive dysfunction to occur.

panencephalitis Panencephalitis, more properly *subacute sclerosing panencephalitis* (*SSPE*), also known as *inclusion body encephalitis* and by other similar names, is a special form of ENCEPHALITIS normally seen in children before the age of 10 years. There is generally a history of measles at an unusually early age. There are three stages to the illness over a course of up to six months: first mood change with some intellectual impairment, followed by akinetic mutism and involuntary movements, and finally decortication. The condition usually, but not invariably, leads to death, although it may be that milder and less serious forms also occur. For the neuropsychologist, the importance of this condition lies in its early presentation by disorders of cognition and mood.

Papez circuit The Papez circuit, described by James W. Papez in 1937, contains many of the elements which constitute the LIMBIC SYSTEM. The circuit consists of a loop of connections running from the THALAMUS through the CINGULATE GYRUS, ENTORHINAL CORTEX, HIPPOCAMPUS, SEPTAL AREA, HYPOTHALAMUS, MAMMILLARY BODIES, returning to the thalamus. Papez called this circuit "the stream of feeling," and it is still accepted that the Papez circuit is a major functional component in emotional experience, although it is now clear that a number of other structures also contribute to this function.

paracusia Paracusias are all forms of auditory illusion with an organic basis. Such auditory illusions may be considered similar to METAMORPHOPSIAS in the visual modality, so that sounds appear softer or louder than normal, nearer or more distant, modified in rhythm or

tone, possess strange qualities, or perseverate. Such sensory illusions, and visual and auditory disturbances may occur together, are typically found in toxic states, particularly if drug-induced, or in association with an epileptic event. Rarely, these auditory distortions may be less transient and represent a relatively permanent modification of perception, when they may be difficult to distinguish from, for example, true amusias.

paragrammatism Inaccuracies of grammatical construction in speech output are termed paragrammatisms. While grammatical errors may occur as part of a primary disorder of speech output, motor disorders of spoken language are often so disordered that paragrammatisms are a minor or unobservable problem. They are also to be observed in patients with a sensory form of APHASIA, where they can be conceived of as resulting from a disorganization of semantic relations. In such patients, speech output is fluent and speech segments may be accurately produced, but the segments are poorly assembled, with abnormal semantic substitutions which together form the abnormal syntactic structure of paragrammatism.

paragraphia Paragraphias are errors in written language which are the signs of AGRAPHIA. These paragraphias, more properly *literal paragraphias*, are the main feature of writing disorders and consist of omissions, distortions, additions, and substitutions of graphemes; the correct generation of individual graphemes is preserved. Similar errors may also be seen if the patient types. The term may also be used in cases of neglect when the patient writes on only one side of the paper or does not type with keys to one side of the keyboard, or alternatively when a word perseverates in written output. The term therefore indicates no more than a dysgraphic error.

parageusia Parageusia is a disturbance of taste in which many substances are perceived to have the same unpleasant flavor. While rather poorly understood, this phenomenon has been linked to irritative lesions of the region of the uncus.

paralexia Paralexias are errors in reading. Patients with receptive disorders of language in which comprehension of spoken language is severely impaired make numerous paralexic errors in reading aloud. Paralexias also occur in literal alexia, where there is an inability to read individual letters, although the ability to read words is relatively preserved. The frequency of paralexias may relate to the grammatical class of the word, and both semantic and visual paralexias may occur, depending upon the form of the underlying DYSLEXIA.

paralysis of gaze Originally referred to as *psychic paralysis of gaze*, it is the inability to displace the gaze voluntarily from the present point of fixation, now more commonly termed BÁLINT'S SYNDROME. In this syndrome, the disturbance of gaze is linked with OPTIC ATAXIA and impaired visual attention.

paraparesis Paraparesis indicates incomplete paralysis of both lower limbs, while *paraplegia* strictly indicates total paralysis of these limbs, although the latter term is sometimes used more loosely to indicate less than total paralysis. The alternative term *incomplete paraplegia* is also sometimes employed.

paraphasia Paraphasia is the production of unintended syllables, words, or phrases during the effort to speak. The speech produced is, however, lawful in terms of the language being spoken, and is correctly articulated. Paraphasic errors are commonly phonemic in that they sound similar to the intended syllable or word; or they are semantic in that they have a similar meaning to the intended word or phrase. Other paraphasic errors do, however, occur. Paraphasia is naturally more common in the fluent forms of APHASIA, but may also occur in milder forms of Broca's aphasia, where it is typically phomenic in character.

parapraxia Parapraxia is the production of an unintended movement during the effort to produce voluntary movement. Such movements are well executed although not the action intended. The relationship between the parapraxia and the intended movement is not well understood, but the occurrence of parapraxias has been considered by some writers to be the critical feature of a true APRAXIA.

paratonia Paratonia is an alternative term for GEGENHALTEN.

paresthesia Any abnormality of sensation is a paresthesia (also *paraesthesia*), although it is normally a partial loss of sensation short of the total loss which is anesthesia. However, the term may also be used for abnormal sensations, such as these of pain, which are not attributable to a reduction of normal sensation. Subjective disorders of sensation which are permanent are rare following cortical lesions, although transitory phenomena are quite commonly reported. These are frequently of a paroxysmal character and associated with migraine or EPILEPSY. In certain forms of epilepsy the Jacksonian sensory march represents a particular characteristic form of paresthesia.

parietal lobe In his classic work on the subject, Critchley (1953) describes the parietal lobe as "a topographical convenience pegged out empirically on the surface of the brain," emphasizing the lack of natural landmarks demarcating its boundaries and the fact that it cannot be "equated with any narrowly defined physiological function." He goes on to point out that the term "parietal lobe," which derives from the overlying parietal bone, was not used in English anatomical teaching until the late 1870s and speculates that it will eventually be replaced by more relevant terminology that would include the "three-dimensional temporo-parieto-occipital territory as a functional unit." Critchley's point is well taken; although one can distinguish functional subunits within the posterior half of the brain, none of them is coextensive with the anatomically defined parietal lobe and the more arbitrary anatomical boundaries of the parietal lobe are also those which are less functionally significant.

Thus the anterior boundary of the human parietal lobe is clearly marked on the lateral surface of the brain by the central sulcus, but no

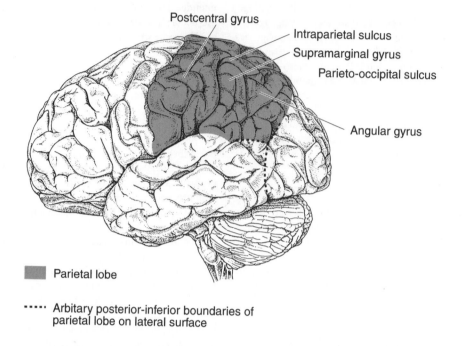

Postcentral gyrus

Intraparietal sulcus

Supramarginal gyrus

Parieto-occipital sulcus

Angular gyrus

Parietal lobe

⋯⋯ Arbitary posterior-inferior boundaries of parietal lobe on lateral surface

Figure 55 The parietal lobe (shaded) showing the arbitrary posterior–inferior boundaries of the parietal lobe on the lateral surface.

clear gross anatomical landmarks distinguish the parieto-occipital boundary posteriorly or the parieto-temporal boundary inferiorly beyond the end of the lateral sulcus. Rather, these boundaries are approximately determined by drawing an imaginary line horizontally backwards from the posterior end of the lateral sulcus until it meets another imaginary line drawn from the superior limit of the parieto-occipital sulcus to the preoccipital notch, a small indentation in the inferior surface of the brain. On the medial surface, the position is reversed: the parieto-occipital sulcus clearly marks the posterior limit of the parietal lobe but its anterior and inferior boundaries are vague.

The area within these boundaries, comprising roughly a fifth of the cerebral cortex, can be divided into three segments: the postcentral gyrus immediately posterior to the central sulcus; the inferior parietal lobule lying posterior to the postcentral sulcus and below the intraparietal sulcus; and the superior parietal lobule lying above it. The latter two lobules are sometimes collectively designated as the posterior parietal

lobe. The postcentral gyrus comprises Brodmann's areas 3, 1, and 2, consisting mostly of neurons with fixed sensory receptive fields on the contralateral side of the body. It constitutes the primary somesthetic area or sensory cortex where tactile and kinesthetic sensations are somatotopically represented.

The anatomic parcelling of the posterior parietal lobe differs between Man and monkey and, in the opinion of different anatomists, reflects the greater development of this region in the human brain. In both species, the superior parietal lobule includes Brodmann's area 5, in which neurons receive predominantly somatosensory input and allow it to function as a sensory association area. In humans, the superior parietal lobule is also usually judged to include the much larger Brodmann area 7 that is sometimes designated as inferior parietal in the monkey. Neurons can be found in area 7 that respond to both visual and tactile input, code position in space independent of eye and head position, and are modulated by attention. They have been implicated in the direction of selective attention, spatial mapping,

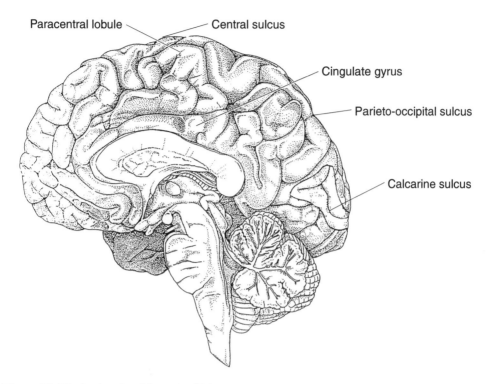

Paracentral lobule

Central sulcus

Cingulate gyrus

Parieto-occipital sulcus

Calcarine sulcus

Figure 56 The landmarks of the parietal lobe.

and the guidance of manual reaching and eye movements.

In humans, the inferior parietal lobule is comprised of the angular and supramarginal gyri, including most of Brodmann's areas 39 and 40, which are not apparent in the monkey brain. The evolutionary expansion of this part of the parietal lobe is probably related to the capacity for language and hemispheric specialization which, if not uniquely human attributes, are at least far more developed than in infra-human brains. The inferior parietal lobule merges anteriorly into Wernicke's area and together these areas around the posterior end of the lateral sulcus constitute the posterior speech zone. This region, including the parietal operculum on the upper bank of the lateral sulcus, is at once the most functionally asymmetrical part of the human brain, the region in which most anatomical asymmetries have been reported, and an area in which damage has very different effects in the left and right hemispheres.

The effects of damage to the parietal lobe reflect its role in the mediation of visually guided

behavior that, in turn, is a function of its location and physiology. Located in the posterior, predominantly sensory half of the brain and being the only lobe that shares a border with the other three lobes and with the limbic system, the parietal lobe is well placed to coordinate visual behavior and integrate spatial information from different sensory modalities. The properties of parietal neurons also clearly suit them for such a role. Even the language-related functions of parietal cortex can be seen as predominantly sensory (or at least receptive) and integrative in that they involve language comprehension and the multimodal language-related activities of writing and reading.

Bilateral parietal lesions may cause severe impairments of visually guided behavior, including the inaccurate reaching for visual targets, impaired redirection of gaze to new targets, and inattention to peripheral stimuli that together constitute BÁLINT'S SYNDROME or the syndrome of visual disorientation. Bilateral lesions can also cause faulty judgment of distance, difficulty appreciating the relative position of visual targets leading to, for example, inability to count

557

scattered objects, simultanagnosia affecting the ability to process two visual stimuli simultaneously and thus to perceive all the elements of a complex scene, and topographical disorientation affecting the ability to find one's way around. These disorders are most frequently caused by trauma, by infarcts in the parietal border-zone area between the middle and posterior cerebral artery territories, or by damage in the territory of the posterior cerebral artery, sometimes as a stage in recovery from cortical blindness. As such lesions are not routine, these disorders are not commonly seen in their full bilateral form, but many occur in lesser degree after unilateral lesions, when the disorder is usually confined to the contralateral half of space. The more common disorder of CONSTRUCTIONAL APRAXIA, affecting the ability to copy geometrical drawings or assemble patterns from blocks, may also be seen after unilateral damage to either parietal lobe, but is more frequent and usually more severe after right, nondominant lesions.

The predominance of right parietal lesions in constructional apraxia is attributable to the right hemisphere's specialization for visuospatial and perceptual ability. The right parietal lobe's contribution to the specialization is specifically spatial, presumably because of the separation of the cortical visual systems analyzing "where" and "what" information, the former taking an occipital-parietal route while the latter flows to the temporal lobe. Consequently, the right parietal lobe takes a leading role in the appreciation of spatial relationships, spatial thinking, and the supramodal representation of external space, probably at several levels.

Thus the syndrome of spatial agnosia and impaired performance on such spatial tasks as maze learning, mental rotation in space, and other tasks requiring spatial thinking is a strong indicator of right parietal damage. Lesions in the right temporo-occipital or parieto-temporo-occipital area, roughly analogous to the posterior language area on the left, are more likely to be implicated in other forms of perceptual disorder affecting visual closure, figure ground discrimination, object recognition, and FACE RECOGNITION. Unilateral NEGLECT of the left after right hemispheric lesions is also much more frequent and more severe than the converse and this too is probably a reflection of the right hemisphere's dominance for spatial representation and possibly ATTEN-TION, although the lesion responsible for neglect is not invariably parietal.

Posterior parietal lesions in the dominant, usually left, hemisphere can affect the spatial organization of the representation of the affected individual's own body. Disorders of this kind have been described as disturbances of the body schema and include the rare syndrome of AUTO-TOPAGNOSIA (literally "unawareness of the topography of oneself"), RIGHT/LEFT DISORIENTA-TION, and FINGER AGNOSIA. The latter two disorders, together with ACALCULIA and DYS-GRAPHIA, constitute the GERSTMANN SYNDROME. Though it is not clear that the four Gerstmann symptoms actually occur together and form a true syndrome, it is generally agreed that they tend to be individually associated with left inferior parietal lesions, particularly around the angular gyrus. Dominant parietal lesions are also frequently implicated in the APRAXIAS, in dysgraphia when this is not simply the motor difficulty experienced when right hemiplegic aphasic patients attempt to write with the nonpreferred hand, and in some of the DYSLEXIAS. Lesions causing APHASIAS characterized by fluent but sometimes empty paraphasic speech and impaired language comprehension frequently include the dominant inferior parietal lobule. In particular, conduction aphasia has been specifically associated with lesions in the angular gyrus or the underlying arcuate fasciculus and transcortical sensory aphasia frequently involves the parieto-temporal junction. However, with these possible exceptions, it makes more sense to treat the posterior language areas as a whole in this context than to separate parietal and nonparietal contributions to fluent aphasia.

In summary, the parietal lobes include a relatively discrete area functioning as the somatosensory cortex, a subregion involved in eye–hand coordination and visual exploration that integrates information from visual and somatosensory cortex, lateralized subsystems representing personal and extrapersonal space, and parts of lateralized functional units processing language (especially visible language) in the left hemisphere and higher-level perceptual functions in the right hemisphere. To the extent that these functions have something in common, one can agree with Critchley's suggestion that the whole temporo-parieto-occipital area be regarded as a functional unit. However, it seems more appropriate to think of the region as a collection of related and interconnected functional units, some of which are parietal, some nonparietal, and some straddling the traditional boundaries between lobes.

BIBLIOGRAPHY

Andersen, R. A. (1987). Inferior parietal lobe function in spatial perception and visuomotor integration. In V. B. Mountcastle, F. Plum, & S. R. Geiger (Eds), *Handbook of physiology* (pp. 483–518). Bethesda, MD: American Physiological Society.

Carpenter, M. B. (1991). *Core text of neuroanatomy*, 4th edn. Baltimore, MD: Williams & Wilkins.

Colby, C. L., Duhamel, J. E., & Goldberg, M. E. (1993). The analysis of visual space by the lateral intraparietal area of the monkey: the role of extraretinal signals. *Progress in Brain Research*, 95, 307–16.

Critchley, M. (1953). *The parietal lobes*. London: Edward Arnold.

De Renzi, E. (1982). *Disorders of space exploration and cognition*. Chichester: Wiley.

Mesulam, M.-M. (1985). *Principles of behavioral neurology*. Philadelphia: Davis.

Newcombe, F. G., & Ratcliff, G. (1989). Disorders of visuospatial analysis. In F. Boller & J. Grafman (Eds), *Handbook of neuropsychology*, Vol. 2 (pp. 333–56). Amsterdam: Elsevier.

Paillard, J. (1991). *Brain and space*. Oxford: Oxford University Press.

Petersen, S. E., Corbetta, M., Miezin, F. M., & Shulman, G. L. (1994). PET studies of parietal involvement in spatial attention: comparison of different task types. *Canadian Journal of Psychology*, 48, 319–38.

Ratcliff, G. (1982). Disturbances of spatial orientation associated with cerebral lesions. In M. Potegal (Ed.), *Spatial abilities: Development and physiological foundations* (pp. 301–31). New York: Academic Press.

G. RATCLIFF

Parkinson's disease Parkinson's disease, also known as *paralysis agitans*, is a degenerative disorder of the brain that affects the extrapyramidal system and is mainly characterized by progressive tremor, bradykinesia (slowness of movement), and rigidity. Its prevalence (the number of existing PD patients over the total population) has been estimated from 84 to 187 per 100,000 population. Degeneration of the substantia nigra (located in the midbrain) with subsequent decrease of striatal dopamine is responsible for the motor and cognitive disturbances seen in these patients. Besides the nigrostriatal dopaminergic loss, involvement of mesocortico-limbic dopaminergic, subcortico-cortical serotoninergic, noradrenergic, and cholinergic pathways are also seen in this disorder. Damage to these latter pathways also contributes to the impaired cognition seen in some PD patients.

The dorsal striatum (putamen and caudate), with the limbic striatum (nucleus accumbens and olfactory tubercle) and pallidum, compose the BASAL GANGLIA. Not all parts of the basal ganglia are equally affected in Parkinson's disease. Alexander and colleagues (1990) suggested that the basal ganglia were connected with different parts of the frontal lobe via five parallel and functionally distinct circuits thought to be the substrates for aspects of motor control, cognition, oculomotor control and affect. It is hypothesized that PD differentially impairs the functioning of these loops with the "motor loop" the most compromised.

Motor but not cognitive deficits are improved with dopaminergic replacement therapy. Initially, most PD patients are stable responders to dopaminergic therapy but, with the course of the disease, fluctuations in responsiveness to therapy eventually appear. Fluctuations are defined by when patients switch between "on" (symptoms controlled by medication) and "off" (symptoms no longer adequately controlled by medication). When in the "off" state, PD patients may be unable to freely move, and demonstrate tremor, hypophonia, and rigidity.

In the original description by Parkinson in 1817, depression was noted in one out of six patients, but no cognitive disturbance was reported. Mental status changes in PD were initially described in the early 1860s by Charcot and were thought to occur only in the late stages of the disease. More recent research has begun to focus on carefully characterizing the cognitive problems in PD (Dubois et al., 1991). Intellectual deficits are currently recognized as a feature of Parkinson's disease, but their incidence, severity, and characteristics are still controversial. Memory, visuospatial, and executive functions can be jointly or individually affected in PD patients. Neuropsychological evaluation routinely identifies three PD subgroups. One subgroup is behaviorally intact, a second has specific deficits, and a third subgroup appears demented. There are no solid data to indicate what the risk factors are for a patient to fall into a particular subgroup, or which patients are likely to change subgroup membership over the course of the disorder.

Mood disorder, specifically depression, is commonly seen in Parkinson's disease and its prevalence varies between 20 and 90 percent, depending on the methods used for evaluation. Most investigators would agree with a ratio of 40 percent, with equal numbers of subjects suffering from major and minor depression.

In most studies (including untreated PD patients) motor dysfunction does not correlate with global or selective cognitive deficits, suggesting that there are different pathological mechanisms underlying each problem. Characterizing the selective and global cognitive deficits that may accompany PD is necessary for a better understanding of its course and treatment.

SELECTIVE DEFICITS

Executive functions include reasoning, problem-solving, planning, concept formation, set-shifting, and social cognition. These functions have been regularly found impaired following damage to the frontal lobes. Executive functions also appear impaired in some nondemented PD patients. In the Tower of London or Toronto tasks, subjects are required to move a series of beads from an initial state array to a goal state array, obeying certain rules. Movement times are recorded in the computerized versions and allow for the evaluation of pre-move planning time. PD patients' difficulty with planning and execution is seen in the increased number of rule violations they make on the Tower of Toronto task and increased planning time on the Tower of London task. PD patients also have problems in forming concepts. In the Wisconsin Card Sorting Test, subjects are presented with a set of cards to be sorted according to one category (color, form, or number) at a time. They must deduce the category from examiner feedback. The total number of categories achieved reflects concept formation

ability. In general, PD patients achieve fewer categories than controls. This deficit is seen early in the disease.

PD patients also have problems in shifting, as well as forming, established conceptual sets, as can be seen in their performance on the Wisconsin Card Sorting Test, the Trail Making Test, part B compared to part A, or in the Stroop Test. PD patients are slower and make more errors in the Trail Making Test part B (which requires alternately connecting numbers and letters) compared to part A (which requires connecting only numbers). This deficit is also seen early in the disease. On the Stroop Test, subjects are required to read color names, then name colors, and finally name the printed color of words that spell a different color. In this third condition, subjects need to inhibit reading the word in order to name the color. PD patients only have difficulty in performing this last condition. Consistent with this deficit, these patients also have trouble in dividing their attention.

PD patients also have difficulty in remembering the order of events. This has been shown on word-list learning tasks and in ordering cartoon pictures to tell a story. Initiation and fluency are also impaired. This can be demonstrated on phonological and semantic fluency tasks (by letter or category). Perseveration errors are also occasionally made by PD patients across tasks.

In summary, nondemented Parkinson's disease patients, early in the course of the disease, may demonstrate impaired executive functions. It is not clear at the present time how frequently they occur, or if these abnormalities progressively deteriorate over the course of the disease.

The "executive" deficits observed in PD patients may be caused by the frontal deafferentation secondary to interruption of the striato-thalamo-frontal circuits or by interruption of the innominato cortical pathways secondary to basal forebrain lesions.

Brown and Marsden (1990) proposed an explanation for these executive function deficits. They studied PD patients when performing the Stroop Test with and without the help of external cues. Their data show that patients were unimpaired when given *external* cues but were deficient when they had to rely on *internal* cues. This inability to rely on internal cues may also be seen in other "executive" tasks, i.e. forming and maintaining a conceptual set probably requires the continuous activation of internal schemas. Brown and Marsden proposed that PD patients had reduced central processing resources which result in a lack of internally generated supervisory schemas. The problem with this "theory" is that it is so general; it is hard to test counter-examples.

MEMORY DYSFUNCTION

Short-term memory, the limited capacity data-driven store, is preserved in nondemented PD patients, as evidenced by their performance on digit span or block-tapping tasks. However, older PD patients appear to have a slowed search of information held in short-term memory, as indicated by their performance on the Sternberg memory scanning task. Furthermore, PD patients recall information less well when the recall follows an interference-filled delay (Brown–Peterson Task). It is not clear whether this impaired recall following interference is indicative of a forgetting or recall deficit. Further studies using this paradigm in conjunction with recognition and implicit retrieval measures are required to resolve this controversy.

Long-term memory, the large capacity conceptually driven store, can be accessed both explicitly and implicitly. *Explicit processing*, which refers to information learned and accessible through conscious recollection, is impaired in PD patients. An aspect of long-term memory which stores *episodic or context-bound information* (as measured by learning lists of unrelated word or paired associates) is particularly impaired. Patients even have difficulty learning semantically organized material such as a story. In contrast, PD patients have normal or near-normal recognition memory, which suggests that encoding and storage processes are preserved. Their recall deficit has been characterized as affecting the more effortful aspects of retrieval of newly learned information and stored knowledge. The explanation for this effortful retrieval deficit may be linked to frontal lobe dysfunction, that is, the inefficient use of conceptual strategies could be accounted for by an impaired supervisory attention system which may be subserved by prefrontal cortex. In demented PD patients (see below), a more pervasive memory deficit is observed that includes encoding, forgetting, and recall. This global memory deficit may be due to more widespread neuropathology.

Implicit memory, or memory without awareness, has been studied in nondemented PD patients using procedural learning (the capacity to acquire a motor skill through repetitive practice) or priming (previous exposure to a stimulus produces temporary facilitation that can be measured in faster reaction times or recognition) tasks. In nondemented PD patients, implicit memory is sometimes impaired (skill learning of fragmented pictures, Tower of Toronto puzzle) and sometimes spared (mirror reading, pursuit rotor learning task, lexical priming). Procedural learning (pursuit rotor learning) and priming (word stem completion) were impaired in demented PD patients. Perhaps implicit memory testing may prove to be clinically helpful in differentiating *demented* PD patients from Alzheimer's disease (AD) patients (preserved procedural learning) and from Huntington's disease patients (preserved verbal priming).

Visuospatial impairment was initially thought to be characteristic of PD patients. Boller and others (1984) defined visuospatial functions as the appreciation of the position of stimuli in space, their integration into a spatial framework, and mental operations such as stimulus rotation and transformation. Some studies have reported that PD patients were impaired on visuomotor (making complex gestures and drawing complex figures) and visuoperceptual (judgment of orientation and of line orientation in space, pattern tracing and construction, mental imagery) tests. Other studies showed no impairment in the ability to manipulate spatial relationships and concepts, right–left discrimination, judgment of spatial displacement, directional forecast, imaginary route-walking tests, mental rotation, matching line orientation or angle, and visuospatial thinking.

Several investigators have questioned if these "visuospatial" deficits primarily reflected PD patients' difficulty with shifting sets and planning and could be considered consistent with their prefrontal lobe dysfunction. This hypothesis was tested using pure visuospatial tasks versus visuospatial set-shifting and planning tasks. PD patients were impaired only on those visuospatial tests in which "executive" functions such as set-shifting or planning were necessary. However, when demented, PD patients' visuospatial impairments were more widespread and almost as severe as the ones found in AD.

Bradyphrenia, or slowness of thought, was considered a cardinal characteristic of PD patients. Initially it was described as a lethargy of the mind with lack of initiative, attention, and vigilance. Several investigators attempted to quantify mental slowness in PD patients, using paradigms that can distinguish between information processing speed, response execution, and movement time. These studies have, in general, failed to show mental slowing in PD patients. Parkinsonians are slowed in initiating and executing movements. Curiously, simple but not choice reaction time is impaired in PD.

Speech is impaired in PD patients. Their DYSARTHRIA (difficulty in articulating words) is linked to a failure of motor control and includes aphonia (severe loss of voice), ANARTHRIA (severe loss of articulation), reduced loudness level, imprecise articulation, tachiphemia (accelerated rate of speech) and less commonly PALILALIA (repetition of words). On the other hand, *language processing and comprehension* is preserved in non-demented PD patients except for the occasional "tip-of-the-tongue phenomenon." Their mild anomia can be overcome by cueing.

DEMENTIA

The prevalence of dementia among PD patients (the proportion of demented individuals over the total number of PD patients) is greater (8 to 93 percent) than in the general population. The variability in prevalence depends on the criteria used to define dementia. Criteria have varied from a Mini Mental State Examination cut-off score, an operational psychometric definition, to the frequently used definition from the Diagnostic and Statistical Manual of Mental Disorders (DSM III/III-R). In the DSM III-R, dementia is defined as a deficit in memory and in at least one other mental function that is severe enough to interfere with the individual's performance in their working and/or social activities, without evidence of confusion. Brown and Marsden (1987) critically reviewed the literature over the last 60 years, using the DSM III criteria, and estimated the prevalence of dementia among PD patients to be approximately 15–20 percent. Pillon and others (1991) favored an operational psychometric definition of dementia (which they defined as a global intellectual performance of at least 2 standard deviations below the mean of a normal population on a battery of psychometric

tests) when studying patients with movement disorders. They argued that the DSM III-R criteria of dementia were adequate for patients with Alzheimer's disease, but in PD the motor disorder alone may preclude the patient from engaging in social or work-related activities. Using the psychometric definition, 18 percent of a nonselected PD population was found to be demented, compared to 93 percent of the Alzheimer's population (Pillon et al., 1991) – a figure similar to that estimated by Brown and Marsden. As noted above, *selective* neuropsychological deficits may occur in PD patients *early* in the course of the disease. We cannot yet predict which of those patients may eventually become demented.

A longitudinal study of newly diagnosed and untreated patients reported dementia in only 8 percent of the early onset PD patients (< 70 years) but in 32 percent of the late onset patients (> 70 years). At three years follow-up, 18 percent of the early onset group and 83 percent of the late onset group now suffered from dementia. This study confirmed previous suggestions of an increase in the frequency of dementia in the older PD population and in the late onset PD group. It also suggests a progressive decline of intellectual functions throughout the course of the disease.

In studies of cognitively impaired but non-demented PD patients, language, praxis, and gnosis were spared while "executive functions" were affected. This profile resembled a "subcortical" as opposed to a "cortical" dementia. *Subcortical dementia* was initially described in patients with progressive supranuclear palsy, who had difficulty in manipulating learned knowledge, were forgetful but not amnestic, slow to process information, and demonstrated changes in mood state or personality. Language, praxis, and gnosis were normal in these patients.

In carefully controlled studies, the differences between demented PD patients and other populations of demented patients are less apparent as language, memory, executive and visuospatial functions may all be impaired to different degrees across demented groups. In these studies, relative more than absolute differences are found. For example, in one study, semantic and episodic verbal memory and visuospatial memory appear to be relatively less impaired in demented PD patients compared to AD patients. On the other hand, executive functions, visuospatial abstraction, and reasoning are relatively more affected in PD compared to AD patients.

This classification of cortical vs subcortical dementias is still controversial, since "cortical" dementias have subcortical lesions and "subcortical" dementias have cortical involvement. Furthermore, the neuropsychological distinction is also fuzzy. In PD, three neuropathological processes may be responsible for the dementia. One is related to the subcortical-cortical dopaminergic, cholinergic and noradrenergic losses mentioned above. Another cause may be the increased association of PD with Alzheimer's disease (either due to the co-occurrence of two degenerative disorders or to a predisposition of patients with one neurodegenerative disease to subsequently have another). The third cause of dementia is due to other Parkinsonian disorders that are mistaken for PD (mainly cortical Lewy body disease, and to a lesser degree, multisystem atrophy and progressive supranuclear palsy) where Parkinsonism and cognitive changes are both present and may occasionally be difficult to differentiate from those found in PD. Despite this confusion regarding the identification of PD as a subcortical dementia, that classification still seems to be clinically useful since progressive supranuclear palsy and Huntington's disease can be differentiated from "cortical" dementias such as Alzheimer's disease on the basis of their *pattern* of cognitive disturbance.

Hemiparkinsonism applies to patients who have the disease restricted to one side of their body. It reflects an early stage of the disease and is accompanied by deficits in cognitive functions considered to be lateralized to one cerebral hemisphere. Studies have shown that right hemiparkinsonians have a poorer performance on verbal tasks such as word fluency and digit supraspan. In contrast, studies with left hemiparkinsonians are inconclusive.

METHODOLOGICAL ISSUES

Several *methodological issues* must be considered when reviewing neuropsychological studies of PD patients. How was dementia defined and what proportion of patients in the study are demented? Was overall level of dementia controlled for across comparison groups in dementia studies (e.g. AD vs PD)? If the study is concerned with selective deficits, have patients with global

dementia or low intelligence been excluded? Has patient age, onset, and duration of disorder been controlled for? If the study is targeting cognitive processes, has movement time been eliminated as a potential confounder? Have the effects of mood disorder (e.g. depression) been accounted for when interpreting the results of cognitive tests? Are the patients being treated? If so, is dopaminergic therapy adequate or is the treatment supplemented with other antiparkinsonian agents, e.g. anticholinergic medication that could affect cognition?

Although dopaminergic therapy may improve motor performance on timed tasks, it has only a mild influence on the patients' cognitive performance (when patients are "off" (see above) there is a reported decrease in verbal fluency and alertness and an increase in choice reaction times). Higher doses of dopamine can produce confusion and hallucinations, as well as making patients' performance deteriorate. Anticholinergic therapy may worsen attention, memory, and executive functions – even in patients who are not demented.

CONCLUSION

In summary, investigators have identified three subgroups of patients with Parkinson's disease: (a) those with normal cognition; (b) those with selective deficits; and (c) those who are demented. Neuropsychological symptoms appear to progress over the course of the disease in many, but not all patients. Variables predicting long-term neuropsychological outcome have not been found. Selective executive, memory, or visuospatial dysfunctions seem to be related to the underlying basal ganglia-thalamo-frontal pathology and not to treatment. Older PD patients and those with late onset of the disorder appear more cognitively impaired. No association between cognitive and motor deficits is apparent. An overlap in neuropathological and neurochemical findings in demented PD and AD patients suggests that differences in neurobehavioral patterns between the two groups are relative rather than absolute. Carefully controlled longitudinal studies combining neuropsychological with neurochemical and neuropathological investigations will continue to advance our knowledge of PD.

BIBLIOGRAPHY

Alexander, G. E., Crutcher, M. D., & DeLong, M. R. (1990). Basal ganglia-thalamocortical circuits: parallel substrates for motor, oculomotor, "prefrontal" and "limbic" functions. In H. B. M. Uylings, C. G. Van Eden, J. P. C. De Bruin, M. A. Corner, & M. G. P. Feenstra (Eds), *The prefrontal cortex: its structure, function and pathology* (Progress in Brain Research, Vol. 85, pp. 119–44), Amsterdam: Elsevier.

Boller, F., Passafiore, O., Keefe, N. C., Rogers, K., Morrow, L., & Kim, Y. (1984). Visuospatial impairment in Parkinson's disease: role of perceptual and motor factors. *Archives of Neurology*, *41*, 485–90.

Brown, R. G., & Marsden, C. D. (1987). Neuropsychology and cognitive function in Parkinson's disease: an overview. In C. D. Marsden & S. Fahn (Eds), *Movement disorders 2* (pp. 99–123). London: Butterworth.

Brown, R. G., & Marsden, C. D. (1990). Cognitive function in Parkinson's disease: from description to theory. *Trends in Neuroscience*, *13*, 21–9.

Cooper, J. A., Sagar, H. J., Jordan, N., Harvey, N. S., & Sullivan, E. V. (1991). Cognitive impairment in early, untreated Parkinson's disease and its relationship to motor disability. *Brain*, *114*, 2095–122.

Dubois, B., Boller, F., Pillon, B., & Agid, Y. (1991). Cognitive deficits in Parkinson's disease. In F. Boller & J. Grafman (Eds), *Handbook of neuropsychology*, Vol. 5 (pp. 195–240). Amsterdam: Elsevier.

Litvan, I., Mohr, E., Williams, J., Gomez, C., & Chase, T. N. (1991). Differential memory and executive functions in demented patients with Parkinson's and Alzheimer's disease. *Journal of Neurology, Neurosurgery and Psychiatry*, *54*, 25–9.

Pillon, B., Dubois, B., Ploska, A., & Agid, Y. (1991). Severity and specificity of cognitive impairment in Alzheimer's, Huntington's, and Parkinson's diseases and progressive supranuclear palsy. *Neurology*, *41*, 634–43.

Taylor, A. E., Saint-Cyr, J. A., & Lang, A. E. (1988). Idiopathic Parkinson's disease: revised concepts of cognitive and affective status. *Canadian Journal of Neurological Science*, *15*, 106–13.

IRENE LITVAN

paroxysmal disorders Any disorder which produces a fit or convulsion or seizure; a paroxysm. The essential feature is a relatively severe disturbance of behavior during a defined period of short duration following which recovery occurs. Such disorders are most commonly termed EPILEPSY. While epilepsy is the most common cause of such paroxysms, they also occur in other disorders. Hysterical convulsions may imitate true epilepsy to some degree, and features of severe anxiety attacks may also be similar to epileptic fits. Similarly, vasovagal attacks may be paroxysmal in nature and may simulate epilepsy, as may migraine, aural vertigo, and hypoglycemia. In CATALEPSY and NARCOLEPSY convulsions do not occur, but the onset of the loss of voluntary power and consciousness respectively for a defined period leads them to be regarded as paroxysmal disorders.

peduncle The cerebral peduncles are large fiber bundles which lie in the ventral portion of the BRAIN STEM, essentially covering the midbrain in this area. These bundles carry descending fibers from the cortex which include, most importantly, the PYRAMIDAL TRACT and so serve voluntary movement. It has been suggested that the peduncles act as an interface between the motor systems of the brain and those of the spinal cord, organizing the integrated outflow from the brain. Gross disorders of movement such as CHOREA, ATHETOSIS, and HEMIBALLISMUS may be relieved by surgical division of the peduncles (pedunculotomy).

The cerebral peduncles should not be confused with the cerebellar peduncles, which are the three paired structures, also in the ventral brain stem, through which fibers enter and leave the CEREBELLUM.

pelopsia Pelopsia is a form of visual illusion or METAMORPHOPSIA in which objects appear to be nearer to the observer than they actually are. The illusion may be combined with a sense of the object being larger than normal (MACROPSIA). It may involve selected objects in the visual array, and occasionally selected parts within the object. As with other metamorphopsias it may be an epileptic phenomenon, associated with migraine attacks or, when persistent, present in the acute phase following cerebral trauma.

perception *See* AUDITORY PERCEPTUAL DISORDERS; OLFACTION; TACTILE PERCEPTION DIS-

ORDERS; TASTE; VISUOPERCEPTUAL DISORDERS; VISUOSPATIAL DISORDERS.

perseveration Perseveration is the tendency to repeatedly emit the same behavioral response when it is no longer appropriate. It may occur in a number of neuropsychological contexts.

Perseveration occurs in association with focal lesions of the FRONTAL LOBES, so that a response which is correct at one point in time will be repeated as the response to subsequent items irrespective of the stimulus demands, so it will be incorrect. This is often interpreted as a loss of flexibility in thinking, as responses remain bound to previous stimuli so that new stimuli cannot properly be assimilated into thinking. The perseveration may be apparent in the response to abstract semantic material, as in the responses to consecutive items in a cognitive test, or to relatively simple patterns of motor response, so that the patient asked to repeatedly open and close the eyes will be unable to stop when instructed to do so. At a high level the perseveration is often assessed by the Wisconsin Card Sorting Test, in which the subject has to deduce a principle of sorting from feedback which the examiner provides on each trial. After the current principle has been attained by the subject, the examiner changes the principle without warning, and the subject must accommodate to the new principle on the basis of the feedback provided. Classically, patients with frontal lesions are able to attain the first principle of sorting (so their deficit does not lie in the ability to extract the principle of sorting from feedback), but they are unable to accommodate to the change of principle, continuing to sort by the first principle despite the evidence that their method of sorting is now incorrect. This demonstrates a failure of the ability to shift from one strategy to another, and to overcome an established response set. The lesion which may result in perseverative failure on this task is normally extensive bilateral frontal damage, commonly, but not exclusively, involving the prefrontal cortex rather than other areas of the frontal lobe.

Perseveration may also be seen in DEMENTIA, where it occurs in language expression, in the form of part-sentences or single words or phrases which may be repeated. In this form it is similar to ECHOLALIA. However, it may also occur at a higher level so that groups of sentences, or accounts of events, may be repeated endlessly in a rather stereotyped fashion. Some studies have reported this form of perseveration to be present in almost every case of dementia of the Alzheimer type, and it is very common in all dementias. Motor perseveration may also occur so that movements, or sequences of movements, are similarly repeatedly executed (*see* ECHOPRAXIA). Perseveration in dementia is presumed to have a similar causation to the perseveration seen following focal frontal lobe lesions in that diffuse degeneration of the frontal cortex is thought to be responsible. However, the contribution of memory deficits may also be a factor in dementia, which it has been shown not to be with the focal frontal lesions.

Visual perseveration is also seen in the METAMORPHOPSIAS, where it is termed PALINOPSIA, occurring with relatively mild defects of the visual fields, being the illusory reappearance of a visual perception after removal of the object which was the basis of the original perception. It is important to distinguish perseveration of visual percept (true palinopsia) and perseveration of the verbal response which reports the current percept; accurate and normal perceptions may give the appearance of palinopsia if the patient perseverates in the verbal description which is employed.

J. GRAHAM BEAUMONT

personality disorders Although a large and heterogeneous number of definitions (usually consistent with a particular viewpoint) have been used to define the term "personality," most authors agree on two basic points: (1) the term personality refers to the integrated set of psychological traits which characterize a given individual; (2) the most important personality features are those motivational, social, and dynamic traits which determine the character of an individual. The ability traits, which form a separate cluster of features, are not usually included in the definition of personality. The stress put on motivational, social, and dynamic features, rather than on ability traits, has both methodological and anatomo-clinical implications for the neuropsychological study of personality disorders.

The methodological implications stem from the fact that very few advances have been made in recent years in the construction of clinical instruments allowing a better assessment of personality disorders (just as few advances have been made toward a more articulated and theoretically defensible model of personality). The clinical tools used to evaluate personality changes resulting from brain damage are therefore much less sophisticated, precise, and reliable than those used to evaluate disorders of specific cognitive abilities. The anatomo-clinical implications stem from the idea that brain structures critically involved in the organization and the disorganization of personality should be the cortical areas intimately linked with the LIMBIC SYSTEM, namely the prefrontal areas and the mesial parts of the temporal lobes, rather than the cortical convexity structures which are crucially involved in language and in other cognitive abilities. This idea comes from the fact that the limbic structures, and in particular the AMYGDALA, play a leading role in various aspects of emotional and social behavior, whereas the mesial temporal and prefrontal areas modulate and integrate these basic emotional and motivational traits.

METHODOLOGICAL PROBLEMS

The tests more commonly used by clinical psychologists to evaluate different aspects and disorders of personality can be roughly classified into two major groups: (a) projective personality tests, whose best-known exemplar is the Rorschach test; (b) objective personality tests, whose best-known and more frequently used representative in medical settings is the Minnesota Multiphasic Personality Inventory (MMPI). The advantages and limitations of these methods for the evaluation of personality features and personality disorders in subjects free from brain damage are well known and will not be discussed here. What is worth stressing in this context is rather the fact that none of these instruments was constructed with the specific problems of patients with cerebral lesions in mind, therefore their use with brain-damaged patients can be highly problematic and often misleading.

If we consider, for example, the MMPI (which has been used much more frequently than the Rorschach test to evaluate behavioral and personality disorders of brain-damaged patients) we can make two general remarks:

1 There is no reason to believe that personality changes resulting from damage to a specific

brain structure must correspond to the psychiatric diagnostic categories used by the MMPI, a test which was originally constructed for and standardized on psychiatric populations.

2 Since many items included primarily in scales Hs (hypochondriasis), Hy (hysteria), and Sc (schizophrenia) of the MMPI refer to questions tapping common symptoms or manifestations of neurological damage, patients with central nervous system disease tend to have higher than average scores on these scales, simply as an artifact of the test items and scale composition (Lezak, 1983).

In order to avoid these methodological shortcomings, several authors have constructed behavioral rating scales, aiming to document the behavioral and social consequences of specific forms of brain damage. Thus, Dodrill and colleagues have developed the Washington Psychosocial Seizure Inventory (see Lezak, 1983) to investigate the social maladaptation associated with chronic epilepsy, whereas Lezak and colleagues have constructed the Portland Adaptability Inventory (see Lezak, 1983) to provide a systematic record of personality and social maladaptation resulting from severe head trauma. All these rating scales, however, can hardly help us to understand the mechanisms (or at least to evaluate the specificity) of personality changes resulting from damage to specific brain structures, since they were conceived as simple inventories or shorthand methods of reporting systematically some clinical judgments in a particular clinical domain.

CLINICAL PROBLEMS

From the clinical point of view, the suggestion that the brain structures subserving both the development and the disorders of personality may be the cortical areas more strongly connected with the limbic system is strongly supported by the observation that two pathological conditions usually considered as involved in personality disorders are evident in patients with frontal lobe lesions and patients with temporal EPILEPSY.

Personality disorders resulting from frontal lobe lesions
The classic description of personality disorders resulting from FRONTAL LOBE damage was provided more than a century ago by Harlow (1868)

in his often quoted description of the profound personality change shown by patient "Gage," who had survived, without neurological defects, a major traumatic injury to the frontal lobes. According to Harlow (1868) this patient, who was described before the accident as a well balanced, energetic, family-oriented construction foreman, "was no longer Gage" after the frontal lesion:

> The equilibrium between his intellectual faculties and animal propensities seems to have been destroyed. He is fitful, irreverent, impatient of restraint or advice when it conflicts with his desires; at times pertinaciously obstinate, yet capricious and vacillating ... A child in his intellectual capacity and manifestations, he has the animal passions of a strong man.

Although subsequent authors have questioned the specificity of this kind of personality disorder, the links between frontal lobe damage and personality disturbances have been confirmed by both clinical and experimental investigations. From the experimental point of view, two basic lines of research have tried to clarify this issue, looking on one hand at the anatomical connections of the frontal lobes and, on the other hand, at the social behavior of animals submitted to frontal lobectomy.

The first line of research was pursued by Nauta (1971), who tried to infer the functional significance of the frontal lobes from the special features of their anatomical relationships. According to Nauta (1971), two characteristics of the neural circuitry of the frontal lobes are very relevant. The first is the importance of the reciprocal relationship between the frontal lobes and the limbic system. The richness of these connections suggests that the frontal lobe might be considered as the major neocortical representative of the limbic system and that one of its main functions might consist in monitoring and modulating limbic mechanisms. The second is the convergence in the frontal lobes of information coming from the external environment (through associations with the visual, auditory, and somatic sensory areas) and from the internal milieu, through the connections of the frontal lobe with the HYPOTHALAMUS and various structures of the limbic system. A massive injury to the frontal lobes, disrupting this convergence of exteroceptive and interoceptive information, could dissociate the appreciation of external events from the concomitant affective response. A consequence of this dissociation could be the development of inappropriate social and emotional behaviors, due to the inability to associate the internal response with the external outcomes of personal acts. Another consequence would be the "loss of foresight" which is so typical of frontal lobe patients, since behavioral anticipation presupposes that external and internal consequences of a given act are linked together at the representative level, a synthesis precluded by frontal lobe injury.

The second line of research has been followed by Myers (1972), who studied in the field, under natural conditions, the behavior of monkeys trapped, subjected to frontal ablation, and then released close to their social group. Several aspects of social interaction, social communication, and maternal behavior were profoundly affected by frontal lobectomy. Almost all these animals showed a marked reduction in the frequency of threat gestures, grooming, facial expression, and vocalization in a social context. Some of them failed even to approach their own social group when released close to it and remained solitary or disappeared into the underbrush. Finally, females with infants ignored or rejected their young in the laboratory or deserted them upon release in the field. These observations consistently show that frontal lobectomy produces in monkeys a range of behavioral changes that can readily be associated with personality disorders in humans.

If we come back now from this basic research to the clinical studies which have investigated personality disorders in frontal lobe patients, we find that a very large array of behavioral abnormalities have been described using the term "frontal lobe personality."

Some patients show unrestrained and tactless behavior with sexually disinhibited humor or a childish tendency to joke. Other patients show a diminution of spontaneity and initiative, with apathy, dullness, indifference, and slowness of thought. Still others look capricious, unstable, and egocentric, with a total lack of concern for others. This heterogeneity of personality disorders and of behavioral disturbances could be due in part to the variety of etiologies that can produce frontal lobe damage and in part to the methodological problems met while trying to study, under controlled conditions, personality disorders in brain-damaged patients. According to some authors, however, part of this variability might be due to the precise location of the lesion within the frontal lobes. Anatomically the prefrontal cortex constitutes a very large part of the whole cortical mantle, and can itself be further subdivided into at least three main sections (the dorsolateral, the medial, and the orbital cortex). It is therefore not unlikely that different kinds of personality disorders may result from damage to these different parts. Thus Blumer and Benson (1975), following a classification originally proposed by Kleist and Kretschmer, have described two different types of personality changes following structural damage to different parts of the frontal lobes: (a) a pseudo-depressed personality, characterized by apathy, lack of drive, inability to plan ahead, and total unconcern, which might be typical of patients with a lesion located in the dorsal-lateral convexity; and (b) a pseudo-psychopathic personality, characterized by a puerile, jocular attitude, by sexually disinhibited humor, and by total unconcern for others, which might be seen in patients with lesions located in the orbital parts of the frontal lobes.

In addition to the clinical studies of personality and behavioral disorders resulting from frontal lobe lesions acquired during adulthood, some authors have investigated the influence on the development of personality of frontal lobe lesions acquired early in life. Price and others (1990) recently reported two such cases and reviewed the available literature.

They maintain that patients who suffered bilateral prefrontal damage early in life are prone to develop a particular type of learning disability in the areas of social and moral judgment, insight, foresight, empathy, and abstract reasoning. In adulthood they usually display impulsive behaviors, triggered by immediate stimuli, are unable to learn from punishment and negative experience, remain socially isolated, have few friends, and show little empathy, and no sense of remorse or fairness toward others. The salient personality features of these patients are therefore similar to those emerging as a consequence of bilateral frontal lobe lesions acquired in adulthood.

Interictal personality changes associated with temporal lobe epilepsy

Although specific personality changes are usually not observed in other forms of epilepsy, several authors have suggested a characteristic constella-tion of changes in temporal lobe EPILEPSY (TLE). These changes are interictal, in that they are manifest between those events that are clinically designated as seizures and they are less pervasive and striking than the personality disorders resulting from frontal lobe damage. The changes most frequently described in TLE concern particular aspects of behavior, such as sexual behaviors or more specific behaviors such as a tendency toward extensive writing, or discrete aspects of personality, such as lack of humor, moralism, or religiosity. Waxman and Geschwind (1975), who have stressed the clinical and theoretical interest of these changes (which provide an example of a human behavioral syndrome resulting from dysfunction of brain areas strongly connected with the limbic system) have also rightly noted that these modifications are not necessarily maladaptive. The discrete and non-maladaptive nature of these changes explains why they do not immediately capture the attention of the observer, and also why their very existence has been questioned by some authors. Investigations conducted with standardized and validated methods of measuring psychopathology, such as the Minnesota Multiphasic Personality Inventory (MMPI) have also failed to reveal significant differences between TLE and other forms of epilepsy. As was pointed out in the methodological section, these instruments, designed to evaluate standard aspects of psychopathology, might be insensitive to the specific personality changes described in TLE. With this problem in mind, Bear and Fedio (1977) developed an ad hoc personality inventory, based on behavioral features supposedly associated with TLE, and gave this test to TLE patients and neuromuscular control subjects. They showed: (a) that TLE patients scored higher on almost all these traits, (b) that laterality differences emerged when patients with right and left temporal lobe foci were taken separately into account. Emotional traits were in the foreground in epileptics with right temporal foci, whereas ideational traits prevailed in patients with left-sided foci. They interpreted these findings as suggesting a cortico-limbic hyperconnection, i.e. a reinforcement, mediated by the temporo-limbic intercritical activity, of the information processing style typical of each hemisphere. These results, however, have been confirmed only in part by other investigations which used the same personality inventory to compare TLE patients with other forms of epilepsy (see Trimble, 1983; Hermann & Whitman, 1984; and Dodrill & Batzell, 1986, for different viewpoints on this subject). The problem of the specificity of the personality traits shown by TLE patients therefore remains unsettled.

In our opinion, the most convincing explanation for these contrasting results has been advanced by Dodrill and Batzell (1986), who suggested that some behavioral features typical of TLE do indeed exist, but occur infrequently. These characteristics may therefore be washed out completely in evaluations based on large group studies, but they may be prominent and of considerable interest when they occur in single patients.

CONCLUDING REMARKS

Personality disorders seem to emerge when a brain lesion impinges upon limbic structures or cortical areas intimately connected with the limbic system. In particular, both a major and a minor behavioral syndrome are described in the neuropsychological literature. The major syndrome, under the heading of "frontal lobe personality," can be observed when the lesion bilaterally disrupts the prefrontal areas, leaving unchecked elementary limbic mechanisms and hampering the integration between cognitive and emotional experience. The minor (and more controversial) syndrome can be observed interictally in a few patients with TLE who show a stereotyped pattern of personality features characterized by viscosity with obsessionalism, moralism, or hyperreligiosity, deepened emotionality, and reduced or altered sexuality. The meaning of these personality features is still controversial, but the hypothesis that they may be due to the establishment of abnormally strong links between certain aspects of experience and the reinforcement produced by the limbic system seems worth considering.

BIBLIOGRAPHY

Bear, D. M., & Fedio, P. (1977). Quantitative analysis of interictal behaviour in temporal lobe epilepsy. *Archives of Neurology*, *34*, 454–67.

Blumer, D., & Benson, D. F. (1975). Personality changes with frontal and temporal lobe lesions. In D. F. Benson & D. Blumer (Eds), *Psychiatric aspects of neurologic disease* (pp. 151–69). New York: Grune & Stratton.

Dodrill, C. B., & Batzel, L. W. (1986). Interictal behavioral features of patients with epilepsy. *Epilepsia*, *27* (suppl. 2), S64–S76.

Harlow, J. M. (1868). Recovery from the passage of an iron bar through the head. *Publications of the Massachusetts Medical Society*, *2*, 327–46.

Hermann, B. P., & Whitman, S. (1984). Behavioral and personality correlates of epilepsy: a review, methodological critique, and conceptual model. *Psychological Bulletin*, *95*, 451–97.

Lezak, M. D. (1983). *Neuropsychological assessment*, 2nd edn. New York: Oxford University Press.

Myers, E. (1972). Role of prefrontal and anterior temporal cortex in social behaviour and affect in monkeys. *Acta Neurobiologiae Experimentalis*, *32*, 567–79.

Nauta, W. J. H. (1971). The problem of the frontal lobe: a reinterpretation. *Journal of Psychiatric Research*, *8*, 167–87.

Price, B. H., Daffner, K. R., Stowe, R. M., & Mesulam, M. M. (1990). The comportmental learning disabilities of early frontal lobe damage. *Brain*, *113*, 1383–93.

Trimble, M. R. (1983). Personality disturbances in epilepsy. *Neurology*, *33*, 1332–4.

Waxman, S. G., & Geschwind, N. (1975). The interictal behavior syndrome of temporal lobe epilepsy. *Archives of General Psychiatry*, *32*, 1580–6.

GUIDO GAINOTTI

PET scan The PET (*positron emission tomography*) scan is a form of physical investigation which permits functional rather than anatomical imaging of the brain (*see* BLOOD FLOW STUDIES; LOCALIZATION; SCAN).

In order to obtain a PET image, the patient is administered a compound of glucose which is chemically unstable and has a limited half-life in terms of minutes. Glucose being the energy source of the brain, it is rapidly taken up by brain tissue, with the more active areas taking up more than the less active areas. The result is that there is an excess of protons over electrons in these areas of the brain, which are then released as neutrons and positrons. A proportion of the positrons collide with electrons, resulting in the annihilation of both, but with two gamma rays being given off in opposite directions. These gamma rays can be detected as they pass out through the skull, and a computer-based image of the brain built up over a period of recording, with the more functionally active areas of the brain being identified. The technique is expensive and therefore not widely available. While it is limited in its neuropsychological application by the time required to build up an image, it has nevertheless permitted the development of an exciting and important area of research.

petalia Petalia is an asymmetry of the configuration of the frontal lobes, so that one lobe significantly protrudes further than the other. It is not necessarily abnormal, and may reflect one aspect of the complex pattern of natural cortical asymmetries which are now recognized.

phantom limb The phantom limb is a form of BODY SCHEMA DISTURBANCE in which the patient perceives the normal presence of a limb following an amputation. The sense of the presence of the limb is vivid, and the full range of tactile and somatosensory perceptions may be registered as if from the missing limb. The patient may, for example, reach to scratch an area of an absent leg, or complain about pain in a foot which is no longer present. It is assumed that the internal representation of the body remains intact following the amputation, so that sensory information may continue to be internally mapped to the absent body part, even though it cannot have originated in the place at which it is perceived.

The phantom limb phenomenon occurs in over 90 percent of cases of amputation and may persist for a considerable period of time, even over years, with recovery being typically a gradual shrinkage back to the operation stump.

The term is also, less commonly, used for the perception of an additional supernumerary limb in certain forms of EPILEPSY, with additional upper limbs being more common than lower limbs.

phenylketonuria Phenylketonuria (PKU) (*see also* CONGENITAL DISORDERS) is a condition of childhood determined by a single gene inherited in an autosomal recessive pattern. The metabolic defect is an inability to convert the amino acid *phenylalanine* (PHE) to *tyrosine*, owing to the

absence of the liver enzyme *phenylalanine hydroxylase* (PAH) (Jervis, 1947). As a result of the block in metabolism, phenylalanine (found in protein foods) builds up to large concentrations in blood and tissues; if untreated the high concentrations of PHE affect normal brain development. Before a treatment was developed the disorder manifested itself as profound motor and mental retardation. The majority of affected infants did not learn to talk, did not progress beyond a mental age of 2 years, exhibited behavioral problems, and abnormally increased muscle tone led to a characteristic "tailor's position" being assumed; most were institutionalized. In addition to the nervous system disorders, anomalies of bone (small skull, growth retardation) occurred; around 75 percent died before the age of 30 years.

Early detection and treatment begun within the first two months of birth with a well-controlled low-PHE diet is very effective; given these conditions prognosis is excellent for normal brain development, and mental retardation is prevented. Phenylketonuria affects about 1 in 10,000 births in the USA and Europe, is more frequent in certain northern European populations and their descendants but is less common among Finns, southern and eastern Europeans, and Asians (Mange & Mange, 1990). The frequency of carriers varies with the group; among Caucasians it is around 1 in 50–60 which is not particularly uncommon, but due to the recessive pattern of inheritance the likelihood of two carriers reproducing is extremely small at about 1 in 2,000–3,000, which explains the low incidence of PKU births.

Phenylketonuria was first described in 1934 by Asbjørn Folling, a Norwegian biochemist and physician. Two children aged 7 and 4 years with mental retardation were presented; the mother noted that they exuded a peculiar "mousy" odor. Excessive phenylpyruvic acid, a type of ketone, was discovered in the urine of the children. Large-scale testing of institutionalized retarded children led to the discovery of others who secreted the same substance. High concentrations of PHE that accumulate in the body fluids (cerebrospinal fluid, blood plasma, and sweat) are converted to phenylpyruvic acid, which is metabolized to several other derivatives; these phenylketones appear in the urine. Because the metabolic block prevents conversion of PHE to tyrosine these individuals are deficient in the derivatives of tyrosine as well. The pathway for tyrosine metabolism includes DOPA, dopamine, noradrenaline, and the pigment melanin. Many untreated phenylketonurics were fair-skinned, with blond hair and blue eyes.

Twenty years after Folling's discovery, treatment by dietary protein restriction was attempted by Bickel and colleagues. PHE intake was restricted and synthetic mixes of amino acids supplemented with vitamins, minerals, fats, and carbohydrates were developed. Neonatal screening became possible in 1963 when Guthrie and Susi developed a simple test for excess serum PHE.

SUBCLASSIFICATIONS OF PHENYL-KETONURIA

It has become apparent that the defective activity of phenylalanine hydroxylase leads to a spectrum of clinical presentations and this has in turn led to various subclassifications of PKU. Over 40 different mutations of the phenylalanine hydroxylase (PAH) gene, which is on chromosome 12, have been identified. The PAH deficiency leads to a wide range of clinical and biochemical severity, from a symptomless disorder with plasma PHE accumulation near normal levels, to a potentially severely handicapping condition with plasma PHE levels over 20 times normal. A proportion of affected individuals are therefore compound heterozygotes rather than homozygotes.

Type I – classic phenylketonuria This form is due to a virtually complete absence (less than 1 percent) of PAH liver enzyme activity, accounting for around 60 percent of all cases of hyperphenylalaninemia (a term for excessively elevated phenylalanine blood-levels). Blood PHE levels greater than 1200 mumol/L usually indicate severe deficiency of PAH.

Persistent mild hyperphenylalaninemia This results from a partial deficiency of PAH (2–35 percent activity); and a *transient* form results from a maturational delay rather than from a defect in the PAH enzyme. These two forms may require either no treatment or only early dietary restriction; they account for around 35 percent of all cases of hyperphenylalaninemia. Blood PHE levels between 600 and 1200 mumol/L lead to "atypical PKU." Cases where blood PHE remains between 120 and 480 mumol/L on a normal diet are termed "benign hyperphenylalaninemia" (Matalon & Michals, 1991).

Type II – atypical hyperphenylalaninemia or dihydropteridine reductase (DHPR) deficiency The PAH enzyme is normal but the DHPR enzyme is nonfunctional, and there is inadequate synthesis of the cofactor BH4, which is required for PAH activity and for the enzymatic hydroxylation of tyrosine and tryptophan. There is an abnormal response to dietary treatment, and despite the control of PHE levels there is progressive deterioration of brain function; in some cases treatment with BH4 appears to slow neurological deterioration, in other cases the outcome is unclear (Mange & Mange, 1990). This form accounts for around 3 percent of all hyperphenylalaninemia cases.

Type III – dihydrobiopterin synthetase deficiency This form comprises 1–3 percent of all hyperphenylalaninemia cases and involves a defect of the dihydrobiopterin synthetase enzyme. There is progressive neurological deterioration even after dietary treatment, although some cases respond to treatment with BH4 and neurotransmitter precursors.

IDENTIFICATION AND MANAGEMENT OF PHENYLKETONURIA

Nationwide neonatal screening programs for the early identification of PKU have been established in many countries since the 1960s. There has been some controversy over the success rates claimed for these screening programs; for example, Smith and colleagues claimed that national coverage in the UK "approaches 100%" (Smith et al., 1991, p. 333); Elliman and Garner (1991) point out that national averages can obscure large individual variations. In a review of the procedures for neonatal biochemical screening in the London borough of Wandsworth, they discovered that results were not readily available for 5 percent of babies born in the first eight months of 1990, and that around 2 percent of infants appeared not to have been tested.

A report from the Medical Research Council Working Party on Phenylketonuria (MRC, 1993) concluded that the availability of complex diets has virtually eliminated severe mental handicap resulting from the disease. The main goal of successful treatment has been the achievement of normal intelligence, involving extensive dependence on measurement of IQ, and there continues to be much debate about the appropriate age at which to relax the controlled diet, with some authors favoring life-long metabolic control for maximizing scores on intelligence tests.

There is some evidence that the diets themselves may be harmful (MRC Working Party, 1993). It is acknowledged that a low PHE diet cannot fully substitute for the fine tuning of PHE turnover normally exerted by PAH. The dietary control of plasma PHE requires rigorous restriction of natural protein and regular intake of unpalatable substitutes for protein, minerals, and vitamins, together with regular biochemical monitoring. Control is difficult to maintain, and investigations of the functioning and coping of families with PKU children have demonstrated positive correlations among perceived family cohesion, dietary adherence associated with metabolic control, and IQs of PKU children.

In a retrospective study of 34 early treated, normally intelligent adolescents with PKU, Weglage and colleagues (1992) found the patients characterized by less autonomy, a more negative evaluation of their scholastic ability, less achievement motivation, low frustration tolerance, more negative self-description, a feeling of being not quite healthy, more grave, and a higher level of dependency on their families; they saw their whole social situation as being distinctly restricted. In addition, their knowledge concerning PKU and diet was alarmingly poor and the majority had great difficulty in managing the diet satisfactorily without parental help. These aspects may account to some degree for the finding that up to the age of 15 years the serum PHE levels of this group were persistently above the desired range. Further evidence suggests that the underlying reason why some parents deviate from the diet and do not always apply it strictly is their adoption of a compromise between an ideal attitude towards the diet, which may lead to an experience of loss and guilt, and the goal of undisturbed personality development of the child. Discussion of the interaction between psychological and social aspects of treatment control and PHE levels is largely absent in the literature.

There is a high risk of fetal damage in offspring of women with PKU. When blood PHE levels are elevated during pregnancy a *maternal PKU syndrome* may result; infant pathology is independent of fetal genotype, but is directly correlated with excessive phenylalaninemia throughout pregnancy. Most reported cases document severe pathological consequences of maternal PKU;

mental retardation, microcephaly, congenital heart defects, and low birth weight. A comparison of PKU and non-PKU sibs from untreated pregnancies in a mother with PKU provided the opportunity to compare the degree of damage from maternal PKU between genotypically different fetuses (Levy et al., 1992). Both offspring were microcephalic at birth and had congenital anomalies, esophageal atresia in the PKU child, and congenital dislocation of the hip in the non-PKU child. Both children also had hypoplasia of the CORPUS CALLOSUM and enlarged cerebral VENTRICLES. Levy and colleagues conclude that residual liver PAH activity of a non-PKU fetus offers little or no protection from damage in untreated maternal PKU. These adverse outcomes can be prevented by a low-PHE diet started before conception and continued throughout pregnancy; however, attempts at dietary management are often unsuccessful, and more abnormal than normal births have been reported (Fisch et al., 1993).

GENETIC ADVANCES AND DEVELOPMENTS

Recent advances in somatic cell gene therapy, a new field of biomedical research, have the potential to prevent, treat, or cure a variety of inherited and acquired diseases. PKU is a possible candidate for the first clinical trials using autologous cell transplantation as an approach to the correction of inherited disease (Raper & Wilson, 1993). A segment of liver from the affected individual is genetically corrected by using recombinant retroviruses to transduce normal genes into the patient's own hepatocytes, which are then transplanted back into the patient. Normal mouse genes for PAH have been successfully inserted into cultured liver cells from a mutant mouse. The modified liver cells were then reimplanted, they remained healthy within the liver parenchyma and corrected the PHE defect for the normal life span of the mouse (MRC Working Party, 1993).

Fisch and others (1993) suggest that currently available methods provide a viable alternative treatment to a low-PHE diet in maternal PKU. They propose in vitro fertilization using the parental gametes, followed by implantation of the pre-embryo in a surrogate mother, in order to avoid the maternal metabolic environment impairing normal development.

NEUROPSYCHOLOGICAL ASPECTS OF PHENYLKETONURIA

The benefits of early treatment in ameliorating the clinical impact of PKU have been well established and documented. However, it is claimed that early-treated subjects as a group exhibit various detectable abnormalities (MRC Working Party, 1993). Most published follow-up studies investigating the consequence of early-initiated dietary treatment have focused on IQ scores of school-age children. Several factors have emerged as important aspects of treatment (Allen, 1990). Neonatal diagnosis is essential, although there is some controversy concerning the time frame for diagnosis; excessive dietary restriction of amino acids is harmful to infant growth and development; and termination of diet before 10 years of age has been followed by "IQ deterioration" in *some* studies both in the UK (MRC Working Party, 1993) and the National Collaborative Study in the USA (Michals et al., 1988). In addition, the issue of diet termination has been extended to include concerns that termination of diet may lead to neurological deterioration in young adults (Thompson et al., 1990). Allen (1990) claims that these caveats lack scientific support. Allen argues that there are no case-control cohort data, such as meta-analyses, which examine hypotheses affecting PKU health-care attitudes; and ethical concerns prevent controlled scientific cohort studies in infants and children.

Studies report that children and adults with PKU have mean intelligent quotients (IQs) half a standard deviation lower than those of unaffected siblings and population norms. Beasley and colleagues (1994) report intellectual status at 18 years of 192 PKU young adults born in the UK between 1964 and 1971. Mean IQs expressed as standard deviation scores (IQ-SDS) showed a small decrease from 14 to 18 years. However Beasley and others found that general ability in young adults with PKU, although related to PHE control in early childhood, was not directly influenced by PHE control in the four years preceding the eighteenth birthday. They conclude that the apparent fall in IQ-SDS between 14 and 18 years may be due to methodological problems in the analysis of longitudinal data without a control group, rather than providing evidence of intellectual decline. Further methodological problems associated with data collection have been highlighted by Beasley and colleagues (1988), who reported a 28 percent error rate in the computation of IQs assessed as part of a national longitudinal follow-up study of PKU children born in the UK.

Problems reported to be associated with PKU have included slower acquisition of language, a higher frequency of learning difficulties, hyperactivity, anxiety, and poor concentration. However, it has been stressed that most early-treated children fall within the normal range of general ability.

Neurological deterioration has been investigated in young adults with PKU by Thompson and others (1990). They report 7 patients with PKU who developed signs and symptoms of upper motor neuron dysfunction; MRI of 6 patients indicated that all had abnormal high-signal areas restricted to white matter. Thompson and colleagues suggest diet termination as the most likely cause of the neurological symptoms. However, Allen (1990) points out that three of the patients were diagnosed and treated at ages well beyond the average age of neonatal screening and delay in treatment may be the cause of the damage. Further, two patients had infantile spasms, which may be associated with permanent brain injury from some unknown origin. PKU infants may develop secondary disorders even while under dietary control, and the findings in late-treated adults are difficult to differentiate from MULTIPLE SCLEROSIS. White matter abnormalities have been shown to be more severe in patients with poor dietary control and high current plasma PHE levels, and there has been marked regression of abnormalities after three months of strict diet control; normal MRI has been found in patients with well-controlled PHE levels.

Gourovitch and colleagues (1994) report that, in a reaction time task employing lateralized visual stimuli, early-treated PKUs demonstrated slowed interhemisphere transfer from the left to the right hemisphere compared with two other control groups. However, the control groups failed to demonstrate the normal pattern of faster reaction times with the ipsilateral hand than with the contralateral hand, and the data are difficult to interpret. In addition, studies of EEG have shown significant, reversible, generalized EEG slowing during PHE loading (dietary supplementation) in both PKU children *and* normal adults; however, comparisons between normal children and PKU children were not made (Epstein et al., 1989).

Welsh and others (1990) hypothesized that mild dopamine (DA) depletion causes subtle prefrontal dysfunction, which in turn affects executive functions such as set maintenance, planning, and organized search. Group comparisons demonstrated that pre-school early-treated PKU children ($n = 11$) were significantly different from controls on executive function task performance, but not on a recognition memory task. Executive function task scores were significantly negatively correlated with concurrent PHE levels; this finding offers support for a biochemical mechanism underlying the specific cognitive deficits. Finally, Schmidt and colleagues (1994) suggest a sustained ATTENTION deficit in adult PKU patients, which varies according to the concurrent PHE level. They conclude that their demonstration of a partial reversibility of the deficits provides support for the hypothesis that biochemical mechanisms, rather than structural changes of the brain, underlie the relationship between concurrent PHE level and sustained attention.

CONCLUSION

In summary, there is unequivocal evidence that neonatal screening and early dietary treatment are essential factors in preventing brain damage in PKU. Metabolic control in adulthood may be important in preventing neuropsychological impairment and cognitive deficits, which appear to be related to biochemical mechanisms and concurrent PHE levels in PKU, rather than to structural changes of the brain; but the available research is limited with regard to these issues.

Although the current recommendation concerning dietary treatment of PKU is that metabolic control should be retained into adulthood in order to avoid decreases in IQ scores (albeit within the normal range in some cases) full account has not been taken of all the relevant issues. The cost in psychological terms of being maintained on a highly restricted diet has to be weighed against the relatively small average loss in IQ which may follow abandonment of the diet on reaching adulthood, a loss which may not be of functional psychological significance in some cases. Clearly, in cases of late identification and poor dietary control in PKU, continuing dietary adherence into adulthood may have significantly more

impact on IQ. However, ethical and moral issues concerning quality of life and manipulation of IQ within the normal range have not been considered, and issues concerning individual variation in IQ scores within the PKU population have not been adequately discussed (*see also* ASSESSMENT). Recent recommendations acknowledge that there should be further studies on the neurological status of early-treated children at all ages. In addition, a more precise measure of *individual* patients' progress should be developed, including brain imaging and neuropsychological and neurophysiological assessments.

BIBLIOGRAPHY

Allen, R. (1990). Neurological deterioration in young adults with phenylketonuria. *Lancet, 336*, 949.

Beasley, M. G., Lobasher, M., Henley, S., & Smith, I. (1988). Errors in computation of WISC and WISC-R intelligence quotients from raw scores. *Journal of Child Psychology and Psychiatry, 29*, 101–4.

Beasley, M. G., Costello, P. M., & Smith, I. (1994). Outcome of treatment in young adults with phenylketonuria detected by routine neonatal screening between 1964 and 1971. *Quarterly Journal of Medicine, 87*, 155–60.

Elliman, D., & Garner, J. (1991). Review of neonatal screening programme for phenylketonuria. *British Medical Journal, 303*, 471.

Epstein, C. M., Trotter, J. F., Averbook, A., Freeman, S., Kutner, M. H., & Elas, L. J. (1989). EEG mean frequencies are sensitive indices of phenylalanine effects on normal brain. *Electroencephalography and Clinical Neurophysiology, 72*, 133–9.

Fisch, R. O., Tagatz, G., & Stassart, J. P. (1993). Gestational carrier – a reproductive haven for offspring of mothers with phenylketonuria (PKU): an alternative therapy for maternal PKU. *Journal of Inherited Metabolic Disorders, 16*, 957–61.

Gourovitch, M. L., Craft, S., Dowton, S. B., Ambrose, P., & Sparta, S. (1994). Interhemispheric transfer in children with early-treated phenylketonuria. *Journal of Clinical and Experimental Neuropsychology, 16*, 393–404.

Jervis, G. A. (1947). Phenylpyruvic oligophrenia deficiency of phenylalanine-oxidizing system. *Society for Experimental Biology and Medicine. Proceedings, 82*, 514–15.

Levy, H. L., Lobbregt, D., Sansaricq, C., & Snyderman, S. E. (1992). Comparison of phenylketonuric and nonphenylketonuric sibs from untreated pregnancies in a mother with phenylketonuria. *American Journal of Medical Genetics, 44*, 439–42.

Mange, A. P., & Mange, E. J. (1990). *Genetics: Human aspects*, 2nd edn. Sunderland, MA: Sinauer.

Matalon, R., & Michals, K. (1991). Phenylketonuria: screening, treatment and maternal PKU. *Clinical Biochemistry, 24*, 337–42.

Medical Research Council (MRC) Working Party on Phenylketonuria. (1993). Phenylketonuria due to phenylalanine hydroxylase deficiency: an unfolding story. *British Medical Journal, 306*, 115–19.

Michals, K., Azen, C., Acosta, P., Koch, R., & Matalon, R. (1988). Blood phenylalanine levels and intelligence of 10-year-old children with PKU in the National Collaborative Study. *Journal of the American Dietetics Association, 88*, 1226–9.

Raper, S. E., & Wilson, J. M. (1993). Cell transplantation in liver-directed gene therapy. *Cell Transplantation, 2*, 381–400.

Schmidt, E., Rupp, A., Burgard, P., Pietz, J., Weglage, J., & Sonneville, L. de (1994) Sustained attention in adult phenylketonuria: the influence of concurrent phenylalanine-blood-level. *Journal of Clinical and Experimental Neuropsychology, 16*, 681–8.

Smith, I., Cooke, I., & Beasley, M. (1991). Review of neonatal screening programme for phenylketonuria. *British Medical Journal, 303*, 333–5.

Thompson, A. J., Smith, I., Brenton, D., Youl, B. D., Rylance, G., Davidson, D. C., Kendall, B., & Lees, A. J. (1990). Neurological deterioration in young adults with phenylketonuria. *Lancet, 336*, 602–5.

Weglage, J., Funders, B., Wilken, B., Schubert, D., Schmidt, E., Burgard, P., & Ullrich, K. (1992). Psychological and social findings in adolescents with phenylketonuria. *European Journal of Pediatrics, 151*, 522–5.

Welsh, M. C., Pennington, B. F., Ozonoff, S., Rouse, B., & McCabe, E. R. B. (1990). Neuropsychology of early-treated phenylketonuria: specific executive function deficits. *Child Development, 61*, 1697–713.

PAMELA M. KENEALY

phonetic disintegration syndrome Phonetic disintegration appears as an articulatory disorder of speech, and is more commonly described as an acquired disorder of language during childhood. It may be associated with impaired writing and poor comprehension of both written and spoken material. As comparison of phonemes occurring at the initial, middle, or final position in words during word repetition has shown that errors occur more commonly at the initial position than at subsequent positions, it has been concluded that the disorder is not of the speech musculature or of the articulatory apparatus, but of the process by which phonological units are encoded prior to speech production.

phosphene Phosphenes are the small flashes of light perceived when the primary visual cortex is stimulated.

If the primary visual cortex of the occipital lobe, the striate cortex, is stimulated electrically, chemically, or mechanically, then points of light (phosphenes) will be briefly perceived at the location in visual space which is represented at the stimulated site on the cortex. The fact that this effect can be produced by mechanical stimulation leads to the common report of "seeing stars" following a blow to the head, and it is also a common representation in cartoon images. This report results from pressure being applied to the occipital cortex (which is not perceived, the brain itself having no sensory receptors) as it is forced against the adjacent skull. Attempts, only partially successful, have been made to make use of the phenomenon to restore vision following damage to the eyes or visual tracts through a prosthesis which directly and appropriately stimulates the visual cortex.

phrenology Once it became generally accepted that it was the brain and not the heart that controlled behavior, the next major point of debate was localization of function. During the eighteenth century mental processes were grouped into specialized functions which were eventually to lead to the search for the neural substrates of these abilities. Franz Josef Gall (1758–1828) and Johann Casper Spurzheim (1776–1832) founded the system they termed phrenology, which was to evolve into the first real attempt to relate specific mental processes to discrete parts of the brain.

The idea that formed the foundation of the theory was that the brain is comprised of many separate organs, each of which governs a particular mental faculty. The belief was that the relative development of these areas correlated with prominences and depressions on the skull that could be identified by palpation. A palpable bump on the head suggested that the organ beneath the skull at that spot was well developed, so the trait for behavior governed by that area was likely to play a significant role in that person's overall character or personality. Conversely, a depression at that particular location on the skull would suggest that the trait played only a minor role. A phrenological map of the skull was produced which identified the traits associated with the different areas of the skull and so by inference with the underlying brain. Ideality, Hope, and Destructiveness are examples of the type of traits allegedly associated with different parts of the skull. Gall and Spurzheim produced little empirical evidence to substantiate their theories, but nevertheless they received considerable support and interest in their ideas.

The most significant opponent of the theory was Pierre Flourens (1794–1867). He rejected the theory of phrenology and its assumption of strict localization of function. His experiments involving the lesioning of the brains of animals led him to conclude that there is no discrete localization of function but that the brain functions as an integrated whole. His work, in seeking to disprove the theory of phrenology, led him to develop ideas that were to form the foundation of later holistic theories of brain function.

MARCUS J. C. ROGERS

Pick's disease   Pick's disease is a degenerative dementia that first appears in late middle life. It is significantly less common than Alzheimer's DEMENTIA and, at least in the early stages, the pathological changes are more circumscribed and the onset more insidious.

Although the clinical picture varies from patient to patient, the first clinical signs frequently involve changes suggestive of frontal lobe involvement. There is an alteration in personality and social behavior, with the person becoming socially disinhibited and engaging in previously unchar-acteristic behaviors such as sexual indiscretions and other ill-judged social activities. Lack of insight and concern for these changes is also common. In tandem with personality changes, there is a gradual reduction in drive. As the condition progresses lack of interest is superseded by indolence and apathy.

During the early stages of the disease cognitive impairments are relatively insignificant relative to the behavioral changes. However, as the condition progresses this pattern alters. Language changes can be an early feature with scant and empty speech, ANOMIA, and CIRCUMLOCUTIONS, progressing to impaired comprehension with echolalic or perseverative tendencies. Disruption of intellect and memory frequently follow until a stage is reached when the clinical features of the condition cannot be distinguished from other advanced dementing processes such as Alzheimer's disease.

The incidence of Pick's relative to Alzheimer's disease varies significantly in different reports, but is consistently lower, with a rate of 50 to 1 often being reported. There is also some inconsistency with regard to relative incidence in males and females; the consensus appears to be that females are affected more frequently than males. Etiology remains unclear, but studies of affected families suggest a strong genetic component with an autosomal dominant pattern.

Pathologically, the disease has a very particular appearance. There is frequently marked atrophy of the frontal and temporal lobes, consistent with the characteristic behavioral and cognitive changes. The atrophy chiefly involves the association areas with relative sparing of the primary projection areas. The atrophy is rarely symmetrical across the two hemispheres. Microscopy shows cell loss in the cortex, astrocytic proliferation, and fibrous gliosis with characteristic balloon-shaped cells that contain irregularly shaped argentophilic inclusions (Pick bodies). These changes gave the disease its original name of "lobar sclerosis." Death invariably follows within 3 to 12 years post onset. There is no effective treatment.

Although there can frequently be some confusion between Alzheimer's and Pick's disease, particularly during the later stages, there are a number of clinical features that can make differentiation possible. In Pick's disease the first clinical signs tend to involve personality and behavioral changes, whereas in Alzheimer's disease the first signs generally involve cognitive, particularly memory impairments. Parietal lobe functions are generally preserved in Pick's but often not in Alzheimer's disease, and incontinence beginning early in the course of the decline is often indicative of Pick's disease. CT or MRI scans will help to confirm diagnosis and distinguish between the two disorders by revealing their characteristic patterns of atrophy.

MARCUS J. C. ROGERS

Pickwickian syndrome The Pickwickian syndrome, named after the "fat boy" of Charles Dickens' *The Pickwick Papers*, is a form of hypersomnia in which there is an increased tendency to episodes of sleep but which, unlike NARCOLEPSY, is not irresistible. It is similar to the KLEINE–LEVIN SYNDROME, but in this case is associated with periodic respiratory insufficiency and obesity. It is not clear whether the obesity contributes to the respiratory insufficiency or whether both are features of some primary constitutional disturbance.

pineal gland The pineal gland, *pineal body*, or *pineal*, is a midline structure at the caudo-dorsal extremity of the third ventricle and is attached to the dorsal THALAMUS. Despite this, it has no direct neural connection with the central nervous system, although it forms part of the autonomic nervous system. In lower animals, where the pineal gland is not so deeply buried within the brain, it is known to release the hormone melatonin in relation to daylight; less during daylight, and less during summer than during winter months. A large amount of melatonin is produced in the years preceding puberty. Some consider the functions of the pineal gland in humans vestigial, but it has been linked to the age of menarche and to SEASONAL AFFECTIVE DISORDER.

pituitary tumor Various TUMORS may arise in the pituitary gland, the gland contained in a pit (the sella) in the base of the skull which acts as a master gland for the control of the entire endocrine system and is the only endocrine gland to have direct neural connections, principally with the HYPOTHALAMUS. These tumors result in specific behavioral disorders.

Pituitary tumors occuring before normal growth is complete may result in *gigantism*, and subsequently in *acromegaly*, due to overproduction of growth hormones (hyperpituitarism). Acromegaly is characterized by changes in the skin, overgrowth in the bones of the skull, face, jaw, and at the extremities, enlargement of the viscera, changes in physical systems, and impairment of sexual function. Alternatively, hypopituitarism may result, also with a decline in sexual function, loss of body hair, softening of the skin, and other metabolic changes.

Other than these hormonal changes, there are other sequelae of pituitary tumors. Besides the generalized pressure changes which may result in headache, there may also be disturbances in visual function as the OPTIC CHIASM lies almost directly above the pituitary sella. Bitemporal HEMIANOPIA is most commonly an early sign as the tumor compresses the decussating fibers of the chiasm, although the effect is not necessarily symmetrical. Optic atrophy may also result. Further pressure changes, in the direction of the third ventricle, may also result in psychological changes with mental slowing, apathy, emotional instability, and personality changes. Changes in memory function may also be prominent, but all these effects depend upon the actual nature of the pressure changes which follow development of the tumor and their location within the subcortical brain systems.

planatopokinesia, planotopokinesia The loss of the ability to conceptualize topographical relationships or form mental maps has been given the name planotopokinesia, although the term strictly indicates a disability of orientation in a two-dimensional plane. Subjects with this disability are unable to orient themselves on a map, to indicate locations on a map, or to indicate directions of travel from one point to another, even if they are familar with the geographic area represented by the map. While these subjects may be able to produce a verbal description of the relationships they are unable to indicate on the map, such descriptions are impoverished. Dressing apraxia, the inability to correctly dress oneself despite not being otherwise apraxic, may also be a feature of the disorder. The deficit is associated with defective maze learning and is more common following right posterior cerebral lesions, although frontal lesions may produce a similar deficit, which is attributable to perseveration or faulty rule-adherence rather than to a spatial disorder.

planum temporale The planum temporale is an area of cortex in the superior and posterior part of the temporal lobe where it turns into the lateral fissure. Its association with HESCHL'S GYRUS and its proximity to other auditory areas have long suggested a link with auditory function. Furthermore it is an area of cortex in which there is a pronounced lateral asymmetry in humans, with measurements of brains at autopsy showing it to be longer and larger in the left hemisphere than in the right in about two-thirds of the brains examined. The finding has been extended to infants and found consistently in a number of studies.

Research employing MAGNETIC RESONANCE IMAGING in a group for whom language lateralization had been previously established by INTRACAROTID SODIUM AMYTAL has confirmed the hypothesis that the enlarged planum temporale is associated with language lateralization in humans, there being complete concordance between the hemisphere subserving language and the side of the larger planum temporale. That the asymmetry is found in infants as well as adults, and that it is only found to a very considerably reduced degree in other primates, suggest that this asymmetry is a phylogenetic development in some way associated with human competence for spoken language.

plaque A plaque is an area of pathological cortical tissue which may be revealed by silver staining, appearing as an irregular mass of about 50–100 microns in diameter. The result of a metabolic disturbance in the neurons and their supporting structures, which leads to neuronal degeneration, they are found much more commonly in gray than in white matter, and in the cortex rather than in subcortical gray matter. Plaques are seen universally and densely in the DEMENTIA of Alzheimer's disease, where the overall result is a grossly atrophied brain.

plasticity The term "neural plasticity" has been used to characterize so many real and putative neural phenomena that it is now all but useless as a scientific concept. Virtually everything from neural repair to neural reorganization and vicarious functioning has been offered as a primary example of neural plasticity. And, while neural repair, compensatory and collateral sprouting, are probably real phenomena, strong evidence for neural reorganization and vicarious functioning, at least with regard to the adult mammalian brain, is thin to the point of vanishing. It would also seem somewhat curious to speak of sprouting, which is neural restoration, as neural plasticity, for when functions are restored in other organs after injury or disease, the event is not labelled as plasticity but more likely as healing.

Notwithstanding these caveats, it is possible to define neural plasticity as any change in the normal structure of the nervous system or its specific functions which is induced by injury or disease. The major issue which then evolves is whether this plasticity may or may not be of benefit to behavioral recovery of function, here defined, as suggested by Alimi and Finger (1988), as "a theoretical construct that implies a complete regaining of the identical functions that were lost or impaired after brain injury." Within this framework, there are two major parameters which set the conditions which allow neural plasticity to occur and influence behavior, namely the patient's age at the time the neural pathology occurs and the physical extent or size of the pathology.

AGE AND NEURAL PLASTICITY

The developing brain is perhaps the most fertile ground for the occurrence of neural plasticity, simply because the nervous system is undergoing rapid change. Unfortunately, the behavioral consequences of this plasticity are not always beneficial to the individual and are never without cost. A most salient and most sobering example of this comes from the classic work of Schneider and his colleagues at the Massachusetts Institute of Technology.

Margaret Kennard (1938), some years prior to Schneider's studies (1979), observed a degree of behavioral recovery from injuries to the motor cortex in very young subhuman primates, which appeared to be substantially greater than the motor recovery which occurred with similar lesions in adult animals. She interpreted this as an example of the developing nervous system's capacity for plasticity. From this came what has been called the Kennard Principle, which, in paraphrase, states "if you are going to have a brain injury, it is better to have it while you are young." The logic behind this principle is complex but hinges upon many observations of the proliferation of neural processes known to occur in the developing brain, which might shelter the nervous system from insult and through plasticity enable a reorganization which would yield normal adult behavior. Notwithstanding the intuitive appeal of the Kennard Principle, later empirical findings raised interesting and distressing questions.

One set of these findings which is of particular interest, if only because it was one of the first, is Schneider's observations on the consequences of unilateral lesions of the superior colliculi in neonatal hamsters. The results clearly demonstrated that this brain, at this time, possessed an amazing degree of neural plasticity, but that this plasticity, in point of fact, was of questionable benefit to the hamster. In the normal hamster the visual system is crossed, with the right eye projecting its visual nerve and tract to the left superior colliculus and the left eye projecting to the right superior colliculus. A unilateral lesion to, say, the left superior colliculus did not prevent the right eye from sending its fibers to the brain but rather induced the eye to project unilaterally, i.e. to the right, undamaged, superior colliculus. Moreover, and more important, this aberrant unilateral visual pathway was functional, as indicated by electrophysiological maps of the visual projection fields of the surviving superior colliculus when either eye was stimulated with spots of light.

Yet, anatomically and physiologically impressive as this neural plasticity is, from the hamster's point of view it is not part of a cure but part of a problem. Normally, visual stimuli presented in the visual field of one eye will induce the hamster to turn toward that stimulus. In the hamster with the unilateral superior colliculus lesion, stimuli presented in the visual field with the aberrant visual projection did not cause the animal to turn toward the stimulus but rather turn *away* from it, that is, stimuli presented in the right visual field of a hamster with a left superior colliculus insult caused the hamster not to turn to the right but to turn to the left. Thus the visual location of food or predators is severely compromised and the neural plasticity and reorganization that occurred, following the infant lesion, was anything but beneficial to the behavioral recovery of function, as far as the hamster was most likely concerned.

A somewhat more positive outcome occurs with the relocation of language functions following destruction of the normal language areas in the brains of very young humans. Human brains are asymmetrical and language functions are usually, but not always, localized in two discrete areas in the left hemisphere, namely Broca's area in the inferior frontal region and Wernicke's area in the temporal parietal region. There is a third speech area in the dorsal medial supplemental motor area, which can be defined electrophysiologically, but it is apparently not critical to overt speech functions. If the language areas are completely destroyed in the young human who is less than about 6 years of age, then language functions will be relocated in the opposite hemisphere. The amount of this relocation, and the consequent recovery of speech function, is inversely correlated with the age of the individual when the injury occurs. Nevertheless the recovery of speech is often impressive and, save for impairments in (1) understanding speech when meaning is conveyed by syntactic diversity, (2) integration of semantic meaning and syntax to replace missing pronouns, and (3) detection and correction of errors of surface syntactic structure, the observed recovery can be virtually complete.

Yet there is a less trivial cost associated with this relocation of speech functions in the contralateral hemisphere. The cost is that the functions normally mediated by the "nonlanguage hemisphere" are severely compromised, if not lost altogether. There are detectable deficits, in this regard, on tasks characterized as visuospatial, which are typically mediated by brain areas in the nonlanguage hemisphere, and the severity of the deficit is directly related to the amount of speech that is recovered. On the other hand, no such relocation of visuospatial functions, and consequent compromising of speech, occurs with lesions to the nonlanguage hemisphere. Hans-Lukas Teuber (1974) summarized this cost of relocation most succinctly:

> All in all, these findings suggest a definite hemisphere specialization at birth, with a curiously greater vulnerability to early lesions for those capacities that depend, in the adult, on the right hemisphere – as if speech were relatively more resilient or simply earlier in getting established. Yet this resilience is purchased

at the expense of nonspeech functions as if one had to admit a factor of competition in the developing brain for terminal space, with consequent crowding when one hemisphere tries to do more than it had originally been meant to do. (p. 73)

Teuber's summary makes clear an important but often overlooked point, that is, when functions are relocated in some brain area that does not usually contribute to those functions but now begins to operate vicariously, what happens to the behaviors normally mediated by the vicariously functioning brain area?

ADULT BRAINS, LESION SIZE, AND NEURAL PLASTICITY

The adult central nervous system is considerably more stable or static than its neonatal counterpart. While the neural reorganization capacities which may occur in the developing brain are difficult to substantiate in the adult brain, some amount of neural plasticity does occur under some conditions.

Small subtotal lesions If the lesion or pathology is small and involves only some limited portion of a component of a functional neural system, then the adult mammalian nervous system is capable of what may be called neural plasticity. This plasticity can take the form of compensatory or collateral sprouting to and within the injured brain area and denervation supersensitivity involving spared synapses in the injured brain area.

However, at a minimum, 10 percent of the affected brain area must be spared and sprouting follows certain rules, as outlined by Cotman and his colleagues (Cotman & Nieto-Sampedro, 1982), namely:

The first rule is that the new synapses completely restore the synaptic input lost following partial denervation. The second rule is that an afferent will reinnervate a denervated zone only if its terminal field overlaps that of the damaged afferent. The third general rule is that reactive growth causes only a quantitative increase or rearrangement of previously existing connections. Qualitatively new pathways are not created during lesion-induced synaptogenesis in the adult organism . . . A fourth general rule may be formulated: when a neuron receives more than one type of afferent, there is a definite hierarchy in the relative capacity of the various afferents to grow in response to synapse loss. It seems that "like" afferents, i.e., those from similar cell types, have growth preference. (p. 375)

The phenomenon of denervation supersensitivity was classified in the late forties and describes a set of events where there is an increase in the sensitivity of muscle and neural tissue when it is deprived of some of its afferent input. In some cases, as documented by Marshall (1984), this increase in sensitivity can mediate behavioral recovery by reversing, for example, the somatosensory deficits produced by interrupting the mesostriatal dopaminergic projection. Thus both sprouting and the biochemical modification of synapses clearly demonstrate what may be called neural plasticity and show that the adult mammalian CNS is not totally lacking resources to deal with injury, although the injuries must be limited.

In fact, recent evidence has demonstrated neural plasticity, in the form of neural regrowth, in the aged mammalian brain. This regrowth is similar to sprouting although, as in the case of the hamster, it may not lead to the normalization of behavior following neural pathology but may rather add to a problem. For example, there is evidence for neural regrowth in Alzheimer patients that appears to be a response to the cell loss that is associated with this disease. Unfortunately, the Alzheimer brain also evidences many amyloid plaques and there is evidence that it is the protein in these plaques, possibly the 42-amino acid fragment form of B-amyloid, which stimulates the neural growth of fibers into the plaques. However, the plaques cannot support the new fibers and the sprouting neuron dies for lack of synaptic termination, thus further contributing to the neural degeneration characterized by Alzheimer's disease.

All in all, the adult and aged mammalian brain does possess some degree of neural plasticity and in certain cases this plasticity may support behavioral recovery of function. However, the pathology must be limited and the restricted plasticity does not produce any dramatic reorganization of the structure or operation of the nervous system that might mediate recovery through a redefinition of the usual operations supported by any particular brain area.

Large complete lesions The situation is much less optimistic with respect to large injuries that encompass all of some particular brain area. Large lesions in the adult mammalian brain simply do not induce any sort of neural plasticity which will mediate behavioral recovery (see LeVere, 1975, 1988).

This is not meant to imply that recovery is impossible after large brain injuries in adult individuals. Rather, it means that if behavioral recovery does occur, it does not do so spontaneously by the sort of neurotrophic response that may follow restricted injury. The reason for this is simple, no part of the brain area sustaining the damage remains to support sprouting or synaptic modification. The nature of the deficit following large injuries must be conceptually quite different from the deficit associated with subtotal injuries and whatever recovery does occur cannot be mediated by mechanisms such as neural plasticity and neural reorganization. To be sure, the behavioral deficit following both subtotal and complete lesions is precipitated by the loss of neural tissue. However, with subtotal lesions the deficit reflects a loss which may be corrected either by sprouting afferents or a change in synaptic sensitivity in the surviving tissue of that brain area, i.e. neural repair. This is not the case with complete lesions and the behavioral deficit is more likely to result from a shift in the normal balance and interaction between different functional neural systems which serves to inhibit the damaged system's influence on overt or covert behavior (see LeVere 1980, 1988). Behavioral recovery, if it occurs following large complete lesions, then depends not upon any inherent plasticity possessed by the nervous system but rather upon therapeutic intervention, which can facilitate greater utilization of whatever is spared of the afflicted functional system.

SUMMARY

Does plasticity occur in the mammalian brain? Yes. Is the plasticity good for or of benefit to behavioral recovery? Yes and no. The negative is precipitated by aberrant neural connections that may occur in the developing and aging brain, where data tempers the initial optimism that the nervous system can reorganize its fundamental operation. With regard to the adult mammalian brain and large complete lesions, Cajal's comment "Everything may die, nothing can regenerate," appears to be still valid. It is hopeful to think otherwise, but the consistency of the empirical findings suggests that this is little more than the fantasies spun around wilderness campfires on cold nights.

BIBLIOGRAPHY

Almli, C. R., & Finger, S. (1988). Toward a definition of recovery of function. In S. Finger, T. E. LeVere, C. R. Almli, & D. G. Stein (Eds), *Brain injury and recovery: Theoretical and controversial issues* (pp. 1–14). New York: Plenum Press.

Cotman, C. W., & Nieto-Sampedro, M. (1982). Brain function, synapse renewal, and plasticity. *Annual Review of Psychology, 33*, 371–401.

Kennard, M. A. (1938). Reorganization of motor functions in the cerebral cortex of monkeys deprived of motor and premotor areas in infancy. *Journal of Neurophysiology, 1*, 477–96.

LeVere, T. E. (1975). Neural stability, sparing, and behavioral recovery following brain damage. *Psychological Review, 82*, 344–58.

LeVere, T. E. (1980). Recovery of function after brain damage: a theory of the behavioral deficit. *Physiological Psychology, 8*, 297–308.

LeVere, T. E. (1988). Neural system imbalances and the consequence of large brain injuries. In S. Finger, T. E. LeVere, C. R. Almli, & D. G. Stein (Eds), *Brain injury and recovery: Theoretical and controversial issues* (pp. 15–28). New York: Plenum Press.

Marshall, J. R. (1984). Brain function: neural adaptations and recovery from injury. *Annual Review of Psychology, 35*, 277–308.

Schneider, G. E. (1979). Is it really better to have your brain lesion early? A revision of the "Kennard principle." *Neuropsychologia, 17*, 557–83.

Teuber, H.-L. (1974). Why two brains? In F. O. Schmitt & F. G. Worder (Eds), *The neurosciences, third study program* (pp. 71–4). Cambridge, MA: MIT Press.

T. E. LEVERE

pneumoencephalography An alternative term for AIR ENCEPHALOGRAPHY.

polyopia Polyopia (also occasionally *polyopsia*) is a form of METAMORPHOPSIA in which multiple images are seen. The images may be replicated in the frontal plane (side by side) or in the sagittal plane (one behind another), and occasionally may be concentric, differing in size. The most common number of replications is three (triplopia), but monocular diplopia and quadriplopia also occur and, more rarely, higher numbers of images. One theory of the generation of polyopia suggests that with a change of fixation there is rapid and repeated stimulation of extrafoveal retinal positions which correspond to a series of functional centers in relation to each of which an image is generated.

pons The pons is the portion of the BRAIN STEM which lies immediately rostral to (above) the MEDULLA. Its name as the "bridge" is derived from the thick fiber bundles which run across its ventral surface and turn up into the CEREBELLUM. The area of the pons includes fibers, mostly with motor functions, which pass between all areas of the cerebral cortex and the cerebellar cortex, and there are fibers which originate in cerebral cortex and terminate in the pons. Other fibers represent the corticospinal tract and the descending PYRAMIDAL TRACT, which passes downward through the PEDUNCLES at this point. Several CRANIAL NERVES originate in the pons and the RETICULAR FORMATION is also prominent as it passes through this region.

porencephaly Porencephaly is an abnormality of development of the brain in which symmetrical cavities are present in the cerebral hemispheres where both cortex and white matter should normally occur. As an acquired abnormality, a *porencephalic cyst* may arise as a single cavity in one of the cerebral hemispheres, associated with cortical atrophy and commonly the result of an INFARCT.

positron emission tomography *See* PET SCAN.

postconcussion syndrome Postconcussion syndrome (not infrequently shortened to PCS) is the most commonly used term referring to the late symptoms of CLOSED HEAD INJURY, usually of minor degree. It is, however, a term not without its difficulties. The word "syndrome" is defined in the *Oxford Companion to Medicine* as "A collection of symptoms and signs which tend to occur together and form a characteristic pattern, but which may not necessarily be always due to the same pathological cause." There are quite a few symptoms which follow closed head injuries. Those who have attempted to search for some pattern have been largely unsuccessful. The term "syndrome" may have been more appropriate when the nature and causation of the symptoms were less clear, but the word "symptoms" seems to have the advantage of simplicity and clarity.

The term "concussion" also has its difficulties. Its lay meaning of "the act of violently shaking or agitating" (*Oxford English Dictionary*) is clear. When we turn to medical dictionaries to find the meaning of the term applied to concussion of the brain, we usually find that one of its components is "temporary impairment of function of the brain" (*Churchill Medical Dictionary* and *International Dictionary of Medicine and Biology*). Many writers state or imply that this impairment is a loss of consciousness. The difficulty in practice is that, in order to establish whether or not there is a loss of consciousness, it is necessary to have an observer, preferably one with medical training. All that the patient can tell is whether or not he or she has memory for the events. An observer like an ambulance man, who arrives 15 minutes after the event, is often unable to say whether or not there has been a period of brief unconsciousness. It is when the patient arrives at hospital in a state of altered consciousness that the fact is likely to be detected and recorded. Occasionally a good witness is available from whom it is possible to get a sufficiently detailed history to make an informed guess, but, with the great majority of patients, the only source of information is the patient, and then only when he or she has recovered sufficiently to explain what they remember before and after the injury. It would seem proper to define concussion in terms of amnesia as well as unconsciousness.

Many authors use the term "concussion" as if it were synonymous with a period of unconsciousness or AMNESIA. The symptoms which follow are then described as postconcussion symptoms. In this case it becomes very difficult to describe the same symptoms following a blow on the head which did not result in unconsciousness or amnesia. The difficulty can be overcome if the term "concussion" is used for both the period of unconsciousness or amnesia and the whole associated illness, including the ensuing symptoms. "Concussion" may then be defined as "an acceleration/deceleration injury to the head, almost always associated with a period of amnesia and followed by a characteristic group of symptoms such as headache, poor memory, and vertigo."

The idea that concussion is a temporary condition may partly be employed to distinguish it from the kind of head injury which leaves the patient with a permanently altered state of consciousness. It may also derive in part from an early pathological classification where concussion was distinguished from contusion, extradural, subdural, subarachnoid, and intracerebral hemorrhages. Concussion was then said to be a head injury with no associated organic damage to the brain. It was thought that the blow to the head might well cause some temporary electrical upset, but there was no macroscopic or microscopic damage to brain tissue. This perception was due to the limitation of histological techniques at the time. It is now clear that concussive blows to the head do damage neurons, and that this damage is permanent. As in the case of strokes, the fact that patients may make a complete functional recovery does not prove that no organic damage took place. As long as the perception remained that there was no organic damage, it was natural that doctors treating patients after concussion should feel that any symptoms ought to be of a temporary nature, and that if they did not resolve the fault lay with the patient, who was either culpably neurotic or flagrantly malingering.

Many studies of the postconcussion syndrome, especially the early ones, concentrated entirely on the late symptoms. In fact there are relatively few studies relating directly to the early symptoms. However, there is an early phase during the first week or two following the end of post-traumatic amnesia and recovery to full consciousness, when the patients' complaints differ significantly from those later on. Table 14 lists symptoms which most would agree to be typical of the two phases.

The early symptoms are typically experienced immediately on return to consciousness and over the following few days. Two of them, headache and dizziness, are also features of the late symptoms. The other four virtually always disappear. Patients who complain of vomiting, nausea, drowsiness, or blurred vision at a late stage may often be found to be involved in claims for compensation and appear to be exaggerating their disability.

The remaining "late" symptoms may appear within a few days, though sometimes they may present only after an interval of weeks or even months. It seems likely that they are not complained of in the first day or two because it takes a little time for the patient to become aware of how he or she has changed. As long as the patient is removed from the stresses of daily life, he or she may feel well. When it becomes necessary to cope with the demands of small children in the house, the minor irritations of daily life, and the added strains of returning to work, the patients may then discover that their faculties are no longer as sharp as they used to be. It may be that, where the neuronal damage has been comparatively small, the brain's ability to process information, to think, feel, and remember will return to normal.

Table 14 The early and late symptoms of concussion.

Early	Late
Headache	Headache
Dizziness	Dizziness
Vomiting	Irritability
Nausea	Sensitivity to noise
Drowsiness	Anxiety
Blurred vision	Depression
	Poor memory
	Poor concentration
	Insomnia
	Fatigue
	Poor hearing
	Poor vision

Symptoms will disappear, and even under the pressure of considerable stress they will not reappear. However, where the damage has been more extensive it is possible that recovery will not be complete. Here stress, especially when combined with a loss of self-confidence, may lead to the recurrence of old symptoms or the emergence of new ones.

WHAT ARE THE LATE SYMPTOMS OF CONCUSSION?

A survey of the literature shows that there is no exact agreement as to which symptoms are considered to make up the postconcussion syndrome. Among 19 papers published between 1962 and 1987 the most commonly mentioned symptoms (in decreasing order of frequency) are headache, irritability, dizziness, poor concentration, fatigue, anxiety, poor memory, depression, sleeplessness, and sensitivity to alcohol. One difficulty is that in some papers the symptoms described may be subdivisions of those mentioned in other papers. Thus sensitivity to noise may be a subgroup of irritability, and apathy may be a subgroup of depression. Among less frequent late symptoms are deafness, anosmia, diplopia, aggression, epilepsy, blindness, loss of libido, personality change, and diabetes insipidus. Both blindness and diabetes insipidus may be quite severe for days or weeks and then resolve completely. It is difficult to say whether all of these symptoms should be counted as part of a syndrome or only

the most common ones. It is simpler to state that they are all symptoms of which patients who have sustained concussion may later complain.

Some people have attempted to classify these symptoms in groups. Keshavan and his colleagues (1981) divided them into somatic and psychological. In their view the somatic symptoms were headache, fatigue, dizziness, intolerance to noise, loss of libido, blurred vision, diplopia, and poor hearing. The psychological ones were sleeplessness, anxiety, irritability, poor memory, poor concentration, aggression, euphoria, and apathy. Levin and colleagues (1987) subdivided symptoms into three groups, somatic (including headaches, dizziness, and blurred vision), cognitive (including memory deficit and loss of concentration), and affective (including anxiety, depression, and sleep disturbance).

HOW FREQUENT ARE SYMPTOMS AND FOR HOW LONG DO THEY PERSIST?

Table 15 shows the results of 11 prospective studies. We will focus first on symptoms six weeks after injury. The studies by Rutherford (1977, 1978), Flynn (1984), and Montgomery (1991) were all carried out in the same department of the same hospital in Belfast, but in different years and with different doctors documenting the symptoms. There is close agreement between these studies in that approximately 50 percent of patients sustaining concussion and only requiring admission for one or two nights for observation

Table 15 Percentage frequency of symptoms at various intervals following concussion.

Author, date	1 mon.	6 wks	3 mon.	6 mon.	1 yr	2 yr	Major/ minor	Number of patients
Lidvall, 1974			24				Minor	83
Rutherford, 1977		51					Minor	145
Rutherford, 1978				15			Minor	131
Cartlidge, 1978/9		(headache)	27	18	24		Minor and	372
	19	(dizziness)	22	14	18		major	
Rimel, 1981			84				Minor	424
Wrightson, 1981			60				Minor	66
Keshavan, 1981 (psychological)		80	65				Minor and major	60
MacFlynn, 1984		53		47			Minor	45
Levin, 1987	89		47	(headache)			Minor	57
Lowdon, 1989		90					Minor	114
Montgomery, 1991		12		54			Minor	26

complained of symptoms at six weeks. The total number of patients was divided almost equally among three groups, based on length of post-traumatic amnesia (PTA), 0–14 minutes, 15–59 minutes, and over one hour. In Keshavan's study 80 percent of patients had symptoms at six weeks, but this series included patients with both minor and severe head injuries.

In Lowden's (1989) series all the patients had PTAs of less than 15 minutes, yet 90 percent complained of symptoms at 6 weeks. Two factors may have influenced this high figure. First, the follow-up was conducted by questionnaire. In the Belfast studies great care was taken not to suggest symptoms, as it was felt that suggestion might have the effect of creating symptoms and artificially inflating their frequency. Second, 34 patients did not reply to the questionnaire. This seems much more likely to have been the case in patients who did not have symptoms, and if all were symptom-free the percentage with symptoms would drop to 62 percent. (This does not invalidate the study, the purpose of which was to compare results between minor head-injured patients admitted to hospital and those allowed to go home.)

In comparison with these estimates for symptoms at 6 weeks, Levin's finding that 89 percent of subjects had symptoms at 4 weeks seems high, though it is possible that early on the incidence is very high and during the early weeks there is a gradual reduction. Turning next to the three-month estimates, Lidvall's figure of 24 percent appears to be relatively low. However, when we look at the severity of the injuries of the patients in this series, we find that over 50 percent had PTAs of under 5 minutes and only 20 percent had PTAs of over 45 minutes. Rimel's (1981) figure of 84 percent is relatively high. Wrightson (1981), whose studies are characterized by care not to suggest symptoms and by active therapeutic endeavors, gives a figure of 60 percent for fit men in active employment. Keshavan, whose series includes major head injuries, gives a figure of 65 percent. Levin gives a figure of 47 percent for headaches.

By six months after injury MacFlynn and others (1984) and Montgomery and others (1991) have figures a little below and a little above 50 percent – not greatly changed from their figures for six weeks. Cartlidge gives a figure of 27 percent for headaches, and from other series it appears that the incidence of headaches is approximately 50 percent in all patients with any complaint. Extrapolating from the figure of 27 percent with headache, one might roughly estimate that 50–55 percent of patients would have suffered from some symptom. This series has patients of all grades of severity, although the great majority have minor injuries. The figure is also that reached after the patients have been questioned against a checklist of symptoms. When merely asked to relate their symptoms only 9 percent complained of headache, which in this case can be extrapolated to roughly 18 percent.

Rutherford's (1978) figure for incidence of headaches in a one-year follow-up was 15 percent, with Cartlidge's (1978/9) figure being 18 percent (equivalent to 36 percent for any symptom). At two years Cartlidge found that 24 percent of subjects complained of headaches. The lack of improvement from the one-year figure is worrying and suggests that patients left with symptoms at this stage may suffer for many years, if not for life. This suspicion is reinforced by a retrospective study by Amphoux and others (1977). Among their construction workers who remembered having had a head injury 16 years or more before questioning, 42 percent were complaining of symptoms of headache. These were men who had returned to work, and any litigation or claims must have been settled many years previously.

While at first sight there appear to be considerable discrepancies between the findings of these different studies, these can usually be explained by the severity of the injuries, the method of questioning employed, or the amount of therapeutic endeavor.

POSTCONCUSSION SYNDROME: AN ORGANIC OR PSYCHOGENIC CONDITION?

For over a hundred years a debate has raged as to whether the postconcussion syndrome is essentially an organic or a psychogenic condition. A spirited correspondence in the *Journal of the Royal Society of Medicine* in 1981 shows that there are still some devoted backers of both views. The last major statement in favor of the psychogenic case is to be found in papers by Henry Millar on accident neurosis in 1961 and on the mental sequelae of head injuries in 1966. He believed that postconcussion symptoms did not occur among head-injured doctors or sportsmen, and that their frequency was inversely proportional to the severity of the injury. His views were based on a review of his experience in examining 200 head-injured patients for the purposes of medicolegal assessment. It is doubtful whether his paper would be accepted for publication today because of weaknesses in the statistical presentation and argument. He showed no awareness that his patients may have been a small and highly unrepresentative group. However, he was a man held in very high esteem both by his colleagues and by the general public, and he argued his case with great emotional fervor.

Some of the prospective studies were examined to see if there was a relationship between post-traumatic amnesia and symptoms. Lidvall's (1974) study found no evidence of a relationship, but the study was based on a small number and all the patients had very short amnesic periods. It is not surprising that no relationship was found. Rutherford's (1977) study had a larger number of patients with a wider scatter of PTA. There seemed to be a trend towards more symptoms in those with longer PTA, but it did not reach significance. Keshavan's (1987) study, which included a complete spectrum of patients from very minor to very severe, showed a significant relationship, those with longer PTAs having more symptoms. Guthleck's (1980) study, which is based entirely on patients involved in compensation claims, showed a significant relationship between longer PTA and longer time off work. The one study which seems to confirm Millar's thesis is the Newcastle one reported by Cartlidge and Shaw (1981). Here headache at discharge, six months, one year, and two years was more frequent in those with PTA < 1 hour and less frequent in those with PTA >‹ 1 hour. The same was true for dizziness. It is possible that this result may be associated with the high percentage of people pursuing claims in this series (25 percent).

Rutherford's studies in 1977 and 1978 showed evidence that both physiogenic and psychogenic factors were at work in the production of late symptoms. Other prospective studies since then have confirmed one or both of these influences.

Several studies have now shown that it is possible to measure reductions in memory, concentration, and attention after minor head injuries. Gronwall and Wrightson (1974) used the PASAT test as a measure of the brain's ability to process information and MacFlynn and others (1984) and Montgomery and others (1991) used a four-choice action time recorder. In both cases the deterioration is marked in the early weeks and by six months returns to normal or even slightly above normal levels. It is easy to see how symptoms may partly be caused by demands being made of the brain at a time when it is not fully functioning.

Lishman (1988) suggested that the early symptoms are more likely to be physiogenic in nature, whereas the longer the symptoms persist the higher the percentage of psychogenic symptoms. Cartlidge and Shaw (1981) found this kind of difference between patients whose headaches and dizziness present shortly after the injury and those where these symptoms appear for the first time some months later. However, normal performance after six months on tests like PASAT and four-choice reaction time does not mean that the brain has returned to normal and all symptoms after this date can be deemed psychogenic. Patients who have concussion for the second or third time have cumulative deterioration. This is most clearly seen in the case of the "punch drunk syndrome." Histological studies in both humans and experimental animals have revealed neurological damage which is unlikely ever to resolve. Recent epidemiological studies of Alzheimer's disease have shown an association with a previous head injury, and so far with no other disease or injury.

It seems therefore that acceleration/deceleration head injuries probably always result in some permanent damage to the brain. Where this is minimal, most patients can compensate and live apparently normal symptom-free lives. Some permanent symptoms may be due to damage to end organs or specific neuronal pathways. Some patients may have a very slight drop in general performance. Those with premorbid psychological weakness or those subject in their daily lives to very considerable strain may complain of persisting or newly emerging signs. Lack of understanding of what is happening to them, compounded by medical advice from doctors who do not understand, can increase feelings of guilt and worthlessness.

The percentage of patients who complain because they are involved in claims for compensation or litigation is small. Some of these are deliberately malingering for financial advantage, but in others the deceptions and exaggerations appear to take place at a subconscious level.

BIBLIOGRAPHY

Amphoux, M., Gagey, P. M., Le Flem, A., & Pavy, F. (1977). Le devenir du syndrome post-commotionnel. *Revue du Médecin du Travail*, *5*, 53–75.

Cartlidge, N. E. F., & Shaw, D. A. (1981). *Head injury*. London: W. B. Saunders.

Gronwall, D., & Wrightson, P. (1974). Delayed recovery of intellectual function after minor head injury. *Lancet*, *2*, 605–9.

Guthleck, A. N. (1980). Post traumatic amnesia, post concussional symptoms and accident neurosis. *European Neurology*, *19*, 157–60.

Keshavan, M. S., Channabasavanna, S. M., & Narayanreddy, G. N. (1981). Post-traumatic psychiatric disturbances: patterns and predictors of outcome. *British Journal of Psychiatry*, *138*, 460–9.

Levin, H. S., Matis, S., Eisenberg, H. M., Marshall, H. F., Tabbador, K., High, W. M. Jr, & Frnakoski, R. F. (1987). Neurobehavioural outcome following minor head surgery: a three-centre study. *Journal of Neurosurgery*, *66*, 234–43.

Levin, H. S., Eisenberg, H. M., & Barton, A. L. (Eds). (1989). *Mild head injury*. New York: Oxford University Press.

Lidvall, H. F., Linderoth, B., & Norlin, B. (1974). Causes of post-concussional syndrome. *Acta Neurologica Scandinavica*, *50*, Supplement 56.

Lishman, W. A. (1988). Physiogenesis and psychogenesis in the "post-concussional syndrome." *British Journal of Psychiatry*, *153*, 460–9.

Lowdon, I. M. (1989). Post-concussional symptoms following minor head injury. *Injury*, *20*, 193–4.

MacFlynn, G., Montgomery, F. A., Fenton, G. W., & Rutherford, W. H. (1984). Measurement of reaction time following minor head injury. *Journal of Neurology, Neurosurgery and Psychiatry*, *47*, 1326–31.

Millar, H. (1961). Accident neurosis. *British Medical Journal*, *5231*, 919–25, 992–8.

Millar, H. (1966). Mental sequelae of head injury. *Proceedings of the Royal Society of Medicine*, *59*, 257–66.

Montgomery, E. A., Fenton, G. W., McClelland, R. J., MacFlynn, G., & Rutherford, W. H. (1991). The psychobiology of minor head injury. *Psychological Medicine*, *21*, 375–84.

Rutherford, W. H. (1989). Concussion. In W. H. Rutherford, R. N. Illingworth, A. K. Marsden, P. G. Nelson, A. D. Redmond, & D. H. Wilson (Eds), *Accident and emergency medicine* (pp. 427–38). Edinburgh: Churchill Livingstone.

Rutherford, W. H., Merrett, J. D., & McDonald, J. R. (1977). Sequelae of concussion caused by minor head injuries. *Lancet*, *1*, 1–4.

Rutherford, W. H., Merrett, J. D., & McDonald, J. R. (1978). Symptoms at one year following concussion from minor head injuries. *Injury*, *10*, 225–30.

Symonds, C. (1962). Concussion and its sequelae. *Lancet*, *1*, 1–5.

Walker, A. E., Caveness, W. F., & Critchley, M. (1969). *The late effects of head injury*. Springfield, IL: C. C. Thomas.

Wrightson, P., & Gronwall, D. (1980). Time off work and symptoms after minor head injury. *Injury*, *12*, 445–54.

W. H. RUTHERFORD

postural control Postural control is often taken to refer simply to the maintenance of an erect stance. However, it can be more accurately and comprehensively defined as the process of orienting the body with respect to the environment in such a way as to support ongoing activity. In order to maintain balance and provide a stable frame of reference, the orientation of the eyes, head, trunk, and limbs must be simultaneously controlled and coordinated. Control is achieved by feedforward commands generated at many levels of the nervous system, guided by information from the visual, somatosensory, and vestibular systems.

In the early part of the twentieth century, research into postural control focused principally upon automatic reflex responses. Magnus identified a number of reactions triggered by head movement or by the orientation of the head with respect to gravito-inertial force (registered by the vestibular system) or relative to the trunk (signalled by neck proprioceptors). The "labyrinthine (vestibular) righting reflex" acts to maintain the head upright despite movement of the trunk (e.g. when walking heel to toe), while the "tonic labyrinthine reflex" and "tonic neck reflex" promote extension or flexion of the limbs, depending upon head position. Although these subcortical reflexes are largely suppressed in normal adult humans, their latent influence may nevertheless be detectable in natural and athletic poses (Fukuda, 1984).

Stability of the head and eyes is maintained by means of relatively automatic responses to eye and head movement: information about eye/head orientation and motion is derived from the visual and vestibular systems and neck proprioceptors, integrated at the level of the vestibular nuclei and the cerebellum, and coordinated with cortically processed information concerning the desired direction of gaze and slippage of the retinal image (*see also* NYSTAGMUS). Upright stance is sustained by preprogrammed (but modifiable) synergistic contractions of leg and trunk muscles, also triggered and regulated by proprioceptive, visual, and vestibular information. At the highest level of the motor control hierarchy, the sensorimotor cortex and basal ganglia are chiefly involved in the development of action plans and strategies, the initiation of preparatory postural adjustments prior to voluntary activity or other anticipated perturbations of posture, and the adaptation and modification of programmed activity. The cerebellum and brain stem contribute to the implementation of postural plans by helping to coordinate the timing and amplitude of multiple muscular responses, and to adjust the threshold and gain of lower-level stretch reflexes in accordance with current circumstances. The way in which different levels of the central nervous system contribute to the various elements and forms of postural control, and the precise role of each of the sensory systems, have been the subject of extensive (and continuing) investigation and debate.

The dominant model of postural control, developed by Gurfinkel and elaborated by Nashner (1985), conceptualizes the human body as an inverted pendulum. The early investigations inspired by this model treated the body as a single-link pendulum hinged around the ankle joint, and examined muscle activity during quiet standing and following perturbations of the surface of support. Initially, interest focused on the "ankle stretch reflexes" triggered proprioceptively by a change in the angle of the ankle joint. The ankle synergies consist of a successive sequence of

muscular reactions, radiating from the ankle to the lower trunk, which serve to reverse the direction of body sway by exerting torque against the surface of support. Three bursts of muscle activity are observed following an imposed perturbation of posture: the short latency monosynaptic spinal responses; the middle latency responses, which are probably polysynaptic spinal responses under supraspinal control; and the long latency responses, which are believed by most researchers to be trans-cortical. The short latency reflexes are generally weak and can even be inappropriate for sway stabilization, which is effectively achieved by means of the long latency responses (often termed the "long-loop" or "functional stretch" reflexes).

Long-loop responses serve to coordinate intended motor plans with immediate internal and external circumstances, but they act at a preconscious level, and occur earlier than voluntary corrections to motor activity can be initiated. The functional ankle stretch reflex was first characterized as a relatively stereotyped preprogrammed response to movement at the ankle, although adaptive changes in the amplitude of the response were noted when posture was repeatedly perturbed in a predictable manner. However, as the number of studies of the response multiplied, each employing slightly different experimental procedures, it became increasingly clear that the response was stereotypic only under stereotypic conditions. The nature of the long latency responses can be influenced by factors such as the amplitude, direction, and velocity of the perturbation, attributes of the support surface, the tilt of the body prior to the perturbation, and expectations or motor set.

In order to determine the contribution of each perceptual system to postural control, various manipulations of the available perceptual information have been employed. The visual information has been removed, degraded, or transformed by eye closure, stroboscopic lighting, visual field motion, and vision-distorting goggles. The effects of changes in the proprioceptive information from the lower limbs have been studied by vibrating the calf muscles, anesthetizing the feet, or by examining stance on a moving or compliant surface. The results of these manipulations suggest that automatic compensation for very rapid disruption to postural stability is mediated principally by proprioceptive reflexes. However, there is evidence that under certain conditions both visual and vestibular information can modulate the amplitude of even rapid muscular reactions to perturbation of posture. In addition, vision appears to play an important role in the control of low-frequency sway (which the vestibular system can less easily monitor), and the continuous fine-tuning of orientation and postural adjustments. The vestibular system, according to Nashner, provides an internal orientation reference against which the accuracy of the other two sources of information can be assessed, and also contributes to the regulation of continuous sway.

In recent times there has been growing interest in postural strategies, and the constraints and functional goals which determine their use and effectiveness. The ankle synergy previously described is not the only method of maintaining balance; a compensatory shift in the center of gravity is also commonly achieved by a rotation

about the hips which exerts a shear force against the support surface (the "hip strategy"). Whereas the hip strategy is optimal for balancing on narrow or compliant support surfaces, or for correcting deviations of the center of gravity too great to be neutralized by ankle torque, it is ineffective when standing on slippery or sloping surfaces. The choice of postural strategy is also influenced by characteristics of the individual; for example, people with poor lower limb proprioception or weak ankle muscles are obliged to resort more frequently to the hip strategy.

Although the relatively stereotyped muscular synergies which characterize the ankle and hip strategies have previously received most attention, in practice, a mixture of these and other strategies can be employed. Stability may be maintained by bending at the knees, stepping, anticipatory leaning, or bracing, or the use of the upper limbs for counterbalancing. Emerging themes in research

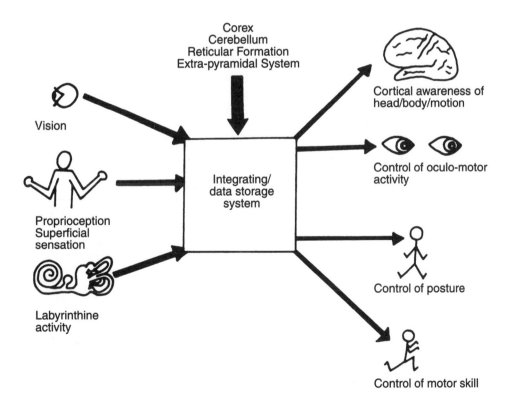

Figure 57 Mechanisms subserving balance in Man. (Reproduced with permission from L. M. Luxon, The anatomy and physiology of the vestibular function. In M. R. Dix & J. D. Hood (Eds), *Vertigo*, Chichester: Wiley, 1984.)

589

into postural control concern the flexible, skilled nature of postural strategies, and the identification of higher-order functional, biomechanical, and perceptual variables which can guide and simplify this complex activity. The choice and timing of the compensatory adjustments may depend upon perception of variables, such as predicted time-to-contact with the boundary of the region of stability, which are simultaneously determined by the biomechanical properties of the individual in relation to the environment, and by neurophysiological constraints (e.g. the limitations of perceptual discrimination and response latency). Functional goals could vary, and might include maximizing stability, security, and automaticity, optimizing the performance of voluntary activity, minimizing muscular effort and neural processing, or some combination of any of these aims. Hence this new approach to postural activity allows for a significant influence of cognitive and affective factors; for example, fear of falling might motivate adoption of a conservative perceptual criterion for initiating postural adjustments, and a postural strategy which emphasized security at the cost of increased effort and reduced movement flexibility.

DISORDERS OF BALANCE

Balance, locomotion, and spatial orientation are thus achieved through complex interactions of sensory inputs, motor output, and sensory motor integration within the central nervous system (CNS) (Figure 57). Not surprisingly, a plethora of diverse pathologies, including otological, neurological, cardiovascular, hematological, endocrine, musculoskeletal, metabolic, ophthalmological, and psychiatric disorders may give rise to dysfunction of this complex system and, by the age of 65 years, 30 percent of people have experienced episodes of dysequilibrium, while between 20 and 40 percent of elderly people living at home fall each year. Vestibular studies in patients with either dizzy or vertiginous episodes or recurrent falls have demonstrated vestibular dysfunction.

In normal circumstances, the resting neural activity generated from the physiologically paired vestibular receptors in each labyrinth is identical. Head movement produces an equal but opposite alteration in this activity within each labyrinth. This asymmetry in neural information provides the basis for vestibular induced compensatory eye and muscle movements, which maintain gaze and posture and allow for cortical awareness of head motion. Pathology affecting the labyrinth or its central nervous system connections may give rise to an asymmetry of vestibular information, which in the absence of a movement leads to a false perception of motion and inappropriate vestibulo-ocular and vestibulo-spinal activity (Luxon, 1987a).

Table 16   General medical causes of imbalance.

	Type of cause	Examples
1	Infective	Syphilis
		Endocarditis
2	Hematological	Anemia
		Hyperviscosity syndromes
3	Vascular disease	Postural hypotension
		Cardiac dysrhythmias
4	Metabolic	Hypoglycemia
		Hyperventilation
5	Neoplastic	Nonmetastatic complications
		Metastases
6	Skeletal	Paget's disease
		Cervical abnormalities
		Osteoarthritis
7	Visual	Bifocal spectacles
8	Iatrogenic	
9	Psychogenic	
10	Multiple causes	Multisensory dizziness syndrome

CLINICAL ASSESSMENT

Clinically, postural instability may be the result of pathology primarily affecting the labyrinth or central nervous system, but it may also result from a multiplicity of disorders which secondarily involve these sites, such as cardiovascular disease (Table 16) (Luxon, 1987b). The differential diagnosis relies on a detailed clinical history, diagnostic clinical signs, and objective investigation of vestibular function.

History

"Vertigo," which may be defined as "a hallucination of movement," is associated classically with disordered vestibular activity. However, patients who are confused and alarmed by non-physiological sensations may describe their symptoms as "dizziness," "lightheadedness," "swimminess," "giddiness," or even "confusion in the head" or "difficulty with the legs." Vertigo of labyrinthine origin is characterized by sudden onset, an episodic nature, short duration (minutes to hours), and associated vegetative symptoms of nausea, vomiting, and diarrhea, while vertigo of central nervous system origin is more insidious in onset, constant in duration, and less likely to be associated with nausea and vomiting. The time course of the disorder is therefore of importance, as is the episodic nature of symptoms. Associated symptoms are of particular relevance, as hearing loss and/or tinnitus suggest involvement of auditory and vestibular elements in the labyrinth or eighth nerve: a constellation of brain-stem symptoms and signs (diplopia, dysarthria, dysphagia, facial weakness, facial numbness, drop attacks, ATAXIA) would suggest brain-stem dysfunction; incoordination and dysarthria would point to a cerebellar lesion, while general motor slowing with tremor and stiffness would point to a basal ganglion disorder, for example, PARKINSON'S DISEASE. Outside the vestibular system, angina,

intermittent claudication, or strokes would raise the suspicion of vascular disease. It cannot be overemphasized that in cases of postural instability, a detailed drug history must be taken, as iatrogenic dizziness related to polypharmacy, poor drug compliance, impaired drug metabolism, side effects of drugs, and ototoxicity are common.

Clinical examination of a patient with imbalance requires a full general medical examination to exclude pathology outside the vestibular system (Table 16). In every case of vertigo, otoscopic examination is essential to exclude chronic middle ear disease with labyrinthine erosion. A detailed assessment of eye movements enables disordered vestibulo-ocular activity to be identified and labyrinthine/eighth nerve vestibular disorders to be differentiated from disorders within the central nervous system. Indeed, the assessment of spontaneous vestibular nystagmus is the most valuable clinical sign in the assessment of dysequilibrium (Table 17).

There is no clinical test of vestibulospinal function, but the Romberg test and GAIT assessment are in part dependent on vestibular activity and may provide valuable contributory, but non-specific, clinical information.

Investigation of vestibular function is dependent upon galvanic testing, which is reported to enable differentiation of vestibular receptor from eighth cranial nerve pathology. Caloric testing, which is the simplest and most readily available vestibular test, enables identification of pathology in one or other labyrinth. Rotation testing, which has the disadvantage of requiring expensive equipment, assesses both labyrinths simultaneously (Kayan, 1987).

DISORDERS OF THE PERIPHERAL LABYRINTH

A variety of pathological processes may affect the vestibular labyrinth and/or the eighth cranial

Table 17   Features of spontaneous vestibular nystagmus.

	Peripheral origin	Central origin
Duration	Short-lived	Permanent
Direction	Unidirectional in horizontal plane	Multidirectional, horizontal, vertical, or rotatory
Type	Conjugate	Conjugate or dysconjugate
Effect of optic fixation	Suppression	Little or no effect

nerve (Luxon, 1987b). Otological causes of imbalance include:

1 Menière's syndrome
2 Post-traumatic syndrome
3 Positional nystagmus
4 Vestibular neuronitis
5 Infection
6 Otosclerosis and Paget's disease
7 Vascular accidents
8 Tumors
9 Autoimmune disorders
10 Drug toxicity

The commonest conditions are head injury which, if severe and associated with a fracture, may result in total loss of vestibular and auditory function, but if mild may give rise to the clinical syndrome of benign positional vertigo of paroxysmal type, characterized by momentary severe spells of vertigo on change of head position; viral labyrinthitis characterized by an acute episode of rotational vertigo and vomiting, lasting for several days, with the resultant dysequilibrium improving over several weeks to months. Vascular labyrinthitis may follow a similar cause. Menière's disease is characterized by the clinical triad of severe episodes of vertigo associated with nausea and vomiting of less than 24 hours' duration, with a fluctuating hearing loss and troublesome tinnitus.

Important but rare causes of vestibular dysfunction and imbalance are acoustic neurinoma and ototoxic drug damage. Whatever the pathological process giving rise to damage in the peripheral vestibular apparatus, vestibular compensation takes place such that symptoms of dysequilibrium gradually subside. It has been shown that there is reactivation of activity in the ipsilateral vestibular nucleus following labyrinthine destruction and cerebellar inhibition upon vestibular activity on the unaffected side. Both these mechanisms tend to redress the asymmetry of neural activity within the vestibular system and thus reduce imbalance. Vision, cervical input, and somatosensory input have all been demonstrated to be of importance in this process. Central reprogramming has also been observed in monkeys following vestibular damage; it is therefore apparent that vestibular compensation is dependent upon a multiplicity of sensory inputs and plastic changes within the central nervous system.

CAUSES OF CENTRAL VESTIBULAR DYSFUNCTION

Central disorders of dysequilibrium are most commonly the result of pathology at the level of the brain stem, CEREBELLUM, or BASAL GANGLIA, although FRONTAL LOBE disorders may also be associated with postural instability (Luxon, 1987b). The following disorders of the central nervous system cause imbalance:

1 Vertebro-basilar ischemia
   Occlusive
   Reduced flow, e.g. migraine
2 Inflammatory disorders
   Bacterial meningitis
   Syphilis
   Polyneuropathies
3 Epilepsy
4 Multiple sclerosis
5 Trauma
6 Drugs and toxins
   Antibiotics
   Anticonvulsants
   Alcohol
   Heavy metals
7 Degenerative disorders
   Hereditary ataxias, e.g. Friedreich's ataxia
   Other spino-cerebellar disorders
   Basal ganglia disorders, e.g. Parkinson's disease, Huntington's disease
   Hereditary neuropathies
8 Congenital malformations
   Arnold Chiari malformation
   Basilar impression
9 Tumors
   Cerebello-pontine angle, e.g. acoustic neuroma
   Brain-stem tumors, e.g. glioma secondaris
10 Frontal lobe pathology

Brain stem and/or cerebellar abnormalities are common in multiple sclerosis, which is a disorder characterized by plaques of demyelination disseminated in time and space within the central nervous system. Vascular lesions of the vertebrobasilar system, which supplies the peripheral labyrinth, the eighth nerve, and the central vestibular connections, may give rise to central vestibular dysfunction as a result of ischemia of major lateral branches, e.g. posterior/anterior inferior cerebellar arteries or perforating arteries arising directly from the basilar artery and supplying the brain stem. Cerebello-pontine angle tumors, most commonly acoustic neuronomata, give rise to a constellation of eighth nerve and brain-stem symptoms and signs, including tinnitus, hearing loss, facial weakness, facial numbness, ataxia, and dysarthria.

Cerebellar dysfunction is commonly seen in foramen magnum lesions, inherited spinocerebellar degenerations, atrophies secondary to metabolic and non-metastatic complications, vascular disease, and tumors.

The commonest BASAL GANGLIA disorder giving rise to postural instability is PARKINSON'S DISEASE, which is characterized by tremor, bradykinesia, and rigidity. However, the multisystem atrophies, Huntington's disease, a dominantly inherited condition characterized by involuntary movements beginning in the face and trunk and accompanied by intellectual deterioration, and frontal lobe lesions giving rise to apraxic postures are other causes of central postural instability.

BIBLIOGRAPHY

Bles, W., & Brandt, Th. (1986). *Disorders of posture and gait*. Amsterdam: Elsevier.

Brooks, V. B. (1986). *The neural basis of motor control*. Oxford: Oxford University Press.

Fukuda, T. (1984). *Statokinetic reflexes in equilibrium and movement*. Tokyo: University of Tokyo Press.

Kayan, A. (1987). Diagnostic tests of balance. In S. D. G. Stephens (Ed.), *Adult audiology. Scott Brown's otolaryngology*, 5th edn (pp. 304–67). London: Butterworths.

Luxon, L. M. (1987a). Physiology of equilibrium and its application in the giddy patient. In D. Wright (Ed.), *Basic sciences. Scott Brown's otolaryngology*, 5th edn (pp. 105–37). London: Butterworths.

Luxon, L. M. (1987b). Causes of balance disorders. In S. D. G. Stephens (Ed.), *Adult audiology. Scott Brown's otolaryngology*, 5th edn (pp. 157–202). London: Butterworths.

Nashner, L. M., & McCollum, G. (1985). The organization of human postural movements: a formal basis and experimental synthesis. *Behavioral and Brain Sciences, 8*, 135–72.

Woolacott, M. H., & Shumway-Cook, A. (1989). *Development of posture and gait across the life span*. Columbia: University of South Carolina Press.

LUCY YARDLEY AND LINDA M. LUXON

Prechtl's syndrome *See* CHOREIFORM SYNDROME.

prefrontal cortex *See* FRONTAL LOBE.

prehension reflex An alternative term for the GRASP REFLEX.

premotor cortex *See* FRONTAL LOBE; SENSORIMOTOR CORTEX.

prosopagnosia Prosopagnosia is a specific form of visual AGNOSIA in which there is a deficit of facial recognition (*see* FACE RECOGNITION). Prosopagnosia may occur in the absence of agnosia for objects and of other failures of visual recognition, and in turn facial recognition may be preserved when these other functions are affected. Prosopagnosia is therefore a specific and isolable form of visual agnosia, which may be a reflection of the early development and biological significance of the recognition of faces.

protopathic innervation Protopathic innervation is one of the two systems (with EPICRITIC INNERVATION) of innervation of the skin. Protopathic sensitivity depends upon specific endorgans grouped together in the skin and characterized by a high threshold and a tendency to radiate and refer sensation to other regions. The sensations associated with the protopathic system are proposed as heat, cold, and pain.

pseudobulbar palsy Pseudobulbar palsy is the result of diffuse cerebrovascular disease affecting both the cerebral hemispheres and the brain stem, often with small areas of softening of tissue, and is characterized by spastic speech, pyramidal signs, and emotional lability. It may be the consequence of repeated episodes of cerebral infarction. Speech becomes slurred and uncontrolled and there are exaggerated reflexes of the mouth and jaw. The emotional impairment results in inappropriate paroxysmal bouts of laughing or crying which are not under voluntary control. As a result of the underlying pathology, dementia, incontinence, and abnormalities of gait are associated with the condition. In the past, the term *atherosclerotic Parkinsonism* has been applied to the disorder.

psychomotor epilepsy *See* EPILEPSY.

psychosurgery Also called *psychiatric neurosurgery* or *functional neurosurgery*, psychosurgery refers to a variety of operations that destroy a part of the brain for the purpose of alleviating mental illness. Psychosurgery has always been surrounded by controversy. Those who support its practice describe psychosurgery as a brain operation capable of alleviating crippling and otherwise intractable mental illness, while those opposed consider it a mutilating brain operation that makes difficult patients more manageable by stunting their emotions and intellect.

The definition of psychosurgery needs further elaboration in order to distinguish it from other procedures. Psychosurgery involves the destruction of normal brain tissue, or at least structures that are not pathological in any demonstrable way. Therefore, brain surgery performed to alleviate symptoms resulting from tumors, strokes, traumatic accidents, infections, or any other pathological condition would not be considered psychosurgery, even if there are symptoms indistinguishable from those of a mental illness. Moreover, an operation that destroys normal brain tissue is not considered psychosurgery if it is performed primarily to alleviate neurological problems, such as movement disorders (Parkinson's disease, spastic conditions, and tremors) or epileptic seizures. Such distinctions, however, may become fuzzy, for example, when an apparently normal brain area is destroyed to alleviate both seizures and mental illness. In such cases, it may not always be clear – even to the neurosurgeon – whether the operation was performed primarily to alleviate the seizures or the mental illness.

EARLY HISTORY

Psychosurgery is usually said to have begun with the publication of the 1936 monograph (*Tentatives opératoires dans le traitement de certaines psychoses*) by the Portuguese neurologist Egas Moniz. Moniz reported that 14 of 20 otherwise intractably ill mental patients were either cured or

significantly improved following "prefrontal leucotomy" (later, also called "prefrontal lobotomy"), an operation that destroys part of the prefrontal area. Moniz, who was 61 at the time, was already well known for having pioneered cerebral angiography.

Within a few months, prefrontal leucotomies were being tried in Italy, Romania, Brazil, Cuba, and the United States. Despite the intervention of the Second World War, by 1948 some form of psychosurgery was being performed in more than 30 countries. It is estimated that during the ten-year period between 1946 and 1956, approximately 60,000–80,000 psychosurgical operations were performed around the world. Obviously, the practice of psychosurgery was widely accepted and, in 1949, Moniz was awarded the Nobel Prize for Physiology and Medicine "for his discovery of the therapeutic value of prefrontal leucotomy in certain psychoses."

There are several reasons why, despite the controversy surrounding it, psychosurgery was so widely and rapidly adopted around the world. Perhaps foremost among these reasons was the lack of any effective treatment for mental illness. Psychiatrists at large public psychiatric institutions, where the accretion of chronic patients far exceeded the resources available, were willing to try almost anything that might alleviate chronic mental illness and make it possible to discharge patients. Somatic therapies were perceived as especially promising, partly because they were not labor-intensive, and it was not mere coincidence that insulin coma, metrazol, and electroconvulsive treatments, as well as prefrontal leucotomy, were introduced within a five-year period.

Moniz was not in fact the first person to try psychosurgery. In 1891 Gottlieb Burckhardt, the Director of the Psychiatric Clinic at Préfargier, Switzerland, cut channels between sensory and motor areas of the cortex in an attempt to reduce the mania of psychotic patients. During the intervening years between Burckhardt's early psychosurgery and Moniz's first prefrontal leucotomy, there were a number of other attempts to explore psychosurgery, but for various reasons none was widely adopted (Valenstein, 1986, 1990).

EVOLUTION OF PROCEDURES AND RATIONALE

Moniz's rationale for performing psychosurgery was, to be kind, not tightly reasoned. He wrote that mental illness occurred when patients could not free themselves from "fixed ideas," which he hypothesized were being sustained by neural pathways that had become "abnormally stabilized." Moniz selected the prefrontal area as the location of the "abnormally stabilized" pathways, partly because it was the most highly developed in Man and partly because it was widely considered to be the seat of mental capacities such as judgment and reflection, which were impaired in the mentally ill.

Prefrontal leucotomy was designed to sever neural fibers in the prefrontal area by inserting a leucotome (an instrument for cutting "white" matter or nerve fibers) through burr holes in the skull. Once inserted to the desired depth, the leucotome was rotated, leaving behind a core of tissue that would soon die. As many as nine separate cores were made in the prefrontal area of some patients. The operations were performed by Almeida Lima, a young neurosurgeon in Moniz's Neurology Department in the University of Lisbon.

Although the Moniz–Lima "core operation" was tried in many countries, it was relatively quickly replaced by other procedures judged to be more accurate. Walter Freeman and James Watts of the George Washington University Medical School Hospital in Washington did much to promote psychosurgery because they developed a surgical procedure (the Freeman–Watts "standard lobotomy") that was widely adopted, and also a rationale much more convincing than the one offered by Moniz. Freeman and Watts promoted their procedure and their explanation of how psychosurgery alleviated mental illness in numerous lectures, articles, and their widely read book, *Psychosurgery*, originally published in 1942 and revised in 1950.

Freeman and Watts claimed that psychosurgery was most successful when the connections between the prefrontal area and the dorsomedial thalamus were severed. At the time, there were several "thalamic theories" of emotion and the dorsomedial nucleus, in particular, was thought to play a major role in modulating emotional state. Freeman and Watts argued that in mental illness intense emotional states disrupt thought processes. Walter Freeman was often quoted in the popular press as stating that psychosurgery "separates the thinking brain from the emotional brain."

The Freeman–Watts theory had much more appeal than Moniz's vague hypothesis about "fixed ideas." In the first place, the theory shifted the emphasis from ideas to emotions, which was consistent with the impression that was emerging, that patients with exaggerated emotional states benefited most from psychosurgery. Secondarily, the theory seemed to be supported by the anatomical studies of A. E. Walker on the primate thalamus, which had demonstrated the specific pathways by which the dorsomedial thalamic nucleus and the ventromedial ("orbital") prefrontal brain area were connected.

By the mid-1940s, evidence was beginning to accumulate from anatomical and clinical studies that damage to the ventromedial prefrontal area often produced a general disinhibition of behavior and the emotions, while damage to the dorsolateral convexity of the prefrontal area was more likely to produce intellectual impairment. Neurosurgeons began to develop psychosurgical procedures that made it easier to restrict the damage imposed to the ventromedial prefrontal area. In England E. Cunningham Dax, Geoffrey Knight, and other neurosurgeons reported that their highest percentage of successful prefrontal leucotomies followed damage restricted to the ventromedial area. In the United States, the Freeman–Watts operation was eventually replaced by the Lyerly–Poppen operation, which made it easier to restrict damage to the ventromedial area, and William Scoville developed a "suborbital undercutting" procedure for destroying the orbital area on the ventral surface of the brain by suction. Thus, during the latter half of the 1940s psychosurgery became increasingly directed toward the ventromedial area and the bundle of fibers connecting this prefrontal area with the dorsomedial thalamic nucleus.

By the early 1950s, however, it had become increasingly evident that many of the patients who had been judged to be significantly improved following prefrontal lobotomy were intellectually and emotionally impaired. The disinhibition that followed destruction of the ventromedial area might help to alleviate introversion, inertia, indecision, obsessiveness, and depression, but it could also produce restlessness, impulsiveness, and lack of judgment. It was starting to be asked whether psychosurgery was not substituting the impairment of an organic brain syndrome for the disruptive behavior of a psychosis.

595

The criticism of psychosurgery had relatively little effect on its practice, as there still was no alternative treatment available, and because there were large numbers of professionals who, for one reason or another, were committed to its practice. Moreover, it was argued that the psychosurgical procedures had changed and that the criticism applied only to the massive and diffuse brain damage imposed by the earlier lobotomies.

John Fulton of Yale University was particularly influential in arguing that psychosurgery should be restricted either to the ventromedial prefrontal area or to certain areas within the so-called LIMBIC SYSTEM. By the early 1950s the hitherto neglected "limbic theory of emotions" advanced by James Papez was beginning to be accepted. In agreement with Papez, evidence was accumulating that was consistent with the view that the emotions were regulated by the subcortical structures comprising the limbic system. Several experimental reports demonstrated that the emotional temperament of animals was dramatically altered following destruction of the amygdala, the septal area, and the cingulum. These limbic structures seemed to regulate emotionality through connections to the hypothalamus and the ventromedial area too had recently been shown to affect visceral emotional reactions through connections to the hypothalamus. A seemingly more sophisticated logic and a body of supporting evidence was emerging. Fulton even predicted that the brain target of the psychosurgery of the future might be tailored to a patient's symptoms.

Neurosurgeons began to report success following cingulotomies, a psychosurgical procedure which targeted the anterior portion of the cingulum. Others explored the amygdala as a target, following Heinrich Klüver and Paul Bucy's report that monkeys became tame following temporal lobe ablations. The growing impression that more selective destruction of targets in the prefrontal area and the limbic system could alleviate specific emotional problems without causing intellectual impairment helped to sustain the practice of psychosurgery at a high level, despite growing criticism. With the introduction of neuroleptic and antidepressant drugs in the mid-1950s, however, the amount of psychosurgery performed worldwide dropped precipitously to approximately 10 to 20 percent of what it was during the peak years of 1949–52. Nevertheless, drugs do not alleviate all mental illness and a low level of psychosurgery continued to be performed throughout the 1960s on intractable cases. Psychosurgery was used in relatively few centers. Many psychiatrists were not even aware that it was still being practiced, and many of those who knew about it were adamant about not being willing to refer patients for such a procedure.

By the 1970s a few neurosurgeons had suggested that the time was ripe to take a "second look" at psychosurgery. It was claimed that knowledge of the anatomy and function of fronto-limbic-diencephalic pathways had significantly increased and that modern neurosurgical technique made it possible to produce small focal brain lesions with great precision. Stereotaxic instruments were more commonly being used and additional precision could be achieved by on-line monitoring of X-ray pictures during the insertion of electrodes into the brain. Lesions were generally made with radio frequency waves, but at a few institutions freezing (cryogenics), radioactive cobalt, or yttrium were used. The era when psychosurgery would be performed with hand-held leucotomes was coming to a close.

An increase in interest in psychosurgery was evident during the 1970s. Following the convening of the First International Congress of Psychosurgery in 1948, no other comparable meeting took place until the one that was held in Copenhagen in 1970. This was followed by the Third International Congress, held only two years later in England, and a fourth in Madrid in 1975. The number of psychosurgical procedures performed did not increase, however, as opposition to the resurgence of interest in psychosurgery became quite militant. In some quarters, the growing interest in psychosurgery was perceived as a plan to perform brain surgery to control "deviant" behavior. The ensuing controversy became political and legislation was passed in several states and countries that either prohibited or seriously restricted the practice of psychosurgery. As a result, the amount of psychosurgery performed began to decline even further during the 1980s.

There developed during the 1970s and there still exists an almost bewildering array of different brain targets used in psychosurgery. A partial list of psychosurgical procedures in use today would include: basofrontal tractotomy, capsulotomy, innominate tractotomy, subcaudate tractotomy, limbic leucotomy (combined subcaudate and cingulum lesions), cingulotomy, cingulotractotomy, and a medial mesoloviolotomy (a subrostral cingulotomy that invades the genu of the corpus callosum), posterior hypothalalotomies, and amygdalectomies. The list is not complete and, even where two surgeons call their psychosurgical procedure by the same name, a close examination of the procedure reveals that the targets are not identical. However, the prediction made by John Fulton in the 1950s that psychosurgical targets would be tailored to patient's symptoms has not been fulfilled, as surgeons generally have their favorite target, which is used for all patients on whom psychosurgery is performed.

Summarizing the results of psychosurgery must be done separately for the earlier prefrontal lobotomies and current psychosurgery but, even so, the task presents great difficulties for a number of reasons. Most psychosurgery is not described in professional journals, so it is impossible to judge the representative quality of the published results. Moreover, the criteria for evaluating improvement are often vague, subjective, and even anecdotal, and the judgments are not usually made by uninvolved observers. Furthermore, it is only the rare psychosurgical publication that includes an adequate control group to make comparisons. Lastly, so many different psychosurgical procedures are used on different patient populations that the results are difficult to summarize.

Despite the poor quality of the literature, it is probably true that many agitated and anxious patients who underwent the earlier prefrontal lobotomy did experience relief – in some instances striking relief – from their most troublesome symptoms. In the best cases, this led to a normalization of behavior. In the worst cases, patients became either childishly impulsive or so inert that they rarely talked or exhibited any spontaneity. The latter cases seem to justify the "zombie" label that was used to describe them. Some patients became careless, indifferent to errors, generally slovenly, and lacking in motivation, insight, and foresight.

The emotional and intellectual impairments could vary enormously in magnitude, from tolerable to devastating. There were also neurological consequences of the operations that were not insignificant. A number of patients (estimated to be about 15 per cent) developed epileptic seizures as a consequence of the surgery and the mortality

figures hovered around 5 percent. Furthermore, if a major blood vessel in the brain was severed during surgery, the patient might deteriorate into an organic demented state.

There definitely were cases where, for whatever reason, a good recovery followed the surgery and, in some instance, people who were lobotomized were able to assume the responsibility of high-level positions. In most cases, however, the outcome was intermediate. There was generally some reduction in the severity of the most troublesome symptoms, making for a somewhat more normal life. A price was generally paid for the improvement as many of those who underwent a lobotomy exhibited some decrease in drive, desire to excel, capacity to think abstractly, imagination, and capacity for deep emotional experiences. As seriously disturbed patients were rarely demonstrating any of these capacities, many psychiatrists concluded that what was lost was not real as it would never have been realized. This conclusion, however, was not undisputed.

The psychosurgery performed today differs in a number of respects from the prefrontal lobotomies performed during the 1940s. As mentioned above, the damage imposed by modern psychosurgery is much smaller and better localized. Whereas almost any intractable psychiatric condition might have provided the justification for prefrontal lobotomy, the patients considered candidates for psychosurgery today constitute a much more restricted group. In general, modern psychosurgery is performed only on patients with serious depression, obsessive-compulsive symptoms, or pain, who are judged to have proven intractable to other treatments. With respect to outcome, the available evidence supports the conclusion that, following psychosurgery today, the neurological complications are minimal with almost no deaths, epilepsy, or other adverse physical consequences. Although the evidence of effectiveness has not been undisputed, the conclusion of several independent studies is that somewhere between 50 percent and 70 percent of the patients who undergo modern psychosurgery experience a substantial improvement. In some cases the improvement is lasting, but in others patients may relapse after a period of time. One persistent problem in evaluating these relatively positive conclusions about modern psychosurgery is that it is difficult to evaluate such attributes as motivation, and also the selection of candidates for psychosurgery may be introducing a bias.

The explanations of how psychosurgery alleviates intense emotional states remain unconvincing and there exists no consensus. Other than *post hoc* statements that psychosurgery modifies activity in the limbic system, diencephalon, and now even the basal ganglia, the arguments for psychosurgery are basically empirical and atheoretical. Reduced to their essence, it is claimed that patients improve, the adverse consequences are minimal, all other treatments have been tried, and the risk of doing nothing is great.

Finally, it might be added that even those who practice psychosurgery today generally agree that it is a stop-gap treatment that will eventually be replaced by drugs or by some surgical procedure that does not require destruction of tissue. Some recent technical advances suggest a possible alternative surgical treatment of mental illness. Previously, the existence of brain pathology has been linked primarily to evidence of infections, tumors, or structural damage due to traumatic or vascular accidents. With the advances in non-invasive, brain-imaging techniques, such as positron emission tomography (PET), it will be possible to detect regional functional abnormalities based on abnormal activity or biochemistry. In epileptic patients, PET has been able to detect local "pathophysiology" responsible for the occurrence of seizures, where traditional pathology would have found nothing abnormal. It is conceivable that a similar linkage might be found between local brain "pathophysiology" and some mental illness. Under such circumstances, it is possible that electrical or chemical stimulation delivered through implanted electrodes or chemotrodes might alleviate symptoms. If that should prove feasible, it will have to be decided whether the definition of psychosurgery should be revised to include what might be called "brain physiotherapy."

BIBLIOGRAPHY

Freeman, W. J., & J. W. Watts (1950). *Psychosurgery in the treatment of mental disorders and intractable pain*, 2nd edn. Springfield, IL: Charles Thomas. (First published in 1942.)

Moniz, E. (1936). *Tentatives opératoires dans le traitement de certaines psychoses*. Paris: Masson.

Valenstein, E. S. (Ed.). (1980). *The psychosurgery debate. Scientific, legal, and ethical perspectives*. San Francisco: W. H. Freeman.

Valenstein, E. S. (1986). *Great and desperate cures. The rise and decline of psychosurgery and other radical treatments for mental illness*. New York: Basic Books.

Valenstein, E. S. (1990). The prefrontal area and psychosurgery. In H. B. M. Uylings, C. G. Van Eden, J. P. C. De Bruin, M. A. Corner, & M. G. P. Feenstra (Eds.), *The prefrontal cortex: Its structure, function and pathology*. (*Progress in Brain Research*, Vol. 85, pp. 539–54). Amsterdam: Elsevier.

ELLIOT S. VALENSTEIN

pulvinar The pulvinar is a region of the THALAMUS that receives projections from the visual cortex and the superior COLLICULUS and sends connections to regions of temporal and parietal cortex. It is therefore implicated in the integration of visual input with other intelligent functions in the cortex.

putamen The putamen is the outer division of the lentiform nucleus which lies ventrolateral to the head of the CAUDATE NUCLEUS, and is at one point continuous with it. It is one element in the extrapyramidal motor system which controls tone rather than movement in normal subjects. It receives input from all regions of the cortex and relevant areas of the THALAMUS and sends fibers to the GLOBUS PALLIDUS. Damage to the putamen contributes to extrapyramidal disorders which include changes in muscle tone and the various forms of "spontaneous" movement: tremor, ATHETOSIS, and CHOREA.

PVS (persistent vegetative state) *See* VEGETATIVE STATE.

pyramidal tract The pyramidal tract is the bundle of fibers descending longitudinally along the ventral surface of the medulla oblongata in the brain stem. The outline of the tract, in transverse sections of the brain stem cut at this level, has a distinctive pyramidal appearance. The existence of the tract has been recognized since the time of Hippocrates.

The tract represents the major descending pathway through which the cerebral cortex communicates with the lower brain stem and spinal cord. It is derived from a number of different cortical areas and has a widespread influence on both sensory and motor structures. Its fibers descend in the internal capsule of the forebrain, pass through the cerebral peduncle into the midbrain and pons, and emerge as a pair of easily identifiable tracts on the ventral surface of the medulla oblongata. In the caudal medulla, close to the junction with the spinal cord, many of its fibers decussate (cross over) and descend throughout the spinal cord as the corticospinal tract. Some of its fibers are highly branched, allowing the same descending commands to be distributed to a number of different parts of the CNS. Rather than having a single role, it is likely that the pyramidal tract carries out a number of important functions, including the execution of fine, skilled movements and the control of transmission through sensory pathways.

Origin of the pyramidal tract

The cerebral cortex is composed of two neuronal cell types, pyramidal and nonpyramidal. Pyramidal cells make up around 70 percent of the total. It is important to point out that these cells are called pyramidal because of their shape, and the term should not be confused with that applied to the profile of the whole pyramidal tract described above. All of the neurons giving rise to the tract are of the pyramidal type, and are located exclusively in the fifth layer of the cortex (lamina V). These cells are referred to as pyramidal tract neurons (PTNs). They have extensive dendrites which collect as many as 60,000 inputs per neuron from all layers of the cortical column in which they are located.

Anatomical studies show that the pyramidal

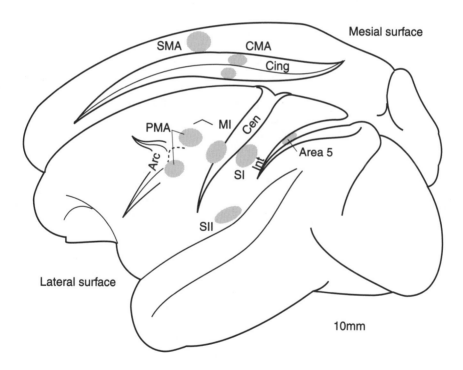

Figure 58 Areas of the macaque cerebral cortex giving rise to the pyramidal tract projections to the arm. Sulci: cing, cingulate; cen, central; arc, arcuate; SMA, supplementary motor area; MI, primary motor cortex; CMA, cingulate motor area; PMA, premotor area; SI, SII, primary and secondary somatosensory area.

tract is derived from an extensive cortical territory. In the *frontal* lobe it originates from the primary motor cortex (M1), the premotor cortex, the supplementary motor cortex (SMA), and the cingulate motor areas, lying in the mesial wall of the hemisphere. In the *parietal* lobe, the tract is derived from the primary and secondary somatosensory cortices (SI, SII) and from higher-order parietal regions (areas 5 and 7). Up to 10 percent of the lamina V pyramidal cells within these different cortical areas give rise to the tract; the cells of origin include some of the largest neurons in the cortex, the giant pyramidal cells or Betz cells which are found in M1. In the macaque monkey and in Man around 60 percent of the fibers come from the frontal lobe, of which about half are derived from M1.

Course of the pyramidal tract

The corticofugal fibers that ultimately form the pyramidal tract descend from the cortex through both the anterior and posterior limbs of the internal capsule; most of the fibers from M1 travel through the posterior limb. The fibers then pass through the cerebral peduncle and descend through the brain stem (see Figure 59). It is important to note that, when considering the effects of capsular lesions following stroke in Man (see below), the pyramidal fibers make up only a small proportion of the fibers passing through the capsule. At the level of the cerebral peduncle they make up only 5–18 percent of the fibers; the proportion for the capsule is probably even lower.

Bundles of fibers pass through the pons and finally emerge as the pyramidal tract, running along the ventral aspect of the medulla oblongata. The cross-sectional area of the tract is larger on the left side than on the right in around 75 percent of brains studied. At the caudal end of the medulla most of the fibers (around 90 percent in Man) decussate and pass into the spinal cord as the lateral corticospinal tract, which descends in the lateral funiculus to all levels of the spinal cord. Some of the uncrossed fibers also travel in the lateral tract, but most descend in the anterior funiculus as the anterior corticospinal tract. Few of these fibers descend below upper thoracic levels.

Numbers and size of fibers

In Man, each pyramidal tract comprises over a million fibers. A wide range of fiber sizes exists,

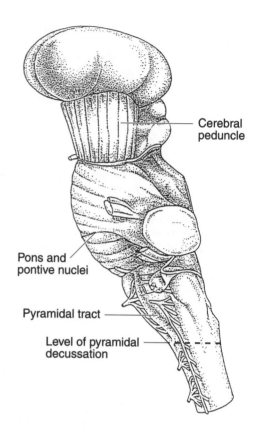

Cerebral peduncle

Pons and pontive nuclei

Pyramidal tract

Level of pyramidal decussation

Figure 59 The corticofugal fibers.

ranging from unmyelinated fibers (< 1 μm in diameter) up to 22 μm. The largest fibers have a conduction velocity of around 70 m.s^{-1}. Small fibers predominate: 92 percent are $<$ μm, and only 2.6 percent are larger than 6 μm. There is no topographic organization within the tract: fibers destined for the cervical cord (arm and hand) seem to be completely intermingled with those terminating more caudally (leg and foot).

Branching of pyramidal tract axons

The pyramidal tract exhibits a substantial degree of branching. Within the cortical gray matter, intracortical collaterals provide for both recurrent inhibitory and excitatory inputs to other layer V pyramidal neurons. Subcortically, its fibers branch to innervate the red nucleus, the pontine precerebellar nuclei, and the reticular formation, including the cells of origin of descending reticulospinal pathways. Corticobulbar projections to cranial motor nuclei are particularly pronounced for those nuclei supplying the muscles of facial expression, tongue, and larynx. There are heavy projections to the dorsal column nuclei; these nuclei are part of the ascending dorsal funiculus-medial lemniscal system, and the pyramidal fibers are concerned with inhibitory control of sensory transmission through this system. Such actions are central to theories of "efference copy," in which a motor command cancels out the sensory input generated by the movement itself.

Destination and termination within the spinal cord

The pyramidal tract supplies fibers to all parts of the spinal gray matter. It is probable that 50 percent or more of its fibers terminate within the cervical spinal cord. The heaviest projections are to the intermediate zone of the gray matter and are concerned with the control of spinal interneurons concerned with transmission of spinal reflexes. Some of these projections are bilateral. Those from the anterior corticospinal tract are mainly bilateral and are thought to influence interneurons concerned with control of muscles acting on the trunk and shoulder girdle.

There are projections to the dorsal horn, which are again concerned with sensory transmission; these arise principally from the sensory cortical areas of the postcentral gyrus. Projections are strongest to those parts of the dorsal horn dealing with input from cutaneous mechanoreceptors and proprioceptors. Finally there are projections to the motoneuronal cell groups in the ventral horn, including τ-motoneurons supplying muscle spindles.

Properties of cortico-motoneuronal projections

Direct cortico-motoneuronal projections are a feature unique to the primate species. The cortico-motoneuronal projection is strongest to the motoneuronal cell groups which supply the most distal muscles (hand and finger, foot and toe muscles) and in some species (e.g. the macaque) there are few cortico-motoneuronal projections to motoneurons supplying more proximal muscles. In Man there appear to be projections to all upper limb motoneurons. Cortico-motoneuronal connections appear to be entirely excitatory, and probably utilize glutamate as a neurotransmitter. However, powerful inhibitory effects on muscular activity can be elicited from the pyramidal tract, and these are relayed through inhibitory interneurons. Inhibition of spinal motoneurons is an important prerequisite for all skilled movements.

Single pyramidal tract neurons have axons which arborize and terminate within several motor nuclei. In general, each neuron tends to facilitate small groups of functional synergist muscles that are used together when performing a given motor action (e.g. wrist flexion) and some of them produce reciprocal inhibition of the group of muscles producing the opposite movement (e.g. wrist extension). Some neurons innervate a specific set of muscles which may serve as task groups for performance of more complex motor acts.

Functional significance of cortico-motoneuronal connections

Several lines of evidence support the idea that cortico-motoneuronal connections are important for the performance of relatively independent finger movements, which are essential for most hand skills, including gesture, tool-making, drawing, and writing. The cortico-motoneuronal system bypasses spinal reflex circuitry and allows the cerebral cortex direct access to the motoneurons. Both anatomical and electrophysiological studies show that this input is of most importance for the hand. Its function is probably to allow discrete control of levels of activity in the many different muscles controlling the hand and fingers, and thereby the production of relatively independent finger movements.

There is a significant correlation between the digital dexterity of a particular species and the density of cortico-motoneuronal connections in that species. Sub-primates in which these connections are lacking show only limited capacity for independent digit control. From New World to Old World monkeys and from great apes to Man there is a progressive increase in the density of cortico-motoneuronal connections and the index of digital dexterity. In Old World macaques, bilateral pyramidal tract lesions produce permanent deficits of relatively independent finger movements.

Finally, there is evidence that cortico-motoneuronal connections are absent at birth and develop over a protracted period, which is up to one year in the macaque and probably longer in human infants. The establishment of these connections is probably one of the essential factors in

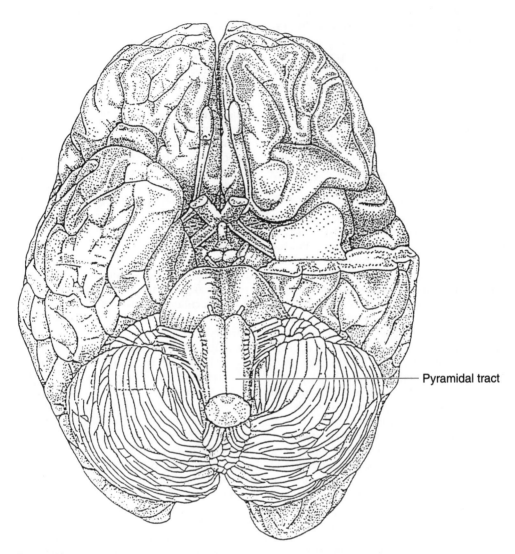

Pyramidal tract

Figure 60 The pyramidal tract.

the acquisition of skilled hand and finger movements.

Development of the pyramidal tract

The projections and connections of the pyramidal tract are immature at birth. In the neonate, fibers have reached all spinal levels, and terminations are seen in the intermediate zone. However, many of these fibers are very small and poorly myelinated; myelination of the tract is largely postnatal. The most rapid phase occurs over the first two years of life, and is accompanied by large increases in the conduction velocity of the tract. Further changes in myelination probably continue up to the time of puberty. As pointed out above, the direct cortico-motoneuronal connections are scarce at birth and develop over a protracted period.

Noninvasive activation of the pyramidal tract in Man

Transcranial magnetic stimulation (TMS) makes it possible to activate the pyramidal tract in Man. This technique involves the delivery of a large, brief current pulse to a coil mounted over the head. This induces a strong magnetic field in the underlying tissues, which in turn generates electrical fields within the cortex. The technique is completely painless. Because the induced fields fall off rapidly with distance from the coil, it is unlikely that deeper CNS structures are activated by TMS.

Natural activity of motor cortex pyramidal tract neurons during movement

Pyramidal tract neurons (PTNs) in the motor cortex are typically active around 50–100 ms before the onset of voluntary muscle activity. Most neurons fire repetitively, and optimal discharge is observed during movement of a particular joint. The pattern of PTN activity appears to be an important determinant of the timing of movement onset. The discharge activity of PTNs can also code the velocity, force, and direction of a voluntary movement. PTNs show particularly marked activity changes during production of low forces, emphasizing their importance for skilled movement. It is unlikely that single neurons

contribute to the control of only one parameter of movement, and specification of these parameters probably involves the cooperation of a large population of PTNs.

The majority of PTNs are sensitive to sensory inputs arising in the periphery. Neurons typically respond at short latency to joint movement or tactile stimuli. Receptive fields are small and most neurons show a close correspondence of output and input activity. For example, a PTN active during flexion of the wrist joint is excited by passive extension of the wrist, a movement which would excite the intramuscular receptors located in the wrist flexor muscles. Sensory inputs can act via a transcortical reflex circuit, involving rapid transmission to the sensorimotor cortex and excitation of PTNs projecting to motoneuron pools. Transcortical reflexes exert their effects at latencies longer than expected for spinal reflex pathways, but are still shorter than the voluntary reaction time. Such reflexes may be important in load compensation (automatic adaptation of muscular force to compensate for unexpected

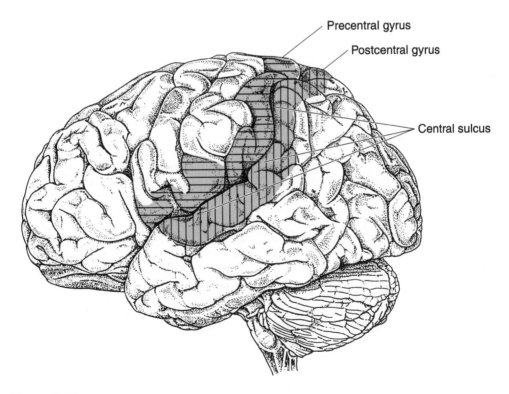

Figure 61 The motor map.

changes in the load) and for increasing the grip force when objects slip unexpectedly from the grasp.

Far less is known about the functions of PTNs in other cortical regions, but there is some evidence that they can function as parallel outputs to the motor apparatus. PTNs in somatosensory cortex are active after rather than before a voluntary movement.

Mapping of motor outputs in the primary motor cortex

It has long been known that electrical stimulation of different regions of M1 results in movements of different parts of the contralateral body half. This observation, made by Fritsch and Hitzig in 1870, was fundamental to the theory of cortical localization of function. The motor map is often shown superimposed upon the exposed surface of the human precentral gyrus, i.e. immediately anterior to the central sulcus (see Figure 61). In this motor map, the foot and leg lie medially, the arm and hand occupy the middle third of the gyrus and the face and mouth lie laterally. There is a disproportionately large representation of the lips, tongue, hand, and foot, with far less tissue devoted to the more proximal parts of the limb and the trunk. The motor effects produced by low-threshold cortical stimulation are probably mediated by the pyramidal tract, since section of the tract abolishes these effects.

Within each major subdivision of the motor map (face, arm, leg) there is no strict somatotopic representation of muscles, as originally proposed, but rather an overlapping mosaic of outputs to different muscles. A single muscle is represented many times over, and these representations are often discontinuous. This pattern of output probably reflects the facts that (a) most voluntary movements require coordinated activity in many different muscles and (b) a given muscle can be used in many different combinations with other muscles.

The output map is a dynamic feature of the motor system. Deafferentation of the cortex (e.g. by amputation of a limb) or damage to other parts of the system can lead to a dramatic reorganization of intracortical influences and connectivity. This capacity for reorganization may be important in recovery from brain damage, although this is not yet firmly established.

Motor maps have been shown to exist in other cortical motor areas, such as the premotor cortex and SMA. The effects elicited from these areas require higher intensities of stimulation, and the outputs to different body parts show a greater degree of overlap than in M1.

BEHAVIORAL CONSEQUENCES OF PYRAMIDAL TRACT LESIONS IN MAN

The devastating effects of stroke on hand movement have been known since Egyptian times. The classical picture of damage to the pyramidal tract at or below its cortical origin is one of impairment of movement in the opposite body half, especially severe in the arm and leg. This impairment is characterized by muscular weakness, spasticity, and hyperreflexia, and the loss of discrete hand and finger movements. Babinski's sign (dorsiflexion of the toes in response to mechanical stimulation of the sole of the foot) is associated with this condition of hemiplegia (paralysis or weakness on one side of the body). The weakness is usually more pronounced in facial than in jaw muscles, and in hand than in shoulder muscles. This may reflect the importance of bilateral cortical projections from the undamaged hemisphere to the less affected muscle groups. In most cases, recovery of movement progresses from proximal joints (shoulder) to distal (hand); in many patients fine, independent movements of the digits are permanently lost, and they experience severe difficulty with such activities as writing or doing up buttons. There is certainly no evidence that all voluntary movement is abolished by pyramidal tract lesions.

The effects of lesions in Man are difficult to interpret because the lesions rarely affect the pyramidal system alone. Infarctions within the internal capsule, which are the most common cause of hemiplegia, affect many other descending and ascending fiber systems. Given the small proportion of fibers within the capsule that enter the pyramidal tract (see above), it is unlikely that all the features of hemiplegia after stroke can be attributed to them. In a few cases, discrete lesions of the pyramidal tract do occur; in these patients there are some deficits of individual finger movements but no marked spasticity. Recovery in such cases has been attributed to alternative motor pathways.

Pyramidal tract lesions in experimental animals

The behavioral consequences of pyramidal tract lesions are generally far more devastating in primates than in nonprimates. In the macaque monkey, complete bilateral section of the tract causes a permanent loss of the ability to perform fine, independent movement of the digits. Effects on more proximal muscle systems are limited, and this may reflect the paucity of cortico-motoneuronal connections to proximal motoneurons in the monkey. In apes, where such projections involve all muscle groups, pyramidal tract lesions affect all upper limb muscle groups.

In the macaque there is also a permanent loss of contactual hand-orienting responses; this illustrates the importance of the pyramidal tract for sensorimotor functions such as active touch. The capacity to perform an active tactile exploration of an object depends on both the pyramidal (motor) and medial lemniscal (sensory) systems. The interpretation of tactile and other sensory inputs is critically dependent upon the CNS receiving copies of the motor commands used to obtain the sensory information.

These effects are only seen after complete lesions; the effects of subtotal lesions of the tract (up to 85 percent of the fibers cut) are usually transitory.

LESIONS OF THE PYRAMIDAL TRACT DURING DEVELOPMENT

Lesions during the early developmental period lead to substantial reorganization of the pyramidal projection. Unilateral pyramidal tract or sensorimotor cortex lesions occurring during development lead to the establishment of a much larger ipsilateral projection from the intact side, a phenomenon which is not seen in the adult organism. The time of occurrence of the lesion in the developmental period is critical. In the macaque, little or no recovery is seen when the lesion is made at birth. In Man the most striking changes are seen as a result of lesions sustained before 29 weeks, the time at which the tract has reached all spinal levels (see above). Hemiplegic patients of this type often show reasonable recovery of hand function but exhibit pronounced mirroring of voluntary hand movements: unwanted activation of the intact hand whenever the affected hand is moved. This is thought to reflect the dominance of the surviving cortex and tract over both sides of the body, and this can be demonstrated by the presence of bilateral responses to TMS of the surviving hemisphere.

PYRAMIDAL AND EXTRAPYRAMIDAL SYNDROMES

Much confusion has arisen in the literature over the use of the terms "pyramidal" and "extrapyramidal" to describe clinical disorders of movement, and the attempt to relate these terms to the anatomy and physiology of the pyramidal tract. Clinically, it is important to distinguish the classic syndrome of hemiplegia following stroke, usually referred to as "pyramidal," from other movement disorders, such as tremor, rigidity, ballism, and athetosis, which are referred to as "extrapyramidal." At one time it was thought that, just as unilateral interruption of the pyramidal tract resulted in hemiplegia, these "extrapyramidal" disorders resulted from disruption of descending pathways other than the pyramidal tract. The term "extrapyramidal tracts" was a collective term describing pathways which mediate cortical control of motor actions, but which do not pass through the pyramidal tract. This included the cortico-reticulospinal projections.

It is now clear that, while the term "extrapyramidal" may be clinically useful for describing *syndromes*, there is no evidence that these syndromes do result from disruption of nonpyramidal *pathways*. These syndromes result from lesions of the basal ganglia, whose influence over the motor output depends chiefly on projections which pass to the premotor cortex and SMA and thence to the primary motor cortex and pyramidal tract. In other words, we can understand these disorders better in hierarchical terms, in which "extrapyramidal signs" are produced by lesions affecting structures, including the basal ganglia, which lie upstream of motor cortex. Most authorities have agreed that the use of the term "extrapyramidal" should be discontinued.

BIBLIOGRAPHY

Armand, J. (1982). The origin, course and terminations of corticospinal fibers in various mammals. *Progress in Brain Research*, *57*, 330–60.

Hepp-Reymond, M.-C. (1988). Functional organization of motor cortex and its participation in voluntary movements. In H. D. Seklis & J. Erwin (Eds), *Comparative primate biology*, Vol. 4 (pp. 501–624). New York: Liss.

Humphrey, D. R., & Freund, H.-J. (1991). *Motor control: Concepts and issues*. Chichester: Wiley-Interscience.

Kalaska, J. F., & Crammond, D. J. (1992). Cerebral cortical mechanisms of reaching movements. *Science, 255,* 1517–23.

Kuypers, H. G. J. M. (1981). Anatomy of the descending pathways. In J. M. Brookhart & V. B. Mountcastle (Eds), *Handbook of physiology: The nervous system II* (pp. 597–666). Bethesda, MD: American Physiological Society.

Lemon, R. N. (1993). Cortical control of the primate hand. The 1992 G. L. Brown Prize Lecture. *Experimental Physiology, 78,* 263–301.

Porter, R., & Lemon, R. N. (1993). *Corticospinal function and voluntary movement.* Oxford: Oxford University Press.

Wiesendanger, M. (1981). The pyramidal tract. Its structure and function. In A. L. Towe & E. S. Luschei (Eds), *Handbook of behavioral neurobiology,* Vol. 5 (pp. 401–90). New York: Plenum.

R. N. LEMON

pyriform cortex   Pyriform cortex (also *piriform cortex*) is the primary olfactory cortex. It receives input from the olfactory tract and projects in turn to the entorhinal area from which fibers also lead to the HIPPOCAMPUS. Pyriform cortex also projects to the AMYGDALA, and in both cases the connections are made without reference to the cerebral neocortex. Projections are also present to the hypothalamus. Together, these links are believed to represent the role of smell in evoking memory, in sexually significant responses, and in potentiating other appetitive behaviors, but these functional associations have not all been directly demonstrated in humans. Olfactory information is also passed to the frontal lobes, where information about smell may be integrated with other modalities for the execution of higher intellectual functions.

Q

quadrantanopia *See* HEMIANOPIA.

quadriplegia Paralysis of all body regions below the neck, therefore including all four limbs, is known as quadriplegia and results from "high" spinal lesions, in the cervical portion of the spine. Although spinal reflexes may continue to operate, no body sensation is received from below the point of the lesion and no motor control, other than that of a reflexive nature, is possible below it. It is interesting to note that emotional experience is preserved in quadriplegic patients, but without the bodily expression of the emotion, although it is not possible to conclude that the emotional experience is of an entirely normal character.

R

rage response The rage response is a period of uncontrolled violent and destructive behavior. Commonly with an appropriate external trigger, it has the appearance and affective qualities of normal anger, but occurs in an extreme form beyond any control on the part of the subject. However, the valid existence of the rage response is controversial. The concept is derived from experimental work with animals in which lesions to the SEPTAL AREA produce a rage-like reaction. It has been inferred that dysfunction of the septal region and associated elements of the LIMBIC SYSTEM in humans may produce similar behavioral consequences, including the rage response. Episodic dyscontrol in children, manifest as outbursts of explosive violent behavior, has been argued to have a similar origin. It is certainly the case that poorly controlled aggressive behavior may follow cerebral lesions; it is whether this is sufficiently similar to the phenomenon seen in experimental animals to be termed the "rage response" that is still a matter for debate.

rCBF *See* BLOOD FLOW STUDIES.

reading disorders *See* DYSLEXIA.

recovery of function In neuropsychology, "recovery of function" is generally taken to mean that cognitive, sensory, or motor deficits normally occurring after brain damage are reduced or eliminated. In the clinic, measures of functional recovery are usually taken at the behavioral level of analysis and the underlying physiological mechanisms are not well understood. Despite growing interest and research in the field of neural plasticity, both "function" and "recovery" are terms that still are not very clearly defined

except in a strictly operational sense. For example, spatial "functions" of the rat are routinely examined in the radial arm maze and performance of that task is used to define "spatial function." If the brain-damaged rat performs well on this defined task, then that is the definition of "recovery." Thus the laboratory investigator defines recovery when an animal can achieve a particular goal in a maze, regardless of how the task is accomplished by the subject.

From one behavioral perspective that is critical of the concept of recovery, it has been argued that recovery need not be identical to the function(s) lost as a result of the injury. In this model, one can argue that subjects simply substitute new behavioral strategies for those that were lost following their CNS damage. Sometimes the tricks employed for such substitution are very subtle and, at first glance, the behavior(s) would seem to be quite normal. Here deficits would only be revealed under very careful scrutiny or by sophisticated testing techniques. It has also been argued that focusing on the achievement of a goal (ends) rather than how the goal is achieved (means) can lead to false conclusions about the substrate of recovery – if indeed it can be said to occur at all. This latter position is one that has been used by those who argue that brain damage always results in permanent and irreversible loss of function. Unfortunately, the issue is made more complex when scientists, clinicians, and health-care professionals disagree on what they mean by "recovery of function." The trauma surgeon may define recovery when the patient emerges from coma and can be removed from intensive care. The social workers or nursing staff may report recovery when the patient no longer requires hand feeding or other personal attentions, while the workman's compensation insurance company representative may define recovery when the patient is capable of returning to the job. On top of

608

all this the patient's lawyer may have yet another definition based on whether the client can function exactly as he or she did before they suffered the trauma. Which of these is the most appropriate definition of functional recovery?

Part of the historical resistance to the concept of recovery from brain damage is that evidence for return of function is quite difficult to reconcile with the long-held doctrine of cerebral localization of function – especially if the doctrine is taken in its most literal sense (Lashley, 1933). For example, if the adult brain is considered to be hard-wired, with each specific and discrete anatomical area responsible for the mediation of a given behavior, extensive removal or significant damage to an area must lead unequivocally to loss of that particular function. Poppel (1989) recently defined CNS functions "as those that, in principle, can be lost after circumscribed injuries of the brain." Another recent example of the localization perspective can be taken from a highly popular textbook of contemporary neuroscience. Here Kandel and Schwartz (1990) write that:

> Clinical studies and their counterparts in experimental animals suggest that all behavior, including higher (cognitive as well as affective) mental functions, is localizable to specific regions or constellations of regions within the brain. (p. 15)

In order to localize function it is first necessary to define what the term itself means; however, it should be noted that the actual definition of the term "function" is rarely provided. Both functions and recovery are inferred from alterations from normal behavior in animals with lesions or, more recently, by the metabolic or electrophysiologic activation of CNS areas which can now be measured by use of computer assisted tomography (CAT), by cerebral blood flow measures, or by magnetic resonance imaging. These techniques do not measure behavior per se but, instead, they are indirect measures of molecular activities that are taken to represent complex cognitive processes. While it is true that much inferential data can be generated with these new tools, they do not measure or define behavioral function. They are, however, a good reflection of how the paradigm permits the development of methods specifically designed to support its hypotheses.

Patricia Churchland (1986) argues that the concept of localization of function is not quite as straightforward as it seems. "If A is the lesioned [sic] area and the patient can no longer do Y, then A is the center for Y? For many reasons, the answer must be no" (p. 163). As Churchland points out, an area could be a necessary link in the mediation of behavior without its being sufficient for the behavior in question to occur. Also damage to area A could have far-reaching consequences on other structures whose changes in activity could be responsible for the behavioral alterations. Churchland states that:

> Breezy use of the [concept of localization] will yield a bizarre catalogue of centers – including for example, a center for inhibiting religious fanaticism, since lesions in certain areas of the temporal lobe sometimes result in a patient's acquiring a besotted religious zeal ... the willy-nilly nature of Gall's phrenological catalogue comes back to haunt us. (p. 164)

Until very recently the strict localization perspective was the prevailing paradigm in the field of clinical neuropsychology and indeed served as a very useful diagnostic and simplified didactic tool for developing a concept about how the brain works. It was also the basis for most of the diagnostic testing of patients with brain lesions, i.e. determination of the locus of the lesion and the behavioral symptoms that were likely to ensue from the loss of that specific tissue. In the laboratory, lesion research was concerned with the experimental creation of injury, the precise measurement of the lesion parameters (e.g. locus and extent of the damage, tracing of neural degeneration, and alterations of pathways) and the careful description of behavioral deficits caused by the damage to provide support for the clinical observations. For the most part, recovery of function, when and if noticed, was considered to be a curious "anomaly" outside the pale of serious, scientific inquiry (Finger & Stein, 1982, Chapter 1).

Despite the problems I have only briefly addressed above, there is now an extensive literature demonstrating functional recovery in the adult mammalian central nervous system. Although there have been consistent clinical reports of patients who seem to show dramatic improvement after traumatic brain damage, recovery of function usually does not occur spontaneously, i.e. in the absence of a specific context or without some form of therapeutic intervention. With respect to the former, one example of how context can influence the functional outcome of traumatic brain damage is provided by the work of Anderson and others (1990). These investigators carefully matched patients with slow-growing tumors localized to the anterior left hemisphere with patients who suffered stroke-induced lesions of the same area. Thus, in one case, the injury to cerebral tissue was induced slowly, while in the other the injury occurred with rapid onset. To use a Jacksonian term, the "momentum of the lesions" was very different although the extent of damage was the same. After careful matching of lesion parameters the patients received a variety of neuropsychological tests to evaluate verbal and nonverbal intellect, verbal and visual memory, speech and language. Anderson and colleagues found that the patients with cerebral tumors had dramatically different neuropsychological profiles from patients with the same locus and extent of damage caused by stroke. All of the subjects with stroke in the left hemisphere had much more severe language impairments than the patients with tumors, and some of the tumor patients had no impairments at all on any of the tests, despite the extensive brain damage.

The data from Anderson and others can be taken as a direct extension of animal research in rats, cats, and monkeys on what has been characterized as the "serial lesion effect" (reviewed in detail by Finger and Stein, 1982) in which slowly inflicted brain lesions (aspiration, neurotoxins, electrocoagulations) in a wide variety of structures (for example: frontal cortex, hippocampus, visual cortex, hypothalamus, reticular formation) result in markedly reduced or no impairments compared to intact counterparts or those with identical damage created in a single stage. In the animal literature the context is simply the momentum of the lesion, since all damage is inflicted using the same technique. With respect to the clinical data, the "contexts" of the injuries are twofold: the type of injury (tumor versus stroke) and the momentum of the damage (slow versus rapid onset).

Another example of a "contextual factor" influencing recovery is the gender of the subject. Although there is a growing awareness that there are sexually dimorphic structures in the brain (e.g. Juraska, 1991), virtually nothing is known about whether there are systematic gender differences in response to brain damage. In one study, Attella

and others (1987) found that, by manipulating the levels of circulating progesterone and estrogen at the time of brain injury, they could dramatically reduce the deficits caused by bilateral removal of the frontal cortex. If female rats received injury when high levels of estrogen were present, the behavioral deficits in spatial learning were long-lasting. When other females were made "pseudo-pregnant" to reduce estrogen and to increase progesterone just prior to surgery, the behavioral impairments were dramatically reduced.

More recently, Roof and colleagues (1992a) were able to show that progesterone can eliminate the cerebral edema that often accompanies brain damage and that the presence of this hormone may account for why normally cycling female rats given contusion injuries of the frontal cortex have much less edema than males. When pseudopregnancy is introduced to increase the level of progesterone, contusion-induced edema is completely eliminated in females. Surprisingly, edema can also be dramatically reduced in male rats given injections of progesterone at the time of injury (Roof et al., 1992b). Aside from the therapeutic implications, considered together, these different studies can be taken to indicate that the outcome of traumatic brain damage is not just a question of which area is damaged, but depends to a very great extent on the "various contextual factors" present at the time injury occurs.

It may very well be the case that certain brain regions in adult subjects are incapable of showing any kind of recovery or "plasticity" no matter what maneuvers are attempted. Such questions need to be empirically tested, but failure to find recovery after a short period of time, after a single manipulation, or even a series of experiments may only indicate that the right maneuver has yet to be found rather than that there is no inherent capacity for recovery. The neurologist Norman Geschwind (1985) made this point when referring to recovery from the aphasias. He stated that:

> Most neurologists are gloomy about the prognosis of severe adult aphasias after a few weeks and pessimism is reinforced by a lack of prolonged follow-up in most cases. I have, however, seen patients severely aphasic for over one year, who then made an excellent recovery. One patient returned to work as a salesman, the other as a psychiatrist. Furthermore there are patients who continue to improve over many years, for example, the patient whose aphasia is still quite

evident six years after onset, cleared up substantially by 18 years. (p. 3)

As evidence pertaining to the "plasticity" of the adult CNS began to accumulate, i.e. that functional recovery could occur under appropriate conditions, the localization doctrine has been slightly modified by introducing the concept of "serial and parallel processing circuits" (and areas). Simply stated, recovery can now be accepted by redefining structure–function relationships in the CNS. For example, instead of a single structure or a small aggregate of areas mediating function, it is now argued that complex functions may require the simultaneous integration of a network of structures acting in unison to produce the behavior.

One way to examine functional reorganization in patients is with the use of positron emission tomography (PET). This technique allows investigators to make comparisons of regional blood flow which are then taken to indicate the role of different brain structures in recovery from stroke, ischemia, or injury. Weiller and colleagues (1992) used PET to examine motor recovery after striatocapsular infarction in adult patients. These clinicians were able to show that there were widespread changes in the pattern of cerebral blood flow in the brain ipsilateral and contralateral to the injured side. As recovery of hand movements and use proceeded, cerebral activation was noted in both hemispheres. Rather than observing localized changes in blood flow, there was widespread distribution of networks affected by the localized lesion and a very complex pattern of functional reorganization concomitant with the behavioral recovery. The authors suggested that "major mechanisms for the restoration of function may include bilateral activation of the motor system with use of ipsilateral pathways and recruitment of additional motor areas" (p. 471). In a similar study using the PET technique, Chollet and others (1991) studied cerebral blood flow and functional recovery in patients with unilateral stroke in the area of the middle cerebral artery. Alterations in cerebral blood flow associated with the return of hand movements were seen in the sensorimotor cortex, the inferior parietal cortex of both hemispheres and cerebellum, to name some of the affected structures. One might ask, in the face of such complexity, what then is **not** interrelated, and what "functions" are, indeed, critic-

ally localized without possibility of recovery? Concepts of serial and parallel processing are certainly a step in the right direction for models of CNS plasticity; however, the addition of more and more blocks to already complex structures still does not address the issue of how the pieces work together or how compensation occurs when the system is injured.

METHODOLOGICAL AND CONCEPTUAL ISSUES REMAINING IN RESEARCH ON RECOVERY

1. Although considerable progress is being made, we do not yet understand all of the conditions that mitigate against recovery from brain injury. When recovery is observed, we do not know whether it is permanent or whether, with aging or other systemic changes, the deficits might return.

2. There is no agreement on what is meant by the terms "function" and "recovery." However, we do know that brain damage itself is not a monolithic event limited to a highly focalized region. Instead, it is generally agreed that injury causes a cascade of biochemical and structural changes, beginning immediately after damage and progressing for days, weeks and perhaps even years after the initial trauma.

3. Injury-induced regenerative events such as axonal sprouting, neurogenesis, dendritic hypertrophy, membrane receptor reorganization, etc., are good examples of CNS "plasticity" but they may not be good examples of functional recovery. If traumatic brain damage or degenerative diseases can produce reorganization of neural pathways, such reorganization can be either beneficial or detrimental. Only functional assessments of the organism's behavior can determine if new synaptic connections are adaptive or dysfunctional. For example, new collateral axonal growth or the emergence of new pathways and receptive fields may be a sign of plasticity, but if such events result in disordered perception, muscular spasticity, or impaired cognition they can hardly be considered beneficial. Only long-term behavioral follow-ups can determine whether functional recovery is attained and maintained to the benefit of the organism. Since only approximately 10 percent of current neuroscience research in the field of neuroplasticity is concerned with behavioral outcomes, this is not a trivial problem.

4. The effects of localized damage need to be viewed in the context of how the injury alters

611

cerebral organization. Functional recovery is likely to be the result of multiple processes distributed throughout the central nervous system rather than coming about through local changes in small neural networks. New technologies such as PET, MRI, and SPECT (*see* LOCALIZATION) and even fetal brain-tissue grafts, give us the opportunity to examine these complex processes in living beings so that correlations between "behavioral functions" and physiological processes can be evaluated systematically. From these technologies we can perhaps gain some insight into the patterns of disruption leading to expression of symptoms as well as the potential mechanisms underlying recovery.

5. In some circles there is growing awareness that the study of the mammalian central nervous system and its capacity for functional recovery may not be amenable to the same methods traditionally applied to the examination of small, orderly systems. Much of current neuroscience research is still predicated upon the paradigm that one can understand all the complexity of the brain by studying its molecular components individually and then predicting functions (and recovery) from detailed analysis of the individual parts. Bak and Chen (1991) use chaos theory to describe highly complex, self-organizing systems (European monetary systems, economics and banking, avalanches, *and the brain*). They argue that such systems exist in very dynamic balance so that even a minor event (loss of confidence in the lire, or a focal stroke in the motor cortex, for example) can affect any number or even all elements in the system. Applying this thinking to recovery of function, it needs to be reiterated that it is likely to be the result of multiple events and dynamic changes throughout the brain, although the processes may be initiated by relatively local events. Just as bricks alone are not a building, the physiological substrates we carefully describe are not the recovery itself but rather components of it. Although molecular neuroscience has much to contribute to our understanding of CNS plasticity and to our development of effective treatments, the only way to examine recovery of *function* is to examine what organisms are capable of doing before, during, or after treatment. Behavior is just as much a product of nervous system activity as alterations in receptor binding sites, regulation of neurotransmitters, or the generation of evoked potentials. In the final analysis it may be the best measure we have of functional recovery after damage to the central nervous system.

Note The author would like to express his appreciation to Dr Revital Duvdevani and Ms Marlou Glasier for their help and advice in the preparation of this essay.

BIBLIOGRAPHY

Anderson, S. W., Damasio, H., & Tranel, D. (1990). Neuropsychological impairments caused by tumor or stroke. *Archives of Neurology*, *47*, 397–405.

Attella, M., Nattinville, A., & Stein, D. G. (1987). Hormonal state affects recovery from frontal cortex lesions in adult female rats. *Behavioral and Neural Biology*, *48*, 352–67.

Bak, P., & Chen, K. (1991). Self-organized criticality. *Scientific American*, 41–53.

Chollet, F., Di Piero, V., Wise, R. J. S., Books, D. J., Dolan, R. J., & Frackowiak, R. S. J. (1991). The functional anatomy of motor recovery after stroke in humans: a study with positron emission tomography. *Annals of Neurology*, *29*, 63–71.

Churchland, P. S. (1986). *Neurophilosophy: Toward a science of the mind/brain*. Cambridge, MA: MIT Press.

Finger, S., & Stein, D. G. (1982). *Brain damage and recovery: research and clinical perspectives* (pp. 153–74). New York: Academic Press.

Finger, S., LeVere, T. E., Almli, C. R., & Stein, D. G. (1988). Recovery of function: sources of controversy. In S. Finger, T. E. LeVere, C. R. Almli, & D. G. Stein (Eds), *Brain injury and recovery: Theoretical and controversial issues* (pp. 351–62). New York: Plenum Press.

Geschwind, N. (1985). Mechanisms of change after brain lesions. In F. Nottebohm (Ed.), *Hope for a new neurology. Annals of the New York Academy of Science*, *457*, 1–11.

Juraska, J. M. (1991). Sex differences in "cognitive" regions of the rat brain. *Psychoneuroendocrinology*, *16*, 105–19.

Kandel, E., & Schwartz, J. H. (Eds). (1990). *Principles of neuroscience*. New York: Elsevier.

Lashley, K. (1933). Integrative functions of the cerebral cortex, *Physiological Review*, *13*, 1–42.

Poppel, E. (1989). Taxonomy of the subjective: an evolutionary perspective. In J. W. Brown (Ed.), *Neuropsychology of visual perception* (pp. 219–32). Hillsdale, NJ: Erlbaum.

Roof, R. L., Duvdevani, R., & Stein, D. G. (1992a). Progesterone treatment attenuates brain edema following contusion injury in male and female rats. *Restorative Neurology and Neuroscience*, 6, 425–8.

Roof, R. L., Duvdevani, R., & Stein, D. G. (1992b). Gender influences outcome of brain injury: progesterone plays a protective role. *Society for Neuroscience Abstracts* (80.6), 179.

Weiller, C., Chollet, F., Friston, K. J., Wise, R. J. S., & Frackowiak, R. S. J. (1992). Functional reorganization of the brain in recovery from striatocapsular infarction in Man. *Annals of Neurology*, 31, 463–72.

DONALD G. STEIN

reduplication Patients experiencing reduplication are convinced that people or things have exact or nearly exact duplicates. This can involve believing that relatives have been replaced by impostors (Capgras delusion), the hospital is a replica of the one everyone else claims to be in (reduplicative paramnesia), objects are being replaced by copies, or that the patient has an extra arm or leg.

The duplicated items usually have strong emotional significance (Weinstein & Burnham, 1991). Patients can be otherwise well oriented; although the delusions are subjectively convincing, they may acknowledge how absurd their claims must seem.

Reduplication is not as rare as was once thought, at least as a transitory phenomenon; 5 percent of outpatients with Alzheimer's disease had suffered the Capgras delusion (Mendez et al., 1992) and 8 percent of alcoholic inpatients had reduplicative paramnesias (Hakim et al., 1988).

REDUPLICATIVE PARAMNESIA

The term comes from Pick (1903). Both of Pick's patients duplicated the hospital environment, but for patient 1 the hospital staff and patients had been duplicated as well, while when patient 2 was asked how the same staff and patients could be in both clinics she replied that "They come from one place to the other."

CAPGRAS DELUSION

This delusion was identified in the 1920s by the French psychiatrist Capgras (Ellis et al., 1994). An early hypothesis was that conflicting feelings of love and hate are resolved by the delusion, since the double can be hated without guilt, but reports of brain damage in many patients show that psychodynamic accounts do not offer a full explanation.

Physical violence has been noted, including murder (Silva et al., 1989). However, violence is not the norm. Most Capgras patients do not show much concern about what has happened to the real relatives, and many are friendly toward the duplicates.

REDUPLICATION AND THE RIGHT HEMISPHERE

Reduplicative delusions are linked to brain injury affecting the right cerebral HEMISPHERE: for patients suffering delusional misidentification (including Capgras delusion) with focal lesions the injuries were right-sided in 19 of 20 cases reviewed by Förstl and others (1991), and in Hakim and others' (1988) prospective study 3 of 4 patients with reduplicative paramnesias had right hemisphere lesions and none had a left hemisphere lesion.

ACCOUNTING FOR REDUPLICATION

Right hemisphere damage does not in itself explain the strange content of reduplicative delusions. They probably reflect an interaction of impairments, in which some form of anomalous experience created by a cognitive or perceptual deficit is misinterpreted (Young et al., 1993). For example, the Capgras delusion may follow damage to pathways responsible for appropriate emotional reactions to familiar visual stimuli. On this hypothesis, the delusion involves the patients' mistaking a change in themselves for a change in others.

BIBLIOGRAPHY

Ellis, H. D., Whitley, J., & Luauté, J.-P. (1994). Classic text no. 17. Delusional misidentification. The three original papers on the Capgras, Frégoli and intermetamorphosis delusions. *History of Psychiatry*, 5, 117–46.

Förstl, H., Almeida, O. P., Owen, A. M., Burns, A., & Howard, R. (1991). Psychiatric, neurological and medical aspects of misidentification syndromes: a review of 260 cases. *Psychological Medicine*, 21, 905–10.

Hakim, H., Verma, N. P., & Greiffenstein, M. F. (1988). Pathogenesis of reduplicative paramnesia. *Journal of Neurology, Neurosurgery, and Psychiatry*, 51, 839–41.

Mendez, M. F., Martin, R. J., Smyth, K. A., & Whitehouse, P. J. (1992). Disturbances of person identification in Alzheimer's disease: a retrospective study. *Journal of Nervous and Mental Disease*, *180*, 94–6.

Pick, A. (1903). Clinical studies: III. On reduplicative paramnesia. *Brain*, *26*, 260–7.

Silva, J. A., Leong, G. B., Weinstock, R., & Boyer, C. L. (1989). Capgras syndrome and dangerousness. *Bulletin of the American Academy of Psychiatry and the Law*, *17*, 5–14.

Weinstein, E. A., & Burnham, D. L. (1991). Reduplication and the syndrome of Capgras. *Psychiatry*, *54*, 78–88.

Young, A. W., Reid, I., Wright, S., & Hellawell, D. J. (1993). Face-processing impairments and the Capgras delusion. *British Journal of Psychiatry*, *162*, 695–8.

ANDREW W. YOUNG

reflex epilepsy *See* EPILEPSY.

reflexes Reflexes are important forms of reaction or movement in animals and Man, often misconceived as the stereotyped automatic responses to some sensory input.

The term "reflex" goes back to the seventeenth-century philosopher and scientist René Descartes, who described animal and human behavior in mechanistic terms. In his example of a typical reflex response, a man's foot inadvertently hits a hot object, whereupon the foot is involuntarily withdrawn by flexing the leg. Descartes provided a mechanistic and in part an ingenious explanation of how this reaction is brought about by the nervous system and its executive instruments (muscles, etc.). Very often it is this type of "nocifensive" avoidance reaction that everyday language refers to as a reflex, but there are many others involved in various aspects of the control of motor behavior and internal body states. Descartes borrowed the term "reflex" from optics, suggesting that motor output is a simple (mirror-like) "reflection" by the central nervous system (CNS) of some sensory input. This view is simplistic. It will be made clear that the term "reflex," as currently used, encompasses quite complex behaviors. This is already demonstrated

by the above example, because withdrawing a foot requires stabilization of equilibrium, which amounts to setting in action a complex set of postural adjustments, which in turn depend on initial conditions.

Reflexes are closely tied to sensory input generated by specialized sensory receptor cells. Roughly, since this sensory input may originate inside or outside the body, i.e. be generated by "proprioceptive" or "exteroceptive" sensory receptors, reflexes may be classified likewise (Hasan & Stuart, 1988). But in various cases these classes overlap. For example, cutaneous receptors may be excited by external stimuli (pressure, touch, vibration) subserving TACTILE PERCEPTION, but they are also activated by the body's self-generated motions. Thus they are proprio- as well as exteroceptors and can be involved in both classes of reflex.

From the *vast multitude of reflexes*, a few examples have been chosen to elucidate several *basic principles*. These principles, albeit applying – mutatis mutandis – to Man, have most intensively been worked out in ANIMAL STUDIES. It will therefore be necessary to draw upon this work in some detail. For simplicity, the examples are taken predominantly from somatic sensorimotor control systems.

THE SIMPLEST REFLEXES: MONOSYNAPTIC TENDON REFLEX

The simplest possible mirror-like reflexes may be assumed to be the ones *including the least number of synapses* between the neurons involved. A well-known specimen is the so-called "tendon reflex," which in neurology is used to test the excitability of the CNS. It is evoked by a tap on a muscle tendon, which briefly stretches the muscle and its in-dwelling length receptors, so-called "muscle spindles." The spindles are innervated by thick sensory nerve fibers, classified as "Ia" afferents. A set of these Ia afferents is excited by the brief stretch and transmits the excitation via a single synapse (monosynaptically) to a set of alpha motor neurons in the CNS. The motor neurons in turn innervate, excite, and make contract the skeletal muscle fibers of the ("homonymous") muscle originally stretched. Hence the muscle stretch stimulus causes a delayed muscle contraction. The reflex appears to simply stabilize muscle length in face of external perturbations (which might classify it as an exteroceptive reflex).

Indeed, Sherrington (1924) thought that an assembly of such reflexes, one for each skeletal muscle, stabilizes the lengths, especially of extensor muscles, and thus maintains upright posture against gravity. However, there are problems with this view.

1. Monosynaptic connections of Ia afferents from one muscle are not confined to homonymous motor neurons, but are also made in a *divergent* manner with motor neurons innervating functionally related (synergist) muscles, even those acting around other joints. Conversely, motor neurons receive *convergent* input from Ia afferents from other muscles. This *divergence–convergence connectivity pattern*, representing a more general principle of CNS networks, may contribute to organizing *synergies of muscle activations* during various motor acts.

2. Muscle spindles are not passive length sensors, but – consisting of specialized muscle fibers themselves – they receive motor innervation from so-called gamma motor neurons. This efferent receptor control – not the only example – serves to excite and change the sensitivity to length and velocity of the receptors. This design led Merton (1953) to propose the *follow-up length servo loop hypothesis*: In slow voluntary movements, the motor commands descending in the spinal cord impinge primarily on the gamma motor neurons. These then activate muscle spindles which in turn reflexly excite alpha motor neurons, causing a muscle contraction. On this view, the *reflex is used as a tool ("servo")* in self-generated voluntary movement. The main advantage of this indirect muscle activation could lie in its insensitivity to internal and external disturbances, such as changes in internal system properties (e.g. muscle fatigue) and unexpected interference from the external world with the intended movement (Houk & Rymer, 1981). This is a well-known feature of *negative feedback systems*, of which there are many in the nervous system (e.g. the Breuer–Hering reflex contributing to the regulation of respiration, and many others regulating internal body state variables). However, Merton's hypothesis – although initiating a flood of fruitful experimental work – turned out to be untenable, one reason being that gamma motor neurons do not start firing – as they should – before alpha motor neurons.

3. The synaptic effects of Ia afferents on alpha motor neurons are subject to change by "presynaptic inhibition," a widespread means to *modulate synaptic transmission*. It is exerted by inhibitory interneurons which receive many other inputs from peripheral afferents and spinally descending pathways conveying motor commands. Ia afferent-to-motor neuron reflex transmission is modulated during voluntary movement and different phases of gait. In general, then, the monosynaptic tendon reflex as well as most other reflexes are *state- and task-dependent*, i.e. variable in their gain and possibly other parameters. Another means to achieve this are *interneurons*. For instance, muscle stretch elicits not only monosynaptic spinal actions, but also effects transmitted through *long-latency neural pathways*, which in part may be localized in the spinal cord and in part may traverse the SENSORIMOTOR CORTEX (*long-loop reflexes*). Transmission through the cortex is highly dependent on a subject's "set" (e.g. ATTENTION, arousal, motivation, instruction; see Prochazka, 1989).

4. There are further muscle receptor afferents monitoring mechanical variables. For instance, Ib fibers from *muscle force-sensing tendon organs* exert reflex effects on motor neurons mediated via interneurons. Since these interneurons again receive many inputs from other afferents and descending motor tracts, their signal transmission properties are highly variable. Therefore, *the balance between force and length feedback* can be varied in a context- and task-dependent manner. For instance, during a *grasping movement*, length and velocity feedback is primarily important during the unloaded approach of the object; force feedback becomes prevalent upon grasping it (Prochazka, 1989). This demonstrates that individual reflexes that can be artificially singled out on account of their special receptor origin are usually embedded in an ensemble of parallel ones which act together in a motor act, albeit with shifting weights. Parallel distributed processing of different variables through parallel pathways is a common principle in the nervous system.

REFLEX GATING

The effect of reflexes is also changed rhythmically during *locomotion*. In vertebrates, the basic locomotor rhythm and appropriate pattern of muscle activations can be generated without sensory feedback by spinal neuronal networks (*central pattern generators: CPG*). The activity of these CPG's can completely alter the effect of some reflexes. For instance, during cat locomotion, cutaneous input excited by obstacles interfering with the flexion movement (swing phase) of a limb causes additional limb flexion to obviate the obstacle, but during the stance phase the same stimulus causes enhanced extension. Thus, depending on the step phase, the elicited *reflexes can be reversed* (or otherwise "*gated*") by the CPG, in a behaviorally meaningful way.

Another example of phase-dependent reflex reversal is provided by the reflexes elicited by excitation of the above-mentioned muscle force-sensitive tendon organs. Whereas in quiescent preparations, Ib afferents from extensor muscles exert widespread inhibition on leg extensor motor neurons, this effect is reduced or abolished during locomotion. Instead, extensor Ib afferents activate extensor motor neurons and inhibit ipsilateral flexor motor neurons, effects that vary in size according to the phase of the locomotor step cycle. During the stance phase, then, this positive feedback reinforces force production. Moreover, in the late stance phase extensor force and Ib afferent discharge decline and may thus release flexors from inhibition and facilitate initiation of the swing phase (Pearson, 1993).

REFLEXES INCORPORATING PATTERN GENERATORS

Many reflexes incorporate neuronal networks which generate *more or less complex sequential patterns of muscle activations*. Examples are the scratch reflex of the cat and the wiping reflex of the frog.

In cats, the scratch reflex is "switched on" by an irritating stimulus to a defined skin area of the anterior body (Gelfand et al., 1988). The reflex consists of two components: the hindlimb is first flexed into a starting position, while postural adjustments are being carried out by the other limbs to stabilize the body; the scratching limb then goes through a sequence of oscillations. The *spinal pattern generator* of this activity has been shown to be distributed along the lower spinal cord and is autonomous insofar as it does not depend on sensory feedback except on the triggering stimulus. The neuronal network defining the pattern generator has not yet been identified, but its operation has been clarified by modelling techniques (Gelfand et al., 1988). If, in the frog, a small noxious stimulus is applied to its dorsal skin surface, it will wipe it off with one (usually the

nearest) hindlimb, whose movement goes through a *sequence of well coordinated stages* (flexion, placement, aiming, whisking, extension; Berkinblit et al., 1986). The precise execution of this reflex is adaptable to initial conditions such as the positions of stimulus and hindlimb and the load on the latter.

These behaviors are entirely generated in the spinal cord which therefore must incorporate a partial body schema, for in both reflexes the well coordinated motor act has to be, and is, spatially related to the location of the stimulus.

INTERNAL MODELS AND SENSORI-MOTOR TRANSFORMATIONS

A reflex fundamental to spatial orientation is the vestibulo-ocular reflex (VOR). At least temporarily, it stabilizes the image of the external world on the retina during involuntary head acceleration about some axis (GAZE stabilization). To achieve this, the EYE MOVEMENT has to be as large as, but opposite to, the head movement. If this is the case, the gain of the reflex (opposing eye movement amplitude vs eliciting head movement amplitude) has the value of 1. Head acceleration is sensed by receptors in the semicircular canals of the vestibular labyrinth (*see* VESTIBULAR STIMULATION). The shortest pathway from these afferents to oculomotor neurons is disynaptic, involving only secondary vestibular neurons as interneurons. The VOR demonstrates well the important features of several reflexes: the construction of *internal models representing the properties of the plant operated on*, and the performance of *sensorimotor transformations*.

The internal model of the VOR organizing the compensatory eye movement must incorporate two features: (1) It must take into account the viscoelastic properties of the plant (bulbus moved in orbit by extraocular muscles). Since the afferent vestibular signal reflects head velocity, eye velocity can easily be derived from it by an appropriate amplification. This component of the motor command to the eye muscles has to compensate for viscosity. The eye position, however, needs to be maintained against an elastic force, for which a tonic command component is necessary. This can be derived from the vestibular signal by a *neuronal integrator* (Robinson, 1981); (2) To rotate the eye about the opposite axis to that of the head, each semicircular canal must establish appropriate weighted connections to each eye motor neuron pool. Since rotations of the head about different axes activate canals differently, different combinations of muscle activity result. Thus, an array of sensory inputs must be converted into an array of motor outputs by a matrix *transformation between different frames of references*: the sensory one spanned by the planes of the semicircular canals and the motor frame spanned by the pulling directions of the extraocular muscles.

PLASTICITY OF REFLEXES

The VOR gain is highly modifiable at a short and a long time scale. When human subjects with eyes closed are sinusoidally rotated on a chair, performance of *arithmetic tasks* reduces the gain to 0.65; imagining a gaze target stationary in external space raises it to 0.95, while imagining a target moving with the subject lowers the gain to 0.35 (Robinson, 1981). Hence, this reflex exhibits the same *short-term task- and context-dependent characteristics* as the spinal and supraspinal reflexes discussed above. In addition to its short-term, state-dependent variability, the VOR shows a pronounced *longer-term plasticity* and therefore is a much investigated paradigm for "*motor learning.*" Its gain can be drastically altered by changing the magnification or direction of image projection onto the retina (using goggles or reversing prisms). Within hours to days, the reflex adapts to the new situation and functions perfectly well. The three-neuron reflex arc does not appear to be complex enough to provide for a PLASTICITY involving visual processing. However, there are longer parallel pathways including the flocculus of the CEREBELLUM, which could provide the required plasticity by modification of the parallel fiber–Purkinje cell synapse. Yet it has recently been proposed that, while the flocculus is indispensable for plasticity, it is not the locus of the gain change in the VOR; rather, synapses of BRAIN STEM neurons receiving vestibular inputs as well as inhibitory Purkinje cell and excitatory climbing fiber inputs are proposed as the targets of plasticity; the flocculus provides the visual information necessary to guide the learning process.

CELLULAR AND MOLECULAR MECHANISMS OF REFLEX PLASTICITY

Defensive reflexes such as the limb flexion reflex are able to be modified over time, exhibiting

habituation, dishabituation, and sensitization. These are considered *basic forms of learning and memory* (Hawkins et al., 1987). However, in vertebrates, the underlying cellular mechanisms could not hitherto be studied because the neuronal network has not yet been identified. By contrast, this is often the case in simpler invertebrate nervous systems (such as that of the sea mollusk *Aplysia californica*), which have therefore been used as models to study cellular and molecular mechanisms of learning and memory, in the hope that the basic processes will turn out to be similar to those in mammals, including humans. Aplysia's gill- and siphon-withdrawal reflex to skin stimulation has been studied most intensively.

Habituation (referred to by Pavlov as EXTINCTION) implies that, upon repeated stimulation, the reflex response becomes weaker. Its *short-term form*, lasting for minutes to an hour, comes about primarily through a progressive depression of NEUROTRANSMITTER release at the receptor-to-motor neuron connection. There is also a *long-term form*, which may involve morphological changes at the sensory neuron–motor neuron synapses. Habituation is primarily restricted to the particular receptor–motor neuron pathway stimulated, with little generalization to parallel ones ("homosynaptic" effect; Hawkins et al., 1987).

Dishabituation denotes the fast recovery of a habituated response upon strong, often noxious, stimulation of another reflex pathway. It involves both a removal of habituation and development of sensitization.

Sensitization designates the enhancement of a defensive response by a strong stimulus to another skin region. It thus involves *heterosynaptic* facilitation of one reflex pathway by another and bears some resemblance to classical conditioning, although temporal contingencies are not crucial. Again there is a short- and a long-term form. Even these simple learning processes occur at several different synaptic sites, representing again a form of parallel distributed processing. As long-term habituation, the equivalent form of sensitization may be based in part on morphological changes at the facilitated sensory neuron–motor neuron synapses (Hawkins et al., 1987).

The above forms of plasticity are referred to as *nonassociative* forms of learning, from which associative forms have traditionally been distin-

617

guished, in which a specific stimulus eliciting a reflex response is associated with and can later be replaced by a nonspecific conditioning (unconditioned) stimulus. To these forms belongs the *classical conditioning* of reflexes, of which Pavlov's dog salivating and producing gastric fluid in response to a tone or the rabbit's nictitating response to some auditory stimulus are well-known examples. However, nonassociative and associative classes may share common cellular and molecular mechanisms, e.g. classical conditioning may utilize the molecular mechanism of sensitization (Hawkins et al., 1987).

MULTIPLICITY OF REFLEX EFFECTS

In parallel to its "specific" reflex effect, a particular stimulus usually evokes a number of other effects, from postural adjustments to changes in vegetative variables such as heart rate, blood pressure, respiratory rate and volume, etc. This will involve great numbers of neurons, in particular interneurons. There are essentially two extreme ways in which the sensory neurons may be coupled to the various output neurons: via separate reflex pathways ("*labelled or dedicated lines*") or via a fairly random *divergence–convergence meshwork of connections*, in which, for instance, defined groups of neurons participate in different reflex actions. Probably there is a mixture of these extremes because, as mentioned above, habituation is essentially restricted to a particular reflex pathway, but there are also interneurons activated in various reflex responses. Some "privacy" of reflex pathways may still be obtained by – probably variable – weighting of synaptic connectivity. This type of organization almost certainly prevails throughout the nervous system up to the cerebral cortex of primates (Abeles, 1982; Windhorst, 1988).

CONCLUSIONS

In general, reflexes are nothing less than simple stereotyped "reflections." By contrast, they may be complex and sequenced actions, making use of and being integrated in intricate neuronal networks; they are versatile, modifiable, "gatable," and plastic responses capable of "learning" from past experience.

BIBLIOGRAPHY

Abeles, M. (1982). *Local cortical circuits: An electrophysiological study*. Berlin and New York: Springer-Verlag.

Berkinblit, M. B., Feldman, A. G., & Fukson, O. I. (1986). Adaptability of innate motor patterns and motor control. *Behavioral and Brain Sciences*, *9*, 585–99.

Gelfand, I. M., Orlovsky, G. N., & Shik, M. L. (1988). Locomotion and scratching in tetrapods. In A. H. Cohen, S. Rossignol, & S. Grillner (Eds), *Neural control of rhythmic movements in vertebrates* (pp. 167–99). New York: Wiley.

Hasan, Z., & Stuart, D. G. (1988). Animal solutions to problems of movement control: the role of proprioceptors. *Annual Review of Neuroscience*, *11*, 199–223.

Hawkins, R. D., Clark, G. A., & Kandel, E. R. (1987). Cell biological studies of learning in simple vertebrate and invertebrate systems. In F. Plum (Ed.), *Handbook of physiology*, Sect. 1: *The nervous system*, Vol. V: *Higher functions of the brain*, Part 1 (pp. 25–83). Bethesda, MD: American Physiological Society.

Houk, J. C., & Rymer, W. Z. (1981). Neural control of muscle length and tension. In V. B. Brooks (Ed.), *Handbook of physiology*, Sect. 1: *The nervous system*, Vol. II, Part 1 (pp. 257–323). Bethesda, MD: American Physiological Society.

Merton, P. A. (1953). Speculations on the servo-control of movement. In G. E. W. Wolstenholme (Ed.), *The spinal cord* (pp. 247–55). London: Churchill.

Pearson, K. G. (1993). Common principles of motor control in vertebrates and invertebrates. *Annual Review of Neuroscience*, *16*, 265–97.

Prochazka, A. (1989). Sensorimotor gain control: a basic strategy of the motor system? *Progress in Neurobiology*, *33*, 281–307.

Robinson, D. A. (1981). Control of eye movements. In V. B. Brooks (Ed.), *Handbook of physiology*, Sect. 1: *The nervous system*, Vol. II: *Motor control*, Part 2 (pp. 1275–310). Bethesda, MD: American Physiological Society.

Sherrington, C. S. (1924). Problems of muscular receptivity. *Nature*, *113*, 929–32.

Windhorst, U. (1988). *How brain-like is the spinal cord? Interacting cell assemblies in the nervous system*. Berlin and New York: Springer-Verlag.

UWE R. WINDHORST

rehabilitation Neuropsychological rehabilitation can be neatly subsumed within a general definition of rehabilitation offered by the World Health Organization which stated, at a meeting held in Finland (1986), that "Rehabilitation implies the restoration of patients to the highest level of physical, psychological and social adaptation attainable. It includes all measures aimed at reducing the impact of disabling and handicapping conditions and at enabling disabled people to achieve optimum social integration" (p. 1).

Although, for the most part, neuropsychological rehabilitation is concerned specifically with cognitive deficits, there are obvious areas of overlap involving the treatment of emotional, personality, and physical deficits resulting from injury or insult to the brain. The effects these deficits have on behavior are of paramount interest to the neuropsychologist involved in rehabilitation. Indeed, neuropsychology is recognized as the study of the relationship between brain and behavior.

The term "neuropsychological rehabilitation" began to be widely used as late as the 1980s, and consistent reference to it as a term referring to a specific area of rehabilitative work appeared in a book entitled *Neuropsychological Rehabilitation after Brain Injury*, by Prigatano and others, in 1986. A further book, simply entitled *Neuropsychological Rehabilitation*, appeared in 1987 and was edited by Meier, Benton, and Diller. A journal of the same title began to be published in 1991.

The term "cognitive rehabilitation" also gained popular usage in the 1980s, and in the latter half of the decade a journal of this title was first published. While it is true that there is much overlap between the two areas, neuropsychological rehabilitation can be said to differ from cognitive rehabilitation in that it encompasses the broader range of disorders outlined above.

Despite the apparent youthfulness of the discipline, attempts to rehabilitate brain-injured people go back as far as ancient Greece and Egypt. The earliest known treatment for head injury is found in an Egyptian document of 2500–3000 years ago, discovered by Smith in Luxor in 1862 (quoted by Walsh, 1987).

Many of the techniques used in rehabilitation today were anticipated by Itard in the eighteenth century in his work with Victor, the Wild Boy of Aveyron (Lane, 1977), but modern rehabilitation of brain-injured people probably began in Germany during World War I as a result of improvements in the survival rates of head-injured soldiers, due to the introduction of more effective neurosurgical techniques. A further impetus came during World War II with developments in Germany, the Soviet Union, the United States, and Britain. Oliver Zangwill's (1945) review recounts the work at the Brain Injuries Unit in Edinburgh. Boake (1989) reports on the history of cognitive rehabilitation for head-injured patients from 1915 to 1980.

Luria and his colleagues were active in neuropsychological rehabilitation in the Soviet Union and the publications of Luria and others (1963; 1969) have offered a rich source of material for contemporary neuropsychologists.

Current interest in neuropsychological rehabilitation is growing rapidly and is reflected in numerous conferences, debates, books, and papers. This interest has been stimulated by both scientific research and improved clinical practice. There is increasing interest in research that seeks answers to questions aimed at improving the quality of life for brain-injured people.

MAJOR CONCERNS OF NEUROPSYCHOLOGICAL REHABILITATION

While it is true that natural recovery and PLASTICITY are important areas in the field of neuropsychological rehabilitation, they are of less *direct* interest than assessment and treatment, and this entry will concentrate on the latter. Readers interested in natural recovery after head injury are referred to Thomsen (1987). Bamford and others (1990) discuss the long-term outcome after stroke; Wade and Hewer (1987) discuss recovery from aphasia; Kertesz (1979) considers recovery from visual object agnosia; and Wilson (1991) reviews the long-term prognosis of patients with severe memory disorders.

Assessment

Appropriate assessment for neuropsychological rehabilitation is of paramount importance and is a prerequisite for effective treatment and management. Assessment is carried out in order to answer questions. Neuropsychological assessment can answer questions about a person's current intellectual functioning, probable premorbid level, areas of cognitive strengths and weaknesses, type of specific cognitive disorder (e.g. "Is the subject with acquired DYSLEXIA suffering from deep dyslexia, phonological dyslexia, or letter-by-letter dyslexia?"), and the subject's comparative standing with others of the same age or diagnostic group.

Bearing in mind our initial definition of neuropsychological rehabilitation fitting within the requirements of the World Health Organization when it stated that rehabilitation should enable "disabled people to achieve optimum social integration," then it is essential that workers in the field consider the everyday implications for patients with brain injuries. Despite the fact that some assessment tools are specially designed to predict possible difficulties likely to be experienced by brain-injured people in their daily lives, it remains true that neuropsychological assessment does not provide detailed information about the nature, frequency, or severity of problems faced by brain-injured people in their daily lives. Indeed, there is often a poor correlation between test performance and ability to function at home or work.

Everyday problems can be assessed more effectively and accurately by direct observation, interviews, role playing, or the recording of behavior in analogue situations designed to be similar to those encountered in real life (e.g. an office, shop, or restaurant). Therapists working in the field of neuropsychological rehabilitation may also be called upon to assess the physical and social environment in which the patient lives in order to assess its effect on learning or to determine whether environmental change can reduce or bypass certain cognitive, social, or emotional difficulties. Rating scales, checklists, or questionnaires may be used to pinpoint everyday manifestations of neuropsychological problems.

Caution must be exercised in interpreting results, as there may be a wide gap between what people *think* they experience and what they actually experience. Wilson and colleagues (1989) show, for example, that severely memory-impaired people underestimate the extent of their problems. This discrepancy has also been demonstrated in people who are not brain-injured. It has been shown, for example, that patients with rheumatoid arthritis thought they had changed their joint-protection behavior as a result of attending a group aimed at learning about joint-protection principles, but videotapes of their real-life behaviors demonstrated no significant change in their behavior before and after treatment.

When planning a treatment program in neuropsychological rehabilitation it is necessary to combine information from both formal, standardized assessments and observational or direct assessments. Although an inability to perform a particular test is not an area for treatment, it is nevertheless essential to understand and appreciate the cognitive, emotional, and physical status of each client in order to maximize the chances of success, at the same time avoiding impossible demands. Complementary assessments should be employed to design effective rehabilitation programs.

Treatment and therapy

Treatment is something *given* to a person to help them recover from an illness or injury, or at least to feel better than they did prior to treatment. Therapy, on the other hand, is an *interactive process* in which the patient works together with the therapist to overcome, reduce, or bypass a disability. While both treatment and therapy are essential components of neuropsychological rehabilitation, it is the latter which is more frequently the province of the neuropsychologist working in rehabilitation.

The five major approaches available to a therapist working in neuropsychological rehabilitation are as follows:

1 Attempting to restore lost functioning.
2 Anatomical reorganization by using an undamaged part of the brain to "take over" the functions of a damaged area.
3 Bypassing or avoiding the problem areas by changing or restructuring the environment.
4 Functional adaptation or finding another way to achieve a particular goal or compensatory path.
5 Helping a patient use residual skills more effectively.

These approaches are not mutually exclusive and can be used in combination. For example, a memory-impaired person may be helped in the following ways:

1 Using signposts and labels, i.e. reorganizing the environment.
2 Teaching appropriate use of compensatory memory books.
3 Enhancing learning by the use of mnemonics, i.e. using residual skills more effectively. (But note that severely memory-impaired people are not expected to use mnemonics spontan-

eously. It is usual for the therapist or a relative to supply the mnemonics in order to encourage learning by the patient.)

Evaluation of therapy and treatment is also an integral part of neuropsychological rehabilitation. Such evaluation can be achieved by the application of conventional group designs and other experimental procedures. Evaluation of an individual patient's response to treatment can be achieved through the use of single-case experimental designs. These enable therapists to determine whether any change is due to spontaneous recovery (or other nonspecific effects) or therapeutic intervention.

THEORETICAL INFLUENCES ON NEUROPSYCHOLOGICAL REHABILITATION

Neuropsychological rehabilitation does not rely upon theoretical input from one discipline, namely neuropsychology, and cannot therefore be classified as a "pure" discipline. As a branch or division of rehabilitation in its most general sense, neuropsychological rehabilitation will be influenced by neurology, geriatric medicine, physical medicine, clinical psychology, occupational therapy, speech therapy, physical therapy, social work, psychotherapy, education, physiology, and any other areas that might shed light on specific problems encountered by patient and therapist. As far as theoretical models are concerned, however, there are probably three major branches of psychology that have contributed most to neuropsychological rehabilitation. These are neuropsychology, cognitive psychology, and behavioral psychology. Each of these provides different and complementary contributions. Neuropsychology has provided understanding of the organization of the brain through the localization model. Modern neuropsychology began with Broca's (1861) publication of his findings on the patient "Tan." Localization of function is still an abiding concern of many eminent neuropsychologists, such as Brenda Milner in Montreal, who has published extensively on localization of functions such as memory (1968) and frontal lobes (1982), and Mesulam (1985), who has provided localization models of attention and unilateral neglect.

A knowledge of the function and organization of the brain enables workers in the field of neuropsychological rehabilitation to anticipate certain deficits and link them with damage to certain skills; it influences the design and selection of assessment tools, and may sometimes influence decisions concerning, for example, the choice of treatments, such as restoration of function or compensatory approaches.

As far as actual rehabilitation is concerned the localization model is limited in its application. It cannot specify particular areas for treatment; neither can it provide guidance as to *how* a patient should be treated or a deficit tackled. In these respects it shares a certain lack of relevance that is found in other models, such as the biochemical or physiological ones. While neuropsychological assessment can help to pinpoint deficits more clearly (for example, identifying unilateral neglect or Broca's dysphasia), and can provide a description of a patient's cognitive strengths and weaknesses, it cannot contribute to knowledge that might be used in actual rehabilitation or treatment.

Models from cognitive psychology and cognitive neuropsychology are proving to be increasingly influential in neuropsychological rehabilitation (see Seron & Deloche, 1989). These models are not concerned with localization but with cognitive function. Models are representations which enable us to understand and explain related phenomena and, in this respect, the cognitive (neuro)psychological models have advanced neuropsychological rehabilitation considerably. The working memory model of Baddeley and Hitch (1974) has proved to be very influential in understanding, explaining, and predicting the pattern of deficits seen in amnesic people. The dual route model of reading (Coltheart, 1985) has led to advances in assessment and treatment planning, and the logogen model of Morton and Patterson (1980) has led to similar advances in language therapy.

In the field of memory therapy, theoretical explanations of the amnesic syndrome have resulted in some general principles or guidelines for the rehabilitation of memory-impaired people. Three major theoretical explanations claim that amnesia is a deficit of (a) *encoding*, (b) *storage*, and (c) *retrieval*. While none of these can account for all characteristics seen in the amnesic syndrome, all provide some help in therapy. For example, therapy can improve the *encoding* stage by simplifying information, reducing the amount presented at any one time, checking that the information has been understood, and using the "little and often" rule. *Storage* can be improved by testing regularly and rehearsing or practicing the information to be recalled. *Retrieval* can be enhanced by presenting information in different contexts during the learning stage, thus avoiding context-specificity; and, where necessary, providing a retrieval cue in the form of a first letter or sound.

For more detailed treatment programs, however, neither neuropsychological nor cognitive models are sufficiently helpful. Once again, they inform with some precision which part of the brain is damaged and which functions are intact or impaired, but they are unlikely to provide sufficient guidance as to how to remedy the deficit.

The third major influence is behavioral psychology, where many of the current treatment approaches originated. Behavioral psychology is not simply concerned with classical and operant conditioning, although these techniques have certainly played a role in the management of severely disruptive behavior problems following brain injury. Behavioral psychology also encompasses assessment, task analysis (identifying the antecedents and consequences of specific behaviors), and numerous techniques from behavior modification and behavior therapy. Methods have been devised to increase and decrease behavior, i.e. teach new skills and reduce or eliminate undesirable behaviors. The richness and complexity of behavioral approaches allows for their wide application in many areas of neuropsychological rehabilitation.

It is essential that the neurological and neuropsychological status of the individual is taken into account when implementing behavioral techniques or strategies that may require modification accordingly. However, the techniques readily lend themselves to such modification. Perhaps the most influential model from behavioral psychology is Kanfer and Saslow's (1969) SORKC model which considers the *stimulus, events, organism, responses, contingencies,* and *consequences* of behavior. This model allows therapists to take into account the prior history, motivation, physical and cognitive limitations of the patient, and reinforcement schedules that have been operating.

To illustrate the strength of the SORKC model we shall examine the case of Mrs Brown, a 56-year-old woman who, as a result of a right hemisphere stroke in the parietal region, has a left

hemiplegia, left visual field loss, and neglect of the left part of space. Her physiotherapist is trying to teach her how to transfer, that is, move herself from her wheelchair to (a) an ordinary chair, (b) her bed, and (c) to the toilet. Because Mrs Brown has difficulty learning to transfer she is referred to the neuropsychologist to see if a successful solution can be found. Applying the SORKC model during observations of attempts to transfer provides the following information:

S = Stimulus Events (may be physical, social, or internal)
Physical stimuli include the wheelchair, the bed, the chair, and the toilet. Social stimulus is the physiotherapist's request for such a transfer. Internal stimulus – Mrs Brown feels tired and confused.

O = Organism (i.e. biological condition)
Mrs Brown has a hemiplegia and visual field loss. Neuropsychological assessment has also identified unilateral neglect and problems with depth and distance which make it difficult for her to determine how far away she is from objects or places. She also ignores the brakes on the left-hand side of her wheelchair, thus making any transfer unsafe.

R = Responses (these may be motor, cognitive, or physiological)
Motor response – Mrs Brown trembles.
Cognitive responses – Mrs Brown is unwilling to attempt the task of transferring and complains.
Physiological response – sweating occurs.

K = Contingencies between behavior and consequences (i.e. schedules of reinforcement)
Partial reinforcement has been occurring – sometimes the physiotherapist or a nurse lifts Mrs Brown to her chair, bed, or toilet. Sometimes the physiotherapist or nurse persuades Mrs Brown to attempt the transfers alone. Partial reinforcement is more resistant to extinction than continuous reinforcement. Mrs Brown's complaints are therefore likely to be harder to overcome than if she had always been persuaded to transfer alone.

C = Consequences (may be physical, social or self-generated)
Physical – Mrs Brown is frequently helped when transferring.

Social – Mrs Brown receives a lot of attention from staff when transferring.

The above information forms the basis on which decisions about Mrs Brown's treatment are made. It might be decided to take any number of the following steps in a treatment program:

1 Control of both left and right wheelchair brakes should be placed on the right side of the wheelchair.
2 Mrs Brown should be given a list of steps involved in transferring, written in large print on the right-hand side of a card.
3 Mrs Brown should be encouraged to touch the chair (bed, toilet seat) to reassure herself that it is not beyond her reach.
4 Occupational therapists should work on depth and distance perception.
5 Therapists and others in the unit should be encouraged to refrain from lifting Mrs Brown when she complains. Instead, they should provide encouragement and reassurance during the transfer sequences and praise each success.

The SORKC model can apply to numerous situations and can take account of the neuropsychological and biological status of the patient when planning treatment.

Behavioral psychology also teaches that generalization should not be expected to occur spontaneously. Many neuropsychological programs fail because generalization has not been built into therapy or treatment. For example, many memory-impaired people have been given tape recorders, computers, or personal organizers which, although they may be used in therapy sessions, are not used elsewhere. Generalization has to be planned as part of therapy, as indeed it is by those working in mental handicap. Techniques to teach generalization to people with mental handicap, such as those described by Zarkowska (1987), can be adapted for use with brain-injured people in neuropsychological programs.

Finally, it is worth pointing out that at this stage in its development there is no right or wrong way to conduct neuropsychological rehabilitation. The discipline is in its early stages and, as yet, very few exact guidelines can be obtained from theoretical principles or models. What is called for is ingenuity on the part of workers in the field, and a willingness to combine and synthesize principles and models from a number of disciplines. A hopeful sign is that academics and theorists are themselves alert to the possible theoretical issues that arise from the study and treatment of people suffering from neuropsychological impairment of one kind or another. Both theoretical input and pragmatic attempts to alleviate, reduce, or bypass problems must continue to feed off each other if progress is to be made.

COMPUTERS IN REHABILITATION

In the early part of the 1980s there was considerable excitement over the possible use of computers in rehabilitation. It was hoped, indeed expected, that cognitive rehabilitation programs would revolutionize rehabilitation and enhance the memory, attention, language, perception, and problem-solving ability of brain-injured people. It was believed, for example, that microcomputers could assist the management of memory disorders through assessment, monitoring treatment effectiveness and retraining. Numerous software programs appeared, although as Robertson and colleagues (1988) pointed out, "the role of microcomputers in cognitive rehabilitation has not been subjected to controlled investigation until recently" (p. 151).

Robertson (1990) published a review of computerized cognitive rehabilitation, looking at programs for language, memory, visuospatial/ visuoperceptual and attention deficits. He focused on programs designed for adults with non-degenerative acquired brain damage and excluded computers used in assessment, recreation, or as prostheses or teaching aids. He found no evidence that computerized memory or visuoperceptual training produced significant changes in cognitive function. Language training programs for highly specific disorders fared a little better, but there was no published evidence of more general effectiveness of computerized language training. Only in attention training programs were there any positive results, although even here the evidence was contradictory, some studies showing positive results while others showed negative ones. Importantly, no computerized procedures were shown to generalize to real-life tasks.

It is therefore hardly surprising that computers have had little effect in cognitive retraining programs. Memory is not like a muscle which improves or strengthens with exercise. Practice at a particular task or activity, such as that performed in a computer-assisted exercise, may well improve performance on the specific items involved in that task or activity, but will not necessarily improve general cognitive functioning.

To emphasize the limitations that surround generalization from *any* practice, be it computer-assisted or not, I refer to the experiments conducted by Ericsson and colleagues (1980), who demonstrated that students could increase their digit span with practice. One student, an athlete, increased his span from an average of 7 to a phenomenal 80 by associating the digits with running times and other athletic performances. When given a similar letter-span task, however, he once again reverted to an average score of 7, thus demonstrating that no improvement of memory functioning per se had occurred.

Computers can of course be of considerable assistance in rehabilitation in other ways. Computerized assessment procedures may be time-saving and extra efficient. Computers as feedback devices also have a role, as Mackey (1989) showed when children with cerebral palsy performed a spasticity inhibiting exercise more efficiently when they were given feedback from a computer than when they were given feedback by a physiotherapist. Training in the use of computers has led to some exciting results (Glisky & Schacter, 1989). The authors taught a number of amnesic people computer terminology. One of their subjects was able to obtain employment subsequently as a computer operator.

Computers as prostheses for people with cognitive difficulties are likely to play an increasingly important role in neuropsychological rehabilitation. Bergman and Kemmerer (1991), for example, describe how they designed a text-writer (a computer-based prosthesis) for a 54-year-old head-injured woman with numerous cognitive difficulties. Instructions for the text-writer were simple and avoided dependence on memory, attention, and learning. Because of the woman's left-sided neglect, only the right side of the screen was used. An audible tone enhanced arousal and attentiveness. The woman learned to use the text-writer after three one-hour training sessions. She used the text-writer thereafter to write lists of things to do or purchase or remember. She now writes instructions and requests to

her companion helper, and makes notes about telephone calls during their progress so that she is helped to remember the topic and the caller. She also writes letters and is able to express her feelings to some extent. The authors suggest that her self-sufficiency has been enhanced and her emotional distress reduced.

FUTURE DIRECTIONS

Interest in neuropsychological rehabilitation continues to grow and, from the outset of the year 1992, much of this interest has centered on areas such as computerized programs, new theoretically driven rehabilitation techniques, group training for cognitively impaired people, and treatment of people in coma or persistent vegetative state.

Despite the relative pessimism of Robertson's (1990) review of published evidence for computerized cognitive training, he nevertheless pointed out that there are promising signs that effective therapies are on the horizon, particularly in the field of language therapy. Gianutsos (1991), a long-standing advocate of computerized cognitive rehabilitation, argues that it is as premature to rule out the possibility that computers will ever be effective in neuropsychological rehabilitation as it is to make too great a claim for their effectiveness. As already suggested, computers as prosthetic aids would seem to have great potential. Many of the problems brain-injured people have in accepting and learning to use microcomputers may be overcome through appropriate teaching methods, such as those used by Sohlberg and Mateer (1989), and through improved designs that will make the hardware and software easier to use.

Among theoretically driven rehabilitation techniques currently being developed is the *errorless learning procedure* that is employed in a series of studies at the Applied Psychology Unit in Cambridge, England. Influenced by *errorless discrimination* learning in *behavioral psychology* and by *implicit learning* in *cognitive neuropsychology*, errorless learning involves the prevention of errors by memory-impaired people during the learning process. Trial and error learning appears to retard the acquisition of information, probably because once an error has been made it tends to be repeated or strengthened. Amnesic people tend to rely on their implicit learning systems (i.e. learning without awareness), and this memory system is poor at error elimination. Thus, by avoiding errors during learning, the acquisition of new material or information is enhanced. Studies investigating this phenomenon are in their infancy but are looking promising (Wilson et al., 1994).

Treating people in groups has potential advantages, both in terms of cost effectiveness and in the reduction of some of the undesirable emotional effects that can accompany cognitive impairment. Two recent papers by Berg and others (1991) and Von Cramon and others (1991) report respectively on group training for memory-impaired people and for people with the dysexecutive syndrome.

In 1992 the journal *Neuropsychological Rehabilitation* devoted a special issue to rehabilitation of *coma* and the *vegetative state*. The subject of coma arousal and sensory stimulation gives rise to heated debate among those who argue that damaged brains need rest and that stimulation is at best ineffective and at worst harmful. Others argue that appropriate stimulation can lead to faster or better recovery. Wood (1991) is of the opinion that sensory stimulation programs have not been guided by a concept of how the brain assimilates and processes such input and, as a consequence of this, a set of clinical procedures has been developed that lacks scientific credibility. Over the next few years we can perhaps expect to see a partial or complete resolution of these arguments concerning the effectiveness or otherwise of coma stimulation.

A few areas of current interest in neuropsychological rehabilitation have been mentioned. Other areas that stimulate active interest are the rehabilitation of brain-injured children; the possibility of slowing cognitive decline in people with dementia; and combining neuropsychological therapies with pharmacological and surgical ones. The next decade will no doubt throw much light on these and perhaps many other areas that hold the attention of those who work in the field.

BIBLIOGRAPHY

Baddeley, A. D., & Hitch, G. J. (1974). Working memory. In G. A. Bower (Ed.), *The psychology of learning and motivation*, Vol. 8 (pp. 47–89). New York: Academic Press.

Bamford, J., Sandercock, P., Dennis, M., Burn, J., & Warlow, C. (1990). A prospective study of acute cerebro-vascular disease in the community: the Oxfordshire Stroke Project 1981–1986. *Journal of Neurology, Neurosurgery and Psychiatry*, 53, 16–22.

Berg, I. J., Koning-Haanstra, M., & Deelman, B. G. (1991). Long term effects of memory rehabilitation: a controlled study. *Neuropsychological Rehabilitation*, 1, 97–111.

Bergman, M. M., & Kemmerer, A. G. (1991). Computer-enhanced self sufficiency: Part 2. Uses and subjective benefits of a text writer for an individual with traumatic brain injury. *Neuropsychology*, 5, 25–8.

Boake, C. (1989). A history of cognitive rehabilitation of head-injured patients, 1915 to 1980. *Journal of Head Trauma Rehabilitation*, 4, 1–8.

Broca, P. (1861). Nouvelle observation d'aphémie produite par une lésion de la moitié postérieure des deuxième et troisième circonvolutions frontales. *Bulletin de la Société Anatomique de Paris*, 6, 398–407.

Coltheart, M. (1985). Cognitive neuropsychology and reading. In M. Posner & O. S. M. Marin (Eds), *Attention and performance*, Vol. 11 (pp. 3–37). Hillsdale, NJ: Erlbaum.

Ericsson, K. A., Chase, W. G., & Falcon, S. (1980). Acquisition of a memory skill. *Science*, 208, 1181–2.

Gianutsos, R. (1991). Cognitive rehabilitation: a neuropsychological specialty comes of age. *Brain Injury*, 5, 363–8.

Glisky, E. L., & Schacter, D. L. (1989). Extending the limits of complex learning in organic amnesia: computer training in a vocational domain. *Neuropsychologia*, 27, 107–20.

Kanfer, F. H., & Saslow, G. (1969). Behavioural diagnosis. In C. Franks (Ed.), *Behaviour therapy: Appraisal and status* (pp. 417–44). New York: McGraw-Hill.

Kertesz, A. (1979). Visual agnosia: the dual deficit of perception and recognition. *Cortex*, 15, 403–19.

Lane, H. (1977). *The Wild Boy of Aveyron*. London: Paladin-Granada.

Luria, A. R. (1963). *Recovery of function after brain injury* (pp. 368–433). New York: Macmillan.

Luria, A. R., Naydin, V. L., Tsvetkova, L. S., & Vinarskaya, E. N. (1969). Restoration of higher cortical function following local brain damage. In P. J. Vinken & G. W. Bruyn (Eds), *Handbook of clinical neurology*, Vol. 3 (pp. 368–433). Amsterdam: North Holland.

Mackey, S. (1989). The use of computer-assisted feedback in a motor-control task for cerebral palsied children. *Physiotherapy*, 75, 143–8.

Meier, M., Benton, A., & Diller, L. (1987). *Neuropsychological rehabilitation*. Edinburgh: Churchill Livingstone.

Mesulam, M.-M. (1985). Attention, confusional states and neglect. In M.-M. Mesulam (Ed.), *Principles of behavioural neuropsychology* (pp. 125–68). Philadelphia: F. A. Davis.

Milner, B. (1968). Visual recognition and recall after right temporal-lobe excision in man. *Neuropsychologia, 6*, 191–209.

Milner, B. (1982). Some cognitive effects of frontal-lobe lesions in man. *Philosophical Transactions of the Royal Society of London B, 298*, 211–26.

Morton, J., & Patterson, K. E. (1980). A new attempt at an interpretation or, an attempt at a new interpretation. In M. Coltheart, K. Patterson, & J. C. Marshall (Eds), *Deep dyslexia* (pp. 91–118). London: Routledge and Kegan Paul.

Prigatano, G. P., Fordyce, D. J., Zeiner, H. K., Roueche, J. R., Pepping, M., & Wood, B. C. (1986). *Neuropsychological rehabilitation after brain injury*. Baltimore, MD: Johns Hopkins University Press.

Robertson, I. (1990). Does computerised cognitive rehabilitation work? A review. *Aphasiology, 4*, 381–405.

Robertson, I., Gray, J., & McKenzie, S. (1988). Microcomputer-based cognitive rehabilitation of visual neglect: 3 multiple-baseline single-case studies. *Brain Injury, 2*, 151–64.

Seron, X., & Deloche, G. (Eds). (1989). *Cognitive approaches in neuropsychological rehabilitation*. Hillsdale, NJ: Erlbaum.

Sohlberg, M., & Mateer, C. (1989). Training use of compensatory memory books: a three-stage behavioral approach. *Journal of Clinical and Experimental Neuropsychology, 11*, 871–91.

Thomsen, I. V. (1987). Late psychosocial outcome in severe blunt head trauma: a review. *Brain Injury, 1*, 131–43.

Von Cramon, D. Y., Matthes-von Cramon, G., & Mai, N. (1991). Problem solving deficits in brain injured patients: a therapeutic approach. *Neuropsychological Rehabilitation, 1*, 45–64.

Wade, D., & Hewer, R. L. (1987). Functional abilities after stroke: measurement, natural history and prognosis. *Journal of Neurology, Neurosurgery and Psychiatry, 50*, 177–82.

Walsh, K. (1987). *Neuropsychology: A clinical approach*, 2nd edn. Edinburgh: Churchill Livingstone.

Wilson, B. A. (1991). Long term prognosis of patients with severe memory disorders. *Neuropsychological Rehabilitation, 1*, 117–34.

Wilson, B. A., Baddeley, A. D., Evans, J. J., & Shiel, A. (1994). Errorless learning in the rehabilitation of memory impaired people. *Neuropsychological Rehabilitation, 4*, 307–26.

Wilson, B. A., Cockburn, J., & Baddeley, A. D. (1989). Assessment of everyday memory following brain injury. In M. E. Miner & K. A. Wagner (Eds), *Neurotrauma: Treatment, rehabilitation and related issues 3* (pp. 83–99). London: Butterworths.

Wood, R. Ll. (1991). Critical analysis of the concept of sensory stimulation for patients in vegetative states. *Brain Injury, 5*, 401–9.

World Health Organization. (1986). *Optimum care of disabled people*. Report of a WHO meeting, Turku, Finland.

Zangwill, O. L. (1945). A review of psychological work at the Brain Injuries Unit, Edinburgh, 1941–5. *British Medical Journal, 2*, 248–50.

Zarkowska, E. (1987). Discrimination and generalization. In W. Yule & J. Carr (Eds), *Behaviour modification for people with mental handicaps* (pp. 79–94). London: Croom Helm.

BARBARA A. WILSON

restless legs syndrome Also known as Ekbom's syndrome, the restless legs syndrome is characterized by restless, fidgety movements of the legs, which may also be described as *akathisia*. The syndrome is most commonly a side effect of treatment by neuroleptic drugs, but it may also be associated with iron deficiency, although cases also occur in which no clear cause can be identified. The pathological mechanism is presumed to result in hyperexcitability of spinal cord motor neurons.

reticular formation The reticular formation constitutes the core of the BRAIN STEM. It extends from the junction between the spinal cord and the medulla to the interface between the mesencephalon (midbrain) and the diencephalon.

The neurons of the brain stem reticular core are morphologically characterized by their very long dendrites which are the targets of inputs arising in multiple heterogeneous structures, from the spinal cord up to the cerebral cortex. Reticular neurons are *not* specialized for relaying and analyzing messages that are exclusively transmitted along a specific sensory modality, such as vision, audition, or touch. The brain stem reticular cells innervate, by means of ascending and/or descending axons, many regions of the central nervous system and thus represent the sources of general regulatory systems of brain excitability. This is the reason why the brain stem reticular formation was viewed as a nonspecific structure. There is, however, a certain specificity within this nonspecificity, and this is mainly achieved by the diversity of chemical codes used by various cell aggregates located within the reticular formation (see below).

The reticular formation was described long ago by anatomists. However, its functional importance for the regulation of brain excitability was only discovered during the late 1940s by the Italian and American physiologists Moruzzi and Magoun (1949). In an article which remains a classical work in neurophysiology, they reported that stimulation of the brain stem core induces a change in electroencephalogram (EEG) activity resembling that accompanying the shift from resting sleep, with slow EEG waves of high amplitude, to arousal, when sleep rhythms are obliterated and the EEG activity has a lower amplitude. We now know that the pattern of EEG arousal does not exclusively consist of the blockage of sleep oscillations, but also includes the appearance of distinct, fast (20–40 Hz) waves, which characterize a state of increased alertness when information can be processed.

While during the late 1940s there was no direct evidence that the changes in EEG rhythms induced by brain stem reticular stimulation were indicative of an enhanced excitability of the brain, Moruzzi and Magoun decided to go far beyond their data. They suggested that the alteration of spontaneous EEG waves, from sleep to arousal rhythms, was the signature of an *activated* brain, that is, a brain with an enhanced capability to respond to afferent signals. A decade later, Bremer and Dell, a Belgian and a French physiologist, independently demonstrated that electrical potentials elicited in the cerebral cortex by stimuli applied to central nervous system pathways were indeed potentiated during the EEG-activated response to brain stem reticular stimulation.

FROM A RETICULAR MONOLITH TO A RETICULAR MOSAIC

In their original article, Moruzzi and Magoun elicited an EEG response, similar to that associated with arousal, by stimulating many sites in the brain stem, from the medulla to the rostral mesencephalon. Although these authors emphasized that the responses with the lowest threshold (i.e. requiring the lowest intensity of stimulation) were evoked from the rostral mesencephalon, the general view prevailed during the early 1950s that most reticular areas have the same activating properties. In other words, it was thought that various areas of the reticular formation do not qualitatively differ as far as their arousing effects upon the thalamus and cortex are concerned. This concept of the reticular formation as a monolith reinforced the idea of a nonspecific structure. We now know that, far from being a monolith, the brain stem reticular formation consists of a variety of cell aggregates, using different neurotransmitters, having different projections, and exerting different actions upon target neurons (see below).

During the late 1950s Moruzzi and his pupils conducted in Pisa a series of elegant experiments that were the starting point toward the demonstration that reticular areas located in the lower (medullary) and the upper (mesopontine) parts of the brain stem have different functional properties. In fact, the general idea that the brain stem does not function as a whole was introduced in 1935 by Bremer, who was Moruzzi's mentor during the late 1930s. Bremer showed that a cat with a transection between the spinal cord and the medulla undergoes normal transitions from sleep to wakefulness, whereas a cat with a transection at the midbrain level is comatose.

What Moruzzi and his team reported in a series of papers published between 1958 and 1960 was the precise location of the brain stem area having arousing properties. Again, this was achieved by transections. A cat with a transection at the midbrain level was comatose, in support of Bremer's earlier findings. By contrast, a transection only a few millimeters more posterior, in the middle of the pons, led the animal to be almost continuously awake. The inescapable conclusion was that the neurons with arousing and activating properties are located within this restricted area of the brain stem, at the mesopontine junction. At that time, nothing precise was known about

627

the neurotransmitters used by those brain stem neurons.

Twenty-five years later, the neurons using acetylcholine (ACh) as a neurotransmitter were identified by immunohistochemical methods and were found to be located in two nuclei, in the region between the two transections that gave opposite effects on states of sleep and waking.

Cholinergic neurons are not the only ones with activating properties on the forebrain. Other brain stem neurons, located quite closely to cholinergic cells, use glutamate (GLU), norepinephrine (noradrenaline) (NE), and serotonin (5-HT) as neurotransmitters. Whereas all these cellular types, releasing ACh, GLU, NE, and 5-HT at their axonal terminals, are conjointly participating

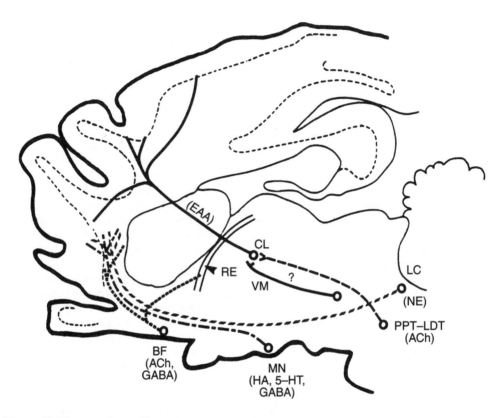

Figure 62 Diagram of ascending activating systems shown on a parasagittal section of the brain of a cat, a species that was the subject of most experimental studies in this field. The cerebral cortex is at left and the upper part of the brain stem is at right: between them is the thalamus with two of its nuclei projecting widely to cortex (CL, centrolateral nucleus; and VM, ventromedial nucleus). Thalamocortical cells use excitatory amino acids (EAA) as neurotransmitters. The arousing systems are schematically drawn with just one cell. Neurons of the pedunculopontine tegmental and laterodorsal tegmental (PPT–LDT) nuclei use acetylcholine (ACh) as a transmitter and project it to the thalamus. In front of PPT–LDT nuclei, a brain stem reticular neuron with thalamic projection is also depicted; its transmitter is not yet precisely known but is thought to be EAA. Above brain stem cholinergic PPT–LDT nuclei is shown the locus coeruleus (LC) whose neurons use norepinephrine (NE) as a transmitter. At the ventral (lower) surface of the brain are located mammillary nuclei (MN) of the posterior hypothalamus. Near that region are neurons using histamine (HA) as a transmitter, as well as other cells using serotonin (5-HT) and GABA (gamma aminobutyric acid). The basal forebrain (BF) area has neurons using ACh or GABA and projecting directly to the cerebral cortex. Some neurons in the BF also project to the reticular thalamic (RE) nucleus.

in the induction of activation processes during the state of arousal, only cholinergic and glutamatergic neurons are quite active during both states of waking and rapid-eye-movement (REM) sleep when dreaming episodes occur. It is known, from recordings of single-cell activity in the thalamus and cerebral cortex, that waking and REM sleep are very similar behavioral states from the point of view of the enhanced neuronal excitability (see BRAIN STEM). Therefore, brain stem cholinergic and glutamatergic neurons are the best candidates to trigger and maintain activation processes during both arousal and REM sleep.

CHOLINERGIC, GLUTAMATERGIC, AND AMINERGIC NUCLEI

The effects of brain stem transections on sleep and arousal, discussed above, were discovered in acutely prepared animals, that is, experiments usually lasting for less than 24 hours. Other investigators attempted to keep alive the transected animals for a long period (7–15 days) after the midbrain transection, although this needed difficult procedures. Having succeeded in doing so, those experimenters observed that the lethargic or comatose state, appearing immediately after the midbrain transection, was replaced 7–10 days later by a behavioral state during which at least some rudimentary signs of wakefulness were recovered. This result led to a new concept according to which the arousing systems are not exclusively located in the brain stem, but also in some supramesencephalic structures. It is now definitely established that there are a series of activating or arousing systems, some in the brain stem, others in different structures representing the rostral continuation of the reticular formation, such as thalamic nuclei with diffuse cortical projections, the posterior part of the hypothalamus, and the basal forebrain. Some of these systems are schematically depicted in Figure 62 and are discussed below.

1. Mesopontine and basal forebrain cholinergic nuclei. The brain stem cholinergic cellular groups are termed pedunculopontine and laterodorsal tegmental nuclei. They are located at the junction between the caudal part of the mesencephalon and the rostral part of the pons. Their inputs mainly arise in the spinal cord, other areas of the brain stem, hypothalamus, basal forebrain, and cerebral cortex. In turn, mesopontine cholinergic

neurons overwhelmingly project to various types of thalamic nuclei. After this synaptic relay, glutamatergic thalamic cells transfer to the cortex the modulatory signals of brain stem origin. On the other hand, basal forebrain cholinergic cells directly project to the cerebral cortex; a minority of these neurons send projections to some thalamic nuclei. Therefore, while the cholinergic innervation of the thalamus is provided by the brain stem, the cholinergic innervation of the cortex originates in the basal forebrain.

The electrical activity of brain stem cholinergic neurons with thalamic projections was recorded by Steriade and colleagues across the natural waking–sleep cycle of behaving animals. The conclusion was that the discharge frequencies of cholinergic neurons are higher during wakefulness and REM sleep than during slow-wave sleep. Moreover, the increase in firing rates precedes by half a minute to one minute the most precocious signs of cerebral activation during either arousal or REM sleep. These neurons were also found to be more reactive to incoming messages during waking and REM sleep, both compared to slow-wave sleep. These data support the idea that cholinergic neurons are effective in inducing and maintaining the enhanced excitability of neurons in higher structures, during both alert and dreaming states (Figure 63).

2. Brain stem glutamatergic nuclei. The immunohistochemical identification of brain stem cholinergic and aminergic neurons showed that these cellular types merely represent a minority of the brain stem core population. What about the other neurons in the remaining parts of the reticular formation? Although the complete identification of the chemical code(s) defining these non-cholinergic, non-aminergic brain stem reticular cells still awaits clarification, there is accumulating evidence that a great majority of them use GLU as a neurotransmitter. Thalamic-projecting glutamatergic neurons recorded from the rostral area of the midbrain reticular formation show activity patterns which are similar to those displayed by mesopontine cholinergic cells, namely increased firing rates during both arousal and REM sleep, as compared to EEG-synchronized sleep. Until quite recently it was believed that GLU is a transmitter with phasic excitatory actions, which could not account for the prolonged activation processes characterizing enduring states of increased alertness. It has now been

629

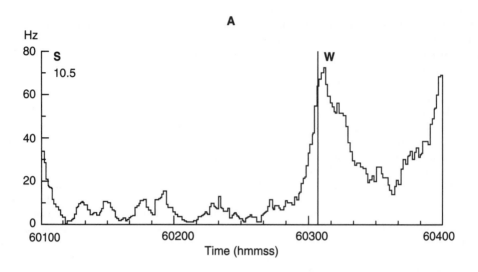

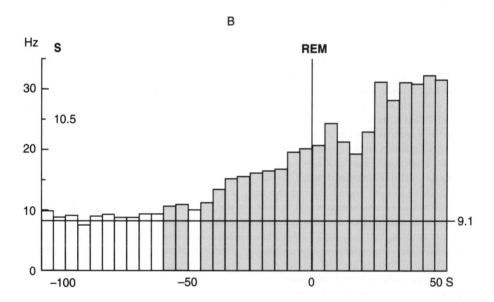

Figure 63 Brain stem cholinergic neurons increase discharge rates in advance of time 0 with transition from slow-wave sleep (S) to waking (W) or rapid eye movement (REM) sleep. A. Neuron increasing discharge rate 20 s before the most precocious sign of brain activation during transition from EEG-synchronized sleep (S) to waking (W). B. Group of neurons (n = 21) increasing discharge rates 60 s in advance of a transition between S and REM sleep.

demonstrated, however, that thalamic and other central neurons have GLU metabotropic receptors which mediate prolonged excitatory actions, very similar to those induced by ACh. Brain stem neurons using GLU may be as effective as cholinergic and aminergic cells in their activating actions. Moreover, in the light of this recent discovery, thalamocortical and corticothalamic neurons, which both use GLU, may be regarded as systems underlying long-term activation processes.

630

3. Brain stem and posterior hypothalamic aminergic nuclei. The neurons which release NE are located in the locus coeruleus and the neurons which release 5-HT are mainly located in the dorsal raphé nucleus. In addition, other aminergic neurons using histamine (HA) are found in the tubero-infundibular region of the posterior hypothalamus, a region which by other lines of evidence is known to be implicated in brain arousal. By contrast to cholinergic and glutamatergic cells, which increase their activity during both arousal and REM sleep, all these three types of aminergic cells using NE, 5-HT, and HA are active during waking, but progressively slow down their discharge rates during sleep, and eventually become silent during REM sleep. Thus the latter neuronal types are conjointly acting with cholinergic and glutamatergic cells during arousal, but they cannot underlie the highly activated state of the thalamus and cerebral cortex during dreaming sleep.

ACTIONS OF ACTIVATING SYSTEMS ON THALAMIC AND CORTICAL NEURONS

The best-known actions of neurotransmitters implicated in activation processes of thalamocortical systems are those elicited by ACh. During the past few years, these effects have been studied in vitro by McCormick (1992) and colleagues. The application of different substances in brain slices allows the investigation of their effects after blockage of synaptic transmission and therefore the differential action of transmitters on various types of neurons can be deciphered. ACh depolarizes (excites) most thalamic neurons with cortical projections. On the other hand, ACh inhibits thalamic cells using GABA as a neurotransmitter and exerting inhibitory actions on thalamocortical neurons. Thus, any condition associated with an increase in firing frequencies of cholinergic neurons projecting to the thalamus will excite thalamocortical cells in two ways: directly as well as indirectly, by removing the dampening actions of inhibitory cells (Figure 64). This is the case in arousal and REM sleep, when brain stem cholinergic cells tonically fire with increased discharge frequencies (see Figure 63). At the level of the cerebral cortex ACh excites both pyramidal-type neurons (having long axons projecting to subcortical structures and to adjacent or distant cortical areas) and local-circuit neurons. To a certain extent, the actions exerted

by NE, HA, and 5-HT are similar to those of ACh. However, the whole range of neurotransmitter actions has not been fully investigated. Future studies should explore the interactions between different transmitters used by activating systems because, during natural states of vigilance, all these substances are released and their combined actions on postsynaptic cells in the thalamus and cerebral cortex are not yet understood.

What also remains to be investigated is the mechanism by which the long-lasting inhibitory potentials of thalamic neurons during sleep develop into shorter periods of inhibition upon awakening and the cellular substrates of the preserved inhibitory efficacy upon arousal. Here the emphasis is on the fact that, however arousal disrupts the prolonged oscillatory periods of inhibition characterizing sleep, it does not completely block inhibitory processes during waking. Indeed, inhibition is needed during wakefulness for shaping the incoming signals, for finely tuning the neuronal responses, and for achieving highly complex integrative processes. All this complexity, which defines the adaptive state of alertness, has now to be explored at the cellular level in performing animals.

BIBLIOGRAPHY

Bremer, F. (1935). Cerveau isolé et physiologie du sommeil. *Comptes Rendus de la Société de Biologie, 118*, 1235–41.
McCormick, D. A. (1992). Neurotransmitter actions in the thalamus and cerebral cortex and their role in neuromodulation of thalamocortical activity. *Progress in Neurobiology, 39*, 33–88.
Moruzzi, G. (1972). The sleep-waking cycle. *Ergebnisse in Physiologie, 64*, 1–165.
Moruzzi, G., & Magoun, H. W. (1949). Brain stem reticular formation and the activation of the EEG. *Electroencephalography and Clinical Neurophysiology, 1*, 455–73.
Steriade, M., & Biesold, D. (Eds). (1990). *Brain cholinergic systems*. Oxford and New York: Oxford University Press.
Steriade, M., Curró Dossi, R., Paré, D., & Oakson, G. (1991). Fast (20–40 Hz) oscillations in thalamocortical systems and their potentiation by mesopontine cholinergic nuclei in the cat. *Proceedings of the National Academy of Science, USA, 88*, 4396–400.

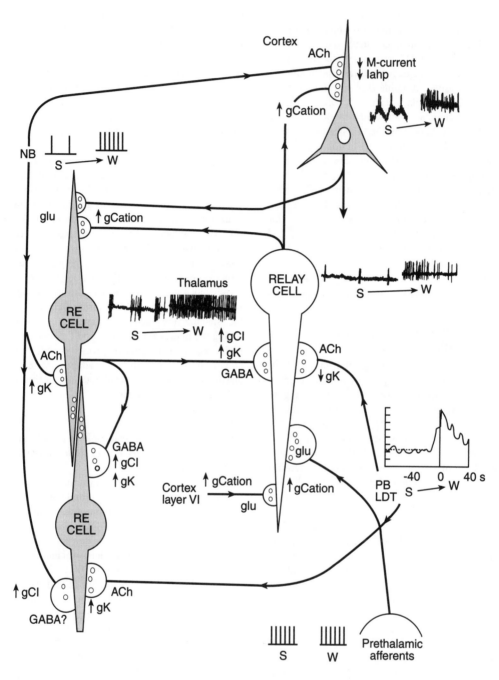

Figure 64 Schematic diagram of ascending cholinergic actions upon thalamocortical (relay) neurons, reticular thalamic (RE) GABAergic neurons, and pyramidal-shaped neurons of the cerebral cortex. Direction of axons is indicated by arrows. Acetylcholine (ACh) is released in the thalamus by peribrachial (PB) neurons of the pedunculopontine tegmental and laterodorsal tegmental (LDT) neurons (Ch 5–Ch 6 groups). In the cortex, ACh is mostly released by nucleus basilis (NB) neurons. In relay and RE thalamic cells as well as in cortical pyramidal neurons, EEG-synchronized sleep (S) is characterized by

Steriade, M., Datta, S., Paré, D., Oakson, G., & Curró Dossi, R. (1990). Neuronal activities in brain stem cholinergic nuclei related to tonic activation processes in thalamocortical systems. *Journal of Neuroscience, 10,* 2541–59.

Steriade, M., Jones, E. G., & Llinás, R. R. (1990). *Thalamic oscillations and signaling.* New York: Wiley-Interscience.

Steriade, M., & McCarley, R. W. (1990). *Brain-stem control of wakefulness and sleep.* New York: Plenum Press.

MIRCEA STERIADE

retrograde amnesia *See* AMNESIA; AMNESIC SYNDROME.

Reye's syndrome Reye's syndrome is associated with liver failure and in its early stages presents as clouding of consciousness which may lead to coma, with vomiting and fever. The second stage of the illness may produce inappropriate verbalization and combative or stuporous behavior, while normal posture is maintained. The syndrome normally has an infective cause, although it may also be produced by aspirin overdose, and a median onset of 14 months, with over 90 percent of cases having an onset before 12 years of age.

Riddoch effect First described in 1917, the Riddoch effect refers to residual ability associated with cortical blindness, in which immobile objects cannot be seen but mobile objects may be grasped and the direction of motion may be indicated. Nevertheless, there may be no awareness of either mobile or immobile objects, and the effect is therefore a form of BLINDSIGHT.

right–left disorientation People are often confused or disoriented with respect to right and left, sometimes (but not always) as a consequence of neurological damage. This confusion may take subtly different forms that are not always clearly distinguished: it may reflect a difficulty in telling right from left, a difficulty with the actual *words* "right" and "left," or a difficulty in superimposing an egocentric sense of right and left onto the right and left sides of other people or objects. There are also cases that suggest a systematic reversal of the right–left sense of stored information or stored habits.

TELLING RIGHT FROM LEFT

In the most general sense, the ability to tell right from left is the ability to map events that differ only with respect to right–left orientation onto events that do *not* differ in this respect. It is demonstrated by a person who says "right" when touched on the right hand and "left" when

---

rhythmic inhibitory periods and bursts of action potentials within the frequency range of spindle oscillations (≈ 14 Hz). The information transfer of thalamocortical cells is dramatically reduced during the oscillatory mode of S. In cortical cells, the activity evoked by prethalamic afferents is further reduced due to relatively uninhibited potassium currents (M-current and I_{ahp}) which underlie spike frequency adaptation. Upon transition from sleep to waking (W), the cholinergic PB/LDT cells increase their rates of discharges. Similar increase is seen in NB neurons. Note that no change in firing rate from S to W is seen in neurons recorded from specific prethalamic relays. Increased activity of cholinergic PB/LDT and NB cells disrupts sleep rhythm generation in the thalamus by depolarizing relay neurons (through a decrease in potassium conductance, g_k). As well, cortical pyramidal cells are activated through a decrease in M-current and I_{ahp}. There is in addition an excitatory action on cortical cells by glutamatergic thalamocortical neurons (increase in cationic permeability). The hyperpolarization of RE cells by PB/LDT cholinergic cells as well as by NB neurons underlies the blockage of sleep spindle generation in the pacemaking RE neurons. Although PB/LDT cholinergic afferents hyperpolarize RE thalamic cells by an increase in g_k, these neurons are brought upon arousal toward single-spike firing, with increased firing rates, because they are subject to excitatory influences from both relay thalamic and cortico-RE neurons using GLU as a transmitter. Schemes of changes in ionic conductances in various neuronal types are from work by McCormick and colleagues, and data related to S–W behavior of brain stem, thalamic, and cortical cellular classes are from work by Steriade and collaborators.

touched on the left hand. However, it need not involve the words "left" and "right" at all, and is also demonstrated by, for example, a child who correctly labels the mirror-image letters *b* and *d* as "bee" and "dee," or by a pigeon that pecks a key when it displays a 45-degree oblique line but not when it displays a 135-degree line. These are examples of *right–left mirror-image discrimination*, in which the stimuli are right–left mirror images but the responses are not. It is not necessary to be able to tell right from left in order to copy these stimuli, say, or to point to the straight side of a *b* or a *d*, since in these cases the left–right sense of the response merely mimics that of the stimulus.

The ability to tell right from left is also demonstrated by the ability to give right–left mirror-image responses to stimuli that do not differ with respect to right and left. This may be termed *right–left response differentiation*, as when a person turns right or left according to verbal command, or a rat turns right in a maze when a buzzer sounds and left when a bell sounds. Again, tests in which the direction of response is directly indicated in the stimulus, as in turning in the direction of a pointing arrow or following a winding road, do not draw on the ability to tell right from left.

A perfectly bilaterally symmetrical organism would be unable to tell right from left according to the above criteria. Most animals, including humans, are to a large degree bilaterally symmetrical, especially with respect to external body shape, the placement of sense organs and motor apparatus, and the organization of the central nervous system. Consequently, tasks requiring the ability to tell right from left are typically more difficult, for both humans and nonhuman species, than are comparable tasks that do not require this ability, such as those requiring a distinction between up and down (Corballis & Beale, 1976). Indeed the problem may be so severe for some otherwise normal people that Elze (1924) coined the term "right–left blindness," suggesting an analogy with color blindness. There is also some evidence that women have greater difficulty than men in telling right from left, and this has been attributed to a lesser degree of functional asymmetry in the female brain (*see* SEX DIFFERENCES).

Bilateral symmetry is itself probably an evolutionary consequence of the fact that, to a freely moving animal, right and left are essentially *equivalent*. Environmental events are equally likely to impinge from either side of the body or with either right–left parity; for example, predators, prey, or environmental landmarks may appear on either side, and the faces or bodies of other animals may appear in either right or left profile. In a general evolutionary sense, therefore, right–left confusion may be not so much a pathological condition as an adaptation to right–left equivalence in the natural world.

However, there are certain exclusively human activities that do require the ability to tell right from left. These include following and giving verbal directional instructions, and, in some cultures at least, the processing of scripts (such as English) that are set out in a consistent left–right direction. It follows that these activities require a structural asymmetry.

Most young children have difficulty telling right from left, and this often creates difficulties in early efforts to read and write. This is manifest in a tendency to write letters, words, or even whole sentences backwards, and in a confusion between mirror-image letters, such as *b* and *d*, or near mirror-image words, such as *was* and *saw*. Orton (1937) argued that the problem was especially persistent in children with poorly established cerebral dominance, and was the major cause of developmental DYSLEXIA. At one time this theory enjoyed a wide currency, and among lay people especially there are still many who regard dyslexia as more or less synonymous with "seeing things backwards." Recent analyses of developmental dyslexia have tended to focus on other sources of difficulty, such as a lack of phonological awareness (a problem that Orton also recognized), although right–left confusions and anomalies of dominance are still quite commonly reported.

One reason that Orton's theory lost favor is that it was based on an implausible neurological theory. Orton argued that the cerebral hemispheres would necessarily record spatial representations, or *engrams*, with opposite left–right orientations simply because they are themselves structural mirror images of one another. Children with poorly established cerebral dominance would therefore have difficulty learning to read and write because they would be as likely to access the reversed engram in one hemisphere as the veridical one in the other. As it stands, this theory makes little sense, since it is difficult to envisage how experiences could be recorded in one hemisphere *as though* right–left reversed. Moreover, bilateral symmetry of itself does not force engrams to be registered with opposite right–left orientation in the two hemispheres, just as it does not follow that a symmetrical camera lens causes photographs to be recorded with opposite orientation on the two sides of an exposed film.

A more plausible hypothesis is that engrams are laid down in veridical fashion as a result of direct experience, but are then right–left reversed in *interhemispheric transfer*. There is some evidence for such a process in nonhuman species, although it is not unequivocal (Corballis & Beale, 1976). There is also evidence that changes induced by peripheral denervation in one cerebral hemisphere are almost immediately mirrored in the other hemisphere, suggesting a general commissural mechanism for preserving structural symmetry. It is conceivable that this process may play a more prominent role than normal in at least a subgroup of developmental dyslexics, possibly in that minority whose difficulties are visuospatial rather than phonological. However, it is probably also responsible for the *general* tendency to treat right–left mirror images as equivalent, and underlies the right–left confusion shown by normal as well as dyslexic children.

MORE COMPLEX TESTS OF RIGHT–LEFT ORIENTATION

More complex tests of right–left orientation have been devised, primarily for testing neurological patients, most notably by Head (1926) and Benton (1959). These are composed of items of varying complexity, and typically require knowledge of the actual *words* "right" and "left." Head (1926) included some items requiring that the subject imitate the examiner's actions, but as we have seen, such items do not actually require the ability to tell right from left. In Benton's test, and variants of it, subjects are asked to name the sides of their own body parts touched by the examiner, or to point to particular parts of their own bodies on the side named by the examiner. They are also asked to name or point to parts on one or other side of the confronting examiner, or of a picture of a person. Some items involve double commands (e.g. "Touch your right ear with your left hand"). The test may be given with the subject's eyes either open or closed.

The performance of children on tests of this sort typically shows three clear developmental stages (Benton, 1959; Clarke & Klonoff, 1991).

Up to the age of about 5, children perform more or less randomly. This is probably because of a general inability to tell right from left, since their difficulty with right–left mirror-image tasks is generally not restricted to those involving the terms "right" and "left." However, Benton has noted that some children show systematic reversal, such as showing their left hands when asked for their right ones and so on. This demonstrates clear ability to tell right from left, as defined above, but does suggest a difficulty with the labels themselves. As one might expect, these children are often deficient in language development (see Benton, 1979). Benton has also observed that some 5-year-olds can respond correctly to single commands relating to the sides of their own bodies, but have difficulty with double commands, especially when they involve crossing the midline; for instance, when asked to touch the right ear with the left hand, the child will typically touch the *left* ear with the left hand.

After the age of 5, most children master the use of the labels "right" and "left" with respect to their own bodies, but cannot reliably label the right and left sides of other bodies or objects. This may occur even in trying to imitate the actions of a confronting person, and probably reflects a failure of mental rotation rather than one of telling right from left or of understanding the labels. At this stage, children often systematically reverse "right" and "left" with respect to a confronting person, presumably because they refer to their own egocentric reference frame rather than to that of the other person. By the age of about 9, however, they reach the final stage of being able to correctly label the right and left sides of other people, and this coincides at least roughly with the development of mental-rotation ability.

Clinically, poor performance on tests of right–left discrimination has been associated with general mental impairment. It has also long been associated with damage to the left cerebral hemisphere (e.g. Head, 1926). It was regarded by Gerstmann as one of the symptoms of a syndrome (*see* GERSTMANN SYNDROME) resulting from damage to the left PARIETAL LOBE, the others being finger AGNOSIA, AGRAPHIA, and ACALCULIA. Although these disorders are no longer regarded as constituting a true syndrome, an ingredient they share is that they all involve verbal or symbolic processes that are acquired relatively late in development, which might therefore be especially vulnerable to a general but mild language impairment (Benton, 1979). Consequently, the problem is probably often one of using the *labels* "right" and "left" rather than one of telling right from left in the sense described above. This is generally corroborated by Head (1926), who found that right–left disorientation was often associated with APHASIA. However, there is also evidence that left cerebral damage may induce systematic right–left reversals; this is discussed separately below.

Right–left disorientation may also result, although less commonly, from right hemispheric damage. But whereas the problem in patients with left hemispheric damage may include difficulty in identifying the sides of their own bodies, in those with right hemispheric damage it is largely restricted to labelling the sides of other people or objects (Benton, 1979). This again suggests a problem of mental rotation, and there is indeed other evidence that mental rotation itself depends primarily on the right posterior cerebral hemisphere. It is worth noting that the great majority of laboratory studies of mental rotation have involved the discrimination of right–left mirror-image stimuli presented in varying angular orientations, again revealing the close connection between right–left discrimination and mental rotation.

TURNER'S SYNDROME provides another example of a disorder that is said to include right–left disorientation among its manifestations, but again the problem is probably a more general one of spatial transformation. The main evidence for right–left disorientation in these patients is their poor performance on a road-map test requiring them to indicate whether the turns on a path drawn on a road map are to the right or left (Alexander & Money, 1966). They typically have normal verbal skills and can read and write normally, indicating little difficulty in right–left discrimination per se. The problem must therefore be one of making the transformation between their own bodily coordinates and those of the path on the map – a problem, in other words, of mental rotation.

RIGHT–LEFT REVERSALS

Sometimes, a person's behavior suggests that right and left have been systematically reversed. As noted above, this may occur as a consequence of adopting an inappropriate reference frame, as when a child uses an egocentric reference frame

to judge the right and left sides of a confronting person. In other cases, though, reversal may have a more fundamental neurological origin. A common example is mirror-writing, and it may be observed in normal as well as in brain-injured people and in some cases of developmental dyslexia. In his 1928 treatise on mirror-writing, Critchley noted that it sometimes occurs spontaneously in states of "dissociation," such as light anesthesia, hypnosis, trance, hysteria, or daydreaming. Left-handers appear to be more prone to it than right-handers, the most celebrated example being Leonardo da Vinci. In most cases of mirror-writing following brain injury, patients who were right-handed prior to the damage switch to left-handed mirror-writing, and the damage typically involves the left parietal lobe.

A possible explanation is that there is a natural tendency for the limbs on opposite sides of the body to make mirror-image movements, so that a skill learned with one hand, for example, is right–left reversed if the person is forced for some reason to use the other hand (Critchley, 1928). A more specific possibility is that representations might be stored independently of right–left orientation, and that reversals occur in converting them to action. In support of such a theory, Chia and Kinsbourne (1987) describe the case of a right-handed Chinese man who mirror-wrote with his left hand following a hemorrhage of the left BASAL GANGLIA, but who showed no reversal tendency in reading.

However, motor reversal cannot easily account for all of the evidence. In one classic case a patient with right HEMIPLEGIA who wrote backwards with the left hand continued to do so with the right hand when she had regained control of it (Ireland, 1881). Some reversals have a strong perceptual as well as a motor component. Orton (1937) observed that many developmental dyslexics not only habitually wrote backwards, but were better at reading script if it were held up to a mirror. One report describes a left-handed woman with a history of EPILEPSY who showed a variety of spatial reversals, including reversing the bases on a baseball field, and reversing the sense of which is the hot and which the cold faucet; she also mirror-wrote with her dominant left hand and was faster and more accurate at reading mirrored than normal script (Wade & Hart, 1991). Another patient, a bilingual woman, after suffering concussion showed mirror-writing and mirror-reading for a sinistrad script (Hebrew) but not for a dextrad one (Polish), was right–left disoriented with respect to her own body as well as the examiner's, and on being discharged from hospital believed her own flat to have been mirror-reversed (Streifler & Hofman, 1976). Luria (1966) described a patient with damage to the *right* parietal lobe who drew a right–left reversed map of Russia.

Such observations have suggested that the two hemispheres, and especially the parietal lobes, may record spatial engrams with opposite right – left orientations, so that unilateral damage may "release" a reversed engram from the uninjured hemisphere. While this idea is reminiscent of Orton's theory, it may be more plausibly linked to the notion of reversal in interhemispheric transfer, outlined earlier. If a representation is initially laid down more strongly in a dominant hemisphere, then transfer may result in the reversed engram being more strongly represented in the non-dominant one. This may explain why it is left hemispheric damage that produces mirror-writing, while it was right hemispheric damage that produced the reversed map of Russia from Luria's patient.

Right–left disorientation following unilateral brain damage may therefore take different forms that reflect different underlying deficits. Damage to the left parietal lobe, in particular, may create difficulty with the use of the actual words "right" and "left," while damage to the right parietal lobe is more likely to create problems with spatial transformations, resulting in right-left disorientation within reference frames that do not coincide with the patient's egocentric frame. Besides these deficits, unilateral damage may "release" reversed engrams, resulting in specific right–left reversals. For a thorough understanding of the significance of right–left disorientation in individual cases, these subtle distinctions may need to be carefully drawn.

BIBLIOGRAPHY

Alexander, D., & Money, J. (1966). Turner's syndrome and Gerstmann's syndrome: neurologic comparisons. *Neuropsychologia, 4*, 981–4.

Benton, A. L. (1959). *Right-left discrimination and finger localization: development and pathology*. New York: P. B. Hoeber.

Benton, A. L. (1979). Body schema disturbances: finger agnosia and right-left disorientation. In K. M. Heilman & E. Valenstein (Eds), *Clinical neuropsychology* (pp. 141–58). Oxford: Oxford University Press.

Chia, L., & Kinsbourne, M. (1987). Mirror-writing and reversed repetition of digits in a right-handed patient with left basal ganglia hematoma. *Journal of Neurology, Neurosurgery, and Psychiatry, 50*, 786–8.

Clark, C. M., & Klonoff, H. (1990). Right and left orientation in children aged 5 to 13 years. *Journal of Clinical and Experimental Neuropsychology, 12*, 459–66.

Corballis, M. C., & Beale, I. L. (1976). *The psychology of left and right*. Hillsdale, NJ: Erlbaum.

Critchley, M. (1928). *Mirror writing*. London: Kegan Paul, Trench, Trubner.

Elze, K. (1924). Rechtslinksempfinden und Rechtslinksblindheit. *Zeitschrift für angewandte Psychologie, 24*, 129–35.

Head, H. (1926). *Aphasia and kindred disorders of speech*. Cambridge: Cambridge University Press.

Heilman, K. M., Howell, G., Valenstein, E., & Rothi, L. (1980). Mirror-reading and writing in association with right–left disorientation. *Journal of Neurology, Neurosurgery and Psychiatry, 43*, 774–80.

Ireland, W. W. (1881). On mirror-writing and its relation to left-handedness and cerebral disease. *Brain, 4*, 361–7.

Luria, A. R. (1966). *Human brain and psychological processes*. New York: Harper & Row.

Orton, S. T. (1937). *Reading, writing, and speech problems in children*. New York: W. W. Norton.

Streifler, M., & Hofman, S. (1976). Sinistrad mirror writing and reading after brain concussion in a bi-systemic (oriento-occidental) polyglot. *Cortex, 12*, 356–64.

Wade, J. B., & Hart, R. P. (1991). Mirror phenomena in language and nonverbal activities – a case report. *Journal of Clinical and Experimental Neuropsychology, 13*, 299–308.

MICHAEL C. CORBALLIS

Rolandic area   The Rolandic area is the region of the cerebral CORTEX which lies immediately anterior and posterior to the central or Rolandic fissure. Anterior to the central fissure, in the frontal lobe, lies the primary motor (or *precentral*) cortex and anterior to that the secondary premotor cortex. Posterior to the central fissure, in the parietal lobe, lies the primary somatosensory cortex and behind that the secondary somatosensory cortex.

The central fissure is an important line of demarcation in the cortex as lesions simply described as "anterior" or "posterior" are so described by reference to this structure. Functionally this distinction has implications so that, for example, all fluent paraphasic APHASIAS occur with lesions posterior to the central fissure, while nonfluent aphasias are associated with lesions anterior to it.

S

SAD *See* SEASONAL AFFECTIVE DISORDER.

scan A scan is a technique for collecting information about brain structure or function using one of a variety of neuroimaging techniques that have become available during the 1970s and 1980s. The four major scanning techniques are Computerized Tomography (CT), Magnetic Resonance Imaging (MRI), Single Photon Emission Computed Tomography (SPECT), and Positron Emission Tomography (PET). Each of these provides a particular type of information about brain structure and function, and each has its own advantages or disadvantages as a clinical or research tool. Two of the techniques, CT and MRI, provide information about brain structure and anatomy, while the other two, SPECT and PET, are functional imaging techniques that provide information about brain metabolism, physiology, and biochemistry.

CT

CT is the oldest of the neuroimaging techniques. The first clinical data were published by Hounsfield in 1973. CT scanning remains the most widely available scanning technique for assessment of the structural integrity of the brain, because of its relatively low cost and ease of use. Compared with the other techniques, however, it provides a relatively limited amount of information, so it is now being steadily surpassed as an assessment tool.

A CT scan is produced by passing an X-ray beam through brain tissue and measuring the degree to which it is attenuated. The image created by CT depends on the fact that attenuation by cerebrospinal fluid is relatively low, attenuation by bone is relatively high, and brain attenuation intermediate. The degree of tissue attenuation is converted to a gray scale, so that CSF appears black, bone white, and brain tissue an intermediate shade of gray. The principle of visualizing the internal structure of organs by slicing through them (i.e. tomography) has been recognized for many years and was employed by Leonardo da Vinci in his anatomical illustrations. The application of tomography to scanning the brain was not possible, however, until high-speed computers became available to store and process the large quantity of information that is generated by scanning procedures.

The image produced by the scanning procedure depends on both slicing the tissue (done by the position of the X-ray beam and the detectors that measure the attenuation) and by the superimposition of a grid on the tissue within the slice, which divides the tissue into tiny cubes, referred to as "volume elements" or "voxels." The actual scan is a dot matrix of gray scale values, which are smoothed through image reconstruction techniques in order to produce a relatively attractive image that visually resembles brain tissue, CSF, and bone. The gray scale dots within the picture are referred to as "picture elements" or "pixels." The first CT scanner used an 80×80 matrix of 6,400 pixels for a given slice. Newer scanners use a 160×160 matrix, which produces 25,600 pixels. Typically, eight to ten one-centimeter slices are collected in the transaxial plane in order to scan the bulk of brain tissue. The amount of data involved, and the need for high-speed computers to process it, are obvious. When CT was in its early developmental era, a complete scan required nearly 30 minutes of data collection and image reconstruction. In the 1990s a much higher quality of scanning data is acquired in seconds to minutes.

CT scanning has been used in order to study many aspects of brain structure. When it was first developed, it was the only technique available for visualizing the brain in vivo, and it represented an exciting advance for clinical neuroscience. It is particularly useful for visualizing lesions produced by stroke or brain tumors. Its capacity to clearly distinguish between CSF and brain tissue permits visualization of neurodegenerative processes occurring in the brain, including the consequences of normal aging and of disorders such as Alzheimer's disease or Huntington's disease. Because its resolution is poorer than MR, MR is usually preferable for identifying small lesions or other more subtle changes that are difficult to visualize with CT, such as the plaques of multiple sclerosis. CT scanning has been used to conduct research on a variety of clinical and neuroscience questions, such as the relationship between lesion localization and clinical presentation in aphasia, the relationship between handedness and cerebral asymmetries, or the structural brain abnormalities of schizophrenia.

MAGNETIC RESONANCE IMAGING

MRI, the other major structural imaging technique, first became available in the early 1980s and began to enjoy wide availability by the late 1980s. The basic principles of tomography and the imposition of a grid of voxels and pixels in order to generate a visual picture are also used in MRI, and indeed in SPECT and PET as well. MR differs from CT, however, in the origin and nature of the signal that produces the image. The MR signal is produced by placing the brain in a magnetic field, aligning the hydrogen protons that are widely dispersed in brain tissue so that they are concentrated to produce a net magnetic moment, altering the energy of that magnetic moment by stimulation with a radio frequency signal, and measuring the relaxation or return of the magnetic moment to its original direction and energy state. The physics of MR are considerably more complex than for CT, in that the nature of the image can be dramatically varied, depending on the timing and intensity of the radio frequency pulse signals, and this complexity makes MR both a more challenging structural imaging technique and a more powerful and flexible one. MR has many advantages over CT. It does not involve the use of any ionizing radiation. While CT scans are generally limited to the transverse or transaxial plane, MR data can be acquired in three dimensions and represented in multiple planes (e.g. coronal, sagittal, transaxial). MR images can also be displayed visually in three dimensions if appropriate computer software is employed. MR has superb anatomic resolution. It permits excellent discrimination between gray matter and white matter, permitting visualization of relatively small structures, such as cranial nerves, nuclei of the basal ganglia, limbic structures such as the hippocampus, or very small areas such as the substantia innominata. The resolution is of such high quality, in fact, that the slices of an MR scan have a close visual resemblance to post-mortem brain slices.

MR has greater power for visualizing most types of brain pathology. Small tumors, multiple sclerosis plaques, and tiny areas of infarction can be clearly identified. Bone is poorly seen with MR (although the marrow is visualized), making MR an inappropriate technique for evaluating possible skull abnormalities such as fractures. The other major drawbacks of MR are its cost and a correlated limitation in availability. At present MR installations are primarily located in larger university medical centers and urban areas.

Because of its flexibility and power, MRI lends itself to research in both basic and clinical neuroscience. Basic neuroscience investigations have examined the quantitative volume of gray matter, white matter, and cerebrospinal fluid in the brain, demonstrating through the study of large groups of normal individuals from a broad age range that the percentage of CSF increases steadily as a consequence of the aging process, while the quantity of gray matter declines. Issues previously explored through study of post-mortem brain tissue (e.g. left versus right asymmetries of the planum temporale, callosal size in right versus left-handers, gender differences in callosal shape) have all been reevaluated with MRI, which permits the in vivo study of the brain in large numbers of people whose physical and mental health can be evaluated and documented. The relationship between cerebral size, gray-matter volume, and intelligence has also been explored. As MR is more widely used as a basic technology in cognitive neuroscience, many other applications are likely to emerge.

MR has also documented many different types of brain lesions in different clinical disorders. For example, MR elicits a distinctive signal from tissue containing a paramagnetic substance such as iron, permitting the study of disorders that have an abnormal concentration in the extrapyramidal system, such as WILSON'S DISEASE. Caudate atrophy in HUNTINGTON'S DISEASE can be clearly visualized and carefully monitored. The relationship between lesion localization and clinical presentation in neurological and psychiatric conditions associated with stroke can be carefully measured and monitored. Abnormalities in temporolimbic regions (e.g. the hippocampus) can be visualized in some patients with schizophrenia. Cerebellar and other abnormalities have been described in autism.

SINGLE PHOTON EMISSION COMPUTED TOMOGRAPHY

SPECT is a functional imaging technique that permits visualization and quantification of regional cerebral blood flow within the brain. Blood flow is an indirect indicator of metabolic activity. Two types of tracers are currently used for the measurement of blood flow. ^{133}Xenon is a low-energy tracer that clears rapidly; it can be administered through inhalation and its clearance curve monitored through a probe over the lungs. Its clearance characteristics permit it to be used for quantitative measurements of cerebral blood flow (milliliters per gram of tissue per minute) and for paired back-to-back studies that can involve a baseline and a cognitive challenge condition. Its major limitation is the relatively poor resolution of the images produced (2- to 3-centimeter range). Xenon SPECT imaging is a relatively inexpensive technique. Although a dedicated head unit is required, it uses commercially available tracers, making it a less costly alternative to PET for the study of cognitive function.

Static tracers such as TC99^m HMPAO are the major alternative to xenon in SPECT studies. They are currently widely used because their higher photon energy produces improved tissue resolution. SPECT images can be obtained with commercially available HMPAO and imaging equipment widely available in most nuclear medicine facilities (i.e. rotating gamma cameras). Resolution can be substantially improved through the use of three-headed gamma cameras, which are becoming steadily more available. Static tracers such as HMPAO are removed in a single first-pass extraction; the scan produced is an image of the distribution of the tracer in the brain during the 2- to 30-second time window when the tracer passes through the brain. These tracers were initially used to visualize flow during the resting state, either to localize lesions produced by

stroke or tumor or to explore the possibility of abnormalities in regional blood flow in illnesses such as schizophrenia or Alzheimer's disease. Specific patterns of abnormality have been noted in Alzheimer's (decreased flow in temporoparietal regions); decreased flow in prefrontal regions has been described in schizophrenia. New strategies are also being developed to apply static tracers to cognitive challenge paradigms through multiple back-to-back injections and image addition and subtraction techniques. The major limitation of the static tracers is that they do not produce quantitative data; numerical analysis must use ratio measures (e.g. frontal: cerebral flow).

The majority of the research and clinical applications of SPECT have involved measurement of regional cerebral blood flow. Although the basic conceptual principles involved in SPECT were introduced by Kety in 1948, dedicated head units for xenon studies or high-energy tracers for gamma camera studies have become widely available only in the 1980s. Tracers have been developed for the evaluation of neurotransmitter systems; specific tracers exist for visualization of acetylcholine and dopamine$_2$ receptors. Clinical and research applications of tracer agents for neurotransmitters are still developing.

POSITRON EMISSION TOMOGRAPHY

PET is similar to SPECT, in that it is a technique that permits the study of brain function. Unlike SPECT, however, it does not employ commercially available tracers, since it is dependent on the use of positron-emitting substances which must be generated in an on-site cyclotron. The positron-emitting tracers used for PET have a relatively short half life: 2 minutes for ^{15}O, 20 minutes for ^{11}carbon, 110 minutes for ^{18}fluorine. These positron emitters are then joined to an informative ligand in an on-site radiochemistry laboratory, administered to a subject through intravenous injection, and mapped distributionally in the brain using a special tomograph designed specifically for PET studies. The tomograph consists of rings of scintillation detectors and photomultiplier tubes, which collect the data in transaxial slices; reconstruction is achieved through the use of voxel/pixel grids and filtering, as in all other neuroimaging techniques.

Since SPECT and PET scans both measure radioactivity counts, the images are usually portrayed in the hot/cold color scale employed in

641

nuclear medicine studies, with red tones representing high areas of activity and blue tones representing low areas of activity. In PET, as in SPECT, the measured counts are photons. In PET the photons are generated through the annihilation event that occurs when the positron strikes an electron in the area of functional activity, thereby producing two 511 Kev photons that are emitted at an angle of 180 degrees, producing a two-point "coincidence line" that can be simultaneously detected by the scintillation counters in the PET camera ring. The use of two points to identify the site of activity accounts in part for the improved resolution that occurs in PET studies as compared to SPECT studies. PET studies now have a resolution in the 5-millimeter range, while the resolution of SPECT is approximately 8 millimeters with the best possible equipment (three-headed gamma cameras) and 12 millimeters with a single-headed gamma camera.

^{18}F deoxyglucose (FDG) is the ligand that has been most widely used in PET research. FDG is a measure of glucose utilization and therefore an indicator of tissue metabolism. FDG is typically used in a single study. It can identify seizure foci (which are hypometabolic), areas of infarction (also hypometabolic), areas of increased activity due to auditory, visual, or cognitive stimuli (which are hypermetabolic), areas of decreased metabolism due to neuronal loss or decreased neuronal activity (hypometabolism in temporoparietal regions in Alzheimer's disease), or abnormal areas observable during resting conditions in other pathological states (e.g. increased metabolic activity in the prefrontal cortex and basal ganglia in obsessive-compulsive disorder).

^{15}O H$_2$O is a ligand that is increasingly widely employed in PET studies. Because ^{15}O has only a two-minute half-life, it can be used for repeated back-to-back studies over a relatively short time. The subject is typically given seven or eight different cognitive stimuli, which are carefully selected in order to break a particular cognitive system or operation down into its component parts: e.g. seeing a nonverbal stimulus, seeing a word, saying a word, or mentioning a use for the word. A sequential study of this type permits mapping of the components in a particular cognitive system, such as memory, language, or attention. The different task components are subtracted from one another using "image math"

techniques. Studies of this type are being used to map cognitive systems in the brain. An eight-injection PET study can be completed in two to three hours; quantitative measurement of regional cerebral blood flow can be obtained if an arterial line is placed. The major strength of this design is that it reduces intersubject variation by using a within-subject design for a series of related cognitive tasks.

Techniques for applying PET to the study of neuroreceptors are also well developed. Ligands are available for measuring dopamine, serotonin, cholinergic, benzodiazapine, and opiate receptors. Development of appropriate modelling techniques has permitted not only visualization of receptors in order to localize their site in the brain, but also quantitative measurement. This particular application of PET permits the investigation of neuronal response to short- and long-term pharmacologic stimulation.

BIBLIOGRAPHY

Andreasen, N. C. (1988). Brain imaging: applications in psychiatry. *Science, 239*, 1381–8.

Brant-Zawadzki, M., & Norman D. (Eds). (1987). *Magnetic resonance imaging of the central nervous system*. New York: Raven Press.

Hounsfield, G. N. (1973). Computerized transverse axial scanning (tomography). *British Journal of Radiology, 46*, 1016–47.

Kety, S. S., & Schmidt, C. F. (1948). The nitrous oxide method for the quantitative determination of cerebral blood flow in Man: theory, procedure and normal values. *Journal of Clinical Investigation, 27*, 476–83.

Petersen, S. E., Fox, P. T., Posner, M. I., Mintun, M., & Raichle, M. E. (1988). Positron emission tomography studies of the cortical anatomy of single-word processing. *Nature, 331*, 585–9.

Sedvall, G., Farde, L., Persoon, A., & Wiesel, F. A. (1986). Imaging of neurotransmitter receptors in the living human brain. *Archives of General Psychiatry, 43*, 955–1005.

NANCY C. ANDREASEN

schizophrenia Schizophrenia is the general term for a group of psychiatric disorders of a psychotic nature with various cognitive, emotional, and behavioral manifestations. Perhaps better regarded as "the schizophrenias," arguments continue about the precise nature and definition of these disorders, with complete agreement not being found among the various international classification systems. However, all forms of schizophrenia are characterized by deterioration from previous cognitive and social functional levels, an onset before midlife, and a pattern of psychotic features which may include thought disturbances, bizarre delusions, hallucinations which are more commonly auditory, a disturbed sense of self, and a loss of contact with reality.

While schizophrenia is normally regarded as a functional rather than an organic psychiatric disorder, neuropsychological interest in the condition has increased in recent years. Studies have reported certain gross brain changes in schizophrenic patients, which include an increase in the size of the CORPUS CALLOSUM, and enlargement of the cerebral ventricles; these effects do not appear wholly attributable to long-term psychotropic medication. Research has also focused on possible abnormalities in the pattern of LATERALIZATION in schizophrenics, with competing hypotheses that either propose a deficit in interhemispheric integration, or else a more specific disorder of lateralization relating to the organization of the anterior left hemisphere. There is evidence to support each of these hypotheses. Other studies have suggested independent evidence for a left-sided frontal deficit affecting specific cognitive and emotional processes, derived from both psychological and behavioral assessments, BLOOD FLOW STUDIES, and other forms of physiological SCAN. At the present time all these hypotheses have received partial support, but none seems entirely adequate to provide a full neuropsychological explanation for schizophrenia. However, it can be concluded that very promising research continues, which may lead to the identification of a clear cerebral abnormality associated with schizophrenic disorder. A biochemical abnormality has for some time been accepted by many as present in schizophrenic states. Although complete agreement has not yet been reached as to its precise nature, it seems probable that this abnormality may be associated with dopaminergic systems in the cerebral cortex and other cerebral centers, and may link with the grosser anatomical changes suggested above.

Schizophrenic states may be more directly associated with organic syndromes. Any form of psychotic illness may accompany cerebral TUMOR, and although schizophrenia-like states are relatively uncommon, they occur at a rate higher than the incidence in the general population. When they do occur they are more likely to be associated with TEMPORAL LOBE and PITUITARY TUMORS and may feature the complex hallucinations which may occur with temporal lobe lesions. Similarly, schizophrenic-like states may follow head injury and, while the incidence may be only in the region of 3 percent, this is again higher than the rate in the general population and is not necessarily associated with a premorbid schizoid personality. Following head injury, paranoid states and states prominently featuring hallucinations are the more common form, but no particular location of damage is associated with the development of the schizophrenic symptoms. Lesions which produce BODY SCHEMA DISTURBANCE may particularly lead to schizophrenia-like states.

Disorders similar to the functional forms of schizophrenia may also follow cerebral infections, and post-encephalitic states (*see* ENCEPHALITIS) may include paranoid and hallucinatory features in up to 30 percent of cases. Similarly GENERAL PARALYSIS OF THE INSANE has a strong association with such states, and rheumatic fever with cerebral involvement may result not only in a distinct form of CHOREA, but also in a schizophrenic state. Alcoholic hallucinosis can also be confusable with schizophrenia.

The association of EPILEPSY with schizophrenia has been much debated, but it is clear that the association is stronger than the chance expectation of the combination of these disorders, and especially temporal lobe epilepsy may produce hallucinations, disorders of the integrity of the self, and even delusional states. DEMENTIA may be difficult to distinguish from chronic schizophrenic deterioration of cognition and personality.

While the diagnostic differentiation of "functional" schizophrenia from organically based schizophrenia-like psychoses may be a significant problem for the psychiatrist and neurologist, it is generally accepted that hallucinations which are visual rather than auditory, a relatively shallow affect in the presence of delusional beliefs, and a vague, inconsistent, and changeable quality to delusions are all evidence in favor of an organic rather than a functional basis to the disorder, but this is no more than a very imperfect generalization.

J. GRAHAM BEAUMONT

sclerosis   Sclerosis is a lesion in which demyelination occurs, followed by gliosis of white matter. It is characteristic of a number of neurological conditions including amyotrophic lateral sclerosis, MULTIPLE SCLEROSIS, temporal lobe sclerosis, and tuberose sclerosis.

scotoma   Scotoma is the term for any isolated area of defective vision within the visual field. Scotomas may have various causes, but these include small lesions of the cortex of the occipital lobe in the primary visual area. When the scotoma is present in the region around and including the point of fixation, it is a *central scotoma*, and occurs in optic neuritis, a disorder of the optic nerve.

A surprising aspect of scotomas is that the patient may be entirely unaware of them. This may simply be because, as in HEMIANOPIA, there is a concomitant loss of visual attention for the relevant region. However, with small scotomas it is even more likely that *completion* occurs across the region of the scotoma, partly a purely perceptual process, but assisted by the continual movement of the eyes, bringing the "hidden" area into a region of normal vision.

seasonal affective disorder   Seasonal affective disorder (SAD) (*see also* DEPRESSION; EMOTIONAL DISORDERS) is a syndrome characterized by affective episodes (depression, hypomania, or mania) recurring regularly during certain seasons of the year. Rosenthal and colleagues (1984) described a form of the condition where fall–winter depressions alternate with nondepressed periods in the spring and summer. Depressive symptoms often include hypersomnia, anergia, fatigue, carbohydrate craving, and weight gain. Spring–summer months are characterized by euthymia (normal moods) or hypomania. Exposure of SAD patients to bright artificial light has been found to improve depressive symptoms.

Jacobsen and others (1987) studied 156 SAD patients at the National Institute of Mental Health from 1981 to 1985. They reported a small percentage of SAD patients (7 percent) who were more severely affected, becoming manic during the spring or summer (Bipolar I), while 10 percent had winter depression without summer symptoms (Unipolar). The majority of SAD patients (83 percent) had depressive episodes that generally ended in the spring and were followed by a constellation of mild symptoms opposite to those seen in the winter (Bipolar II). Wehr and others (1987) reported a variant of the syndrome with the opposite pattern, namely depression in the summer and nondepressed periods in fall and winter, a condition they have called reverse SAD.

CLINICAL ASPECTS OF SEASONAL AFFECTIVE DISORDER

Diagnosis of SAD was based on the validated Research Diagnostic Criteria (RDC) for major depression from which the American Psychiatric Association's DSM is derived. SAD diagnostic criteria were originally described by Rosenthal and colleagues (1984):

1   A history of depression fulfilling RDC criteria (Spitzer et al., 1978) for major affective disorder, depressed.
2   A history of at least two consecutive years of fall/winter depressive episodes remitting in the spring or summer.
3   The absence of any other DSM-III-R Axis I major psychiatric disorder.
4   The absence of seasonal psychosocial stressors which might provide an explanation for the seasonal mood changes (Rosenthal & Blehar, 1989).

Most researchers have used these criteria in studies of the condition. The consistent recurrence of seasonal depression has led to the conclusion that SAD may be a distinct subgroup of depressive illness. The incidence of SAD is difficult to evaluate as formal epidemiological studies have not been reported; Thase (1986) estimated that 15.6 percent of a large clinical population ($n = 115$) with recurrent depressive disorders met the criteria for SAD, as defined above.

More recently the criteria have been revised and incorporated into DSM-III-R as "seasonal pattern." The new criteria of DSM-III-R allow more rigorous classification, and seasonality is viewed as a dimension rather than a category; in

addition the timing of symptoms is more specifically defined:

1 A DSM-III-R diagnosis of recurrent mood
   disorder with "seasonal pattern."
2 At least three episodes of mood disturbance in
   three separate years that demonstrate a regular temporal relationship between onset and a
   particular 60-day period of the year, and full
   remission (or a change from depression to
   hypomania or mania) within a 60-day period
   of the year. At least two of the three years
   consecutive.
3 Seasonal episodes of mood disturbance out-
   number nonseasonal episodes by more than
   three to one.
4 No obvious effect of seasonally related psychosocial stressors, e.g. regularly being unem-
   ployed every winter (Rosenthal et al., 1989a).

DSM-IV states that both bipolar and unipolar
depressive disorders can be subdiagnosed as
"seasonal" if there is a regular relationship between an episode and a particular time of year.

The validity of SAD has been discussed extensively; reports from many different groups in the
United States, Europe, and Australia have corroborated the existence of most of the clinical
features of the condition; the unipolar–bipolar
distinction remains mildly controversial (Rosenthal et al., 1989a). Bauer and Dunner (1993)
review data regarding the validity of seasonal
pattern (SP), according to DSM-III-R, as a
modifier for recurrent mood disorders. They
conclude that, while the definitions of SP and
SAD are similar and available data support a
distinct clinical syndrome, it is not yet clear
whether SP or SAD represents a distinct affective
syndrome, a subtype of recurrent affective illness,
or the most severe form of a widely distributed
population trait (Bauer & Dunner, 1993).

NEUROBIOLOGICAL EXPLANATIONS OF SEASONAL AFFECTIVE DISORDER

There are several reports that symptoms of SAD
increase with the distance from the equator and in
climatic conditions of low light. Recent studies
have shown that modification of the physical
environment may be used to treat affective
episodes; these studies have established that
phototherapy with full-spectrum light is effective
in ameliorating the depressive symptoms of SAD.

the response to bright light has been extensively
documented (Rosenthal et al., 1984; 1989b).
However, the mechanism for the antidepressant
effect of light remains unclear, as does the
biological basis for the diverse psychological and
biological changes associated with SAD. Several
hypotheses have been proposed to explain the
effects of phototherapy on SAD and these will be
discussed; to date none provides a completely
satisfactory explanation of all the phenomena
associated with SAD and its treatment.

Melatonin hypothesis

The melatonin hypothesis proposes that bright
light treatment exerts its antidepressant effects by
modifying melatonin secretion, which is responsible for the symptoms of SAD. Melatonin is a
hormone secreted at night by the PINEAL GLAND.
In the 1980s, Lewy and colleagues reported that
nocturnal melatonin secretion in humans could
be suppressed by bright environmental light but
not by ordinary room light. Their findings
suggested that light could affect functions mediated by pathways traversing the HYPOTHALAMUS,
and led to the hypothesis that other brain-
mediated functions might also be influenced by
bright environmental light.

It is suggested that changes in the photoperiod
(the period between the first and last exposure to
light on a given day) initiate winter depression by
changing the pattern of nocturnal melatonin
secretion, which acts as a chemical indicator of
darkness. Phototherapy should only be effective
when administered before dawn or after dusk,
thus extending the photoperiod and shortening
the phase of active melatonin secretion.

Strong supporting evidence for the melatonin
hypothesis has not been provided by research
findings. A number of studies have failed to
demonstrate a statistical difference between
bright and dim light; this contrast is important in
order to demonstrate that the treatment is distin-
guishable from that of a placebo.

Other studies have shown phototherapy to be
effective when administered during daylight
hours, also failing to support the importance of
photoperiod extension in modifying the pattern of
melatonin secretion. Research has also demonstrated that restoring high plasma levels of melatonin only partially reversed the antidepressant
effect of light. Finally, drugs which suppress
melatonin secretion have not been effective in

ameliorating symptoms in patients with SAD; Rosenthal and colleagues failed to find any therapeutic difference between the beta-adrenergic blocker, atenolol, which inhibits melatonin secretion, and placebo in a double-blind crossover design study.

Findings suggest that patients with SAD do not have physiological responses to light that are significantly different from controls, except perhaps in cerebral blood flow. Murphy and colleagues (1993) report a small pilot study into the effect of light on cerebral blood flow in four SAD patients and four controls. There were no initial differences between patients and controls in global, regional or cerebral hemispheric blood flow; however, after exposure to 1,500 lux artificial light the SAD patients and controls had a significantly different percentage change in cerebral blood flow.

These findings taken together lead to the conclusion that, while melatonin may play some role in the symptoms of SAD and the effects of phototherapy, the melatonin hypothesis by itself cannot account for these phenomena.

Circadian rhythm phase-shift hypothesis

This hypothesis proposes that patients with SAD have a phase delay of circadian rhythms in winter which causes their depression. Circadian rhythm phases become abnormally delayed relative to sleep patterns in winter due to the increasing lateness of dawn. As morning light advances the phase position of circadian rhythms it should improve winter depression, whereas evening light delays the phase position and should have the opposite effect. Evidence that patients with SAD can have their rhythms reset by bright light in the morning, but are made worse by bright light in the evening, has been provided by Lewy and colleagues (1987). However, other investigators have provided contrary evidence that mood changes do not accompany alterations in circadian timing in phase-delayed normal subjects during the Antarctic winter. Further studies have failed to demonstrate a superior effect of morning over evening light; indeed, evening light, which according to the hypothesis should worsen depression, has been shown to improve it.

The hypothesis has received only partial support; Checkley's group provided some evidence that the antidepressant effect of phototherapy is more than a placebo response but concluded that

a phase advance is clearly not a prerequisite for an antidepressant effect of light. Lewy has reformulated the hypothesis as an internal phase alteration between sleep and other rhythms; in other words, the mechanism relates to an endogenous biological rhythm rather than to a direct response to the environment.

Sleep is thought to be less delayed than other circadian rhythms in winter depression; when sleep time is held constant, morning light exposure corrects the abnormality by causing a phase advance in the other circadian rhythms. Future research may resolve these issues.

Photon-counting hypothesis

In this hypothesis the reduction in the total amount of available light in winter is thought to generate SAD; however, the emphasis is on the *total* amount of light available, that is the number of photons hitting the retina, and the simple replacement of light in phototherapy is thought to be the therapeutic agent. The timing of phototherapy is not critical and photoperiod extension is not necessary. This hypothesis is compatible with the data from a number of research groups; but it is more conservative than the other hypotheses and has less explanatory power.

Other hypotheses

A number of other hypotheses exist, including the view that artificial light may act as a conditioned stimulus (Thompson & Silverstone, 1989, p. 165). Patients with SAD associate the lack of light with the observation that their depression occurs in winter; bright artificial light acts as a conditioned stimulus leading to the response of elevation of mood. Sensitivity to light is another hypothesis which has been investigated following Lewy's finding that manic depressive patients may be supersensitive to light. SAD patients may either be supersensitive, like the manic depressives, whom they resemble clinically, or subsensitive, explaining their greater need for light. The available data fail to support either of these explanations (Thompson & Silverstone, 1989).

Cognitive impairments in patients with SAD have been reported by O'Brien and colleagues (1993). Attention, memory, and learning were assessed in SAD patients and matched controls. When depressed, patients were impaired on spatial memory and learning but showed no deficit in attention. Patients were significantly slower to respond than controls; however, O'Brien and others (1993) suggest that the pattern indicated slowed information processing centrally, rather than simple sensory or motor slowing. On recovery from depression, an impairment remained in response latency on a test of spatial memory; this continuing impairment correlated with residual depressive symptoms, but not with ventricular brain ratio.

Animal studies have indicated that serotonin (5-HT) is a major neurotransmitter involved in the control of numerous central nervous system functions, including mood. Biological studies of depression have focused on the monoamine neurotransmitters and these have been examined in SAD patients as well, but the available information is limited. Of the neurotransmitter systems examined so far, the serotonin system appears most likely to be dysregulated (Skwerer et al., 1989; Thompson & Silverstone, 1989).

PHOTOTHERAPY

The efficacy of phototherapy treatment for SAD has been widely demonstrated and generally acknowledged. Phototherapy with full-spectrum light held great promise as a non-pharmacological antidepressant treatment, providing rapid remissions with minimal side effects. The portal of entry of the therapeutic effect is thought to be the eyes rather than the skin. Although side effects are uncommon, patients sometimes complain of irritability, eyestrain, headaches, or insomnia.

Full-spectrum light is used in phototherapy because it produces the closest replication of natural light, which contains a relatively even distribution of *all* the frequencies of the visible spectrum. Full-spectrum lighting operates on the same basis as fluorescent tubes (which give off a high level of yellow-green light), but the compounds lining the tubes are designed to emit *all* colors of the spectrum in virtually the same proportions as natural daylight. Several factors have been shown to influence the efficacy of phototherapy with full-spectrum light, most notably the *intensity, timing,* and *duration* of light.

The intensity of light necessary for mood improvements to occur was initially thought to be 2,500 lux with no improvements occurring with dim light of less than 300 lux. Later studies demonstrated that intensity levels of 2,500 and 300 lux were equally effective for mood improve-

ment, and that for some people intensities of up to 10,000 lux may be significantly superior to 2,500 lux when used for only 30 minutes a day (Rosenthal et al., 1989b). Rosenthal and colleagues (1993) investigated the treatment of 55 winter SAD patients with a light visor, a newly developed portable light-delivery system. They compared the efficacy of two different light intensities: a dim 400 lux visor and a bright 6,000 lux visor for either 30 or 60 minutes in the morning for one week (a controlled parallel design). They concluded that there was no evidence that the brighter visor was superior in efficacy to the dimmer one. An alternative explanation of their failure to obtain a difference was that the light visor acted as a placebo, or that the light visor was equally effective over a wide range of intensities (Rosenthal et al., 1993).

There is considerable controversy regarding the timing of phototherapy. Some studies report a superiority of morning over evening phototherapy treatment; others report no significant difference between morning and evening treatments. It appears that some patients are differentially sensitive to phototherapy at different times of the day. Lafer and colleagues (1994) investigated the outcome of an alternating time schedule versus two fixed schedules (either morning or evening) and found no significant difference among patients in the three groups for response criteria after one week of treatment; they conclude that these results support the use of more flexible phototherapy schedules.

Further inconsistencies are apparent in the literature with respect to the duration of phototherapy. Early studies used five to six hours of treatment per day; later studies found two hours of treatment per day to be effective, and others found no difference between two hours and half an hour of treatment a day.

In an attempt to address the equivocal nature of these findings, Terman and colleagues (1989) conducted a meta-analysis of the data collected from 332 patients in 14 research centers over a five-year period. The analysis of 29 light therapy studies reported between 1984 and 1987 showed considerable variability in treatment outcome as a function of time of day and duration of light administration. Data pooled across studies indicated that, overall, 2,500 lux intensity light exposure for at least two hours daily for one week resulted in significantly more remissions;

morning, midday, and evening light exposures were all significantly more effective than dim light alone. A clear positive treatment effect for early morning bright light exposure was found; however, results regarding the effectiveness of midday and evening exposures were equivocal. The highest remission rates were found among mildly depressed patients, who as a group showed a differential response favoring morning over evening light (Terman et al., 1989).

CONCLUSION

In summary, there is agreement among researchers that SAD is a recognizable clinical condition and that in a large percentage of cases the symptoms respond well to treatment with bright environmental light. Phototherapy has been shown to be effective in SAD as a viable clinical treatment and, in some cases, the treatment of choice. The efficacy of phototherapy in nonseasonal depression has not been established and further research is required. Apart from these fundamental points of agreement, the many other aspects of this area remain highly controversial.

Brain-mediated functions are clearly influenced by bright environmental light, but the mechanism for the antidepressant effect of light remains unclear, as does the biological basis for the diverse psychological and neurobiological changes associated with SAD. Several hypotheses have been proposed to explain the effects of phototherapy on SAD, but none provides a completely satisfactory explanation of all the phenomena associated with SAD and its treatment; individual variation in response to treatment has been shown to contribute significantly to the equivocal nature of findings from research in this area. A further complication, pointed out by Thompson and Silverstone (1989), is that with the demise of the melatonin hypothesis there is no way of devising a properly double-blind placebo-controlled trial of the treatment that would convincingly demonstrate that phototherapy is more effective than a placebo.

BIBLIOGRAPHY

Bauer, M. S., & Dunner, D. L. (1993). Validity of seasonal pattern as a modifier for recurrent mood disorders for DSM-IV. *Comprehensive Psychiatry, 34*, 159–70.

Jacobsen, F. M., Wehr, T. A., Sack, D. A., James, S. P., & Rosenthal, N. E. (1987). Seasonal affective disorder: a review of the syndrome and its public health implications. *American Journal of Public Health, 77*, 57–60.

Lafer, B., Sachs, G. S., Labbate, L. A., Thibault, A., & Rosenbaum, J. F. (1994). Phototherapy for seasonal affective disorder: a blind comparison of three different schedules. *American Journal of Psychiatry, 151*, 1081–3.

Lewy, A. J., Sack, R. L., Miller, L. S., & Hoban, T. M. (1987). Antidepressant and circadian phase shifting-effects of light. *Science, 235*, 352–4.

Murphy, D. G., Murphy, D. M., Abbas, M., Palazidou, E., Binnie, C., Arendt, J., Campos, C. D., & Checkley, S. A. (1993). Seasonal affective disorder: response to light as measured by electroencephalogram, melatonin suppression, and cerebral blood flow. *British Journal of Psychiatry, 163*, 327–31.

O'Brien, J. T., Sahakian, B. J., & Checkley, S. A. (1993). Cognitive impairments in patients with seasonal affective disorder. *British Journal of Psychiatry, 163*, 338–43.

Rosenthal, N. E., & Blehar, M. C. (Eds). (1989). *Seasonal affective disorders and phototherapy*. New York: Guilford.

Rosenthal, N. E., Kasper, S., Schulz, P. M., & Wehr, T. A. (1989a). New developments in seasonal affective disorder. In C. Thompson & T. Silverstone (Eds), *Seasonal affective disorder* (pp. 97–132). London: CNS (Clinical Neuroscience) Publishers.

Rosenthal, N. E., Moul, D. E., Hellekson, C. J., Oren, D. A., Frank, A., Brainard, G. C., Murray, M. G., & Wehr, T. A. (1993). A multicenter study of the light visor for seasonal affective disorder: no difference in efficacy found between two different intensities. *Neuropsychopharmacology, 8*, 151–60.

Rosenthal, N. E., Sack, D. A., Gillin, J. C., Lewy, A. J., Goodwin, F. K., Davenport, Y., Mueller, P. S., Newsome, D. A., & Wehr, T. A. (1984). Seasonal Affective Disorder: a description of the syndrome and preliminary findings with light therapy. *Archives of General Psychiatry, 41*, 72–80.

Rosenthal, N. E., Sack, D. A., Skwerer, R. G., Jacobsen, F. M., & Wehr, T. A. (1989b). Phototherapy for seasonal affective disorder. In N. E. Rosenthal & M. C. Blehar (Eds), *Seasonal affective disorders and phototherapy* (pp. 273–94). New York: Guilford.

Skwerer, R. G., Jacobsen, F. M., Duncan, C. C., Kelly, K. A., Sack, D. A., Tamarkin, L., Gaist, P. A., Kasper, S., & Rosenthal, N. E. (1989). Neurobiology of seasonal affective disorder and phototherapy. In N. E. Rosenthal & M. C. Blehar (Eds), *Seasonal affective disorders and phototherapy* (pp. 311–32). New York: Guilford.

Spitzer, R. L., Endicott, J., & Robbins, E. (1978). Research diagnostic criteria: rationale and reliability. *Archives of General Psychiatry, 35*, 773–82.

Terman, M., Terman, J. S., Quitkin, F. M., McGrath, P. J., Stewart, J. W., & Rafferty, B. (1989). Light therapy for seasonal affective disorder: a review of efficacy. *Neuropsychopharmacology, 2*, 1–22.

Thase, M. (1986). Interview: defining and treating seasonal affective disorder. *Psychiatric Annals, 16*, 733–7.

Thompson, C., & Silverstone, T. (Eds). (1989). *Seasonal affective disorder.* London: CNS (Clinical Neuroscience) Publishers.

Wehr, T. A., Sack, D. A., & Rosenthal, N. E. (1987). Seasonal affective disorder with summer depression and winter hypomania. *American Journal of Psychiatry, 144*, 1602–3.

PAMELA M. KENEALY

seizure epilepsy *See* EPILEPSY.

semantic access disorder A semantic access disorder is a deficit in auditory word comprehension which may be demonstrated by poor performance in word–picture matching.

An important aspect of the performance of patients considered to have a semantic access disorder is that performance with respect to particular words shows variability. From this it is inferred that it is the processes of access to semantic information, rather than the semantic representation itself, which are at fault. When performance is consistent with respect to particular items, the disorder is referred to as *semantic degradation*, indicating a loss from the semantic knowledge base.

These semantic disorders also show important category specificity, that is, that performance with respect to particular semantic classes of item (for example: fruit, animals, inanimate objects), which is evidence that it is the semantic system which is affected.

Individuals with semantic access disorders may be very sensitive to the timing of item presentation, requiring more time than would be normal to recover from the stage of single word comprehension, a phenomenon known as *refractoriness*. The inference is that additional time is required to complete the word comprehension processes which may then interfere with the process of object or picture identification within the matching task; if these stages are temporally separated, then the deficit demonstrated by the patient may be reduced. Patients with a semantic access disorder may also experience greater difficulty in performing word to picture matching when the items are drawn from a single semantic category than when the items are drawn from different categories (or have a greater semantic distance within the category). This observation, however, is open to alternative theoretical explanations.

Semantic access disorders may also be relevant in considering individuals who habitually read by sight vocabulary, patients who employ a logographic route and are unable to rely on grapheme-to-phoneme conversion processes (being therefore unable to read novel words or nonwords; *see* DYSLEXIA). Such individuals depend upon semantic access and disorders of this system will naturally have an impact (which is potentially semantic category-specific) upon their reading performance.

J. GRAHAM BEAUMONT

sensorimotor cortex Sensorimotor cortex includes a large portion of frontal and parietal cortex of all mammals, where electrical stimulation produces body movements and cortex is activated by receptors in skin, muscles, and joints. Thus subdivisions of sensorimotor cortex have anatomical connections that include both somatosensory inputs and motor outputs. Traditionally, sensorimotor cortex has been divided into motor cortex of the frontal lobe and somatosensory cortex of the parietal lobe, but early investigators, especially Woolsey (1958), emphasized that the sensory areas also have a motor component and the motor areas have a sensory component, the difference being largely one of degree or proportion. Woolsey modified the symbols for sensorimotor areas to reflect the balances of sensory and motor functions so that primary motor cortex, M-I, became Ms-I and primary somatosensory cortex became Sm-I. This style has been largely abandoned, and formal recognition of the motor components of sensory areas and the sensory components of motor areas is often neglected. Current terminology, reflecting the useful distinction between parietal areas which are more clearly sensory and frontal areas which are more obviously motor, is used here, yet it is important to recognize that these sensory and motor areas are all sensorimotor in function.

In all mammals, sensorimotor cortex includes a number of subdivisions or areas, but the number varies across species (Kaas, 1987). In addition, the exact number and arrangement of areas for any species is typically uncertain because regions of cortex have not been adequately studied. Part of the reason for uncertainty is that cortical areas, as "organs of the brain" (Brodmann, 1909), were first recognized by often subtle differences in histological structure. This anatomical approach is often unreliable by itself, and modern efforts to subdivide cortex combine histological and electrophysiological procedures. Thus sensorimotor areas are more adequately defined by multiple criteria. Histologically distinct fields that are coextensive with systematic maps or representations of body receptors and movements, and have distinct patterns of anatomical connections, are most likely to be valid subdivisions of the brain.

SENSORIMOTOR CORTEX IN RATS AND OPOSSUMS

The organization of sensorimotor cortex in rats and opossums appears to be simpler than in primates, and the organization in these small-brained mammals may more closely reflect the basic mammalian plan. Sensorimotor cortex has been most extensively studied in rats, and a number of conclusions seem well supported by experimental results (Figure 65). First, an irregularly shaped region of parietal cortex represents mechanoreceptors of the skin from foot to face in a mediolateral pattern across cortex that identifies the field as primary somatosensory cortex, S-I (Kaas, 1983). In brain sections stained by the Nissl procedure for neurons, S-I has architectonic characteristics typical of primary sensory areas, including small or granule-sized neurons

densely packed in layer IV. Hence S-I is clearly called granular cortex. S-I is also revealed by a number of other histological procedures, such as stains for the metabolic enzyme, cytochrome oxidase. Thus there are several ways to histologically identify S-I in rats with a high degree of assurance. In addition, S-I has a very detailed and systematic representation of tactile receptors of the body that is highly similar across individuals. Recordings with microelectrodes reveal that neurons in the foot region have small receptive fields on various parts of the foot, the paw region on the paw, and so on. The behaviorally important long whisking vibrissae of the upper face are represented individually in the specialized so-called "barrel-field" of lateral S-I. Finally, S-I has a motor component. Electrical stimulation with penetrating microelectrodes produces body movements in a somatotopic pattern that matches the somatosensory map. However, higher current levels are typically needed to evoke movements in S-I than more rostrally in motor cortex. Thus foot movements are produced by stimulations of foot cortex, and vibrissae movements follow stimulation of vibrissae cortex.

Other subdivisions of somatosensory cortex in rats are less understood. Cortex with a less granular layer IV, the so-called dysgranular cortex, separates the representations of major body parts in S-I. While S-I receives sensory input from the main thalamic nucleus for the relay of cutaneous information, the ventroposterior nucleus, dysgranular cortex receives inputs from a more dorsal sensory nucleus, the posterior nucleus, which may relay information from muscle receptors to cortex. Muscle receptor information is especially important in the sensory control of movements, and dysgranular cortex may distribute muscle receptor information to other cortical areas, including primary motor cortex.

Most of the cortex lateral to S-I has generally been considered to be the second somatosensory area, S-II. More recent evidence suggests that this cortex contains two separate, systematic representations of body receptors, S-II and the parietal ventral area, PV (Li et al., 1990; Krubitzer et al., 1990). A third parietal rostral area, PR, appears only crudely to represent the body. Finally, a narrow strip of parietal medial cortex, PM, receives somatosensory information from S-I and crudely represents body receptors. All of these sensory areas in rats project to neurons in

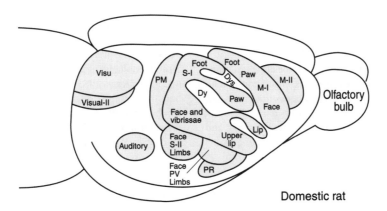

Domestic rat

Figure 65 Subdivisions of sensorimotor cortex on a dorsolateral view of the brain of a rat. The general arrangement of cortical areas and the somatotopic organization within areas probably reflects the pattern found in many small-brained mammals. Somatosensory areas include the primary field S-I, the secondary field S-II, the parietal ventral field PV, and the parietal rostral region or field PR. Dysgranular somatosensory cortex (Dys.) may be the homologue of area 3a (Figure 61) of monkeys. In frontal cortex, a primary motor field (M-I) and a second motor field (M-II) exist. M-II may correspond to the supplementary motor field of primates (Figure 61). First and second visual areas, primary auditory cortex, and the olfactory bulbs have been identified for reference.

the gray of the spinal cord (Li et al., 1990), implicating these fields in the modulation of motor outflow from neurons in the ventral horn of the spinal cord.

Cortex just rostral to S-I has no clear sensory layer of granule cells, and thus is known as agranular cortex. Electrical stimulation of this cortex produces movements of vibrissae and other body parts at relatively low levels of current. Inputs are from the ventral anterior thalamus, which only indirectly gets sensory information from the cerebellum. These characteristics and relative position identify this "lateral" agranular field as primary motor cortex, M-I. A second largely agranular medial field just rostromedial to M-I constitutes a second motor area, M-II, where higher levels of electrical stimulation are needed to evoke movements. By position, M-II of rats appears to correspond to the supplementary motor area of primates, but this suggested homology is as yet uncertain. Both M-I and M-II project to the spinal cortex and may directly affect motor neurons (Li et al., 1990).

An interesting feature of S-I in rats and perhaps a number of other rodent species is that the hind foot region contains more large pyramidal neurons than other parts of S-I, and thus

more closely resembles motor cortex. In addition, electrical stimulation of the hind foot representation of S-I produces movements at lower thresholds than in other parts of S-I. Because of these motor-like characteristics, some investigators portray S-I and M-I as overlapping in the foot region. Nevertheless, agranular M-I does have its own foot representation. Thus M-I and S-I each contain separate representations of the body, as in other mammals, but the foot representation of S-I has more pronounced motor characteristics.

The subdivisions of sensorimotor cortex found in rats may be typical of sensorimotor cortex in a range of small-brained mammals (see Kaas, 1987). However, opossums and other marsupials may have an even simpler organization in that early investigators failed to find a separate motor field rostral to S-I. Because body movements could be easily evoked by electrical stimulation of S-I, they described S-I as a sensorimotor amalgam (e.g. Lende, 1963). More recent research has identified S-II, PV, dysgranular, and parietal medial fields in North American opossums, but there are still uncertainties about the existence of a separate M-I, as well as other motor fields. Yet there is evidence for M-I in some marsupials and, with further investigation, opossums and other marsupials may turn out to resemble rats more closely in cortical organization.

MONKEYS AND HUMANS

The organization of sensorimotor cortex in monkeys (Figure 66) and humans is more complex than in mammals such as rats and opossums (see Kaas, 1990). Most notably, anterior parietal cortex contains four strip-like fields termed 3a, 3b, 1, and 2 after Brodmann (1909). Each of four parallel

fields contains a separate, parallel representation of body receptors in a tail to tongue somatotopic pattern in a mediolateral cortical sequence. Area 3b, with a well-developed layer IV of granule cells, is the homologue of granular S-I in rats and other mammals (Kaas, 1983). Area 3b receives information from rapidly adapting and slowly adapting mechanoreceptors in the skin via a projection from the ventroposterior nucleus of the thalamus. Area 3b distributes sensory information to other areas,

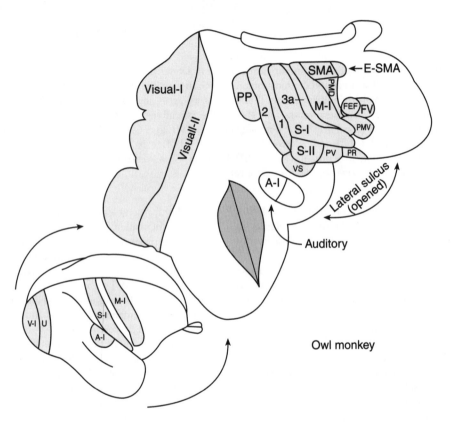

Figure 66 Subdivision of sensorimotor cortex in an owl monkey *(Aotus)*, a small New World monkey. The pattern of areas in this monkey appears to be similar to that found in other higher primates, including humans. A few subdivisions of cortex are shown on a dorsolateral view of the brain on the lower left. Because some of the sensorimotor areas are hidden from view in fissures in the intact brain, cortex of one hemisphere is shown with sulci opened and flattened on the upper right. Subdivisions of somatosensory cortex include areas 3b (S-I), 3a, 1, and 2 of Brodmann (1909), the second area S-II, the parietal ventral area PV, the parietal rostral area PR, the ventral somatosensory area VS, and posterior parietal cortex PP. Motor areas include primary motor cortex M-I, the supplementary motor area SMA, the dorsal premotor area PMD, and the ventral premotor area PMV. The frontal eye field FEF and the rostral eye portion of the supplementary motor area E-SMA are devoted to producing eye movements, while the frontal visual area FV receives inputs from visual cortex and helps control eye movements. First and second visual areas and auditory cortex are identified for reference.

especially areas 1, 2, and S-II, but also somewhat to area 3a and primary motor cortex, M-I.

Area 1 also receives some input from the ventroposterior nucleus, but its primary drive comes from area 3b. Thus area 1 is a higher station in a processing sequence for information from skin receptors. Receptive fields for neurons in area 1 are larger than for neurons in area 3b, and receptive field properties are more complex. Rats, opossums, and even prosimian primates do not have a region of cortex that has the characteristics of area 1, and the small marmoset monkeys have a poorly developed area 1. Thus area 1 appears to be a subdivision of sensorimotor cortex that first emerged in monkeys. We are not certain how area 1 evolved in primates, but it seems to have differentiated from the less responsive PM zone of somatosensory cortex that exists caudal to S-I in rats and most mammals.

Area 2 is another field that seems to exist only in monkeys and other higher primates. Area 2 receives information about skin receptors from areas 3b and 1, and merges this information with inputs from muscle receptors relayed from the ventroposterior superior nucleus of the thalamus. Thus area 2 is a higher-order processing field that integrates highly analyzed tactile information with inputs from muscles so that manipulated objects can be identified.

Area 3a is largely activated by muscle receptors via inputs from the ventroposterior superior nucleus of the thalamus. Area 3b and, to some extent, areas 1 and 2 provide other inputs that relate to skin receptors. The main outputs of area 3a are to motor cortex, and thus area 3a is considered the major source of information about movement and limb position for guiding motor control in motor areas.

All four of the areas of anterior parietal cortex (3a, 3b, 1, and 2) distribute to a number of other cortical fields. Most important, they all project densely to S-II and PV, and these fields depend on this input for activation. S-II in turn projects most densely to PV and both fields project to PR, which accesses limbic structures important for long-term memory. This lateral pathway involving S-II, PV, and PR is critically important in the identification of objects by touch, and lesions in this pathway severely impair object recognition by touch.

Area 1 and especially area 2 also project to subdivisions of posterior parietal cortex. Various proposals are currently in use for how to subdivide posterior parietal cortex into functionally significant fields, but considerable uncertainty remains. Posterior parietal cortex appears to be largely involved in the sensory control of motor behavior. Connections of posterior parietal cortex with more medial cingulate cortex may be important in involving motivation and attention in sensorimotor behavior, while the major connection of posterior parietal cortex with premotor and supplementary motor areas, and to a lesser extent with primary motor cortex, provides an avenue for guiding motor behavior. Parts of posterior parietal cortex receive visual information, and have a role in the visual control of reaching and other motor behavior.

The sensory areas of anterior, lateral, and posterior parietal cortex interconnect to form a highly complex network. Each area connects with several others, providing varying degrees of influence, and each area receives inputs of several different stages of analysis. Outputs from this complex network are to the extrapyramidal motor system, motor and premotor neuron clusters in the brain stem and spinal cord, and motor and premotor cortex. Electrical stimulation of these sensory fields with microelectrodes produces movements, although current levels typically need to be higher than in motor cortex. Stimulation thresholds vary, so that, for example, more current is required to elicit movements from area 3b and less current from area 3a. Normally, stimulation effects probably depend in part on the projections to motor cortex and rather indirect access to subcortical motor neurons, but movements can be evoked from these sensory fields after motor cortex lesions. Thus the sensory areas are sensorimotor in function, and they can mediate motor behavior independently of motor cortex.

Much progress has been made in understanding the organization of the motor cortex of the frontal lobe of primates in recent years (see Stepniewska et al., 1993). The general consensus is that the major fields include primary motor cortex (M-I), the supplementary motor area, (SMA), a dorsal premotor area (PMD), and a ventral premotor area (PMV). Movements can be evoked by electrical stimulation with microelectrodes from all of these fields, and under light anesthesia, most of these fields are also activated by stimulation of skin and muscle receptors, though the sensory inputs are less direct than for areas of parietal cortex.

Primary motor cortex is also known as area 4 of Brodmann. A layer IV of granule cells is not apparent, and hence area 4 is called agranular cortex. Large pyramidal cells in layer V project subcortically, and provide direct access to motor neurons of the brain stem and spinal cord. Hence low levels of current are capable of evoking movements from M-I. The representation of body movements in M-I is complex in that the same or similar movement can be evoked from several nearby but separate locations. The gross organization of M-I resembles that of area 3b and other areas of anterior somatosensory cortex in that movements of the foot are evoked from most medial M-I, leg and trunk movements are from more lateral cortex, hand and forelimb are next, and the most lateral parts of M-I relate to face and tongue movements. Sensory inputs are congruent with this motor map. However, in contrast to the global somatotopy, the local organization of M-I is less systematic and is individually variable. The local organization is reasonably characterized as a mosaic of narrow columns of tissue, each evoking a specific movement upon stimulation. Several nonadjacent columns relate to the same movement, and adjacent columns relate to nearby but not necessarily adjoining body parts. Thus thumb movements can be evoked from several nearby locations in M-I, and these sites can be next to sites where different finger or wrist movements are evoked, but adjacent sites are less likely to evoke arm or shoulder movements. There is some evidence that M-I is divided into rostral and caudal halves having somewhat different functions. Similar body movements are represented in both halves, but fine digit movements are concentrated in the caudal half. In addition, stimulation thresholds are somewhat higher rostrally, and densities of connections differ, with area 2, for example, contributing more to rostral M-I. Besides major sensory inputs, M-I is activated by inputs from premotor and supplementary motor areas, and these areas appear to mediate much of their control on motor behavior through M-I. M-I also receives major inputs from the cerebellum via the ventrolateral nucleus of the thalamus. Lesions of M-I produce a profound but partially recoverable motor impairment.

The supplementary motor area, SMA, is a large medially located premotor area of primates. As for other sensory and motor areas, SMA represents contralateral body movements and contralateral sensory receptors in the somatotopic pattern. In a cortical sequence extending rostrally from the foot representation in M-I, SMA represents the foot, trunk, hand, face, and finally the eyes in cortex along the curvature of dorsomedial cortex as it forms the medial wall of the cerebral hemisphere. SMA has dorsal and ventral subdivisions differing somewhat in connections and presumably function. SMA receives major inputs from posterior parietal cortex, and may normally function in conjunction with posterior parietal cortex. Other connections are with M-I, premotor fields, and cingulate cortex. SMA also receives inputs from parts of the ventrolateral thalamus that relay information from the basal ganglia and cerebellum. Studies of increases in regional blood flow in humans during different behaviors indicate that SMA is active both in the execution of complex movement sequences and in the planning and mental rehearsal of such sequences without actual movement. Unilateral lesions of SMA produce deficits in bimanual coordination between the two hands. These observations support the view that SMA has a major role in the programming of sequences of movements, and in the relay of instructions to motor cortex of both hemispheres.

The most rostral part of SMA is devoted to eye movements, and it is sometimes called the supplementary eye field, E-SMA. The other major eye movement field is the frontal eye field, FEF, which is just rostral to M-I and a narrow strip of premotor cortex. FEF may be an eye movement portion of M-I that is highly differentiated and somewhat displaced from the M-I border.

Premotor cortex has been defined as cortex immediately rostral to M-I where body movements are elicited by typically higher current levels than in M-I. This premotor region has been divided in various ways, but the bulk of the evidence supports the now prevailing opinion that the region is best divided into dorsal and ventral premotor fields. The dorsal premotor area, PMD, occupies a narrow strip of cortex within lateral area 6 of Brodmann that is just rostral to M-I, lateral to SMA, and extends laterally to the level of the frontal eye field. Histologically, this cortex is dysgranular or agranular, but the field does not have the large pyramidal cells of M-I. Microstimulations reveal a lateromedial sequence of representation of face, hand, and foot representations. Recordings in monkeys suggest that PMD is involved in the preparation and performance of motor activity, perhaps mediated via its major connections with M-I. Other cortical connections are with SMA and PMV. The ventral premotor area, PMV, is just rostral to the face representation of M-I. The cortex has dysgranular features of lateral area 6 of Brodmann, and stimulation studies reveal movements of face, hand and digits, and, to a much lesser extent, other body parts. A representation of the leg may be missing. Neurons in PMV respond to tactile and visual stimuli, and this area may be involved in using sensory information to prepare for and guide hand and arm movements, and perhaps guide hand and mouth coordinations. The mouth movement portion of PMV is in the approximate location of Broca's area, and Broca's area in humans may constitute a major enlargement of PMV of monkeys. As for PMD, the ventral premotor area is densely interconnected with M-I, and many of its functions may be mediated through M-I. Studies of patients with lesions suggest that premotor cortex is important in the generation of sequences of movement from memory and in the precise timing of patterns of movements.

Much less is known about the organization and connections of sensorimotor cortex in humans than in monkeys, but what is known suggests that this cortex in humans is very similar to that in monkeys. Stimulations and recordings in anterior parietal cortex have consistently demonstrated a foot-to-tongue somatotopic sequence comparable to those in areas 3a, 3b, 1, and 2 in monkeys, and more recent evidence supports the conclusion that these areas also contain separate representations in humans. Primary motor cortex has also been mapped in humans and its gross mediolateral organization corresponds with that in monkeys. The supplementary motor area was first described in humans, and SMA has a similar somatotopic organization in humans and monkeys. As imaging procedures in humans improve and are more frequently used, a more detailed understanding of sensorimotor cortex will emerge, and we will better determine similarities and differences.

BIBLIOGRAPHY

Brodmann, S. K. (1909). *Vergleichende Lokalizationlehre der Grosshirnrinde.* Leipzig: Barth.

Donoghue, J. P., & Wise, S. P. (1982). The motor cortex of the rat: cytoarchitecture and microstimulation mapping. *Journal of Comparative Neurology, 212,* 76–88.

Kaas, J. H. (1983). What, if anything, is S-I? The organization of the "first somatosensory area" of cortex. *Physiological Reviews, 63,* 206–31.

Kaas, J. H. (1987). The organization of neocortex in mammals: implications for theories of brain function. *Annual Review of Psychology, 38,* 124–51.

Kaas, J. H. (1990). The somatosensory system. In G. Paxinos (Ed.), *The human nervous system,* (pp. 813–44). New York: Academic Press.

Krubitzer, L. A., & Kaas, J. H. (1990). The organization and connections of somatosensory cortex in marmosets. *Journal of Neuroscience, 10,* 952–74.

Lende, R. A. (1963). Cerebral cortex: a sensorimotor amalgam in the Marsupialia. *Science, 141,* 730–2.

Li, X.-G., Florence, S. L., & Kaas, J. H. (1990). Areal distributions of cortical neurons projecting to different levels of the caudal brain stem and spinal cord in rats. *Somatosensory and Motor Research, 7,* 315–35.

Nudo, R. J., & Masterton, R. B. (1990). Descending pathways to the spinal cord, III: sites of origin of the corticospinal tract. *Journal of Comparative Neurology.*

Stepniewska, I., Preuss, T. M., & Kaas, J. H. (1993). Architectonics, somatotopic organization, and ipsilateral cortical connections of the primary motor area (M-I) of owl monkeys. *Journal of Comparative Neurology, 330,* 238–71.

Woolsey, C. N. (1958). Organizational sensory and motor areas of the cerebral cortex. In H. F. Harlow & C. W. Woolsey (Eds), *Biological and biochemical bases of behavior* (pp. 63–81). Madison: University of Wisconsin Press.

JON A. KAAS

sensory deprivation Sensory deprivation describes a situation, occurring either naturally or experimentally, in which exposure to sensory stimulation is dramatically curtailed. It is of importance in two contexts within neuropsychology.

Infants who are sensorily deprived, if this is during a CRITICAL PERIOD of development, may fail to establish normally functional cerebral sensory and perceptual systems. While much of the relevant data have come from animals, there is evidence from selective exposure in infants, and from individuals who are for some reason incidentally deprived of stimulation during infancy, that the same principles apply: that exposure to appropriate stimuli during the critical period is essential for normal neural development. While sensory functions may subsequently be partly gained following the end of the deprivation, it may be that a normal level of function is never established. The inference is that there is a critical period for the formation of the cortical systems which relies on exposure to relevant stimulation.

Sensory deprivation in adults, if it is prolonged, may be extremely aversive, with distortions of time sense, bizarre images and ideas, and hallucinations. The reason why these phenomena occur is unclear, but it is presumed that the brain is dependent upon the normal inflow of information for the regulation of mental processes, and that discomfort will occur if the normal level of sensory stimulation cannot be maintained. There may be implications for the reduced sensory experience of severely disabled adults who lack motor and communication capacities, and are often confined to a relatively unchanging and understimulating environment, but these have not been systematically explored.

septal area   The septal area indicates the region which includes the septum (septum pallucidum), a nucleus within the LIMBIC SYSTEM. The septum is continuous with the anterior part of the HYPOTHALAMUS, and it runs between the under surface of the corpus callosum and the upper surface of the fornix, running between the medial surfaces of the two lateral ventricles. In rats, lesions of the septal area produce SHAM RAGE. By contrast, septal stimulation appears to produce a pleasant state, in that animals will continue to self-stimulate this area without additional reward.

sex differences   Sex differences – differences between men and women or between girls and boys – exist in several areas in neuropsychology. The term "sex difference" is used, not "gender difference," although use of the latter term is increasing, particularly in the public domain. "Gender" is a grammatical term referring to the

sex (masculine, feminine, or neuter) of nouns or pronouns. Fowler's *Modern English Usage* (1983, p. 221) states: "to talk of persons or creatures of the masculine or feminine gender, meaning of the male or female sex, is either a jocularity or a blunder." The use of the term "gender" as a euphemism for sex is probably considered politically correct at this time because it appears to negate or de-emphasize the possible role of biology as a factor in the etiology of any psychological differences between the sexes. The proponents of the term "gender" define it as referring to culturally determined sex differences in cognition and attitudes. However, such usage assumes that the origins of sex differences are known.

Sex differences occur in brain structure, in neuroendocrinology (the hormones influencing the brain), in behavior and cognition, in the patterns of hemispheric functional specialization or LATERALIZATION, and in the incidence of various neuropsychological or neuropsychiatric disorders.

Research in the last decade has provided a still small but compelling body of evidence of sex differences in brain structure. The consequences of these neuroanatomical sex differences are not yet elucidated, but they may underlie some of the sex differences in behavior and cognition and in patterns of lateralization. Sex differences in cognition and lateralization have been reviewed in numerous publications and will be only briefly summarized here. The focus will be on the neuroanatomical sex differences and their possible relation to function.

COGNITION

In general, women do better than men on various tests of verbal fluency, phonetics, verbal memory, perceptual speed, and fine-motor manual tasks, and such differences are often evident in young children (Halpern, 1992). Men do better on various tests of spatial cognition and mathematical reasoning, and again some differences appear in the prepubertal years (Harris, 1978). There are also sex differences in personality traits (Maccoby & Jacklin, 1974). At the level of complex real-life social behavior, such as career choice, lifestyle, or interpersonal relationships, the sex differences may, in part, be built upon the sex differences in smaller units of perception, cognition, and personality. The difference in mean performance on specific cognitive tests between the sexes is sometimes not large, and there is considerable overlap between the groups, as there is, for example, for body height, but the differences are statistically significant and may be biologically important. If selection is made for high scores, then one sex will be selected more frequently than the other. The differences may have little practical significance for any one person, but they may be theoretically important in elucidating the mechanisms of individual differences.

A prevalent interpretation of the sex differences in behavior and cognition is that they are due to learning and the environment: the result of different socialization. This is probably a factor, but it does not preclude the operation of biological influences. Sex differences in the behavior of newborns are difficult to attribute to learning (e.g. Hittleman & Dickes, 1979). Performance on tasks for which there are sex differences has been shown to fluctuate in women with changes in the levels of sex hormones across the menstrual cycle (Hampson & Kimura, 1988). Patients with various disorders associated with atypical levels of sex hormones early in development (such as congenital adrenal hyperplasia, which results in higher testosterone levels) show sex-atypical patterns of cognitive skills compared to matched control groups (e.g. Hines, 1993). Sex differences are evident in non-reproductive behavior in other animals where socialization cannot be a factor and sex hormones have been demonstrated to affect these behaviors, for example, MAZE LEARNING in rats (Williams & Meck, 1991). These findings and considerations suggest that a search for neurobiological factors underlying sex differences may be fruitful.

LATERALIZATION

When studies of brain-damaged people first started to include female patients, and performance of each sex was assessed separately, the results of many studies suggested that men showed greater lateralization, that is, a greater separation of function between the two hemispheres. For example, men showed greater and more persistent deficits than women with comparable unilateral brain damage (McGlone, 1980). More recently, the pattern of intrahemispheric LOCALIZATION of function has been suggested to be different between men and women, with women having some aspects of

language represented more focally in the anterior than posterior regions of the left hemisphere, compared to men, who showed more widespread representation of language in both anterior and posterior regions (Kimura, 1987). Many of the studies using lateral perceptual techniques to study lateralization in neurologically intact subjects have shown sex differences early in life (see Witelson, 1987). In addition, the groups of patients with atypical sex chromosomes and/or atypical early levels of sex hormones mentioned previously, also show atypical patterns of lateralization (e.g. Hines, 1993). The origin of the sex differences in lateralization has not been elucidated. One of the main issues to be resolved in neuropsychology is whether individual differences in lateralization have any consequence for level of cognition.

SEX DIFFERENCES IN ANATOMY OF THE HUMAN BRAIN

Size of the male brain (measured by weight or volume) is about 10 to 15 percent larger than the female brain. This sex difference has been clearly documented for decades. What this difference could reflect microscopically or physiologically, or what it could mean for function has not been resolved. It is interesting that brain size is similar in girls and boys until age 2 to 3 years; it then increases at a faster rate in boys until about age 6 years, when almost full brain weight is reached in both sexes. The sex difference in brain size emerges well before the sex difference in height, which starts around age 8 years.

One of the first parts of the brain for which a sex difference was observed was the MASSA INTERMEDIA. It is a band of tissue which connects the right and left halves of the THALAMUS (see Figure 67). It is not always present in the human brain, and it is absent more frequently in men than women (Lansdell & Davie, 1972). In addition, its presence may be associated with particular patterns of verbal and spatial skills. It may also be larger in cross-sectional area in women than men.

Some subcortical nuclei show sex differences. In the anterior regions of the HYPOTHALAMUS (the preoptic area or the interstitial nuclei), nuclei were found to be about twice as large in men as in women and to contain twice as many cells (Allen et al., 1989). In the rat, development of the preoptic area is under the control of

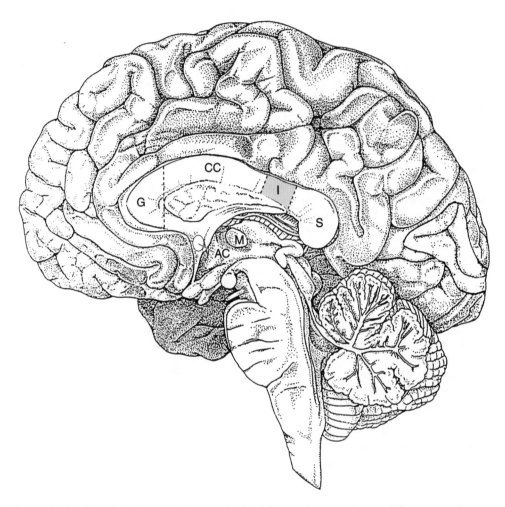

Figure 67 A midsagittal view of the human brain: AC, anterior commissure; CC, corpus callosum; G, genu; I, isthmus; M, massa intermedia; S, splenium.

gonadal hormones early in life and is involved in the sexual behavior of both males and females and in the regulation of the neural control of endocrine functions (Gorski et al., 1978). One of the interstitial nuclei of the anterior hypothalamus was recently reported to be smaller in homosexual than heterosexual men (LeVay, 1991). This result bears replication but has important implications for the role of sexual differentiation of the brain with respect to the origins of sexual orientation.

The CORPUS CALLOSUM (CC) has received much attention regarding possible sex differences in its size and shape (morphology). It is the main interhemispheric commissure connecting neurons of the right and left cortex (see Figure 67). Early large-sample studies at the turn of the century noted that the area of the CC in the midsagittal plane was larger in men than women. Since the overall brain is larger in men, it would not be surprising to find that certain parts are also larger. However, about 10 years ago, a study of 14 brain specimens reported that the posterior bulbous region of the CC (the SPLENIUM, see Figure 67) was larger in area and in maximal breadth in women than in men (de Lacoste-Utamsing and Holloway, 1982). This finding captured the interest of many neuroscientists, as it appeared compatible with greater bihemispheric representation of cognitive functions in women than in men. This result has not been replicated in numerous subsequent studies. In almost all reports, the splenium was found to have a larger area in men (e.g. Witelson, 1989). However, there may be some subtle increase in the size of the splenium in women. The area of the splenium expressed as a ratio of the area of the total CC shows a slightly larger (but not statistically significant) value for women in several studies. Detailed reviews of more than a dozen studies are available (Clarke et al., 1989).

The CC may be divided into regions which have some topographic representation to cortical regions. For example, the splenium contains axons which originate from and terminate in mainly occipital and inferior temporal cortex (visual regions). The genu (the anterior part; see Figure 67) serves the connections between the prefrontal regions. A sex difference has been found for the region referred to as the isthmus (see Figure 67). The isthmus contains axons serving the superior TEMPORAL LOBE and posterior PARIETAL cortex. It is particularly these regions, which mediate linguistic and visuospatial functions, which are asymmetrically represented in the two hemispheres. The area of the isthmus has been found to be larger in women than in men, both in the study of post-mortem brain specimens and through MAGNETIC RESONANCE IMAGING. This result indicates that, even though the total CC is larger in men, the isthmal region is larger in women.

What this could mean for function remains to be elucidated. Some preliminary possibilities have been observed. The sex difference in the size of the isthmus is complicated by the finding that it interacts with the effect of HANDEDNESS. Among men, those who were consistently right-handed were found in several studies to have a smaller isthmal area than men who showed some left-hand preference. Among women, there was no difference in isthmal area between right- and left-handers. The larger isthmus in left-handed men and all women compared to right-handed men may underlie greater bihemispheric representation of speech and motoric functions. Similarly, only in men was handedness observed to be

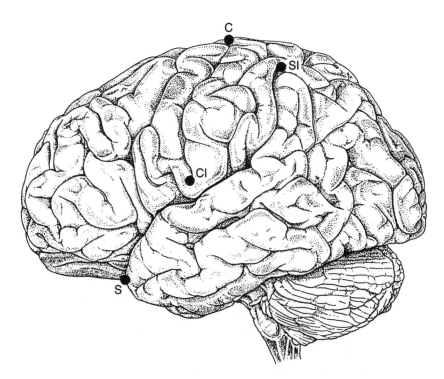

Figure 68 The lateral view of the human brain. S–S$_1$, extent of the Sylvian fissure; C–C$_1$, extent of the central sulcus.

associated with the anatomy of another region, the postcentral region of the lateral or SYLVIAN FISSURE (see Figure 68) and associated cortical regions, such as the PLANUM TEMPORALE (Witelson & Kigar, 1992). These results suggest that the anatomical substrate relating to asymmetry in motor programming (including handedness) is not the same in women as in men. If one brain region serves different functions in the two sexes, then other regions still undetected must also serve different functions. This hypothesis of sex differences in structure–function relationships is consistent with some of the findings from neuropsychology, namely that speech and praxic (motoric) functions in women are more localized in the left frontal lobe region compared to men, who show more widespread representation in anterior and posterior regions of the left hemisphere. Sex differences have also been observed in the patterns of brain activation in functional imaging studies.

The small commissure, the anterior commissure (see Figure 67), has also been found to show a sex difference. It appears to be larger in women than men (Allen et al., 1991). Interestingly, both the callosal isthmus and anterior commissure interconnect right and left temporal lobe regions. They have also both been found to be larger in homosexual than in heterosexual men.

A sex difference regarding the size of the CC and AGING has been reported. Area of the total CC decreases with advancing chronological age in men, but no such decrease has been found in women, at least up to age 70 years (Witelson, 1991). Similar sex differences were found for frontal and temporal lobe regions (Cowell et al., 1994). Such results raise the question of whether CC changes may be an indicator of cognitive changes and whether the cognitive changes with age may be different between the sexes.

Macroscopic differences may reflect microscopic differences. Most recently a sex difference in cell packing density was found in the cortex of the planum temporale. Women had a greater number of neurons per unit volume than men (Witelson et al., 1994). This is unlikely to be due merely to the same total number of cells being packed into a smaller volume. The sex difference was found only in specific layers of the cortex, layers II and IV, which are input layers, the layers receiving sensory input from the thalamus. The possible association of this histological difference

with function remains to be determined. Further studies of the role of sex hormones in brain development and function, and of the relationship between sex differences in neurobiological factors and cognition, will help to shed light on the origins of the sex differences in behavior.

BIBLIOGRAPHY

Allen, L. S., Hines, M., Shryne, J. E., & Gorski, R. A. (1989). Two sexually dimorphic cell groups in the human brain. *Journal of Neuroscience, 9*, 497–506.

Clarke, S., Kraftsik, R., Van der Loos, H., & Innocenti, G. M. (1989). Forms and measures of adult and developing human corpus callosum: is there sexual dimorphism? *Journal of Comparative Neurology, 280*, 213–30.

Cowell, P. E., Turetsky, B. I., Gur, R. C., Grossman, R. I., Shtasel, D. L., & Gur, R. E. (1994). Sex differences in aging of the human frontal and temporal lobes. *Journal of Neuroscience, 14*, 4748–55.

de Lacoste-Utamsing C., & Holloway, R. L. (1982). Sexual dimorphism in the human corpus callosum. *Science, 216*, 1431–2.

Gorski, R. A., Gordon, J. H., Shryne, J. E., & Southam, A. M. (1978). Evidence for a morphological sex difference within the medial preoptic area of the rat brain. *Brain Research, 148*, 333–46.

Halpern, D. F. (1992). *Sex differences in cognitive abilities*, 2nd edn (Chapter 3). Hillsdale, NJ: Erlbaum.

Hampson, E., & Kimura, D. (1988). Reciprocal effects of hormonal fluctuations on human motor and perceptual-spatial skills. *Behavioral Neuroscience, 102*, 456–9.

Harris, L. J. (1978). Sex differences in spatial ability: possible environmental, genetic, and neurological factors. In M. Kinsbourne (Ed.), *Asymmetrical function of the brain* (pp. 405–522). New York: Raven.

Hines, M. (1993). Hormonal and neural correlates of sex-typed behavioral development in human beings. In M. Haug, R. E. Whalen, C. Aron, & K. L. Olsen (Eds), *The development of sex differences and similarities in behavior* (pp. 131–49). London: Kluwer.

Hittelman, J. H., & Dickes, R. (1979). Sex differences in neonatal eye contact time. *Merrill Palmer Quarterly, 25*, 171–84.

Kimura, D. (1987). Are men's and women's

brains really different? *Canadian Psychology*, *28*, 133–47.

Lansdell, H., & Davie, J. C. (1972). Massa intermedia: possible relation to intelligence. *Neuropsychologia*, *10*, 207–10.

LeVay, S. (1991). A difference in hypothalamic structure between heterosexual and homosexual men. *Science*, *253*, 1034–7.

Maccoby, E. E., & Jacklin, C. N. (1974). *The psychology of sex differences*. Stanford, CA: Stanford University Press.

McGlone, J. (1980). Sex differences in human brain asymmetry: a critical survey. *Behavioral and Brain Sciences*, *3*, 215–27.

Williams, C. L., & Meck, W. H. (1991). The organizational effects of gonadal steroids on sexually dimorphic spatial ability. *Psychoneuroendocrinology*, *16*, 155–76.

Witelson, S. F. (1987). Neurobiological aspects of language in children. *Child Development*, *58*, 653–88.

Witelson, S. F. (1989). Hand and sex differences in the isthmus and genu of the human corpus callosum: a postmortem morphological study. *Brain*, *112*, 799–835.

Witelson, S. F. (1991). Sex differences in neuroanatomical changes with aging. *New England Journal of Medicine* (letter), *325*, 211–12.

Witelson, S. F., Glezer, I. I., & Kigar, D. L. (1995). Women have greater numerical density of neurons in posterior temporal cortex. *Journal of Neuroscience*, *15*, 3418–28.

Witelson, S. F., & Kigar, D. L. (1992). Sylvian fissure morphology and asymmetry in men and women: bilateral differences in relation to handedness in men. *Journal of Comparative Neurology*, *323*, 326–40.

SANDRA F. WITELSON

sexuality In sharp contrast to its importance in the life of men and women, sexuality is relatively poorly documented in the field of neuropsychology. This may be due to the fact that scientists have focused their attention mainly on the reproductive function of sexuality and its associated hormonal changes. Large amounts of data have been amassed concerning the pharmacology, endocrinology, and even psychology and sociology of impaired sexual behaviors such as impotence, frigidity, homophilic gender orientation, and paraphylics or perversions; these will not be considered here. However, recent advances have been made in understanding how sex hormones may modify certain cognitive skills; these studies have given particular insight into sex differences. Even if the great hysteria described by Charcot is now outmoded, many psychiatric disorders are related to sexuality, including the role of sex in Freudian psychopathology. However, very little is known about the role of brain lesions or local dysfunctions in the specific impairment of sexuality in men and women.

HYPOTHALAMUS

The so-called sexual centers are located within the hypothalamus. The evidence for this comes from a number of different experimental approaches: ablation, electrophysiological stimulation with observation of effects, and electrophysiological recordings under various circumstances related to sexual behavior, morphology, and biochemistry.

Ablation studies have suggested that the medial preoptic area (towards the front of the hypothalamus) plays an important role in male sexual behavior; its destruction leads to a reduction or cessation of copulatory behavior with females. This reaction is apparently independent of sex drive, as monkeys who have undergone such an operation continue to masturbate and often even show increased "female-typical" behavior such as lordosis, especially when the operation is combined with estrogen treatment.

As would be expected, the opposite type of operation, consisting of electrical stimulation of the same area in the male, induces copulatory behavior with females, as long as the females are in heat. If this is not the case, the stimulation is without effect. This implies that the medial preoptic area is responsible for a receptive sexual state of the animal, making it sensitive to signals from females.

We have little information on the relays of information between the medial preoptic area and other brain regions. No doubt information is converged to the dorsomedial nucleus, known to play a role in ejaculation, as well as to the motor regions of the cerebral cortex to generate the voluntary movements required for pelvic thrusting, and to lower centers in the BRAIN STEM for the sexual reflexes such as erection.

As for incoming information, the medial preoptic area receives inputs from the olfactory system, underlining the importance of odor in sexual behavior, and from the cerebral cortex via the amygdala, probably mediating other sensory influences on the state of sexual arousal. Electrophysiological experiments have shown that certain neurons in the visual cortex, for instance, discharge when the animal is viewing faces, and that some of these only respond to one particular face. It is easy to base a hypothesis on this information by saying that the activity of such neurons may mediate the sexual arousal induced by a partner or a potential partner.

Other than neuronal connections, the medial preoptic area is also subject to the influence of sex hormones, showing a higher concentration of androgen receptors than any other brain region, as well as estrogen receptors and aromatase activity (the enzyme responsible for converting androgens to estrogens).

The role of androgens in sexual behavior has been shown in castration experiments, which lead to reduced male sex drive in parallel with decreased electrophysiological activity of medial preoptic neurons. Mounting behavior can be restored by direct application of testosterone to the medial preoptic area. The action of sex hormones on a neuron, as on other cells, involves a modification of gene expression. There is evidence that the genes affected include many coding for enzymes and neurotransmitters; thus the steroid activity changes the resting activity or responsiveness of a neuron to incoming signals.

The effects of testosterone provide one reason why males show more male-specific sexual behavior than females. A second reason could be provided by a size divergence between males and females in the medial preoptic area. This region is sexually dimorphic, containing at least one nucleus that is larger on average in males than in females; the second and third interstitial nuclei of the anterior hypothalamus, especially the latter, showing approximately a threefold difference between sexes.

Furthermore, a third reason for differences in sexual behavior between males and females is revealed in electron-microscopic studies, which show sex-related differences in the size and position of synapses between neurons in the medial preoptic area, and by immunohistochemistry, which shows differences in the distribution of several neurotransmitters in this region.

Close to the medial preoptic area, a second hypothalamic nucleus seems to be more largely implicated in female-typical sexual behavior, i.e. the ventromedial nucleus. The functions of this nucleus are not exclusively sexual – it is also involved in the regulation of feeding behavior, but the ventrolateral portion of the nucleus is more specifically involved with sex, although there is no evidence for the same type of sexual dimorphism in this nucleus as that seen in the medial preoptic area.

Sex drive in females seems to be due more to the action of the testosterone liberated by the adrenal glands than estrogen and progesterone, and to olfactory signals emanating from the female which affect the male's approach behavior. Despite the amassing of these different types of information, the level of control of the hypothalamus in sexual function remains to be determined: whether it acts as a low-level initiator of simple behavioral acts or whether it generates sexual feelings. Animal research cannot shed much light on this problem as it is difficult to question animals about their sexual feelings. A certain amount of information has been obtained from human subjects, following controlled lesions of the medial preoptic and ventromedial nuclei as a treatment for pathological or sociopathic sexual behavior in West Germany in the 1960s. These men reported an overall loss of sexual desire as well as of sexual behavior, implying a "high-level" role for the hypothalamus in the generation of sexual feelings. The same effects have been observed following treatment by androgen-blocking drugs, although the conclusions to be drawn from this type of experiment are less clear, given the relative ubiquity of androgen receptors.

In all interpretations it is important to bear in mind the two-way information flux between the hypothalamus and the cortex, which acts in conjunction with olfactory inputs, sensory inputs from genitalia, and circulating sex hormones to set the level of activity of neurons in the medial preoptic and ventromedial nuclei. These neurons in turn send signals to the brain stem and spinal cord to influence the mechanics of sex, but also to the cortex, probably influencing complex sexual behavior by a cortico-hypothalamo-cortical circuit, and possibly including other structures such as the amygdala.

AMYGDALA

When electrically stimulated in patients, the

amygdala induces an erection or its inhibition, according to the place of the electrodes. Studies in animals have shown that the amygdala is involved in emotion and social behavior, but with conflicting data concerning sexuality. Local destruction of the amygdala by neurosurgery in patients presenting with aggressive behavior or in hyperkinetic children apparently did not cause any sexual dysfunction. A recent observation of a patient suffering from Urbach–Wiethe disease, which causes a complete bilateral destruction of the amygdala, has shown that this brain region plays a specific role in the recognition of emotion in facial expression and apparently does not affect sexuality.

SEPTUM

Hypersexuality is an uncommon consequence of septum lesions. Two cases have been reported of markedly increased sexuality following septal damage sustained in the course of placement of ventroperitoneal shunts. These observations, together with experiments in rodents, suggest that the septum has an inhibitory action on sexual behavior. Conversely, the electrical stimulation of the septum in patients receiving stereotaxic exploration induced sexual arousal or, more exceptionally, an orgasm. In its reductionist version, orgasm is presented as a kind of "reflex epilepsy." Indeed, sustained discharges of spike and wave activity have occasionally been recorded in the septum during orgasm.

TEMPORAL LOBES

The ablation of the anterior part of the temporal lobes induces the KLÜVER–BUCY SYNDROME. Monkeys whose temporal lobes have been removed showed spectacular changes in their social and emotional behavior. These previously wild animals became gentle and tame, and they were no longer afraid of a human presence. They were submissive and did not react when attacked by other monkeys. Their sexual and feeding behavior was caricatural, excessive, and inappropriate, and they sought to eat anything within reach, whether it was edible or not, and showed an incongruous sexual inclination for the most unlikely objects. This condition was called "psychic blindness," as the monkeys were incapable of interpreting visual stimuli correctly.

In an adult man the Klüver–Bucy syndrome is characterized by psychic blindness, blunted affect, hypermetamorphosis, hyperorality, bulimia, and sexual behavior alterations. It is commonly associated with neurodegenerative conditions, exceptionally with frontal lobe degeneration of a non-Alzheimer type but more often with verified Alzheimer's disease, presenting severe loss of large neurons in the parahippocampal gyrus. In children the Klüver–Bucy syndrome has been recognized almost exclusively in association with acute bitemporal injury or dysfunction.

FRONTAL LOBES

Frontal lobe damage in patients is frequently associated with a decrease in sexual activity and with impotence. The observed sexual disinhibition consists more often in verbal obscenity and absence of bashfulness than in acting out. Compared with the sexual dysfunction observed in temporal lesions, which consist of behavioral misdemeanours, the sexual symptoms of frontal damage concern nearly exclusively moral attitudes. A famous example is given by the case of Phineas P. Gage, a brave and hard-working foreman who, following destruction of his frontal lobes by a metal rod, became a depraved child, capricious, lacking in respect, and proferring obscenities. In contrast with observations describing anhedonia and lack of sexual emotion in the case of lesion or disconnection of the prefrontal cortex, a case of hypersexuality with altered sexual preference has been observed after frontal cortex injury.

Another approach to the role of different brain regions in sexuality is given by the observation of rare sexual seizures. Two different groups of seizures can be observed. The first one is characterized by unilateral sensory symptoms. It consists of abnormal sensations in the genital regions, sometimes producing hypersexual cravings and nymphomania – priapism is exceptionally associated with the genital sensations. The EEG shows sharp waves and spiking activity located unilaterally on the parietal regions.

The second type of seizure is less systematized. The sexual components of seizures can be analyzed as follows: (1) generalized seizures symptomatic of a diencephalic dysfunction which are exceptionally accompanied by other associated paroxysmal manifestations, particularly priapism; (2) seizures originating from the convexity of the hemispheres (sensory cortex in the paracentral lobule) manifested by paroxysmal erotomania related to abnormal sensations in the genitalia; and (3) seizures originating from the temporal lobe, which may be accompanied by temporary or permanent sexual manifestations of a hypersexual type. Some may manifest as priapism, erotomania, or exhibitionism and be associated with lesions in the perifalciform area, amygdala, and gyrus hippocampus. The sexual manifestations may accompany or follow psychomotor seizures. Decreased sexuality has been reported in the interictal period in patients with temporal lobe epilepsy. Unilateral temporal lobe ablation in patients with temporal lobe seizures has been followed by an improvement in sexual adjustment in patients who were previously hyposexual. Several reports of abnormal sexual behavior associated with temporal lobe seizures show fetishism, transvestism, and exhibitionism. Some patients undergo the movements and behavior of sexual intercourse with orgasm during their seizures. It should be noted, as Currier and others (1971) claimed, "that in none of the observed cases, was the sexual motor activity appropriate and purposeful. Therefore, it seems unlikely in sexual acts such as rape that seizures or seizure activity could legally be used as an explanation for the behavior. They are as different from appropriate sexual functions as running epilepsy is from the 100 yard dash."

The sexuality of patients suffering from temporal seizures has been well analyzed. The majority of them show hyposexuality with a loss of sexual desire, and a decrease of sexual fantasies and genital excitability. It has been suggested that these patients present a syndrome opposite to that of Klüver and Bucy.

Among the few other brain diseases which involve troubles of sexuality, special attention must be given to the KLEINE–LEVIN SYNDROME. It is a rare and probably underdiagnosed syndrome. It is characterized by periodic attacks of the triad: hypersomnia, vegetative disturbances such as hyperphagia and hypersexuality, psychopathological changes in the level of consciousness and control of emotions. Boys and young men in the age group 10–20 years are most commonly affected. Spontaneous remission with a tendency to relapse is observed and the disease "burns out" after a prolonged period of years. The etiology and pathogenesis are unknown. Theories have been propounded suggesting dysfunction of the hypothalamus. No pathognomonic findings have been observed in the early phase of sleep during the daylight hours. Central stimulating drugs have been reported to have some effect on the hypersomnia. The diagnosis is based on the clinical picture. Frequently a long period elapses before the diagnosis is established and some cases are never diagnosed.

NORMAL SEXUALITY AND THE BRAIN

The functional anatomy of human sexuality has remained poorly understood, mainly because invasive experiments in humans are not acceptable.

The expectation wave observed on the EEG during the seconds which precede a specific and identified stimulus is increased before the presentation of an image of a person of the other sex. In right-handed patients, the EEG recordings showed a larger activation of the right hemisphere in response to visual erotic stimuli. An activation of the right temporal lobe was correlated with the degree of penile tumescence as measured by a strain gauge. It may be noted that during REM sleep the penile erection is associated with major activation of the nondominant hemisphere.

It has also been reported that during orgasm the nondominant hemisphere exhibits slower EEG with increased amplitude. This effect is independent of the hand used for masturbation. The regional cerebral blood flow has been measured by single photon emission computed tomography in healthy, right-handed, heterosexual males during orgasm. The results showed a decrease of cerebral blood flow during orgasm in all cortical areas except the right prefrontal cortex, where the cerebral blood flow increased significantly.

The psychological control of sexual arousal remains a major topic of sex research. The clinical implications of this are particularly salient to the treatment of paraplulias and impotence. Research shows that imagery can be used to modify sexual behaviors. In particular, presentation of stimuli via imagination has been found to be effective in modifying sexual function. A number of studies have been reported on various treatments of sexual deviation using sexual fantasy and operant conditioning techniques. However, since most of the studies concern masturbatory fantasy, the role of sexual fantasy in sexual interactions with a partner has yet to be experimentally documented.

HOMOSEXUALITY

Homosexuality is the expression of a sexual orientation towards a partner of the same sex and is not supposed to be considered in the frame of neuropsychology. Above all, "atypical" sexual orientation, or the choice of a partner of the same sex, should be distinguished from sexual differentiation disorders. The latter result in sexual dimorphism, which influences not only bodily appearance but also certain behavior patterns such as: violent games, physical and verbal aggressiveness, parental imitation games, choice of friends, a tomboy or effeminate character. Sexual differentiation depends on the sex steroids. Established mainly from experiments in rodents, heterotypical behavior or homosexuality would seem to be due to insufficient secretion of testosterone in the fetuses of mothers under stress. These observations challenge the general opinion that sexual orientation is totally different from sexual differentiation.

Recently, it has been claimed by Le Vay (1992) that a difference exists in the volume of interstitial nuclei of the hypothalamus between homosexual and heterosexual men. Another brain structure, the anterior commissure examined in postmortem brains, has been revealed to be larger in homosexual men than in heterosexual men and women. This anatomical difference, which correlates with gender and sexual orientation, may, according to Allen and Gorski (1992), underlie differences in cognitive function and cerebral lateralization in homosexual men, heterosexual men, and heterosexual women. Preliminary results concerning an eventual genetic link support the "theory" of biological factors in male homosexuality. Nevertheless, even if genetics and neuroanatomical traits turn out to be correlated with sexual orientation, causation is far from proved. In an alternative model, temperamental and personality traits interact with the familial and social milieu as the individual's sexuality emerges. Because such traits may be heritable or influenced by hormones, it is possible that homosexuality appears heritable without requiring that either genes or hormones directly influence sexual orientation per se.

Finally, a lot of terra incognita remains in the brain concerning human sexuality. Simple observation confirms the primacy of the brain in sexual activity and that desire and its fantasies are in the head, not in the heart or the genitals. The new functional imaging techniques, such as PE and SPEC tomographies, will make it possible to study the brain in relation to sexual activity. Nonetheless, it seems that sex and love will remain subjects more appreciated in the mysterious garb of poetry than under the harsh light of scientific facts.

BIBLIOGRAPHY

Adolphs, R., Tranel, D., Damasio, H., & Damasio A. (1994). Impaired recognition in facial expressions following bilateral damage to the human amygdala. *Nature, 972,* 669–72.

Allen, L. S., & Gorski, R. A. (1992). Sexual orientation and the size of the anterior commissure in the human brain. *Proceedings of the National Academy of Sciences of the United States of America, 89,* 7199–202.

Currier, R. D., Little, S. C., Suess, J. F., & Andy, O. J. (1971). Sexual seizure. *Archives of Neurology 25,* 260–4.

Heath, R. G. (1972). Pleasure and brain activity in man: deep and surface electroencephalograms during orgasm. *Journal of Nervous and Mental Diseases, 154,* 3–18.

Le Vay, D. S. (1993). *The sexual brain.* Cambridge, MA: MIT Press.

Vincent, J. D. (1990). *Biology of the emotions.* Oxford: Blackwell.

J. D. VINCENT

shaft vision Shaft vision, which is one of the characteristics of BÁLINT'S SYNDROME, is a disorder of visual attention which mainly affects peripheral vision and so results in a narrowing of the effective field of vision. The phenomenon may occur only when the patient concentrates upon the visual environment, and so not be detected by standard perimetry.

sham rage A state of pathological and enduring rage, known as sham rage, has been described in decorticate animals (in which the cerebral cortex has been removed). The behavioral components of intense rage are exhibited in the absence of an appropriate stimulus likely to provoke rage. The caudal HYPOTHALAMUS appears to mediate this response, together with its inputs from the SEPTAL

AREA. Surgical attempts to modify aggressive behavior in humans have involved the placement of lesions in the septal area.

sign language Sign language is a form of gestural communication employed by those individuals unable to speak. In North America the predominant form is Ameslan (American Sign Language), but other forms are employed in other parts of the world, with British Sign Language (BSL) being used in Britain. Its use as a form of therapy for aphasic patients has met with only limited success (*see* APHASIA).

simultanagnosia The first report of simultanagnosia was made by Bálint in 1909, and concerned a patient with bilateral lesions of the anterior regions of the occipital cortex who appeared to have a decreased range of visual perception. The patient was completely unable to perceive two or more objects simultaneously, although there was no difficulty in seeing one object at a time (regardless of its size). Bálint argued that there appeared to be a constriction of visual attention. Not only was Bálint's patient able to perceive only one item at a time, he also showed a gross disturbance in eye movements and was unable to transfer his gaze smoothly from one object to another. Bálint's patient had bilateral lesions, but similar problems may also result from unilateral lesions. Kinsbourne and Warrington (1962, 1963) described four cases with unilateral left-side lesions; in all cases the lesion was posterior (in the region of the occipital lobes). All four had marked difficulties in reading, which was slow and error-prone. They also found it very difficult to describe the contents of a complex picture and appeared to process it item by item. This led them to fail to grasp the "semantics" of the scene; for example, one was able to describe the figures in a picture but did not appreciate that one of the boys had broken a window and was being castigated by a woman.

Farah (1990) has argued that there may be different varieties of simultanagnosia. She distinguishes between dorsal and ventral simultanagnosias; dorsal simultanagnosia results from bilateral lesions affecting occipital and/or parietal regions, while ventral simultanagnosia results from left temporo-occipital lesions. According to

Farah, both dorsal and ventral simultanagnosics are able to recognize single objects, but impairments are shown if more than one object is presented. In the case of dorsal simultanagnosics, unattended objects are not seen at all, with the result that such patients experience extreme difficulty in everyday life (tending to bump into objects). On the other hand, ventral simultanagnosics do not appear to have any difficulty in negotiating their environment and, while they may be unable to *recognize* multiple visual objects they are able to *see* them. However, other evidence suggests that dorsal simultanagnosics may process apparently "unseen" stimuli to a high level (even if that processing is not available for conscious report). Thus, Coslett and Saffran (1991) have shown that their patient was better able to identify pairs of words if they were related in some way, for instance, if they could be joined to form a compound word (such as NEWS and PAPER), or if they were associatively related (such as HOT and COLD) relative to unrelated pairs.

It is probably premature to attempt to classify different varieties of simultanagnosia. There is a paucity of reported cases, and in many instances testing of visual function is relatively crude. It seems likely that there are dissociations, but until more cases are reported and tested in sufficient detail with similar tests it seems unwise to speculate. Dorsal and ventral simultanagnosia may constitute two different syndromes or ventral simultanagnosia may simply exemplify a less severe form of dorsal simultanagnosia.

Early writers have suggested that the problems experienced by patients with simultanagnosia may be due to impaired eye movements or defective visual fields. Bay (1953) proposed that the essential defect in simultanagnosia is "shaft vision," which prevents the patient surveying the field as a whole. Bay argued that the patient is initially able to perceive the object as a whole, but that continued viewing causes apparent fragmentation of the object with the patient being able to perceive only single fragments. Bay argues that this is caused by a "certain type of distribution of pathologically increased local adaption in the paracentral area." As the patient continues to look at the object, there will be increased local adaption of the paracentral area and shaft vision results. According to this argument we might expect differences in the ability to see large and small objects (large objects being relatively disadvantaged). However, this does not seem to be the case; large objects are seen as effectively as small objects. Furthermore, both Coslett and Saffran (1991) and Humphreys and Price (1994) have shown the visual fields of some patients with simultanagnosia to be full (in that the patient was able to detect peripherally presented stimuli).

While the impairment may not be accounted for in terms of defective visual fields, it may be accounted for in terms of defective eye movements (in at least some cases of simultanagnosia). Thus Luria in 1963, reporting the case of a patient with bilateral occipital lesions, revealed that while tracking movements were normal, as was the ability to fixate a single light source in an otherwise dark field, the ability to shift fixation from one point to another was very impaired and eye movements became "chaotic." Again, this is not true of all cases; Coslett and Saffran's case had both normal visual fields and normal eye movements, and was able to shift fixation in response to a cue. Reports of defective eye movements may also be associated with cases of unilateral lesions. For instance, Levine and Calvanio (1978) reported a normal range of eye movements, and normal saccades, although their patient did have difficulty in following objects into the right field and convergence to approaching objects was poor.

Since defective visual fields and/or eye movements cannot account for the deficits shown in all cases of simultanagnosia, other impairments of visual processing are implicated. Both dorsal and ventral simultanagnosics appear to be impaired in the speed of processing of visual stimuli. Kinsbourne and Warrington (1962) and Levine and Calvanio (1978) have shown that patients with unilateral lesions are abnormally slow in identifying two or more items relative to a single item. More recently Humphreys and Price (1994), reporting the cases of two patients, have shown impairments in the speed of processing, even in the processing of single items. While the patients showed that recognition was reasonably intact when viewing time was unlimited, when exposure time was reduced (to 500 ms in one case and 100 ms in the other), impairments were shown in both cases. These data suggest that speed of processing is not normal in cases of simultanagnosia.

In addition to problems concerned with the speed of visual processing, basic visual processes may in themselves be impaired. Humphreys and Price (1994) showed that performance is poor if two overlapping pictures are presented (even if they are of different colors) and if pictures are masked (by being overlaid with a grid of circles). The patients appear to demonstrate a deficit in figure-ground segmentation. Coslett and Saffran (1991) argued that the ability to detect simple features was intact in their case of simultanagnosia. Their patient performed at a similar level to control subjects in a visual search task *in terms of accuracy of detection*. Coslett and Saffran's task involved the ability to detect an oriented line from distractor elements. Humphreys and Price (1994) employed a much more extensive series of visual search experiments with two simultanagnosic subjects and demonstrated that, while the patients were able to detect a salient color-defined target in parallel across a display, their performance was slow relative to age-matched controls. Furthermore, detection of less salient targets of color and size, and the detection of all form-defined targets was impaired. Humphreys and Price conclude that this elementary deficit in feature discrimination may underlie the simultanagnosia manifest in their two cases.

Since Bálint's original report of simultanagnosia, some form of attentional impairment has been suggested. Luria (1966) gives an account of a lecture by Pavlov in 1949. Pavlov suggested that the effect of the lesion was to weaken the cerebral cortex. The effect of processing one stimulus would have an inhibitory effect on other areas of the cortex, and other stimuli could not then be simultaneously processed. Luria put this theory to the test in 1959 by investigating the effects of caffeine on performance (assuming that caffeine would affect the general tonic state of the cortex, i.e. general arousal). Following an injection of caffeine, the patient stated

> that all of a sudden everything appeared to him in a "brighter light" and he was able to accomplish in a new and direct way many tasks which normally gave him very considerable difficulty. These changes manifested themselves 15 to 20 minutes after the injection, and reached their maximum level in 30 to 35 minutes. Thereafter they gradually declined, performance returning to the previous level after about one hour to one hour and a half. (p. 447)

More recent accounts of the attentional problem have been proposed by Humphreys and Riddoch (1992). They have argued that patients with simultanagnosia may suffer from different underlying attentional deficits according to which components in an attentional network have been impaired. At least three components have been identified: the ability to maintain attention at its current locus, the ability to orient attention in response to appropriate data-driven signals; and the ability to voluntarily orient attention to new locations; these components will mutually inhibit each other. Humphreys and Riddoch assessed the performance of two simultanagnosic patients on two tasks: a cueing task and a visual selection task. One patient showed impaired orienting but a relatively intact ability to detect multiple targets (particularly when items were close rather than spaced). The reverse pattern was shown in the other patient. Humphreys and Riddoch argued for an impairment in the orienting component of an attentional network in one of their cases, and a problem due to the over-maintenance of visual attention in the other.

Reports of cases of simultanagnosic patients are relatively rare, and no real consensus as to the underlying deficits has yet been achieved. With more detailed case studies, we may begin to gain some insight into the nature of this disorder.

BIBLIOGRAPHY

Bálint, R. (1909). Seelenlähmung des "Schauens", optische Ataxie, räumliche Störung der Aufmerksamkeit. *Monatschrift für Psychiatrie und Neurologie, 25,* 5–81.

Bay, E. (1953). Disturbances of visual perception and their examination. *Brain, 76,* 515–51.

Coslett, H. B., & Saffran, E. (1991). Simultanagnosia: to see but not two see. *Brain, 114,* 1523–45.

Farah, M. J. (1990). *Visual agnosia.* Cambridge: Cambridge University Press.

Humphreys, G. W., & Price, C. J. (1994). Visual feature discrimination in simultanagnosia: a study of two cases. *Cognitive Neuropsychology, 11,* 393–434.

Humphreys, G. W., & Riddoch, M. J. (1992). Interactions between object and pace systems revealed through neuropsychology. In D. E. Meyer & S. Kornblum (Eds), *Attention and Performance XIV: Synergies in experimental psychology, artificial intelligence and cognitive science,* (pp. 143–62). Cambridge, MA: MIT Press.

Kinsbourne, M., & Warrington, E. K. (1962). A disorder of simultaneous form perception. *Brain, 85,* 461–86.

Kinsbourne, M., & Warrington, E. K. (1963). Limited visual form perception. *Brain, 86,* 697–705.

Levine, D. L., & Calvanio, R. (1978). A study of the visual defect in verbal alexia-simultanagnosia. *Brain, 101,* 65–81.

Luria, A. R. (1959). Disorders of "simultaneous perception" in a case of bilateral occipito-parietal brain injury. *Brain, 82,* 437–49.

Luria, A. R. (1966). *Higher cortical functions in man.* New York: Basic Books.

Luria, A. R., Pravdina-Vinaskkaya, E. N., & Yarbus, A. L. (1963). Disorders of ocular movement in a case of simultanagnosia. *Brain, 86,* 219–28.

M. JANE RIDDOCH

sleep Sleep is a state of motor quiescence associated with raised thresholds to internal and external stimuli. It should be distinguished from coma because of its rapid reversibility.

From a behavioral point of view, sleep is further characterized by the preliminary acts of choosing the place and posture for sleep, its onset at about the same time each day, and its stability in time. Finally, sleep shows some attributes of typical instinctive behaviors: the need to sleep (appetitive phase) precedes sleep itself (consummatory act) which is thereafter followed by a feeling of "satisfaction" and "satiety."

Homeothermic animals and Man display two different types of sleep: non-REM (REM = rapid eye movements) or quiet, synchronized sleep, and REM or agitated, desynchronized, paradoxical sleep.

PHENOMENA OF SLEEP

From a neurophysiological standpoint, the transition from wakefulness to NREM sleep is gradual. During drowsiness (Stage I) EEG alpha rhythm (8–13 c/sec) is replaced by low-voltage theta activities (4–7 c/s). True sleep (stage II) begins with the appearance of characteristic electroencephalographic elements: the sigma spindles (spindle-shaped bursts of 11.5–15 c/s waves lasting 0.5–15 sec) and the K-complexes (sharp biphasic EEG waves followed by a high-voltage slow wave). The appearance and progressive increase in high-amplitude delta waves (less than 3 c/s and more than 75 μV) indicate the transition to deep sleep (stages III and IV), also called slow wave sleep (SWS) or delta sleep. The presence of bursts, rapid eye movements (REMs), and inhibited muscle tone, evident on polygraphic recordings, distinguish REM sleep from stage I NREM sleep (Figure 69).

The cycles of sleep

In Man sleep usually begins with an episode of NREM sleep, followed after about 90 minutes by a first short episode of REM sleep. NREM and REM sleep then alternate about every 90 minutes, four to six times, until waking in the morning.

In the first cycles of sleep (each cycle comprises an episode of NREM sleep and the following REM stage) deeper sleep stages are prevalent (stages III and IV), and in the last cycles light (stages I and II) and REM sleep are prevalent.

Falling asleep takes a few minutes (2–10). In an adult subject total sleep duration is about 8 hours. There are, however, people who need to sleep fewer than 5 hours a day (short sleepers) whereas others need at least 10 hours (long sleepers). The relative duration of each stage of sleep is constant, within some limits. As a mean, light sleep (stages I–II) represents 50–60 per cent, deep sleep (stages III–IV) and REM sleep 20–25 per cent each. People may go to sleep and wake up early (so-called "larks") or instead go to sleep late at night and wake up late in the day (so-called "owls"). Young "owls" often become "larks" with age.

Sleep and aging

In the newborn, sleep alternates with wakefulness every 3–4 hours and has a total duration of about 16 out of the 24 hours. It comprises over 50 percent of agitated sleep (the equivalent of REM sleep in the adult). During the third month of age, sleep becomes a mainly nocturnal event.

Duration of sleep quickly diminishes in the course of the first years of life: at 4 years of age it lasts about 10 hours, at 14–15 years about 9 hours. With increasing age it continues to diminish, but very slowly. A young adult sleeps about 8 hours, an elderly subject about 7 hours. Sleep in the child is distinguished from the adult's by rapidity in falling asleep, the high percentage of delta sleep, and the scarcity and short duration of nocturnal awakenings. In the elderly it takes longer to fall asleep, nocturnal awakenings are more frequent and more prolonged, and delta sleep is scant (Figure 70).

Depth of sleep

Stimuli must progressively increase in strength to provoke a behavioral arousal from stage I to stage IV of NREM sleep.

In REM sleep the threshold of arousal varies. Verbal stimuli are effective more for their meaning (tone of voice, ideational and affective content of speech) than their intensity.

Awakening from slow-wave sleep is gradual, often associated with memory and speech

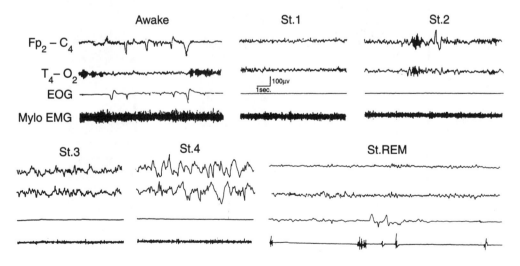

Figure 69 Polysomnographic recording: electroencephalogram of fronto-central and ($F_{p2}-C_4$) and temporo-occipital (T_4-O_2) regions; electro-oculogram, EOG; electromyogram of a chin muscle, EMG.

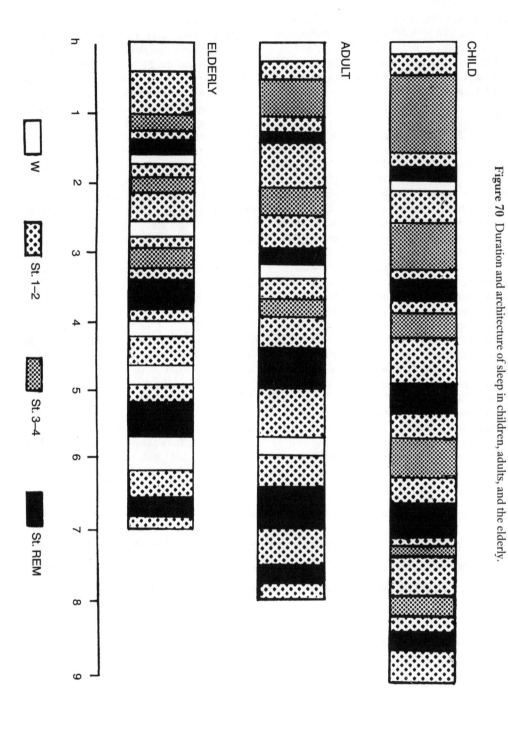

Figure 70 Duration and architecture of sleep in children, adults, and the elderly.

CHILD

ADULT

ELDERLY

h

W

St. 1–2

St. 3–4

St. REM

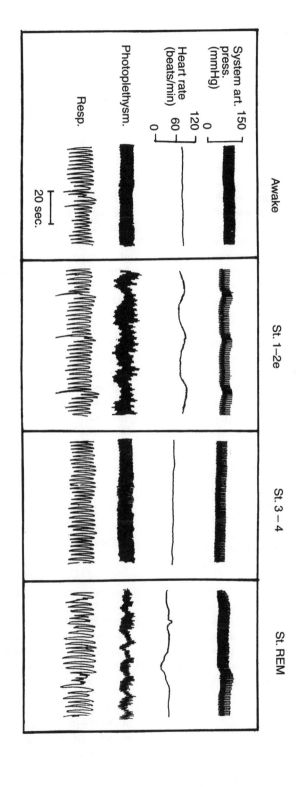

Figure 71 Systemic arterial pressure, heart rate, and peripheral vasomotor tone (photo–plethysmo) and breathing (respiration) in wakefulness, light (stages I–II), deep (stages III–IV), and REM sleep.

difficulties. Awakening from REM sleep is quick: subjects appear clear-headed, immediately well-oriented, and able to recall what they were dreaming.

Motor phenomena of sleep

The main motor features of sleep are represented by:

1 *Physiological hypnic myoclonus:* small, irregular arrhythmic and asynchronous muscle twitches, not associated with arousal. They are present during every stage of sleep, but are more abundant during REM sleep.
2 *Hypnic jerks* (or sleep startles): sudden bodily jerks, which prevail in axial and proximal limb muscles and may involve the entire body or a major limb. Hypnic jerks appear sporadically during drowsiness or during light sleep and are associated with EEG arousal and autonomic activation. Sometimes they provoke a behavioral arousal, associated with a feeling of anguish or of "falling into the void."
3 *Postural shifts:* slow changes in the posture of the trunk and limbs, more frequent at the beginning and end of an REM sleep episode. They may protect against the onset of palsies, due to prolonged compression of nerve trunks.
4 *Mimic and gestural motions:* smiling, grimacing, sighs, scratching the head and genitalia may sporadically appear during every sleep stage, but especially so during light sleep. Their meaning and origin are unknown.
5 *Periodic leg movements (PLM) or nocturnal myoclonus (NM):* a rapid flexion of the foot at the ankle, occurring in light sleep with a periodicity of 20–60 seconds in a stereotyped pattern lasting 0.5–5.0 sec. PLM are absent in the young, they show up in 30 percent of people over 50 years of age, and in 70 percent of those over 65 years. In the RESTLESS LEGS SYNDROME, PLM may be present throughout every sleep stage and even in the waking ones preceding sleep or following awakening from sleep.

Sleep and the autonomic system

Breathing and cardiocirculatory functions are closely integrated with sleep. A progressive reduction in breathing and heart rate and systemic blood pressure occurs with drowsiness and as sleep deepens.

In the transition from wakefulness to sleep (stages I–II), cycles of autonomic activation and deactivation alternate every 20–60 seconds. Phases of activation (with sympathetic prevalence) are associated with EEG signs of arousal (K complexes) and increased muscle tone. With the transition from light to deep sleep, heart and breathing rates and systemic blood pressure stabilize.

REM sleep is characterized by great respiratory and cardiocirculatory instability: tachy- and bradycardia and tachy- and bradypnea alternate irregularly. Systemic blood pressure shows phasic hypertensive peaks; the peripheral vascular tone undergoes rapid variations (Figure 71).

During REM sleep transient penile erections and tumescence of the clitoris appear. Penile erections, frequent since the first month of age, but more constant and consistent from the third year, persist until 70 years of age and after. Erections are not related to dreams with an erotic content, even though they may become stronger and more persistent during such dreams.

Motor and secretory activities of the gastrointestinal system also oscillate during the 24 hours, but in a way unrelated to the wake–sleep cycle.

Sleep and circadian rhythms

More than 100 physiological and behavioral functions oscillate within the 24 hours, including body temperature and hormonal secretions (Figure 72).

Sleep and body temperature

Body temperature oscillates between a trough of about 36.5 °C, which is reached 5–6 hours after the start of sleep, and a peak of about 37.5 °C, reached in the early afternoon. In physiological conditions, sleep begins with a decreasing body temperature and terminates when body temperature is on the increase.

The propensity to fall asleep is particularly strong when body temperature reaches its nadir, at about 4–6 o'clock in the morning, but is also pronounced in the first hours of the afternoon, when the temperature reaches its highest values. This has suggested the existence of a circasemidian (of about half a day) rhythm which

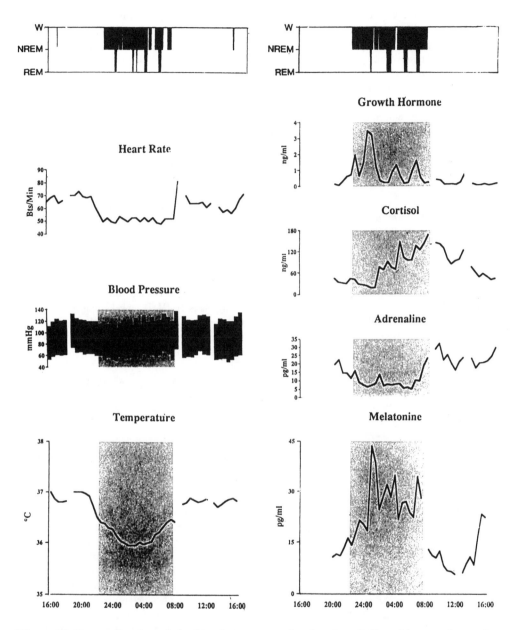

Figure 72 Twenty-four hour behavior of some vegetative functions (left) and hormonal secretions (right). See text for explanation.

could justify the custom of some peoples (those of the Mediterranean area) and some well-known celebrities (Churchill and Kennedy, for instance) to take an afternoon nap habitually.

The circadian oscillations of body temperature do not correlate directly with the variations induced by the wake–sleep cycle (for instance in shift workers or in transmeridian flyers). Perturbation of such biological rhythms is accompanied by peculiar psychic and physical ill feelings.

When sleep is lacking the night-time temperature drop is often less than expected: sleep thus provokes a decrease in body temperature, independently of the circadian oscillations of the latter.

As regards the relationship between sleep and environmental temperature, the farthest one is from a condition of thermal neutrality (which, for a fully dressed man, is about 21°C), the worse sleep becomes. Cold impedes falling asleep, increases the number of body movements, and shortens the total duration of sleep, especially at the expense of light sleep (stage II) and REM sleep, whereas a high environmental temperature mainly decreases the percentage of delta sleep (stages III–IV).

Sleep and hormones

In Man, growth hormone (GH) and prolactin (PRL) secretions are closely related to sleep. GH is secreted especially in the first hours of sleep when delta sleep is well represented. PRL is secreted mainly during the last hours of sleep, when REM sleep episodes are particularly prolonged and body temperature lower.

Catecholamine, especially adrenaline, secretion

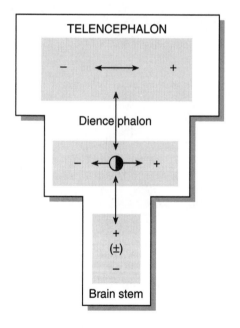

Figure 73 Schematic representation of activating (+) and deactivating (−) brain structures inducing wakefulness and sleep respectively. The centers responsible for paradoxical sleep (±) are located in the brain stem. The circadian pacemaker (◑) regulates the wake–sleep rhythm.

diminishes greatly during sleep. ACTH and cortisol secretion increase in the hours preceding and following waking in the morning. ACTH and cortisol circadian oscillations are linked more to body temperature than to sleep. Melatonin secretion increases considerably during the night, related more to darkness than sleep (Figure 73).

Mental activities during sleep

Thought processes persist during sleep, but they assume different features in relation to the type and stage of sleep. During drowsiness (stage I of NREM sleep), the loss of relationship with the environment and the waning of consciousness favor a flux of thoughts and images, deprived of any coherence or logic. Those subjects who are awakened in this sleep stage are often able to report a dream, differing from those experienced during REM sleep only because it is more fragmentary and less elaborate.

In stages II–III–IV, awakening is more often followed by the recall of thought-like activities, the simpler the deeper the sleep. Emotional participation in the mental activities recalled is usually poor.

During REM sleep, awakenings are followed by referring complex and articulated dream activity in 85–90 percent of cases. Dreaming is common to everyone, even though some people may recall their dreams while others do not. Poor sleepers, having more awakenings during the night, have a better recollection of their dreams. Dreams are particularly rich in visual imagery, but they also include auditory and tactile sensations, which are particularly abundant in those who are born or become blind in their first years of life.

Dreaming is rich in sensory perceptions, especially in very imaginative people; it has pessimistic overtones in depressives and optimistic ones in euphoric people. Dreams reported to a psychoanalyst are usually much more complex, rich, and articulated than those reported immediately after a provoked awakening in the laboratory. Subsequent elaboration may intervene, enriching the content and imagery of dreams. It may also be that the oneiric content of REM sleep is much more complex than that of NREM sleep because memory recall following these two types of sleep is different: faster and more complete after REM sleep, slower and imperfect after NREM sleep.

Finally there are people who seem to become aware that they are dreaming and who can continue dreaming and also control the content of their dreams (lucid dreams).

ANATOMO-PHYSIOLOGICAL AND BIOCHEMICAL MECHANISMS OF SLEEP

Basic anatomo-physiological mechanisms

Since the early twenties, the anatomo-clinical observations of Von Economo and the experimental work of Hess have offered some basic understanding of the anatomical and physiological basis of sleep.

Nervous structures whose ablation impedes and whose stimulation favors sleep are located in the lower BRAIN STEM, the anterior HYPOTHALAMUS, and the basal forebrain. The upper brain stem and posterior hypothalamus contain those nervous structures whose stimulation favors and whose ablation impedes wakefulness. The nervous structures whose ablation suppresses REM sleep are instead located in the pontine tegmentum. Ablation of the cerebral cortex and the THALAMUS (Villablanca et al., 1972a, b) and a selective lesion of some thalamic nuclei (Lugaresi et al., 1986) provoke severe and persistent insomnia in experimental animals and in Man respectively. This suggests that cortical and thalamic structures also play an active role in regulating wakefulness and sleep. The wake–sleep rhythm therefore seems to be regulated by an intricate and complex neuronal network stretching from the brain stem to the cerebral cortex, and including gray structures located in the hypothalamus, basal forebrain, and the thalamus.

This complex system has probably developed according to a phylogenetic hierarchy: the ability to alternate active and restful behavior also belongs to archaic neuronal structures located in the lower brain stem. With the evolution of the species, other structures with executive and control functions have become superimposed in the diencephalon. The richness and intricacy of instinctive and social life, and the parallel development of the telencephalon in mammals and in Man, are mirrored in the control of more and more complex behaviors at the level of the limbic cortex. Such a complex system, regulating the homeostasis of the organism, works in a unitary and integrated fashion.

The circadian organization of sleep and wakefulness according to a cycle determined by the alternation of darkness and light seems linked to the functioning of a small number of nervous cells, located in the suprachiasmatic nucleus (SCN). The SCN is equipped with an intrinsic rhythmicity, which is continuously set on a 24-hour rhythm by the stimuli directly or indirectly following from the retina. In the darkness and in the absence of other environmental time cues (*Zeitgebers*), the biological day in Man tends to increase until it may reach 36 or 48 hours.

The neurochemical mechanisms

At the beginning of the century it was proposed that sleep is favored by a "hypnotoxin" produced during wakefulness. Since then, many data have been gathered and numerous theories postulated, but a convincing neurochemical interpretation of sleep has yet to be formulated. We know nowadays that the cholinergic cells of the pontine tegmentum are particularly active during REM sleep ("REM on" cells). It has also been suggested that cortical arousals are also related to a cholinergic system. A catecholaminergic system also seems to intervene in the mechanisms of arousal, and the role of the serotoninergic neurons placed in the raphé nuclei is discussed. They are thought to stimulate wakefulness but, at the same time, they favor secretion of a sleep-promoting neurohormone. Adenosine seems to exert a favoring effect on sleep. The neurotransmitters regulating sleep- and wake-promoting structures of the hypothalamus seem to belong to the prostaglandin group. Finally, a role of the GABAergic systems in the promotion of sleep and of the glutaminergic ones in the maintenance of wakefulness has also been hypothesized. Much more numerous, however, are the neurotransmitters, neuromodulators, and hormones which seem able to regulate waking and sleep. It is still therefore impossible, at the moment, to have an integrated view of sleep and waking mechanisms which takes all these variables into account.

THE BIOLOGICAL MEANING OF SLEEP

Any researcher involved in the study of sleep has, at one time or another, wondered about the purpose of sleeping every day for a number of hours. Sleep deprivation could answer such a question from the effects it provokes.

The effects of sleep deprivation

Trying to deprive an experimental animal or a human being of sleep means giving repeated, severe, and often painful stimulations. It may thus be difficult to differentiate the effects which are induced by stress from those provoked by sleep deprivation instead.

In experimental animals, these methodological problems were overcome by Rechtschaffen and others (1983). In the rat either total sleep deprivation (TSD) or a paradoxical sleep deprivation (PSD) provoked a complex syndrome characterized by debilitated appearance, skin lesions, increased food intake, increased energy expenditure, at first an increase and thereafter a decrease in body temperature, increased plasma norepinephrine (noradrenaline), and decreased plasma thyroxine. Death supervenes in a state of severe cachexia, within 14–19 days in TSD rats, 16–54 days in PSD rats.

The most relevant biological effect is the increase in caloric expenditure, which largely overtakes that related to continuous waking and movement. Energy expenditure may reach values more than double the basal levels during the final quarter of survival. Such an abnormal increase in energy expenditure, which is the primary mechanism responsible for progressive debilitation and death, is related both to an increase in the processes generating heat (increased thermoregulatory setpoint) and a greater loss of energy (excessive heat loss).

Sleep therefore serves to adjust thermoregulation decisively and effectively; it also exerts, of course, other relevant biological functions (Rechtschaffen et al., 1989). In Man, total sleep deprivation cannot, for various reasons, be prolonged for more than 100–200 hours. It provokes drowsiness, fatigue, difficulties in mental concentration, mood depression, muscle fatigue, apathy, and irritability. It may, more rarely, cause psychotic reactions, delusions, or hallucinations. Sleep-deprived subjects show difficulties in psychomotor performances related to vigilance and attention, and occasional short-term memory lapses. Sleep deprivation may finally worsen physiological or postural tremor, slur speech, and cause epileptic fits in predisposed subjects. Selective REM sleep deprivation may improve, albeit transiently, a depressive state (Vogel et al., 1980).

In a disease termed fatal familial insomnia (FFI), total loss of sleep precedes death by some months. Insomnia was associated with fever, tachycardia, and increased circulating catecholamines, as in Rechtschaffen's TSD rats,

though not with the same weight loss and cachexia. In patients affected with FFI, coma associated with autonomic impairment precedes death by some weeks (Lugaresi et al., 1986). There is therefore no proof that TSD in Man provokes the same effects seen in the rat.

Theories on the function of sleep

The biological function of sleep and dreaming has been considered in several hypotheses, but still without firm scientific evidence. It has been proposed that slow-wave sleep is needed for bodily restitution and musculoskeletal recovery and that REM sleep is a period of brain restitution (Oswald, 1974). Undoubtedly sleep is energy-saving in that it intervenes in the thermoregulatory processes (Rechtschaffen et al., 1989).

REM sleep, in itself an endogenous phenomenon of cerebral activation, promotes brain maturation and ontogenic development through the learning of acquired behaviors (Roffwarg et al., 1966). Dreams could represent an escape for the instinctive impulse accumulated during wakefulness (Vogel, 1979). Sleep could however also represent a behavioral control mechanism in living beings which has evolved to enhance waking survival patterns (Meddis, 1975).

Finally, sleep could represent an instinctive pattern of behavior with the purpose of maintaining body homeostasis (McGinty & Beahm, 1984). The problem with all these theories of sleep is that nowadays we know many things about the anatomofunctional mechanisms of sleep, but we do not yet have any clear idea of the essential biological function sleep serves.

BIBLIOGRAPHY

Kryger, M. H., Roth, T., & Dement, W. C. (Eds). (1989). *Principles and practice of sleep medicine*. Philadelphia: W. B. Saunders.

Lugaresi, E., Medori, R., Montagna, P., Baruzzi, A., Cortelli, P., Lugaresi, A., Tinuper, P., Zucchini, M., & Gambetti, P. (1986). Fatal familial insomnia and dysautonomia with selective degeneration of thalamic nuclei. *New England Journal of Medicine, 315*, 997–1003.

McGinty, D. J., & Beahm, E. K. (1984). Neurobiology of sleep. In N. A. Saunders & C. E. Sullivan (Eds), *Sleep and breathing* (pp. 1–89). New York and Basel: Marcel Dekker.

Meddis, R. (1975). On the function of sleep. *Animal Behaviour, 23*, 676–91.

Oswald, I. (1974). *Sleep*. Harmondsworth, Middlesex: Penguin.

Parkes, J. D. (1985). *Sleep and its disorders*. London: W. B. Saunders.

Rechtschaffen, A., Bergmann, B. M., Everson, C. A., Kushida, C. A., & Gilliland M. A. (1989). Sleep deprivation in the rat. X. Integration and discussion of the findings. *Sleep, 12*, 68–87.

Rechtschaffen, A., Gilliland, M. A., Bergmann, B. M., & Winter, J. B. (1983). Physiological correlates of prolonged sleep deprivation in rats. *Science, 221*, 182–4.

Roffwarg, H. P., Muzio, J. N., & Dement, W. C. (1966). Ontogenetic development of the human sleep-dream cycle. *Science, 152*, 602–19.

Thorpy, M. J. (Ed.). (1990). *Handbook of sleep disorders*. New York and Basel: Marcel Dekker.

Villablanca, J., & Markus, R. (1972a). Sleep-wakefulness, EEG and behavioral studies of chronic cats without neocortex and striatum: the "diencephalic" cat. *Archivio Italiano Biologico, 110*, 348–82.

Villablanca, J., & Salinas-Zeballos, M. E. (1972b). Sleep-wakefulness, EEG and behavioral studies of chronic cats without the thalamus: the "athalamic" cat. *Archivio Italiano Biologico, 110*, 383–411.

Vogel, G. W. (1979). A motivational function of REM sleep. In R. Brucker-Colin, M. Mhkurovich, & M. B. Sterman (Eds), *The functions of sleep* (pp. 233–50). New York: Academic Press.

Vogel, G. W., Vogel, F., McAbee, R. S., & Thurmond, A. J. (1980). Improvement of depressions by REM sleep deprivation. *Archives of General Psychiatry, 37*, 247–53.

ELIO LUGARESI

smell *See* OLFACTION.

snout reflex Also known as the *pouting reflex*, the snout reflex is a form of primitive reflex, and, as with other primitive reflexes, is a pathological neurological sign in adults. It may be evoked by a sharp tap on the center of the closed lips, and can be associated with either focal or generalized brain damage.

social behavior Social behavior requires many skills and abilities. Cognitive, language, and memory skills are all important. Emotional regulation and inhibition, and other aspects of fine tuning of emotional reaction, are also important underpinnings of social behavior. Higher-level cognitive and behavioral skills, involving the integration of many different inputs, enable sensitivity to and understanding of feedback from others, an essential requirement for skilled social behavior. The underpinnings of social skills and behavior have been considered extensively. For example, Tajfel and Fraser (1978) state: "The subtleties of social interaction would not be possible if we were not able to monitor, skilfully and continuously, the effects of our own and others' social actions" (p. 21).

Argyle (1967) also brings out the breadth of skills necessary for social behavior in describing social techniques as: "all the things we do, verbally or non-verbally, deliberately or unconsciously, in the course of social encounters to influence others" (p. 31). He lists these techniques as: bodily contact; physical proximity and position; gestures; facial expression; eye movements; non-linguistic aspects of speech; and speech.

Brain damage or injury may cause a wide range of physical, cognitive, and emotional changes and deficits (e.g. Brooks, 1984). It is not surprising therefore that social behavior should be especially vulnerable to brain injury, depending as it does on the integration of a wide range of abilities. Physical limitations (e.g. hemiparesis) may affect how an individual leads his or her life, including effects on social relationships with others: for example, loss of employment because of an acquired physical disability may have a considerable impact on social life (and may produce affective change, such as depression). However, it is not physical disabilities, or even depressive reaction to disability, which are at the heart of changes in social behavior after brain injury. Many individuals who have physical disabilities continue to lead active and varied social lives; such disability does not in general produce the change in personality, the fundamentally altered way of relating to others, which is the key element in changed social behavior.

Changes in social behavior resulting from brain injury are bound up closely with disinhibition, with cognitive deficits, with emotional behavioral changes, with "loss of insight" or "denial," and with reduced sensitivity to the social signals of others. Changes in social behavior may take many forms. Slight disinhibition may be manifested initially by relatively subtle changes in social behavior (e.g. reduction in tact, outspokenness, irritability). This is sometimes one of the first signs heralding the onset of a degenerative disorder, and is often associated with deterioration of the frontal lobes. More severe frontal damage will produce more severe disinhibition and/or a loss of overall regulation of thinking and behavior. Many of the problems of social behavior seen clinically are related to disinhibition.

Cognitive changes are also relevant. Memory deficits, especially if severe, present problems for recollecting the shared experiences which give meaning to our friendships and other relationships. Language disorders have obvious implications for communication, and if severe can make even simple social exchanges slow and difficult.

"Denial" and "loss of insight" are terms which relate to the phenomenon known as ANOSAGNOSIA or unawareness, whereby the individual is unaware of his/her deficits. Unilateral NEGLECT is a classic instance of this, representing most often neglect of the left side of the body and of the external world in individuals with right-sided brain lesions. This of course does not have an effect on social behavior per se. However, somewhat similar phenomena appear to arise in a more general sense, so that it is fairly common for individuals who have suffered brain injury to deny or lack insight into the changes they have suffered.

Very often deficits of the kind mentioned above occur in combination. Traumatic brain injury (TBI) is the most common single cause of acquired disability in early life; and since most survivors' life expectancy is near normal, it accounts for very many years of "disabled surviving." In TBI, and indeed in another of the most common neurological events to strike people of all ages, the subarachnoid hemorrhage, the injury to the brain is generally fairly widespread and patchy rather than tightly focused, resulting in a mixture of deficits of various degrees of severity. It follows that the effects on social behavior are not uniform, but there are changes which are common; these are described later.

SPECIFIC CHANGES
Disinhibition
While it is obvious that major deficits in cognition and/or emotional regulation will have an impact on

social behavior, it is also the case that even fairly subtle and/or specific deficits may have an impact. For example, subtle changes in personality, representing a degree of disinhibition, may be one of the first mental changes in some conditions. An instance is a case seen some years ago by the first writer in which a minister of religion alluded (honestly) at a funeral to the unpopularity of the deceased when a more anodyne formula would have been more tactful and acceptable. Such early signs may take the form of isolated incidents of this sort, with a progression to what are seen as changes in personality or character, such as outspokenness, tactlessness, swearing, and boastfulness.

Of course, as such degenerative conditions progress, what was initially a seemingly isolated change will become part of a pattern of extensive mental deficits and behavioral changes. Such a progression has been described, for example, in PICK'S DISEASE (a rare form of dementia):

> the early abnormalities often concern changes of character and social behaviour rather than impairment of memory and intellect. Drive becomes diminished and episodes of tactless or grossly insensitive behaviour may occur. Lack of restraint may lead to stealing, alcoholism, sexual misadventures or other ill-judged social conduct. From an early stage the expression becomes fatuous and vacant, manners deteriorate and indolence may become extreme. A tendency to indulge in foolish jokes and pranks has often been noted. Insight is impaired early and to a severe degree. (Lishman, 1987, pp. 391–2)

In the above description, the changes reflect frontal lobe changes in particular. The role of the frontal lobes has attracted much attention and research endeavor. These lobes, especially the prefrontal areas, were thought at one time to be "silent" (i.e. without significant function) but they are in fact crucial to the highest levels of judgment and subtle regulation of behavior. Luria (1973) has described the role of the frontal lobes in planning behavior in general, something which is obviously crucial to social interaction with others:

> The disturbance of plans and intentions in patients with massive lesions of the frontal lobes can be clearly seen by carefully observing their general behaviour. Patients with the largest frontal lobe lesions . . . usually lie completely passively, express no wishes or desires and make no requests . . . patients cannot complete their tasks, cannot reply to questions and

apparently do not pay proper attention to anyone speaking to them. (p. 198)

However, it is not only in planning and driving behavior that the frontal lobes are crucial. They also, perhaps paradoxically, inhibit behavior. In this context it is especially important to remember that the frontal lobes – like other brain areas – cannot be viewed in isolation from a functional viewpoint. The intactness of many of the brain's other systems (e.g. the limbic system or structures) is also crucial. The limbic structures have extensive frontal connections and the whole fronto-limbic system is considered essential for the regulation of emotional reaction. This is obviously highly relevant to social behavior. The limbic system may be viewed as a phylogenetically more primitive area of the brain, among other things a sort of engine of the emotions, with the cortex and especially the frontal lobes providing the regulatory mechanisms. Individuals with frontal damage may be disinhibited so that they are prone to gross and sometimes violent over-reaction, something that is likely greatly to disrupt normal social relationships. Luria (1973) notes that such changes are often greatest where there are orbital lesions. The orbital cortex is especially richly connected to the midbrain structures (including limbic structures), and damage often produces disinhibition: "The phenomena of disinhibition . . . [have] often been described . . . lack of self-control, violent emotional outbursts and gross changes in character, arising in lesions of the orbital cortex are among the clearest symptoms of such lesions" (p. 223).

Other behavioral changes

It is important not to over-ascribe changes in the direction of aggressiveness to frontal lobe dysfunction, and there are certainly other potential causes. Mark and Ervin (1970) have put forward an argument that aggression in humans is (at least sometimes) linked to (subictal) temporal lobe seizures. This argument has the beginnings of some clinical support in that anticonvulsant medication has reportedly been effective in a small number of brain-injured individuals who show unpredictable aggressive outbursts (presumed to represent subcortical epileptic events) (Lewin & Sumner, 1972).

Examples can also be given of the impact of much more circumscribed deficits on social behavior. An example is in Parkinsonism, where changes in outward behavior, especially facial expression, occur in the absence of changes in internal mood state (Pitcairn et al., 1990). It has been shown that these external appearances in Parkinson patients cause misleading judgments to be made, with their "mask-like countenance" (Pentland et al., 1987) leading to judgments that they are cold, withdrawn, unintelligent, and moody, whereas it is the Parkinson sufferers' limitations in producing facial expressions which impacts on how they are judged in social contexts. Cases have also been reported in which specific brain lesions appear to be associated with a deficit in the interpretation of facial expressions by individuals without other more general cognitive deficits (Adolphs et al., 1994).

A variety of behavioral problems, some of which may be fairly specific, may affect social behavior. An unusual but not isolated example is an increase in sexual activity (decrease being more common but less socially disruptive). In the case of hypersexuality the individuals involved may be sexually explicit in exposing themselves, disinhibited in touching or kissing – usually members of the opposite sex – or by invading others' personal space (Zencius et al., 1990). All of this may seriously affect normal social relationships. Although these cases demonstrate a specific behavioral problem it did not occur in isolation, and some individuals also demonstrated cognitive problems, for example, memory deficits or poor concentration, and other problems of general impulsivity.

Cognition

While behavioral changes may seem to have the most direct impact on social life, cognitive changes may also be important. Clearly, language disorders may have a very great impact on social behavior. In language disorders, understanding and use of "pragmatics," including nonverbal aspects of communication such as gesture, facial expression, and turn-taking, may be preserved to varying degrees. However, deficits in the decoding and production of speech and language have the potential to cause major limitations in social interaction. For example, Angeleri and others (1993) found in their population of stroke patients under 65 years that, as regards return to work, "the main discriminating element was the ability to understand language" (p. 1478).

More general cognitive changes experienced as

a result of brain injury or damage may also have effects on social interaction. Limitations in memory and concentration are very common brain-injury sequelae, as also are deficits in divided attention, in which affected individuals have problems in applying themselves to any task, including, for example, holding a conversation when there is background noise or indeed any distraction. More generally, such individuals find it very hard to keep track of more than one task or topic at a time. Other cognitive impairments may result in a lack of understanding of the world, or understanding of others' reactions. If memory problems are present (and there is a very high probability of this after brain injury), individuals may forget names (which may *seem* to reflect lack of interest in others), may forget appointments and arrangements (again *seeming* to reflect indifference), and may lose shared memories of events. For example, one report (Oddy et al., 1985), commenting on the symptoms reported by individuals who had suffered brain injury and their relatives 7 years after head injury, found that 28 percent of individuals with TBI had difficulty following conversation, and 53 percent of individuals with TBI reported "trouble remembering things" – although when relatives were asked, 79 percent of them reported this as being present in the injured parties. Slowness and concreteness of thought, again common brain-injury sequelae, may also bear on social relationships.

Lack of insight

A particular issue which has received a good deal of attention is "lack of insight" or "denial." Those who lack insight fail to appreciate or acknowledge (i.e. they deny) that they have limitations arising from brain injury or damage, or at least fail to realize the extent of them. It is a difficult topic: sometimes an individual with TBI who has gross deficits will maintain that he or she is fully fit and well, and this is a clear instance of lack of insight. However, more commonly, at assessment the individual with TBI reports rather few problems while a close relative (e.g. a parent or spouse) paints a very different picture, and often one more consistent with the nature and severity of injury. However, it would plainly be naïve to assume that relatives are always accurate informants while individuals with TBI are not. Moreover, there is evidence that the reports of relatives are related to their own personality characteristics, with those

who have higher N (neuroticism) scores painting a worse picture as regards the effects of head injury on the individuals affected (McKinlay & Brooks, 1984).

In contrast to this are the findings of Sunderland and others (1983, 1984). They compared the self-reporting of memory failure by individuals who had suffered head injuries with the reports of relatives and with neuropsychological tests. The self-reports of everyday memory were found to be an underrepresentation of memory failure when compared to tests and relatives' reports, not surprising, considering that this constitutes a memory test in itself. They found that self-reports were demonstrated to be more reliable when a memory checklist (a record made at the time of memory failure) was used daily.

These findings suggest that relatives' accounts are more accurate than the accounts of individuals with TBI, at least as regards memory failures, and that the accounts of individuals with TBI can be improved by contemporaneous recording – suggesting that their underreporting is at least in part driven by memory limitations.

Langer and Padrone (1992) have provided an interesting discussion of how unawareness arises. Among other things, they consider whether it arises from a neurological deficit or whether it arises in the form of emotionally driven denial. They suggest that a tripartite model is useful: that unawareness may arise due to lack of information, implication, and integration. Contributors to lack of awareness, in their view, may include the details that the individual concerned:

1 does not have the information regarding a particular impairment;
2 does not understand the implications;
3 is in a state of denial – as if he or she cannot "believe" what has happened.

Implicit in their discussion is that unawareness (or whatever term is used) is not an "all or none" phenomenon.

GENERAL CHANGES

Having discussed a number of elements which may affect social behavior, it is important to remember that, while damage to certain brain areas produces a characteristic "flavor" of change, most cases of acquired brain damage are due to conditions which do not produce precise and limited lesions. The most common causes of acquired brain damage in adults are TBI and stroke, which produce damage which is often widespread and patchy. For example, in TBI the effects are a mixture of primary effects (damage directly due to trauma) and secondary effects (including infection, swelling, impaired perfusion, raised intracranial pressure, etc.). Given that the damage in such cases is not precisely localized in a particular brain area, the changes characteristic of brain damage in general will be described. However, there is a caveat: not all effects described will apply in all cases, and the balance will be influenced by the locus or loci of greatest insult to the brain.

Personality change

A key notion is "personality change," which is commonly reported after brain injury, and is really a way of saying that an individual's whole social interaction with others has changed. In a study examining the changes resulting from head injury, Brooks and others (1986) found that at 5 years post-injury the change most commonly reported by relatives of the individual with TBI was personality change. This was reported in 74 percent of a sample of individuals with "very severe" brain injury (median post-traumatic amnesia 21 days). This finding is similar to the 71 percent of relatives reporting personality change in the individuals with TBI at 2 years post-injury in a study by Oddy and others (1985) and 80 percent at 2.5 years and 65 percent at 10–15 years reported by Thomsen (1984). McKinlay and others (1981) not only found relatives reporting a high incidence of emotional changes, but also that the amount of stress in relatives was related to the incidence of mental and emotional changes in the individual with TBI.

In another study (Brooks & McKinlay, 1983), an attempt was made to identify the particular changes that went to make up an overall "personality change." Many particular changes were reported in those cases where personality change was said to occur, and those most strongly associated with reported personality change were:

- a lack of control of temper;
- poor regulation of mood (rapid mood changes);

- irritability;
- violent outbursts;
- reduced motivation ("sitting around", "staring at the walls");
- extreme tiredness;
- depressed mood;
- increased anxiety.

There have also been reports of more specific social changes after TBI. In a follow-up of individuals with TBI (Brooks et al., 1987), assessed between 2 and 7 years post-injury, relatives reported that 38 percent of the brain-injured sample talked excessively, 38 percent behaved in a socially embarrassing way (for example, showing impaired perception of and use of body language or being outspoken, perhaps swearing or boasting), 30 percent tended to withdraw from social interaction, and 22 percent of family members reported that the individual with TBI had become more intrusive or prying. (In these studies, relatives were interviewed to reduce the problem of limited insight and memory on the part of some individuals with TBI.)

Social isolation

As a result of these changes, individuals with TBI no longer perform adequately in social situations and they may begin to avoid them. The loss of ability to recognize people, or remember their names, or the rejection from previous friends who have lost patience with inappropriate social behavior, can all lead to social withdrawal by the individual with TBI and result in social isolation. Ponsford and others (1995) reported that 50 percent of individuals who had suffered TBI reported social isolation as a behavioral change at 2 years post-injury. Thomsen (1984) investigated the late outcome of traumatic brain injury, examining individuals at between 10 and 15 years post-injury (her second follow-up). She found that:

> At the second follow-up two-thirds had no contact outside the close family, and social isolation remained the patients' severest burden ... Several preferred to make friends with old people, since they were kind and patient. (p. 265)

Finset and others (1995) report on a similar finding in a sample of individuals with TBI at 2 years after admission to a rehabilitation hospital. Fifty-seven percent of the sample reported that

681

their social networks had "markedly declined" since their injury. Where social support remained, it was mainly received from family members rather than from friends or neighbors. Finset and colleagues propose that the degree of support received from family members is reflective of the family's perception of the severity of the injury sustained. This is based on the finding that those individuals with a shorter length of coma perceived their social networks and support from family as being poorer than those with a more severe injury (a longer period of coma). Of course, those individuals who have sustained a more severe injury may be exaggerating the support they receive and the networks that remain as a result of a lack of insight or as a result of a more severe memory impairment.

Thomsen (1984) did not just comment on the psychosocial experiences of the individuals with TBI but also commented on the corresponding effects on the families:

> While lack of social contact at the former [first follow-up, average 2.5 years post-injury] was the greatest subjective burden to the patients, changes in personality and emotion presented the severest problem to the families. The spouses of the seven patients who had a divorce declared that their wives or husbands had become complete strangers. Loss of emotional control, with rapid changes between apathy and aggression, irritability, and childishness were the main complaints. The relationship between the patients and their children developed badly in all cases and the spouses considered themselves the only grown-ups in the families. (p. 264)

The relatives' view

The position of the relatives of the head injured is an important consideration. Brooks and others (1986), in examining the 5-year outcome after head injury, found that the relatives were under considerable strain. This increased rather than decreased over time – family members were reporting more strain 1 year post-injury than at 3 months, and more still at 5 years. The best predictor of the relatives' strain was the magnitude of behavioral and personality change in the individual with TBI. The burden on families has been reported widely, with Thomsen (1974) reporting the finding that spouses of the injured seem less able to cope than parents.

This whole area has received more recent examination by Kreutzer and others (1994a, b). They found that spouses were significantly more likely than parents of the individual who had suffered brain injury to report elevated depression. Of all their sample population (62 families with a member having suffered traumatic brain injury and another member caring for the injured) approximately 50 percent of carers reported elevated distress, 33 percent elevated anxiety, and 25 percent elevated depression, with spouses especially prone to depression. Feelings of burden and alienation were common.

Return to work

The above changes in social behavior have far-reaching effects. One of the key problems after receiving brain damage is an inability to return to previously held work positions. In a recent study (Teasdale et al., 1993) it was found that 95 percent of subjects (individuals with TBI and stroke victims) were in employment pre-injury, whereas 22 percent were in employment post-injury. The position taken up after the injury may not be of the same nature and may only be a mundane, manual position. However, the benefits to an individual with TBI of being able to work are, for example, in providing a structure and meaning to daily life, providing social contact, giving relief to carers, and there may also be economic benefits (although, of those returning to work, many individuals have been demoted, and some receive only a nominal wage in a supported work placement).

It is the cognitive and emotional-behavioral changes which are particularly predictive of the ability to return to work. Brooks and others (1987b) found that 86 percent of individuals with TBI in their study were employed before their injury and only 29 percent afterwards. Six key predictors were identified which most strongly differentiated those who did and those who did not return to work (up to 7 years post-injury): from the cognitive test battery, verbal memory, and mental speed/concentration; and from the interview with relatives, a disturbance in self care; behavioral disturbance; emotional disturbance; and language/speech disturbance (mainly a problem in keeping track of conversations with several participants). All are related to social factors and emphasize the restrictions placed on individuals experiencing social problems.

Community re-entry

In order to achieve community reintegration for

individuals who have suffered a brain injury or brain damage, it is necessary to provide rehabilitation and retraining relevant to their reduced social skills. This can concentrate on, for example, anger management programs to control bad temper (McKinlay & Hickox, 1988; Wood, 1990; Uomotu & Brockway, 1992); training in the use of memory aids and techniques; vocational retraining to assist in finding a job that is suitable; occupational therapy to assist in relearning simple skills and planning social activities.

Increasingly, rehabilitative approaches are directed at community re-entry and learning and practicing compensatory skills in the "real-life" social environment in which they will be used. More recently, for example, vocational retraining operates on a job-coaching basis where following training a job coach attends work placements with the patient (Wehman et al., 1989, 1993; Skord & Miranti, 1994). The idea is to return the individual to as close a social environment as would be considered "normal." The implementation of case management, on the other hand, aims to enable individuals with TBI to live in the community by providing potential sources of help available, including sheltered work schemes or tolerant employers with simple work available, and support/voluntary groups. The individual with TBI may also need help to find suitable carers or housekeepers, who should be briefed in the limitations the individual has and how best to help them (e.g. what to do for them and what to prompt them to do). The case manager's overall remit is to identify possible local sources of help, explore just what may be available, and help the injured individual to structure his or her time to provide an appropriate social program.

In an editorial, Brooks (1991) commented on the importance of transferring skills and techniques learned in rehabilitation to the normal milieu of the individual with TBI. He observes that "generalization . . . seems not to take place unless specifically built (into rehabilitation programmes)." The importance of ensuring that social skills learned (or relearned) in rehabilitation are transferred to the everyday social world of the patient is increasingly recognized.

BIBLIOGRAPHY

Adolphs, R., Tranel, D., Damasio, H., & Damasio, A. (1994). Impaired recognition of emotion in facial expressions following bilateral damage to the human amygdala. *Nature, 372,* 669–72.

Angeleri, F., Angeleri, V. A., Foschi, N., Giaquinto, S., & Nolfe, G. (1993). The influence of depression, social activity, and family stress on functional outcome after stroke. *Stroke, 24,* 1478–83.

Argyle, M. (1967). *The psychology of interpersonal behaviour.* London: Penguin.

Brooks, D. N., & McKinlay, W. W. (1983). Personality and behavioural change after severe blunt head injury – a relative's view. *Journal of Neurology, Neurosurgery and Psychiatry, 46,* 336–44.

Brooks, D. N., McKinlay, W. W., Symington, C., Beattie, A., & Campsie, L. (1987b). Return to work within the first seven years of severe head injury. *Brain Injury, 1,* 5–19.

Brooks, N. (1984). *Closed head injury.* Oxford: Oxford University Press.

Brooks, N. (1991). The effectiveness of post-acute rehabilitation. *Brain Injury, 5,* 103–9.

Brooks, N., Campsie, L., Symington, C., Beattie, A., & McKinlay, W. (1986). The five year outcome of severe blunt head injury: a relative's view. *Journal of Neurology, Neurosurgery, and Psychiatry, 49,* 764–70.

Brooks, N., Campsie, L., Symington, C., Beattie, A., & McKinlay, W. (1987a). The effects of severe head injury on patient and relative within seven years of injury. *Journal of Head Trauma Rehabilitation, 2,* 1–13.

Finset, A., Dymes, S., Krogstad, J. M., & Berstad, J. (1995). Self-reported social networks and interpersonal support 2 years after severe traumatic brain injury. *Brain Injury, 9,* 141–50.

Kreutzer, J. S., Gervasio, A. H., & Camplair, P. S. (1994a). Primary caregivers' psychological status and family functioning after traumatic brain injury. *Brain Injury, 8,* 197–210.

Kreutzer, J. S., Gervasio, A. H., & Camplair, P. S. (1994b). Patient correlates of caregivers' distress and family functioning after traumatic brain injury. *Brain Injury, 8,* 211–30.

Langer, K. G., & Padrone, F. J. (1992). Psychotherapeutic treatment of awareness in acute rehabilitation in traumatic brain injury. *Neuropsychological Rehabilitation, 2,* 59–70.

Lishman, W. A. (1987). *Organic psychiatry.* Oxford: Blackwell Scientific.

Lewin, J., & Sumner, D. (1992). Successful treatment of episodic dyscontrol with

Carbamazepine. *British Journal of Psychiatry*, *161*, 261–2.

Luria, A. R. (1973). *The working brain*. London: Penguin.

McKinlay, W. W., & Brooks, D. N. (1984). Methodological problems in assessing psychosocial recovery following severe head injury. *Journal of Clinical Neuropsychology*, *6*, 87–99.

McKinlay, W. W., Brooks, D. N., Bond, M. R., Martinage, D. P., & Marshall, M. M. (1981). The short-term outcome of severe blunt head injury as reported by relatives of the injured person. *Journal of Neurology, Neurosurgery, and Psychiatry*, *44*, 527–33.

McKinlay, W. W., & Hickox, A. (1988). How can families help in the rehabilitation of the head injured? *Journal of Head Trauma Rehabilitation*, *3*, 64–72.

Mark, V. H., & Ervin, F. R. (1970). *Violence and the brain*. New York: Harper and Row.

Oddy, M., Coughlan, T., Tyerman, A., & Jenkins, D. (1985). Social adjustment after closed head injury: a further follow-up seven years after injury. *Journal of Neurology, Neurosurgery, and Psychiatry*, *48*, 564–8.

Pentland, B., Pitcairn, T. K., Gray, J. M., & Riddle, W. J. R. (1987). The effects of reduced expression in Parkinson's disease on impression formation by health professionals. *Clinical Rehabilitation*, *1*, 307–13.

Pitcairn, T. K., Clemie, S., Gray, J. M., & Pentland, B. (1990). Non-verbal cues in the self-presentation of Parkinsonian patients. *British Journal of Clinical Psychology*, *29*, 177–84.

Ponsford, J. L., Olver, J. H., & Curran, C. (1995). A profile of outcome: 2 years after traumatic brain injury. *Brain Injury*, *9*, 1–10.

Skord, K. G., & Miranti, S. V. (1994). Towards a more integrated approach to job placement and retention for persons with traumatic brain injury and premorbid disadvantages. *Brain Injury*, *8*, 383–93.

Sunderland, A., Harris, J. E., & Baddeley, A. D. (1983). Do laboratory tests predict everyday memory? A neuropsychological study. *Journal of Verbal Learning and Verbal Behaviour*, *22*, 341–57.

Sunderland, A., Harris, J. E., & Gleave, J. (1984). Memory failures in everyday life following severe head injury. *Journal of Clinical Neuropsychology*, *6*, 127–42.

Tajfel, H., & Fraser C. (1978). *Introduction to social psychology*. London: Penguin.

Teasdale, T., Christensen, A.-L., & Pinner, E. M. (1993). Psychosocial rehabilitation of cranial trauma and stroke patients. *Brain Injury*, *7*, 535–42.

Thomsen, I. V. (1974). The patient with severe head injury and his family. *Scandinavian Journal of Rehabilitation Medicine*, *6*, 180–3.

Thomsen, I. V. (1984). Late outcome of very severe blunt head trauma: a 10–15 year second follow-up. *Journal of Neurology, Neurosurgery, and Psychiatry*, *47*, 260–8.

Uomoto, J. M., & Brockway, J. A. (1992). Anger management training for brain injured patients and their family members. *Archives of Physical Medicine and Rehabilitation*, *73*, 674–97.

Wehman, P., Kreutzer, J., West, M., Sherron, P., Diambra, J., Fry, R., Groah, C., Sale, P., & Killam, S. (1989). Employment outcomes of persons following traumatic brain injury: pre-injury, post-injury, and supported employment. *Brain Injury*, *3*, 397–412.

Wehman, P., & Kregel, J., Sherron, P., Nguyen, S., Kreutzer, J., Fry, R., & Zasler, N. (1993). Critical factors associated with the successful supported employment placement of patients with severe traumatic brain injury. *Brain Injury*, *7*, 31–44.

Wood, R. Ll. (1990). *Neuro-behavioral sequelae of traumatic brain injury*. New York: Taylor & Francis.

Zencius, A., Wesolowski, M. D., Burke, W. H., & Hough, S. (1990). Managing hypersexual disorders in brain-injured clients. *Brain Injury*, *4*, 175–83.

WILLIAM W. MCKINLAY AND ANNA J. WATKISS

somatosensory evoked potential *See* EVOKED POTENTIAL.

somesthetic system The somesthetic system is the system by which somatic sensory information is passed up to the brain. The precise neuroanatomy of the system depends to some degree on which aspect of somatic sensory function is being considered.

All peripheral sensory receptors pass information into the central nervous system via the dorsal roots of the spinal cord. From this point there are two major routes to the THALAMUS, but each eventually reaches the thalamus in the cerebral hemisphere contralateral to the side of the originating stimulus. These two routes are the spinothalamic and the dorsal column routes.

The spinothalamic route runs from the dorsal horn of the spinal cord at the level of the dorsal nerve root, crosses immediately to the opposite side of the cord, and travels up through the spinothalamic neuron to the ventrobasal nucleus of the thalamus. This route is used for pain and temperature sensation, and is as concerned with reflex reactions organized across adjacent levels of the spinal cord as it is with the transmission of information up to the brain.

The dorsal column route does not synapse on entry into the spinal cord, but runs upwards through the dorsal columns of the spinal cord on the same side as the dorsal root of entry. Within the MEDULLA (at the cuneate nucleus where the dorsal column nuclei are located) the pathway synapses and at this level crosses to the contralateral side of the BRAIN STEM from where it runs through the medial lemniscus to the ventrobasal nucleus of the thalamus. Fibers in the dorsal column route serve proprioception.

The sensation of touch is served by both routes. From the thalamus both routes project upwards to the primary somatosensory cortex through the posterior part of the internal capsule. Within each of the somatosensory routes there is a laminar organization of the fibers, so that a topographic representation of the body surface is preserved up to the cerebral cortex.

J. GRAHAM BEAUMONT

spasticity A clinical term alluding to a complex of symptoms disturbing the movements of patients with lesions of the central nervous system (CNS). Lance (1980) has formulated a more explicit and commonly used definition: spasticity is "a motor disorder characterized by a velocity dependent increase in the tonic stretch reflexes ('muscle tone') with exaggerated tendon jerks, resulting from hyperexcitability of the stretch reflex." The key sign is the velocity-dependent increase in passive stretch resistance of a muscle, which separates the spasticity from other forms of muscle hypertonia, e.g. rigidity and dystonia. Although disputed, there is clear evidence that stretch of the spastic muscle elicits pathological

muscle activity, which is due to an increased gain of the stretch reflex, and which contributes to the increased resistance.

Increased stretch reflexes and muscle hypertonia constitute only one aspect of the multiple deficits in the motor behavior of patients with spasticity. Other symptoms are often more impairing, e.g. paresis (i.e. muscle weakness) with impaired voluntary control, slowness of movements, lack of dexterity, and fatigability all contribute significantly to the patients' inability to function. Movements are commonly restrained by co-contraction of agonist and antagonist muscles and by inadequate coordination of muscle activation patterns. Spasticity is usually associated with an irradiation of tendon reflexes to other muscles. Clonus, flexor spasms (involuntary flexion reflexes), mass reflexes, and the BABINSKI RESPONSE are often present. The clasp-knife phenomenon, which is characterized by a sudden release of the passive muscle force during ongoing stretch, is only rarely present.

Pathology Spasticity is a consequence of lesions of corticofugal pathways, including the upper motor neuron at any level during its passage down to the spinal cord, i.e. motor cortex, internal capsule, brain stem, or spinal cord. A lesion at any of these levels has essentially the same functional result, although the clinical presentation of the symptoms depends on the locus and extent of the injury to the CNS. Interestingly, selective section of the corticospinal tract (see PYRAMIDAL TRACT) at the medullary pyramids or cerebral peduncles produces no or only minor spasticity in humans and nonhuman primates (Bucy, 1957). There is only a permanent loss of manual dexterity and independent finger movements. Such discrete lesions rarely occur as a result of disease, and generally involve "parapyramidal fibers." Hence it is not correct to refer to spasticity as a sign of a pyramidal tract lesion, which is often done in clinical practice.

Various diseases may damage the upper motor neurone and lead to spasticity. STROKE is the most common disease causing spasticity after cerebrovascular accidents. It usually affects one hemisphere, producing HEMIPARESIS and spasticity in the contralateral limbs. CEREBROVASCULAR ACCIDENTS or hypoxia during fetal or perinatal life leads to CEREBRAL PALSY, which can be divided into various syndromes depending on the distribution of the symptoms, i.e. QUADRIPLEGIA,

HEMIPLEGIA, DIPLEGIA, and monoplegia. Tumors may occur at any level of the upper motor neuron. Traumatic transection of the spinal cord produces paresis and spasticity below the lesion, i.e. PARAPLEGIA. Muscles innervated from the damaged segment are flaccid due to destruction of the motor neurons. Several DEGENERATIVE DISEASES may also affect the upper motor neuron. MULTIPLE SCLEROSIS may affect various parts of the CNS and produce a multifocal distribution of paresis and spasticity in various body parts. Amyotrophic lateral sclerosis mainly destroys the motor neurons, but also produces spasticity, indicating involvement of the upper motor neuron.

Pathophysiology The stretch reflex elicits activity in a stretched muscle after a short latency. The reflex response is generated from a lengthening of muscle spindles within the stretched muscle and is monosynaptically transmitted to the α-moto neuron of the stretched muscle via large afferent nerve fibers, i.e. Ia afferents. The sensitivity of the muscle spindle is controlled by a smaller γ-motor neuron innervating intrafusal muscle fibers. Several spinal pathways control the stretch reflex excitability (Figure 74). The spinal interneurons and synapses involved in these pathways are controlled by descending pathways, e.g. the corticospinal tract, and normally modify the gain of the stretch reflex during various motor behaviors. An abnormality in the supraspinal control can therefore alter the function in any of the spinal pathways and produce an exaggeration of the stretch reflex. Many concepts about the pathophysiology of human spasticity are based on

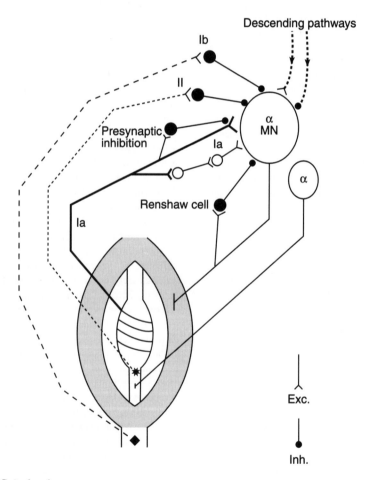

Figure 74 Spinal pathways.

deductions drawn from experiments on decerebrate cats. It was thought that the abnormalities responsible for the muscle hypertonia present in decerebrate rigidity also underlay the increased muscle tone in human spasticity. Accordingly, hyperactivity of the γ-motor neuron (see (b) below) was considered as the major cause of the spasticity. However, recent electrophysiological experimentation using microneurography (i.e. single-unit recordings from afferent nerve fibers in the peripheral nerves) and H-reflexes (i.e. the Hoffman reflex when the afferent Ia fibers are activated by electrical stimulation) has allowed studies in healthy humans and patients with spasticity and revealed some other abnormalities in the spinal cord circuits:

(a) Hyperexcitability in the α-motor neurons,

caused by changed intrinsic properties of the moto neurons or by an imbalance between excitatory and inhibitory input from descending tracts, may produce spasticity. Yet this has not been demonstrated in humans since it would require intracellular recordings.

(b) Hyperactivity of the γ-motor neurons could also cause a stretch reflex exaggeration, since it controls the sensitivity of the muscle spindle receptors. In spastic patients the increase of the tendon jerk, i.e. when the reflex is elicited by the muscle spindles following a tendon tap, is larger than that of the H-reflex. However, the electrical stimulation also evokes activity in Ib afferents which inhibits the α-motor neurons. The Ib afferents originate from Golgi tendon organs, which are normally sensitive to the tension

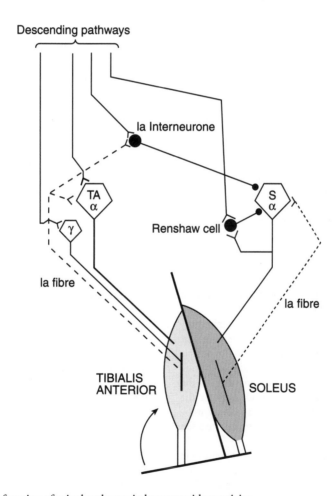

Figure 75 Dysfunction of spinal pathways in humans with spasticity.

developed by the muscle fiber contraction. It has not been possible to demonstrate an increase of the Ia discharge produced by a given stretch in patients with spasticity by means of microneurographic recording. Thus there is so far no satisfying evidence for an increased drive of the γ-motor neurons in human spasticity.

(c) Ia impulses, i.e. the afferent volley following a muscle stretch (tendon tap), reach the α-motor neurons not only via the classical monosynaptic pathway but also through polysynaptic pathways. A facilitation of the transmission in these pathways, subsequent to altered supraspinal influence, could contribute to spasticity.

(d) Signals from the Ia afferent are normally reduced by presynaptic inhibition before exciting the α-motor neurons. A decrease in presynaptic inhibition of Ia fibers is found in most patients with spasticity, although there is no significant correlation between the decrease and the intensity of the stretch reflex exaggeration.

(e) The discharge of the α-motor neuron is opposed by recurrent inhibition via Renshaw cells, and a decrease of this effect would enhance the firing of the motor neurons. In most patients with spasticity, changes in recurrent inhibition are not responsible for the exaggeration of passively induced stretch reflexes. On the other hand, the supraspinal control of the Renshaw cells, which normally accompanies voluntary movement, is lacking in spastic patients (Figure 75). This control is important to depress the activity in antagonistic muscles during a movement, i.e. reciprocal inhibition. It is likely that the disturbance of voluntary movements in spastic patients is partly due to the lack of supraspinal control of the Renshaw cells, e.g. triggering of stretch reflexes of antagonistic muscles during the active stretch induced by the agonist contraction.

(f) The supraspinal control of the Ia inhibitory interneuron does not influence the passively induced stretch reflex, but prevents reflex activation of the stretched antagonistic muscles during active movements in a similar manner to the Renshaw cell. A lack of supraspinal control of the Ia inhibitory interneuron in spastic patients probably contributes to the antagonistic coactivation during voluntary movements.

(g) Muscle stretch evokes impulses not only in Ia afferents but also in Ib fibers from Golgi tendon organs and group II fibers from muscle spindles' secondary endings. The net effect is an inhibition of the stretched muscle. It has been shown that Ib inhibition is markedly depressed in spastic patients, which could contribute to the exaggerated reflexes, while there is no evidence that decreased inhibition from group II afferents contributes to the increased stretch reflexes in spasticity.

In conclusion, until now a dysfunction has been observed at four instances of the spinal pathways in human patients with spasticity: (i) presynaptic inhibition of Ia fibers; (ii) Ib inhibition during passive stretch; (iii) recurrent inhibition (Renshaw cells); and (iv) reciprocal Ia inhibition during active movements (see Pierrot-Deseilligny, 1990).

Spasticity is not an acute symptom, but rather a syndrome that in most cases develops gradually and persists indefinitely. Over time, a complex series of plastic changes may alter the neuronal circuits and pathways in the otherwise intact spinal cord by means of (i) sprouting of axon terminals and the formation of new synapses, (ii) synaptic degeneration and induction of synapses that normally are ineffective, or (iii) synaptic degeneration and enhanced sensitivity of the remaining receptors (DENERVATION HYPERSENSITIVITY). Although these mechanisms are well known in the mammalian CNS, their significance for the development of human spasticity is not known.

Investigations of stance, GAIT, and arm movements have shown a discrepancy between exaggerated stretch reflexes and the degree of impaired movements in patients with spasticity, supporting the fact that other mechanisms are underlying the spasticity. Alteration of the muscle fiber properties has been suggested to directly enhance the resistance to stretch. This is supported by morphological and biomechanical changes in spastic muscles (see Dietz, 1987).

CLINICAL MANAGEMENT

Good nursing and active physiotherapy are important to reduce the spasticity (see Katz, 1988). Avoidance of noxious stimuli, such as urinary tract and bowel complications, contracture, and pressure sores are crucial, since these have a tendency to enhance the spasticity. Regular ranging of a patient's limb helps to prevent contracture and often reduces the muscle tone for several hours. Casting and splinting techniques, positioning the limb in a tonic stretch, have a more sustained effect by elongating the elastic components and increasing the numbers of sarcomeres within a muscle fiber. The application of cold packs to the affected limb has been reported to decrease tendon reflex excitability, reduce clonus, and increase the range of motion of the joint, probably due to decreased sensitivity in cutaneous receptors and reduced nerve conduction. The cold treatment can be used to improve motor functions for short periods of time. Various schools of physical therapy have suggested that reflex inhibition or reflex facilitation may reduce the muscle hypertonia and unmask underlying movement patterns. Disregarding the mechanisms behind the treatment, active motor training often improves the movement capacity in adult patients after STROKE and in children with CEREBRAL PALSY. Biofeedback techniques have also been observed to modify the spastic hypertonia, but they have not been extensively used. Functional electrical stimulation, e.g. stimulation of the peroneal nerve during walking to induce dorsiflexion of the foot during the swing phase, may also lead to sustained decrease of the tonic muscle activity in both agonist and antagonist muscles.

Today there are several drugs potentially useful to treat patients with spasticity (see Davidoff, 1985). Several drugs act outside the CNS. Dantrolene curtails the activation of the contractile process and decreases the mechanical force of the contraction of the muscle fibers, by reducing the release of calcium ions from the sarcoplasmic reticulum. Botulinum-A toxin, produced by the bacterium *Clostridium botulinum*, can be locally injected into spastic muscles and reduces the release of acetylcholine at the neuromuscular junction. Both these drugs have a general effect on the strength of the contraction independent of the source of the activation, e.g. local injection of Botulinum-A toxin selectively controls abnormal muscle activity in TORTICOLLIS, DYSTONIA, and BLETHAROSPASM. The anticonvulsants phenytoin and carbamazepine have a more specific action, decreasing the sensitivity of the muscle spindles and thereby reducing the afferent input from Ia fibers.

Glycine and γ-aminobutyric acid (GABA) have been identified as major inhibitory transmitters in the spinal cord, and drugs enhancing the effect of these transmitter systems often have a good effect on spasticity. GABA mediates the presynaptic inhibition at the terminals of Ia afferents as well as other afferents. The benzodiazepines bind to specific receptors linked to (GABA$_A$) receptors located on the terminals of the Ia afferents. This binding results in an increased affinity for GABA to the GABA$_A$ receptor, inducing an augmented flux of chloride ions across the terminal membrane, and an increase in the amount of presynaptic inhibition. Baclofen activates GABA$_B$ receptors located on the same nerve terminals. Activation of these receptors delays the influx of calcium ions into the terminals, thereby reducing the evoked release of excitatory amino acids and possibly other transmitters. Progabide and its metabolites act on both GABA$_A$ and GABA$_B$ receptors. Glycine seems to be the transmitter released by inhibitory Ia interneurons responsible for reciprocal inhibition and by Renshaw cells responsible for recurrent inhibition. Glycine is one of the few pharmacologically active amino acids that pass through the blood–brain barrier. It acts at the specific glycine receptors located on spinal interneurones and motor neurons. The phenothiazines act on the brain stem to alter the drive of the γ-motor neurons and may reduce the sensitivity of the muscle spindles. Usually the drugs are orally administered, but intrathecal administration (i.e. in the cerebrospinal fluid surrounding the spinal cord) of benzodiazepines, baclofen, and morphine sulfate with mini-pumps, has also been used to produce a high concentration of the drug in the spinal cord while keeping the systemic and brain concentrations low. Selective posterior rhizotomy has long been used for the treatment of spasticity. Recently this method has become popular again, especially for children with cerebral palsy. The dorsal roots from L2–S2 are partially sectioned, thereby cutting a majority of group Ia afferents. The reduced Ia input decreases the muscle tone, while the sensory information from the limbs is left intact via the remaining dorsal rootlets.

BIBLIOGRAPHY

Bucy, P. C. (1957). Is there a pyramidal tract? *Brain, 80*, 376–92.

Davidoff, R. A. (1985). Antispasticity drugs: mechanisms of action. *Annals of Neurology, 17*, 107–16.

Dietz, V. (1987). Role of peripheral afferents and spinal reflexes in normal and impaired human locomotion. *Revue Neurologique (Paris), 143*, 241–5.

Katz, R. T. (1988). Management of spasticity. *American Journal of Physical Medicine and Rehabilitation, 67*, 108–16.

Lance, J. W. (1980). Symposium synopsis. In R. G. Feldman, R. R. Young, & W. P. Koella (Eds), *Spasticity: Disordered motor control* (pp. 485–94). Chicago: Year Book Medical Corporation.

Pierrot-Deseilligny, E. (1990). Electrophysiological assessment of spinal mechanisms underlying spasticity. In P. M. Rossini & F. Mauguière (Eds), *New trends and advanced techniques in clinical neurophysiology (EEG Suppl. 41)* (pp. 264–73). Amsterdam: Elsevier.

HANS FORSSBERG

speech disorders   *See* APHASIA; SPEECH THERAPY FOR APHASIA.

speech therapy for aphasia   Therapeutic approaches to communication impairments of neuropsychological and neurological origin will be discussed here. The main interest is in REHABILITATION for impairments of the expression and comprehension of language, whether through speech or writing, especially impairments that can be described in terms of the core components of a linguistic model – features like semantics, syntax, morphology and phonology. Such impairments are generally referred to as APHASIA, although the term should be viewed as generic. While "aphasia" describes a problem of cognitive processing, for the patient it is a problem of communication.

People with acquired neurological damage can suffer from a range of communication problems which do not directly affect straight linguistic aspects of language. We shall not look at therapy for the motor speech disorders, i.e. those disorders which affect articulation and voice due to impaired muscle tone and/or coordination in neurological disease – DYSARTHRIA.

APHASIA THERAPY

Aphasia therapy has a relatively long history, and currently there are a range of approaches in use. We can group these in various ways: under functional approaches, linguistic or cognitive approaches, or neuropsychological approaches. To some extent approaches vary around the world, but in general treatment aims either for the restitution or reestablishment of lost functions or for substitution or compensation for lost functions. The therapist may employ specific reorganizational methods to achieve reestablishment or substitution. Developments in aphasia therapy have emerged from developments in other areas. Thus it is no surprise that aspects of education, learning theory, counselling, linguistics, neuropsychology, and cognitive psychology have been introduced and modified.

In their historical survey Howard and Hatfield (1987) classify approaches to aphasia therapy into several main "schools." To a large extent there is an overlap between these broad approaches, but this general structure will serve as a useful introductory starting point for discussion. For those of the *didactic school* the approach is to reteach language, using a mixture of the traditional and intuitive educational methods used with children and foreign-language learning. While historically therapists worked in a didactic tradition, in practice, these days, most aphasia therapists all over the world make use of general teaching techniques and methods. Overlapping didactic methods is the approach adopted by *the behavior modification school*, where the techniques of behaviorist psychology are used in reteaching language. Examples of programmed instruction approaches to treatment can be found from the 1960s and contemporary computer-based methods use systematic behavioral methods. Behaviorist methodology, such as imitation and modelling, prompting and cueing, and the use of reinforcement, is widely used by many therapists who would not take kindly to being called "behaviorists." Indeed, the approach is essentially atheoretical and crosses theoretical boundaries. Some methods use highly systematic hierarchical techniques, such as MELODIC INTONATION THERAPY (see Helm-Estabrooks & Albert, 1991, and chapters in Chapey, 1987), and hierarchically organized approaches for APRAXIA of speech (see Helm-Estabrooks & Albert, 1991, and chapters in Code & Muller, 1989).

For those who support *the stimulation school* the patient has not lost language functions, but brain damage has caused these functions to become inaccessible. Language competence has survived and it is language performance which is impaired.

Therapy essentially entails facilitating and stimulating language use in the patient. Improvement, if it occurs, comes about through a recovery process where the patient does not learn new vocabulary or grammatical forms, but facilitates and integrates what he or she already knows. The stimulation approach is most widely associated with Wepman and Schuell. The general techniques and methods advocated by this approach are still used fairly widely. For Schuell, intense auditory stimulation and maximum response from the patient are essential and fundamental features of the approach, with repetition, facilitation, and various forms of cueing being general features. Studies have shown that the widely used facilitation techniques of repetition and phonemic cueing (i.e. providing the patient with the first sound of a target word) have a marked effect on picture-naming performance, but the effect wears off 30 minutes later and the patients are just as poor at naming pictures as they were before the stimulation (see chapters in Code & Muller, 1989).

The neuropsychological model of Luria (1970) is the basis for *the reorganization of function school*, where intact functional subsystems can be used to substitute for impaired subsystems. For instance, for patients with severe apraxia of speech, Luria (1970) advocated using humming (something the patient can do) to elicit an /m/, or shaping the blowing out of a candle into a /p/. Also for severely apraxic patients, Luria (1970) developed "articulograms," which are drawings of the lips producing particular combinations of speech sounds. Here the patient makes use of an intact visual route into the speech production system. Intact visual and kinesthetic channels can be used to treat sensory aphasic deficits where the deficit is due to impairment of the acoustic analyzer. Lurian approaches have had their main impact in Eastern Europe.

Reorganizational approaches exist which are based on surviving right hemisphere modes of processing information. These, reviewed by Code (1987, 1994), are mostly reorganizational methods which aim to compensate for lost functions. Melodic intonation therapy (Helm-Estabrooks & Albert, 1991), for instance, aims to re-establish some speech in patients with motoric problems by reorganization of the speech production process, using melodic intonation as a vehicle. Artificial languages have been developed and tested with groups of severely impaired aphasic subjects. These languages are made up of visual arbitrary shapes, or idiographic and iconographic symbols. These approaches have reported remarkable success with globally impaired patients, being able to use propositional communication. The heightening of visual imagery mediated by the right hemisphere and the use of hypnosis have been advocated in aphasia therapy. Also reported in Code (1987, 1994) are two separate attempts to directly influence cognitive processing in the right hemisphere and stimulate latent right hemisphere language processes using LATERALIZATION techniques of DICHOTIC LISTENING, DIVIDED VISUAL FIELD TECHNIQUES, and DICHHAPTIC processing. The single Wernicke's subjects of both studies were reported to have improved significantly over an 18-month period on the basis of performance on standardized batteries, but neither design was capable of determining whether improvement was actually due to the right hemisphere completing tasks or other uncontrolled factors.

Aphasia for the patient, and therefore also for the therapist, is a communication problem. Therapists recognize this and approaches have been developed which are concerned with enhancing and improving functional communication. These developments form the foundations of *the pragmatic school*, which has advanced in parallel with progress in theoretical and applied pragmatics. For most aphasic individuals, problems affect linguistic levels primarily and pragmatic aspects of language and communication are spared. For the large number of patients whose problems are so severe that they fail to make any progress with treatment aimed at restitution, therapists have developed methods to compensate for lost functions. An approach which has gained a large following from therapists disappointed in the effectiveness of methods of restitution in recent years is the PACE (Promoting Aphasics Communicative Efficiency) approach (Davis & Wilcox, 1985; Carlomagno, 1994). Here the emphasis is on successful communication, not precise oral naming or correct syntax. The main features of PACE therapy are: (i) the therapist and patient participate equally as sender and receiver of messages; (ii) therapeutic interactions between patient and therapist entail the exchange of new information; (iii) the patient chooses the modality or methods of communication; (iv) feedback is based on the patient's success in communicating

691

the message (Davis & Wilcox, 1985; Carlomagno, 1994). Typically, patients are encouraged to use writing, gesture, drawing, or pointing, in fact any means at their disposal to communicate their message. There are a range of treatment studies using GESTURAL BEHAVIOR and drawing (Helm-Estabrooks & Albert, 1991) as well as studies of the efficacy of PACE. Group therapy for aphasia is often considered by its advocates to be particularly relevant for functional and more natural communication (see chapters in Chapey, 1987, 1994; Code & Muller, 1989, 1995; Howard & Hatfield, 1987).

In the United States methods have been developed by therapists working in association with the Boston Aphasia Research Center. Howard and Hatfield (1987) call these approaches *the neoclassical school* because they are partly inspired by, and to some extent tied to, the Wernicke–Lichtheim–Geschwind model. Perhaps what many of these approaches have in common is that they are designed for specific types of aphasia, like melodic intonation therapy (MIT) and visual action therapy (VAT) (Helm-Estabrooks & Albert, 1991), for patients with Broca's or global impairments. MIT is based on the observation that many globally aphasic individuals have remarkably retained abilities to hum, whistle, and sing. Most noted is an ability to render the lyrics of over-learned songs, often in the context of severe expressive problems and apraxia of speech. MIT exploits these retained abilities in patients with severe motor speech difficulties. The training method again uses a systematic behavioral hierarchy, organized into steps and levels. VAT uses a fairly systematic approach to training severely aphasic patients to use gesture to communicate, and it is divided into a proximal form (this uses grosser arm, elbow, and wrist movement-based gestures, which are easier for most globally impaired patients) and a distal form (using finer movements of hands and fingers), which is more difficult. Improved performance on gestural components of standardized tests are reported in severely impaired patients.

The *neurolinguistic school* describes a predominantly Western European approach which grew mainly out of the linguistics revolution in the 1960s. This approach began to take linguistic theory and linguistic characterizations of aphasia seriously. There are many studies where treatment has concentrated on a linguistic analysis of the patient's problems and targeted specific impaired linguistic features. In practice this has meant linguistically inspired treatment for the various manifestations of AGRAMMATISM, as found in Code and Muller (1989, 1995), Helm-Estabrooks and Albert (1991), and Howard and Hatfield (1987). To some extent the distinctive features of the neurolinguistic approach form the major part of cognitive neuropsychological approaches to treatment.

Assessing aphasia *for treatment* is an issue in the clinical field, where assessment of aphasia purely for diagnosis and localization of damage is of less concern. The concern of cognitive neuropsychology for single-case research has strongly influenced the development of a hypothesis-driven single-case assessment process based on the information processing model (e.g. Lesser, 1995). The argument is that standardized psychometric batteries can provide only inadequate information on the specific deficits underlying an individual impairment profile. Hypotheses concerning the deficit areas must be stated and tested, accepted or rejected, on the basis of performance on specific psycholinguistically controlled tests. This view has resulted in the development of a psycholinguistically controlled battery of assessment resources (see Lesser, 1995, for review). The counter argument is that standardized and reliable test batteries can provide information on type and severity of aphasia and provide a baseline against which to measure change in performance (Shallice, 1979). From the perspective of assessment for treatment, batteries are perhaps best seen these days as standardized and reliable screening procedures, which can fairly quickly provide a basic profile to compare areas of impairment and preservation and to highlight areas for detailed investigation, as well as to give information on severity and type, and by extension, localization of damage. Comprehensive assessment for treatment should also entail functional communication. This is particularly important for the more severely impaired. Assessments available range from functional communication profiles, everyday language tests, to profiles which take account of discourse, speech acts, and other pragmatic aspects of communication. In addition, there is now a standardized Right Hemisphere Language Battery (Bryan, 1994) for the assessment of impairments of language and communication in right hemisphere-damaged patients.

The cognitive neuropsychology school has had, and is continuing to have, an important impact on developments in aphasia therapy. In recent years there has developed a fundamentally different way of thinking about research into treatment for aphasia, based on the principles of cognitive neuropsychology. The view is that a "theory-driven" approach to the investigation of individual patients is preferable to attempts to compare heterogeneous groups of patients categorized according to the classical syndrome models. It has been recognized by clinicians for some time that no two aphasic individuals present with the same pattern of impaired and preserved abilities at a detailed level of analysis. Many argue that the syndrome approach to research in neuropsychology has outlived its usefulness, and this view has been embraced by many therapists.

One of the main features of cognitive neuropsychology is that it assumes that components of cognition, for instance, language processing, are organized and represented in the brain in a modular fashion. These modules are seen as domain-specific (in the sense that computations performed by a module are specific to that module only), associated with circumscribed neural structures, genetically determined, and computationally autonomous, being independent of other cognitive processes. The model adopts the information processing paradigm as the core framework of the approach for the interpretation of deficits in brain-damaged individuals.

Analysis entails using the boxes and arrows of a processing model to represent the stages and routes involved in such activities as reading single words aloud, writing single words to dictation, and naming objects. A model can be built specifying what is impaired and what is retained by detailed hypothesis-driven assessment of individual patterns of deficit. Through such a process of fractionation, it is suggested, we can gain detailed knowledge of the patient's specific problems in terms of impaired functioning of interconnecting processing routes.

The approach has attractive features for the aphasia therapist as it comes with a promising model of assessment for treatment, and an important feature for the therapist is its emphasis on the individual patient and his or her problems. Its impact on British aphasia therapy has already been significant (Howard & Hatfield, 1987). Howard and Patterson (1988) make a detailed

case for the adoption of the cognitive neuropsychological approach in treatment. For them, three broad strategies for therapy logically flow from cognitive neuropsychological research: (1) re-teaching of the missing information, missing rules or procedures based on a detailed hypothesis testing approach to assessment; (2) teaching a different way to do the same task; (3) facilitating the use of defective access routes. There are promising signs that patient-specific and deficit-specific treatment can improve performance in patients which cannot be accounted for in terms of spontaneous recovery or non-specific effects like attention or novelty (Code & Muller, 1995; Howard & Hatfield, 1987).

Cognitive neuropsychology does not have a model which can cope with the complexity of human language; its realm is cognitive processing of language and it is still limited to single-word processing. For an aphasic individual, and for an aphasia therapist, aphasia is more than a cognitive problem. It is a communication problem and models to deal with these central aspects of therapy are needed. But it contributes to therapy a single-case study approach to research, a detailed investigation of impairments through psycholinguistically controlled tests, and characterization of underlying patterns of deficit in terms of information processing. What is required in addition is a model of therapy for aphasia which allows replication. This entails developing, not only models of cognitive processing and materials for psycholinguistic assessment, but methods which allow replication of patient–therapist interaction (see chapters in Code & Muller, 1992).

RIGHT HEMISPHERE LANGUAGE IMPAIRMENTS

Impairments in language use following right hemisphere damage are less well documented. It is the problems of the left hemisphere-damaged aphasic individual which appear the most severe. The right hemisphere-damaged person often appears relatively normal, in a superficial conversational setting. For this reason, probably, therapy for aphasia has been more developed. The impairments in communication which can arise from right hemisphere damage appear to affect extralinguistic and paralinguistic aspects of language, as well as complex linguistic entities which entail humor appreciation, and metaphor narrative interpretation (Code, 1987). However, there has been little development in therapy for the communication impairments of right hemisphere damaged individuals (Bryan, 1994). Emphasis has been put on the experiential problems of those with right hemisphere damage and the need to treat problems of using contextual information, understanding, inferring and integrating meaning, and difficulties understanding complex linguistic entities like metaphors and jokes. Treatment may also need to consider nonverbal and pragmatic features of communication.

APRAXIA OF SPEECH

Impairments in the initiation, coordination, and programming of speech in the absence of impaired muscle tone – *apraxia of speech* – is common following left frontal damage, often occurring in combination with buccofacial APRAXIA and some of the characteristics of Broca's aphasia. While the patient does not have the problems of DYSARTHRIA, apraxia of speech is seen as a motor speech disorder. Treatment for apraxia of speech usually either aims to compensate when the motor speech problems are very severe, or takes an articulatory drill approach. Compensation methods include gesture and melodic intonation, whereas drilling usually entails a behavioral hierarchy of stages and levels tied to knowledge of articulatory complexity and disintegration.

BIBLIOGRAPHY

Bryan, K. (1994). *The right hemisphere language battery*, 2nd edn. London: Whurr.

Carlomagno, S. (1994). *Pragmatic approaches to aphasia therapy*. London: Whurr.

Chapey, R. (Ed.). (1981). *Language intervention strategies in adult aphasia*. Baltimore, MD: Williams & Wilkins.

Code, C. (1987). *Language, aphasia and the right hemisphere*. Chichester: Wiley.

Code, C. (1994). The role of the right hemisphere in the treatment of aphasia. In R. Chapey (Ed.), *Language intervention strategies in adult aphasia*, 3rd edn (pp. 380–6). Baltimore, MD: Williams & Wilkins.

Code, C., & Muller, D. J. (Eds). (1989). *Aphasia therapy*. London: Whurr.

Code, C., & Muller, D. J. (Eds). (1995). *The treatment of aphasia: From theory to practice*. London: Whurr.

Davis, A., & Wilcox, J. (1985). *Adult aphasia rehabilitation: Applied pragmatics*. Windsor: NFER-Nelson.

Helm-Estabrooks, N., & Albert, M. L. (1991). *Manual of aphasia therapy*. Austin, TX: Pro-Ed.

Howard, D., & Hatfield, F. M. (1987). *Aphasia therapy: Historical and contemporary issues*. London: Erlbaum.

Howard, D., & Patterson, K. (1990). Models for therapy. In X. Seron & G. Deloche (Eds), *Cognitive approaches in neuropsychological rehabilitation* (pp. 39–64). London: Erlbaum.

Lesser, R. (1995). Making psycholinguistic assessments accessible. In C. Code & D. J. Muller (Eds), *The treatment of aphasia: From theory to practice* (pp. 164–72). London: Whurr.

Luria, A. R. (1970). *Traumatic aphasia*. The Hague: Mouton.

Shallice, T. (1979). Case study approach in neuropsychological research. *Journal of Clinical Neuropsychology, 1*, 183–211.

CHRIS CODE

spelling disorders The term "spelling" is ambiguous and may refer to two quite different cognitive processes: those involved in the production of written language or those involved in the letter-by-letter representation of words in the mind. The term *spelling disorders* also conveys this ambiguity. When we think of spelling as referring to the production of written words, then spelling problems encompass many aspects of writing: difficulties in generating ideas, difficulties in programming motor movements, as well as difficulties in remembering spellings of words. In young children who are learning to read and write, spelling problems are often difficult to separate from handwriting problems. On the other hand, when we think of spelling as referring to internal orthographic representations, then spelling problems encompass reading difficulties. The internal representation of words, which in the skilled reader are specified in letter-by-letter order, is equally vital for accurate recognition *and* for accurate spelling production.

SCRIPTS AND WRITING

There are several fundamentally different systems of script, briefly described as ideographic (e.g. Chinese), syllabic (e.g. South Indian languages), and alphabetic (e.g. Western languages). Alphabetic scripts are based on the idea that speech sounds can be segmented into phonemes and that phonemes can be represented by graphemes. Different languages have differently sized sets of phonemes, while the set of graphemes is usually restricted to 26 letters and particular combinations of letters, e.g. ou, ch, th, ai, ee. Japanese has a script which combines aspects of two major script systems and is therefore of great interest to those studying neuropsychological patients with problems in written language. Dissociations have been reported between Kanji (ideographic script) and Kana (syllabic script) such that patients may retain command over one but not both of their script systems.

Most alphabetic scripts also have a component in their orthography which is not based on speech sound. This component is negligible only in those scripts where there have been recent and vigorous spelling reforms promoting the principle of unambiguous sound-letter relationships. English spelling, in particular, has many ambiguous and exceptional words (e.g. fir/fur, gaol/jail, aisle/isle) which do not obey this principle. Thus spelling depends on word-specific as well as alphabetic knowledge.

SPELLING DISORDERS AND OTHER LANGUAGE IMPAIRMENTS

Although it seems intuitively plausible that reading and spelling a word draw on the same internal representation, this assumption is undermined by the fact that reading and spelling disorders can exist as separate problems. Nevertheless, reading and spelling difficulties frequently occur together. Moreover, disorders of written language are often accompanied by impairments in spoken language. This has been known for a long time and is true for acquired as well as for developmental disorders (Joshi & Aaron, 1991). In the following section only specific disorders will be discussed, that is, those which exist either without or over and above more general problems with spoken language.

CHARACTERISTICS OF SPELLING DISORDERS

Spelling disorders in alphabetic scripts, whether acquired or developmental, tend to fall into two very broad categories. Most spelling problems are assumed to originate from a particular type of phonological disorder, given the anchoring of written language in subsyllabic speech sound,

which is the basis of alphabetic scripts. Spelling disorders can, however, exist in the absence of phonological problems. This type of disorder is commonly held to reflect visuospatial or specific memory problems, given that skilled spelling depends to a large extent on word-specific knowledge. Each of two aspects of spelling, the speech-based (phonological) and that based on visual memory for specific letter-sequences (lexical), can serve as a means of compensation if the other is not functioning. This pattern has been documented in single-case studies which provide evidence for a double dissociation of lexical and phonological routes in the processing of written language.

ACQUIRED SPELLING DISORDERS

English orthography has a long and complex history and learning the letter-by-letter representations of words is no mean achievement. The acquisition of extensive spelling knowledge therefore takes many years. Breakdown of such knowledge occurs as a result of particular types of brain injury, and loss of previously automatized spelling skills (AGRAPHIA) is painfully noticeable to sufferers. They may complain of this loss before complaining of more insidious memory or language problems, which they may also experience. English-speaking patients with acquired agraphia have therefore provided a rich testing ground for theories about the cognitive components of reading and spelling. The results of such research are reflected in two excellent review chapters of agraphias by Shallice (1988), and by McCarthy and Warrington (1990). In these reviews the information on published cases with specific spelling disorders following brain insult is systematically compared and discussed. Shallice examines the implications for cognitive process models, while McCarthy and Warrington emphasize the localization in the brain of specific processing components.

In all the cases of agraphia reported by McCarthy and Warrington, areas of varying size in the left parietal lobes are lesioned. This is not the case in disorders of handwriting, as opposed to spelling. Errors in handwriting might look like spelling problems, since they can take the form of neglect, repetition of strokes, and changes in letter orientation and spacing, but they have a different origin, and are associated with right hemisphere posterior lesions. The underlying

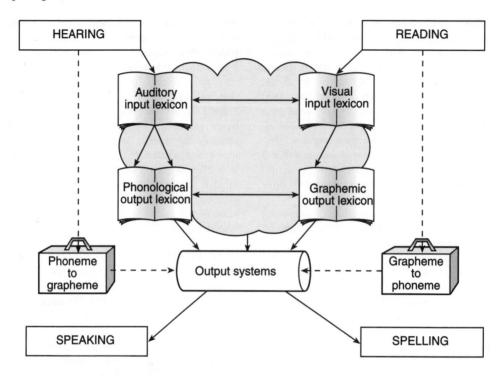

Figure 76 Main features of the Logogen model.

disorder is not related to either language or memory problems but can be considered as a subtype of apraxia.

MODELLING THE SPELLING PROCESS

Morton's (1980) Logogen model successfully unifies diverse data from many different patients with acquired reading and spelling disorders, and furthermore is based on experimental evidence gathered from skilled readers. Its main features are illustrated in Figure 76. Alternative models of the spelling process can be found in a collection of highly readable and informative papers in Brown and Ellis (1994).

In Morton's model the distinction between phonological and lexical systems is made explicit, as is the modality-specific nature of lexical and sublexical components. Bold lines in the figure denote systems commonly used by skilled spellers (and readers), while broken lines indicate the back-up procedures for translating sound to spelling (and vice versa) in the case of novel stimuli. Figure 76 shows that the predominant system serving skilled spelling provides a link

between the representations of words in our spoken vocabulary (phonological output lexicon) and the representations of words in our spelling vocabulary (graphemic output lexicon). A sublexical component is also shown, connecting auditory input with output systems. Use of this sublexical route requires that the target word is first segmented into its constituent phonemes, an appropriate grapheme is assigned to each phoneme, and the resulting information synthesized so that the entire word can be written correctly. As indicated, output systems receive input from both lexical and sublexical routines, and it is at this point that an appropriate representation of the graphemic string is organized, ready for use in handwriting, printing, typing, etc.

Spelling disorders in English can be categorized according to whether they affect one or more of the components illustrated in Figure 76. There is the ability to spell from memory either specific words or parts of words according to their orthographic conventions (lexical processing). There is also the ability to spell novel words by the phoneme-to-grapheme conversion route (sublexical processing), and the ability to realize the spelling of a word in writing or typing or oral spelling (output systems). Dissociations between the ability to spell a word by writing and by saying the letters have in fact been observed, and McCarthy and Warrington refer to these as modality-specific spelling impairments.

Impairment of the graphemic output lexicon in Figure 76 corresponds to lexical agraphia, in Shallice's terminology. This is therefore characterized by errors that follow rule-governed phoneme-to-grapheme conversion and hence a tendency to render irregular words in English as if they were of a simplified phonetic spelling (spelling "yacht" as "yot"). Nevertheless, very common irregular words, even in these patients, are often preserved, suggesting that the orthographic lexicon is not completely destroyed. Patients can sometimes use their semantic knowledge in order to access the spelling of a word (for "time" they might write "clock"), an error reminiscent of those committed by deep dyslexic patients when reading words.

By contrast, phonological agraphia is characterized by very poor nonword spelling and relatively successful word spelling. The standard interpretation of such a disorder is that the sublexical route in Figure 76 is impaired or abolished, while the lexical system is relatively intact. Thus irregular word spellings can often be successfully realized and regularity effects are not apparent. Again, these patients can often master simple nonwords, suggesting that the sublexical system is still functioning to some extent. That high levels of word spelling can be achieved in the absence of routines for assembled spellings is part of the evidence which suggests that a graphemic output lexicon is the primary processing mechanism for skilled adult spellers, with a phonologically based assembled spelling routine serving merely as a back-up system when spellings are unknown, half-remembered, or when stimuli are nonwords.

The dissociations identified by those studying acquired agraphias have enabled the development and clarification of theories of word recognition and spelling. However, "pure" cases of phonological and lexical agraphia are rare, and distinctions between different subtypes of spelling (and reading) disorders are becoming increasingly fragmented. Clearly discernible clinical syndromes may exist, but those patients with either a mixture of symptoms, or with unclassifiable disorders, are likely to continue to challenge our understanding of spelling processes (Ellis, 1987).

DEVELOPMENTAL SPELLING DISORDERS

While evidence from agraphic patients points to a major separation of lexical and phonological spelling processes, in children the two processes are less clearly separated. Phonology, while demonstrably playing a minor part for skilled adult spellers, who can rely on a graphemic output lexicon, is a crucial factor in the acquisition of spelling skills (Treiman, 1993). Frith's (1985) model of reading and spelling acquisition explains the central role of phonology in terms of three strategies, logographic, alphabetic, and orthographic. Because the strategies are contingent on each other, the graphemic lexicon can only be established when a minimum of alphabetic knowledge has been acquired, which in turn enables the orthographic strategy to be developed. Thus intact phonology is critical to the development of both assembled and lexical spelling routines. The logographic strategy is assumed to be available to the pre-reader and to those who fail to acquire alphabetic skills.

Dyslexic children (at least a particular subgroup) are thought to suffer from some subtle and specific brain abnormality which disrupts phonological processing and hence impedes the normal acquisition of a sound-based script system. Lacking alphabetic skills, they find it hard to establish orthographic lexicons sufficiently well specified to support accurate word spelling. Therefore neither lexical nor sublexical routines work very well. Nevertheless dyslexic individuals may develop effective, albeit effortful, compensation strategies, so that some form of lexical spelling is eventually possible. Developmental dyslexics also show phonological problems outside the area of written language, for instance, in word naming and word repetition. Their underlying difficulty is highlighted in reading and spelling problems, particularly with unfamiliar words for which a lexical representation does not exist. Spelling errors in these children are notable for their dysphonetic properties. Consonant clusters (e.g. spl, nt) are often misspelled in reduced form. Repetition of spoken words rich in consonant clusters is similarly problematic.

Developmental dysgraphics exist who read well

but spell badly, although in the majority of cases reading ability imposes an upper limit on spelling ability (Snowling, 1994). Some developmental dysgraphics may be partially compensated dyslexics, others may have a neurological problem specific to spelling, while still others may be poor spellers for strategic rather than neurological reasons. While dyslexic children's phonemic analysis skills are poor (hence the number of dysphonetic features of their errors), dysgraphic children seem to have a problem at the stage of grapheme selection; that is, a phonemic analysis has been performed successfully via the sublexical route (see Figure 76), but difficulties arise when particular (correct) graphemes have to be selected from a pool of phonetically plausible ones. Dysgraphics do not have available sufficiently exact letter-by-letter representations in their graphemic output lexicon and thus detailed specifications are unavailable at the level of output systems. Furthermore, their handicap persists into adulthood. That this problem coexists with good reading skills reflects the fact that English sound-to-spelling rules are even less consistent than spelling-to-sound rules. Good readers who have yet to perfect their spelling skills usually make errors which are phonetically plausible, and which often reflect knowledge of lexical/orthographic constraints (e.g. "nasion" rather than "nashun"). Consonant doubling rules, silent letters, and rendering of schwa-vowels (e.g. sep*a*rate) tend to be particular trouble spots.

The question of whether there are specific subtypes of developmental spelling problems (with correspondingly different underlying difficulties) is still a matter of debate. Spelling error analyses have not always shown qualitative differences between dyslexic and dysgraphic spellers. However, developmental dysgraphics can be very successful with nonword spelling since they are able to produce an appropriate/legal graphemic string which captures the sound structure of English words, while dyslexics generally find this hard. Difficulties with selecting correct graphemic representations for real words may reflect a lexicon containing orthographic representations of insufficient degrees of specificity. The reason for this lack of specificity is unknown. It could be that these individuals have incomplete orthographic representations because they use a less efficient form of "partial cue" reading. Effective orthographic strategies for reading and spelling,

leading to complete orthographic representations, may require relatively dense sampling of text, at least at a critical stage of acquisition.

While it is possible that specific visual problems for analysing and remembering letter-strings play a role in developmental dysgraphia (Goulandris & Snowling, 1991), the prevailing opinion is that phonology is by far the most critical component in the development of alphabetic literacy. Thus phonological problems may manifest themselves either directly as difficulties with a phonological analysis of speech sounds leading to slow learning of alphabetic skills and/or, more indirectly, as a relatively underspecified orthographic lexicon, an impairment which may be apparent only in children's spelling.

THE BIOLOGICAL BASIS OF DEVELOPMENTAL SPELLING DISORDERS

Procedures for mapping developmental disorders onto their neurological substrates are still in their infancy, although there is evidence from twin studies that underlying phonological deficits, as assessed by nonword spelling tests, have an important genetic component (DeFries et al., 1991). It has been suggested that the cerebral hemispheres of developmental dyslexics fail to demonstrate the asymmetry typical of the human brain (Galaburda et al., 1989); more precisely, exhibiting symmetry where asymmetry would be anticipated (a larger left temporal language region). Detailed studies of acquired agraphias have considerably advanced our understanding of localization of spelling components and there is every likelihood that similar advances will be made in our understanding of developmental spelling disorders.

BIBLIOGRAPHY

Brown, G. D. A., & Ellis, N. C. (Eds). (1994). *Handbook of spelling: Theory, process and intervention*. New York: Wiley.

DeFries, J. C., Stevenson, J., Gillis, J. J., & Wadsworth, S. J. (1991). Genetic aetiology of spelling deficits in the Colorado and London twin studies of reading disability. *Reading and Writing, 3,* 83–95.

Ellis, A. W. (1987). Intimations of modularity, or, the modelarity of mind: doing cognitive neuropsychology without syndromes. In M. Coltheart, G. Sartori, & R. Job (Eds), *The cognitive neuropsychology of language* (pp. 397–497). London: Erlbaum.

Frith, U. (1985). Beneath the surface of developmental dyslexia. In K. Patterson, J. Marshall, & M. Coltheart (Eds), *Surface dyslexia: Neuropsychological and cognitive studies of phonological reading* (pp. 301–30). London: Erlbaum.

Galaburda, A. M., Rosen, G. D., & Sherman, G. F. (1989). The neural origin of developmental dyslexia: implications for medicine, neurology and cognition. In A. M. Galaburda (Ed.), *From reading to neurons* (pp. 377–88). Cambridge, MA: MIT Press.

Goulandris, N., & Snowling, M. J. (1991). Visual memory deficits: a possible cause of developmental dyslexia? *Cognitive Neuropsychology, 8*, 127–54.

Joshi, R. M., & Aaron, P. G. (1991). Developmental reading and spelling disabilities: are these dissociable? In R. M. Joshi (Ed.), *Written language disorders* (pp. 1–24). Dordrecht: Kluwer.

McCarthy, R. A., & Warrington, E. K. (1990). *Cognitive neuropsychology: A clinical introduction*. London: Academic Press.

Morton, J. (1980). The logogen model and orthographic structure. In U. Frith (Ed.), *Cognitive processes in spelling* (pp. 117–34). London: Academic Press.

Shallice, T. (1988). *From neuropsychology to mental structure*. Cambridge: Cambridge University Press.

Snowling, M. J. (1994). Towards a model of spelling acquisition: the development of some component skills. In G. D. A. Brown & N. C. Ellis (Eds), *Handbook of spelling: Theory, process and intervention* (pp. 111–28). New York: Wiley.

Treiman, R. (1993). *Beginning to spell*. Oxford: Oxford University Press.

UTA FRITH AND ALISON GALLAGHER

sphincter control Disturbance of the control of the sphincters, which may result in either retention or incontinence of either urine or feces, is common in neurological disease, and may be a significant nursing concern in a patient who is unconscious or in a VEGETATIVE STATE. Problems of sphincter control may be associated with paraplegia by lesions which affect the operation of spinal neurons, but may also result from higher lesions which affect the perception of the state of the bladder, bowel, or condition of the sphincters, or which affect the central control of the voluntary sphincters.

splenium More properly the *splenium of the corpus callosum*, the splenium is the posterior portion of the CORPUS CALLOSUM, comprising roughly a third of its extent, and being rather thicker than the more anterior portions. The splenium interconnects the right and left cortices of the occipital lobes, and its function is therefore primarily concerned with the integration of vision in the left and right visual half-fields.

After section of the splenium in the COMMISSUROTOMY operation, visual motor coordination may be affected and there may be a deficit in visual learning, although these effects have been more clearly demonstrated in the monkey than in humans. However, visual spatial AGNOSIAS may result from interference with splenial fibers. Alexia without agraphia (*see* AGRAPHIA, DYSLEXIA), or pure word blindness in which the patient is unable to read, although both speech and writing may be normal, is also associated with lesions of the occipital lobe and the splenium, presumably as the lesion disconnects the visual perceptual mechanisms of reading from other normally functioning language systems.

It is incidentally remarkable that no clinical condition, including section of the splenium, produces a dislocation of the two visual half-fields in humans, although this may be a consequence of visual integrity being maintained by more basic, lower-level brain mechanisms.

split brain   *See* COMMISSUROTOMY.

status epilepticus Status epilepticus is a form of EPILEPSY in which recurrent convulsive episodes occur without any intervening recovery of consciousness. This is a life-threatening condition and demands emergency intervention. Certain epileptic patients appear particularly prone to develop status epilepticus, and the condition may also be precipitated by abrupt withdrawal of barbiturate medication or, to a lesser degree, other anticonvulsant medications.

stenosis Stenosis refers to the pathological narrowing of any vessel, so that its normal function is affected. It may commonly be applied to partial blocking of the ventricular system, usually in the aqueduct, or to the main arterial blood supply to the brain, as in carotid stenosis, due to the accumulation of material on the walls of the carotid artery.

stereognosia Stereognosia is one of the forms of tactile agnosia (*see* TACTILE PERCEPTION DISORDERS), and is the inability to identify the category to which a stimulus belongs from tactile information alone. It is therefore considered a secondary disorder of touch, in distinction from the primary disorders of MORPHAGNOSIA and HYLOAGNOSIA.

stereopsis *See* VISUOSPATIAL DISORDERS.

stereotypy The repeated use of a small number of words or brief phrases over and over again (verbal stereotypes) is termed stereotypy. It is common in the speech of dementing patients, particularly those with PICK'S DISEASE, and those with subcortical DEMENTIA. It is normally accompanied by other aphasic disturbances.

striate cortex The striate cortex is known by a variety of names. "Striate" derives from a gross anatomical feature, which was identified by Gennari in 1776 (see Glickstein, 1988). This feature is a white band, composed of myelin, within the middle layers of the cortical gray matter itself. The termination of this band coincides well with the transition from striate cortex to neighboring areas of the cortex. The transition is also marked by a change in the density of cortical blood vessels, which are so obviously more numerous in striate cortex that the difference in coloration can be seen with the naked eye. Other names for the striate cortex are: the *primary visual cortex* (which implies a functional priority for this area, primarily because it receives the vast majority of the input from the lateral geniculate nucleus), *area 17* (which derives from the classification of the cortex by Brodmann on the basis of differences in the distribution of neurons visualized by Nissl staining and light microscopy), and most recently *cortical area V1* (a term which is shorthand for

Visual 1 and derives from the identification of a multiplicity of neighboring cortical areas all concerned with visual processing, the other members of which comprise the extrastriate visual areas). The striate cortex is located on the OCCIPITAL LOBES of the cerebral hemispheres. In humans it mostly occupies a position on the medial surfaces of the hemispheres within the calcarine fissure and on its borders, but a smaller area that receives input from the retinal FOVEAE is exposed on the extreme posterior part of the occipital pole.

The identification of striate cortex as preeminently visual in function came much later than its anatomical determination. Munk in 1892 correctly proposed a visual function of the occipital lobes on the basis of an experimental study of lesions in primates. The clinching evidence was the demonstration that the visual scene is systematically mapped onto the striate cortex. This conclusion was the culmination of almost half a century of observation by clinical neurologists. Notably, Inouye (Japan), and Holmes and Lister (UK) examined the consequences of relatively restricted lesions of the occipital lobes caused by gunshot wounds to soldiers in the Russo-Japanese war (1904–5) and in World War 1 (1914–18). They were able to demonstrate a systematic relationship between the exact site of the lesion and the position and spatial extent of a part of the visual field in which the patients exhibited the symptoms of CORTICAL BLINDNESS. This work established that the visual scene maps onto the cortex in a non-uniform way because much more of the striate cortex is devoted to the central (foveal) region of the visual field. It also established the topographical order of the projection, so that, for example, the upper visual field projects to the inferior regions of the striate cortex. The organization of the input from each eye was also revealed. The loss of vision caused by cortical lesions is binocular; a lesion of the right visual cortex gives rise to a loss of vision in the left visual field in both eyes and the vertical meridian that marks the boundary between left and right visual fields is precisely defined.

TOPOGRAPHY

A more accurate map of the central region of the visual cortex was obtained by Talbot and Marshall in the 1940s by recording with silver ball electrodes visually evoked electrical potentials on the exposed cortical surface of anesthetized macaque

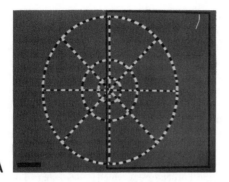 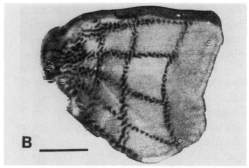

A   B

Figure 77 The visuotopic map of the striate cortex of a primate (rhesus macaque). The visual system was exposed for 30 minutes to a flickered version of the pattern illustrated in the upper part of the figure, while a continuous infusion of radioactively labelled 2-deoxyglucose was made. The radioactively labelled material is taken up by brain cells as if it were glucose, but then cannot be broken down any further by the cells. Thus the 2-deoxyglucose accumulates in cells that are metabolically active. Sections of fixed brain are made after the animal has been killed painlessly with a lethal overdose of anesthetic. These sections of tissue are placed next to photographic plates so that the pattern of high radioactive labelling can be visualized as dark regions of the final image. A sample section is presented in the figure on the right (scale bar = 1 cm).

The pattern of uptake reflects the pattern of visual stimulation. On the surface of the striate cortex, which has been flattened out, the pattern shows that regions serving foveal vision are expanded relative to those serving more eccentric locations. Thus the cortical map is highly non-uniform. The three circumferential lines in the visual pattern transform to the three approximately vertical stripes in the pattern of radioactive labelling. The vertical meridian of the visual field is transformed into a long arc beginning in the upper region of the visual cortex, moving round to the left of the illustration and then to the lower region. The other radial lines in the visual field are also radial on the cortex and converge to the position occupied by the foveal projection at the left of the picture, which was provided by Dr Roger Tootell (Harvard) and is reproduced with the permission of the American Association for the Advancement of Science.

monkeys. More recent techniques have used a microelectrode (active tip sizes of 5–30 μm), which is moved systematically through the cortex in small steps and from which the electrical activity of single nerve cells can be recorded. Each nerve cell is excited by light only if it is presented in a highly localized region of the visual field, which is termed the receptive field for the neuron. As the electrode moves across the cortex, the shifts in spatial position of the visual receptive fields can be established. Near the foveal representation, the receptive fields are small and there is only a relatively small shift in visual field location for a given shift in position across the cortex. Away from the FOVEA, the receptive fields become steadily larger and the shift in visual field location for the same-sized shift in cortical position is correspondingly larger.

These changes can be summarized by expressing them as a cortical magnification factor, which is a ratio:

mm distance across the cortical surface:
shift in visual field position expressed in
degrees of visual angle

The cortical magnification factor, when it is estimated by these techniques, changes from 12–18 mm/degree in the foveal region to c.1.6mm/degree at an eccentricity of 8 degrees in the periphery and continues to decline. (These values are for the macaque monkey, whose basic spatial visual performance in terms of acuity, contrast sensitivity, and anatomical density of retinal cone photoreceptors is very close to that of humans – exact human values are hard to obtain but could be about 2–3 times these values (Horton & Hedley-Whyte, 1984).) Another method for estimating the cortical magnification factor is illustrated in Figure 77, which shows clearly the distortions of visual field locations that are induced by having a cortical magnification factor that varies with spatial position in the visual field. The distortions are clearly irrelevant in one sense for perceptual processing (since there is no internal observer, or homunculus, to look at the distorted cortical visual map), but they do reflect the distribution of cortical resources devoted to each portion of the visual field. In fact, the changes in cortical magnification factor are almost completely accounted for by changes in the density of innervation from the retina and lateral geniculate nucleus. Thus equal cortical areas are devoted to approximately equal numbers of inputs from the earlier stages of visual processing. Any deviations from this principle will certainly be of great interest, but are very hard to establish securely.

One phenomenon of neuropsychological concern that can be interpreted in the light of these results is the visual appearance of the fortification illusions often suffered in migraine. These appear as radial or spiral patterns, which are fixed in retinotopic coordinates and are composed of repeating elements of similar shape, but whose size increases with eccentricity from the fovea. Although the patterns are visually complicated, it has been shown that they probably correspond to rather simple linear waves of excitation on the cortex. The complexity is largely a consequence of the projection of cortical coordinates back into the visual world (Richards, 1971). Similar patterns have been reported after the use of hallucinogenic drugs.

FUNCTIONAL PROPERTIES OF STRIATE NEURONS

The most striking aspect of the neurophysiology of the striate cortex in the higher mammals is the great diversity of receptive field types that is encountered. The pioneering work of Hubel and Wiesel established the properties of orientation selectivity (most cortical cells respond best to elongated contours whose orientation must be within a limited range), binocularity (many cortical cells receive input from both left and right eyes), and direction selectivity (some cells respond only to contours moving at certain speeds in a particular direction). Subsequent work has added stereoscopic depth, color (in primates), and spatial frequency to the list. This diversity is much

greater than that seen at earlier stages in the visual pathway and the more limited results from extrastriate visual areas suggest a trend towards some degree of specialization of receptive field types in each of those areas. Thus striate cortex is in many respects unique.

These experimental studies suggest that striate cortex processes elementary tokens of visual information over a limited spatial extent. There are also results from focal electrical stimulation of human striate cortex (carried out during neurosurgical procedures), which indicate that stimulation causes humans to perceive isolated contours, movements, and visual "phosphenes," but not perceptually organized forms or complete objects or visual scenes.

Hubel and Wiesel divided the orientation selective cells of the striate cortex into two types: simple and complex. Simple cells have spatially discrete *on* and *off* regions of their receptive fields that summate in a predictable fashion, whereas complex cells do not. Within *on* regions increases in firing rate are obtained by applying a stimulus that is brighter than the background illumination, while in *off* regions increases in firing rate can be obtained by applying a stimulus that is darker than the background. Simple cells were so called because mapping these *on* and *off* regions of the receptive field with one type of stimulus, such as a thin bar, allows a reasonably accurate prediction of the cell's response to other stimuli, such as a luminance contrast edge. Complex cells tend to show both *on* and *off* responses at multiple positions within their receptive fields and their responses are not straightforwardly predictable on the basis of a receptive field map.

FUNCTIONAL ARCHITECTURE OF THE STRIATE CORTEX

The basic pattern for the connections of the striate cortex is a modified version of the general pattern for neocortical connectivity. The neocortex is a 6-layered structure about 2 mm in depth from layer 1 at the pial surface to the bottom of layer 6, which overlies the white matter. The major input from the lateral GENICULATE BODY arrives via the optic radiation to layer 4 in the middle of the cortical lamination. There are weaker inputs to layer 6 and to the upper cortical layers (2 and 3). The significant outputs are from layers 2 and 3 (to other cortical areas, notably the extrastriate visual areas), from layer 5 (to the superior COLLICULUS) and from layer 6 (which projects back to the lateral geniculate body). A great deal is now known about these extrinsic connections and the extensive and systematic patterns of intrinsic connections (Lund, 1988).

Within the striate cortex, many of the functional properties of neurons are systematically organized. Again, the early work of Hubel and Wiesel was critical in recognizing this. They adopted the idea of columnar organization of cortical modules to summarize the important features. Particularly in layer 4 of the cortex, there is a systematic pattern of stripes, which are about 0.5 mm in width and are alternately devoted to input from the left eye and then the right eye. The pattern of stripes is fairly uniform in width across the cortical area, but the stripes curl and swirl in a pattern not unlike that of the dermal ridges of a human finger. Certain expected deviations from this general pattern are readily observed: there are no stripes in the region of the visual field where the input from one retina would correspond to the blind spot in the other retina; there are no stripes in the parts of the striate cortex that represent the far periphery of each visual field, since this is exclusively monocular. The visual angle corresponding to these stripes varies markedly, owing to the magnification factor discussed above, but in the foveal representation each stripe in the cortex corresponds to a distance on the retina that is occupied by the linear dimensions of about 4 or 5 cones.

Neurons in the striate cortex also show a systematic representation of preferred orientation such that the preferred orientation of the receptive fields changes from vertical round the clock to horizontal and then back to vertical, as location on the cortical surface is changed. These changes are most marked in the upper layers (2 and 3), but are apparent throughout the cortex. The distance corresponding to a complete rotation of orientation is about 0.7 mm, but there are many interruptions and therefore incomplete sequences. These observations gave rise to the conjecture that a complete cortical module (hypercolumn) might contain, within a $1 \times 0.7 \, mm^2$ area, all the neuronal machinery for analyzing the input from a small patch of the retina. The neighboring columns serve neighboring patches of retina (with some degree of overlap) so that the retinotopic mapping mentioned above is preserved and the functional organization of receptive field properties is made on a finer scale.

Many of the details remain to be worked out. Current investigations include the exact nature of the correspondence, if any, between the stripes representing each eye and the changes of orientation, the possibility that other receptive field properties (such as color, motion, depth, or spatial frequency) are also mapped in a systematic way onto the striate cortex, and the extent to which outputs to other cortical areas are made selectively from different parts of the hypercolumnar structures. Unfortunately, the columnar structures are just smaller than the present spatial resolution of the newer techniques for mapping brain activity, such as PET (POSITRON EMISSION TOMOGRAPHY).

VISUAL CORRESPONDENCES

The studies of the visual properties of neurons and the realization that these properties are organized anatomically in a columnar fashion have given rise to a large number of experiments to investigate whether there are any perceptual phenomena that can be related to the underlying neural organization. Naturally, such experiments have most closely examined simple stimuli that would correspond in a straightforward way to the visual properties of the neurons. Thus, experiments involving judgments about the orientation of lines, the detection thresholds for patterns that approximate the receptive field structures, and investigations of the binocular properties of vision have been the most popular. Some striking correspondences have been found. More recently, attention has also turned to the possibility that careful measurement of the neurons' properties might provide a basis for making predictions about the outcome of psychophysical experiments.

Perhaps the most interesting example from the current perspective of neuropsychology is that it may be possible to account for the losses of vision in the neuro-ophthalmological condition called amblyopia by appealing to abnormalities in the organization of neurons in the striate cortex (Movshon & Kiorpes, 1990). The relevant evidence has come from a careful analysis of clinical cases, an extensive experimental study of animal models of the condition, and more recently the initiation of longitudinal studies of visual development from infancy through to childhood. Losses of visual performance in amblyopia are by definition not associated clinically with retinal disease or other retinal conditions, but are often associated developmentally with defects of focus or defects of visual alignment of the eyes (strabismus). Sometimes, the two eyes will have markedly different visual acuities, even after optical correction; in other cases, the subjective reports are that details (especially text) are "scrambled" when viewed with one eye. Defects of binocular vision are almost always found. Animal studies strongly suggest that the primary site of disturbance is the cortex rather than earlier stages of vision. The evidence from both animal and clinical studies is that inequalities between the eyes (such as in anisometropia, where both eyes cannot be in focus simultaneously) may so significantly affect the visual experience received by the cortex during a specific CRITICAL PERIOD that its synaptic connections become abnormally distributed.

INFORMATION PROCESSING IN THE STRIATE CORTEX

The general conception of the functional role of striate cortex is pre-eminently that of a stage for the initial processing of visual information and the redistribution of this information to other parts of the visual cortex. Its central nature can be confidently asserted on the basis of the phenomenon of CORTICAL BLINDNESS (see also BLINDSIGHT). The striate cortex is also a major cortical location for the processing of fine-detailed pattern information: in particular, it has been accorded a special role in so-called hyperacuity tasks, in which humans can show acuities for changes in the spatial configuration of stimuli (such as tilt or width judgments) with a resolution better than the distance between neighboring cone photoreceptors. Although this proposal would fit with some of the evidence from studies of amblyopic vision (see above), the idea remains controversial, as there is little evidence that the striate cortical processing actually elaborates the signals necessary for these tasks over and above the processing of the earlier stages in the retina and lateral geniculate nucleus.

The columnar architecture of the striate cortex suggests that the information processing that it carries out must take place on relatively local, discrete patches of the scene. The patches may overlap to cover the visual image in a moderately efficient manner, neither leaving gaps nor duplicating the efforts of the available cortical

resources. The obvious neuropsychological correlate of this fine-grain vision in the striate cortex is the fact that lesions produce SCOTOMA with quite sharply defined boundaries. If each patch of the visual image is analyzed in this fine-grain manner and the patches correspond to the hypercolumns mentioned above (or perhaps more realistically, a hypercolumn and its near neighbors), then there are some obvious limitations in the capabilities of the striate cortex, however powerful we imagine it to be.

If one considers the complete range of tasks that vision needs to serve, for some tasks information needs to be assimilated over wide spatial extents. This may happen with global processing of visual motion information, which needs to be converted into a control signal for an eye movement or other visual guided movement, or it may happen with certain types of spatial judgments (e.g. the edge of a very tall building may be evidently straight and yet extend over a third of the visual field, thus covering scores of hypercolumns and far exceeding the integration zone of a single orientation selective cortical neuron). Perhaps in this regard the extensive pattern of back projections to the striate cortex from extrastriate visual cortical areas may be of importance, as several of these areas are known to have much coarser scale representations of the visual scene, which would permit the integration that is needed.

BIBLIOGRAPHY

Glickstein, M. (1988). The discovery of the visual cortex. *Scientific American* (September), 84–91.

Horton, J. C., & Hedley-Whyte, T. (1984). Mapping of cytochrome oxidase patches and ocular dominance columns in human visual cortex. *Philosophical Transactions of the Royal Society of London B, 304*, 255–72.

Hubel, D. (1988). *Eye, brain and vision.* New York: Scientific American Library.

Lund, J. S. (1988). Anatomical organization of macaque monkey visual cortex. *Annual Review of Neuroscience, 11*, 253–88.

Movshon, J. A., & Kiorpes, L. (1990). The role of experience in visual development. In J. R. Coleman (Ed.), *Development of sensory systems in mammals* (pp. 155–202). New York: Wiley.

Richards, W. (1971). The fortification illusions of migraines. *Scientific American, 224* (May), 88–97.

Tootell, R. B. H., Silverman, M. S., Switkes, E.,

& DeValois, R. L. (1982). Deoxyglucose analysis of retinotopic organization in primate striate cortex. *Science*, *218*, 902–4.

A. J. PARKER

striatum There is potential confusion in the use of this term to refer to a specific structure, and the region surrounding that structure. The *corpus striatum* is the larger region which appears as a distinct subcortical mass anterior to the THALAMUS and below the lateral ventricles, each side of the third ventricle. The posterior end of the corpus striatum passes laterally over the thalamus between it and the lateral ventricles. The corpus striatum is composed of two main structures: the GLOBUS PALLIDUS and the *striatum*. The striatum itself is in turn divided into two main structures by the internal capsule (part of the PYRAMIDAL TRACT), which passes between them: the CAUDATE NUCLEUS and the PUTAMEN. The whole region of the corpus striatum is involved in the extrapyramidal motor system serving involuntary movement. Lesions therefore produce motor automatisms: complex movements which are more elaborate than tremor or twitches, which are outside the patient's volition and control. The clearest example is HUNTINGTON'S DISEASE, in which the pathology is primarily striatal.

stroke A lay term commonly used to describe all varieties of cerebrovascular disease. In general, stroke may be defined as a sudden loss of neurological function due to disruption of the normal vascular supply of the brain. Strokes are associated with increased age, and are the third leading cause of death in North America. In addition, strokes are a major cause of morbidity, and represent the leading cause of focal neuropsychological impairment in adults. Strokes also occur in younger individuals, although the underlying cause tends to be different. The ultimate outcome following stroke is primarily related to the severity of the lesion, but numerous other factors have also been noted to influence the sequelae of stroke, including the patient's age, previous cardiovascular and cerebrovascular disease, etiology, and site of lesion.

CEREBROVASCULAR ANATOMY

The specific nature of neurobehavioral sequelae following strokes is dependent (in large part) upon the specific vessel which becomes compromised. The brain receives its blood supply via two major arterial systems. The anterior circulation originates from the internal carotid artery and bifurcates to give rise to the middle cerebral artery and ANTERIOR CEREBRAL ARTERY. The two anterior cerebral arteries are joined by the anterior communicating artery. The posterior circulation is also referred to as the vertebro-basilar system and is composed of the two vertebral arteries, which merge to form the basilar artery. The vertebro-basilar system is connected with the anterior circulation by the posterior communicating artery, which typically arises from the internal carotid artery. These interconnected vessels constitute a structure at the base of the brain known as the Circle of Willis. Connections between these vessels represent a source of potential collateral vascular supply, which can be important in attenuating the effects of a stroke.

Each of the major cerebral arteries provides the primary blood supply for specific regions of the brain. The nature and severity of neuropsychological deficit in stroke is largely a function of which vascular territory is affected and where in that network blood supply is compromised. Disruption of smaller branches will result in more focal lesions than will abnormalities in the principal arterial trunk. In fact, clinically silent strokes may occur with the smaller branches that supply the basal ganglia, white matter, and parts of the frontal lobe. Strokes that do not produce a hemiplegia (approximately 20–30 percent of strokes) are more likely to be undetected.

The middle cerebral artery supplies approximately 70 percent of the lateral surface of the cerebral hemisphere, the lateral portion of the orbital surface of the frontal lobe, and gives off penetrating branches to the basal ganglia and internal capsule. Strokes in the territory of the middle cerebral artery commonly result in neuropsychological deficit because of the behaviorally important structures which are supplied, including Broca's area, Wernicke's area, pre- and post-central gyri, angular gyrus, and much of the temporal and parietal lobes. The anterior cerebral artery supplies areas in the interhemispheric fissure and supplies the anterior 80 percent of the medial surface of the hemisphere, the corpus callosum, cingulum, and also reaches the most superior portions of the lateral surface of the cerebral hemisphere.

The vertebral arteries enter the skull and give off branches which supply the medulla and parts of the cerebellum. After the two vertebral arteries merge to form the basilar artery, additional branches supply other parts of the cerebellum and pons. The major terminal branch of the basilar artery is the posterior cerebral artery, which supplies the occipital lobe, uncus, and the anterior and inferior surfaces of the temporal lobe.

MECHANISMS OF STROKE

Strokes may be classified into two groups on the basis of the underlying mechanism of disease. Ischemic strokes are caused by the reduction of blood supply and the resulting deprivation of oxygen and glucose. Hemorrhagic strokes are the result of bleeding from a vessel into brain tissue (intracerebral hemorrhage) or at the surface (SUBARACHNOID HEMORRHAGE). Most ischemic strokes are due to ATHEROSCLEROSIS whereas hemorrhagic strokes tend to be caused by ruptured ANEURYSM, ARTERIOVENOUS MALFORMA-TION, or HYPERTENSION. It is not uncommon for both types of stroke to exist in the same patient. For example, in patients with hemor-rhagic stroke the resulting intracerebral hema-toma can act as a space-occupying lesion which can displace adjacent structures (referred to as mass effect). This mass effect can constrict blood flow in nearby and otherwise intact vessels leading to a secondary area of infarction.

The majority (approximately 80 percent) of strokes in adults are caused by THROMBOSIS or embolism and result in ischemic stroke. ISCHEMIA is caused by insufficient blood supply, which deprives the brain of oxygen and glucose and prevents removal of potentially toxic by-products of cerebral metabolism such as lactic acid. Thrombosis and embolism refer to the occlusion of a vessel, but differ in regard to the initial site of pathology. In thrombosis, gradual narrowing and occlusion occurs primarily at the site of actual occlusion. For example, atherosclerotic plaques may develop within an artery and gradually produce complete blockage. In embolic stroke the primary site of pathology is elsewhere in the body, often in the heart, lungs, or extracranial carotid artery. Embolism occurs when portions of a

vascular lesion at some location break off and are carried through the arterial system until they reach a distal part of the arterial system where the vessel becomes occluded. Atherosclerotic plaques tend to occur at points of arterial bifurca-tion (branching). Plaques at the bifurcation of the internal carotid artery (in the neck) are frequent causes of ischemic stroke. Because of the close association between atherosclerosis, thrombosis, and embolism, this type of stroke is sometimes referred to as athero-thrombotic or thrombo-embolic stroke.

Intracerebral or subarachnoid hemorrhage represents the second type of stroke, and tends to be associated with different underlying disease mechanisms. The most common causes of hem-orrhage are hypertension and rupture of vascular abnormalities such as aneurysms or arteriovenous malformations. Hypertension tends to affect the small-caliber penetrating arteries, and thus tends to result in intracerebral hemorrhage. The most commonly damaged areas include the basal gang-lia, thalamus, white matter, pons, and cerebellum. Aneurysms, like atherosclerotic plaques, tend to occur at points of arterial bifurcation and are most often found at the junction of the anterior cerebral and anterior communicating arteries, the junction of the posterior communicating and internal carotid arteries, and at the first intra-Sylvian branch of the middle cerebral artery.

NEUROPSYCHOLOGICAL CHANGES FOLLOWING STROKE

The specific behavioral changes that occur foll-owing stroke depend upon several factors, the most important of which is the particular arterial distribution which is compromised. Disruption of blood supply from a major cerebral artery will produce broad patterns of deficit, whereas dis-ruption of smaller arterial branches will result in more circumscribed behavioral deficits. Patients suffering focal strokes have played an important role in the history of the study of brain–behavior relationships. Many of the classical neurobehavi-oral syndromes were first identified in stroke patients. The patterns of neuropsychological im-pairment associated with abnormalities of the major cerebral arteries are described below.

Strokes in the distribution of the middle cerebral artery Strokes in this distribution cause the most frequent cerebrovascular syndrome, character-ized (in the typical case) by weakness, sensory loss, and homonymous HEMIANOPIA on the side of the body opposite the cerebral hemisphere affected. Because of the organization of the motor and sensory cortex, the arm and face are more severely affected than the leg. In addition, strokes in this territory cause a variety of deficits in higher cognitive function, depending on which hemisphere and which arterial branches are involved. After the acute phase, motor difficulties may be characterized by slowing and clumsiness that appears disproportionate to the level of actual weakness. Higher-order sensory changes, such as a reduced ability to appreciate stimulation of the affected side in conjunction with simultaneous stimulation of the unaffected side, and AS-TEREOGNOSIS are common.

Some strokes in the middle cerebral artery may produce only motor and sensory deficits, and others may produce deficits only in "higher" functions, although most result in both types of symptoms. Strokes in the left hemisphere may lead to a variety of language deficits depending on which arterial branches are involved, and may produce ideational or ideomotor APRAXIA if the parietal lobe is damaged. Right hemisphere strokes (particularly when the parietal lobe is affected) lead to a variety of visuospatial deficits and different types of dyspraxia including constructional or dressing apraxia. Strokes in the right hemisphere are more commonly associated with hemi-inattention syndromes in which patients neglect one side of space (including their own body). Some studies indicate that right hemisphere strokes may produce deficits in the affective components of language which are comparable to the language deficits associated with homologous lesions in the left hemisphere. These disorders are called APROSODIAS and refer to deficits in the ability to express or appreciate the emotional aspects of language.

Strokes in the distribution of the anterior cerebral artery These may result in weakness and sensory loss in a pattern that is different from that caused by middle cerebral artery strokes. The leg is represented in the superior and medial portions of the pre- and post-central gyri, which are supplied by the anterior cerebral artery. Therefore strokes in this distribution will result in motor and sensory changes primarily in the contralateral leg. Perhaps the most neuropsychologically interesting syndrome related to strokes in this vascular territory are those that affect the anterior corpus callosum. This lesion will result in a disconnection syndrome which is referred to as *sympathetic* or *callosal apraxia*. In this syndrome patients may be unable to execute skilled movements with their left hand, although they are able to complete the movements with the right hand.

Strokes in the distribution of the posterior cerebral artery These may result in a homonymous hemianopia because of loss of blood supply to the calcarine cortex. The hemianopia tends to spare central vision (in contrast to the visual loss associated with middle cerebral artery strokes) because the occipital pole is usually supplied by the middle cerebral artery. Strokes in this distribution are also associated with several classical neurobehavioral syndromes. Pure ALEXIA or alexia without agraphia occurs with strokes involving the left posterior cerebral artery, which causes lesions in the left occipital lobe and the splenium of the corpus callosum. Disruptions of blood flow in the branches which supply the medial temporal lobe (including the hippocampus and amygdala) may result in memory deficits.

Strokes in the distribution of the anterior communicating artery These are usually the result of a ruptured aneurysm and may result in a variety of cognitive and emotional sequelae. Some patients will develop a severe anterograde AMNESIA, with relatively less retrograde amnesia. Although the exact mechanism is unclear, the frontal lobe, anterior hypothalamus, and septum, which are supplied by the anterior cerebral artery or its penetrating branches, have been proposed as possible substrates of the memory deficit. Some patients may also exhibit CONFABULATION, which may be due to a combination of frontal lobe "disinhibition" and a memory deficit. Personality changes are also commonly observed with strokes in this vascular territory, and are more common than with aneurysms in other arteries. The personality changes include mood alterations (elevated or, less commonly, depressed), decreased inhibition, or increased irritability and emotional lability. Approximately 40–50 percent of aneurysm patients die within three months following hemorrhage. In those who survive, a severe generalized cognitive deficit is uncommon. In some studies, patients with anterior communicating artery aneurysms have a worse neuropsychological outcome than those with aneurysms elsewhere in the brain.

707

Strokes in the distribution of the basilar artery These often lead to a variety of motor and sensory deficits, cranial nerve palsies, signs of cerebellar dysfunction, or unconsciousness because the primary vascular territory is the brain stem and cerebellum. Occlusion of the basilar artery at the point of origin of the posterior cerebral arteries may produce bilateral lesions that can result in well-recognized neurobehavioral syndromes. Occlusion leading to bilateral occipital cortex lesions may result in a phenomenon called ANTON'S SYNDROME or "cortical blindness," in which the patient fails to recognize that he or she cannot see. Occlusion of the basilar artery at the point of origin of the posterior cerebral arteries may also result in bilateral lesions of the medial temporal lobe structures, resulting in a global amnesia. Temporary disruption of blood supply in this manner is thought to represent the basis for transient amnesia syndromes.

FACTORS WHICH INFLUENCE THE EXPRESSION OF NEUROBEHAVIORAL DEFICIT FOLLOWING STROKE

The primary factors which determine the behavioral deficits in stroke patients include which arterial system is affected and where in that system the disruption occurs. Severe deficits may occur if the main arterial trunk is involved, whereas the occlusions of smaller penetrating branches or the rupture of micro-aneurysms (associated with hypertension) may be clinically silent. There are several other factors which may contribute to the severity and extent of behavioral deficits in stroke patients. One such factor is the availability and viability of collateral blood supply. The Circle of Willis provides a mechanism whereby loss of blood flow in one vessel can be compensated by flow from the other vessels. The Circle of Willis provides potential communication between the anterior and posterior circulations within the hemisphere, as well as between hemispheres. It is not uncommon for the Circle of Willis to be incomplete, and for various anomalous patterns of vasculature to exist (e.g. both anterior cerebral arteries arising from a common trunk). In such cases the normal collateral circulation may not be possible, and the anomalous patterns may result in more severe deficits than would typically be found. Anastomoses between the major vascular territories also occur

and represent another source of collateral blood supply.

The rate and extent of disease progression or development is an important factor, which influences the amount of collateral blood supply that may be available. Most hemorrhagic strokes as well as embolic episodes tend to occur acutely and thus offer no opportunity for the development of collateral flow. In thrombotic stroke the atherosclerotic plaque produces a gradual stenosis or narrowing which may take many years to develop. This slowly progressing occlusive lesion offers the opportunity for intracerebral collateral vessels to develop. These collateral vessels may attenuate the severity of neurobehavioral deficit when the thrombosed artery becomes fully occluded.

As noted above, some intracerebral hemorrhages produce additional neurobehavioral deficits by acting as a space-occupying lesion. In addition to the possible compression of other vessels leading to further ischemic damage, the hemorrhage itself can disrupt normal brain function and create additional deficits. Apart from the "local" effects of hemorrhage, some patients also develop vasospasm in which the cerebral arteries become constricted. This typically affects the major cerebral vessels. This can lead to focal or generalized ischemia, depending on which territories are affected, and can result in additional areas of infarction. In vasospasm the cerebral metabolic rate of oxygen has been shown to be decreased in proportion to the diameter of the constricted vessel, and disproportional to the reduction in cerebral blood flow.

PERMANENCE OF NEURO-PSYCHOLOGICAL DEFICIT FOLLOWING STROKE

Strokes may be classified by a number of criteria, including the underlying mechanism (thrombo-embolic vs hemorrhagic), the vascular territory involved, and severity of damage. In addition, strokes can also be classified in regard to the course and progression of damage. It is estimated that approximately 30 percent of stroke patients may experience a deterioration within the first week of onset which may, in the majority of cases, be due to edema, rebleeding, or recurrent emboli. In contrast to these patients with progressing stroke, many patients experience symptoms that last for only a few hours. Traditionally, patients whose symptoms resolve within 24 hours are classified as having transient cerebral ischemia. The specific neurobehavioral symptoms may refer to any vascular distribution, but are most commonly associated with emboli in the anterior cerebral circulation. Unilateral visual loss (from the ophthalmic artery branch of the internal carotid), language or spatial deficits, and unilateral sensory-motor deficits are the most common symptoms. Recent studies have demonstrated that approximately 50 percent of patients classified as having a transient attack have abnormalities on computed tomography or MAGNETIC RESONANCE scans. Some studies suggest that symptoms which last more than four hours should actually be classified as strokes. In many of these patients the symptoms are completely resolved within 24 to 48 hours. This category of cerebrovascular disease is classified as reversible ischemic neurological deficit.

Effects of surgical intervention on neuropsychological deficit There are a number of surgical treatments that have been developed for occlusive cerebrovascular disease. Carotid endarterectomy involves removal of stenotic lesions at the bifurcation of the carotid artery in the neck. Although stenosis of less than 85 percent does not result in a hemodynamically significant reduction in blood flow, it is theoretically possible that improvement of blood supply in the carotid artery (particularly when the opposite carotid artery is also stenosed or occluded) may result in improved neuropsychological function. Several studies have failed to demonstrate a general neuropsychological improvement, although some studies have identified individual cases of dramatic improvement. Various intracranial to extracranial bypass procedures have been developed to circumvent obstructive lesions that occur within the skull. There have been fewer studies of the neuropsychological impact of these procedures, but again there is no convincing evidence of improved function following these procedures.

BIBLIOGRAPHY

Barnett, H. J. M., Mohr, J. P., Stein, B. M., & Yatsu, F. M. (1986). *Stroke: Pathophysiology, diagnosis, and management.* New York: Churchill Livingstone.

Bornstein, R. A., & Brown, G. (1991). *Neurobehavioral aspects of cerebrovascular disease.* New York: Oxford University Press.

Furlan, A. J. (1987). *The heart and stroke: Exploring mutual cerebrovascular and cardiovascular issues.* New York: Springer-Verlag.

Maurice-Williams, R. S. (1987). *Subarachnoid hemorrhage: Aneurysms and vascular malformations of the central nervous system.* Bristol: John Wright.

Millikan, C. H. (1987). *Stroke.* Philadelphia: Lea & Fibiger.

Reivich, M., & Hurtig, H. I. (1983). *Cerebral vascular diseases.* New York: Raven.

Sundt, T. F. (1987). *Occlusive cerebrovascular disease: diagnosis and surgical management.* Philadelphia: Saunders.

Toole, J. F. (1990). *Cerebrovascular disorders*, 4th edn. New York: Raven.

R. A. BORNSTEIN

stuttering Stuttering is the repetition of parts of a word, especially the initial consonant, in the effort to articulate. It is closely related to and is often confused with *stammering*, in which a similar dysfluency occurs in the form of either hesitations or syllable repetitions within words. In both the pauses are referred to as *tonus*, and the repetitions *clonus*. Neuropsychologically, the two may be considered together. Both are strongly associated with other developmental language disorders and delays, and with other soft neurological signs; as with many of these related phenomena, both are three to four times more common in boys than in girls. It has been claimed that left-handedness (*see* HANDEDNESS) is more common among stutterers, but this is not supported by the available evidence.

There is a hypothesis that stuttering results from an abnormal pattern of LATERALIZATION, which may in turn be the result of some maturational delay, which leads to a failure to resolve the left and right hemisphere competition for motor control of speech. Some initial evidence which showed an abnormally high degree of left ear dominance in a DICHOTIC LISTENING task seems not to have been supported by later work. However, administration of INTRACAROTID SODIUM AMYTAL in the Wada test has revealed bilateral speech representation in a number of stutterers, the condition also being relieved by the amytal depression of one of the hemispheres. Subsequent temporal lobectomy also incidentally relieved the stuttering. Again, however, there have been failures to replicate this finding, but there is at least partial support for the evidence linking stuttering with abnormal lateralization for speech.

subarachnoid hemorrhage Subarachnoid hemorrhage (SAH) is caused by bleeding into the subarachnoid space and is commonly the result of the rupture of a cerebral arterial saccular ANEURYSM. Other less common causes of SAH are ARTERIOVENOUS MALFORMATIONS (AVM). Finally, over 20 percent of SAH has no proven etiology.

Prior to rupture, if size remains moderate (giant aneurysms may occur) and if no compression on CRANIAL NERVES occurs, saccular aneurysms are usually asymptomatic. Aneurysmal bleeding may follow trauma or physical exertion (including coitus). However, a third of SAH occurs in sleep and many others during normal daily activities.

Massive bleeding produces a sudden explosive headache, with the patient falling unconscious almost immediately. These cases have, in general, a very poor prognosis. Loss of consciousness rarely occurs without preceding headache, and again it implies a grave prognosis. In many other cases, the sudden excruciating headache is not accompanied by loss of consciousness. The patient remains alert, often confused and agitated. Other clinical signs and symptoms are nausea and vomiting, neck stiffness, and fever. Neurological signs are not constant. When present, they may point to the site of bleeding.

LABORATORY FINDINGS

Patients with symptoms consistent with SAH should undergo a noncontrast CT or MRI scan. If the scan is obtained within the first 48 hours of aneurysmal rupture, it should show, in approximately 80 percent of the cases, a subarachnoid clot in the basal cistern. AVM and mycotic aneurysms usually present with subarachnoid blood located over the hemisphere. If the CT or MRI scans are negative for subarachnoid blood, then a LUMBAR PUNCTURE should be done.

If either the CT/MRI or the lumbar puncture is positive for SAH, an angiogram should be obtained. The goal of ANGIOGRAPHY is to identify the cause and location of the hemorrhage. Approximately 40 percent of aneurysms arise from the internal carotid artery (ICA), 35 percent from the ANTERIOR CEREBRAL ARTERY (ACA), 20 percent

from the middle cerebral artery (MCA), and 5 percent from the posterior cerebral artery (PCA) or the vertebro-basilar artery (VB). However, a normal angiogram may also be seen in patients with SAH, because occasionally intense spasms can prevent filling of an intracranial aneurysm.

COURSE, PROGNOSIS, AND THERAPY

The major complications of SAH are the tendency for the hemorrhage to recur, cerebral vasospasm, and HYDROCEPHALUS. The peak time for rebleeding and cerebral vasospasm occurs within the first two weeks after the initial bleed.

Data in the literature suggest that when an intracranial aneurysm is identified, surgical clipping should be undertaken as soon as possible in order to avoid the peak times for rebleeding and vasospasm. The incidence of neuropsychological deficits associated with early or late surgery is discussed in the next section. The use of antifibrinolitic agents may decrease mortality from rebleeding, but it also increases thrombotic side effects. When vasospasm occurs, blood volume expansion with plasma is recommended. Recent studies have suggested that calcium antagonists such as Nimodipine may be useful in the prophylaxis and treatment of this condition. Communicating hydrocephalus usually occurs within one to three weeks after hemorrhage; it is often transient and it does not require surgical intervention. If significant neurological deterioration occurs, a shunt may be indicated.

Of those who survive SAH and its complications, more than half are left with neurological, cognitive, and psychiatric sequelae. Generally speaking, the greater the neurological impairment, the higher the cognitive and/or psychiatric disturbances. Furthermore, despite a satisfactory neurological recovery, some SAH patients may show personality changes and cognitive dysfunction that interfere with REHABILITATION and social reintegration.

FACTORS INFLUENCING COGNITIVE DISORDERS

Although a few studies have suggested increased age as a factor negatively influencing neuropsychological outcome, some data in the literature do not confirm this finding. An earlier view was that late surgery was associated with a better neuropsychological prognosis. However, some studies have suggested that the timing of the operation makes no difference to central cognitive functioning. Recent data, though, have suggested that delayed surgery is associated with a worse neuropsychological prognosis, indicating that it is more appropriate to speak of a late surgery disadvantage rather than an early surgery advantage. This disadvantage does not seem to be due to pertinent variables such as vasospasm, suggesting that it may be attributed to "toxic" factors that act diffusely on the cerebral cortex, without producing focal injuries to the brain.

This view is supported by a study made by Sonesson and others (1989), which demonstrates that there are no significant differences in mean test scores involving memory functions, spatial perceptual organization, visuoconstructive abilities, reasoning, perceptual speed and accuracy, and concept formation between SAH patients without any identifiable source of the bleeding and aneurysmal SAH patients. They suggest that, although the final prognosis of patients with SAH of unknown origin is essentially favorable compared to that of aneurysmal SAH, the presence of blood per se anywhere in the subarachnoid space may affect higher brain functions.

Some authors suggest that there is a clear pattern of general agreement between neurological and neuropsychological outcomes, whereas others claim that, when the neuropsychological evaluation is integrated in the final outcome assessment, only a minority of all patients classified as having a "good neurological outcome" may be regarded as having a favorable neuropsychological outcome. On the contrary, a provocative study from McKenna and others (1989) showed that, when SAH patients with a good neurological outcome are compared to myocardial infarction patients without a history of cerebrovascular disease, there is no difference in cognition between the two groups, indirectly suggesting that SAH does not, per se, lead to long-term cognitive changes.

Early CT scan studies suggested a relationship between disturbances of cognition after aneurysmal SAH and the severity of aneurysmal bleed, but more recent MRI scan data do not confirm the finding. Other neuroradiological findings have suggested that the pattern of cognitive deficits may be strongly related to infarctions and brain atrophy revealed by CT scans. Patients with left lateral infarctions should have deficits on performance requiring verbal efficiency, whereas patients with right cerebral infarctions should disclose deficits on visuoconstructional tasks. These deficits should be more pronounced if lateral infarctions are associated with diffuse brain damage. The patients without infarction should not differ from the control group. These data seem to suggest the major role of vasospasm in the neuropsychological outcome of SAH patients. Unfortunately, the role of vasospasm as a factor determining cognitive disorders after SAH has not been confirmed in a number of neuropsychological studies.

Regarding the location of aneurysms, some data have suggested that there are no obvious relationships between the type of cognitive dysfunction and aneurysm location, whereas others have indicated that anterior communicating artery (ACoA) aneurysms are associated with a poorer neuropsychological outcome.

NEUROPSYCHOLOGICAL DEFICITS

Cognitive disorders and aneurysm location

A wide variety of intellectual, emotional, and behavioral deficits are reported among survivors of SAH. Patients who have suffered from SAH frequently show verbal and spatial learning and memory dysfunctions, disturbed spatial organization, and visuoconstructive impairment. Furthermore, deficits in higher mental processes, such as abstract analytic thinking and concept formation, could be discerned in these patients, frequently associated with fluctuations in ATTENTION, lack of mental flexibility, and impairment of the ability to shift between simultaneously operating abstract principles. A deficit in short-term memory for verbal and nonverbal material has been described in about a third of the patients who have suffered from an aneurysmal SAH. Finally, a general slowdown in perceptual speed and/or accuracy is frequent.

It seems that the study of patients who have suffered from SAH, as a group, is likely to be relatively uninformative with regard to the neuroanatomical localization of normal cognitive function. In fact, a number of group studies found no correlation between the location of bleeding and the cognitive disorders shown by the patients. This seems to be due to the coexistence of different factors that may affect cognition in SAH patients, such as the toxic effect of the blood, vasospasm, and so on; alternatively, it may be the result of diffuse cerebral damage rather than any specific characteristics of either the aneurysm itself or the subsequent surgical treatment.

Memory dysfunctions are the most common cognitive deficits after SAH. Detailed neuropsychological studies have shown both short- and long-term memory disorders, mainly for verbal material, in these patients, regardless of the location of the bleeding. These findings therefore seem to contradict the impression derived from case studies that memory dysfunction following SAH is specifically associated with aneurysms of ACoA. In this regard, memory disturbances have also been described after rupture of MCA, VB, or PCA aneurysms. If a general rule might be extracted from a survey of the more recent literature, it would be that the principal residual deficit produced by SAH, regardless of the location of the bleeding, lies in the efficiency of word retrieval.

Nevertheless, it is useful for clinical purposes to divide neuropsychological disorders after SAH on the basis of the location of the aneurysm.

ACoA and ACA aneurysms

In almost all patients, lethargy and agitation are prominent postoperatively. The next stage is frequently dominated by CONFABULATION, confusion, or denial of illness, but it is usually transient, clearing in a few weeks. Later some patients may show behavioral disturbances, including changes in affect and emotion, social judgment, ability to plan, and memory. Personality changes include apathy, fatuousness, socially inappropriate behavior, and unpredictable aggression. These changes depend on a variety of factors, most notably the location of the bleeding, the extent of vasospasm, the presence of a developing hydrocephalus, and the type of surgical repair. These changes are generally interpreted as a manifestation of frontal lobe damage.

In some patients, the memory disturbance is the most salient defect and it is similar in some aspects to that shown by alcoholic Korsakoff patients. ACoA aneurysm AMNESIA is characterized by severely impaired free recall of verbal and visuospatial material, by normal recognition of visual and verbal material, by improvement of the performance with semantic cueing, and by a high susceptibility to proactive interference. In fact, the recall protocols of patients with ACoA contain an abnormal number of intrusions from previously presented material, as well as other signs of sensitivity to interference effects. In general, these patients show difficulties in so-called "contextual chunking," such as a profound impairment in the Brown–Peterson task, sensitivity to interference, and performance at a chance level on temporal discrimination, and they display a release from proactive interference when the dimensional shift is at a semantic level.

Retrograde amnesia is often less important. Only a few earlier studies described SAH patients with retrograde amnesia that extended to several years prior to hemorrhage. In most of the other reports, however, remote memory appears to be intact in patients with ACoA. This finding differs from that in other amnesic diseases, like KORSAKOFF SYNDROME, HUNTINGTON'S DISEASE, herpes ENCEPHALITIS, and Alzheimer's disease. A percentage (about 25 percent) of patients have a defective verbal memory span. Patients with ACoA aneurysm ruptures generally have poorer performance on verbal fluency tasks when the cue is phonological rather than when the cue is semantic. The phonological task probably requires a large deployment of attentional resources, which are defective in ACoA patients because of frontal lobe dysfunction.

Damasio and colleagues (1985) have proposed that amnesic patients with ruptured ACoA aneurysms are able to learn separate modal stimuli, as well as other associated features, but they fail in the computation of the relationship and co-occurrence of stimuli, or perhaps in the storage or evocation of such a computation. In addition, a predominant retrieval deficit is suggested from the fact that cueing strongly benefits recall and recognition of both anterograde and retrograde memories, and that recognition in these patients is normal or near normal.

In summary, all the deficits observed in these patients seem to have to do with contextual material only. The availability of contextual memories depends on the recording of separate stimuli that compose a perceived episode, the computation and recording of relationships between the multiple components, and some form of time-tagging of those records. This failure may also account for the type of confabulation of ACoA patients. In fact, among the two main generally recognized types of confabulation, namely (a) fantastic or spontaneous (fabrication of false memories) and (b) momentary or provoked (actual or real memories displaced in a temporal context), these patients often display the latter.

The anatomic correlate of the disturbance seems to be damage to the basal forebrain region (BFR), a complex area that includes the septal nuclei, substantia innominata, and related white matter connections. The BFR is interconnected with the amygdala via the ventro-amygdalo-fugal pathway and is interconnected with the hippocampus via the fornix.

Evidence from functional neuroimaging indicates that damage in the BFR is associated with diminished activity in medial temporal regions, suggesting that amnesia in ACoA patients may result from interference in the hippocampal formation, amygdala, and parahippocampal gyrus. The partially impaired hippocampal formation would permit the establishment and retrieval of modal memories but would be incompatible with the determination of relationships between stimuli and temporal marking.

ACoA patients, despite being severely amnesic, are able to learn a complex cognitive rule, such as a seven-step algorithm for mentally squaring two-digit numbers (Milberg et al., 1988). This learning occurs despite the patient's inability to accurately describe the steps of the algorithm. It is interesting to underline that both patients described by Milberg and colleagues needed cues (both explicit and implicit) to complete the squaring task. It might be that improvement in the overall performance of the mental algorithm by means of cues is dependent on the impaired capacity to spontaneously initiate its component steps by the patients. This finding may also support the hypothesis of Damasio (1985) on the core of the functional disorder of amnesia in ACoA patients, which is that a derangement of contextual memory may cause, during the learning of a mental algorithm, a disturbance of the recording of the relationships between several functional steps.

Other speculations about the site of damage responsible for the memory disorders following ACoA hemorrhage or surgery have focused on damage to the medial forebrain bundle (MFB), the paraventricular nucleus (PV) of the hypothalamus, and the septum. MFB is a dopaminergic pathway which runs through the lateral hypothalamus, carrying bidirectional pathways from medial frontal regions to the hypothalamus and midbrain. This pathway has been considered important in cerebral arousal. PV produces vasopressin, which may have a role in memory. Some of the patients with a rupture of aneurysmal ACoA have transient or permanent diabetes insipidus. Damage to the septum may impair the cholinergic system in the ventral forebrain, with widespread cortical projections.

ACoA patients also show an impairment, ranging from mild to severe, on intelligence tests. In addition, ACoA patients have shown deficits in constructional and visuoperceptual tasks, generally sensitive to damage in posterior regions of the brain. The source of these deficits may be due to the attentional loading, related to the FRONTAL LOBE involvement, rather than to the spatial loading of the task.

Finally, callosal syndromes following hemorrhage from ACoA aneurysms, with unilateral tactile ANOMIA and dyspraxia, difficulty in interhemispheric transfer, and covert competition between the left and right extremities, have also been reported.

MCA and posterior cerebral artery (PCA) aneurysms

MCA and PCA or PCoA aneurysm patients show a considerable incidence of neuropsychological disorders. In general, their pattern agrees with the competence of the left and right cerebral hemispheres, namely left MCA and PCA or PCoA patients show difficulty on verbal tasks, such as naming, verbal fluency, and verbal short-term memory, whereas right MCA and PCA or PCoA patients evidence deficits in visuoperceptual abilities, such as discrimination of line orientation, and short-term and long-term visuospatial memory.

Young and others (1990) have described the case of a prosopagnosic patient who suffered SAH from a right MCA which caused a right temporal intracerebral hematoma. The patient showed deficits on face processing tasks, such as identification of familiar faces, unfamiliar face matching, and perception of facial expression. Severe disorders were evident on all FACIAL RECOGNITION tasks. In face-name learning tasks, there was evidence of covert recognition of faces that the patient did not recognize overtly.

Despite an adequate insight into other neurological and neuropsychological deficits produced by her illness, including HEMIPLEGIA, HEMIANOPIA, and poor memory, the patient did not think that she had any problems in facial recognition. Young and colleagues suggest that the lack of insight of the patient into her face recognition disorders involved a deficit-specific ANOSAGNOSIA, resulting from a deficit in domain-specific monitoring skills.

BIBLIOGRAPHY

Alexander, M. P., & Freedman, M. (1984). Amnesia after anterior communicating artery aneurysm rupture. *Neurology*, *34*, 752–7.

Barbarotto, R., De Santis, A., Laiacona, M., Basso, A., Spagnoli, D., & Capitani, E. (1989). Neuropsychological follow-up of patients operated for aneurysms of the middle cerebral artery and posterior communicating artery. *Cortex*, *25*, 275–88.

Brown, G. G., Spicer, K. B., & Malik, G. (1991). Neurobehavioral correlates of arteriovenous malformations and cerebral aneurysms. In R. A. Bornstein & G. Brown (Eds), *Neurobehavioral aspects of cerebrovascular disease* (pp. 202–23. New York: Oxford University Press.

Damasio, A. R., Graff-Radford, N. R., Eslinger, P. J., Damasio, H., & Kassell, N. (1985). Amnesia following basal forebrain lesions. *Archives of Neurology*, *42*, 263–71.

McKenna, P., Willison, J. R., Lowe, D., & Neil-Dwyer, G. (1989). Cognitive outcome and quality of life one year after subarachnoid haemorrhage. *Neurosurgery*, *24*, 361–7.

Milberg, W., Alexander, M. P., Charness, N., McGlinchey-Berroth, R., & Barrett, A. (1988). Learning of a complex arithmetic skill in amnesia: evidence for a dissociation between compilation and production. *Brain and Cognition*, *8*, 91–104.

Mohr, J. P., Kistler, J. P., Zabramski, J. M., Spetzler, R. F., & Barnett, H. J. M. (1986). Intracranial aneurysms. In H. J. M. Barnett, J. P. Mohr, B. M. Stein, & F. M. Yatsu (Eds), *Stroke: Pathophysiology, diagnosis, and management*, Vol. 2, (pp. 643–77). New York: Churchill Livingstone.

Richardson, J. T. E. (1989). Performance in free recall following rupture and repair of intracranial aneurysm. *Brain and Cognition*, *9*, 210–26.

Sonesson, B., Saveland, H., Ljunggren, B., & Brandt, L. (1989). Cognitive functioning after subarachnoid haemorrhage of unknown origin. *Acta Neurologica Scandinavica*, *80*, 400–10.

Young, A. W., de Haan, E. D. F., & Newcombe, F. (1990). Unawareness of impaired face recognition. *Brain and Cognition*, *14*, 1–18.

GIAN LUIGI LENZI AND MARCO IACOBONI

subcortical dementia   A group of dementing disorders are commonly referred to as the subcortical dementias. This group includes HUNTINGTON'S DISEASE, MULTIPLE SCLEROSIS, PARKINSON'S DISEASE, and progressive supranuclear palsy. Although the term is intended to indicate DEMENTIAS in which the pathology is subcortical and not cortical, other disorders such as Alzheimer's disease are sometimes included to emphasize subcortical involvement alongside the involvement of the cerebral cortex. Although there are common features in the neuropsychological dysfunction of those who suffer from one of the subcortical dementias, distinct patterns of impairment characterize each disorder.

substantia nigra   The substantia nigra is a cell group in the midbrain close to the cerebral PEDUNCLES. It receives fibers from the STRIATUM and has a return projection, so being a satellite of the striatum. Neurons in the substantia nigra include neuromelanin, which is black in color, giving the structure its name, and employ dopamine as their striatal neurotransmitter. The substantia nigra is part of the extrapyramidal motor system, and extensive loss of the neurons in this cell group is associated with PARKINSON'S DISEASE.

sucking reflex   The sucking reflex is one of the primitive reflexes which are normal in infants but abnormal in adults, re-emerging after damage to the brain. Tactile contact with the lips provokes contractions of the muscles of the lips, tongue, and jaw that are involved in sucking. When the sucking reflex is unilateral and accompanied by a GRASP REFLEX on the same side, it is termed the *rooting reflex*.

superior longitudinal fasciculus   The superior longitudinal fasciculus is one of the large bundles of fibers (fasciculi) which connect distant regions of the cortex within each cerebral hemisphere. This fasciculus, together with the ARCUATE FASCICULUS, which is adjacent and superior, interconnects regions of the frontal lobe with the anterior occipital and posterior temporal regions. It is therefore implicated in the integration of auditory-visual perception with motor performance, and in the link between posterior and anterior language systems in the hemisphere subserving language.

superior occipito-frontal fasciculus The superior occipito-frontal fasciculus is one of the large bundles of fibers (fasciculi) which connect distant regions of the cortex within each cerebral hemisphere. This fasciculus runs above the SUPERIOR LONGITUDINAL FASCICULUS and interconnects the posterior and superior regions of the occipital lobe with the superior regions of the frontal lobe. It is therefore implicated in the integration of primary visual perception with the premotor region of the frontal lobe.

supramarginal gyrus The supramarginal gyrus is a cortical structure close to the ANGULAR GYRUS and the posterior termination of the SYLVIAN FISSURE. These structures lie at the junction of the occipital, temporal, and parietal lobes, and lesions of the supramarginal gyrus are associated with visuospatial dysfunction (especially if the lesion is bilateral), in disorders of FACE RECOGNITION, and in APHASIA.

surface dyslexia *See* DYSLEXIA.

Sylvian fissure The Sylvian fissure is one of the principal landmarks on the cortex and is the most easily recognized. It is the prominent fissure which runs backwards and upwards from below the frontal lobe, so establishing the division between the temporal lobe, which lies below it, and the frontal and parietal lobes, which lie superior to it. An important feature is that the posterior course of the fissure has considerable individual variability, but on average shows an asymmetry between the hemispheres, being longer and turning more upwards on the right.

This has the implication, particularly important in electrophysiology, that homolateral points on the scalp in this region may not lie above truly homolateral points on the cortex, and may even lie above different cortical lobes.

syphilis Syphilis is a contagious disease caused by the spirochete *Treponema pallidum*. It is a systemic disease and can affect any tissue of the body. Its usual mode of transmission is through sexual contact; it passes into the body through mucous membranes or skin. Invasion of the central nervous system (CNS) occurs relatively early after initial infection and can result in two main forms of neurosyphilis: meningovascular neurosyphilis or parenchymatous neurosyphilis, which comprises tabes dorsalis and general paresis.

Meningovascular neurosyphilis generally occurs at about 5 years post infection and involves inflammation of the meninges of either the brain or spinal cord, along with vascular changes in these areas. The symptoms may resemble those of subacute meningitis with headache, dizziness, neck stiffness, and poor concentration. Cranial nerve involvement may lead to hearing or visual changes. Confusion, APHASIA, and mono- or HEMIPLEGIA may also occur. Motor symptoms are more pronounced with involvement of the spinal cord.

Tabes dorsalis is one of the parenchymatous forms of neurosyphilis where the organism has invaded nervous tissue. Onset is gradual and insidious and generally occurs 8–10 years after infection. There is wasting of dorsal spinal roots and the posterior columns of the spinal cord, which results in pain, sensory ATAXIA, sensory changes, and loss of tendon reflexes. This condition is seen in approximately 20 percent of cases of general paresis. Males are four times as likely to suffer from tabes dorsalis and general paresis as females.

General paresis (dementia paralytica, general paralysis of the insane, or GPI) is a progressive DEMENTIA. It is the only form of neurosyphilis where the spirochetes are present in the brain tissue. The dementia is a direct consequence of the action of the organism. Post-mortem reveals a thickened dura mater with the pia mater frequently adherent to the cortex. There is general atrophy of the brain with widening of the sulci and dilated ventricles. There is evidence of inflammatory lesions throughout the cortex, with cell loss being particularly apparent in the parietal and frontal lobes. Onset is signalled by behavioral and cognitive changes. Self-care behaviors may deteriorate, with emotional lability being common. A range of ill-judged behaviors may be engaged in and insight may become impaired. Cognitively there may be evidence of general intellectual inefficiencies, with memory and concentration being the first functions to be impacted. On the whole, symptoms resemble those of a progressive dementia. The face takes on a mask-like expression with voluntary motor control becoming progressively weak as the condition advances.

Since the introduction of penicillin the incidence of neurosyphilis has dropped dramatically. The incidence is higher among some sections of the community, particularly those engaging in promiscuous sexual behaviors. However, it is only a fairly small percentage that now shows evidence of nervous system involvement.

MARCUS J. C. ROGERS

T

tactile perception disorders Tactile perception is the result of the acquisition and processing of information using the sense of touch. The principal tactile organ in primates (including Man) is the hand, which is used in active sensing of multiple object properties such as shape, size, surface attributes, and compliance, leading ultimately to an integrated percept and object recognition (stereognosis).

ANATOMICAL PRINCIPLES

Neural apparatus

Tactile sensation depends on cutaneous mechanoreceptive afferents, of which there are four types in the human hand. Slowly adapting (SA) afferents respond continuously to sustained skin indentation and comprise two types, SAI (Merkel discs) and SAII (Ruffini endings, which are absent in the monkey fingerpad). Afferents responding transiently at stimulus onset or offset comprise rapidly adapting (RA, corresponding to Meissner corpuscles) and Pacinian corpuscle (PC) afferents. The afferent fibers are peripheral processes of dorsal root ganglion cells, whose central processes enter the spinal cord in the dorsal roots. The spinal tracts carrying tactile information rostrally are the ipsilateral dorsal columns and the contralateral spinothalamic tract. Dorsal column axons synapse in the dorsal column nuclei on neurons whose axons cross the midline to form the medial lemniscus, which, along with the spinothalamic tract, terminates in the nucleus ventralis posterolateralis (VPL) of the thalamus contralateral to the origin of the afferent input. From the thalamus, the thalamocortical radiation conveys information to the primary somatosensory cortex.

Cortical organization

Somatotopy is the orderly "mapping" of the receptor sheet onto its neural representation in cortex as well as subcortical nuclei. Cortical somatotopy is organized on a columnar basis, with vertical columns defined by afferent input. There are multiple cortical representations of the body, with differing receptive field properties. Primary somatosensory cortex (SI) comprises four cytoarchitectonic fields in the postcentral gyrus: Brodmann's areas 3a, 3b, 1, and 2. Areas 3b and 1 contain two separate cutaneous representations of the contralateral body surface; area 3a contains a representation of deep receptors, and area 2 yet another map with larger receptive fields and a combination of deep and cutaneous inputs. Further posteriorly in parietal cortex, cells in area 5 receive proprioceptive input arising from movement of multiple joints. SII (second somatosensory cortex), located in the parietal operculum, contains another complete body representation with receptive field characteristics that differ substantially from those in SI (larger receptive fields, often bilateral inputs). The locations of these different cortical areas are shown in Figure 78.

Other cortical areas also receive somatosensory input. These include area 7b in posterior parietal cortex, retro-insular cortex, and granular insular cortex. It is likely that the multiple somatosensory representations are specialized for different functions, as in visual cortex. A hierarchical organization of somatosensory cortical areas, analogous to that in the visual system, has been proposed (Mishkin, 1979). The dependence of SII on SI for its cutaneous mechanoreceptive input (Burton et al., 1990) is consistent with this hypothesis.

Neural plasticity

It has long been recognized that the capacity to

717

A

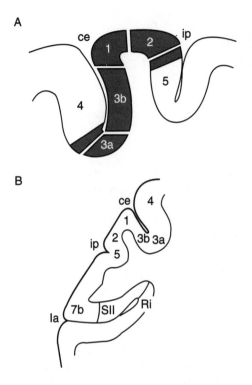

B

Figure 78 A parasagittal (A) and a coronal (B) section of a macaque brain to show the major somatosensory cortical areas; ce, central sulcus; ip, intraparietal sulcus; la, lateral sulcus; SII, second somatosensory cortex; Ri, retroinsular cortex. Numbers designate Brodmann's cytoarchitectonically defined areas. (Modified, with permission, from T. P. Pons, P. E. Garraghty, D. P. Freedman, & M. Mishkin in *Science, 237*, 1987, 417–20.)

reorganize after injury is considerably greater in the infant than in the adult nervous system. Infant monkeys recover tactile capacities much better after lesions of either SI or SII than do adult monkeys (which are seriously impaired by a lesion of either area). The differential recovery after an SI lesion correlates with the greater responsiveness of SII to cutaneous mechanoreceptive input in infants than in adults after an SI lesion (Burton et al., 1990), but the underlying mechanisms remain obscure.

The capacity for somatotopic reorganization after injury, even in adults, has attracted considerable interest over the last decade. Following

de-afferentation of part of the hand by nerve section or digit amputation, the representation of adjacent parts of the hand expands (over millimeters) into the cortical territory that has been deprived of its normal sensory input (Merzenich & Jenkins, 1993). This expansion can be observed immediately after the experimental manipulation and is therefore thought, at least in part, to represent unmasking of pre-existent connections (Killackey, 1989). After more extensive de-afferentation, involving an entire limb, the de-afferented zone of primary somatosensory cortex was found, years later, to be occupied by an expanded face representation (Pons et al., 1991). It has recently been proposed that this "massive" cortical reorganization (over centimeters) underlies the referred sensations that map to the "phantom" limb when humans with upper limb amputations are touched on the face (Ramachandran, 1993). Expansion of adjacent representations into cortex disconnected from its normal input or output has also been reported in motor and visual cortex.

A variety of surgical manipulations of afferent input, as well as some interventions in the CNS, have been shown to modify the details of cortical maps (Merzenich & Jenkins, 1993). Further, cortical somatotopy appears to be dynamically maintained. Evidence for this idea includes the findings that surgical fusion of digits abolishes the normal discontinuity between their cortical representations, and that continued stimulation of one or two fingers expands their cortical representation (Merzenich & Jenkins, 1993). Although these experiments have attracted controversy (Killackey, 1989), observations attesting to the dynamically modifiable nature of cortical representational topography have now been made in motor and visual areas of cortex. The mechanisms responsible for these phenomena are not yet clear. Understanding them is likely to offer crucial insights into the workings of the brain.

PERCEPTION AND ITS NEURAL CODING

The last 25 years or so have witnessed substantial progress in research into the neurophysiology of tactile perception. Stemming from the pioneering work of Mountcastle and his colleagues, the predominant approach has been to define the behavioral capabilities of the system as a whole by classical psychophysical methods, and to explore the neural basis of these behavioral capacities in a quantitative manner. This approach has been successfully applied to many distinct aspects of the tactile sense, with the result that the peripheral neural basis of some tactile abilities is understood fairly well. Research into central neural processes, which has virtually been restricted to the cerebral cortex, has been more limited. Some aspects of touch remain largely unexplored. It is important to realize that skin mechanics impose substantial spatiotemporal filters on stimulus information, so that primary afferent signals reflect significant transforms of stimulus input. A detailed mechanical model of the skin-receptor complexes that fully accounts for these transforms is still lacking.

Vibration

Among punctate stimuli, vibrating probes have been particularly useful in characterizing primary afferents. The capacity to discriminate vibratory frequency (for which the threshold frequency difference is about 10 percent) depends on stimulus-entrained periodicity in the activity of primary afferents, as well as of cortical neurons in areas 3b and 1 (Mountcastle et al., 1990). Such entrained activity appears about 6–8 db above absolute afferent threshold, accounting for an "atonal interval" between the threshold amplitudes for detection and frequency discrimination. U-shaped tuning curves relate threshold amplitudes to frequency, and differ among afferent types. SAs are most sensitive at low frequencies (under 30 Hz), RAs at intermediate frequencies (around 40 Hz), and PCs at high frequencies (over 200 Hz). The overall level of activity in the primary afferent population correlates with judgments of vibratory amplitude.

Texture

Surface texture (roughness) is a property which appears to be better extracted by touch than vision. It has been studied using synthetic periodic surfaces consisting of raised elements, with independently variable element width and spacing in the millimeter range (Johnson & Hsiao, 1992; Sathian, 1989). As element spacing increases, subjective roughness increases, up to about 3 mm, beyond which it decreases. Roughness also increases, though less markedly, as element width decreases. Humans can discriminate between surfaces that differ in spatial period

by as little as 5 percent, and can detect a dot half a millimeter wide that is raised only a few micrometers above a smooth background. Tangential motion between skin and surface is necessary for maximal sensitivity, but it makes no difference whether movement is active or passive. Movement speed (in the range 10–250 mm.s^{-1}) has no effect, and contact force little effect on perceived roughness.

The peripheral neural basis of roughness perception has been studied by examining the responses of single primary afferents innervating the monkey fingerpad. Goodwin, Darian-Smith, and their colleagues showed that the firing rate of all mechanoreceptive afferent types is an increasing function of element spacing up to 3mm. Representations of element spacing independent of movement speed are found in the discharge rate of the SA afferent population and in the ratio of the discharge rates of the RA and PC afferent populations. Further, the afferent discharge occurs in bursts which are time-locked to surface periodicity, and the number of impulses per burst precisely represents stimulus parameters such as element spacing and temporal frequency (Sathian, 1989).

Johnson and colleagues have examined a number of different potential coding mechanisms for roughness. Among these, a neural code based on local spatial variations in afferent discharge emerged as the likely basis of tactile roughness judgments for surfaces with spatial periods between 1–6 mm (Johnson & Hsiao, 1992). SAI afferents have the highest spatial acuity (of about 1 mm) and probably mediate this spatial coding, though RAs, with their somewhat lower spatial acuity, may also contribute. Similar conclusions apply in the human, although the coding mechanisms have not been explored in as great detail. PC innervation density (and spatial acuity) is considered to be too low for them to contribute to this coding mechanism.

LaMotte and others showed that perception of "microtextures" composed of tiny elements appears to depend on different mechanisms. RAs have the lowest threshold for detecting a fine dot (a few micrometers high) on a smooth background, followed by SAs and then PCs; while PCs are the only afferents activated by microtextures with sub-micrometer element height. Interestingly, detection of slip between skin and a surface requires the presence of microtexture that can activate either RAs or PCs, so that slip cannot be detected if the surface is perfectly smooth. These findings (see reviews cited above) underscore the differing, yet overlapping, functional roles of the various afferent types.

Thalamic (VPL) and many cortical (SI: 3b and 1) neurons in awake, behaving monkeys appear to respond in a manner similar to peripheral tactile afferents, with their responses being affected not only by element spacing but also by movement speed and/or contact force. A subset of SI neurons appear to respond solely as a function of element spacing, independent of movement speed or contact force, while some neurons appear to increase their response rate as spatial period decreases. Similar types of responses have recently been reported in SII, although these texture-related responses were noted less frequently than in SI (Sinclair & Burton, 1993). These observations point to the emergence in cortex of response types not seen in the periphery or thalamus, i.e. arising from cortical processing.

Patterns

Braille reading is an everyday instance of the tactile capacity to distinguish spatial patterns. Braille, which can be read at a speed of up to 100 words per minute, is a spatial code using a 3×2 array of 6 cells to represent each letter, where each cell contains 0 or 1 dot. Braille-like dot patterns and embossed Roman letters have been used to study the tactile capacity to assess spatial surface detail (Johnson & Hsiao, 1992). This capacity clearly depends on a detailed spatial representation of the stimulus patterns in the neural discharge.

Neurophysiological studies of primary afferents innervating the fingerpad of monkeys and Man (Johnson & Hsiao, 1992) indicate that, as in the case of texture, the high spatial acuity of SAI afferents renders them the most suited to signal spatial detail, with RAs providing a less acute representation that may also contribute. SAII and PC afferents are not suited to this function, due to their low density. Subjects make consistent errors in tactile letter recognition, which are entirely explicable in terms of the details of their spatial representation in the primary afferent pool. For example, the relative overemphasis of leading edges in the spatial representation of letters scanned across the fingerpad, with a loss of internal and trailing structure, can account for the

confusability of the letters B and D (Johnson & Hsiao, 1992).

Cortical recordings have also provided evidence in support of the spatial coding hypothesis (Johnson & Hsiao, 1992). About a third of SA neurons in area 3b show spatial modulation in response to moving dot arrays, down to and below the threshold for resolution. A similar proportion of these neurons yields isomorphic images of embossed letters scanned across the fingerpads, resembling in detail those of peripheral afferents. These neurons are therefore prime candidates for encoding spatial pattern information, although a detailed analysis of spatial codes has not been presented. Other SA neurons in 3b and 1, and RA neurons in both these areas, show non-isomorphic responses. Some of these, especially in 3b SAs, can be interpreted as the result of cortical inhibitory processes on isomorphic input. Interestingly, many of these responses match those of intermediate-level units in a back-propagation neural network model. The implications of this cortical processing for perception are not clear yet.

Shape

Tactile determination of shape requires ascertaining local object curvature and its changes, as well as a more global determination of three-dimensional shape and size, using the relative position of fingertips and finger joints in space. Local surface contour has been studied in LaMotte's laboratory, using surfaces bearing a step-like transition of constant height between two planes, with step curvature being a controlled variable (Sathian, 1989). The peripheral neural basis for discriminating step curvature is found in afferent discharge rates, which increase with curvature (RAs better than SAs), and in the spatial profiles (SAs better than RAs) of these rates, which are narrower for steeper steps.

The neural coding of 3-D shape is being actively studied. The only report published to date describes neurons in areas 1, 2, and 5 of monkey parietal cortex that responded differently when the monkey palpated a sphere or a cube (Koch & Fuster, 1989).

Other aspects of touch

A number of aspects of the tactile sense, including size, sharpness, softness, thickness, stickiness, and "wetness," remain completely or largely unexplored. Proprioceptive inputs contribute to some aspects of the tactile sense (e.g. size and shape) as well as to control of exploratory and manipulative movements. A detailed discussion of proprioception is beyond the scope of this entry. Suffice it to point out that muscle afferents are important in signalling of joint position and movement, with joint afferents functioning chiefly as "limit detectors" and cutaneous afferents (especially SAIIs) being involved additionally in the hand.

Finally, robotics researchers are interested in "haptic" (active manual) sensing, and interesting insights into the biology of tactile perception are likely to be derived from their approaches to real and "virtual" sensing, particularly in terms of the computational strategies that may be used.

DISRUPTION OF PERCEPTION BY LESIONS

Standard tests of tactile function used in clinical practice include: (1) localization of a punctate tactile stimulus; (2) distinguishing the sharp from the dull end of a pin; (3) determining, for a pair of punctate tactile stimuli, the minimal inter-stimulus distance required for their separate perception (two-point discrimination); (4) extinction of a stimulus when it is paired with a simultaneous contralateral one; (6) graphesthesia or recognition of writing on the skin; and (7) tactile-kinesthetic recognition of form, either by object identification (stereognosis) or by tracing standard shapes. These tests encompass a wide range of tactile abilities, but are largely qualitative. Application of the stimuli of vibration, patterns, shape, and texture, with the insights gained from studies of neural coding, will doubtless lead to refinement of our understanding of the effects of neural lesions on tactile performance. In turn, this can be expected to guide further neurobiological studies.

Spinal cord lesions

According to traditional teaching, dorsal column (DC) lesions impair vibratory and kinesthetic sensation. However, this view has required substantial modification (Davidoff, 1989). A number of studies in humans and experimental animals indicate that DC section alone does not impair tactile sensation as tested clinically. Recent studies suggest that DC lesions impair the ability to discriminate the direction of movement of a stimulus on the skin and to discriminate shape, size, pressure, and vibratory frequency. Adding a lesion of the dorsolateral fasciculus or the spino-thalamic tract to a DC lesion produces a severe and permanent loss of virtually all tactile sensation. The role of these pathways in tactile sensation remains to be elucidated.

Cerebral lesions

In monkeys Experimental ablation of the post-central gyrus in monkeys substantially impairs a variety of tactile capacities, including discrimination of vibratory frequency, roughness, size, shape, orientation and softness. A more restricted removal of area 3b alone reproduces most of these deficiencies (Randolph & Semmes, 1974). This correlates with the denser thalamic input to area 3b as compared to the posterior subdivisions of postcentral cortex, and with the hierarchical organization of connections within the postcentral gyrus, from 3b to 1 to 2. Selective ablation of area 1 reportedly impairs discrimination of roughness and softness but not of size or shape, while a selective lesion of area 2 causes the opposite effect (Randolph & Semmes, 1974). This has been correlated with the differences in peripheral input to these fields, area 1 receiving mainly cutaneous, and area 2 cutaneous and deep inputs.

Removal of SII also severely impairs the ability of adult monkeys to discriminate roughness and size, while lesions of area 5 in posterior parietal cortex produce relatively modest impairments of roughness discrimination (Murray & Mishkin, 1984).

In Man In clinical practice, lesions involving the medial lemniscus, thalamus, and subcortical white matter have been reported to impair tactile sensation. As traditionally taught, lesions of somatosensory cortex impair "discriminative" abilities (tactile localization, two-point discrimination, stereognosis, and graphesthesia) while thalamic lesions profoundly impair touch and pain sensation. This notion has not been carefully tested: in fact, a recent report described a "pseudothalamic" syndrome resulting from inferior parietal lesions involving the operculum and subcortical white matter (Basetti et al., 1993).

Lesions of human postcentral cortex have been found to impair a variety of tactile capacities (as in the monkey) – these include tactile localization and von Frey thresholds, two-point discrimination, kinesthesis, discrimination of roughness, size, and shape, and tactile recognition of objects.

Roland (1987) has performed a detailed analysis of the effects of surgical excision of various cortical regions on a number of tasks. Obviously, these lesions are not necessarily restricted to particular cortical fields as in the experimental material, and cannot be precisely delineated in terms of cortical cytoarchitectonics or physiological characteristics. Roland found that roughness discrimination was severely affected by a lesion of the postcentral gyrus, and less severely by lesions of the supplementary sensory area (the part of area 5 that lies on the medial surface of the hemisphere), of the posterior part of parietal opercular cortex, or of some areas of frontal cortex. Lesions involving the postcentral gyrus also impaired discrimination of size and shape, with lesions of the anterior bank (areas 3a, b) causing a more severe deficit than lesions of the crown of the gyrus (area 1). Mild to moderate deficits of shape but not size discrimination followed lesions of cortex lining the postcentral sulcus (areas 2 and 5), of the supplementary sensory area, and of frontal cortex. While lesions of these areas also impaired kinesthetic discrimination, kinesthetic deficits did not correlate with deficits in discrimination of shape and size. In this study, SII lesions did not affect roughness discrimination, in contrast to studies in monkeys (see above).

These studies of monkeys and humans with cortical lesions suggest that the multiple areas receiving somatosensory inputs are indeed specialized for different functions. However, a clear picture of functional specialization of these areas is still not available. Further studies, guided by neuroscientific insights, are called for.

COGNITIVE PROCESSES AND THEIR IMPAIRMENT

The study of cognitive processes in tactile perception, especially from a neurobiological perspective, has been rather patchy. The majority of reports have been devoted to the effects of lesions. Progress in this area will require multidisciplinary efforts to define the component cognitive operations involved in each behavioral realm, to localize the brain areas performing these operations, to understand their neural implementation, and to characterize their disruption by lesions.

Learning, memory, and recognition

Koch and Fuster (1989) recorded single neuronal responses in parietal cortex of monkeys discriminating between a sphere and a cube in a haptic delayed matching-to-sample task. They found some neurons with transient or sustained activity during an 18 sec delay period (i.e. between manipulation of the two objects in a trial, during which the animal was not actually palpating an object). Some of these neurons responded differentially, depending on whether a sphere or cube had been palpated. These cells were commonest in area 5a, and were believed to mediate tactile short-term memory.

This kind of *immediate memory* is that involved in perceptual discrimination between successive stimuli, which is independent of temporal lobe structures. When a longer delay (of minutes rather than seconds) is interposed between registration and recall, memory is dependent on the temporal lobe. In the tactile realm, this is illustrated by Ross's (1980) report of loss of tactile *recent memory* in 3 patients who had medial temporal lobe lesions contralateral to the deficit. These patients were allowed to palpate a relatively unfamiliar, non-verbalizable object for 10 sec. After a 3-minute verbal distraction time, they were unable to choose this object from among four others, using the affected hand. Since the ability to perform this task with the other hand or immediately (i.e. without a delay period) with the affected hand, the ability to match objects between hands, and stereognosis (presumably tested using previously familiar objects) were all intact, it was concluded that the deficit was specific to tactile recent memory. The deficits were transient, occurring in the setting of acute infarction or post-ictally.

A recent study using PET scanning demonstrated increases of regional cerebral oxidative metabolism in human cerebellar cortex, during tactile *learning* of previously unfamiliar objects (which had to be recognized subsequently). The increases were higher during this learning phase than in the subsequent recognition phase of the task, suggesting a specific role for cerebellar cortex in this type of tactile learning (Roland et al., 1989).

The study of tactile learning has been pursued in Mishkin's laboratory with the use of experimental lesions. Monkeys learned a tactile form discrimination task with one hand and were tested for transfer of this task to the opposite hand. A forebrain COMMISSUROTOMY interfered with the inter-manual transfer. An extensive lesion of sensorimotor cortex in the trained hemisphere produced a similar impairment, as expected. However, a comparable deficit was also created by ablation of the medial temporal and inferior frontal cortices. These experiments led to the concept that learning depended critically on interaction between trained sensorimotor cortex and these limbic areas, either in the same hemisphere or in the opposite one via commissural connections; and to the hypothesis that tactile learning depends on serial processing in a pathway from SI through SII to limbic cortex (Mishkin, 1979). Evidence in favor of this includes the profound impairment of tactile learning produced by a lesion of SII in monkeys, while a lesion of area 5 did not impair learning (Murray & Mishkin, 1984).

In keeping with these studies in monkeys is the recent finding that lesions involving the parietal operculum in humans specifically impaired tactile object *recognition* (Caselli, 1993). Patients with these lesions were unable to name familiar objects, or to describe the objects and their uses, when the objects were presented tactually. The deficit in tactile recognition appeared to be out of proportion to the extent of somatosensory deficits, prompting characterization of the deficit as a *tactile agnosia*. In contrast to these lesions, more medial lesions including (but not restricted to) the supplementary sensory area impaired tactile object recognition only when they were so severe as to cause a profound impairment of more "basic" somatosensory deficits.

A related disorder is *tactile anomia*, where the patient is unable to name objects presented to his left hand. This has been described as a result of disconnection of the left hemisphere language areas from the right hemisphere somatosensory areas by a callosal lesion. A more severe *tactile aphasia* has been described in a patient with a left parieto-occipital lesion (Beauvois et al., 1978). This patient misnamed and was unable to describe without dysphasic errors, objects presented to *either* hand, and also made errors in deciding whether a palpated object fitted a stated name. However, he was able to manipulate the objects appropriately, had no somatosensory impairments as clinically tested, and was not aphasic when cued with non-tactile sensory modalities (vision and hearing). It is not clear whether this deficit was due to destruction of a specific cortical area or to disconnection of the left hemisphere language areas from the somatosensory areas in both hemispheres by the subcortical extent of the lesion.

It should be emphasized that these studies do not strictly localize the relevant cognitive processes, as distinct from more "basic" sensory processes. More rigorous definition of the sensory and cognitive operations involved in each of these behavioral domains is required before we can hope to understand their localization in the brain. By the same token, the precise nature of the disorders described, in terms of their effects on sensory versus cognitive processes, is far from clear. For instance, is the impairment of tactile object recognition in patients with parietal opercular lesions due to a true agnosia – a failure of recognition in the presence of normal perception – or to interference with the higher-order sensory processing necessary for recognition? Questions such as this also highlight the arbitrary nature of the distinction between "sensory" and "cognitive" processes, one that may increasingly blur in the future.

Attention

Attention can be oriented spatially in touch, just as in vision. The requirement for spatially focusing attention is minimal in the detection of an abrupt change in texture (Sathian & Burton, 1991) or of a vibrotactile amplitude change that can occur randomly on one of four digits. In contrast, detecting the absence of such changes (when 3 out of 4 digits encounter them) benefits from a cue focusing attention on the appropriate digit. These experiments suggest that, as in the visual system, some stimuli can be processed "preattentively" or in a state of distributed spatial attention, while other stimuli demand spatially selective attention. The neural substrate of spatially selective tactile attention is unknown. However, when attention is specifically directed to the tactile (as compared to the visual) modality, about half the recorded neurons in monkey SI and SII show an enhanced response to embossed letters scanned across the fingerpad, while nearly a quarter of SII neurons respond in the opposite manner with these cross-modal shifts of attention (Hsiao et al., 1993).

It is well known that lesions of the posterior

parietal cortex produce inattention to the contralateral half of the body. In its milder forms, this may be manifest merely by extinction of a stimulus on the affected side of the body when it is paired with a similar one on the opposite side. When more severe, especially with right parietal lesions, there may be neglect of an entire hemibody, along with neglect of visual and auditory hemispace. Recent studies confirm that patients with such lesions do process somatosensory stimuli contralateral to the lesion, as evidenced by normal cortical SEPs and positive electrodermal skin conductance responses (Vallar et al., 1991), despite appearing to neglect them. More detailed knowledge of tactile attentional mechanisms awaits further research.

As I have pointed out at various places in this entry, the correlated psychophysical-neurophysiological approach to studying the tactile sense has begun to yield dividends. The time is ripe for a concerted, multi-disciplinary assault on the psychology and physiology of tactile perception.

BIBLIOGRAPHY

Note Only selected references are provided, either to a review or a relatively recent publication, which may be consulted for further references.

Basetti, C., Bogousslavsky, J., & Regli, F. (1993). Sensory syndromes in parietal stroke. *Neurology, 43*, 1942–9.

Beauvois, M.-F., Saillant, B., Meininger, V., & Lhermitte, F. (1978). Bilateral tactile aphasia: a tacto-verbal dysfunction. *Brain, 101*, 381–401.

Burton, H., Sathian, K., & Dian-Hua, S. (1990). Altered responses to cutaneous stimuli in the second somatosensory cortex following lesions of the postcentral gyrus in infant and juvenile macaques. *Journal of Comparative Neurology, 291*, 395–414.

Caselli, R. J. (1993). Ventrolateral and dorsomedial somatosensory association cortex damage produces distinct somesthetic syndromes in humans. *Neurology, 43*, 762–71.

Davidoff, R. A. (1989). The dorsal columns. *Neurology, 39*, 1377–85.

Hsiao, S. S., O'Shaughnessy, D. M., & Johnson, K. O. (1993). Effects of selective attention on spatial form processing in monkey primary and secondary somatosensory cortex. *Journal of Neurophysiology, 70*, 444–7.

Johnson, K. O., & Hsiao, S. S. (1992). Neural mechanisms of tactual form and texture perception. *Annual Review of Neuroscience, 15*, 227–50.

Killackey, H. P. (1989). Static and dynamic aspects of cortical somatotopy: a critical evaluation. *Journal of Cognitive Neuroscience, 1*, 3–11.

Koch, K. W., & Fuster, J. M. (1989). Unit activity in monkey parietal cortex related to haptic perception and temporary memory. *Experimental Brain Research, 76*, 292–306.

Merzenich, M. M., & Jenkins, W. M. (1993). Reorganization of cortical representations of the hand following alterations of skin inputs induced by nerve injury, skin island transfers and experience. *Journal of Hand Therapy, 6*, 89–104.

Mishkin, M. (1979). Analogous neural models for tactual and visual learning. *Neuropsychologia, 17*, 139–51.

Mountcastle, V. B., Steinmetz, M. A., & Romo, R. (1990). Frequency discrimination in the sense of flutter: psychophysical measurements correlated with postcentral events in behaving monkeys. *Journal of Neuroscience, 10*, 3032–44.

Murray, E. A., & Mishkin, M. (1984). Relative contributions of SII and area 5 to tactile discrimination in monkeys. *Behavioural Brain Research, 11*, 67–83.

Pons, T. P., Garraghty, P. E., Ommaya, A. K., Kaas, J. H., Taub, E., & Mishkin, M. (1991). Massive cortical reorganization after sensory deafferentation in adult macaques. *Science, 252*, 1857–60.

Ramachandran, V. S. (1993). Behavioral and magnetoencephalographic correlates of plasticity in the adult human brain. *Proceedings of the National Academy of Sciences of the USA, 90*, 10413–20.

Randolph, M., & Semmes, J. (1974). Behavioral consequences of selective subtotal ablations in the postcentral gyrus of *Macaca mulatta. Brain Research, 70*, 55–70.

Roland, P. E. (1987). Somatosensory detection of microgeometry, macrogeometry and kinesthesia after localized lesions of the cerebral hemispheres in man. *Brain Research Reviews, 12*, 43–94.

Roland, P. E., Eriksson, L., Widen, L., & Stone-Elander, S. (1989). Changes in regional cerebral oxidative metabolism induced by tactile learning and recognition in man. *European Journal of Neuroscience, 1*, 1–18.

Ross, E. D. (1980). Sensory-specific and fractional disorders of recent memory in man. *Archives of Neurology, 37,* 267–72.

Sathian, K. (1989). Tactile sensing of surface features. *Trends in Neurosciences, 12,* 513–19.

Sathian, K., & Burton, H. (1991). The role of spatially selective attention in the tactile perception of texture. *Perception and Psychophysics, 50,* 237–48.

Sinclair, R. J., & Burton, H. (1993). Neuronal activity in the second somatosensory cortex of monkeys (*Macaca mulatta*) during active touch of gratings. *Journal of Neurophysiology, 70,* 331–50.

Vallar, G., Sandroni, P., Rusconi, M. L., & Barbieri, S. (1991). Hemianopia, hemianesthesia, and spatial neglect: a study with evoked potentials. *Neurology, 41,* 1918–22.

K. SATHIAN

taste   In relation to hearing and vision, taste is little studied and poorly understood. Receptors in the anterior two-thirds and posterior third of the tongue pass information through different route to the PONS, from which there is a common route to the THALAMUS, with a relay to the cortical representation for taste at the foot of the postcentral gyrus. Loss of taste (ageusia) may occur separately for the two regions of the tongue; facial paralysis may be associated with a deficit for taste in the anterior portion. Disturbances of taste may occur with lesions affecting the pons, MEDULLA, or thalamus, but little is known about loss of taste resulting from cortical lesions. Hallucinations of taste may occur in UNCINATE FITS, and lesions of the uncus may result in *parageusia*, in which all substances have the same unpleasant flavor. Disturbances of taste may be difficult to distinguish from disturbances of smell (ANOSMIA).

telegraphic speech, writing Telegraphic speech or writing occurs in expressive aphasic disorders in which the output is restricted to the essential key nouns and verbs, similar to the abbreviated style employed in telegrams. Function words, syntactic words, and words of an unstressed character are omitted, and the syntax is often indicated by the order of words within the production. This is an agrammatic form of aphasia, and is typical of the classic Broca's aphasic (*see* APHASIA).

teleopsia   Teleopsia is the form of METAMORPHOPSIA in which an object or objects appear to be more distant than they are in fact. The distortion of the perception of distance may occur independently of the perception of actual size.

temporal lobe   The temporal lobes are readily recognizable in a side view of the brain (see Figure 79). When viewed from this angle, the temporal lobe looks like a thumb at the side of a closed fist, extending slightly downwards toward the front of the cranial cavity. However, like the parietal lobes, the "temporal lobe" is more a convenient fiction than an anatomical or functional entity. It is also the case that, in common with the occipital and parietal lobes (but not the frontal lobes, with their central sulcus), the border of the temporal lobe is neither simple nor precise; its margins cannot be clearly defined by functional or anatomical landmarks. The imprecision of defining the functional limits of the temporal lobe raises problems for the organization of this entry, but an attempt has been made to highlight the functions of the various subunits contained in the space within the lobe as currently defined, focusing on work with humans but referring to animal research where relevant. Because excision of the temporal lobe is often used to help control medically intractable seizure disorders, much of what is known about the effects of damage to (or stimulation of) this area comes from investigations with epileptics being considered for surgery.

HEMISPHERIC SPECIALIZATION

In humans, the temporal lobe is one of many cerebral structures that cannot be understood without invoking the concept of lateralization of function. It has been clearly established that important contributions to memory and perception are made by the temporal lobes, and the types of materials for which the relevant temporal lobe mechanisms play a role are appropriate to the side being considered (in order to simplify the description of these functions, references to

725

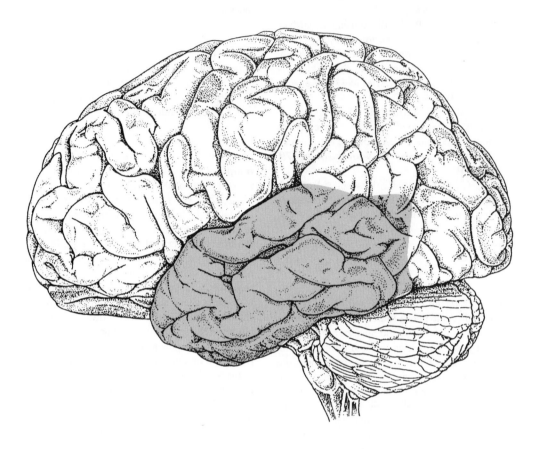

Figure 79 A side view of the brain, showing the temporal lobe.

the right and left hemispheres in the discussion that follows will be based on a "typical" representation, as seen in the majority of both right- and left-handers; *see* HANDEDNESS). This needs to be stated because for the temporal lobes, as well as for significant portions of the frontal and parietal lobes, many of the functions subserved need to be discussed in the context of the functional organization of the hemisphere within which the lobe is located. Evidence for this assertion comes from observations of patients with brain damage, from the effects of direct electrical stimulation during brain surgery, and from functional imaging studies (e.g. positron emission tomography). While discussing structure, it is worth noting that

the striking differences between the functions of the right and left temporal lobes are not reflected in equally striking morphological differences. While it is true that most individuals have a Sylvian fissure that rises more sharply on the left than on the right, this pattern is by no means invariable and its probable underlying cause (the size of the planum temporalis), is only weakly correlated with the side of speech mechanisms (more than 60 percent of right-handers have a larger planum temporalis on the left, while more than 97 percent of normal right-handers appear to have left hemisphere speech mechanisms). Interestingly, these morphological differences between the hemispheres appear to have predated the acquisition of speech abilities. Higher apes show the same pattern of morphological asymmetry and possess lateralized differences in the motor system (preferring the right hand for manipulation tasks and the left for spatial localization: *see* HANDEDNESS), but it is clear that speech is not developed in these animals and "true" language abilities in nonhuman primates remain controversial.

CYTOARCHITECTURE, PATHWAYS, CONNECTIONS

There are only fuzzy structural, functional, or morphological criteria for determining some of the boundaries between the temporal lobe and adjacent lobes. The posterior border is delimited ventrally by area 19 of the occipital lobe. Dorsally, the *Sylvian fissure* (sometimes called *lateral cerebral fissure*) demarcates the border anteriorly, while the posterior border with the parietal lobe is arbitrary and probably best defined by reference to projections of the thalamic nuclei such as the pulvinar, and/or cytoarchitectonic features (Brodmann's classification). Along the border, areas 22 and 37 (laterally) and 27 and 36 (mesially) belong within the temporal lobe: areas 39 (laterally) and 23, 26, 29, and 30 (mesially) belong within the parietal lobe. To some extent, it would have made functional sense to consider the posterior portions of the inferior temporal lobe (especially the fusiform gyrus) as being an extension of the occipital lobe, since functional PET findings in visual tasks and microelectrode recordings from inferior temporal cortex demonstrate activation in selected visual tasks. The *superior, middle*, and *inferior sulci* run parallel to the Sylvian fissure. Above the *superior temporal sulcus* is the *superior temporal gyrus*. In the left hemisphere, electrical stimulation of this gyrus frequently causes speech arrest or other alterations of language abilities; Wernicke's area (involved in language comprehension) lies at the posterior end of this gyrus where it meets the parietal lobe. Bilaterally, just in front of this region is Heschel's gyrus (primary auditory cortex). PET findings show bilateral activation of Heschel's gyrus and unilateral activation of Wernicke's area (left hemisphere only) when subjects listen to a story. Between the middle and superior temporal sulci lies the *middle temporal gyrus*. Islands of areas contributing to speech are occasionally found here as well, although it is not known if such unusual patterns of speech representation are common or are restricted to patients with pre-existing brain damage (e.g. patients with intractable epilepsy).

Mesial structures of the temporal lobe (*amygdala, hippocampus, rhinal cortex*) all have demonstrated roles in some aspects of the establishment of new memories (the relative roles of these portions of mesial temporal lobe are still being worked out; interpretation is difficult because it is unusual for one region to be damaged without a disturbance of the functions of the others, and animal studies, in which precise lesions are possible, do not have exact analogues to the kinds of memory tasks given to humans).

Effects of lesions

Because of its position in the cranium, the temporal lobe is vulnerable to damage from closed head injuries and increased intracranial pressure (sometimes induced during the process of vaginal delivery); its proximity (vascular and metric distance) to the face and to openings into the cranium from the nose leads to a major involvement in diseases such as herpes simplex encephalitis (*see* AMNESIA). Most of what we know about the functional significance of temporal lobe mechanisms comes from the effects of lesions on behavior. While much of this work comes from animal studies, the higher cognitive skills subserved by the temporal lobes mean that it has been more rewarding to work with humans who, in addition to psychometric deficits, can report their subjective impressions of the changes brought about by the damage. Cognitive changes occurring after damage to the temporal lobes are mainly seen in the domains of memory and perception, and again the concept of hemispheric specialization is relevant because of the material-specific nature of some of the deficits.

There is a clinical impression that some patients with right-hemispheric temporal lobe lesions undergo an increase in religiousness, sometimes to such an extent that the term "hyper-religiosity" is applicable. The theoretical basis for such a change has resisted definition but, if the phenomenon does exist, its origin may lie in an attempt by the patient to explain the presence of unusual and "unworldly" feelings that arise from the effects of their lesions or seizure activity, especially if arising from the right hemisphere.

The hemispheric organization of emotion has

received renewed attention since the strengthening of the biological revolution in psychiatry, and the LIMBIC SYSTEM has traditionally been accorded a role in the experience and expression of emotion. The amygdala especially has been seen as contributing to normal and abnormal emotional responses and experiences (leading, in extreme and misguided cases, to psychosurgical excision of these structures in individuals who are seen to have unacceptable emotionally-driven behavior). Bilateral amygdaloid destruction causes a severe disturbance of normal affective behavior (the Klüver–Bucy syndrome); damage in humans is usually unilateral and often incomplete, but even unilateral amygdaloid damage has led to changes in emotional experience and there have been recent suggestions that the amygdala is involved in the manifestations of schizophrenia.

The contribution of the temporal lobe to visual perception has become clarified by the division of visual projections from the occipital lobe in two directions or "streams": a dorsal route into parietal lobes involved in spatial localization; and a ventral route into the temporal lobe involved in the appreciation of the qualities of objects (and their identification) in the visual scene. Early and somewhat controversial evidence from single-cell recordings that neurons in the inferior temporal lobe of monkeys respond to complex visual stimuli has thus been confirmed and extended. Most of the studies have been carried out in primates but PET activation scans confirm the impression that visual analysis extends into the inferior portions of the temporal lobes, probably bilaterally but with a predominance on the left side when the object's name is being sought. In animal work, posterior lesions of inferior temporal lobe tissue disturb visual discrimination, while more anterior lesions disturb visual recognition.

BIBLIOGRAPHY

Ungerleider, J. G., & Mishkin, M. (1982). Two cortical visual systems. In D. J. Ingle, M. A. Goodale, & R. J. W. Mansfield (Eds), *Analysis of visual behavior* (pp. 549–86). Boston: MIT Press.

HENRY A. BUCHTEL

temporal lobe epilepsy *See* EPILEPSY; TEMPORAL LOBE.

temporal lobectomy *See* EPILEPSY; PSYCHOSURGERY; TEMPORAL LOBE.

test battery *See* ASSESSMENT; NEUROPSYCHOLOGY.

thalamic syndrome The thalamic syndrome is an excessive response to affective stimuli, the action of the thalamus having been released from control by cortical inhibitory impulses. The term was introduced by Head in the early years of the present century, and is now essentially obsolete except with regard to thalamic pain (*see* THALAMUS).

thalamus A large mass of gray matter at the rostral end of the central neuraxis, the thalamus relays information to the cerebral cortex and regulates the level of cortical activity related to behavioral states. The left and right thalami are located on either side of the third ventricle, in the dorsal part of the diencephalon, above the hypothalamus. During embryonic development, growth of the internal capsule causes the diencephalon and cerebral hemisphere to fuse. Thus the thalamus, although not part of the cerebral hemisphere, is embedded in it.

The mammalian thalamus evolved in intimate association with the cerebral cortex and functionally it is interposed as an obligatory relay between the sensory and motor pathways of the brain stem and the cerebral cortex and basal ganglia. The thalamus has two fundamental modes of operation: a relay mode and an oscillatory mode. The relay mode is characteristic of the alert, waking state during which sensory and motor information is transferred rapidly and faithfully to perceptive and motor control centers of the cortex. The oscillatory mode is characteristic of the change in behavioral state from alertness to drowsiness and slow-wave sleep, during which thalamic transmission is less efficient and the sense organs are functionally disconnected from the perceptive centers. The anatomical organization of the thalamus and the physiological properties of its neurons reflect its capacity to operate in these two oppositional, state-dependent modes.

DIVISION OF THE THALAMUS INTO NUCLEI

The largest division of the thalamus is into three embryologically distinct components: a small *epithalamus* consists mainly of the habenular nuclei, which are not connected with the cerebral cortex and will not be considered further; a very large *dorsal thalamus* forms the bulk of the thalamus and is divided into subsidiary nuclei connected with the cerebral cortex and/or basal ganglia; a *ventral thalamus* of which the greater part is the *reticular nucleus*, covers the anterior, lateral, and much of the ventral surfaces of the dorsal thalamus and is probably the major structure recruiting cells of the dorsal thalamus into cooperative action. "Thalamus," as loosely applied, customarily refers to the dorsal thalamus.

Divisions of the dorsal thalamus The dorsal thalamus is divided into a number of constellations of neurons called nuclei. The primary division is into *intralaminar nuclei* and *relay nuclei*. The intralaminar nuclei lie within an intrinsic sheet of white matter, the internal medullary lamina, and send axons to the basal ganglia, especially to the striatum (caudate nucleus, putamen, and nucleus accumbens), and to a lesser extent to the cerebral cortex. The relay nuclei are arranged in five large groups: *anterior, lateral, and medial*, plus the *medial* and *lateral geniculate bodies*. Each group of relay nuclei sends axons to a particular region of the cerebral cortex. The anterior group projects to cortex of the cingulate gyrus and cortex continuous with it and is concerned with limbic functions; the medial group projects to prefrontal cortex, basal fronto-temporal cortex, and the hippocampal formation and may play a special role in memory; the lateral group is divided into a dorsal set of nuclei which includes the large pulvinar – itself further subdivided – and a ventral set of nuclei; the pulvinar and associated lateral nuclei project to the association cortex of the parietal, temporal, and occipital lobes and are concerned with higher-order visual and sensory-motor integration; the ventral nuclei project to the premotor, motor, and somatosensory areas of the pre- and post-central gyri; the medial and lateral geniculate nuclei project to the primary auditory and visual cortical areas respectively.

Each subsidiary nucleus of the major, regionally projecting groups, is an entity in its own right. It receives inputs from a major afferent pathway and relays it to one or more functional areas within the large regional cortical territories defined by the projections of the nuclear group. For example, information arising in the cutaneous and deep sensory receptors of the body and carried in the medial lemniscus, is relayed via the posterior nucleus of the ventral group (ventral posterior nucleus) to somatosensory cortex of the post-central gyrus; the output of the cerebellum, carried in the brachium conjunctivum, is relayed via the ventral lateral nucleus to the motor cortex of the precentral gyrus; the output of the retina, carried in the optic tract, is relayed via the lateral geniculate nucleus to the primary visual cortex, and so on. Because there are no connections between nuclei in the dorsal thalamus, each is an independent relay and there is no cross-talk or modality dispersion in the thalamus.

The dorsal thalamus as a relay At a fine level of organization, each relay nucleus shows a high degree of topographic order. The best reflection of this is the possession of a sensory or motor map, that is, the visual field, body surface, and auditory frequency range, are systematically laid out in the appropriate nucleus so that neighboring thalamic neurons represent neighboring parts of the receptive periphery. Such a map is then projected intact onto the relevant cortical area. Within the thalamic map, individual relay neurons, i.e. the neurons that receive synapses from the afferent pathways and project to the cerebral cortex, tend to be functionally distinct. These functional distinctions are commonly reflected in morphological differences, in projections to different cortical layers, or both. In the lateral geniculate nucleus, for example, there is little or no cross-talk between neurons receiving inputs from the principal functional classes of retinal ganglion cells; the geniculate cells show different chemical and structural properties and project to different layers or sublayers of the visual cortex. This is the finest level of organization reflecting the relay capacities of the thalamus. The capacity to transmit information that is a close reflection of the patterns of discharges from the sense organs and motor-related centers of the brain stem resides, however, in the properties of the thalamic relay cell itself. At its normal resting membrane potential (usually about -60 mV), the cell is readily discharged, at low threshold, in response to an afferent volley. The pattern of discharges is a tonic one that faithfully reflects the pattern of afferent input. The ionic basis of the repetitive, fast spikes so discharged is an increased sodium conductance. The precision of organization in the synaptic inputs to the relay cells and their capacity to engage this mechanism are the keys to understanding the thalamic cell as a relay neuron.

CELL TYPES AND ELEMENTARY CIRCUITRY

There are two basic cell populations in the thalamus. Approximately 70 percent of the neurons in the dorsal thalamus are *relay neurons*, that is, they project their axons beyond the thalamus to the cerebral cortex (thalamocortical neurons) and/or to the basal ganglia (thalamostriatal neurons). The other neurons are those whose axons remain confined to the thalamus (*local circuit neurons* or *interneurons*). There are two kinds: small, *intrinsic local circuit neurons* are found in every nucleus of the dorsal thalamus, where they form 25–30 percent of the neuronal population; their axons remain within the nucleus in which the cells lie. Larger local circuit neurons are situated in the *reticular nucleus*, where they form 100 percent of the population. Their axons extend into the underlying dorsal thalamus and spread widely within it.

Afferent fibers entering a dorsal thalamic nucleus terminate in excitatory synapses on both relay neurons and intrinsic interneurons. They probably release the neurotransmitter glutamate. The relationship of a dorsal thalamic nucleus to the cerebral cortex is bi-directional and involves the reticular nucleus: the relay neurons project their axons to the cerebral cortex; as they pass through the reticular nucleus, they give off collaterals which terminate in the reticular nucleus. Axons of cells in the cortex return to the thalamic nucleus and terminate in glutamergic excitatory synapses on both the relay neurons and intrinsic local circuit neurons; as they pass through the reticular nucleus, they too give off collaterals to it.

The principal function of the intrinsic interneurons and of those in the reticular nucleus is inhibition. Their synapses release the inhibitory transmitter, gamma amino-butyric acid (GABA). The intrinsic neurons make synapses on relay neurons and on one another. They appear to refine the patterns of relay cell discharges during transfer of afferent information. The axons of reticular nucleus cells synapse on relay neurons

and on intrinsic neurons and appear to be involved in recruiting groups of relay cells into oscillatory behavior during slow-wave sleep.

Terminating widely in all dorsal thalamic nuclei and in the reticular nucleus are a series of pathways arising in brain-stem nuclei that do not form parts of the sensory or motor pathways. These release the neurotransmitters, acetylcholine, noradrenaline, or serotonin, and appear to exert a modulatory effect on thalamic excitability. Acetylcholine, for example, enhances relay cell excitability by depolarizing the relay cells and by hyperpolarizing the inhibitory cells, thus freeing the relay cells from the inhibitory influence of the latter.

The thalamus as an oscillator Thalamic cells operating in the relay mode transmit information rapidly, faithfully, and with great synaptic security to the cerebral cortex. Operating in the oscillatory mode, they effectively deprive the cortex of the excitatory drive essential for its capacity to respond to stimuli. This appears to serve as the prelude to falling asleep. In the oscillatory mode, large numbers of thalamic cells are recruited into synchronous activity that is reflected in the electroencephalographic (EEG) phenomena characteristic of slow-wave sleep. A number of anatomical pathways and physiological mechanisms are involved in shifting thalamic cells from the relay to the oscillatory mode. A set of so-called nonspecific afferent pathways arise in the brain stem and distribute widely throughout the thalamus. Unlike the sensory and motor-related pathways, these do not respect the borders of the relay nuclei. The chief concentrations of their terminations are in the intralaminar and adjacent nuclei in the medial part of the thalamus. Changes in the activity of these pathways usually precede by several seconds the changes in EEG activity that herald the transition from sleep to wakefulness and vice versa. Enhanced activity, particularly in the pathway in which the neurotransmitter is acetylcholine, precedes the onset of EEG desynchronization that marks the waking state. Then thalamic cells return from the oscillatory to the relay mode and the perceptive centers of the cerebral cortex are again functionally coupled to the sense organs.

Two other sets of anatomical connections appear to play a predominant role in recruiting thalamic relay cells as a group into the oscillatory behavior that accompanies slow-wave sleep and which is also seen under barbiturate anesthesia. These are the connections from the reticular nucleus which extend into all dorsal thalamic nuclei, and the "feedback" or corticothalamic connections. The latter return from all areas of the cerebral cortex to the nuclei providing input to them. The reticular nucleus and the cortico-thalamic projection appear to play an important, although incompletely understood role in recruiting thalamic neurons into rhythmic activity. This makes the thalamus less effective as a relay of information to the cerebral cortex. However, it is the membrane properties of the thalamic relay neuron that permit it to be switched from the relay to the oscillatory mode. At membrane potentials that are hyperpolarized, i.e. more negative to the resting potential (-65 to -70 mV), the same stimulus that generates the fast, repetitive discharge characteristic of the relay mode now generates a low-threshold, slow depolarization crowned by a short, rapid burst of typical action potentials. The slow spike has its basis in the activation of a calcium conductance that is inactivated at membrane potentials nearer the resting level. The superimposed burst of spikes are typical sodium spikes. When a relay cell is hyperpolarized, it will tend to fire in bursts, which cannot be an accurate reflection of the afferent input. This is the key to understanding the thalamic cell as the regulator of cortical vigilance.

The most obvious manifestations of the large-scale oscillations of thalamic neurons that accompany EEG synchronization (slow-wave sleep) are the so-called thalamic spindles. These consist of spontaneously occurring slow, rhythmic, neuronal discharges with a frequency of about 10 Hz and occurring in sequences that last about 1–2 seconds. These discharges form the basis of the spindle waves recorded in the EEG. Rhythmic patterns of discharge with higher or lower frequencies than the spindle discharges are also recorded in the thalamus. Their significance is a subject of continuing interest.

Any condition that drives thalamic relay neurons into a hyperpolarized state will tend to induce spindle oscillations. Spindles identical to the spontaneously occurring spindles can be induced by stimulation of afferent pathways or by stimulation of the corticothalamic fibers. These evoke initial discharges of the relay cells but the discharges are followed by a prolonged hyperpolarization, due to the actions of the GABAergic

intrinsic local circuit and reticular nucleus neurons. This hyperpolarization predisposes to burst firing and oscillation. It is likely that the reticular nucleus is involved as a kind of pacemaker in promoting spindle discharges under both spontaneous and stimulus-dependent conditions because its inhibitory neurons oscillate in reverse phase to the relay cells. They thus produce rhythmic hyperpolarizations in the relay cells. Moreover, relay cells experimentally disconnected from the reticular nucleus no longer show spindle bursts.

The intralaminar nuclei The thalamostriatal pathway is the orphan of the thalamus. It has been neglected in favor of the more intensively studied thalamocortical pathway. Yet it is by no means insignificant and probably accounts for a substantial proportion of the thalamic outflow. The greater part of the thalamostriatal projection arises from relay cells of the intralaminar nuclei. These receive a large variety of inputs from the cerebral hemisphere, brain stem, cerebellum, and spinal cord. Together with the cerebral cortex and substantia nigra, the intralaminar nuclei provide the greater part of the input to the striatum, the afferent side of the basal ganglia. The outflow from the efferent side, the globus pallidus, includes a return projection to the thalamus, primarily to the largest of the intralaminar nuclei, the center median, and to the nuclei of the ventral group that furnish inputs to premotor areas of the cerebral cortex.

At one level, therefore, the intralaminar nuclei and the thalamostriatal projection can be seen as engaged in mechanisms of higher motor control centered in the basal ganglia and premotor cortex. However, in the striatum, thalamic input interacts with input from all functional areas of the cerebral cortex. This is probably an indication of a more general involvement of the basal ganglia in higher cerebral function. In many ways, the basal ganglia stand to the thalamus in much the same relationship as the cerebral cortex. The thalamostriatal and thalamocortical pathways form parallel circuits within the cerebral hemisphere.

Many relay cells in the intralaminar nuclei also project to the cerebral cortex. Unlike the majority of those in the relay nuclei, however, their axons are distributed over relatively widespread areas, unconstrained by functional divisions of the cortex. They terminate in the most superficial layer of the cortex. It is this projection that forms the basis of the *recruiting response*. This is a long latency, initially surface-negative, high-voltage wave that spreads repetitively over the surface of the cerebral cortex in response to low-frequency electrical stimulation of the intralaminar nuclei in experimental animals. Although the functional significance of the recruiting response in the activities of the normal brain remains uncertain, it is generally thought that it indicates the presence of the ascending brain-stem pathways that regulate cortical arousal, probably by actions upon the thalamus.

Clinical and behavioral manifestations of thalamic function Apart from being expressed in terms of an effective sensory-motor relay or a regulator of behavioral state, thalamic function may also be revealed under a variety of clinical and/or behavioral conditions. Generally, these conditions reveal the operations of the different nuclei of the thalamus as parts of integrated brain systems. A thalamic stroke, for example, if it destroys a particular sensory relay nucleus will disconnect the cortical area(s) to which that nucleus projects from the peripheral sense organs, with obvious consequences. One of the most disturbing effects of a stroke involving obstruction or hemorrhage of the posterior thalamic arteries, and resulting in destruction of parts of the pulvinar and ventral nuclei, is the phenomenon of thalamic pain. In this, severe paroxysmal pain of a most unpleasant type occurs spontaneously or is precipitated by trivial, normally non-noxious stimuli. The causes of this *thalamic syndrome* are uncertain. They probably stem from a disturbance in the balance of inputs from peripheral somatosensory receptors to the ventral nuclei as the result of destruction of fiber tracts entering the ventral aspect of the thalamus. This and other forms of *central pain syndrome* that can accompany limb amputation, spinal deafferentation, or involvement of trigeminal nerve pathways in the brain-stem, appear to be accompanied by abnormal paroxysmal discharges of neurons in the ventral posterior nuclei of the thalamus.

The ventral and certain other nuclei of the thalamus that are involved in the relay of sensory messages induced by noxious stimuli to the cerebral cortex have in the past been the targets for surgical destruction in the operation of *stereotaxic thalamotomy*. In this, an electrode is introduced into the thalamus through the overlying brain, guided by radiographic and electro-physiological monitoring, and the target is destroyed. Such operations, usually performed as a last resort in an attempt to alleviate intractable pain, have had mixed success and commonly result in only temporary amelioration.

A greater level of success has perhaps been achieved by stereotaxic thalamotomies aimed at the ventral nuclei that form parts of the central motor pathways, in an effort to alleviate the involuntary movements associated with diseases such as Parkinsonism. The involuntary tremors of PARKINSON'S DISEASE are associated with rhythmic discharges of relay neurons in the ventral lateral nuclei. Although less commonly carried out since the widespread use of drug therapy in Parkinson's disease, the success of this operation in reducing severe tremors is high.

Cerebral functions of an integrative nature that primarily involve cortical areas outside the primary sensory and motor areas can also be revealed by experimental investigations or by pathology involving the thalamic nuclei connected with them. Aphasia of the fluent kind, showing some resemblance to the Wernicke's aphasia that follows destruction of the parieto-temporal speech cortex, has been described following lesions of the pulvinar on the side of the dominant cerebral hemisphere. The pulvinar on this side contains the relay cells projecting to the posterior speech cortex. Transient disturbances of speech performance can also be elicited by electrical stimulation in the ventral thalamic nuclei connected with the dominant hemisphere, probably reflecting the connections between this part of the thalamus and the motor speech areas of the frontal lobe.

The pulvinar also appears to be involved in visual spatial attention, possibly by operating as a filter to separate a visual target from surrounding, potentially distracting, visual images. In performing this function it may intervene in the sequence of successive intracortical connections passing from the primary visual area through other areas of cortex in the temporal lobe. This sequence of connections forms the elaborative machinery for higher-order visual perception.

A number of psychoses are associated with thalamic pathology, although the degree of involvement of the thalamus in the primary condition has sometimes been controversial. The medial nuclei are reported to show loss of neurons in SCHIZOPHRENIA, perhaps reflecting (or being a cause of) the reduced functional activity of the prefrontal cortex revealed by brain imaging studies in this condition. The medial nuclei are also reported to show degeneration in KORSAKOFF'S SYNDROME, among the symptoms of which are confabulation and amnesia for recent events. AMNESIA is regularly reported following surgical, vascular, or traumatic lesions of the medial aspect of the thalamus. In experimental animals, the medial nuclei can be shown to play an important role in olfactory guided behavior. Memory and olfaction may not appear obviously related but both involve frontal lobe function, and the prefrontal cortex is a projection target of the medial thalamic nuclei.

The close proximity of the anterior and medial thalamic nuclei makes it difficult to distinguish them in brain SCANS, and behavioral deficits attributed to involvement of the medial nuclei may in fact reflect damage to the anterior nuclei or their connections as well. *Fatal familial insomnia* is an autosomal dominant disease in the group of diseases that includes CREUTZFELDT–JAKOB DISEASE. It is associated with marked atrophy of the anterior and medial nuclei and is character- ized by untreatable insomnia and disturbances of autonomic and motor function.

The condition in which the capacity of thalamic relay cells to oscillate in collective ensembles is most highly expressed is nonconvulsive EPILEPSY: petit mal or *absence* attacks. In generalized seizures of this kind, high-voltage electroencep- halographic discharges with frequencies of 3–5 Hz spread bilaterally over the cerebral cortex. The spikes and waves of the EEG result from the combined oscillations of large groupings of cort- ical neurons and are temporally coincident with synchronous burst behavior in large groupings of thalamic relay cells. The thalamic bursts are dependent upon generation of the low-threshold calcium spike from a hyperpolarized state (see above) and are probably generated by rhythmic oscillations of the inhibitory neurons of the reticular nucleus. The reticular nucleus has the capacity to become a pattern generator for thalamic oscillations, but how it comes to do so paroxysmically in petit mal epilepsy is not certain. The resting tremor of Parkinson's disease also has a frequency of approximately 3–5 Hz, and this too depends upon rhythmic oscillations of thalamic relay neurons that may be engendered by a similar mechanism.

Over the years the thalamus has been the subject of intensive experimental investigation, much of it involved with relay functions and focused on the sensory and motor relay nuclei. The nuclei connected with the association cortex and the involvement of the thalamus in higher cerebral function have been relatively neglected. In recent years the state-dependent functions of the thala- mus have become topics of renewed interest and the biophysical properties of thalamic cells, and the properties of the thalamic network of which they form a part in mediating these functions, are at the forefront of modern thalamic research.

BIBLIOGRAPHY

Bentivoglio, M., & Spreafico, R. (Eds). (1988). *Cellular thalamic mechanisms*. Amsterdam: Ex- cerpta Medica.

Buzsaki, G. (1991). The thalamic clock: emer- gent network properties. *Neuroscience, 41*, 351–64.

Jones, E. G. (1985). *The thalamus*. New York: Plenum.

La Berge, D., & Buchsbaum, M. S. (1990). Positron emission tomographic measurements of pulvinar activity during an attention task. *Journal of Neuroscience, 10*, 613–19.

McCormick, D. A. (1989). Cholinergic and nora- drenergic modulation of thalamocortical pro- cessing. *Trends in Neuroscience, 12*, 215–29.

McCormick, D. A., & von Krosigk, M. (1992). Corticothalamic activation modulates thalamic firing through glutamate "metabotropic" receptors. *Proceedings of the National Academy of Science of the USA, 89*, 2774–8.

Sherman, S. M., & Koch, C. (1986). The control of retinogeniculate transmission in the mam- malian lateral geniculate nucleus. *Experimental Brain Research 62*, 1–20.

Steriade, M., Jones, E. G., & Llinás, R. (1990). *Thalamic oscillations and spindling*. New York: Wiley.

Steriade, M., & Llinás, R. (1988). The functional states of the thalamus and the associated neuronal interplay. *Physiological Review, 68*, 649–742.

E. G. JONES

thiamine deficiency A deficiency of thiamine (vitamin B$_1$) may have a number of consequences. It may result in a form of peripheral neuropathy including beriberi, Wernicke's encephalopathy, pellagra, and confusional states associated with arteriosclerosis in the elderly. In the peripheral neuropathies the symptoms are usually restricted to sensory and motor changes in the periphery of the limbs, the lower limbs being more affected than the upper, although the facial muscles may also be involved. Optic atrophy may also occur. Central cognitive effects may, however, be associated with Wernicke's encephalopathy, which is commonly a result of alcoholism, when it may be known as KORSAKOFF'S SYNDROME. In this case confusion is usually the sign at onset, with limb ataxia and disordered eye movements, followed by a gross disorder of memory for recent events, confabulation, and disorientation. In pellagra, skin lesions are associated with a variety of psychiatric disturbances: neurotic complaints, emotional instability, and depression; in severe cases intellectual deterioration and memory disturbances may also occur.

thrombosis   A thrombosis is an embolus in a blood vessel caused by coagulation of the blood similar, although not strictly equivalent, to a clot. When the thrombosis is mobile within the arterial system, it may travel down the gradually narrowing arteries until it eventually plugs the supply at the point at which it lodges, resulting in a STROKE. The sudden blocking of an artery in this manner is known as *embolism*, although an embolism may equally be caused by a bubble of air, or an embolus of a mass of fatty tissue or sclerotic cells. The result is the same: a loss of blood supply temporarily (if the thrombosis later dislodges) or permanently beyond the point at which the arterial blood supply has been interrupted.

TIA   *See* ISCHEMIA.

tic   Any brief, repeated, and stereotyped movement may be described as a tic, which is therefore an abnormal involuntary movement. Tics may occur without any cause being identified, but may represent a secondary reaction to certain drugs, or may follow ENCEPHALITIS or trauma. Tics also classically occur in GILLES DE LA TOURETTE SYNDROME.

tonic disorders   Tonic disorders are any abnormal states characterized by abnormal muscle tone. Abnormal muscle tone may develop as a direct or indirect consequence of head injury, and is one of the conditions which physiotherapists specializing in neurodisability seek to correct.

Tonic disorders are also associated with unilateral ASOMATOGNOSIA and have been employed by some in explanations of that disorder. This hypothesis depends upon the concept that somatic integrity results from mechanisms which relate to the control of equilibrium and posture. Any imbalance between the visual image and the kinesthetic image which may be distorted by lateralized tonic changes might result in a disturbance of the internal body representation and a rejection of elements of the body as a part of the self. An alternative hypothesis has also considered the imbalance between tonic approach and avoidance reactions, resulting in an abnormal predominance of one of these motor patterns in reaction to environmental stimuli. Neither of these hypotheses is of great contemporary significance.

A rare form of EPILEPSY, *tonic seizures*, involves periods of sustained muscular spasm. Sometimes these brief episodes may be asymmetrical, resulting in slow twisting writhing movements. Various causes have been proposed for these fits, and some have considered them psychogenic. The more severe form of *tonic postural fits*, temporally producing a picture similar to decerebrate rigidity, can be seen in cases of cerebellar tumor, where they should probably not be regarded as epileptic in nature, but transient attacks of decerebrate rigidity.

topectomy   Topectomy is a term for the removal, or surgical disconnection, of a discrete area of the CORTEX, although the term is not commonly used. It occurs in relation to LOBECTOMY, and is strictly the more correct term employed where a removal is less than a complete lobe of the cerebral cortex. However these terms, together with LOBOTOMY, are all used rather loosely to describe a variety of surgical procedures in which an area of cortex is removed or surgically disconnected from either adjacent cortex or from underlying neural centers.

topographical disorders   A striking disorder

that can follow focal brain lesion is the inability to find one's way in familiar surroundings and to learn new paths. More frequently it is found in the context of a general impairment of consciousness (confusional states), intellectual deterioration (dementia), or global amnesia. In some patients the deficit stands out for its purity in a framework of preserved memory and cognitive functions and affords an opportunity to study the relation of topographical orientation to brain organization.

The full-blown picture is easy to diagnose both from the patient's history and clinical observation. While following a familiar route, the patient suddenly discovers he or she is unable to find his or her way, and roams the streets in search of names or landmarks that may help in taking his or her bearings. Sometimes he or she will keep on walking along the road where his or her house is located, realizing that it must be in the neighborhood but unable to recognize it. When the patient is in hospital, it is soon apparent that whenever he or she leaves his or her room, he or she has trouble finding his or her way back, and desperately looks for verbal tags (e.g. the number of his or her room or other landmarks). The problem is that even when these are recognized, the patient may be unable to remember the spatial information they bear, i.e. whether they mean that he or she must go left, right, upstairs, or downstairs. The clinical examination may be complemented by the request to verbally describe a familiar route, paying particular attention to different aspects of the performance, namely what can be recovered from verbal memory, e.g. reciting the stations of the subway, or the names of the towns crossed when driving from home to work (a function which is often preserved), and information that must be retraced from spatial memory, e.g. the turns of the street connecting two places (a function which is lost). Drawing maps of the patient's home or of how the furniture of a room is arranged, or locating places and tracing paths on a blank map are other convenient means of assessing topographical memory (De Renzi, 1982).

Following the seminal paper of Paterson and Zangwill (1945), two discrete though often concomitant disorders have been identified as responsible for route-finding difficulties, namely *topographical agnosia* and *topographical amnesia*. They correspond to the disruption of the abilities that mostly contribute to finding one's bearings: the recognition of buildings, streets, and landmarks that help in localizing a place in a wider spatial context and are endowed with directional value ("if this is the post office, then I must turn to the left"), and the development of a spatial scheme from previous experience which maps the sections of a route and turns them into a mental representation.

A scrutiny of the literature shows that patients suffering either topographical agnosia or topographical amnesia have been reported, though the majority probably suffers from both deficits and it is for the examiner to weigh their respective contribution to route-finding difficulty.

A typical case of topographical agnosia was Pallis's (1955) patient, who lost his bearings in spite of being able to provide accurate verbal descriptions of paths and draw maps of familiar places, because he failed to identify buildings and places. He clearly verbalized his deficit. "In my mind's eye I know exactly where places are, what they look like. I can visualize the square without difficulty, and the streets that come into it . . . It's when I'm out that the trouble starts. My reason tells me that I am in a certain place and yet I don't recognize it . . . My difficulty with buses is to know where to get off." Note that he had no trouble in recognizing buildings or places as belonging to certain categories and could distinguish, for instance, "terraced council houses from detached villas, a living room from an office, a country lane from a main road." What he failed to identify was that they were a particular house, room, or road and consequently he could not attribute any directional value to them. The patient of Whiteley and Warrington (1978) knew the turns required to reach certain place and was able to make use of a schematic map of the route to be followed, yet he lost his bearings because streets, buildings, and other landmarks looked unfamiliar.

A patient of De Renzi and Faglioni (see De Renzi, 1982) had both topographical agnosia and topographical amnesia. This patient failed to recognize the La Scala theater and the Galleria, famous buildings of Milan; even when they were identified by the examiner, he could not find his bearings, as he had forgotten their location with respect to other nearby, well-known buildings of the city.

The nature of topographical agnosia is still a matter of debate. Is it the consequence of defective processing of visual information, which prevents the patient from discriminating the visual features qualifying a place, in the same way as happens with other categories of objects? A few patients with topographical disorientation have been investigated in sufficient detail to permit an assessment of their fine-grained perceptual analysis to be made. Some of them were also found to be impaired in recognizing other categories of objects, but others were not. It is difficult to relate this performance to the topographical deficit.

Alternatively, the deficit may be conceived as being mnestic rather than perceptual, recognition failing because of the inability to retrieve the mental image of specific buildings and places. Whitely and Warrington's (1978) patient failed to recognize familiar buildings, streets, and landmarks, but performed correctly on a series of perceptual, spatial, and memory tests. The authors speculated that he suffered from a selective visual memory deficit concerning building features, and found some support for their thesis in his poor scores on a test of unknown building recognition. The evidence, however, is somewhat equivocal, since the recognition of well-known buildings was in the normal range.

It is worth stressing that topographical agnosia makes different demands on the patient than object agnosia, in that what is requested is not the identification of a class, but of a unique exemplar of a class. In this respect, it is more like PROSOPA-GNOSIA, in which the failure does not concern the recognition of male or female faces in general, but of the face of a specific person. Topographical disorientation and prosopagnosia often occur together in the same patient, although not with the same degree of severity, and the question remains whether the coincidence reflects the disruption of a common mechanism, or rather the close proximity of the neural substrates underlying the respective abilities.

Probably more common are those patients who recognize familiar places, but are unable to learn or to retrieve from long-term memory the spatial schema that represents, in abstract terms, the route one must cover to arrive at a place. For instance, to go to the doctor's office, first I must turn right, then follow the corridor until the second door, turn left, go upstairs, etc. This memory is integrated by the recall of landmarks, e.g. seeing a clock on the wall means that the next room is the one being looked for, although their orientation value may also be lost. Whenever

Meyer's patient (De Renzi, 1982) had to return to his room he lost his bearings, because at any choice point he did not know whether to go left, right, upstairs, or downstairs. Once he walked from the main floor to the basement instead of going to the first floor. When he eventually entered the room, he recognized it not from its spatial arrangement, but because he noticed some distinguishing feature (e.g. the black beard of his roommate). When he was taken to his own neighborhood, he desperately looked for familiar landmarks, but recognition of them failed to provide him with directional cues. The independence of spatial memory from other aspects of visual memory is attested by patient no. 5 of Aimard and others (1980), who got lost in his apartment and opened the wrong doors in the corridor in search of a particular room, but as soon as he saw it, he recognized it.

Topographical disorientation, if the disease has stabilized, tends to recover with the passage of time. Generally, patients will first improve in their ability to find their bearings in surroundings that were familiar before their illness, while new routes long remain a problem. A trick they use to overcome their difficulty is to rely on verbal descriptions of the itinerary and on salient visual cues.

Pathology and neuroradiological evidence is available in a sufficient number of cases to permit the localization of the lesion responsible for topographical disorientation. The pertinent literature has been reviewed by De Renzi (1982) and Landis and others (1986). In patients who came to autopsy the lesion was found to involve the posterior cortical areas bilaterally or was limited to the right hemisphere. The brunt of damage was borne by the lateral temporo-parieto-occipital cortex or by the medial occipito-temporal cortex. A larger body of evidence has been marshalled with the introduction of neuroimaging techniques, which have confirmed the dominant role played by the right hemisphere. In vascular patients, infarcts in the territory of the posterior cerebral artery are by far the most common correlate of topographical disorientation (Landis et al., 1986).

A peculiar symptom that has occasionally been found in the context of topographical disorders, but which can also appear independently of them, is disorientation for place. This consists of a patient who, though able to identify his or her present whereabouts, maintains that they are located in different geographical areas (Fisher, 1982). The patient's fanciful responses may change from day to day and assume the features of a true confabulation, strictly confined, however, to spatial orientation and not extending to temporal and personal identification. The subjective conviction that a familiar place or person has been duplicated was first described by Pick (1903) in a patient with senile dementia under the name of "reduplicative amnesia," and has since been reported in patients with focal brain lesions. Confabulation is often accompanied by amnesic deficits, but may outlive them, a finding which has led to speculation on its metaphorical, compensatory significance; it has been attributed to frontal lobe damage, although the lesion is more frequently in the right posterior areas.

DISORDERS OF SPATIAL MEMORY

Insight into topographical disorientation is provided by the administration of spatial memory tests, which allow an analysis to be made of the deficit and its constituent components. The tests have also been given to large samples of patients with focal brain lesion, with the aim of unravelling subclinical deficits of spatial memory and garnering evidence on the relation they bear to damage in particular cerebral areas.

A first distinction, analogous to that which holds for verbal memory, is between short-term and long-term spatial memory. Short-term memory stores a limited amount of visuospatial information for brief periods of time to permit its use in mental operations carried out as soon as data have been processed by the perceptual system. It is tested by assessing the maximal number of spatial positions the subject is able to retain and reproduce immediately after their presentation (spatial span). A suitable test is the Corsi block test, where nine cubes, glued on a board in an irregular arrangement, are tapped by the examiner in sequences of increasing length that the patient is asked to reproduce. Clinical evidence that a few patients with topographical disorientation have short-term memory impairment comes from the observation of their inability to recall the position of an object if it is removed from sight for a few seconds, e.g. after folding the page of the newspaper, they are no longer able to find where the article they were reading is located (De Renzi et al., 1982). It has been speculated

that the inability to keep visuospatial information in the short-term memory store prevents its consolidation in the long-term store and is responsible for the route-finding difficulty. This inference, however, is questionable, because the relation of the short-term deficit to topographical disorientation is far from consistent, as shown by two patients, with an exceedingly poor span of 2.5 on the cube test and no difficulty in route-finding, and by patients with topographical disorientation and normal spatial span (De Renzi, 1982).

When the Corsi cube test was given to unselected samples of patients with focal hemispheric damage, spatial span was found to be reduced in patients with visual field defects, independent of the side of lesion (De Renzi et al., 1977a). Though mild, the deficit was genuine and could not be attributed to visuospatial disorders, such as neglect, mislocalization, etc., because right brain-damaged patients were not impaired relative to controls, when the cubes bore a digit on their upper surfaces and the tapping was verbally guided by presenting orally a string of digits.

The lack of hemispheric asymmetry in short-term memory contrasts with the selective impairment shown by patients with damage to the posterior areas of the right brain in learning a supra-span spatial sequence. When the Corsi cube test was given, requiring the reproduction of a sequence two cubes longer than the span and repeating the task until the criterion of three errorless runs was attained, the stable acquisition of a supra-span string proved to be remarkably difficult for patients with right posterior brain damage (De Renzi et al., 1977a).

Another test sensitive to long-term spatial memory disorders is the stepping-stone maze, first introduced in neuropsychology by Milner (1965). The subject is presented with a board bearing a 10 × 10 array of bolt-heads and is requested to discover a path going from a starting point to an end point, both identifiable on the board. He must proceed from bolt-head to bolt-head with a stylus which produces a loud click when a wrong bolt-head is touched and informs the subject that he or she must return to the previous bolt-head and make a different choice. Learning takes place by trial and error and is achieved when all the turns of the path are memorized. This test was given to patient H. M., who, following the bilateral resection of the temporal lobes, had a profound anterograde amnesia that involved the inability to find his bearings in surroundings known after the operation. He was completely unable to learn the path (Milner, 1965). Particularly relevant to the issue of topographical disorders is the performance of M. A. (De Renzi et al., 1977b), a patient with a pure form of route-finding disability, who failed to learn the path after 275 trials. Group studies have provided evidence for the existence of a circuit involving the hippocampus and the parietal lobe of the right hemisphere, specialized in spatial memory performance. Patients with right temporal ablation that included the hippocampus were found to be impaired on the visual stylus maze (Milner, 1965). Right frontal patients also scored poorly, but their deficit appeared to be more dependent on their tendency to break the rules and perseverate than on a true deficit of spatial memory. In Milner's series, patients with parietal ablation were too few to permit conclusive inferences, but they were largely represented in other samples and provided evidence that the maze performance is specifically disrupted by a lesion involving the right parieto-occipital areas.

Memory for position is another aspect of spatial memory that has been investigated in brain-damaged patients. It has been claimed that the location a target occupies in space is part of the contextual information that a normal subject automatically records when he tries to memorize the target, and that performance does not improve if he focuses on position. Smith and Milner (1981) tested incidental recall of location in patients submitted to partial lobectomies for the relief of epilepsy. Toys representing objects were laid down on a grid and the patients were asked to estimate the cost of the corresponding objects. After a delay, they were requested to recall as many toys as they could and were then given the toys and asked to put them in the original positions they occupied on the grid. Patients with left temporal lobectomies were impaired on toy recall but not on toy location, while patients with right temporal lobectomies showed the opposite pattern and the deficit was proportional to the extent of hippocampus removal. Frontal patients had a normal performance.

Memory for position has also been investigated in global amnesics with the aim of testing the hypothesis that they suffer from an inability to automatically process contextual information and

that it is to this defective encoding that the target information amnesia must be ascribed. Since memory for position belongs to contextual information, two predictions were made: (1) that in amnesics spatial memory is poorer than target memory, and (2) that they differ from normal subjects in benefiting from intentional encoding of spatial information. Results have been contradictory. The greater impairment of spatial memory relative to target memory has found support in some experiments, but not in others (MacAndrews et al., 1993), possibly dependent on the paradigm used and the etiology of the amnesia. The improvement with intentional encoding has also not been consistent (MacAndrews et al., 1993). By and large, the evidence in favor of the special status of spatial memory in amnesics is not sufficiently robust to corroborate the context memory deficit hypothesis.

The testing procedures so far considered are intended to assess the ability to acquire new spatial data and the findings are therefore relevant to the study of anterograde memory. Retrograde memory, i.e. the retrieval of information acquired before the onset of disease, is notoriously more difficult to evaluate with a standardized procedure. This is because previous experiences differ across subjects and there is therefore no common background of knowledge. For verbal and visual remote memories the problem has been tackled by questionnaires about public events, pictures of famous faces, and archival recordings of famous voices that are presumed to have been popular in a particular period and then to have disappeared. For spatial memory, geographical facts have been used to assess the ability to recover knowledge acquired before the disease. For instance, Benton and others (1974) required patients with unilateral brain damage to name the state in which a city was located, the direction in which the subject would travel in going from one city to another, and to mark on a blank map of the USA the location of cities and states. No hemispheric asymmetry emerged from this study and only the last part of the test was found to be sensitive to brain damage. The problem with geographical tests is that the score is likely to be influenced not only by the educational background of the subjects, but also by the extent of their travel experience, which is a factor difficult to control. The advantage that can accrue from their use is probably limited to the investigation of patients with retrograde memory deficits, but even in these cases it remains to be ascertained what relation geographical knowledge bears to the inability to find one's way in familiar surroundings.

BIBLIOGRAPHY

Aimard, G., Vighetto, A., Confavreux, C., & Devic, M. (1981). La désorientation spatiale. *Revue Neurologique, 137*, 97–137.

Benton, A. L., Levin, H. S., & Van Allen, M. W. (1974). Geographic orientation in patients with unilateral cerebral disease. *Neuropsycologia, 12*, 183–91.

De Renzi, E. (1982). *Disorders of space exploration and cognition.* Chichester: Wiley.

De Renzi, E., Faglioni, P., & Previdi, P. (1977a). Spatial memory and hemispheric locus of lesion. *Cortex, 5*, 274–84.

De Renzi, E., Faglioni, P., & Villa, P. (1977b). Topographical amnesia. *Journal of Neurology, Neurosurgery and Psychiatry, 40*, 498–505.

Fisher, C. M. (1982). Disorientation for place. *Archives of Neurology, 39*, 33–6.

Landis, T., Cummings, G. L., Benson, D. F., & Palmer, E. P. (1986). Loss of topographical familiarity. An environmental agnosia. *Archives of Neurology, 43*, 132–6.

MacAndrews, S. B. G., Mayes, A. R., & Jones, G. V. (1993). Spatial memory in amnesics: evidence from Korsakoff subjects. *Cortex, 29*, 235–49.

Milner, B. (1965). Visually-guided maze learning in man: effects of bilateral hippocampal, bilateral frontal, and unilateral cerebral lesions. *Neuropsychologia, 3*, 317–38.

Pallis, C. A. (1955). Impaired identification for faces and places with agnosia for colours. *Journal of Neurology, Neurosurgery and Psychiatry, 18*, 218–24.

Paterson, A., & Zangwill, O. L. (1945). A case of topographical disorientation associated with a unilateral cerebral lesion. *Brain, 68*, 188–211.

Pick, A. (1903). On reduplicative paramnesia. *Brain, 26*, 242–67.

Smith, M. L., & Milner, B. (1981). The role of the right hippocampus in the recall of spatial location. *Neuropsychologia, 19*, 781–93.

Whiteley, A. M., & Warrington, E. K. (1978). Selective impairment of topographical memory: a single case study. *Journal of Neurology, Neurosurgery and Psychiatry, 41*, 575–8.

ENNIO DE RENZI

torticollis Torticollis (more properly *spasmodic torticollis*) is a rare condition in which the head is pulled and held turned to either the left or the right by prolonged spasms of contraction of the sternomastoid and trapezius muscles on the appropriate side. The sustained nature of the abnormal posture differentiates this from a TIC. As such, it is one of the DYSTONIAS and may be of unknown cause and without other neurological problems. The onset is insidious, the progression slow, and the outcome is extremely variable. There are arguments and evidence in favor of both a psychogenic and an organic cause of the disorder, which may be treated as either a psychiatric or neurological condition. It seems likely that the condition has an organic, possibly biochemical basis which has yet to be discovered, but which is only precipitated in certain predisposed individuals as a result of emotional or other psychological factors. The range of treatments includes physical therapy, drug therapy, systematic relaxation, psychotherapy, and neurosurgery.

Tourette syndrome *See* GILLES DE LA TOURETTE SYNDROME.

toxicology Neuropsychological toxicology is the study of the psychological effects of poisons on the central nervous system. The scope of the area is broad and, as a developing field, difficult to define precisely. The topic encompasses at least three distinct domains: (1) occupational and environmental neurotoxicology: the study of the effects of exposure to substances at work and incidental exposure to toxins in the environment; (2) the neuropsychology of substance abuse: this area includes the study of ALCOHOLISM, and the effects of abuse of drugs and solvents; (3) psychopharmacology and drug neurotoxicology (drug intoxication): the investigation of both short-term and long-term psychological effects of pharmaceuticals.

Examples of substances which can cause intoxication of the nervous system are shown in Table 18. Although there is a wide variety of substances which cause intoxication, only a selection have been shown to produce neuropsychological changes which outlast the acute effects. This is not a uniformly well-researched field and it is

Table 18   Some representative toxins of the nervous system.

Metals: aluminum, barium, bismuth, cadmium, cobalt, lead, lithium, manganese, mercury, thallium
Arsenic, bromide, cyanide
Methyl alcohol
Organophosphorous and organochlorine insecticides
Phosphorylated phenols (industrial lubricants)
Solvents: carbon disulphide, carbon tetrachloride, chloroform, methyl n-butyl ketone, n-hexane, styrene, toluene,
   trichloroethylene
Drugs:
   Central stimulants: amphetamines, cocaine
   Psychedelic drugs: LSD, mescaline, marijuana
   Sedatives and hypnotics: barbiturates, benzodiazepines, alcohol
   Narcotic analgesics: morphine, heroin, and other opiates
   Antiepileptic drugs: phenytoin
   Other psychotherapeutic drugs: chlorpromazine
   Chemotherapy: vincristine

---

likely that further work will extend the appreciation of the neuropsychological significance of toxins. For example, over 60,000 chemicals are in common use in industry, but only a small number of these have been studied extensively. The effects of some toxins are confined to the peripheral nervous system. For others the issue of whether or not they produce lasting psychological changes is controversial. Some are well known to produce neuropsychological impairment as a result of a large exposure, but it remains a matter of debate whether prolonged exposure to small amounts of the substance leads to measurable impairment.

Exogenous versus endogenous toxins Exogenous neurotoxins originate from outside the human body; however, there are substances occurring naturally within the body which are also neurotoxic. An example of an endogenous neurotoxin is the neurotransmitter glutamate, which is widely distributed in the brain. Glutamate is released in high concentrations after ischemic brain damage (i.e. damage caused by lack of blood flow) and it is neurotoxic in these concentrations. Such endogenous neurotoxins may play an important role in some forms of brain damage, and their significance is an issue of current research.

Acute versus chronic intoxication A distinction is commonly made between acute and chronic intoxication, but it is often not as clear as one would wish. Some confusion arises because the terms "acute" and "chronic" are applied to both the duration of exposure to a neurotoxin and the duration of any effects. Acute exposure results from a single, usually large dose of a poison, while chronic exposure refers to repeated intake, often of small amounts, over an extended period of time. Acute effects are those seen immediately after exposure and which later subside over a period of, at most, a few weeks, while chronic effects are persistent. A further difficulty with this distinction lies in defining precisely which neuropsychological effects persist. Both acute and chronic exposure may lead to acute and chronic effects. A particularly insidious situation arises when exposure does not give rise to any acute problems but leads some time later to chronic effects. The cause of neuropsychological change may be very difficult to establish definitively under such circumstances.

Reversibility Reversibility refers to the potential for recovery of function after cessation of exposure, and is part of the issue of whether the neuropsychological impairment is acute or chronic. After exposure ends the acute effects of the substance will subside more or less quickly. If there is dependence on the substance there may follow a period of withdrawal, during which psychological functions are obviously impaired. However, after these two processes are complete there will also typically be a longer period during which there is some recovery of function. Well-designed studies of recovery of function after exposure to toxins are few and far between, and thus relatively little is known concerning the long-term reversibility of the effects of many toxic substances.

Susceptibility There is a substantial degree of

variation between individuals in their functional responses to similar exposures. It is well recognized in psychopharmacology that individuals may require either larger or smaller doses of a drug to produce the same effect. Furthermore, serious adverse reactions may be seen in some individuals and not in others, for example, in allergy to penicillin. Individual variability is also a feature of other neurotoxins, and is related to differences in absorption, distribution, metabolism, and excretion of the agent. Individual differences in metabolism are a particularly important source of such variability. In some instances there may be an established inherited inability to metabolize a particular substance, e.g. in WILSON'S DISEASE copper metabolism is abnormal and the metal accumulates in toxic amounts. Changes in metabolism also account for drug tolerance whereby some drugs require increasingly large doses to achieve the same effect. It follows that similar levels of exposure to a toxin may lead to much more pronounced neuropsychological effects in some individuals than in others. The idea of inherent individual variability in the response to neurotoxins is important and not always properly appreciated.

ASSESSMENT

Neuropsychological assessment has three contributions to make to understanding the effects of intoxication: monitoring psychological changes in acute intoxication; establishing whether there are lasting effects; and assessment of individual cases, including consideration of the impact on daily living.

Most neuropsychological work has focused on the chronic effects of intoxication. Since this concerns a very heterogeneous group of substances it is probably misleading to propose that a single battery of tests is appropriate for assessment in all conditions. Some batteries have been devised for use in particular settings, for example, the Pittsburgh Occupational Exposures Test battery (POET) consists of a selection of neuropsychological measures designed for use in cases of industrial exposure. Insofar as there is a common picture, it is that of the effects of diffuse brain damage. Typical findings are memory difficulties, slowing on psychomotor tasks, problems of attention and concentration, affective disorders (usually depression), and subtle changes in personality.

Neuropsychological assessment is of particular importance because it may be the only way in which brain damage can be established. Techniques such as EEG and brain scanning are often insensitive to the effects of mild to moderate diffuse brain damage due to intoxication. Neuropsychological assessment therefore plays a central part in detection of the adverse effects of toxic exposure. Neuropsychological evidence has correspondingly come to have an increasingly important role in litigation after industrial or environmental exposure. As in other areas, the use of neuropsychological test results as evidence of organic damage has potential pitfalls: lack of sensitivity of tests; lack of specificity to particular conditions; and problems of motivation or simulation in the person who is assessed. The effects of some toxins may not be obvious on conventional neuropsychological tests, but become apparent only when particularly demanding tasks are used.

EXPOSURE TO METALS

Many of the heavy metals are highly neurotoxic. Concern about environmental exposure to these toxins has increased considerably in recent years. Metals may be excreted only very slowly; for example, cadmium has a half-life in the body of 10 to 30 years, and thus levels may accumulate over a lifetime.

Aluminum Generalized intellectual impairment has been described as a result of exposure to aluminum through renal dialysis. Other problems reported include personality change, seizures, dysarthria, and motor deficits of varying severity.

Arsenic This well-known poison is in wide use in the pharmaceutical and agricultural industry. Arsenic can cause peripheral neuropathy (i.e. loss of peripheral nerve function, resulting in numbness and weakness). It is usually assumed that arsenic may also affect the central nervous system.

Barium Barium is recognized as being neurotoxic, but little appears to be known about the neuropsychological effects of exposure.

Bismuth This metal has been used as a treatment for bowel disorders, and has been shown to result in damage to the central nervous system. Milder symptoms include depression, anxiety, irritability, and tremulousness. In more severe cases intoxication results in confusion, myoclonic jerks, dysarthria, and apraxia.

Cadmium Chronic exposure to cadmium in industry has been linked to impairment on measures of attention, memory, and psychomotor speed.

Lead One of the most widely studied heavy metals, the neuropsychology of LEAD POISONING is described in a separate entry.

Manganese Chronic exposure to manganese can lead to Parkinsonism (mainly exhibited as rigidity and bradykinesia) and generalized intellectual impairment.

Mercury Mercury is highly neurotoxic and can produce widespread nervous-system damage, including narrowing of the visual fields, ataxia, dysarthria, tremor, and intellectual deficits.

VOLATILE SUBSTANCE EXPOSURE

Exposure to volatile substances may occur both through incidental exposure in industry and deliberate abuse of solvents. These form a heterogeneous group of substances, but most solvents are volatile, lipophilic (fat-loving), and have central nervous depressant effects.

Industrial exposure to solvents

Industrial workers may encounter a wide variety of solvents, for example, in boat-building, dry cleaning, painting, printing, and shoe manufacturing. In Scandinavian countries there has been widespread concern that exposure may have toxic effects on the nervous system. The idea of a syndrome of organic changes caused by solvent exposure became established in Scandinavia in the 1970s. However, studies in other countries have sometimes failed to find effects of prolonged exposure to solvents in an industrial setting. There does appear to be a general agreement that, at least in a proportion of the population exposed, solvents produce organic damage. A report from the World Health Organization in 1985 defined two types of disorder due to long-term exposure to solvents: an organic affective disorder and a chronic toxic encephalopathy. The first is marked by depression, irritability, and loss of interest in everyday life. This condition is usually believed to be reversible. The second type of disorder is indicated by fatigability, poor memory, concentration difficulties, loss of initiative, and personality change. The report also distinguished a mild form of the latter syndrome which was usually reversible, and a severe form in which impairment was usually irreversible.

VOLATILE SUBSTANCE ABUSE

The main solvents in glues which are abused for recreational purposes are toluene and acetone. A wide variety of other substances also contain abusable solvents, including dry-cleaning fluids, lighter fluids, nail-polish removers, aerosol fly sprays, hair sprays, typewriter correction fluids, and petrol. Review of the literature on volatile substance abuse suggests that evidence of permanent brain damage in abusers is inconclusive. The literature on solvent abuse is typical of the literature on substance abuse in general. There are isolated reports of clear neuropsychological impairment, but group studies often find little if any difference between users and controls. Studies in this area have often suffered from methodological problems. In part, the failure to find effects of abuse may be because group studies have tended to concentrate on relatively young users who do not have a prolonged history of abuse. In general, when group studies have included individuals with a protracted history of substance abuse, more convincing evidence of psychological impairment has been forthcoming. Thus, for example, toluene abuse has been shown to lead to cerebellar atrophy. It is noteworthy that cognitive and affective disorders found in solvent abusers are often attributed to premorbid factors, while similar disorders observed in industrial workers are attributed directly to the effects of exposure.

Effects of specific solvents

There is a general consensus that the following solvents produce organic damage.

N-hexane and *methyl n-butyl ketone* share the same metabolite and cause sensory, motor, and optic neuropathy.

Toluene exposure is associated with cerebellar dysfunction and cortical atrophy; the ataxia associated with cerebellar damage tends to persist.

Carbon disulphide can cause cortical dysfunction, including psychiatric and personality disorders. It also causes reversible peripheral sensory and motor neuropathy.

Trichloroethylene can cause persistent anesthesia of sensory nerves of the face, mouth, and lips (trigeminal nerve changes), which may spread to the motor nerves.

Future work may well add further substances to this list, and will characterize the psychological effects of exposure to solvents more precisely.

DRUG INTOXICATION

All drugs are toxic to a greater or lesser extent; however, neuropsychological interest focuses on drugs with established effects on the central nervous system.

Drugs of abuse

Apart from alcohol and solvents, the most commonly abused substances are stimulants (amphetamine, cocaine), narcotics (morphine, heroin), psychedelics (LSD), cannabis, and sedatives (barbiturates, benzodiazepines). A detailed description of the classification and acute effects of psychoactive drugs is contained in Julien (1991). There have been few well controlled studies of the neuropsychological effects of chronic drug abuse, and in general, research has not clearly established that abuse of single classes of drugs leads to neuropsychological impairment. This may be because these substances are not individually toxic; on the other hand, it may reflect the difficulty of carrying out research in this area. Most drug abuse is polydrug abuse, and it is therefore difficult to determine the toxicity of specific drugs. The evidence that polydrug abuse is associated with neuropsychological impairment is more convincing than for abuse of single classes of drugs.

The question of whether abuse of psychoactive drugs leads to neuropsychological impairment thus remains open. It is nonetheless the case that there are clinical reports of profound deterioration after prolonged drug use. Such reports may derive from a number of factors: assessment during withdrawal or recovery from acute effects, use of drugs adulterated with toxic substances, failure to allow for premorbid level of functioning, a history of head injury or alcohol abuse, and a history of poor nutrition and health. In the past few years the issue of poor health in this population has come into prominence, and particularly the risk of AIDS among intravenous drug abusers. It is possible that some earlier reports of neuropsychological deterioration in this population reflected unrecognized AIDS-related cognitive impairment.

Patterns of drug abuse are subject to changes with fashion. In recent years there has been a growth in the supply of "designer drugs" which are synthesized to imitate existing drugs of abuse. The lack of proper control over the manufacture of these drugs constitutes an additional hazard. In one incident, users of a synthetic heroin substance MPTP developed irreversible characteristics of advanced PARKINSON'S DISEASE: the drug was found inadvertently to contain a substance which destroyed dopamine-producing neurons.

Drugs of prescription

A wide variety of commonly prescribed drugs have been suspected of producing neuropsychological changes.

The tricyclic *antidepressants* can have neurological side effects, including tremor and blurred vision. However, there is no consistent evidence that they produce neuropsychological impairment.

Antipsychotic drugs, often called "major tranquillizers," are prescribed to control disturbed behavior. When they are administered to alleviate the symptoms of chronic schizophrenia their use may be long-term. Extrapyramidal symptoms are the most troublesome side effects of these drugs. They consist of Parkinson-like symptoms including tremor, dystonia (abnormal face and body movements), and akathisia (restlessness); a further consequence can be tardive dyskinesia (often seen as involuntary movements affecting the face). The Parkinsonian symptoms usually abate when the drug is withdrawn, while tardive dyskinesia may be irreversible. Little is known concerning neuropsychological changes accompanying these motor side effects.

Anticonvulsant drugs prescribed to control epilepsy are often taken for very long periods, if not permanently. Several common antiepileptic agents, including carbamazepine, phenytoin, and sodium valproate, have been suspected of producing impairment in memory and attention. The evidence for lasting neuropsychological effects is strongest for phenytoin, which has been associated with deficits of attention, motor performance, and speeded information processing.

Anxiolytics and *hypnotics*, especially the benzodiazepines, which include valium and librium, are very widely prescribed for their anti-anxiety and sleep-inducing properties. It is recognized that use of these drugs produces an acute impairment of memory and attention. However, apart from isolated cases, there is no consistent evidence for chronic neuropsychological effects which outlast withdrawal.

Lithium is an alkali metal which is used in the treatment of manic-depressive illness. High doses of lithium are associated with acute neurotoxic effects including dysarthria and ataxia. Lithium has been suspected of producing memory impairment, but, the evidence for this remains inconclusive.

The use of *cardiovascular* antihypertensive drugs has been suspected of resulting in memory impairment. Confirmation of neuropsychological effects of these drugs awaits further study. The specific neuropsychological effects of the drugs used in *chemotherapy* are difficult to disentangle from the effects of the disease process itself, and of other treatments, including radiation therapy, which are used in parallel. It is known that vincristine produces peripheral and autonomic neuropathy. Methotrexate is suspected of delaying intellectual development when used as a prophylactic therapy in childhood leukemia.

BIBLIOGRAPHY

Brust, J. C. M. (1993). *Neurological aspects of substance abuse*. Oxford: Butterworth.

Goodman, A. G., Rall, T. W., Nies, A. S. & Taylor, P. (Eds). (1990). *Goodman and Gilman's The pharmacological therapeutics*. New York: Pergamon.

Hartman, D. E. (1995). *Neuropsychological toxicology*, 2nd edn. New York: Plenum.

Hawkins, K. E. (1990). Occupational neurotoxicology: some neuropsychological issues and challenges. *Journal of Clinical and Experimental Neuropsychology, 12,* 664–80.

Julien, R. M. (1991). *A primer of drug action*, 6th edn. New York: Freeman.

Weiss, B. (1983). Behavioral toxicology and environmental health science. *American Psychologist, November*, 1174–87.

J. T. L. WILSON

transcortical aphasia *See* APHASIA.

tumor Tumors, more properly *intracranial tumors*, are neoplasms occurring within the skull, although the term may be extended a little to include any space-occupying lesion of the brain and its surrounding tissues.

There are a variety of forms of tumor, but their effects depend on a number of general factors: speed of growth, invasion of brain tissue, pressure effects, displacement effects, as well as physiological and biochemical disturbances. Different types of tumor grow at different speeds, with the slowest developing at a pace which may mean that they go undetected, producing no functional disturbance, over a period of many years. Indeed, they may never be detected during the life of the individual. A general principle is that the slower the growth of the tumor, the less its functional impact, as the brain presumably has a greater opportunity to accommodate to the changes which are occurring. A slow-growing tumor will have less impact than a fast-growing tumor when the tumors are of equal mass.

Not all tumors invade neural tissue; some grow in the supporting tissues or in the meninges or blood vessels. In general, noninvasive tumors have less impact than invasive tumors, although this effect is not as striking as might be anticipated. The most important processes related to the development of tumors are the consequent changes in intracranial pressure and in the displacement of brain structures. As tumors are space-occupying lesions, they tend to produce an increase in pressure within the skull, resulting in acute disturbances of consciousness and behavior, and headache and sickness, which may be the first signs which bring the tumor to medical attention. Displacement effects will depend on the precise location of the tumor and its mass, but will be in general to compress areas of the brain and produce neuronal stretching, even at some distance from the tumor. Both raised pressure and displacement may result in *tentorial herniation* by which part of the brain is forced past the sharp edges of the tentorium, the flange of the meninges which runs between the cerebrum and the CEREBELLUM, with further neurological consequences.

Tumors are the classic lesions, together with penetrating missile wounds, which produce clearly defined focal lesions in the cerebral cortex, and the consequent neuropsychological effects naturally depend upon the site and extent of the lesion. Whether different types of tumor produce differential neuropsychological effects is difficult to determine, as different types of tumor grow at different rates and have different characteristic distributions over the cerebral cortex. Comparative studies comparing types of tumor are therefore difficult to construct, these factors producing methodologically confounding effects in any comparison.

The principal types of tumor are ASTROCY-TOMAS, GLIOMAS, HEMATOMAS, and MENING-IOMAS, although there are also *angiomas* and *hemangioblastomas*, which are tumors of the blood vessels, and *adenomas* (usually as PITUITARY TUMORS), as well as rarer types. In addition secondary tumors, METASTASES, often associated with primary tumors in the lung or breast, can occur in the brain, when they are usually multiple and diffusely distributed through the cerebrum.

Tumors are usually treated by radiotherapy or by surgical excision, in the latter case incidentally generating very precise information about both the nature of the tumor and the extent of the lesion which exists following the surgery. Even when surgical treatment is not undertaken, the identity of the tumor may be ascertained by brain *biopsy*, in which a small sample is taken from the tumor site. While lesions may apparently be clearly described during a neurosurgical proced-ure, the clinical neuropsychologist should also bear in mind the possible secondary disruption to more distant areas of the brain during the surgical approach to the tumor site, and the effects of retraction of parts of the brain during surgery.

J. GRAHAM BEAUMONT

Turner's syndrome Turner's syndrome is a sex-linked genetic abnormality in which only a single X chromosome is present (XO). It is associated with female gender, short stature, ptosis, NYSTAGMUS, a webbed neck, undeveloped breasts, heart defects, and sterility.

As individuals with Turner's syndrome have reduced levels of both testosterone and estrogen from and before birth, their case is often cited as an example of the importance of early hormonal influences on normal development of the brain. However, the reason why these abnormal influen-ces should produce the specific psychological abnormalities they do is unclear.

Neuropsychologically, individuals with Turner's syndrome show deficits in general intel-lectual function, particularly in spatial construc-tion tasks, as shown by the block design and object assembly subtests of the Wechsler intelligence scales. They may show similar deficits on tasks of spatial and figural retention and route following, as well as showing more general evidence of CONSTRUCTIONAL APRAXIA. Verbal and reading abilities may be significantly superior to these spatial abilities, and the neuropsychological deficit may be characterized as a deficit in percep-tion of extrapersonal space. It has been suggested that the pattern of deficits shown is parallel to the effects of a right parietal lobe lesion.

U

ulegyria Ulegyria is an abnormality arising during the process of neural growth and development. When the cerebral CORTEX is subject to destructive processes such as HYPOXIA or IS-CHEMIA later than 30 weeks of gestational age, death of cerebral tissues may occur with proliferation of glial cells, scar tissue formation, and sclerosis. These processes result in a characteristic shrunken and firm cortex, which may be associated with cognitive and behavioral abnormality, depending on the location and extent of the ulegyria.

uncinate fit Uncinate fits (or *uncinate attacks*) are a form of EPILEPSY which begin with an olfactory or gustatory aura which may be followed by automatic movements of chewing, tasting, or smacking the lips. The attack may or may not end in a generalized convulsion. This a form of complex partial epilepsy, or temporal lobe epilepsy, which results from a lesion in or near the temporal lobes; in this case the lesion is presumed to be in the uncus, which is an area of the pyriform cortex at the anterior end of the hippocampal gyrus on the medial surface of the temporal lobe.

unilateral neglect   *See* NEGLECT.

urinary incontinence   The inability to control emptying of the bladder is a common consequence of severe head injury and a feature of many neurological diseases. The neural pathways concerning bladder function (and sexual function, with which it is closely related) ascend and descend in the lateral columns of the spinal cord, and may be affected in traumatic paraplegia, MULTIPLE SCLEROSIS, FRIEDREICH'S ATAXIA, and spinal cord tumors, among other neurological conditions. Control of the urinary sphincters may also be affected by lesions in the superior FRONTAL LOBE, the midbrain, and the PONS. DEMENTIA, PARKINSON'S DISEASE, and STROKE are all conditions which may result in incontinence of urine. Sedation or confusion may also be associated with loss of bladder control, and loss of the sensation of a distended bladder or of urinary flow may also impair the patient's ability to maintain control. There are many other physical causes of urinary incontinence, including urinary infections, diabetes, and fecal impaction, to which neurologically disabled individuals may be prone.

V

vegetative state Vegetative state is classically defined as absence of function in the cerebral cortex as judged behaviorally. Patients in this condition have spontaneous heartbeat and respiration. Their eyes open spontaneously and they have sleep–wake cycles. They may show reflexive movements. They do not speak but they may grunt or groan. There is an absence of psychologically meaningful responses. A more recent definition provided by the American Medical Association Council on Scientific Affairs (1990) is "a condition in which the body cyclically awakens and sleeps, but expresses no behavioral or cerebral metabolic evidence of possessing cognitive function or of being able to respond in a learned manner to external events and stimuli."

A recently proposed set of criteria for the diagnosis of vegetative state (Multi-Society Task Force on PVS, 1994) are as follows: (1) no evidence of awareness of self or environment and an inability to interact with others; (2) no evidence of sustained, reproducible, purposeful, or voluntary behavioral responses to visual, auditory, tactile, or noxious stimuli; (3) no evidence of language comprehension or expression; (4) intermittent wakefulness manifested by the presence of sleep–wake cycles; (5) sufficiently preserved hypothalamic and brain-stem autonomic functions to permit survival with medical and nursing care; (6) bowel and bladder incontinence; and (7) variably preserved cranial nerve reflexes (pupillary, oculocephalic, corneal, vestibulo-ocular, and gag) and spinal reflexes. They describe the distinguishing feature of the vegetative state as being an irregular but cyclic state of circadian sleeping and waking unaccompanied by any behaviorally detectable expression of self-awareness, specific recognition of external stimuli, or consistent evidence of attention or intention or learned responses.

An earlier set of criteria for defining the vegeta-

tive state patient were put forward by the Japan Neurosurgical Society in 1972 (cited by Fujiwara et al., 1993). They describe the diagnosis of vegetative state as being appropriate for an individual who has led a meaningful daily life prior to brain injury and is able to satisfy all of the following six requirements for more than three months after brain injury: (1) unable to move without assistance; (2) unable to ingest food without assistance; (3) presence of urinary or fecal incontinence; (4) inability to recognize objects even though sometimes traced with the eyes; (5) cannot produce intelligible speech even when vocalization is possible; and (6) failure to respond to even simple instructions such as to open the eyes or grasp a hand.

The report of the House of Lords Select Committee on Medical Ethics (1994) noted (p. 34) that review of the literature indicated possibly significant variations in diagnostic criteria and the report calls for the development of a commonly accepted definition of persistent vegetative state (p. 53), as well as a code of practice relating to its management.

Causes

Vegetative state can occur as the result of acute injury to the brain, whether through traumatic or nontraumatic causes; it can also occur as the consequence of degenerative and metabolic disorders. Developmental malformations, such as anencephaly and severe microcephaly, may prevent the development of awareness and cognition in infants and young children; the diagnosis of vegetative state in the very young may be very difficult to make because of the limited behavioral repertoire at this age. Patients with degenerative disorders such as Alzheimer's disease or CREUTZ-FELDT–JAKOB DISEASE may evolve into vegetative state following the progressive decline of their cognitive abilities. In acute traumatic and nontraumatic injuries, such as motor-vehicle accidents or other forms of direct cerebral injury, near-drowning, and CEREBROVASCULAR ACCIDENTS, vegetative state can evolve from coma. If coma persists, between two and four weeks post injury the patient may evolve into vegetative state and this is marked by the return of spontaneous eye-opening and the resumption of apparent sleep–wake cycles. Patients may recover from this condition or survive in it for years. A small proportion of patients who remain in coma do not resume spontaneous eye-opening.

Terminology

This condition is referred to in the literature by a number of terms. Persistent vegetative state is sometimes used synonymously with vegetative state; on other occasions the term "persistent" is used to convey that the condition has endured over a certain period of time. Some sources consider that vegetative state can be considered persistent after a few weeks; others propose that the term should not be applied until a year has elapsed. Vegetative state has also been referred to in the literature by a number of other names including: apallic syndrome, prolonged coma, post-comatose unawareness, neocortical death, and altered states of consciousness.

There are a number of other causes of reduced responsiveness which should be differentiated from vegetative state. Coma has been defined as "not obeying commands, not uttering words and not opening the eyes" (Jennett & Teasdale, 1981). It results from the dysfunction of the reticular activating system. In LOCKED-IN SYNDROME the patient is rendered tetraplegic and mute by the interruption of pathways in the ventral pons, but is responsive and sentient. Akinetic MUTISM, the extreme form of ADYNAMIA, is characterized by the patient giving a clear impression of being alert and aware, but neither spontaneously saying anything or replying to questions and showing a profound lack of general activity. Complete APHASIA is another condition which may occasionally be mistaken for a state of reduced consciousness; certain psychiatric states, such as schizophrenic catatonic stupor, and hysterical coma, in which EEG and eye movements are incompatible with the apparent unresponsiveness of the patient, may also be confused with it.

In brain death the patient is always dependent on a ventilator and, however much is done, the heart always stops beating within a week or so, usually after a few days. Once brain death is established there is a progressive loss of viability of the organs, beginning with the brain, no matter how much artificial support is provided (Jennett & Teasdale, 1981). In brain death the EEG is described as being flat or isoelectric.

Epidemiology

The incidence of vegetative state (from all causes) has been estimated at 2.5 per 100,000 of the population (Higashi et al., 1977). The annual incidence of vegetative state arising from trauma in the United Kingdom is estimated (Jennett, 1993) at 4 cases per million of the population, and the number of surviving cases at any one time is estimated (Andrews, 1993) at less than a thousand. Jennett estimates that the incidence of vegetative state arising from trauma must be considerably greater in North America and some European countries, where the incidence of severe head injuries is more than twice as great as in Britain. It is difficult to establish the prevalence of vegetative state because of the lack of widely accepted diagnostic criteria.

Pathology

Two major patterns of pathological features have been identified as being associated with acute traumatic or nontraumatic brain injury (The Multi-Society Task Force on PVS, 1994). One pattern is that of diffuse laminar cortical necrosis with almost invariable involvement of the HIPPOCAMPUS and this follows acute, global hypoxia and ischemia. The other pattern is that of diffuse axonal injury, which is usually due to a shearing injury after acute trauma. Severe abnormalities of the BRAIN STEM in vegetative state are rare and lesions confined to the brain stem seldom, if ever, cause long-term unconsciousness.

ASSESSMENT: NEUROPHYSIOLOGICAL MEASURES

EEG studies

In vegetative state, most patients will show diffuse generalized polymorphic theta or delta activity with transistion from wakefulness to sleep being accompanied by some desynchronization of the background activity (Multi-Society Task Force on PVS, 1994). Reported EEG findings can vary from alpha activity to isoelectric; there is some debate about the latter, since it is considered that true isoelectric EEGs are only seen in brain death and what may have been seen in vegetative state patients was EEG of very low voltage. Typical epileptiform and seizure activity are unusual in vegetative state patients. Infants and children are reported as having similar abnormalities to those of adults, but the EEG activity tends to be more discontinuous and of lower voltage.

Whereas conventional EEG has limited diagnostic or prognostic use for patients in vegetative state, compressed spectral analysis of the EEG appears to have more potential. Tsubokawa (1993) reported that, in a study of 31 cases diagnosed as "prolonged deep coma" at three months post insult, those who remained in a chronic comatose state with respiratory assistance showed slow monotonous spectrums and those who emerged into vegetative state showed changeable spectrums. In addition he reported that there was further differentiation among the vegetative state patients, as those with lower neurobehavioral scores showed no desynchronization and those with the higher scores did. Changeable spectrums with desynchronization were also characteristic of the three cases in this group who made a recovery.

EP studies

EVOKED POTENTIAL studies on individual patients can be used to assess sensory functioning and probable sensory deficits, and also to monitor these conditions over time. In prognostic terms they have limited value. Somatosensory evoked responses (SEPs) appear to be the most useful, but it has been noted that patients without SEPs may recover at least minimal cognitive activity and patients with normal somatosensory responses may enter a vegetative state and remain in it (Multi-Society Task Force on PVS, 1994). One study (Tsubokawa, 1993) has found that the pain-related P250 component of the SEP was not recorded in any of a group of patients who remained in chronic coma but was observed in all those who evolved into vegetative state; a correlation was also found between the suppression of the P250 amplitude and the severity of the neurobehavioral score.

Imaging

CT, MRI, and PET scans can all provide diag-

nostic information; in particular, PET scans can provide quantifiable measures of changes within the brain that occur as concomitants of behavior and this may be particularly useful when overt manifestations of behavior may not be discernible. There appear to be no established correlations between the results of neuroimaging studies with MRI or CT and the development of the vegetative state or potential for recovery (Multi-Society Task Force on PVS, 1994). Studies using PET have found that patients in vegetative state following trauma have rates of glucose metabolism at 40–60 percent of those of normal subjects; cerebral blood flow has been found to be similarly reduced (Levy et al., 1987; Tsubokawa, 1993). The Multi-Society Task Force on PVS (1994) has commented that there is not yet sufficient information to warrant the use of PET scanning to determine prognosis.

In general, although neurodiagnostic tests may help to elucidate individual cases, in the present state of knowledge it appears that they alone cannot confirm the diagnosis of vegetative state or predict the potential for recovery (Multi-Society Task Force on PVS, 1994).

ASSESSMENT: BEHAVIORAL MEASURES

The casual observer encountering vegetative state patients may feel there is very little to observe. Changes do occur in these patients but sometimes over a very long time course, and sometimes signs of returning awareness are not always elicited in the first instance by formal assessments but may be picked up by chance observations. The recommendation is not to be dependent on one type of assessment.

Assessments which utilize the more overt components of behavior can be divided into two main types: (1) scales which assess recovery by examining for or eliciting specific aspects of behavior; (2) observational methods that record behaviors which occur spontaneously and include ad hoc observations, interview, and time sampling.

Behavior scales

These can be subdivided into four groups according to their main area of application: acute coma, vegetative state, acute coma and vegetative state, and recovery scales.

The best-known of the scales for acute coma is the Glasgow Coma Scale (GCS) (Jennnett & Teasdale, 1977). This consists of three ordinal subscales: eye opening (four points), motor response (six points), and verbal response (five points). The scores from the subscales can be summed to give a coma score; acute coma is defined by observations summing to eight or less. The use of this scale can be continued into vegetative state but is relatively insensitive to changes in patients in this condition, and it is best used in conjunction with other measures more appropriate to this condition. The ceiling of the eye-opening scale will be reached when the patients emerge into vegetative state. In addition, if patients have a tracheostomy they will be unable to vocalize, or if their injuries have impaired their motor system, which is difficult to assess properly until they have fully regained consciousness, then the use of the coma score may underestimate their recovery. As the verbal response subscale is inappropriate for use with children under 5, a modified version of the GCS, the Adelaide Coma Scale, has been developed for pediatric use (Simpson & Reilly, 1982). There are a number of scales primarily for use with acute coma, including the Glasgow–Liège Scale (Born, 1988), the Reaction Level Scale (RLS85) (Stalhammar et al., 1988), and the Comprehensive Level of Consciousness Scale (CLOCS) (Stanczak et al., 1984). A review of some of the scales developed for use in acute coma is given by Horn and colleagues (1993) and this review also includes examples of scales from the other categories.

There are also a number of scales which have been developed for use with vegetative state patients. The Sensory Stimulation Assessment Measure (SSAM) is administered by giving a graded series of stimuli to each of the senses: auditory, visual, olfactory, gustatory, and tactile. Responses are scored on three six-point subscales: I eye opening, II motor, and III vocalization (Rader & Ellis, 1989). There are also subscale scores derived for each of the senses, as well as a general responsiveness score. The stimuli used are everyday in nature; for example, the protocol for auditory stimulation requires the administrator to clap hands, ring a bell, call the patient's name, give commands such as "blink your eyes," and ask questions such as "If you are a male, move your hand." The authors present data on test-retest and inter-rater reliability and the scale was validated against other scales including the GCS. There are other scales based

on the examination of the functioning of the senses, such as the Visual Response Evaluation (Davis, 1991).

Another type of scale developed for use with vegetative state patients grades their recovery according to the presence or absence of particular behaviors. One example of this is the Nihon University Neurological Grading of the Persistent Vegetative State (Tsubokawa et al., 1990). This is a ten-point scale with the grading as follows: (1) alive with spontaneous respiration; (2) withdrawal response to pain; (3) spontaneous eye opening and closing; (4) spontaneous movement of extremities; (5) pursuit by eye movement; (6) emotional expression; (7) oral intake; (8) producing sounds; (9) obeying orders; (10) verbal response.

Some scales have been developed which are intended for use with both acute coma and vegetative state. One of these is the Coma/Near-Coma Scale (CNC), which is based on the authors' contention that coma and vegetative states phase into one another, can be quantified in an ordinal scale, and need not occur in any fixed-time sequence (Rappaport et al., 1992). The scale is applied by assessing eight different parameters of behavior, each with repeated administration of specified stimuli. The parameters are: auditory, command responsivity, visual, threat, olfactory, tactile, pain, and vocalization. The scale allows for the nonuse of items that are not appropriate for a particular patient, e.g. assessing vocalization when there is a tracheostomy. An average CNC score is obtained from the sum of the scores for individual items and the number of items actually scored and a classification of severity of coma is provided, based on average scores.

The State of the Patient Questionnaire (Freeman, 1987) was written for use by relatives, though it can equally well be applied by professionals. This assesses function in ten areas: vigilance, emotion, drive, vision, audition, touch, limb and body movement, hand movement, vocalization, and swallowing. Sensory function is divided into five stages: no reaction, reflex stage, withdrawal stage, localizing stage, and discriminating stage. Similarly, motor function is also divided into five stages: no reaction, reflex movement, spontaneous movement, controlled movement, and fine controlled movement. The questionnaire does not provide a score; it is intended as a means of establishing the patient's level of function in specified areas and monitoring changes in functional ability.

Some scales have been developed with the purpose of monitoring recovery from severe head injury beyond coma and vegetative state. The Disability Rating Scale (DR) (Rappaport et al., 1982) aims to monitor recovery from "coma to community." It consists of eight items within four categories: (1) arousability, awareness, and responsivity; (2) cognitive ability for self-care activities; (3) dependence on others; (4) psychosocial adaptability. Each item in the DR has its own scoring scale and these vary in length between four and six items, with the higher scores being related to greater disability.

The Western Neuro Sensory Stimulation Profile (WNSSP) was developed to assess patients categorized as "slow to recover," who are candidates for sensory stimulation programs. It consists (Ansell et al., 1989) of 33 items divided into six subscales which assess: arousal and attention, expressive communication, auditory comprehension, visual comprehension, visual tracking, and object manipulation. The scale allows for indication when the use of particular items is inappropriate and normative data are available.

The selection of scales for use in the assessment of patients in vegetative state has to depend on whether frequent or periodic assessment is required, how much time is available for carrying out the assessment, and also who, in terms of skills and numbers of staff, will be responsible for its administration.

Ad hoc observations

The simplest approach is the noting of responses that might indicate increased arousal or returning awareness as and when they occur and by whoever observes them, whether relative, friend, or professional. Freeman (1993) advises that, when a response has been observed by only one person, it should be so documented; the response can be confirmed when it has been seen again, especially by another person.

Interviews

A structured interview has been used by Wilson and others (1993a) which was administered to nursing staff, although it could equally well have been used with relatives or others in frequent contact with the patient. It asked whether improvement or deterioration had been noted in specific areas of behavior over the last week and what incidents had specifically led to that conclusion. The aspects of behavior included were: general arousal level, mood, movement (quantity and/or nature), muscle tone, response to touch, visual tracking, eye contact, response to speech sounds, expressive communication (crying, moaning, laughing, and other vocalizations), response to music, and behavior in social circumstances. As well as giving the opportunity to systematically gather qualitative information, the data can also be represented in a quantitative form (Powell & Wilson, 1994).

Time sampling

More familiarly used in the context of measurement associated with behavior modification, momentary time sampling has been applied both in long-term monitoring of recovery (Powell & Wilson, 1994) and in evaluating the immediate effects of treatment in vegetative state patients (Wilson et al., 1993a, b). In the latter, patients were observed for a period of 10 minutes with behaviors being recorded every 10 seconds. The time-sampling schedule included the following categories of behavior: eyes shut with no body movement, eyes shut with reflexive body movement, eyes shut with spontaneous body movement, eyes open with no body movement, eyes open with reflexive body movement, eyes open with spontaneous body movement, engaged in activity (e.g. scratching), and vocalization. The behaviors were regarded as mutually exclusive apart from vocalization. In analysis, the authors focused on two behaviors, eyes open and eyes open with spontaneous body movement; increases in both these behaviors were considered to be indicative of increased arousal.

TREATMENTS

Several treatments have been advocated for use with vegetative state patients, but establishing their efficacy is beset by a number of methodological issues. First, because of the relative rarity of this condition, the first problem is acquiring sufficient numbers of subjects in the same place within a reasonable time frame. Multi-centered studies may present problems of matching other aspects of care. Treatment effects are usually assessed in terms of variables such as time taken to emerge from vegetative state or changes in functional level; controls for nonspecific effects such as spontaneous recovery are needed. Control subjects need to be matched on variables which may influence recovery or responsiveness and this may be problematic in a group which is so heterogeneous in terms of pathology. One of the treatments, sensory stimulation, presents particular problems in the use of control subjects; since its nature allows its application by relatives, they may well decide to try it for themselves. There is also the ethical issue of withholding a treatment that does no apparent harm when there is the possibility it may be of benefit.

The reader of research literature is also beset by the variations in diagnostic criteria and terminology that are used.

Deep brain stimulation and spinal cord stimulation

Deep brain stimulation involves implantation of electrodes in the RETICULAR FORMATION or the THALAMUS (e.g. Tsubokawa et al., 1990); spinal cord stimulation involves the implantation of electrodes at the C2 level or lower within the cervical vertebrae (e.g. Kanno et al., 1993). The initial studies indicate that these methods may be useful in some patients, but reports on studies incorporating controls are awaited.

Sensory stimulation

Review of the research literature shows that the protocols for sensory stimulation can vary considerably in terms of variables such as content, duration and frequency of treatment, and identity of therapist, but they are consistent in that the stimuli used tend to be of an everyday nature and are applied systematically (Wilson & McMillan, 1993). The rationale for sensory stimulation stems from two research areas: animal studies on the effects of environment on recovery from experimentally induced lesions, and the studies of the psychological effects of environmental deprivation (as vegetative state patients are indeed limited in their capacity to seek stimulation from external sources). Wilson and McMillan (1993) found, in their review of research into sensory stimulation, that relatively few studies had paid attention to control of extraneous factors; where this had been done, the balance of evidence suggests that sensory stimulation could alter

behavior in the patient who is not conscious and can reduce the duration of acute coma. Further research is certainly warranted.

BIBLIOGRAPHY

Andrews, K. (1993). Recovery of patients after four months or more in the persistent vegetative state. *British Medical Journal, 306,* 1597–600.

Ansell, B. J., Keenan, J. E., & de la Rocha, O. (1989). *Western Neuro Sensory Stimulation Profile: A tool for assessing slow-to-recover head-injured patients.* Tustin, CA: Western Neuro Care Center.

Born, J. D. (1988). The Glasgow–Liège Scale: prognostic value and evolution of motor responses and brain stem reflexes after severe head injury. *Acta Neurochirurgica, 91,* 1–11.

Davis, A. L. (1991). The Visual Response Evaluation: a pilot study of an evaluation tool for assessing visual responses in low-level brain-injured patients. *Brain Injury, 5,* 315–20.

Council on Scientific Affairs and Council on Judicial Affairs. (1990). Persistent vegetative state and the decision to withdraw or withhold life support. *Journal of the American Medical Association, 263,* 426–30.

Freeman, E. A. (1987). *The catastrophe of coma.* Buderim, Queensland: David Bateman.

Freeman, E. A. (1993). The clinical assessment of coma. *Neuropsychological Rehabilitation, 3,* 139–48.

Fujiwara, S., Ogasawara, K., Nakasato, N., Shimizu, H., Nagamine, Y., Kohshu, K., & Yoshimoto, T. (1993). Brain MRIs of twenty-five patients with prolonged disturbance of consciousness after head injury: analysis in the chronic stages. In K. Takakura & T. Kanno (Eds), *The Society for Treatment of Coma.* Vol. 2 (pp. 89–98). Tokyo: Neuron Publishing Co.

Higashi, K., Sakata, Y., Hantano, M., Aniko, S., Ihara, K., Katayama, S. et al. (1977). Epidemiological studies of patients with persistent vegetative state. *Journal of Neurology, Neurosurgery and Psychiatry, 40,* 876–85.

Horn, S., Shiel, A., McLellan, L., Campbell, M., Watson, M., & Wilson, B. (1993). A review of behavioural assessment scales for monitoring recovery in and after coma with pilot data on a new scale of visual awareness. *Neuropsychological Rehabilitation, 3,* 121–38.

House of Lords (1994). *Report of the Select Committee on Medical Ethics*. Vol. 1. London: HMSO.

Jennett, B. (1993). Vegetative survival: the medical facts and ethical dilemmas. *Neuropsychological Rehabilitation, 3*, 99–108.

Jennett, B., & Teasdale, G. (1977). Aspects of coma after severe head injury. *Lancet, 1*, 878–81.

Jennett, B., & Teasdale, G. (1981). *Management of head injuries*. Philadelphia: F. A. Davis.

Kanno, T., Kamel, Y., & Yokoyama, T. (1993). Treating the vegetative state with dorsal column stimulation. In K. Takakura & T. Kanno (Eds), *The Society for Treatment of Coma*. Vol. 1 (pp. 67–76). Tokyo: Neuron Publishing Co.

Levy, D. E., Sidtis, J. J., Rottenberg, D. A., Jarden, J. O., Strother, S. C., Dhawan, V., Ginos, J. Z., Tramo, M. J., Evans, A. C., & Plum, F. (1987). Differences in cerebral blood flow and glucose utilisation in vegetative versus locked-in patients. *Annals of Neurology, 22*, 673–82.

Multi-Society Task Force on PVS (1994). Medical aspects of the persistent vegetative state. *New England Journal of Medicine, 330*, 1499–508.

Powell, G. E., & Wilson, S. L. (1994). Recovery curves for patients who have suffered very severe brain injury. *Clinical Rehabilitation, 8*, 54–69.

Rader, M. A., & Ellis, D. W. (1989). *Sensory Stimulation Assessment Measure: A manual for administration*. Camden, NJ: Institute of Brain Injury Research and Training.

Rappaport, M., Dougherty, A. M., & Kelting, D. L. (1992). Evaluation of coma and vegetative states. *Archives of Physical Medicine and Rehabilitation, 73*, 628–34.

Rappaport, M., Hall, K. M., Hopkins, K., Belleza, T., & Cope, D. N. (1982). Disability rating scale for severe head trauma: coma to community. *Archives of Physical Medicine and Rehabilitation, 63*, 118–23.

Simpson, D., & Reilly, P. (1982). Paediatric coma scale. *Lancet, 2*, 450.

Stalhammar, D., Starmark, J.-E., Holmgren, E., Eriksson, N., Nordstrom, C.-H., Fedders, O., & Rosander, B. (1988). Assessment of the responsiveness in acute cerebral disorders. A multicentre study on the Reaction Level Scale (RLS85). *Acta Neurochirurgica, 90*, 73–80.

Stanczak, D. E., White, J. G., Gouview, W. D., Moehle, K. A., Daniel, M., Novack, T., & Long, C. J. (1984). Assessment of level of consciousness following severe neurological insult. A comparison of the psychometric qualities of the Glasgow Coma Scale and the Comprehensive Level of Consciousness Scale. *Journal of Neurosurgery, 60*, 955–60.

Tsubokawa, T. (1993). Persistent vegetative state – the pathophysiological entity and its diagnosis. In K. Takakura & T. Kanno (Eds), *The Society for the Treatment of Coma*. Vol. 1 (pp. 3–12). Tokyo: Neuron Publishing Co.

Tsubokawa, T., Yamamoto, T., & Katayama, Y. (1990). Prediction of outcome of prolonged coma caused by brain damage. *Brain Injury, 4*, 329–37.

Tsubokawa, T., Yamamoto, T., Katayama, Y., Hirayama, T., Maejima, S., & Moriya, T. (1991). Deep brain stimulation, in persistent vegetative state: follow-up results and criteria for selection of candidates. *Brain Injury, 4*, 315–27.

Wilson, S. L., & McMillan, T. M. (1993). A review of the evidence for the effectiveness of sensory stimulation treatment for coma and vegetative states. *Neuropsychological Rehabilitation, 3*, 149–60.

Wilson, S. L., Powell, G. E., Elliott, K., & Thwaites, H. (1993a). Assessing change in vegetative state patients. Paper presented at the *3rd Annual Conference of the International Association for the Study of Traumatic Brain Injury*, Tokyo, September 8–10.

Wilson, S. L., Powell, G. E., Elliott, K., & Thwaites, H. (1993b). Evaluation of sensory stimulation as a treatment for prolonged coma – seven single-case experimental studies. *Neuropsychological Rehabilitation, 3*, 191–202.

SARAH L. WILSON

ventricles The ventricles are the cavities within the brain which contain CEREBROSPINAL FLUID (CSF). There are four ventricles. The pair of lateral ventricles in the forebrain, within which the CSF is produced, connect to the third ventricle in the midline of the brain stem by the interventricular foramen (or foramen of Monro). The third ventricle is in turn connected to the fourth ventricle at the level of the PONS and

CEREBELLUM by the cerebral aqueduct (or aqueduct of Sylvius), from where the CSF flows out around the brain and spinal cord. From Classical times through to the eighteenth century, the ventricles and the fluid which they contain were believed to be the location of psychological functions, rather than the actual substance of the brain matter.

ventriculography Ventriculography is a technique, less commonly employed since the introduction of modern medical imaging (*see* SCAN), which permits the VENTRICLES to be visualized. This may be achieved by either inserting a radiologically opaque medium into the ventricles, or a bubble of air as in PNEUMOENCEPH-ALOGRAPHY (or the AIR ENCEPHALOGRAM). The contrast medium may be injected through a lumbar puncture, or by a cannula directly through the skull and brain substance. The subsequent X-ray images may reveal blockages in the circulation of CSF; enlargement of the ventricles; or shifts in the form or location of the ventricles, indicating the presence of a space-occupying lesion.

Verger–Déjerine syndrome The Verger–Déjerine syndrome is a form of cortical somatosensory loss. It consists of an impairment of the ability to recognize the perceptual qualities of an object by touch, loss of tactile form discrimination, loss of two-point discrimination, loss of tactile localization, loss of position sense for the limbs in space, and stereognosis. Peripheral sensitivities to touch, pressure, temperature, and pain are by contrast only minimally affected, if at all. The syndrome has been associated with lesions of the parietal cortex.

vestibular stimulation Equilibrium may be assessed by vestibular stimulation. The function of equilibrium is supported by parts of the labyrinth in the middle ear: the semicircular canals, the utricle, and the saccule. These structures detect angular acceleration in three planes, the position of the head in space, and the direction of influence of gravity. The resulting information is conducted by the vestibular division of the eighth CRANIAL NERVE to the pons

and the cortex of the cerebellum, and to parts of the posterior temporal lobe. The peripheral elements of this system can be tested by one of two methods which involve vestibular stimulation. The first method involves rotating the patient, which normally produces NYSTAGMUS in the opposite direction. The second employs caloric stimulation (the *caloric test*), irrigating each ear in turn by either hot or cold water, and so investigating each labyrinth separately. The effect is recorded as the latency from the onset of stimulation to the resolution of the resulting nystagmus. Abnormal responses may indicate not only pathology of the eighth cranial nerve and Menière's syndrome (a syndrome of vertigo, tinnitus, and deafness), but also lesions of the cerebral vestibular areas or of the brain stem.

visual acuity, testing The assessment of basic visual functions, including *visual acuity* (the ability to resolve fine detail in the stimulus array), is technically a very difficult process and it rarely attracts the attention or skill it requires from either neuropsychologists or neurologists.

The reason that visual acuity testing is unusually difficult is that a large number of stimulus dimensions need to be considered in undertaking the assessment. Location, size, brightness, contrast, movement, color, temporal distribution, and stimulus complexity may all contribute to whether a particular stimulus is detected or not. In addition, visual perception may fluctuate over time in an individual patient, and the picture may be complicated by the presence of META-MORPHOPSIAS or the phenomenon of BLIND-SIGHT.

The point to be made is that simple confrontational testing of the visual field by moving a poorly specified stimulus such a pen, or waving fingers, gradually into the visual field from the periphery in a variety of directions, as practiced in the standard neurological examination, is no more than the most crude way of assessing the functioning of basic visual processes in the detection of stimuli and the associated extent of the visual fields. Even more formal *visual perimetry*, in which an apparatus is employed to chart more systematically the visual fields, and within which some systematic control of stimulus parameters is possible, may fail to identify problems of visual acuity which the patient suffers.

A full assessment of visual acuity should include the measurement of detection thresholds, local adaptation time, flicker fusion, movement after-effect, tachistoscopic presentation, luminance discrimination, and depth perception. Although these aspects are rather broader than the specific aspect of acuity, acuity interacts with each of the parameters assessed within these paradigms and must be considered together with them in any assessment of abnormality in basic visual function.

visual agnosia *See* AGNOSIA; VISUOPERCEPTUAL DISORDERS.

visual communication (VIC) The VIC system of visual communication is a system of symbols which has been employed in the therapy of global aphasic patients. The approach is derived from the successful training of chimpanzees to recognize and manipulate symbols as a medium of communication. A similar set of nonverbal symbols, or hand signals, may be used to permit globally aphasic patients to express their desires and feelings, commands, or the answers to questions (*see* SPEECH THERAPY FOR APHASIA).

visual evoked potential *See* EVOKED POTENTIAL.

visual field defects Conventionally, a region of blindness (a SCOTOMA) which is restricted to part of the visual field and is the result of disruption of the afferent, geniculostriate pathway from the retina to the STRIATE CORTEX, located on the mesial surface and pole of the OCCIPITAL LOBE. The term is also applied to regions of relative blindness in the visual field where some residual capacity remains.

The geniculostriate pathway proceeds from the retina, via the optic nerves, the OPTIC CHIASM, the optic tract, the lateral GENICULATE BODY, and the visual radiations. Lesions at various stages of the pathway lead to characteristic visual field losses at locations which can be predicted from the retinotopic organization of the projection pathways. Lesions of the retina or optic nerve result in a monocular scotoma. When optic nerve fibers that

cross in the optic chiasm are affected, for example, as a result of tumors in the region of the pituitary gland, bitemporal hemianopia ensues. The left and right visual fields are affected for the left and right eyes respectively. When more lateral portions of the optic chiasm are involved, field defects are confined to the nasal half of the visual field in the eye ipsilateral to the affected side. Lesions to the optic tract, visual radiations, and primary visual cortex lead to homonymous defects where the density and shape of the defect is the same for each eye, although the shape is rarely precisely congruent. The field loss is commonly restricted to one hemifield (HEMIANOPIA) and can occur with or without sparing of the macular field, an area subtending 5–10 degrees which surrounds the fixation point. Restriction of the field loss to the upper or lower quadrant is termed QUADRANTANOPIA.

Assessment of visual field defects

The extent of a visual field defect is charted using conventional perimetry. Subjects are required to detect a spot of light, of specified intensity and angular size, presented at various locations in the visual field while maintaining fixation at the center of a screen. The subject may be required to detect either a briefly presented spot of light (static perimetry) or a light that is moved from the periphery of the visual field towards the center (kinetic perimetry). Colored targets may be used where the subject is required to identify the color of the target and chromatic fields can then be charted. The field for blue is greater than that for either red or green and each field is smaller than for achromatic targets. Color perimetry is used to detect retinal and optic nerve disease and color blindness of cortical origin (ACHROMATOPSIA).

A further method of visual field evaluation is dynamic perimetry, requiring the subject to determine whether small flickering targets appear intermittent or steady. The critical flicker frequency, the minimum flicker rate at which the target appears stationary, is decreased in impaired regions of the visual field. While patients may be unaware of the presence of a scotoma, a recent finding is that, when patients view a pattern of randomly distributed black and white dots flickering at high temporal frequency, the field defect appears as a homogeneous gray and can be readily perceived and described by the observer (noise-field campimetry). This is true for scotomata resulting from retinal, optic nerve, chiasmal, and tract damage but not when scotomata are a result of damage to visual cortex and radiations. In the latter case, unless the damage is of recent origin, the field defect exhibits a "filling-in" (completion) in the same manner as with the natural blind spot.

RESIDUAL VISION IN VISUAL FIELD DEFECTS

Much of the evidence concerning the nature of visual field defects derives from the studies of war veterans who sustained perforating gunshot wounds during the Russo–Japanese War (1905–6) and the First (1914–18) and Second (1939–45) World Wars. Such injuries, unlike vascular lesions or space-occupying tumors, result in local and circumscribed lesions. The correlation between the location of brain damage and the resulting scotomata enabled Gordon Holmes (1918) to construct the map of the visual fields on striate cortex. Holmes believed scotomata to be regions of absolute blindness, while acknowledging that scotomata may be surrounded by a zone of indistinct and partial vision. Residual vision in a field defect is not uncommon and Holmes ascribed this to the result of incomplete lesions resulting in an "amblyopia, colour vision being generally lost and white objects appearing indistinct, or only more potent stimuli, as abruptly moving objects, may excite sensations." In contrast, and during the same period, Poppelreuter (1917) claimed that some rudimentary vision was always present in the blind field and ordered the different levels of visual function in a hierarchy as follows: amorphous light sensitivity, size perception without definite form, amorphous form perception, perception of discrete objects, mild amblyopia, and normal vision. The severity of the visual field defect reflected, he argued, the degree of completeness of the lesion. Teuber and others (1960) also subscribed to the view that the degree of recovery from cortical blindness reflected an "order of fragility" of mechanisms subserving various visual functions. Such a view contrasts with the proposal that specific dissociations of visual abilities result from the brain lesion sparing pathways that are specialized for the processing of different visual attributes. For example, the RIDDOCH EFFECT, described as early as 1917, refers to the observation that a patient may detect a moving target

presented in a scotoma yet be blind to stationary stimuli. Riddoch suggested that motion perception constitutes a "special visual perception" that can be dissociated from the perception of form and color and that preserved motion perception is the result of the sparing of a mechanism specialized for the processing of motion information. Holmes also reported preservation of motion perception in an otherwise blind region of the visual field, but argued that it was the result of hypoesthesia where "stronger and more adequate stimuli" alone excite sensations. The Riddoch effect can also be seen with more anterior lesions to the visual pathway, implicating the optic tract and chiasm.

Other dissociable visual disorders can occasionally occur, notably that of cerebral ACHROMATOPSIA, a disorder that can be confined to a single hemifield, where cerebral damage in Man results in a complete loss of color vision. Patients typically describe the visual scene as appearing in shades of gray and drained of color. They characteristically perform poorly on the Farnsworth–Munsell 100-Hue Test, a task which requires them to order a number of graded colored discs on the basis of their chromaticity. Early authors were sceptical of the existence of achromatopsia, interpreting it as an early or partial case of amblyopia where partial or recovering hemianopic field defects display an order of fragility for the detection of colored, achromatic, and moving targets in perimetry.

Recent studies

Retention or recovery of visual capacity in field defects has repeatedly been demonstrated since the earlier observations. Nevertheless, some field defects remain absolutely and permanently blind when tested with conventional methods, although pupillary reaction to light and OPTOKINETIC NYSTAGMUS to certain patterns of moving stimuli may be preserved.

Two particular issues have been addressed in the last two decades. The first is whether local destruction of striate cortex results in an absolute scotoma and residual vision, where it exists, is the result of an incomplete lesion. Alternatively, complete abolition of visual capacity in a field defect may require accompanying damage to extrastriate areas. Interest in this matter was revived when novel methods of testing uncovered hitherto unexpected visual capacity within field defects (*see* BLINDSIGHT and below). The second issue arose from the discovery that extrastriate cortex in the monkey contains multiple visual areas. This raised the possibility that selective impairments in field defects, for example, for the processing of color or motion, could be the result of disturbance to one or more of these areas.

When is the scotoma absolute? To account for differences in the degree of severity of the impairment requires information about the limits of the lesion. However, striate cortex in Man is largely buried in the calcarine sulcus on the medial surface of the brain, and damage is rarely confined to this region but extends into prestriate and other cortex. In contrast, striate cortex in the monkey is exposed on the lateral surface and lesions can be made with some precision. The extent of residual abilities of animals with total striate cortex ablation had been a question of some controversy since the early years of the century. During the 1960s Cowey and Weiskrantz examined the properties of visual field defects in monkeys with partial lesions of striate cortex, using the perimetric method. The resulting impairments showed some important properties. The field defects were not absolute regions of blindness and the animals' ability to detect light flashes improved markedly over several months of postoperative testing. The size of the defective region decreased over the same period and such improvement did not occur spontaneously but was dependent on the training regime. Finally, flash thresholds were highest at the center of the defective region and diminished towards the periphery.

At first blush these findings appeared to support Poppelreuter's view that no field defect was absolute. Permanent and absolute scotomata could be accounted for by the possibility that the lesion had not only destroyed striate cortex but had encroached into extrastriate regions. Some support for this view had come from earlier observations in the monkey that residual vision is seriously degraded when extrastriate damage accompanies a striate cortical lesion. The matter might have rested there but for studies carried out in the 1970s; most notably, the extensive examination by Weiskrantz of a single case, patient DB, following surgical excision of a tumor, where surgical notes confirmed the tissue removed was confined to striate cortex. Residual ability in such cases has been termed blindsight. The resulting

field defect is perimetrically blind and the patient denies any visual experience. However, when the patient is asked to discriminate or detect visual stimuli presented to the blind field, using a technique of forced-choice guessing, the tasks are performed with remarkable accuracy. The types of residual vision include manual and saccadic target detection and localization, orientation discrimination, and the detection and discrimination of chromatic stimuli. Nevertheless, the paradox persists that the "blindness" reported following striate cortex ablation in Man is of a greater severity than is apparent in the monkey. Whether conscious experience is also absent in the monkey, necessitating a reliance on "guessing" for detection and discrimination, is at present unknown.

Selective deficits The properties of blindsight are consistent with the electrophysiological properties of pathways that survive striate cortex removal, the most conspicuous of which is the midbrain pathway from the retina to the superior COLLICULUS, which projects via the pulvinar to extrastriate areas. Knowledge of the organization of the retino-geniculate pathway, derived from studies of nonhuman primates, has also contributed to an understanding of selective impairments in visual field defects. The cerebral cortex of nonhuman primates contains a patchwork of visual areas, perhaps as many as 30, which are the outcome of a small number of relatively independent processing channels that originate in the retina, maintain anatomical and functional segregation in the lateral geniculate nucleus, and further differentiate in the striate and extrastriate cortices. Anatomical evidence in monkeys for independent channels for the processing of visual information begins in the retina. The channels arise from morphologically and functionally distinct populations of cells, the Pα and Pβ retinal ganglion cells. Pβ cells project to the parvocellular layers of the dorsal lateral geniculate nucleus, which innervate anatomically separate regions of striate cortex (area V1), which project in turn to cortical area V2. From area V2, the P-channel continues to cortical area V4 and has been implicated in the processing of both color and form.

The second pathway, arising from Pα retinal ganglion cells and innervating cortical area V1 via the magnocellular layers of dLGN, constitutes the M channel. From V1, information is relayed to area MT (V5) and areas V3, V3A via area V2. It has been proposed that the M-channel primarily plays a role in the processing of form and motion.

Early authors accounted for relative sparing of visual abilities in terms of striate cortex, disregarding the possibility that specialized areas outside striate cortex subserved separate visual submodalities. More recently, the demonstration of functional specialization in prestriate cortex has led to the view that either lesions in specific visual areas outside striate cortex or selective disturbance of either the P or M channel may result in specific visual defects.

Such specific defects are not readily uncovered using traditional methods of visual field assessment. While conventional perimetry uncovers the shape of a field defect, its size and sensitivity requires greater control over the parameters of target stimuli presented in the perimeter. More recent studies have examined the spatiotemporal contrast sensitivity in patients in whom the Riddoch effect was observed in conventional perimetry. Plant (see Plant, 1991, for review) and his colleagues characterized the residual vision of patients with homonymous hemianopic field defects as a result of ischemic damage to the optic radiations and cases of chiasmal compression. Sensitivity to low spatial and intermediate temporal frequencies was relatively preserved and direction discrimination was possible at contrast levels close to threshold. Such deficits resemble those seen in the nonhuman primate lacking the P-channel.

Recently, the complementary condition to that of the Riddoch effect has been described by Zihl and his colleagues (see Zeki, 1991, for review) where a patient can see a stationary object but is severely defective in her ability to see objects in motion. The lesion did not involve striate cortex but included the presumed homologue of cortical area MT. The exquisite sensitivity of single neurons in MT to the direction and speed of a moving stimulus is consistent with the proposed role of the latter area in visual motion processing.

Selective impairments in color vision can occur in hemianopia and quadrantanopia. Luminance vision is frequently spared. In such cases, performance on arrangement tests is invariably preserved and the deficit can only be detected by color perimetry. The early skepticism of the existence of cerebral achromatopsia has now been resolved (see Zeki, 1990, for review). Postmortem evidence and magnetic resonance imaging in patients indicates that damage to an area in the caudal region of the FUSIFORM GYRUS in the ventral portions of the occipital lobe results in achromatopsia. In addition, positron emission tomography (PET) in normal observers has confirmed that neural activity in this region is heightened during processing of chromatic information. The existence of a localized "color center" in visual cortex has been proposed, which is arguably the homologue of cortical area V4 in the nonhuman primate.

There is, however, a serious objection to the view that damage to specialized cortical visual areas results in selective visual disturbances. A selective disorder following ablation of a single visual area in the monkey has yet to be demonstrated. Lesions to cortical area V4 or MT do not lead to the profound disturbances in the processing of color or motion seen in achromatopsia and akinetopsia (visual motion blindness) respectively. Whether such disturbances can more readily be accounted for in terms of selective destruction of the P and M channels remains to be established. Certainly the recent finding that optic axons subserving the two channels remain segregated in the optic tract may provide the explanation for selective impairments following partial optic tract damage. However, the role in vision of the cortical elaboration of the P and M pathways remains to be elucidated.

BIBLIOGRAPHY

Grusser, O.-J., & Landis, T. (1991). *Vision and visual dysfunction*. Vol. 12: *Visual agnosias and other disturbances of visual perception and cognition*. Basingstoke: Macmillan.

Holmes, G. (1918). Disturbances of vision by cerebral lesions. *British Journal of Ophthalmology, 2*, 353–84.

Plant, G. T. (1991). Temporal properties of normal and abnormal spatial vision. In D. Regan (Ed.), *Vision and visual dysfunction*. Vol. 2: *Spatial vision* (pp. 43–63). Basingstoke: Macmillan.

Poppelreuter, W. (1917). *Die pschischen Schodigungen durch Kapfschuss in Kriege 1914–16. Die Storlungen der miederen und hoheren Sehleistingen durch Verletzung des Okzipitalhirns.* Leipzig: Voss.

Ruddock, K. H. (1991). Spatial vision after cortical lesions. In D. Regan (Ed.), *Vision and visual dysfunction*. Vol. 2: *Spatial vision* (pp. 261–89). Basingstoke: Macmillan.

Teuber, H.-L., Battersby, W. S., & Bender, M. B. (1960). *Visual field defects after penetrating missile wounds of the brain*. Cambridge, MA: Harvard University Press.

Zeki, S. M. (1990). A century of cerebral achromatopsia. *Brain, 113,* 1721–77.

Zeki, S. M. (1991). Cerebral akinetopsia. *Brain, 114,* 811–24.

C. A. HEYWOOD

visuoperceptual disorders   The normal adult lives in a visual world of objects and scenes. These perceived objects are, for the most part, familiar and can typically be named should the occasion arise. They will be seen as a particular shape, size, and color, as having a specific orientation, and as being at a particular distance and direction from the viewer. Some relational properties of objects will change as the perceiver moves in space or as the object itself so moves. Some "intrinsic" properties of objects will appear to change as the conditions of illumination change or as objects are partially occluded by other objects. The "visual constancies" reflect the ways in which the perceiver's world maintains stability despite gross changes in the ambient stimulation that impinges on the retina.

Visual experience, however, is not always dependent upon retinal stimulation. Most normal people can "image" visual objects at will, although there are substantial individual differences in the reported "vividness" of such imagery. Likewise, most people experience complex visual scenes every night of the year when their eyes are firmly closed (dreaming), and it is not uncommon for normal people to have visual hallucinations dependent upon sensory deprivation or drug abuse, for example.

Current views of brain organization (Zeki, 1993) suggest that in higher primates (including Man) there are very many distinct visual areas in the cortex, each of which is primarily (but not exclusively) responsive to a different aspect of visual stimulation and organization. These prestriate regions thus seem to contain "maps" that are differentially sensitive to form, color, orientation, depth, movement, and so forth. That such properties are coded in separate regions of the

brain has been argued to give rise to the so-called "binding problem."

Our phenomenological experience of the visual world is of objects (with particular properties), not of a fragmentary, disorganized chaos of unrelated sensations of shape, size, color, and orientation. (We do not see "qualia" except in the philosophical literature.) As Muller, Humphreys, Quinlan and Donnelly (1989) write: "The question of how independently coded features are bound together into integrated descriptions of objects presents a major problem for current vision research" (p. 411). That illusory conjunctions of features from two objects can be experienced by normal observers in some circumstances shows that some kind of "binding mechanism" must, as it were, hold the visual world together. There is evidence that "the synchronisation of oscillatory responses to spatially distributed, feature selective cells might be a way to establish relations between features in different parts of the visual field" (Gray et al., 1989, p. 334); there is also evidence that "attentional mechanisms" are implicated in "feature integration" across maps of qualitatively distinct stimulus dimensions.

That there are separate informational channels for the perception of visual attributes is attested most strongly by the existence of selective impairments for (relatively) "elementary" stimulus components after (relatively) focal brain damage. Thus, at the most basic level, even figure-ground discrimination can break down in patients with normal visual acuity. In other patients with normal acuity and fair color perception, figure-ground discrimination can be intact (even for figures with subjective or illusory contours) while shape discrimination is so poor that squares cannot be distinguished from much thinner rectangles (Davidoff & Warrington, 1993).

Achromatic (brightness) discrimination can break down with relative preservation of color perception, and vice versa, cortical color blindness can be seen in cases with relatively intact achromatic discrimination. The perception of stimulus orientation (tilt) can be selectively impaired after right posterior damage (McCarthy & Warrington, 1990). In some patients the entire visual world can seem to invert through 180 degrees in a fashion analogous to that produced by wearing inverting lenses. Perceived location in space can also be laterally shifted, as when patients with visual ALLESTHESIA apparently "see" (and point to) objects in left space in the corresponding position in right space. Patients have also been reported who show a double dissociation between form and movement perception. Thus the patient of Zihl, von Cramon, and Mai (1983), with bilateral damage to prestriate cortex, had a severe impairment of the ability to see continuous movement, while the perception of stationary form and color was relatively intact. By contrast, some "agnosic" patients can see shapes as defined by movement in random-dot kinematograms, despite a severe impairment of stationary form and object recognition (Humphreys & Riddoch, 1987).

Normal depth perception is dependent upon a wide range of different cues of which one of the most important is stereopsis – the computation of depth from retinal disparity. Impairments in stereopsis are frequently seen in patients with bilateral posterior damage, and are also found after unilateral (usually right hemisphere) damage. There are occasional reports of patients with normal stereoscopic vision who cannot perceive depth in drawings and photographs; the impairment may reflect a selective inability to use such cues as occlusion and perspective that are involved in monocular depth perception.

The vexed question of "perceptual consciousness" is raised by the existence of BLINDSIGHT. In this condition, patients deny "seeing" anything in the hemianopic field but can nonetheless make fairly accurate discriminations between simple stimulus configurations if forced to "guess." They can also point quite well to objects that they insist they cannot see. A similar dissociation between overt and covert "perception" has been reported by Goodale and colleagues (1991). Their patient had suffered extensive bilateral damage to occipital and occipitoparietal regions, due to carbon monoxide poisoning. On conventional testing, she had a profound impairment of visual form, both shape and orientation. Nonetheless, she could accurately shape and guide her hand and finger movements to "the very objects whose qualities she fails to perceive." Goodale and others (1991) accordingly suggest that "the neural substrates for the visual perception of object qualities such as shape, orientation and size are distinct from those underlying the use of these qualities in the control of manual skills" (p. 154).

The contrary dissociation between "conscious perception" and visually-guided action is seen in ANTON'S SYNDROME. In this condition, patients with profound visual loss consequent upon bilateral occipital damage fail to identify people or objects by sight and bump into stationary objects. Yet, despite behaving like a blind person, the patient will firmly assert that he or she sees perfectly normally. When challenged to explain their poor visual performance, the patients will complain of poor illumination or claim that their glasses need a new prescription. Another form of hyperactive perception is seen in CHARLES BONNET SYNDROME. These patients with entirely normal intellectual functioning experience well-formed visual hallucinations in clear consciousness. The condition can be caused by damage to either the peripheral or central visual system.

The point of visual perception is, of course, to provide observers with accurate information about *what* objects are in their environment and *where* those objects are located; appropriate action can then be taken. There is reasonable agreement that relatively distinct circuits are involved in these two functions. The dorsal visual system (from occipital cortex to posterior parietal cortex) is primarily involved in computing spatial location; the ventral visual system (from occipital cortex to inferotemporal regions) is principally concerned with computing the identity of objects.

Impairments of the latter system (visual object recognition) were first described in the late nineteenth century, when a distinction was drawn between apperceptive and associative agnosias. In the former cases, the disorder of visual recognition was held to result from a combination of numerous "sensory" deficits in conjunction with a more general intellectual impairment. The latter cases (associative visual agnosia) are accordingly of more theoretical interest, as both intellect and visual sensation are relatively intact. Visuoperceptual abilities seem to be sufficiently well preserved to support identification by sight, and the patients may have no difficulties in recognizing (and naming) stimuli presented in other modalities (auditory or tactile, for example). The most striking examples of the condition are seen when the patients are able to copy line drawings (or draw from a three-dimensional model) accurately enough to allow a normal observer to identify the object depicted in the copy. Yet despite such performances, the patients themselves can recognize neither the original nor their own copy; they may, however, identify the object depicted if permitted to trace its outline with the finger. Although these patients may show adequate visual acuity, texture perception, and spatial contrast sensitivity, it is probably mistaken to assume that perception (as opposed to "recognition") is fully intact. Copying, for example, is often very slow and "slavish"; the patients frequently fail to respect the Gestalt properties of a visual configuration, producing their copies in a piecemeal fashion and following contours that do not respect object boundaries (Behrmann et al., 1992). Thaiss and de Bleser (1992) have accordingly suggested that in some of these patients "the spotlight" of maximal focal attention has a diameter that is greatly reduced from its normal size. In other patients, however, global form is available and the deficit resides in an inability to analyze and integrate local features of the visual display (Humphreys & Riddoch, 1987).

There are undoubtedly many distinct varieties of "visual associative agnosia" (Humphreys & Riddoch, 1987), provoked by both bilateral posterior damage and, in some cases, by unilateral left occipital-temporal damage (McCarthy & Warrington, 1986). One important distinction concerns whether or not the patients can visualize objects in the "mind's eye." In some cases of agnosia, there is an inability to describe verbally the visual characteristics of objects and it accordingly seems that the knowledge base of pictorial properties is (partially) destroyed. Although these impairments to "visual semantics" (McCarthy & Warrington, 1990) or a store of "pictograms" are not uncommon in the agnosias, there are patients with relatively intact pictorial knowledge and visual imagery who are nonetheless unable to recognize objects that they can copy adequately (Behrmann et al., 1992; Jankowiak et al., 1992). The generation of visual imagery is primarily dependent upon the integrity of left posterior cortex.

In some cases of damage to bilateral occipito-parietal cortex, there is preserved identification of single objects but an impaired ability to perceive multiple objects or complex scenes. The impairment (SIMULTANAGNOSIA) is not necessarily dependent upon the visual angle subtended by the array; an individual large object may be recognized while only one of two or more objects is perceived. A patient reported by Luria (1959) illustrates the way in which the condition depends upon the pictorial parsing of the stimulus array. Presented with an all-black drawing of a star of David (two superimposed equilateral triangles, one rotated through 180 degrees), the patient correctly reported a star. When one triangle was blue and the other red, only a single component triangle was perceived. Simultanagnosia is usually found in conjunction with "psychic paralysis of gaze" and "optic ataxia," a triad of symptoms known as BÁLINT'S SYNDROME. Observations of the kind reported by Luria (1959) show that the disorder in the perception of multiple objects cannot be entirely due to oculomotor impairment. The condition of simultanagnosia has sometimes been interpreted as a bilateral NEGLECT. In unilateral visual neglect (Robertson & Marshall, 1993), patients with left, or more frequently right, posterior lesions fail to detect stimuli in locations contralateral to the side of the lesion. Hence in "extinction paradigms", patients (without a visual field deficit) who can report a single object shown in either the left or the right visual field will fail to "see" the contralesional stimulus when two objects are presented simultaneously, one in the left and one in the right field. Simultanagnosia is thus similar to this "neglect" phenomenon, but without the lateralized component thereof.

Within the general class of visual stimuli, the faces of members of the same species are crucially important. Some patients have particular difficulty in recognizing the specific identity of known (indeed highly familiar) faces by sight. This condition (PROSOPAGNOSIA) is usually seen after bilateral posterior lesions but is occasionally found after right unilateral hemisphere damage (De Renzi, 1986; Young, 1992). Prosopagnosia can certainly exist in the absence of gross deficits in the recognition of other visual objects, but there has been considerable controversy over whether the problem is truly specific to human faces. On one interpretation, human faces are merely the most extreme example of stimuli where very small physical differences make a large psychological difference. It may therefore be possible to interpret cases of impaired familiar face recognition (without object agnosia) as reflecting no more than the difficulty of perceiving the slight differences between faces that are critical to the identity of the individual. Studies of object agnosia, by contrast, usually involve the recognition of, say, chairs, cups, and cabbages as basic level stimuli, not one cabbage rather than another, or my Queen Anne chair rather than your Queen Anne chair.

Recent evidence does, however, suggest that prosopagnosia may be genuinely specific to the domain of human faces. A patient reported by De Renzi (1986) had severe prosopagnosia but could reliably distinguish between different breeds of cat, and between Italian and foreign coins. He could also identify his own personal belongings (a coin purse, for example) in the context of other objects in the same class. Even more strikingly, a farmer studied by McNeil and Warrington (1993) was also able to learn to recognize and name his individual sheep despite a severe prosopagnosia for human faces after bilateral stroke. Similarly consistent with the notion that prosopagnosia is domain-specific is the fact that some patients with severe visual object agnosia do not show a disorder of familiar face recognition (Behrmann et al., 1992). In some cases of prosopagnosia, there is evidence of covert recognition despite the loss of conscious identification (and naming). Thus patients may show a galvanic skin response to familiar faces, or may be able to learn correct face and name pairs faster than incorrect pairs, without having any overt access to knowledge of the identity of the faces. What is perceived will often demand a motor response (fight or flee in the more dramatic instances). But equally well (in more civilized contexts), the appropriate response may be verbal.

The link between the perceptual system and the language system is broken in the rare syndrome of optic anomia. In these cases, both visual perception and language seem to be intact but the patient nonetheless fails to name objects to visual confrontation. As in other more purely agnosic or aphasic conditions, there is a wide range of different impairments that have sheltered under the general rubric of optic anomia or optic aphasia (Davidoff & De Bleser, 1993). The possible fractionations include impaired object naming with spared action naming (Manning & Campbell, 1992) and a disorder specific to the naming of faces (Carney & Temple, 1993).

BIBLIOGRAPHY

Behrmann, M., Winocur, G., & Moscovitch, M. (1992). Dissociation between mental imagery and object recognition in a brain-damaged patient. *Nature, 359,* 636–7.

Carney, R., & Temple, C. M. (1993). Prosopagnosia? A possible category-specific anomia for faces. *Cognitive Neuropsychology, 10,* 185–95.

Davidoff, J., & De Bleser, R. (1993). Optic aphasia: a review of past studies and reappraisal. *Aphasiology, 7,* 135–54.

Davidoff, J., & Warrington, E. K. (1993). A dissociation of shape discrimination and figure-ground perception in a patient with normal acuity. *Neuropsychologia, 31,* 83–93.

De Renzi, E. (1986). Current issues on prosopagnosia. In H. D. Ellis, M. A. Jeeves, F. Newcombe, & A. Young (Eds), *Aspects of face processing* (pp. 243–52). Dordrecht: Nijhoff.

Goodale, M. A., Milner, A. D., Jakobson, L. S., & Carey, D. P. (1991). A neurological dissociation between perceiving objects and grasping them. *Nature, 349,* 154–6.

Gray, C. M., Konig, P., Engel, A. K., & Singer, W. (1989). Oscillatory responses in cat visual cortex exhibit inter-columnar synchronization which reflects global stimulus properties. *Nature, 338,* 334–7.

Humphreys, G. W., & Riddoch, M. J. (1987). The fractionation of visual agnosia. In G. W. Humphreys & M. J. Riddoch (Eds), *Visual object processing: A cognitive neuropsychological approach* (pp. 281–306). Hove: Erlbaum.

Jankowiak, J., Kinsbourne, M., Shalev, R. S., & Bachman, D. L. (1992). Preserved visual imagery and categorization in a case of associative visual agnosia. *Journal of Cognitive Neuroscience, 4,* 119–31.

Luria, A. R. (1959). Disorders of simultaneous perception in a case of bilateral occipito-parietal brain injury. *Brain, 82,* 437–49.

McCarthy, R. A., & Warrington, E. K. (1990). *Cognitive neuropsychology: A clinical introduction.* New York: Academic Press.

McNeil, J. E., & Warrington, E. K. (1993). Prosopagnosia: a face-specific disorder. *Quarterly Journal of Experimental Psychology, 46A,* 1–10.

Manning, L., & Campbell, R. (1992). Optic aphasia with spared action naming: a description and possible loci of impairment. *Neuropsychologia, 30,* 587–92.

Muller, H. J., Humphreys, G. W., Quinlan, P. T., & Donnelly, N. (1989). Fundamental design limitations in tag assignment. *Behavioral and Brain Sciences, 12,* 410–11.

Robertson, I. H., & Marshall, J. C. (Eds). (1993). *Unilateral neglect: Clinical and experimental studies*. Hove: Erlbaum.

Thaiss, L., & De Bleser, R. (1992). Visual agnosia: a case of reduced attentional "spotlight"? *Cortex, 28*, 601–21.

Young, A. W. (1992). Face recognition impairments. *Philosophical Transactions of the Royal Society B, 335*, 47–54.

Zeki, S. (1993). The visual association cortex. *Current Opinion in Neurobiology, 3*, 155–9.

Zihl, J., Von Cramon, D., & Mai, N. (1983). Selective disturbance of movement vision after bilateral brain damage. *Brain, 106*, 313–40.

JOHN C. MARSHALL AND
PETER W. HALLIGAN

visuospatial disorders The importance of visuospatial disturbances lies in their functional and behavioral consequences. All visual stimuli have position and extension within space relative to the observer. Adequate visual spatial analysis is essential for carrying out most activities of daily living, e.g. dressing, object manipulation, reading, writing, drawing, walking, and generally interacting with people and objects in the everyday environment. Visuospatial disorders are common after brain damage and, in particular, damage to the right hemisphere. They constitute a substantial barrier to functional recovery and can limit the effectiveness of rehabilitation more than obvious motor, sensory, and speech deficits.

Historically, the term "visuospatial disorder" or "visuospatial agnosia" has been used imprecisely in the medical literature to diagnose a wide variety of disorders involving the faulty appreciation and manipulation of visuospatial information. In the absence of any clearly defined conceptual framework of normal spatial functioning, it is difficult to offer a coherent classification of visuospatial disorders. Given the disparate nature of the presenting symptoms and the use of different tests and terminology, there is a great deal of functional and conceptual overlap between the descriptions and interpretations offered. What one study regards as an underlying deficit, another may describe as a defining characteristic or associated feature.

Difficulty in characterizing the spatial mechanisms involved

One of the main problems in defining and classifying spatial disorders remains the difficulty in characterizing and defining the elusive concept of perceptual space itself. In everyday life space is experienced as relatively independent of the head, trunk, and eye movements we make. This implies the transformation from person-centered (or egocentric) information to viewer-independent or allocentric referenced information. Kant, the eighteenth-century German philosopher, envisaged space as an implicit organizing principle whereby all sensations were mentally structured. The abstract conception of space is derived from the analysis of the spatial relationships perceived to exist between an observer and objects in personal and extrapersonal space. From a Kantian position, the difficulty in studying spatial behaviors resides in the fact that, as a phenomenological experience, it is difficult to appreciate and identify the psychological mechanisms underlying spatially orientated behavior. Consequently, spatial disorders do not readily form a well-defined set that adequately represents specific psychological deficits, but rather describes selective features that have been intuitively abstracted from a complex set of behavioral effects that follow focal brain damage. These include the inability to follow routes, difficulty in judging distance, misreaching for objects, and difficulty in localizing objects in space. Some of the discrete classifications currently in use were inherited from clinical case reports originally described in the first half of this century, and as such provide little agreement about the underlying functions impaired.

Difficulty in classifying spatial disorders

Compared with disorders of language and perception, the systematic study of spatial disorders began only in the 1950s with the recognition of the asymmetrical specialization of spatial functions in the right hemisphere. The concept of left hemispheric dominance for language had arisen almost a century before. Aside from contralateral sensory and motor loss, the role attributed to the right hemisphere was that of a mute, unthinking automaton, lacking in independent cognitive capacities. Clinical and experimental research with brain-damaged patients (including COMMISSUROTOMY studies) confirmed a specialization of the "nondominant" hemisphere for visuospatial functions. It took clinicians much longer to specify and characterize the cognitive disorders that followed right brain damage. Unlike language disorders, most visual spatial deficits are less salient and consequently more difficult to identify in a precise manner. Diagnosis can be complicated by primary sensory (visual field deficits) and/or motor (deficit in making saccadic eye movements) impairments, neither of which in their own right are sufficient to account for the emergence of visuospatial disorders. Another difficulty concerns the problem of isolating impaired spatial deficits from the effects of other cognitive deficits involving language, memory, intelligence, and recognition abilities.

Recent attempts to produce a coherent classification of visuospatial disorders have drawn upon information processing theory and knowledge of different spatial coordinate systems, including accounts of internal representation. Newcombe and Ratcliff (1989) distinguish between spatial disorders which result from a disturbance of comparatively early and simple stages of visual analysis and those that involve damage to later more complex processes. They suggest that the early processing levels (e.g. point localization, depth perception, size estimation, line orientation) can be carried out by both hemispheres and primarily in terms of an egocentric coordinate framework (viewer-dependent). By contrast, damage to the later stages (spatial perception, mental rotation, maze learning, short-term spatial memory) can be characterized by functional hemispheric differences and involve allocentric coordinate frames of reference.

Given that any discussion of visuospatial disorders is encumbered by problems of definition and assessment this discussion will limit itself to the main spatial disorders that have received clinical attention. These include ALLESTHESIA, BÁLINT'S SYNDROME, disorders of spatial localization, TOPOGRAPHICAL DISORDERS, constructional APRAXIA, unilateral spatial NEGLECT, RIGHT–LEFT DISORIENTATION, and AUTOTOPAGNOSIA.

ALLESTHESIA

Allesthesia is a clinically elicited phenomenon observed in right brain-damaged patients with left-sided visual neglect. It was first described in the tactile modality whereby a mechanical stimulus applied to the affected side is incorrectly attributed to a position on the other side. The condition suggests that, although the stimulus on the affected side is perceived, it is incorrectly attributed to the good side. When mislocations are reported to occur in a symmetrical position on the unaffected side, the term ALLOCHIRIA is usually applied. The phenomenon has also been described in the visual modality. On drawing a clock face from memory some patients place all the numbers to the right side. Similarly on a pointing or copying task patients may detect objects in the left visual field but erroneously point to or copy them over in right space. Motor transpositions have also been described. It has commonly been regarded as a form of inattention seen after right-hemisphere damage and in association with spatial neglect. A coherent explanation of allesthesia has to account for how the transposition is achieved and why these patients apparently fail to notice the resultant errors on the unaffected side. Allesthesia may also occur in cases of spinal cord injury or in conversion hysteria.

BÁLINT'S SYNDROME

This comparatively rare and striking condition was named after the Hungarian physician Rezzo Bálint, who in 1907 described a constellation of discrete spatial symptoms in a patient with bilateral damage. Such patients complain about (a) objects vanishing from a scene they are looking at; (b) an inability to detect people approaching them; and (c) a difficulty in reaching for or indicating the location of objects around them. The original account by Bálint was expanded by Holmes (1918) who included loss of visual orientation and a disorder of ocular movements as relevant features. The classical presentation of Bálint's syndrome comprises three major components: simultanagnosia, optic ataxia, and ocular-motor apraxia, all of which can occur in isolation or in a modified form. When present, visual field defects usually involve the inferior quadrants.

● *Simultanagnosia* or "piecemeal vision" describes the restriction of visual attention to selective components (usually within macular vision) in a scene and has been likened to a bilateral form of the more common unilateral visual neglect. Bálint noted that, although single elements of a visual scene could be reported, the patient failed to combine the individual components of the scene into a meaningful whole.

Patients fail to notice other objects located close to the fixated parts of the scene. Striking examples include the inability to light a cigarette because the patient could not see both the cigarette and the match at the same time; failure to see cars passing in front while looking at a building or person on the other side of the road. Presented with a star of David comprising two triangles coloured in black and red, patients describe seeing only one of the triangles. Furthermore, in Bálint's case the patient appeared to have unilateral neglect as his attention was biased primarily towards the right-sided features. The consequences of simultanagnosia are as follows: patients fail to detect and orient to new stimuli that appear in the periphery of the visual field; as the center of vision shifts, objects clearly seen may suddenly seem to disappear from view. The deficit can easily be tested by asking the patient to describe a picture of a complex scene. The term simultaneous agnosia has also been used by Wolpert and Luria to describe the patients' inability to grasp the meaning of a complex visual picture or a scene that depicts an event or action.

• *Optic ataxia* or visuomotor ataxia is an impairment of visually guided pointing or reaching skills, i.e. an inability to use visual information to control voluntary hand movements in extrapersonal space. When reaching for a small coin in space a patient's hand may overshoot the target by several inches. Requested to pick up a cup in front of them, patients grope for the target and make contact as if by chance. The same patients usually have no difficulty in pointing accurately to the source of sounds, targets on their own body, or to objects in space when the tasks are carried out under proprioceptive guidance. The disturbance can affect one or both visual fields. On the traditional finger–nose test of visuomotor coordination, the patient can touch his or her nose accurately while missing the examiner's fingers. In most cases the problem involves both hands in all parts of the visual field, although defective reaching in the contralateral visual field can occur after discrete unilateral left or right occipital-parietal lesions. The disorder has been explained as a disconnection of visual input from the motor mechanisms necessary to prepare reaching or pointing movements, or as a disorder of the mechanism responsible for specifying the egocentric positional coordinates of a visual stimulus prior to motor response.

• *Oculomotor apraxia* or "psychic paralysis of gaze" refers to an inability to change or redirect visual gaze so as to bring objects from the periphery into central fixation. There appears to be no difficulty in tracking a moving stimulus. When saccades do take place they are often inaccurate. Since these patients can move their eyes spontaneously or to command, the problem cannot be simply explained as a motor paresis. To complicate matters, some of these patients also have difficulty in maintaining a fixation once achieved. Without the ability to make normal saccades to a novel stimulus originating from the periphery, these patients can appear functionally blind. Some patients resort to artificial means of overcoming this, such as closing their eyes or shaking their head.

Patients with Bálint's syndrome typically have bilateral damage to the occipital-parietal junction. The primary visual cortex is spared, and visual acuity may be unimpaired. Infarction is the most common cause for bilateral occipital-parietal junction damage. Such infarctions may occur after hypotension, cardiac arrest, or cardiac bypass surgery.

CONSTRUCTIONAL APRAXIA

The term "constructional apraxia" is somewhat confusing, as the disorder is not clinically related to the apraxias. The term is considered a misnomer by most clinicians who regard "visuoconstructive impairment" as a more useful designation. The central component of constructional apraxia is a disturbance on tasks which require the active manipulation of objects in space. Evidence of constructional apraxia can involve: failure to perceive the constituent elements of a model or drawing; failure to perceive spatial relationships, or failure to execute the task adequately. A large number of tests have been used to identify and evaluate constructional apraxia. These include drawing geometric shapes, copying block designs, constructing complex figures, and building three-dimensional models. Constructional apraxia can follow from injury to either hemisphere, although most studies report the condition to be more prevalent and more severe in patients with right posterior damage. Furthermore, the nature of constructional apraxia has been shown to differ qualitatively depending on the hemisphere damaged. Right hemisphere-damaged patients show gross alterations in the spatial arrangements of features, whereas the drawings of left hemisphere-damaged patients tend to be over-simplified and manifest less attention to detail. Originally defined as a purely behavioral diagnosis, the condition makes no claim regarding the underlying deficits involved. Recent reviews confirm that there are at least two different types, depending on the laterality of the brain damage. After right hemisphere brain damage the primary impairment is the processing of the spatial relationships involved; after left hemisphere brain damage the key element that is affected is the organization of the actions necessary to carry out the task.

DISORDERS OF SPATIAL LOCALIZATION AND ORIENTATION

Impairments of the ability to perceive the location of single targets in extrapersonal space have been extensively investigated. The right hemisphere plays a special role in the spatial localization of visual stimuli. A distinction is made between "absolute" localization of a single stimulus in relation to the viewer and "relative" localization involving the spatial relationship between two objects as seen by the observer. Examples of the "absolute" form include requiring the patient to touch target stimuli in extrapersonal space, while "relative" forms of localization tasks include the judgment and matching of simultaneous or successive presentation of objects. Impairment of localizing objects in extrapersonal space is commonly seen after posterior lesions. Short-term spatial memory appears to be a dominant function of the posterior right hemisphere (De Renzi et al., 1977). Visual appreciation of the orientation of lines can also be impaired following right parietal damage. Kimura has shown that spatial localization is superior in the left rather than the right visual fields of normal subjects. This is consistent with the view that the right hemisphere is dominant for spatial localization.

DISORDERS OF PERSONAL OR BODY SPACE

These disorders imply a disruption of spatial concepts involving the body image or body schema.

- *Right–left disorientation* refers to the inability to verbally distinguish left from right consistently in the absence of significant comprehension, expressive disorder, or generalized intellectual impairment. The confusion can involve both the patient's own body and that of the examiner.
- *Autotopagnosia* is a selective disorder involving the locating of bodily parts, which cannot be explained by an underlying category-specific language deficit. The inability to *point* to one's own body parts on verbal command can also extend to parts of the examiner's body or photographs of a human body. Although these patients can readily name and describe body parts pointed out to them, they show difficulty in finding the exact location of various body parts in relation to the whole body. For example, they may indicate a wrist for an elbow. The deficit appears to affect those explicit tasks requiring the patient to intentionally locate bodily parts. The patient may exhibit no difficulty in locating bodily parts in everyday situations. The disorder occurs in patients with left hemisphere damage and usually involves the parietal lobe. Evidence of autotopagnosia has been used to support the concept of a mental body image located in the left hemisphere.
- *Anosognosia:* in the acute stage, patients with large right hemisphere lesions may experience a defective appreciation of the consequences of their brain damage. Some patients verbally deny or fail to recognize the physical effects of the brain damage, including the existence of a visual field deficit or left-sided paralysis or gross sensory loss. When the examiner requests the patient with a left-sided hemiparesis to raise the left arm, the patient may indicate that he or she has done so, but without moving the arm. When this is pointed out to patients, they may excuse it by saying that the hand is tired! Some patients attempt to mitigate the obvious effects of their brain damage, while other patients may appear unaware of one side of their body (HEMIASO-MATOGNOSIA). The condition is generally associated with marked sensory loss and has been variously explained as a specific agnosia, a type of neglect, and/or evidence of hemispheric disconnection.

DISORDERS OF TOPOGRAPHICAL ORIENTATION AND MEMORY

This term describes a range of disorders, all of which compromise the patients' ability to recall or find their way about in surroundings previously familiar to them. It can also refer to those patients who fail to learn new routes in unfamiliar places. Patients may show difficulties with visuospatial memory in locating public buildings in their town or in finding specific objects located in rooms in their homes. They may become lost when travelling on familiar routes or when moving between offices or wards in a hospital. Other patients may describe difficulties in constructing a geographic map of their locality or country. Such disorders are frequently associated with disorders of memory, recognition, and other visuospatial disorders, particularly spatial neglect. Explanations of the disorder include an impaired ability to associate intact visual percepts with incomplete visuospatial memories or a selective impairment of forming topographical memories. The condition is strongly associated with bilateral posterior lesions and with unilateral right posterior lesions.

VISUOSPATIAL NEGLECT

Visual neglect is by far the most common visuospatial condition encountered in clinical practice. The ability of eye movements to proceed rapidly from fixating a stationary target in central vision to intercepting and tracking an incoming peripheral target requires an elaborate detection mechanism capable of monitoring and updating changes across the whole visual field. Right-sided brain damage, following stroke or tumor, can produce dramatic and spatially specific inattention for objects and people located on the left side of both personal and extrapersonal space. Patients with neglect may fail to shave, groom, or dress the left side of the body and they may fail to orient to events in left hemispace. There is a marked tendency to direct the head and eyes towards the right side. When asked to copy drawings they omit detail on the left side, and when reading they may fail to read the left half of each sentence. On line bisection they show marked deviations to the right. Clinically, left neglect is more common, more severe, and more lasting than the similar right unilateral neglect after left hemisphere

damage. This has fuelled theories which support a hemispheric specialization account for directed attention. The left hemisphere only contains mechanisms responsible for directing attention to the contralateral right hemispace, whereas the right hemisphere contains mechanisms for attending to both sides of space. Accordingly, left hemisphere injury does not result in chronic unilateral neglect because the ipsilateral attending mechanisms of the right hemisphere are assumed to compensate.

BIBLIOGRAPHY

Benton, A., & Tranel, D. (1993). Perceptual and spatial disorders. In K. Heilman & E. Valenstein (Eds), *Clinical neuropsychology*, 2nd edn (pp. 165–213). New York: Oxford University Press.

Bradshaw, J., & Nettleton, N. (1981). The nature of hemispheric specialisation in man. *Behavioral and Brain Sciences, 4*, 51–63.

Critchley, M. (1953). *The parietal lobes*. London: Edward Arnold.

De Renzi, E. (1982). *Disorders of space exploration and cognition*. London: Wiley.

Halligan, P. W., Marshall, J. C., & Wade, D. T. (1992). Left on the right: allochiria in a case of left visuo-spatial neglect. *Journal of Neurology, Neurosurgery and Psychiatry, 55*, 717–19.

Newcombe, F., & Ratcliff, G. (1989). Disorders of visuospatial analysis. In F. Boller & J. Grafman (Eds), *Handbook of Neuropsychology*, Vol. 2 (pp. 333–56). Amsterdam: Elsevier.

Ogden, J. (1985). Autotopagnosia; occurrence in a patient without nominal aphasia and with an intact ability to point to parts of animals and objects. *Brain, 108*, 1009–22.

Riddoch, J., & Humphreys, G. (1989). Finding the way around topographical impairments. In J. Brown (Ed.), *Neuropsychology of visual perception* (pp. 79–104). London: LEA.

Rondot, P., de Recondo, J., & Ribadeau Dumas, J. L. (1977). Visuomotor ataxia. *Brain, 100*, 355–76.

PETER W. HALLIGAN AND
JOHN C. MARSHALL

W

Wada test *See* INTRACAROTID SODIUM AMYTAL.

Wallenberg's syndrome Wallenberg's syndrome is also known as the *lateral medullary syndrome* and is a rare condition resulting from acute cerebrovascular disease or a CEREBROVASCULAR ACCIDENT involving part of the MEDULLA. Associated with the syndrome are loss of temperature and pain sensation in the face and mouth, loss of taste, disorders of the palate, and loss of the gag reflex. ATAXIA may also occur.

An interesting further feature of the syndrome is that it may be associated with unilateral experience of orgasm, presumably as a result of the fact that the sensory fibers from the genital region pass upward in whole or in part to the medullary region, but that only one lateral half of this projection is affected.

Wernicke's aphasia *See* APHASIA.

Wernicke's encephalopathy This disorder is a form of ENCEPHALOPATHY which is caused by a deficiency of the vitamin B_1 (thiamine or aneurine). The deficiency causes a build-up of pyruvate in the blood, which produces both this disorder and *beriberi*. Common antecedents which lead to the vitamin deficiency are persistent vomiting, possibly in pregnancy, malnutrition associated with cancer of the stomach, and chronic alcoholism when it is associated with KORSAKOFF'S DISEASE. Korsakoff's disease may be the chronic consequence of an acute episode of Wernicke's encephalopathy, which has led some to use the term *Wernicke–Korsakoff syndrome*.

Cerebral lesions in Wernicke's encephalopathy occur in thalamic and hypothalamic nuclei, the MAMMILLARY BODIES, the periaqueductal gray region around the fourth ventricle, and in the cerebellum. The first signs of the disorder are usually confusion and insomnia, with disordered eye movements and ataxia of the limbs. In the acute phase, indifference, variability in arousal, disorientation, and fatigability are prominent, and hallucinations, delusions, perceptual distortions, and agitation are reported in some patients. There may also be emotional abnormalities in the form of apprehension, depression, and emotional lability.

However, the main cognitive concomitant of Wernicke's encephalopathy is a disorder of memory. Disturbance of memory may be apparent in the acute stage of the illness, although it may be difficult to assess memory function in a patient who is highly confused. Thereafter there is commonly a severe memory deficit characteristic of the AMNESIC SYNDROME, and CONFABULATION may be present although it does not invariably occur.

Treatment with thiamine, coupled with other supplements, is highly effective, although those not treated early, or in whom borderline states go unrecognized, as may occur in chronic alcoholism, may be left with enduring amnesic deficits.

Wilson's disease Wilson's disease, which is also known as *hepatolenticular degeneration*, is a progressive disorder of early life. It is due to a recessive autosomal genetic defect which results in the faulty metabolism of copper, so that concentrations of copper increase in the brain and in the liver, leading to cirrhosis of the liver and degeneration of areas of the brain, particularly in the BASAL GANGLIA. It is therefore primarily, but not exclusively, a disorder of movement. A diagnostic sign of the disorder is a ring of corneal pigmentation (the Kayser–Fleischer ring), golden-brown or grayish-green in color, resulting from deposition of copper.

The disorder is rare as the gene only occurs in about 0.1 percent of the population, and the onset of neuropsychological symptoms is usually between the ages of 10 and 25, although it may be later in life. The early signs are choreiform or athetoid (*see* ATHETOSIS; CHOREA) movements of the face and hands while the affected person is at rest, but these are reduced by systematic relaxation. General muscular rigidity, rather similar to that seen in PARKINSON'S DISEASE, follows, together with resting tremor and abnormal dystonic postures of the limbs. Later the expression may become stiff and motionless with a rigid fixed smile. Mental deterioration leading to a generalized mild dementia, within which language functions may be relatively spared, also occurs, often accompanied by involuntary laughing and crying in a picture of general loss of emotional control, with occasional outbursts of rage or destructive behavior. Other forms of antisocial behavior may occur and psychotic states, either as enduring conditions or as episodic manifestations, occur in some cases, there being an intriguing similarity between Wilson's disease and HUNTINGTON'S DISEASE.

Untreated individuals normally survive from one to six years, but treatment by penicillamine, which binds the copper and allows it to be excreted, is highly effective if commenced early and continued.

withdrawal syndrome   The withdrawal syndrome occurs, following the reduction or termination of a drug previously administered to the point of intoxication, as a temporary central nervous system reaction. The pattern of the syndrome may vary according to the specific drug withdrawn, but may include restlessness, anxiety, irritability, insomnia, and impaired attention. The time course also varies according to the drug, but in most cases subsides within a week. Changes in drug regime may be an important factor to be taken into account in performing a neuropsychological ASSESSMENT within the period of the withdrawal syndrome.

witzelsucht   *Witzelsucht* is a term applied to the prankish joking and punning, the inappropriate jocularity, which are often present in the change in personality which follows FRONTAL LOBE lesions.

word blindness   Word blindness (*or pure word blindness*) is one of the two forms of ALEXIA originally described by Déjerine, the other being alexia associated with agraphia. Pure word blindness is associated with a preserved capacity to write (alexia without agraphia) and is generally considered to result from a combination of lesions in the occipital lobe in the hemisphere dominant for language, and the splenium (the posterior portion) of the CORPUS CALLOSUM, although the necessary involvement of the splenium is a matter of debate. Such lesions may follow disturbance of the territory of the posterior cerebral artery.

X

X-rays The use of X-rays forms the basis of the investigative techniques used in neuroradiology. Conventional radiology employs *plain X-ray* images or *films* (in this context, static pictures) which permit not only the bony structures surrounding the nervous system to be visualized, but also certain details of the cerebral structures themselves. The addition of *contrast* by the insertion of either air or a radio-opaque dye into the arterial or ventricular system (ANGIOGRAPHY, PNEUMOENCEPHALOGRAPHY, VENTRICULOGRAPHY) may provide improved delineation of the cerebral structures. However, while plain X-rays are still employed principally to examine the bony structures of the head and spine, the examination of cerebral structures is more usually conducted by the use of X-rays within computerized axial tomography (CT SCAN), or by imaging techniques which do not involve X-radiation (*see* SCAN).

Z

Zellweger malformation The Zellweger malformation is a disorder of abnormal development which is a recessive genetic condition producing complex systemic metabolic effects. In the CORTEX it produces an abnormality of the gyral pattern in the ROLANDIC AREA and around the SYLVIAN FISSURE, with some gyri narrower and some wider than in the normal brain.

Index

Index

amygdala (cont'd)
olfaction 173; personality disorders 566; schizophrenia 728; sexuality 662–3
amygdalectomy 69
analgesia 551; *see also* pain
anarithmetria 2, 69
anarthria 69–70, 499, 562
Andermann syndrome 183
Anderson, S. W. 610
androgens 662
anencephaly 70
anesthesia **70**, 240, 244–5
aneurysm **70–1**, 706, 710, 711–14
angiography **71**, 460, 520, 594, 710, 770
angioma 108
angular gyrus 71–2
anhedonia 31, 265
animal studies **72**, 205–7, 224–5, 579, 596; *see also* macaques; monkeys
animism 489, 491, 492
Annett, M. 368, 374–5
anomia 72–6; aphasia 93, 99; proper names 343, 483; tactile 723
anorexia nervosa 166, 430
anosagnosia: *see* anosognosia
anosmia **77–80**, 252, 547, 725
anosodiaphoria **80**, 265, 513
anosognosia 80–4; auditory perception 129–30; deficit specific 678, 714; denial 81–2, 164, 264–5, 766; insight lacking 343; neglect 513
anoxia **84–5**, 187, 257
anterior cerebral artery 85, 707
anterior commissure 85–6
anterior parietal cortex 652–3
anterograde amnesia: *see* amnesia
antibiotics 521
anticonvulsants 520–1, 743
antidepressants 596, 743
antipsychotic drugs 743
Anton's syndrome **86**, 249, 265, 541, 708, 760
anxiolytic drugs 743
apathy 181, 228, 402, 424
aphasia **86–99**, 692; agrammatism 94; agraphia 21, 22–4, 97–8; amnesic 89; anarthria 69; anomia 93, 99; auditory perceptual disorders 132; Broca's 5, 20, 41, 69, 92, 93, 94, 98, 104, 350, 725; cerebral palsy 212; cognitive neurolinguistics 90–1; contiguity 247; differential 148–9; dysprosody 300–1; echolalia 302; fluency 95, 98–9, 638; gestural behavior 361; global 98–9, 395; localization 525; melodic intonation therapy 319, 476, 690, 691; motor articulatory problems 92; naming disorders 71, 92–4; nonfluent 20, 300, 638; paragrammatism 554; paraphasia 94–5, 555; parietal lesion 558; polyglots 149–50; reading disorders 96–7; recovery of function 610–11; right–left disorientation 636; selective 148; semantic 140; supramarginal gyrus 715; symbolization disorder 362; tactile 723; vegetative state 748
aphasia therapy: *see* speech therapy for aphasia
aphemia 69, 92, 98, 350; *see also* anarthria
apractagnosia 100–1
apraxia 101–6; adiadochokinesia 500; agraphic 24–5, 119; apractagnosia 100–1; avocalia 142; buccofacial

345; constructional 102–3, 558, 745, 765–6; denial 265; dressing 104, 577; frontal lobes 349; ideational 71, 101–2; ideomotor 101, 105, 361; left-sided 248; limb-kinetic 104–5; models of 105–6; oculomotor 547, 765; oral 103–4; parapraxia 555; parietal lesion 558; recovery 106; of speech 694; stroke 707
aprosodia 106–7, 707
ARC (AIDS-related complex) 32
arcuate fasciculus 107
Argyll Robertson pupil 107, 252
arousal 206, 318, 418
arteriosclerosis 107–8
arteriovenous malformation 108
asomatognosia 44, **108**, 376, 377, 734
aspartate 533
asphyxia, perinatal 381
assessment **108–15**, 260, 328
association area 116–17
associationism **117–18**, 365, 482–3
astereognosia 118, 707
asthenopia 118
astrocytoma 118
asymbolia 88, 108, **118**, 361, 363
asymmetries, human/non-human 440–1
ataxia 118–20; cerebellar 118, 119, 120, 499; cerebral palsy 120, 210; Friedreich's 120; frontal 119; of gait 118, 119, 196, 499; general paralysis of the insane 360; optic 119, 143, 547, 555, 761, 765; visuomotor 765
atherosclerosis 121, 706
athetosis 119, **121**, 301, 501, 769
atonia, muscular 176, 178
atrophy, cerebral 121–2, 257
attention **122–7**, 240, 411–13; aging 10; alerting 126; blood flow studies 161–2; brain input/output 172; cingulate gyrus 216; confusional state 226–7, 228, 230–1; consciousness 241–2, 244–5; dyslexia 299; EEG 306, 309–10; event-related potential 336; frontal lobes 125–6, 349–50; hemispheric specialization 281–2; information-processing 122–3; lead poisoning 445; neglect 511, 515–17; orienting reflex 122, 123–6, 548; parietal lobe 558; pattern recognition 124; phenylketonuria 574; tactile perception disorders 723–4; visual 541, 666, 759, 764–5
attention deficit disorder: *see* hyperactivity
Aubert's phenomenon 127–8
auditory agnosia: *see* agnosia; auditory perceptual disorders
auditory evoked potential: *see* evoked potential
auditory perceptual disorders **128–32**, 212, 249, 498
aura: depersonalization 265; epilepsy 257, 327, 345, 367, 443, 457
autism **133–7**, 236; echolalia 302; EEG 309; fragile X syndrome 235; infantile 133–4, 203; MRI 641
autocriticism **137**, 279, 284
automatism 137, 327, 328, 353, 457
autonomism 489, 490
autotomy 552
autotopagnosia 108, **137–41**, 164, 558, 766
average evoked potential: *see* evoked potential
avocalia 142
awareness: in anosognosia 82–3; and attention 126; covert 517; implicit 157; lacking 680; variations 240; see also consciousness

Index

Index

Index

hemorrhage 416; hemiplegia 379, 381; subarachnoid 70, 710–14
Henschen, S. E. 2, 6
Henschen's axiom 395
hepatolenticular degeneration 768–9
herpes simplex encephalitis 424
herpes simplex virus 321, 322, 323, 324
herpes zoster 322
Heschl's gyrus 395, 578
heterotopia 303, **395**, 549
Heubner's artery 395
Hinton, G. E. 295
hippocampus **395–400**; aging 12; Alzheimer's disease 400; amnesia 45, 46, 53, 61, 457; appetite 173; basal ganglia 144; ECT 303; entorhinal cortex 325; limbic seizure 457–8; memory 34, 395; vegetative state 748
histamine 533
HIV infection 32, 238, 261–2, 450–1
Hobson, R. P. 136–7
Hoffman reflex 687
Holmes, Gordon 756, 764
holoprosencephaly 401
homeostasis 418
homosexuality 658, 659, 665
hormones: hypothalamus 416–18; immune system 424; sex hormones 418, 657, 661, 662; sleep 673, 674
Horn, J. L. 9
Howard, D. 690–2, 693
Hunkin, N. M. 53
Huntington's disease 146, 147, 216, **401–6**; emotions 319; extrapyramidal 262; MRI 641; striatum 705
hydrocephalus 215, 237, 303, **406–10**
hyloagnosia 411
hyperactivity **411–14**; anhedonic drive syndrome 31; episodic dyscontrol syndrome 333; fetal alcohol syndrome 238; lead poisoning 446; minimal brain dysfunction 492; phenylketonuria 236
hypergraphia 27
hyperkinetic movement disorders 146
hyperlexic state 415–16
hypermetria 118
hypersexuality 402, 663, 664
hypersomnia 428
hypertension **416**, 437, 706
hypertonia 380
hypnagogic phenomena 367, 416
hypnic jerks 672
hypnosis 245, 743
hypochondriasis 420
hypokinesia 147, 167, 416; see also bradykinesia
hypomania 416
hypometria 118, 499–500
hypophonia 416
hyposexuality 664
hypotension 416
hypothalamus **416–19**, 657–8, 661–2, 665–6
hypotonia 419
hypoxia 85, 685; see also anoxia
hysteria 359, **419–22**, 509

ictal phenomenon 424
ideagraphy 207

idealism 489–90
ideational apraxia: see apraxia
identity 224
ideomotor apraxia: see apraxia
idiopathic epilepsy: see epilepsy
Ignelsim R. J. 385
illusion 367, 477, 554, 702; see also hallucination
imaging techniques: see scan
immune system 424
imperviousness 424
impulsivity 424
incontinence 699, 746
indifference 267, 420, 421, **425**
individual-centered normative approach 526
indoleacetic acid 204
infancy, reflexes 173
infantile hemiplegia 380–1, 382
infantile spasms 327
infarct 217, **425**, 426, 437, 582
inferior parietal lobule 556, 557
information processing 229–30; agraphia 29–30; attention 122–3; cerebellum 198; human/non-human 122–3; methodological issues 478; speed 200, 202; striate cortex 704; visuospatial disorders 764
Ingram, T. T. S. 210
Ingvar, D. H. 207
innervation: epicritic 325, 447; protopathic 447, 593
insight loss 343, 567, 678, 680
insomnia 676, 733
insula 425
intelligence 9, 446, 494, 506
intelligence quotient 9, 425
intention tremor 499
intentionality, and understanding 529, 531
interactionism 489, 491, 492
interhemispheric transfer: see commissurotomy; lateralization
intermanual conflict 221, 279, 284
intermetamorphosis 425
interneurons 730
interthalamic connexus: see massa intermedia
intracarotid sodium amytal 313, **425–6**, 439, 440, 462–3, 709
intoxication, acute/chronic 740
intralaminar nuclei 729, 731–2
ischemia 107, **426**, 706

Jackson, J. Hughlings 65, 88, 103, 117, 313, 362, 522, 525
Jakob–Creutzfeldt disease 256, 323, 510
Jakobson, R. 94, 247
jamais vu 257, 327, **427**
Jones, K. L. 233
Just, M. A. 242

Kahn, R. L. 81, 83
Kandel, E. 609
Kanfer, F. H. 622
Kapur, N. 53, 56
Katz, J. 552
Kennard principle **428**, 462, 578–9
Kety, S. S. 641
Kimura, D. 274, 275, 277

Index

Index

Index

Index